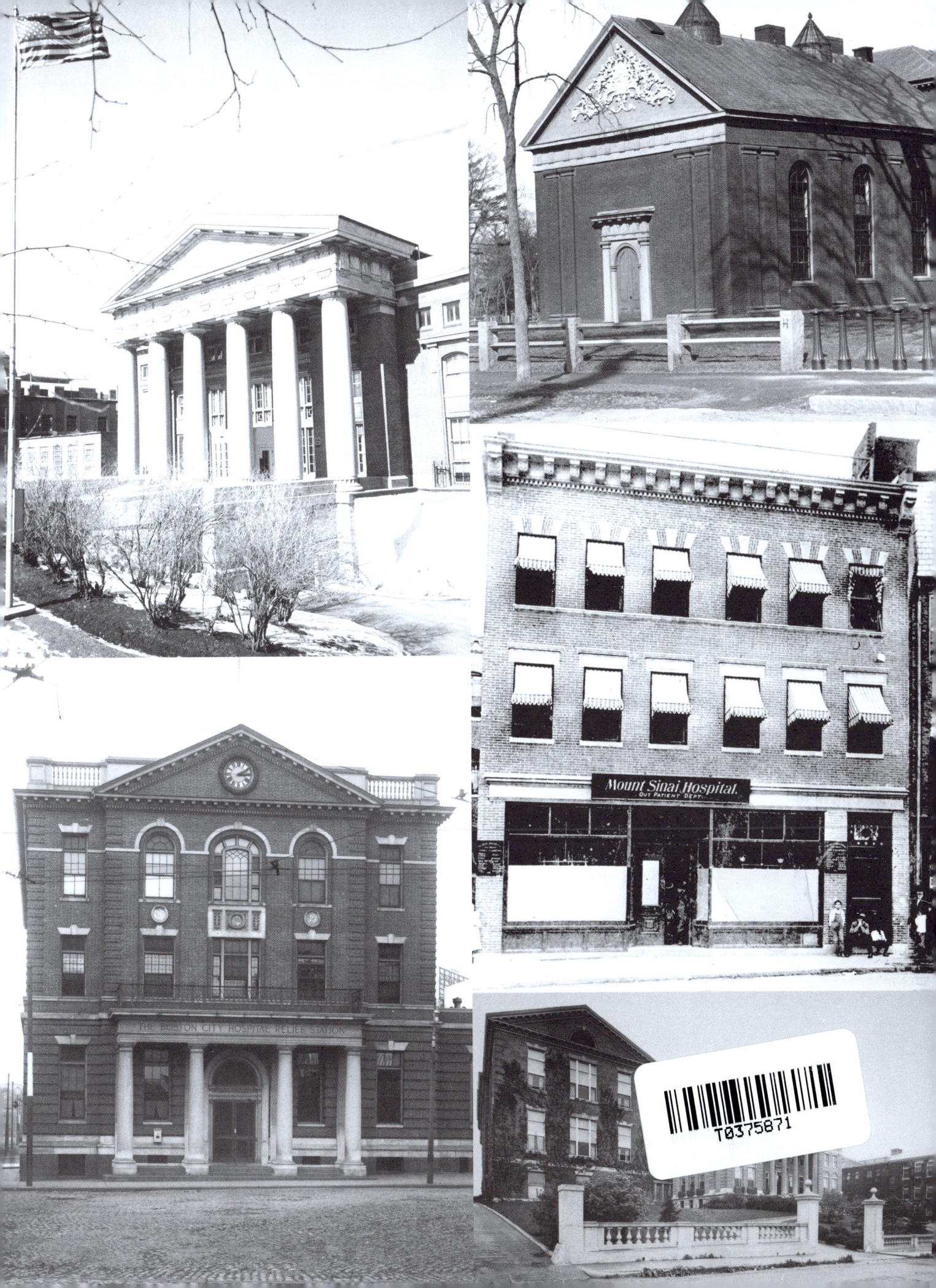

BIRTH of a SPECIALTY

BIRTH *of a* SPECIALTY

A History of Orthopaedics at Harvard and Its Teaching Hospitals

VOLUME 2

by

James H. Herndon, MD, MBA

Peter E. Randall Publisher
Portsmouth, New Hampshire
2021

© 2021 James H. Herndon
All rights reserved.

ISBN: 978-1-942155-36-2
Library of Congress Control Number: 2021916147

Published by
Peter E. Randall Publisher LLC
Portsmouth, NH 03801
www.perpublisher.com

Volume 1: Harvard Medical School
Volume 2: Boston Children's Hospital
Volume 3: Massachusetts General Hospital
Volume 4: Brigham and Women's Hospital, Beth Israel Deaconess Medical Center, Boston City Hospital, World War I, and World War II
Volume 5: Bibliography (available only in PDF form, visit www.birthofaspecialty.com)

Cover images:
Front:
   Volume 1: Boston Medical Library collection, Center for the History of Medicine in the Francis A. Countway Library.
   Volume 2: *Images of America. Children's Hospital Boston.* Charleston, SC: Arcadia Publishing, 2005. Boston Children's Hospital Archives, Boston, Massachusetts.
   Volume 3: Massachusetts General Hospital, Archives and Special Collections.
   Volume 4: Brigham and Women's Hospital Archives.

Back:
   Volumes 1–4: Warren Anatomical Museum collection, Center for the History of Medicine in the Francis A. Countway Library.

Endpaper images:
Front: **Top:** (l) Exterior view of the Old Harvard Medical School, Boston, Mass, ca. 1880. Photograph by Baldwin Coolidge. Courtesy of Historic New England; (cl) Boston Children's Hospital Archives, Boston, Massachusetts; (cr) Brigham and Women's Hospital Archives; (r) Theodore Roosevelt Collection in the Houghton Library, Harvard University.
Center: (l) The Ruth and David Freiman Archives at Beth Israel Deaconess Medical Center; (c) Boston Children's Hospital Archives, Boston, Massachusetts; (r) The Ruth and David Freiman Archives at Beth Israel Deaconess Medical Center.
Bottom: (l) Massachusetts General Hospital, Archives and Special Collections; (c) Boston City Archives; (r) Brigham and Women's Hospital Archives.
Back: All: Kael E. Randall/Kael Randall Images

All reasonable efforts have been made to obtain necessary copyright permissions. Grateful acknowledgment for these permissions is made at point of use (for images) and in Volume 5 (for text). Any omissions or errors are unintentional and will, if brought to the attention of the author, be resolved.

Book design by Tim Holtz

Printed in the United States of America

Contents

Section 4	**Boston Children's Hospital**	
Chapter 14	Boston Children's Hospital: The Beginning	3
Chapter 15	Edward H. Bradford: Boston's Foremost Pioneer Orthopaedic Surgeon	19
Chapter 16	Robert W. Lovett: The First John Ball and Buckminster Brown Professor of Orthopaedic Surgery	45
Chapter 17	James W. Sever: Medical Director of the Industrial School for Crippled and Deformed Children	83
Chapter 18	Arthur T. Legg: Dedicated to Disabled Children	101
Chapter 19	Robert B. Osgood: Advocate for Orthopaedics as a Profession of Physicians and Surgeons Who Restore Function	113
Chapter 20	Frank R. Ober: Caring Clinician and Skilled Educator	143
Chapter 21	William T. Green: Master in Pediatric Orthopaedics	167
Chapter 22	David S. Grice: Advocate for Polio Treatment	207
Chapter 23	BCH: Other Surgeon-Scholars (1900–1970)	217
Chapter 24	Melvin J. Glimcher: Father of the Bone Field	319
Chapter 25	John E. Hall: Mentor to Many and Master Surgeon	333
Chapter 26	Paul P. Griffin: Southern Gentleman and Disciple of Dr. William T. Green	349
Chapter 27	BCH Other Surgeon Scholars (1970–2000)	357
Chapter 28	Boston Children's Hospital: Modernization and Preparation for the Twenty-First Century	427
	Index	441

Volume 1 Contents

Acknowledgements		xiii
Foreword		xv
Preface		xvii
Introduction		xix
About the Author		xxv

Section 1 — The First Family of Surgery in the United States

Chapter 1	Joseph Warren: Physician Before the Revolution	3
Chapter 2	John Warren: Father of Harvard Medical School	21
Chapter 3	John Collins Warren: Co-Founder of the Massachusetts General Hospital	31
Chapter 4	Warren Family: Tradition of Medical Leaders Continues into the Twentieth Century	71

Section 2 — Orthopaedics Emerges as a Focus of Clinical Care

Chapter 5	John Ball Brown: The First American Orthopaedic Surgeon	95
Chapter 6	Buckminster Brown: Founder of the John Ball & Buckminster Brown Chair	105
Chapter 7	The Boston Orthopedic Institution: America's First Orthopaedic Hospital	113
Chapter 8	House of the Good Samaritan: America's First Orthopaedic Ward	123

Section 3 — Harvard Medical School

Chapter 9	Orthopaedic Curriculum	133
Chapter 10	The Evolution of the Organization and Department of Orthopaedic Surgery	171
Chapter 11	The Harvard Combined Orthopaedic Residency Program	183
Chapter 12	Harvard Sports Medicine	245
Chapter 13	Murder at Harvard	291

Volume 3 Contents

Section 5	**Massachusetts General Hospital**	
Chapter 29	Massachusetts General Hospital: The Beginning	3
Chapter 30	Henry J. Bigelow: The First Orthopaedic Surgeon at MGH	23
Chapter 31	Charles L. Scudder: Strong Advocate for Accurate Open Reduction and Internal Fixation of Fractures	53
Chapter 32	Orthopaedics Becomes a Department at MGH: Ward I	67
Chapter 33	Joel E. Goldthwait: First Chief of the Department of Orthopaedic Surgery at MGH	77
Chapter 34	Ernest A. Codman: Father of the "End-Result Idea" Movement	93
Chapter 35	Elliott G. Brackett: His Character Was a Jewel with Many Facets	147
Chapter 36	Nathaniel Allison: A Focus on Research and Education	163
Chapter 37	Marius N. Smith-Petersen: Prolific Inventor in Orthopaedics	179
Chapter 38	Joseph S. Barr: A "Gentle Scholar" and a Great Teacher	201
Chapter 39	William H. Harris: Innovator in Hip Replacement Surgery	215
Chapter 40	MGH: Other Surgeon Scholars (1900–1970)	227
Chapter 41	Henry J. Mankin: Prolific Researcher and Dedicated Educator	381
Chapter 42	MGH: Other Surgeon Scholars (1970–2000)	395
Chapter 43	MGH: Modernization and Preparation for the Twenty-First Century	453

Volume 4 Contents

Section 6 Brigham and Women's Hospital

Chapter 44 Peter Bent Brigham Hospital and Robert Breck Brigham Hospital: The Beginning — 1

Chapter 45 Robert Breck Brigham Hospital and Peter Bent Brigham Hospital: Orthopaedic Service Chiefs — 43
Robert Breck Brigham Hospital — 44
Peter Bent Brigham Hospital — 72

Chapter 46 RBBH and PBBH: Other Surgeon Scholars, 1900–1970 — 79
Robert Breck Brigham Hospital — 80
Peter Bent Brigham Hospital — 104

Chapter 47 Origins of BWH and Organizing Orthopaedics as a Department — 113

Chapter 48 Clement B. Sledge: Clinician Scientist — 125

Chapter 49 BWH: Other Surgeon Scholars: 1970–2000 — 143

Chapter 50 BWH's Modernization and Preparation for the Twenty-First Century — 191

Section 7 Beth Israel Deaconess Medical Center

Chapter 51 Beth Israel Hospital: The Beginning — 199

Chapter 52 Albert Ehrenfried: Surgeon Leader at Mount Sinai and Beth Israel Hospital — 215

Chapter 53 Beth Israel Hospital: Orthopaedic Division Chiefs — 223

Chapter 54 Augustus A. White III: First Orthopaedic Surgeon-in-Chief at Beth Israel Hospital — 257

Chapter 55 Stephen J. Lipson: Chief of Orthopaedics at Beth Israel Hospital and Beth Israel Deaconess Medical Center — 267

Chapter 56 Beth Israel Deaconess Medical Center: A History of New England Deaconess Hospital and Its Merger with Beth Israel Hospital — 273

Chapter 57 BIDMC: Modernization and Preparation for the Twenty-First Century — 283

Section 8 Boston City Hospital

Chapter 58 Boston City Hospital (Harvard Service): The Beginning — 293

Chapter 59 Frederic J. Cotton: Orthopaedic Renaissance Man — 309

Chapter 60 The Bone and Joint Service at Boston City Hospital: Other Surgeons-in-Chief — 333

Chapter 61 Boston City Hospital: Other Surgeon Scholars — 357

Chapter 62 Pedagogical Changes: Harvard Leaves Boston City Hospital — 377

Section 9 Harvard Orthopaedists in the World Wars

Chapter 63 World War I: Trench Warfare — 385

Chapter 64 World War II: Mobile Warfare — 463

Volume 5 Contents

Bibliography

Copyright Acknowledgments

"Military Orthopedic Surgery," World War I by R. W. Lovett

Harvard Faculty Who Served as Presidents of Major Professional Organizations

James H. Herndon, MD, MBA Curriculum Vitae

Volume 5 is available as an electronic version only and is included with purchase. It is available for download at www.birthofaspecialty.com.

To access link directly, go to https://pathway-book-service-cart.mypinnaclecart.com//peter-e-randall/birth-of-a-specialty-bibliography-only/

SECTION 4

BOSTON CHILDREN'S HOSPITAL

"The heritage of the past is the seed that brings forth the harvest of the future"
    Inscription on the south portico of the **Archives Building**, Washington, DC

"I will look upon him who shall have taught me this Art even as one of my parents...
I will impart this Art by precept, by lecture, and by every mode of teaching...
To disciples bound by covenant and oath, according to the Law of Medicine"
    —**Hippocratic Oath**

"The leader in medicine is essentially a self-made man, standing on his own feet,
strong in his own convictions, relying on his own achievement"
    —**Robert Lovett**, President of the Boston Surgical Society
    Address at presentation of the Bigelow Medal to Dr. William
    J. Mayo, June 6, 1921. (BMSJ, 1921; 184:653.)

Boston Children's Hospital
The Beginning

CHAPTER 14

Children's Hospital—founded in 1869 and later named Boston Children's Hospital—is the fourth-oldest pediatric hospital in the United States, following the Nursery for Children in 1854 in New York (renamed the Nursery and Child's Hospital in 1857) and the Children's Hospital of Philadelphia in 1855. When opening their doors, Children's Hospital became the second hospital in Boston dedicated entirely to the care of children. The Children's Infirmary was the first; it had opened in 1846.

THE CHILDREN'S INFIRMARY

Mr. Amos Lawrence, founder of the Children's Infirmary, purchased the medical school's building on Mason Street during a time when Harvard Medical School (HMS) was moving to its new location on North Grove Street. He wrote in his diary that he wanted to support a charitable hospital for children of poor families "to overcome their repugnance to giving up their children to the care of others" (W. R. Lawrence 1855). Lawrence was also a strong advocate for the education of physicians, especially teaching anatomy with human dissection. He even volunteered his body to John Collins Warren, stating, "I would gladly have him use me in the way to instruct the young men" (W. R. Lawrence 1855).

It turned out that the building housing the infirmary was not suitable to care for sick children. Lawrence sold it and refurbished a large house with 30 beds located on Washington Street, in the current Dorchester area and near the Lying-in Hospital. He then re-opened the hospital in 1847 for children ages 2–16 years. Mr. Lawrence's son, Dr. William P. Lawrence, a Harvard Medical graduate and one of the original trustees of City Hospital, served as physician of the Children's Infirmary. Eleven months later, Dr. Lawrence moved the hospital to a third location, returning to Mason Street, and close to its original site. However, one year later, in November 1848, it was closed. It had remained open for 18 months and had treated 192 patients between the ages of 2 and 15. Surprisingly, Dr. Lawrence did not think that lack of resources was responsible for its closure; he believed the poor were averse to accepting help at the hospital because they did not trust that adequate treatment would be provided; instead, they relied upon the care they could provide themselves. After the infirmary's closure, patients and families may have gradually become more accepting of treatment by physicians as other hospitals that provided pediatric care began to open, but it would be another 21 years before the founding of Boston Children's Hospital.

ORIGINS OF CHILDREN'S HOSPITAL

At the time Children's Hospital opened, other hospitals in Boston included the House of the Good Samaritan (founded 1861) and the Massachusetts General Hospital (1821) in the west, and Boston City Hospital (1864) and Carney Hospital (1863) in the south. Each admitted both adults and children; patients were usually over the age of two years. About 14% of the admissions were children at both Massachusetts General Hospital and Boston City Hospital in the late 1860s. Children were treated as small adults; they were admitted to adult wards and received no unique treatments for their care. Other than Lawrence, no one in the United States before 1855 believed infants and children had unique needs or required special care.

However, children younger than five-years-old had a much higher mortality rate in Boston at the time, and almost 50 percent of all deaths in the 1870s were among this age group. Lemuel Shattuck went so far as to say the children of the poor in Boston "seemed literally 'born to die'" (L. Shattuck 1846). Boston was densely populated, much like Philadelphia and other major cities in the United States and Europe, and, at the time, poor ventilation and malnutrition were common. Cities were vectors for infectious disease. In Boston, the majority of deaths occurred from eight infectious diseases: cerebrospinal meningitis, diarrheal disease, diphtheria, measles, scarlet fever, small-pox, typhoid fever, and whooping cough. Death from tuberculosis, bronchitis, and pneumonia were also common.

In 1855, Dr. Frances West Lewis founded the Children's Hospital in Philadelphia with two

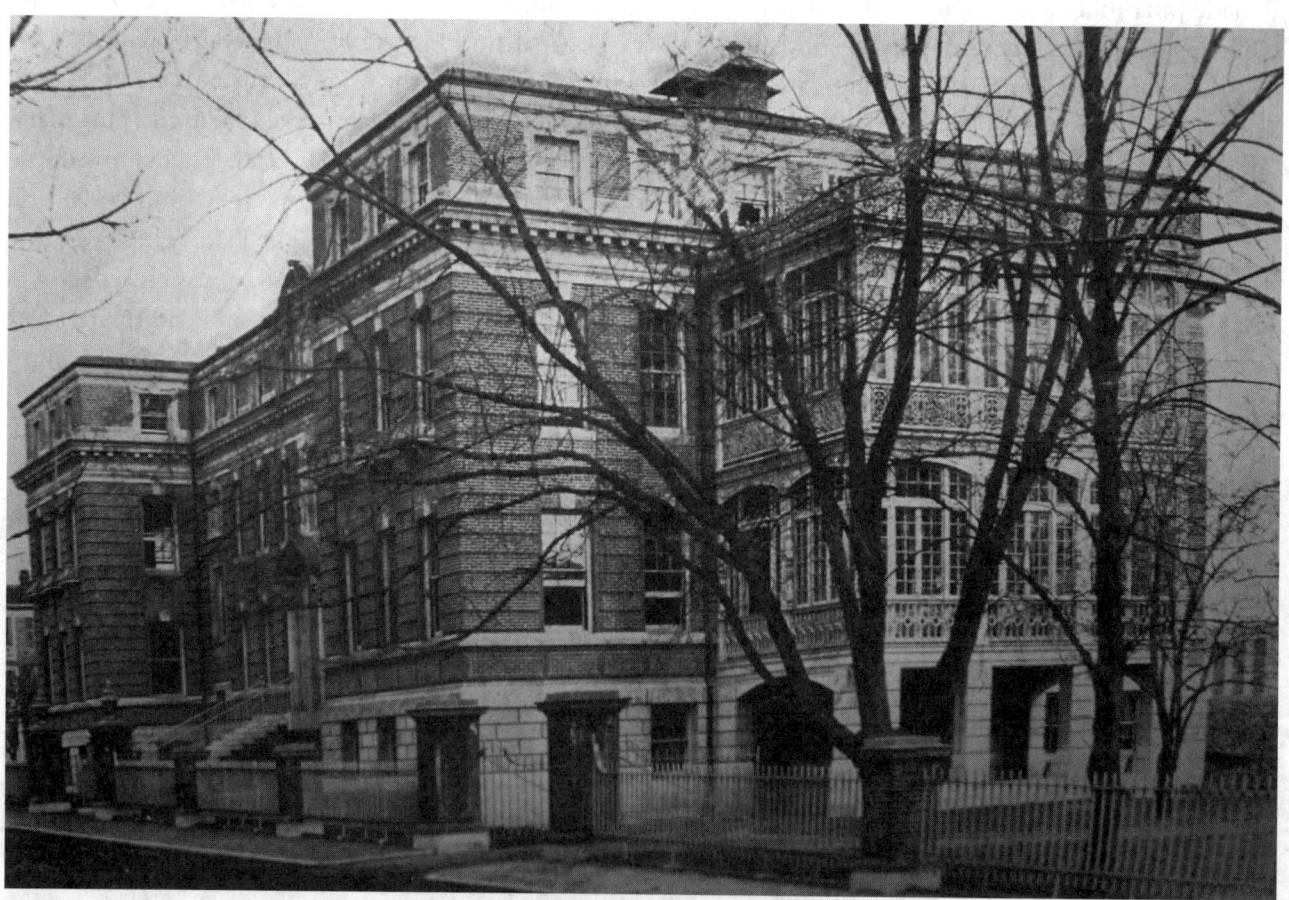

House of the Good Samaritan, 25 Binney Street, ca. 1906. *Images of America. Children's Hospital Boston.* Charleston, SC: Arcadia Publishing, 2005. Boston Children's Hospital Archives, Boston, Massachusetts.

other physicians. They modeled it after the Great Ormond Street Hospital of London, one of the leading children's hospitals in Europe. They had previously visited the Great Ormond Street Hospital in 1854. We do not know whether any of the founders of Children's Hospital visited Dr. Lewis, the Children's Hospital of Philadelphia or the Nursery and Child's Hospital in New York; they did, however, visit St. Luke's Hospital and the Sheltering Arms in New York City and were impressed by what they saw:

> Here was a hip joint case, confined in its little bed…two or three in different parts of the ward, each confined as to the lower extremities by some apparatus…interested in the horse-driving…ball rolling…or all the little games of their more fortunate companions…There were plenty of chairs and tables, and everything for little people…[not] these things in an adult ward or hospital…in one large room were thirty-five or more children, from nine years to…two…scarcely a face among them which it was not pleasant to look upon…there did not seem to be any manifestation of selfishness among them.
> (F. H. Brown et al. 1879 [Countway Medical Library])

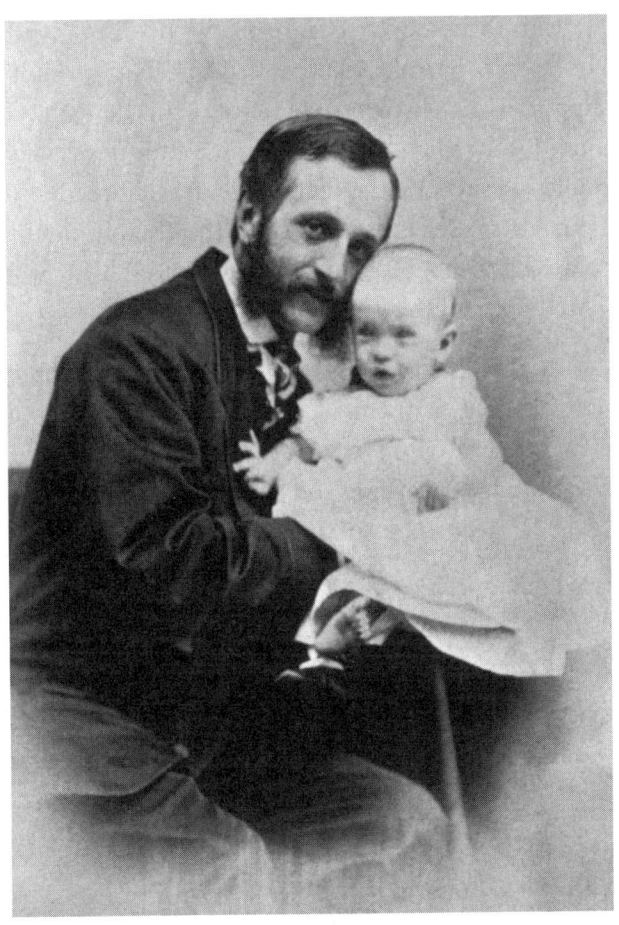

Francis Henry Brown, MD. Founder of BCH.
One Hundred Years at Children's by Lendon Snedeker, MD. Boston: Children's Hospital, 1969. Boston Children's Hospital Archives, Boston, Massachusetts.

Francis Henry Brown (no relation to John Ball or Buckminster Brown) was the leader amongst the physicians who went on to found Children's Hospital; he practiced in Cambridge before the Civil War. In 1864, he was acting assistant surgeon to Dr. William Ingalls (another founder of Children's Hospital) at the 1000-bed United States General Hospital in Readville, Massachusetts. After the war, he resumed his long-standing interest in hospital construction, and he spent about a year traveling throughout Europe studying it. We do not know if he visited the Great Ormond Street Hospital in London, but, given his interests, he may have. In his Harvard thesis in 1861, Dr. Brown had written about hospital construction: "I start with these principia—abundance of air; abundance of sunlight; simplicity of construction. These are the essentials; without these no hospital can exist and perform its proper function in the community; and under these heads may be included all the minutiae of hospital construction" (F. H. Brown 1861). In his bibliography, he mentioned that Florence Nightingale's "Notes on Hospitals" (published in 1859) emphasized that lack of cleanliness was the single most important cause of child mortality in London, closely followed by a lack of adequate ventilation.

In December 1868, Dr. Brown invited two physicians and three private citizens to his home to hear about his plans for a hospital for children in Boston: Dr. William Ingalls, Dr. S. G. Webber, Reverend Chandler Robbins, George H. Kuhn, and J. Huntington Wolcott. They met again in January along with Albert Fearing and Nathaniel

H. Emmons—two community leaders—and Dr. S. G. Langmaid, a surgeon. The group strongly supported Dr. Brown's views for a children's hospital. By the end of the month, the four physicians publicly issued a pamphlet, "A Statement made by Four Physicians in Reference to the Establishment of a Children's Hospital in the City of Boston." The objects of the charity included:

1. The medical and surgical treatment of the diseases of children
2. The attainment and diffusion of knowledge regarding the diseases of children
3. The training of young women in the duties of nurses (F. H. Brown et al. 1879)

They went on to state:

[We] well know the sad fatality of children in our community; medical practitioners are painfully aware that the hygienic influences which surround the children of the poorer classes are of the worse description. We desire to afford these sufferers, for darkness…sunshine; for filth and disorder, cleanliness and system; for the rough word or neglect…chance blow…or threat,

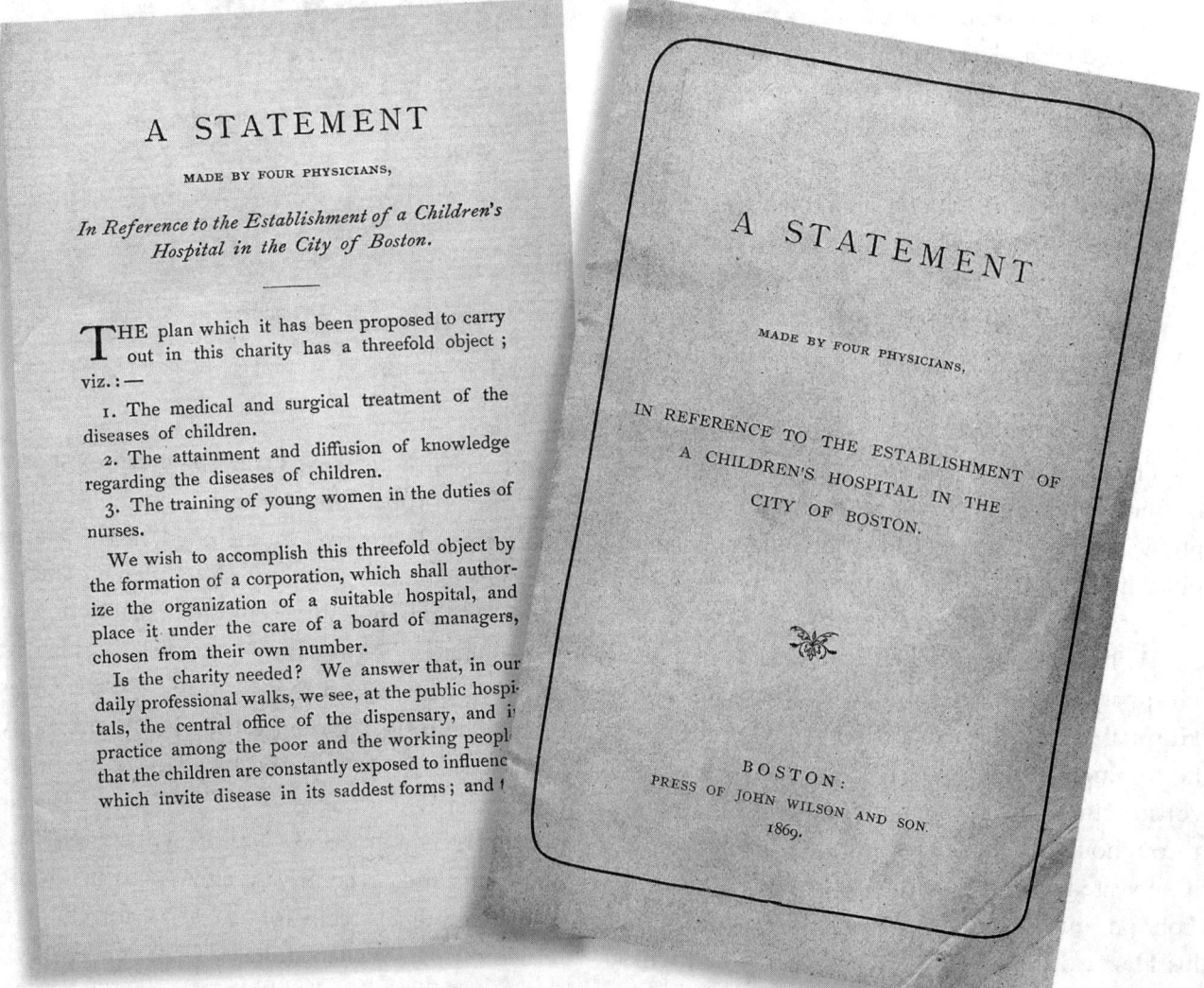

A Statement Made by Four Physicians. *Images of America. Children's Hospital Boston.* Charleston, SC: Arcadia Publishing, 2005. Boston Children's Hospital Archives, Boston, Massachusetts.

gentleness, kindly attention, encouragement… If…the thousand ills to which these children are subject do not cause death, they frequently leave enfeebled frames…We not only desire to treat these cases…successfully, but…also to give a tone to the general health of our patients…Considered undesirable patients… although often received and kindly cared for in our present hospitals…little sick children are entirely out of place among sick adults. Adults can complain if they are neglected; the little fellows cannot do so, or fear prevents them…The liability to neglect exists. The beds and general appliances and conveniences of an adult hospital are not fitted to children. Physicians and nurses for children should have a peculiar adaptedness for the management of their young charges.
(F. H. Brown et al. 1879)

These four physician planners also strongly supported the education of future physicians and nurses. They wrote: "There is a want in our community, long felt in our medical schools, though provided for in foreign cities, namely, an opportunity to study infantile diseases [and] which furnish a distinct branch of medical science, the importance of which can hardly be sufficiently recognized…Still farther, we wish, in connection with the hospital, to initiate a system hitherto unknown in Boston, of instructing young women of the middle and lower classes in the duties of nurses, both for children and adults" (F. H. Brown et al. 1879). At the time, pediatric medical literature was sparse, perhaps nonexistent. The first textbook on pediatrics in the United States was not published until later that same year, *Treatise on the Disease of Infancy and Childhood* by Job L. Smith at the Nursery and Child's Hospital in New York (C. A. Smith 1983). No medical journals were devoted to pediatrics until the *Journal of Pediatrics* was published in 1884.

A petition for a charity corporation was then presented to the Massachusetts Legislature. Approval by the Commonwealth of Massachusetts for incorporation of the Children's Hospital, dated February 26, 1869, stated: "for the purpose of establishing and maintaining, in the city of Boston, a Hospital for the care, treatment and cure of diseased or maimed children…" (F. H. Brown et al. 1879). The Children's Hospital opened on July 19, 1869, in a purchased private house at 9 Rutland Street. It had a capacity of 20 beds (T. M. Rotch 1914).

Despite the overwhelming support from the Massachusetts Legislature and the general public, a strong objection to a hospital for children was expressed in a letter written to the *Boston Daily*

COMMONWEALTH OF MASSACHUSETTS.

In the Year One Thousand Eight Hundred and Sixty-nine.

An Act

To Incorporate The Children's Hospital.

Be it enacted by the Senate and House of Representatives, in General Court assembled, and by the authority of the same, as follows:—

SECT. 1. Chandler Robbins, George H. Kuhn, Nathaniel H. Emmons, their associates and successors, are made a corporation, by the name of The Children's Hospital, for the purpose of establishing and maintaining, in the city of Boston, a Hospital for the care, treatment, and cure of diseased or maimed children; with all the powers and privileges, and subject to all the duties, liabilities, and restrictions set forth in all general laws which now are or may hereafter be in force and applicable to such corporations.

SECT. 2. Said corporation shall have power to hold real and personal estate to an amount not exceeding one hundred and fifty thousand dollars.

SECT. 3. This act shall take effect upon its passage.

House of Representatives, February 24, 1869.
    Passed to be enacted.
                Harvey Jewell, *Speaker.*

In Senate, February 25, 1869.
    Passed to be enacted.
                Robert C. Pitman, *President.*

February 26, 1869.
    Approved.
                William Claflin.

                Secretary's Department,
                Boston, March 2, 1869.
A true copy.
    Attest:
                Charles W. Lovett,
                Deputy Secretary of the Commonwealth.

Act of incorporation, BCH.

The Children's Hospital of Boston: Built Better Than They Knew by Clement A. Smith. Boston: Little, Brown and Co., 1983. Boston Children's Hospital Archives, Boston, Massachusetts.

Advertiser signed by "Benjamin S. Shaw, Resident Physician, Massachusetts General Hospital...April 19, 1869" (C. A. Smith 1983). Dr. Shaw's letter stated in part:

> As there seems to be a general impression that no "adequate provision exists in...Boston for the medical and surgical treatment of the diseases of children," some statement to the contrary is called for. Published reports of the Massachusetts General Hospital show that there is no discrimination made between adults and children in...admission of patients into that institution, chronic and contagious diseases alone being refused.
>
> In 1866 of 1,120 patients [admitted to the Massachusetts General], 118 were children... in 1868, 190 of 1,264...or an average for three years about 14 percent...about the same number were treated...in the City Hospital. The House of the Good Samaritan...has 30 beds, and one-half of them constantly occupied by sick children. The new Carney Hospital... receives patients of all ages...our existing institutions, public and private, provide adequately for the hospital treatment of children.

The managers of the Children's Hospital published a reply the next day in the *Boston Daily Advertiser*:

> The facts stated in yesterday's *Advertiser*... were already well understood and considered by the managers of "The Children's Hospital." It is not their intention to come into collision with, or encroach upon the field occupied by an existing institution. They propose to establish a hospital expressly for children...They also wish to educate young women for the duties of nurses of children and of adults...They are well persuaded that there is a need of such an institution, and room for its beneficent work without prejudice to any other hospital. (F. H. Brown et al. 1879)

Support for the Children's Hospital remained high, including among both the press and the medical community. Editorials published in the first volume of the new *Journal of the Gynaecological Society of Boston* stated:

> Whatever excuse may exist for the jealousies of medical men...there can be no condoning attempts to thwart public charities. The perusal, therefore, of the late letter of the Resident Physician of the Massachusetts General Hospital, in opposition to the establishment of a hospital for children in this city, has caused us regret...There has been far too much of intentional blocking the way, in matters medical and surgical, in Boston and it is high time to file an effective protest.
>
> The evil...has brought discredit in more ways than...at first apparent upon this city... It has caused an undue subservience...of the younger men to supposed authority, a fear to assert one's professional manhood...With the wheat sown by Jackson and Warren, there were also planted tares and...the bad stock has grown apace. Monopolies were established that in their infancy were for the general good [but]...soon attained a controlling power. The Medical School succeeded in destroying that attempted to be established by Brown University...prevented that...at Lowell, [and] persistently endeavored to strangle the Berkshire Medical Institution at its birth and after...to prevent establishment of the City Hospital...
>
> The opposition...displayed by that institution towards The Children's Hospital is not from private misunderstandings...but from...more forceful causes...a fear, on the part of those of the hospital staff in the Harvard employ, that a new hospital may serve as...nucleus of a second medical school...and the fact that two of the... four physicians, whose masterly statement... initiated the movement...are members of the attending staff of the other rival of the General Hospital, the Carney...

The time has passed for petty trifling like that being displayed...It is not for present incumbents of hospital posts to assert so offensively that "adequate provision exists in...Boston for the...treatment of children," or to endeavor to render futile the philanthropic exertions [of the founding physicians] for such a school [St. Luke's in New York] for all that is good in grown people here at home...we heartily give its near-coming God-speed. (F. H. Brown et al. 1879)

All further objections to a children's hospital ceased after this brief public dialogue.

Only three of the original founding physicians (Langmaid, Brown, and Ingalls) were officially listed on the staff of the new Children's Hospital. Dr. Francis Greenough (who was not among the original founders) joined the first appointments to the medical staff; he specialized in dermatology. Dr. Langmaid specialized in diseases of the throat; and Dr. Ingalls and Dr. Brown practiced surgery. Dr. Brown's expertise included some orthopaedics, and in 1870 he published one orthopaedic paper, "Rheumatic Arthritis of Coxofemoral Articulation, Spontaneous Dislocation on Dorsum Ilii, Reduction after Several Months" (C. A. Smith 1983). But he spent the majority of his time—about 25 years—steering the course of Children's Hospital, serving as secretary of the board until 1915 and a member of the board of managers until he died at age 82 in 1917. Dr. Webber was the only founding physician who never practiced at Children's. He was a neurologist who had an adult practice, and he became the first professor of neurology at Tufts Medical School.

Children's Hospital quickly expanded and opened the original convalescent home for children in the United States around 1871—Wellesley Convalescent Home. Wellesley provided "sick children the therapeutic benefits...from fresh air. The Hospital has [since] educated and trained a large group of skilled practitioners who have formed an alumni association" (T. M. Rotch 1914).

ORTHOPAEDIC SURGERY

The first two children admitted to the hospital in 1869 were orthopaedic cases, including a seven-year-old child with a fractured radius and an eight-year-old child with a fractured right femur. Seventeen percent of the children admitted in the first year had tuberculosis with hip disease, spine disease, or consumption (pulmonary tuberculosis). The hospital was very successful, but it soon became too small to accommodate the increasing demand. After just one year, the hospital moved to a leased estate at 1583 Washington Street, where

---

REPORT OF THE MEDICAL STAFF.

The first patient was received in the Hospital on the 20th July, and since that time to this date there have been

Received and treated . . . . 30 patients.

16 males; 14 females.
12 medical; 18 surgical.

The result of treatment has been as follows:—

Discharged well 8
Discharged relieved 2
Discharged not relieved 3
Discharged not treated 3
Remaining 14
— 30

There have been no deaths.

A table of the *cases* is herewith presented. Two patients were removed from Hospital within a day or two, by their parents, contrary to advice.

Of the surgical cases, there have been some excellent results; no doubt there will be, at some future time, special reports, which will embrace the unfavorable as well as the favorable cases.

Of the medical cases, there were *three*, whose condition, upon admission, would have warranted any one, however sagacious and skilful, to prognosticate a fatal result, and that within days, if not hours. This is mentioned because it affords a reasonable belief that their restoration is to be nursing.

Some cases, of course, require more care and attention than others; all have received the care they have needed, and all have seemed to be contented and happy.

For the Medical Staff,

WM. INGALLS,
Secretary.

Report of the Medical Staff.
Images of America. Children's Hospital Boston. Charleston, SC: Arcadia Publishing, 2005. Boston Children's Hospital Archives, Boston, Massachusetts.

Registry of patients admitted to BCH, 1869. Many were orthopaedic patients, including the first patient, who had a fractured radius. *Images of America. Children's Hospital Boston.* Charleston, SC: Arcadia Publishing, 2005. Boston Children's Hospital Archives, Boston, Massachusetts.

it remained for 12 years, until 1882. According to Lovett, "the work was still very light [in 1870], for only 30 medical [43%] and 39 orthopaedic and surgical patients [57%] were treated in that year" (R. W. Lovett 1914). Of the 39 surgical cases, 29 were orthopaedic cases, and most addressed tuberculosis of the joints or spine. Other orthopaedic cases included one or two patients each year who were treated in each one of the following conditions: arm burn, club foot, curvature of the tibiae, foot injury, necrosis of the femur or tibia, hip adductor sprain or fractures of the femur, tibia, or fibula. The medical staff publicly reported the results of treatment: 39 discharged well, 13 discharged relieved, 3 discharged not relieved, 6 discharged not treated, 5 died, and 5 remained hospitalized.

At the new location, the medical staff expanded to six, including Benjamin E. Cotting (physician) and John Homans (surgeon). When Edward H. Bradford replaced Francis Brown on the surgical staff in 1878, there was a major shift to focus on orthopaedic surgery. After retiring from his position, Dr. Brown remained on the consulting board for another 25 years. Bradford—who had previously

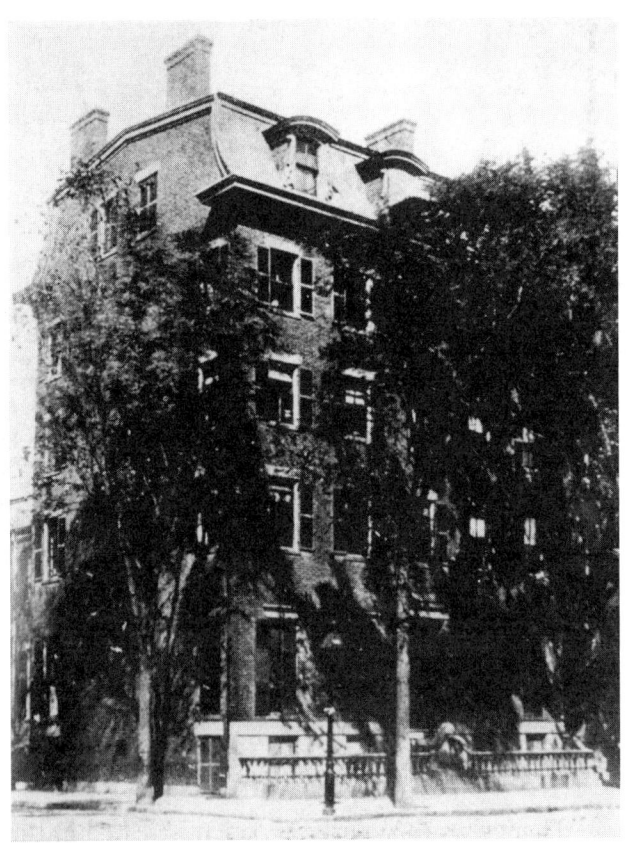

Children's Hospital at Washington and Rutland streets, ca. 1870. *Images of America. Children's Hospital Boston.* Charleston, SC: Arcadia Publishing, 2005. Boston Children's Hospital Archives, Boston, Massachusetts.

limited his own practice to orthopaedic surgery—was joined on the staff by another surgeon, Arthur T. Cabot, who followed Dr. Ingall (and who had switched from the medical to the surgical staff).

Bradford and Cabot led the way for growth and specialization at Boston Children's Hospital, and the hospital saw a new focus on providing surgical treatment where medical remedy could not produce improvement in patient outcomes. The total number of orthopaedic cases increased from 29, in 1870, to 62, in 1881. More patients were also cared for in outpatient clinics, which had opened in 1874. Surgical staff led innovation in treatment for bone and joint tuberculosis—stimulating growth at the hospital, and the majority of pediatric patients admitted were treated for tuberculosis of the spine and extremities. With continued growth, expansion was necessary. Children's Hospital moved again to a building on land purchased just west of Symphony Hall on Huntington Avenue. It was part of the "Flight from the South End" and the "Westward Movement" of Boston institutions described by W. M. Whitehill in his topographical history (1968). It opened the Huntington location

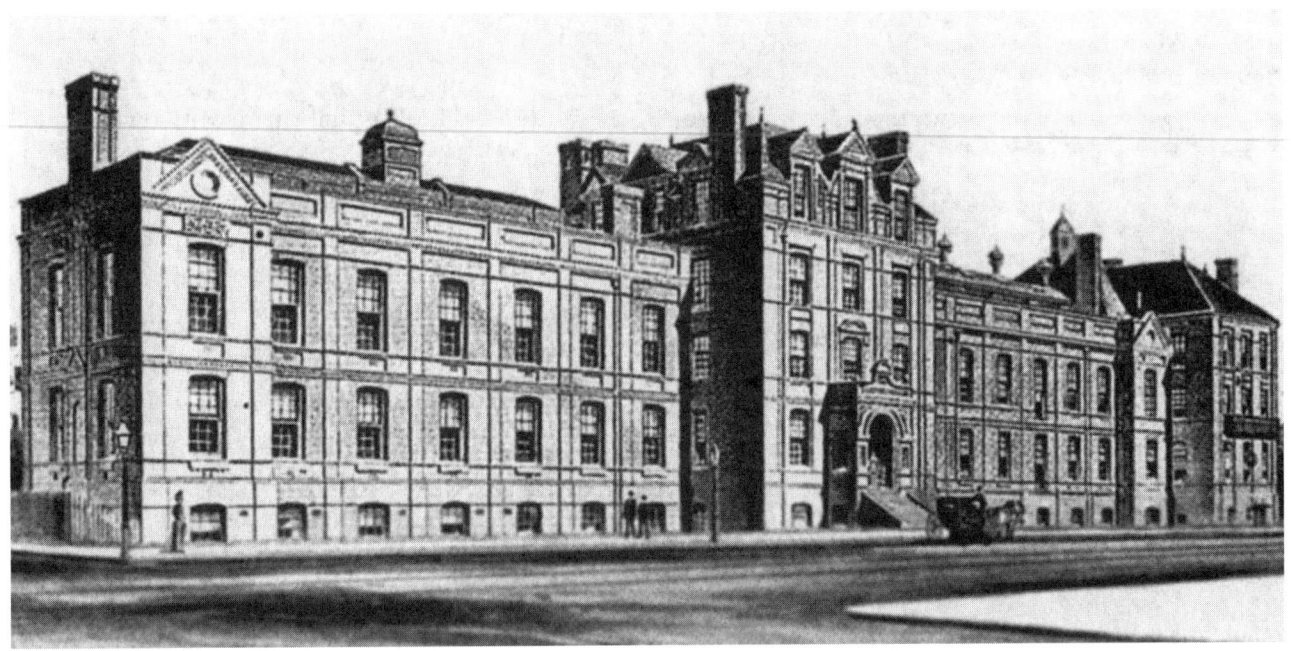

Children's Hospital on Huntington Avenue, ca. 1882. *Images of America. Children's Hospital Boston.* Charleston, SC: Arcadia Publishing, 2005. Boston Children's Hospital Archives, Boston, Massachusetts.

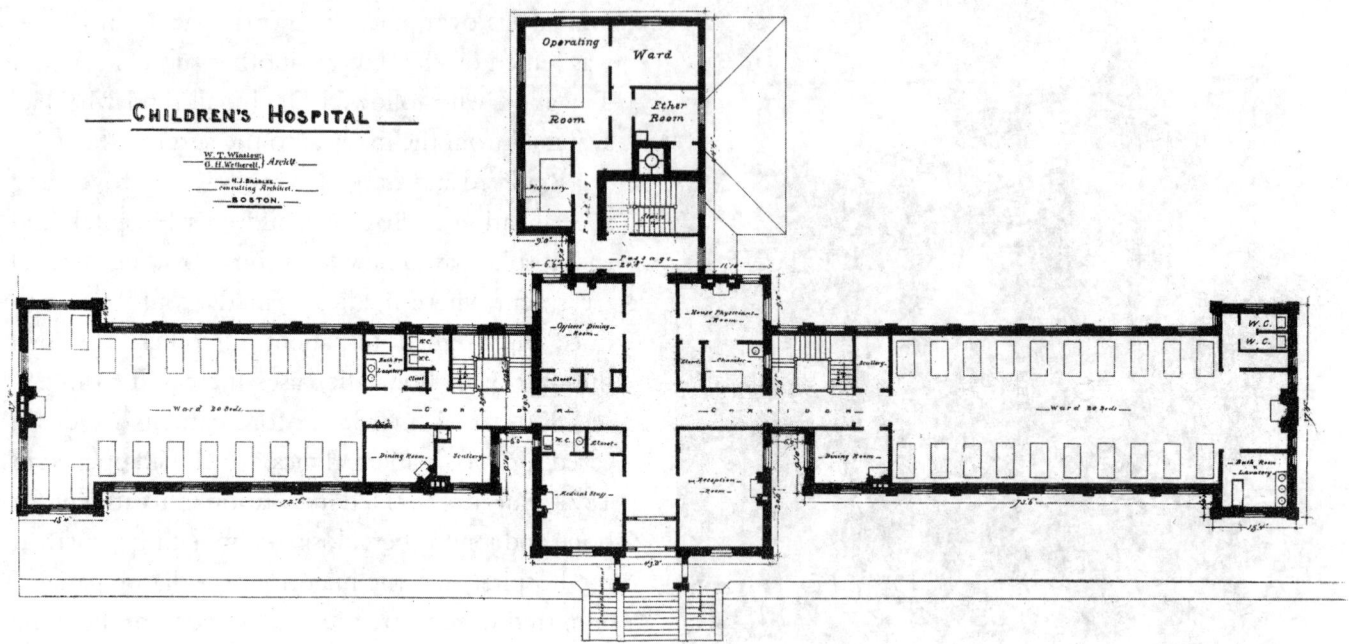

First floor plan, Children's Hospital on Huntington Avenue. *Thirteenth Annual Report of the Children's Hospital, from December 28, 1880 to December 28, 1881.* Boston: University Press: John Wilson and Son, 1882. Boston Children's Hospital Archives, Boston, Massachusetts.

on December 26, 1882, where it now had 60 inpatient beds. That same year, the number of orthopaedic and surgical cases had risen to 178. Of these 178 cases, 62 orthopaedic cases had recorded outcomes (**Table 14.1**).

Table 14.1. Outcomes for Children's Orthopaedic Cases Treated in 1882

DIAGNOSIS	OUTCOME			
	Total	Relieved	Not Relieved	Died Not Treated
Caries, Ankle	2		1	1
Tarsus	3	3		
Club Foot	7	7		
Fracture, Femur	2	2		
Hip Disease	24	18	2	2
Necrosis, Hand	1	1		
Paralysis, Infantile	2	1		
Spastic	2			
Rickets	5	4	1	
Spine, Disease of	10	7	2	1
Lateral Curvature	1	1		
Wry Neck	2	2		

C. A. Smith 1983.

There were 123 surgical patients treated in the Outpatient Department in 1882. A steep increase in outpatient case load occurred over the next few years, with a substantial increase to 421 cases by 1883 and a more than tripling of cases to 1,488 by 1884. The next few years saw the following changes:

- *1884*: The hospital opened its own surgical appliance shop with one technician; within 10 years it expanded to six men and one woman who fitted children for braces, plaster casts, jackets, splints, traction devices, and other appliances.
- *1886*: Dr. Harvey Cushing was appointed as an outpatient assistant.
- *1887*: Cushing was promoted to assistant surgeon and Robert W. Lovett joined the staff as an outpatient assistant.
- *1888*: The managers and the corporation recognized the importance of the outpatient clinics and built a separate facility, the Outpatient Department.

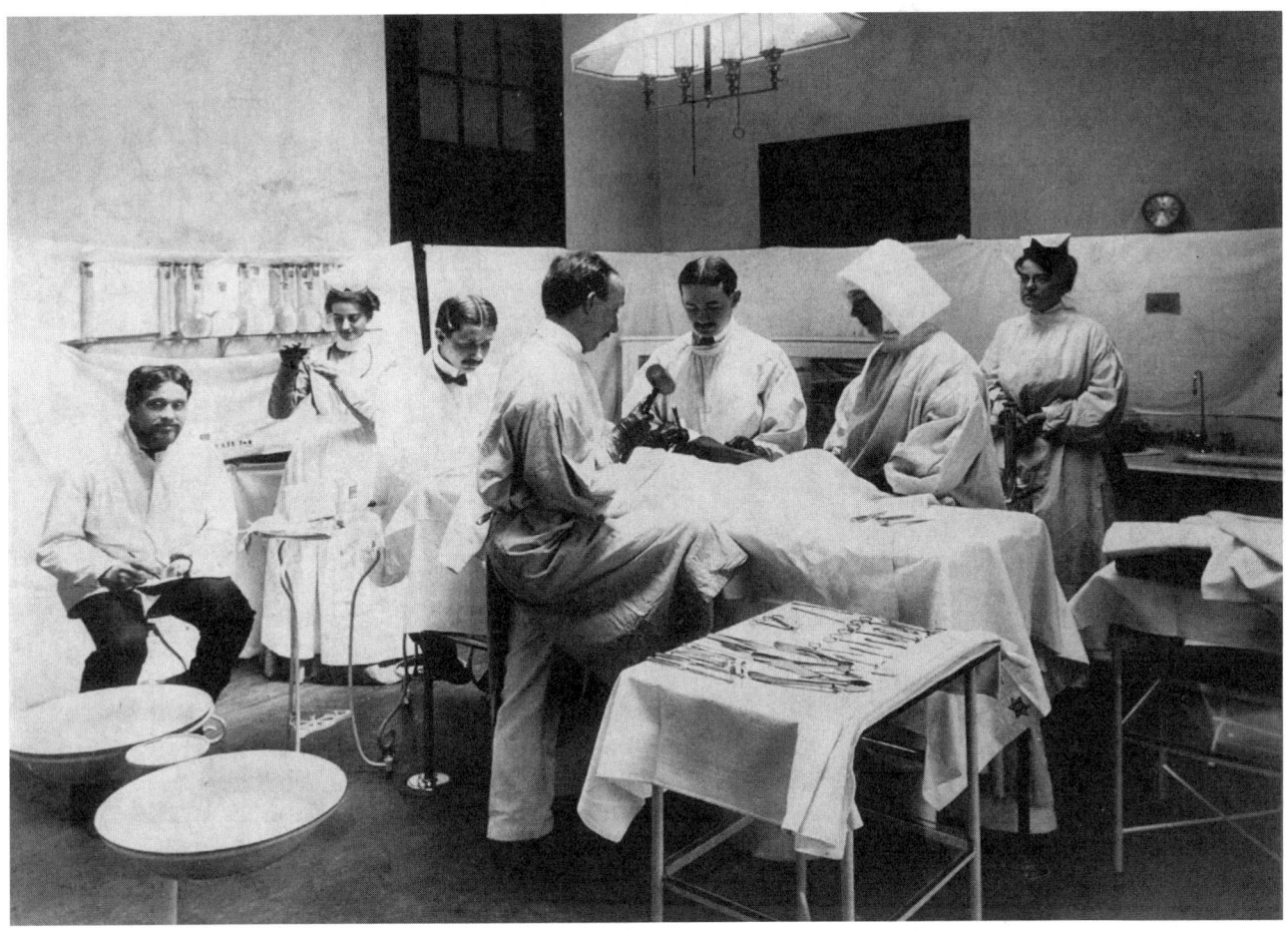

Orthopaedic case in the Huntington Avenue operating room. *One Hundred Years at Children's* by Lendon Snedeker, MD. Boston: Children's Hospital, 1969. Boston Children's Hospital Archives, Boston, Massachusetts.

- *1889*: Dr. Bradford and Dr. Lovett were joined on the staff by Elliott G. Brackett as an outpatient assistant.
- *Subsequent years*: By 1892, Dr. Joel E. Goldthwait was appointed junior assistant orthopaedic surgeon, by 1906, Dr. James Warren Sever as junior assistant orthopaedic surgeon, and by 1908, Dr. Arthur T. Legg (who had previously worked at the hospital as a medical intern and who would later pioneer research on Legg-Calve-Perthes disease) was appointed junior assistant orthopaedic surgeon.

An east wing was added in 1890, bringing the total number of inpatient beds to 96. The new wing was for medical patients, and the west wing contained two wards for surgery. Each year additional physicians and surgeons were added to the medical and surgical staff. In 1891, the third goal of the founding physicians was achieved: a two-year training program for nurses opened. Dr. Thomas Morgan Rotch—the first president of the New England Pediatric Society and the first chair of pediatrics at HMS—recognized these achievements in his paper, "The Development of the Hospital, with Especial Reference to the Medical Service." Rotch (1914) wrote:

> It is well…to call attention to the reputation for excellent work which the institution has deservedly earned throughout the country among the laity as well as the medical profession…this reputation is recognized…by the

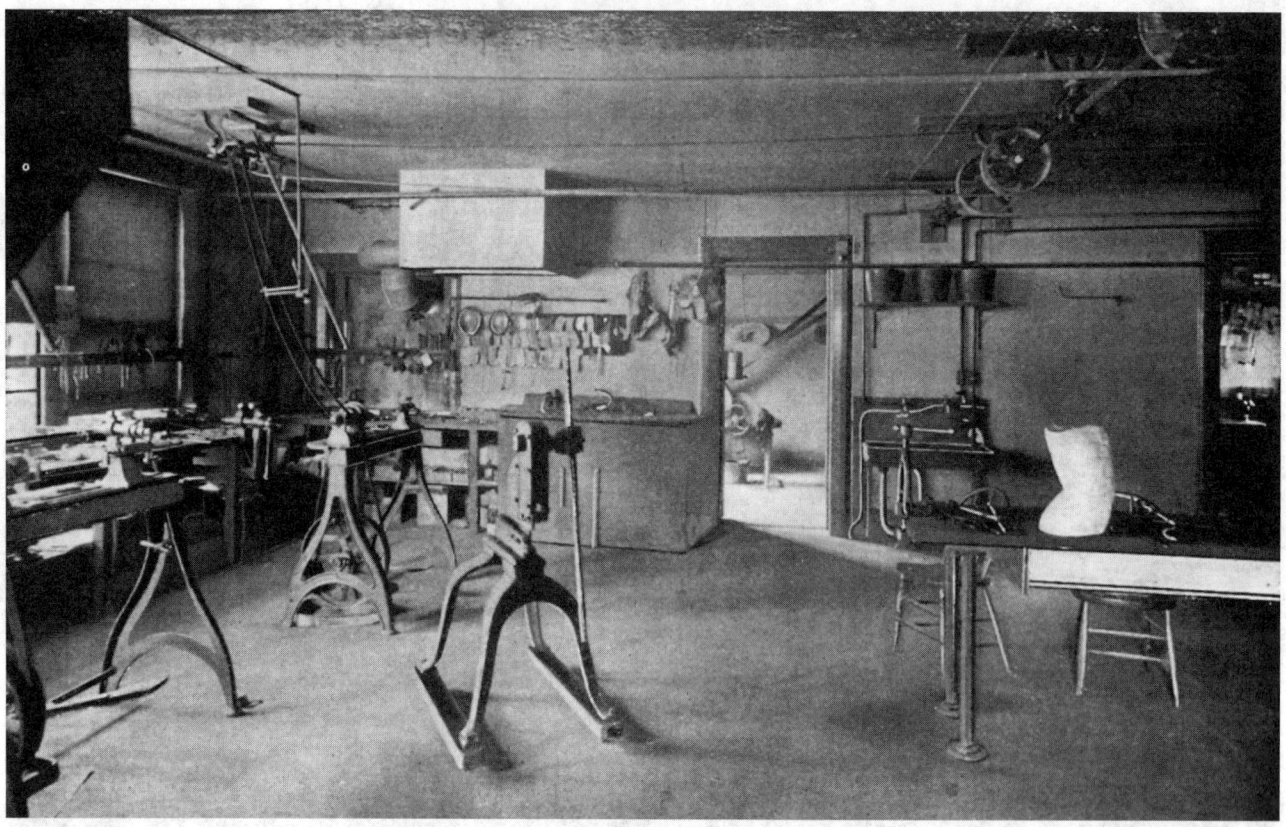

Charitable surgical appliance shop, 1895. *Medical and Surgical Report of the Children's Hospital, 1869–1894*, edited by T. M. Rotch, M.D. and Herbert L. Burrell, M.D. Boston: Children's Hospital Board of Managers, 1895. Boston Children's Hospital Archives, Boston, Massachusetts.

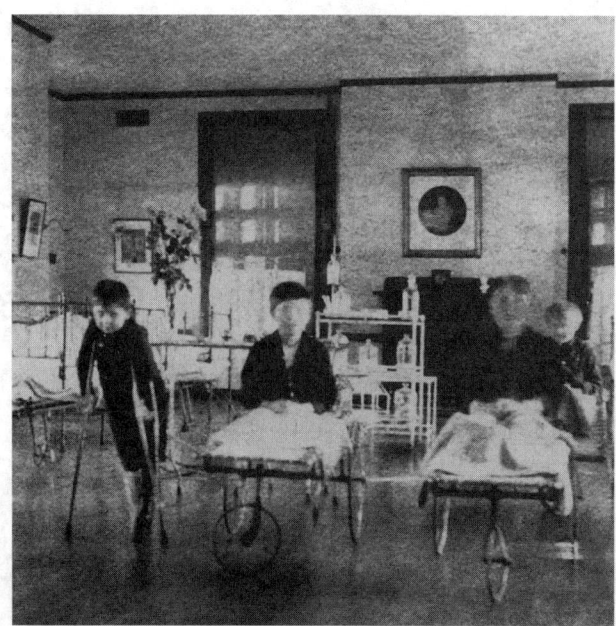

Boy's Ward, ca. 1910.

Images of America. Children's Hospital Boston. Charleston, SC: Arcadia Publishing, 2005. Boston Children's Hospital Archives, Boston, Massachusetts.

fact that during the year 1890 patients came for treatment from all parts of the United States as well as from New Brunswick, Nova Scotia and Aberdeen, Scotland. Another evidence of the superior advantages offered by the institution is the number of physicians who come from afar to avail themselves of the clinical teaching and abundant material to be found in the wards. Interested students esteem it a high favor to be able to work under the physicians and surgeons in charge.

The hospital remained on Huntington Avenue for 32 years, and orthopaedics was their leading specialty in the 1880s and 1890s. **Table 14.2** shows the diagnoses related to these admissions. **Box 14.1** lists the illustrious surgeons who served as department chair. Orthopaedic surgery had continued to advance at a rapid rate, following the

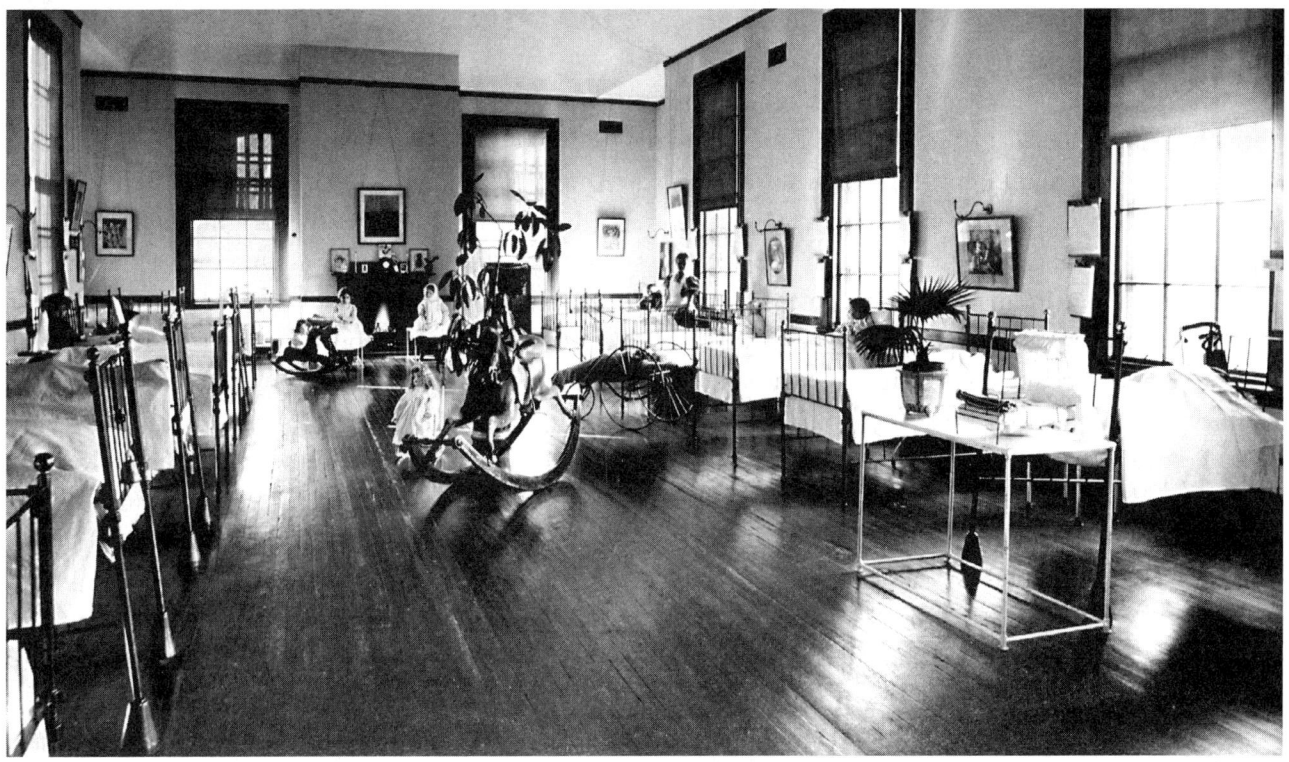

Girl's Surgical Ward. *Medical and Surgical Report of the Children's Hospital, 1869-1894*, edited by T. M. Rotch, MD, and Herbert L. Burrell, MD. Boston: Children's Hospital Board of Managers, 1895. Boston Children's Hospital Archives, Boston, Massachusetts.

discovery of anesthesia and antisepsis. However, the American Pediatric Society described the years from 1889 to 1900 as a "Dark Ages" in pediatrics (H. K. Faber and R. McIntosh 1966). At that time, there was a high infant and neonatal mortality rate, and desperately inadequate public hygiene led to rampant infectious disease among children with few successful treatments available.

Table 14.2. Reasons for Orthopaedic Admissions at Children's Hospital (1883–1898)

	1883–1885	1896–1898
Skeletal tuberculosis	214	442
Spine	66	201
Hip	129	185
Knee	19	56
Clubfeet	37	73
Congenital dislocated hip	3	28
Orthopaedic (other)	12	57

Data originally from the Children's Hospital's annual reports: 1883–1885 and 1896–1898 C. A. Smith 1983, pg. 65.

Box 14.1. Orthopaedic Chairpersons

Edward H. Bradford	1903–1915
Robert W. Lovett	1915–1922
Robert B. Osgood	1922–1931
Frank R. Ober	1931–1946
William T. Green	1947–1968
Interim: Arthur M. Pappas	1969–1970
Melvin J. Glimcher	1970–1981
John E. Hall (Chief of Clinical Services)	1971–1979
Paul P. Griffin	1981–1986
John E. Hall	1986–1994
James R. Kasser	1994–2013
Peter M. Waters	2013–present

Bradford had worked at Children's for almost 35 years before becoming dean of Harvard Medical School in 1912. During his period of service, Bradford "saw the hospital rise from its very small beginnings to an institution of national reputation, and in this progress, he was one of the important factors. No one else had so long a connection with the staff" (R. W. Lovett 1914). Tuberculosis remained the major admitting diagnosis on the orthopaedic service for almost 30 more years until a rapid decline in the early 1920s (**Table 14.3**). Prevention work—including efforts to pasteurize all milk—ultimately led to this decline. They had discovered that tubercular cows were often the source of infection for cases of bone and joint tuberculous. Pulmonary tuberculous was spread through human contact.

Table 14.3. Decline in Admissions for Skeletal Tuberculosis of the Hip and Spine

Year	Number of Admissions
1921	136
1924	80
1925	67
1936	2

C. A. Smith 1983.

RADIOLOGY

Concurrently with the period of specialization in pediatric orthopaedics at Children's, Dr. Ernest Amory Codman was appointed skiagrapher in 1900. Skiagraphy was the original name applied to radiology. Codman, a surgeon at the Massachusetts General Hospital, had become very interested in x-rays after their discovery by Roentgen in 1895. He experimented clinically with the use of a primitive x-ray machine, both at the Massachusetts General Hospital and at Children's Hospital. He is listed in Children's Hospital Annual Report of 1900 as "skiagrapher" (C. A. Smith 1983), but he was not listed as a member of the medical staff. The first official radiologist at HMS was Percy E. Brown, named staff radiologist at Children's Hospital in 1903 after Robert Osgood (1901–1903). He received a teaching appointment at HMS where he taught students on "The Use of the Roentgen Ray" (C. A. Smith 1983). The use of roentgenography spread rapidly, with most examinations ordered for orthopaedic cases (**Table 14.4**).

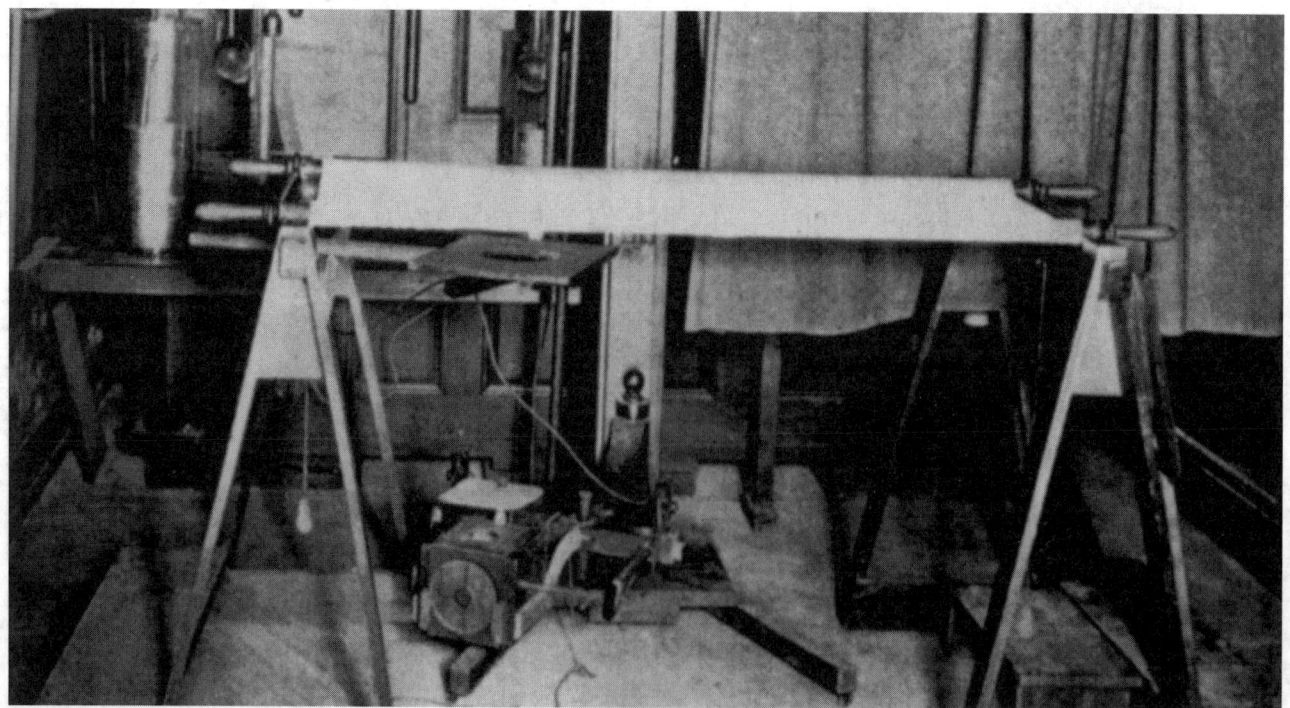

Radiology equipment, ca. 1899. *Images of America. Children's Hospital Boston.* Charleston, SC: Arcadia Publishing, 2005. Boston Children's Hospital Archives, Boston, Massachusetts.

Table 14.4. X-ray Negative (Glass Plates During) 1904–1905 at Children's Hospital

Reason for x-ray	Number taken
Fractures	156
Dislocations	7
Congenital Deformities	175
Tuberculosis of the Hip	191
Tuberculosis of Other Bones and Joints	112
Osteomyelosis (perhaps a misprint for "osteomyelitis")	99
Luetic Conditions	7
Periostitis	3
Paralytic Conditions	7
Lateral Curvature of the Spine	16
Other Diagnoses or No Diagnosis	58
Negative Results	102

Total in 843 cases, 933 negatives N. T. Griscom 1996.

Children's Hospital was later renamed Children's Hospital Medical Center in 1959 and then Boston Children's Hospital in 2012. During the twentieth century, it was unofficially referred to as the Children's Hospital; Children's Hospital, Boston; or the Children's Medical Center. For consistency, I have referred to it as Boston Children's Hospital (BCH) throughout the remainder of this book. BCH from its earliest conception has paved the path forward in the treatment of pediatric diseases. The hospital has been a major contributor to medical education, the development of new knowledge from physician experience, and original basic and clinical research. Through its more than 150-year history, it has continued to be on the forefront of advances in pediatrics and orthopaedic surgery.

CHAPTER 15

Edward H. Bradford
Boston's Foremost Pioneer Orthopaedic Surgeon

Edward Hickling Bradford was born in Boston on June 4, 1848, to Charles Frederick Bradford and Eliza Edes (Hickling) Bradford. He was a descendent of William Bradford, who arrived in Plymouth, Massachusetts, in 1620 on the ship *Mayflower*. William Bradford became the second governor of the Plymouth Colony in 1621; it was a position he held until 1633, after which he was then reappointed governor on four additional occasions: 1635, 1637, 1639, and 1645. He died in office in 1657. *The Boston Medical and Surgical Journal* described Edward Bradford as "by rights a Pilgrim rather than a Puritan" and as one "ruled by the highest personal standards, but tolerant and charitable as regards the rights and opinions of others" ("F. C. S." [F. C. Shattuck], *Boston Medical and Surgical Journal* [*BSMJ*] 1926).

Edward Bradford graduated from the Roxbury Latin School and then Harvard College with an AB degree in 1869, which was the same period that Buckminster Brown was the leading orthopaedic surgeon in Boston and chief of the orthopaedic service at the House of the Good Samaritan. In 1873, Bradford received a medical degree from Harvard Medical School (HMS), which was located on North Grove Street at the time. While a medical student, he also obtained a master of arts degree in 1873. Newly elected Harvard President Charles Eliot had not yet completed his major educational reforms to the medical school curriculum. The students, therefore,

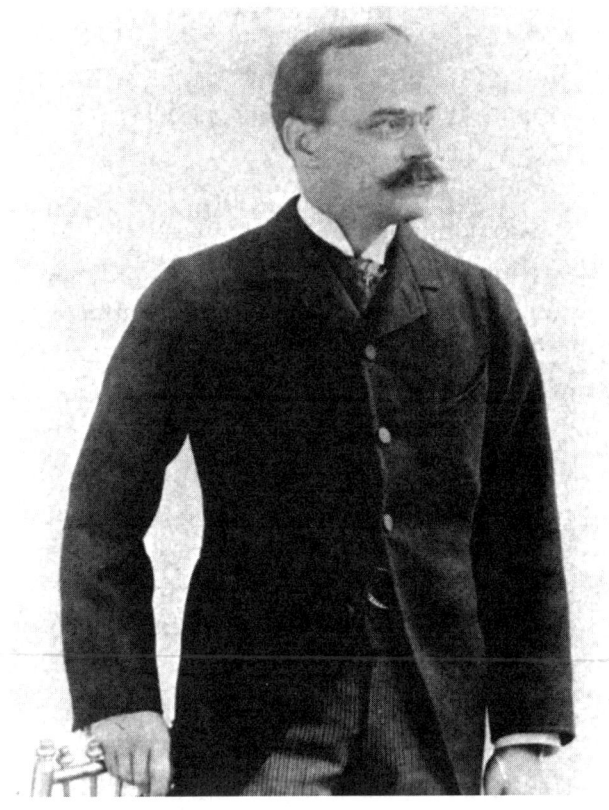

Edward H. Bradford, ca. age 40. *The Early Orthopaedic Surgeons of America* by Alfred Rives Shands Jr. Saint Louis: Mosby, 1970.

Physician Snapshot

Edward H. Bradford
BORN: 1848
DIED: 1926

SIGNIFICANT CONTRIBUTIONS: Surgeon-in-chief in the first orthopaedic department in New England at Boston Children's Hospital; coauthor of the *Treatise on Orthopedic Surgery*; dean of Harvard Medical School could choose the old requirements (the oral examination method) or the new ones (a written exam in all subjects). With some friends, Bradford took all the written exams and passed each one. Bradford spent his last year of medical school as a surgical house officer (pupil) at Massachusetts General Hospital (MGH):

> Dr. Eliot...recommended the election of house pupils at the Massachusetts General Hospital on competitive examinations. Dr. Bradford was chosen from a large number of contestants. Here he came under the direct supervision of those masters in medicine, Henry J. Bigelow and John C. Warren in surgery, James Jackson Putnam in neurology, Henry Jackson in medicine. (J. G. Kuhns and R. B. Osgood, n.d.)

We do not know whether Bradford met Buckminster Brown at HMS or MGH, but it is unlikely because Brown did not have an appointment in either institution. He may not have met him until a later point.

Bradford expressed an early interest in surgery and orthopaedics, and—with his friend Frederick C. Shattuck—he sought additional training in Europe and England; in London, Paris, Strasbourg, Berlin, and Vienna. He was 27 years of age when he visited Liverpool, spending several months with Hugh Owen Thomas, a bone setter well-known for his original contributions to orthopaedics, e.g., the Thomas splint, which saved many lives during World War I. Bradford returned to the United States after two years abroad and spent a short time in general practice in Boston before he pursued further orthopaedic studies in New York with Charles Fayette Taylor—a surgeon well-known in America and Europe for his hip and spine braces. Thomas and Taylor had never met, but Bradford observed similar traits in each. They were both brilliant, dynamic, persistent, and independent in their approach to thinking and deed. Bradford believed it was this unique combination of characteristics that drove forward the rapid advances in orthopaedics at the time. Bradford only worked with Taylor for a few months, however, before Taylor resigned as surgeon-in-chief at the New York Orthopaedic Dispensary and Hospital in 1876 and devoted himself to his large private practice. Taylor also worked at St. Luke's Hospital and operated at a small sanatorium close by, where Bradford most likely also accompanied him.

EARLY YEARS IN ORTHOPAEDIC RESEARCH AND PRACTICE

Bradford returned to Boston in late 1876 and joined Buckminster Brown—whom he had long admired as a pioneer in orthopaedic surgery on the staff at the House of the Good Samaritan, and where he remained for years—becoming chief of surgery upon Brown's retirement. Bradford was influenced by Brown, his mentor, in his decision to focus his surgical career on orthopaedics, and the two became colleagues and friends. During the same period, he had also started his private surgical and orthopaedic practice, and he received an appointment at the Boston Dispensary as well. Opened in 1796, the Boston Dispensary provided free medical care for patients who didn't want to enter the Alms House. Buckminster Brown also worked at the Boston Dispensary between approximately 1876 and 1880. By 1878, Bradford had accepted an appointment as surgeon to outpatients

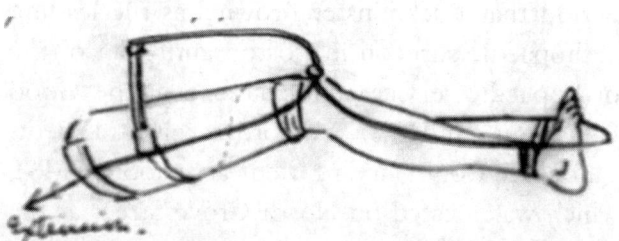

Bradford's sketch of an appliance he designed to correct knee flexion contractures.

The House of the Good Samaritan Records 1860-1966. Archival Collection—AC4. Box 16, volume 24, p. 81. Surgical Records, Nov. 1879-Aug. 1889. Boston Children's Hospital Archives, Boston, Massachusetts. Photo by the author.

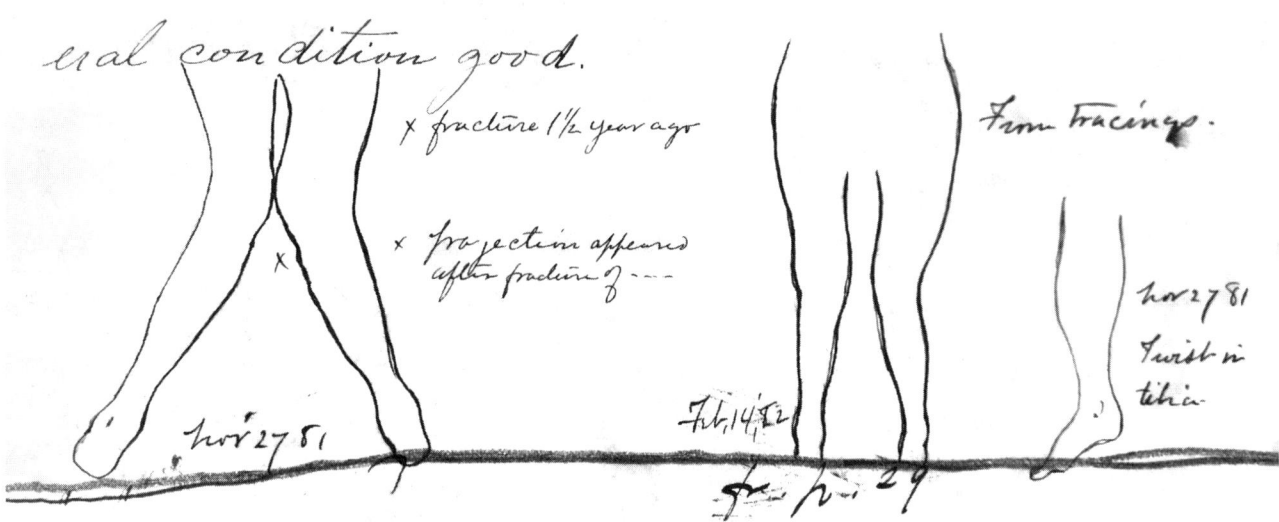

Bradford's sketches of a patient with a knee valgus deformity. Preoperative: November 27, 1881. Postoperative: February 14, 1882.
The House of the Good Samaritan Records 1860–1966. Archival Collection—AC4. Box 16, Volume 24, pg. 52. Surgical Records, Nov. 1879–Aug. 1889. Boston Children's Hospital Archives, Boston, Massachusetts. Photo by the author.

at the Boston City Hospital (which had opened in 1864) and joined the surgical staff at Boston Children's Hospital on Washington Street—where he replaced the founding lead surgeon Dr. Francis Brown (no relation to John Ball or Buckminster Brown).

Hip Disease

Just two years later, Bradford had been appointed chief of surgery at the House of the Good Samaritan after Brown's retirement, and he was also appointed assistant in clinical surgery in the surgical department at HMS where he was assigned to teach orthopaedic surgery. That same year, after having practiced for only four years, he wrote an article on "The Treatment of Hip Disease," in which he studied cadavers on the use of traction of the hip in extension with and without muscle releases. Hip disease in the nineteenth century meant tuberculosis of the hip, with its associated morbidity from pain, spasm, loss of motion, deformity, and a high mortality rate. Bradford had learned this method of traction, which had been

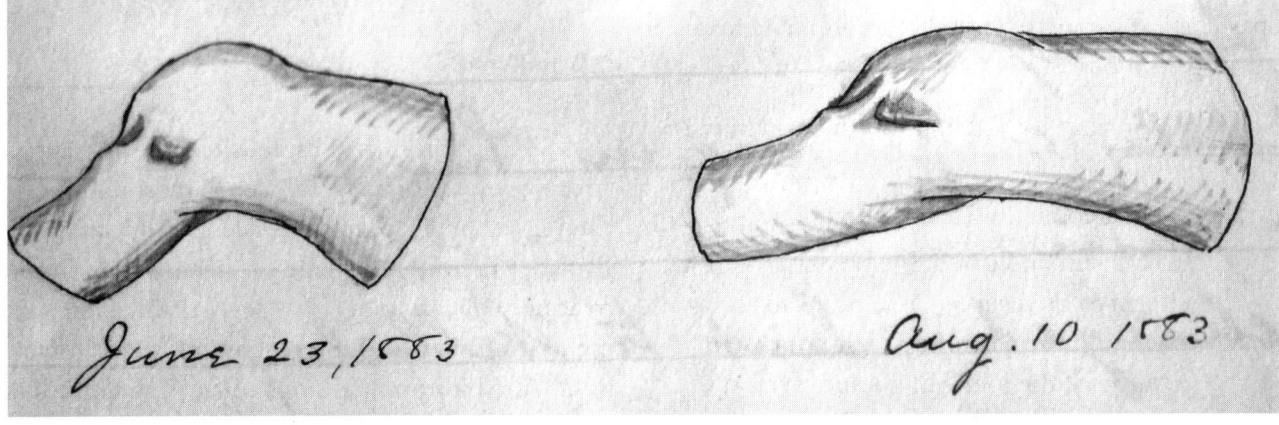

Bradford's drawing of the result he obtained using his appliance to correct a knee flexion contracture.
The House of the Good Samaritan Records 1860–1966. Archival Collection—AC4. Archives of Children's Hospital Boston. Box 16, Volume 24. Pg. 81. Surgical Records, Nov. 1879–Aug. 1889.

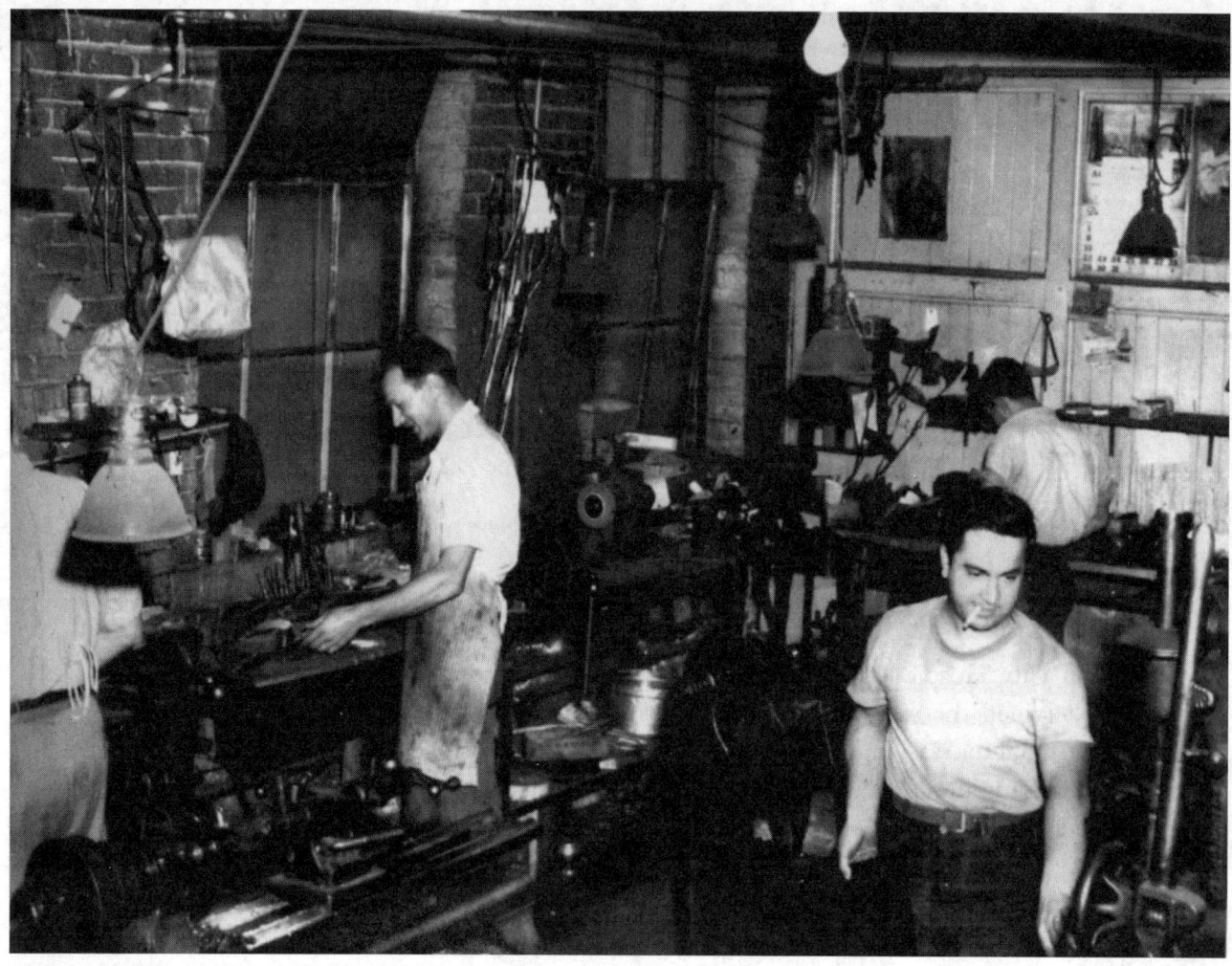

Orthopaedic Brace Shop after WWII. It remained functional for decades after being founded by Bradford. *Images of America. Children's Hospital Boston.* Charleston, SC: Arcadia Publishing, 2005. Boston Children's Hospital Archives, Boston, Massachusetts.

"perfected by C. F. Taylor" (E. H. Bradford 1880). In early cases with patients experiencing spasm, pain, or deformity, he recommended an initial period of rest in traction:

1. To prevent jar and injurious motion at the joint.
2. To overcome muscular contraction.
3. To prevent and correct deformity. Extension is to be regarded as a means for overcoming muscular contraction, for partial fixation of the joint, and, under certain conditions, for "distraction," or actual separation of the bones forming the joint. (E. H. Bradford 1880)

He aspirated or drained tuberculosis abscesses involving the hip and spine.

Club Feet

By 1884, Bradford had established the first appliance shop at Boston Children's Hospital. Continuing the work of his predecessor, Buckminster Brown, Bradford also made further advances in the treatment of club foot. He "devised and employed methods similar to those of Hugh Owen Thomas in the forcible correction of clubfeet" (J. G. Kuhns and R. B. Osgood, n.d.). In addition to Brown, Bradford was undoubtedly influenced by Henry G. Davis in his modern approaches to treating club feet, scoliosis, hip joint disease, limb deformities, and the surgical treatment of abscesses, what some have called the American method of orthopaedic surgery. Davis had practiced for 15 years in Worcester and Millbury, Massachusetts, before moving to New York. He had introduced the use of traction with weights and pulleys for fractures and limb deformities four years before Dr. Gordon Buck introduced his similar traction in 1860. Bradford's approach to orthopaedics can be seen in Davis's description of the American method:

> I insisted from the first on the fact, that mobility is natural to and required by a diseased as well as a healthy joint and introduced that as one of the principles of my treatment. I insisted also from the first on the fact that pressure, mostly owing to muscular contraction, is the most active agent of destruction in the morbid process, which it is the object of my treatment to overcome; and I, therefore, directed my efforts to obviating in all stages of the morbid process, the pressure to which the parts diseased are exposed. To attention to this, I ascribe mainly my success.
>
> The distinctive principle of my treatment is the procuring to the diseased structures support without pressure, and motion without friction. The treatment itself, concisely defined, consists in abtraction [sic] of the joint affected, by continued elastic extension. (H. G. Davis 1863)

Bradford reported in 1884 on a series of 16 cases of resistant club-foot deformities that he had treated at the House of the Good Samaritan, Boston Children's Hospital, and one case at the Boston City Hospital. Because relapsed cases, resistant cases, and "half treated cases of congenital talipes equino-varus may be cured without the expenditure of a great amount of time[,] the operation of excision of the tarsus has probably come into vogue on account of this need...attended by slight risk and followed by excellent results, if equally good results can be obtained by less severe surgical interference the method is certainly to be discarded" (E. H. Bradford 1884). Arguing that the deformity was the result of contracted tissues and not bone deformity, Bradford preferred to avoid tarsectomy by releasing contracted tendons and then obtaining further correction by use of special appliance that he designed to allow gradual correction. He also objected to Phelps's technique of surgical release of all ligaments on the medial side of the foot because of the large open

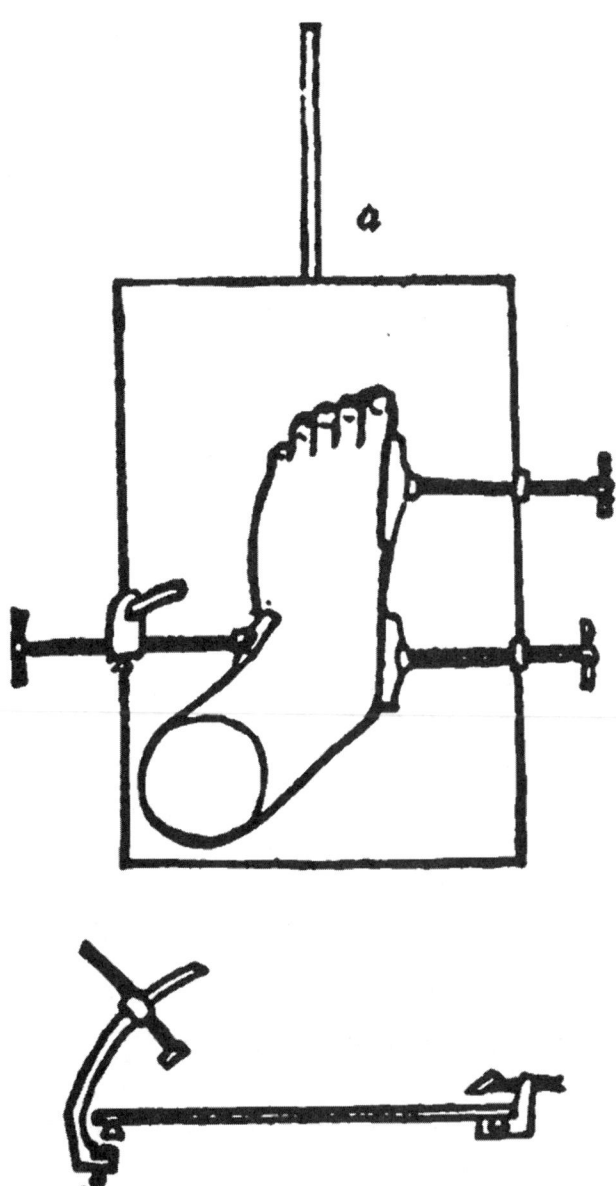

Bradford's device to forcibly correct a severe club-foot deformity. Bradford, "On the Use of Force in the Treatment of Resistant Club-Foot," *Boston Medical and Surgical Journal* 1884; 110: 265.

wound remaining after the foot was repositioned and the subsequent high recurrence rate of the deformity secondary to scar contractures. After surgical releases (tibialis tendons and Achilles tendon), if he was unable to passively correct the foot deformity, he would use his special apparatus, applying braces to correct the foot while the patient was anesthetized. He noted that "sometimes complete correction is not possible at one sitting, and something will have to be left for after treatment or for a second sitting" (E. H. Bradford 1884). Occasionally, he would perform a plantar fasciotomy.

After correction, Bradford would apply a long leg cast (plaster-of-Paris) for up to three weeks, followed by a walking shoe. Of the 16 resistant cases he reported, 10 were what he described as perfect ("patient stands and walks on the whole of the sole of the foot" [E. H. Bradford 1884]), three were nearly perfect ("the heel can be brought to the floor without twisting the foot, but the front of the foot cannot be raised without lifting the heel" [E. H. Bradford 1884]), and three were imperfect ("condition of the foot falling short of this [perfect] standard" [E. H. Bradford 1884]). He believed "the method to be safe, to save time and trouble, to give perfect results" (E. H. Bradford 1884). Shands wrote that Bradford believed "half-cures are practically no cures at all" (A. R. Shands 1970). Bradford's dedication to achieving more permanent cures was prescient; to achieve this goal, he followed his patients for a long time. In his treatise "Orthopaedic Surgery in the United States of America," Leo Mayer stated, "[Bradford's] study of club-feet published sixty years ago might well be used today in an orthopaedic instructional course" (L. Mayer 1950).

Other Surgical Advances

In 1885, Bradford was appointed visiting surgeon at the Boston City Hospital. Although Bradford recognized the importance of orthopaedics as a specialty in the field of surgery, early in his career he practiced surgery in general while increasingly focusing his efforts on orthopaedics. In 1888, he performed the first craniotomy for tumor in Boston, removing a brain tumor measuring 7-by-4-by-3 centimeters. Three months later, Dr. Henry H. A. Beach performed the first craniotomy at MGH. Surgeons determined localization of the tumor preoperatively using the patient's signs and symptoms. Roentgenograms would not be discovered until seven years later, in 1895. During surgery, Bradford located and removed the tumor by pushing his index finger into the cerebral cortex, and he "passed [it] around the whole mass, and [after] separating it from the adjacent parts, the tumor was then turned out of its bed by means of [his] finger, stretching the incision in the cortex slightly" (P. C. Knapp 1889). The operation took 50 minutes, and the nodular mass proved to be tuberculosis. The patient died almost one hour after the operation was completed, and the only recorded observations were the patient's pulse, respirations, and blood loss. At Boston City Hospital, "he was regarded by his associates as a courageous surgeon with excellent judgment, broadminded and generous to his fellow physicians" (J. G. Kuhns and R. B. Osgood, n.d.).

He was also described by peers as "broadminded, generous hearted, free from jealousy, the first to congratulate an associate and the last to criticize his fellows" (R. B. Osgood 1926a). During his time at the Boston City Hospital, Bradford instituted its first orthopaedic ward, but he firmly believed that orthopaedic surgeons must have a strong foundation in general surgery; for Bradford, a specialty must evolve naturally within the field and could not be forced to develop.

Bradford's Presidential Address to the American Orthopaedic Association

The specialty of orthopaedics was changing; it was in transition and was entering a new era of a specialty with new operative procedures as well as medical and mechanical options at its disposal for treating patients with complex musculoskeletal problems, diseases, injuries, and deformities. The year after he performed the craniotomy, Bradford gave the presidential address to the American Orthopaedic Association, and he carefully traced the historical evolution of orthopaedic surgery:

> But though great progress was made in orthopedic surgery, it is not to be overlooked that it fell from the high estate it held in general surgical interest fifty years ago, until it became an almost despised and rejected branch. The orthopedic surgeon was regarded as a man of mere straps and buckles, or the custodian of that surgical chamber of horrors, the orthopedic institute. (E. H. Bradford 1889a)

He does not state which orthopaedic institute or institutes he was referring to, but by this point in time he had worked for about 14 years on the orthopaedic ward of the House of the Good Samaritan in addition to his other early experiences. Most likely, he had also seen or was at least aware of the Boston Orthopedic Infirmary, and he knew that patients had been treated for months—or longer—in traction and they wore various types of mechanical devices to improve deformities. He had treated patients with Pott's disease and tuberculosis of bones and joints with prolonged rest in open-air environments, which was the common treatment of the nineteenth century. He had also read about and most likely had heard Buckminster Brown describe his successful treatment of a young child with bilateral congenital dislocated hips, treated in bed with traction for 13 months. Bradford wrote: "The case reported some years ago by Dr. Buckminster Brown is of so much importance that it would be desirable that the method of treatment be extensively carried out. The difficulty in the method is the prolonged character of the treatment, necessitating confinement to the bed for at least a year" (E. H. Bradford 1891).

In the same address, he further wrote about the development of orthopaedic surgery:

> Fifty years ago the attention of the surgical world was turned to the remarkable feats of the great surgeons who taught us precision, skill, and boldness in the triumphs of the amphitheatre, and that the ambition of all men of energy prompted them to emulate those monarchs of the operating-table. The famous line in the *Iliad*…was interpreted to mean the surgeon whose feats meant so much for humanity.
>
> Following this period came the introduction of anaesthetics, which enormously enlarged the field of possible operations; and subsequently came the introduction and perfection of the antiseptic system, which has enabled the surgeon to perform in his operations veritable marvels. It is not strange that in the active current of progress the less brilliant branch of orthopedic surgery…where the element of patient, persistent work is so important, should have been for the while passed aside by the energetic and ambitious…the natural spirit of mechanical ingenuity became manifest in this branch of surgery…led to mechanical extravagance, but… the tendency is in the right direction. (E. H. Bradford 1889a)

He then briefly reviewed the history of orthopaedics in America. Although he included many of John Ball Brown's publications in his "Bibliography of American Orthopedic Surgery Prior to 1860" from his speech (E. H. Bradford 1889a), he doesn't mention his name in the use of tenotomy. He did mention that Dr. William Ludwig Detmold reported on his first case of tenotomy of the Achilles tendon in club foot in 1837 (only a few months before John B. Brown opened his orthopaedic institution in Boston), noting that two surgeons—Rogers in 1834 and Dickson in 1835—had previously performed the operation but did not publish their results.

Bradford had previously asked Buckminster Brown to write a history of orthopaedics in New England for him, which Bradford included verbatim in his speech:

The history of orthopedic surgery in New England commenced in 1838 when Dr. John Ball Brown, of Boston, treated nine cases of spinal disease and curvature...On February 21, 1839, he did the operation [subcutaneous tenotomy for club foot] on a little girl four or five years of age...The treatment was successful. So far as was known to Dr. Brown, this was the first time that subcutaneous tenotomy had been done in America. He afterward learned it had been done once previously by Dr. Detmold, of New York. Dr. W.J. Little, of London, about this time published his first work on "Club-foot and Analogous Distortions"...a great assistance to the American pioneer...From the date above named, Dr. Brown had an extensive experience in his branch of surgery, and his reputation spread widely...Dr. Brown continued in the practice of orthopedic surgery until his death, which occurred in 1862. (E. H. Bradford 1889a)

Bradford further credited other orthopaedic surgeons who had advanced the field in America:

Dr. Henry G. Davis for the originality and courage of conviction he displayed at a time when originality was needed...whether we know it or not, we are all followers of the teachings of Dr. Davis...It is difficult to do full justice to the great influence and excellence of the work of Dr. C. F. Taylor...perfect adaptation of mechanical appliances to surgical indications, and a force of character enabling him to carry, through years of discouragement, difficult cases of caries of the spine, until ultimate and permanent cures were reached...Without his teachings our specialty would not have attained the perfection in mechanism it has reached... Dr. Sayre...His fame in this regard is worldwide...Orthopedic surgery is no longer— thanks to the surgery of Dr. Sayre, his brilliancy as a writer and teacher—a neglected branch of surgery...he has broadened the field of general surgery...

One other name can be added to the list, for the painstaking, determined courage of his work, and especially for the unusual record of success won through his unparalleled persistence. The records of surgical annals can be searched in vain for a well-established cure of double congenital dislocation of the hip, until we come to the work of Dr. Buckminster Brown...

And though orthopedic surgery today offers many opportunities for the exercise of that surgical sense, and the art of operative interference...yet we should remember always, as our predecessors have done, that our specialty must essentially remain conservative in the best sense of the word. It should seek to obtain results with the least sacrifice of tissue, the least impairment of function. We are bound by our calling not to maim; we must, of all surgeons, be the last to fall victims to the délire operatoire...our duty as surgeons compels us to obtain the best results in the speediest way compatible with safety to our patient and that he certainly is unworthy—a surgical laggard—who trusts to the temporizing expectancy of a mechanical appliance, when an osteotomy, an arthrectomy, an excision is needed. (E. H. Bradford 1889a)

Orthopaedics, in Bradford's opinion, had become a surgical specialty, separate from other branches of surgery and medicine. Perhaps this may have been the reason that he didn't mention Dr. John Ball Brown, leaving the history of orthopaedics in Boston in his presidential address to his mentor, Buckminster Brown. After all, John Ball Brown was an orthopaedist of the past, who specialized mainly in using mechanical devices to correct deformity and only later using tenotomy in the treatment of club foot, scoliosis, and torticollis. Buckminster Brown had advanced the field by adding more surgical treatments— including additional tenotomies in foot deformities (even in adults), tenotomies for hand and wrist contractures, release of hip contractures, release of knee contractures, improving splinting/brace techniques, and by providing careful, detailed postoperative management until the optimal result was obtained. Brown had previously written:

> For twenty-five or more years it has been my practice to operate upon contracted muscles, tendons, or cicatricial tissues connected with the knee or hip joints: first by subcutaneous section in the hip of the adductor longus, tensor vaginae femoris, rectus, or sartorius, and in the knee of the biceps flexor cruris, semi-tendinosus and semi-membranosus, or such of the tissues as required division; followed by forcible rupture of the more deeply-seated adventitious impediments to free movements—this brisement forcé being in all cases carefully gauged and measured as to the degree of power employed by the amount, estimated under ether, of resistance to be overcome. (B. Brown 1881)

Buckminster had trained in many of Europe's leading orthopaedic centers, whereas his father had served apprenticeships locally in general medicine and surgery and only later in his career focused on orthopaedics; John Ball was essentially self-taught.

Bradford's Advances in Orthopaedic Surgery

During his active years in orthopaedic surgery, Bradford saw the introduction of many new orthopaedic surgical treatments which he discovered or enthusiastically supported, and he continued to seek faster, more accurate, and successful treatments. He modified traction methods and designed his famous Bradford Frame, and he favored ambulatory treatments, especially operative ones. "To Bradford, historians say, belongs the credit for establishing orthopaedics as a discipline separate from surgery" (*Harvard Medical School Perspectives* 1990). Although orthopaedic surgeons still used traction, they increasingly replied upon splints, braces, and new plaster casts/jackets to treat musculoskeletal deformities, surgery, and the indications for surgery. Virgil Pendleton Gibney (1897)—the second surgeon-in-chief at the Hospital for the Ruptured and Crippled (later named the Hospital for Special Surgery)—wrote:

> The orthopedic surgeon is prepared to conduct a case from its incipiency to its close; that, if apparatus fails to meet the indications, he is able to conduct an operation, which operation

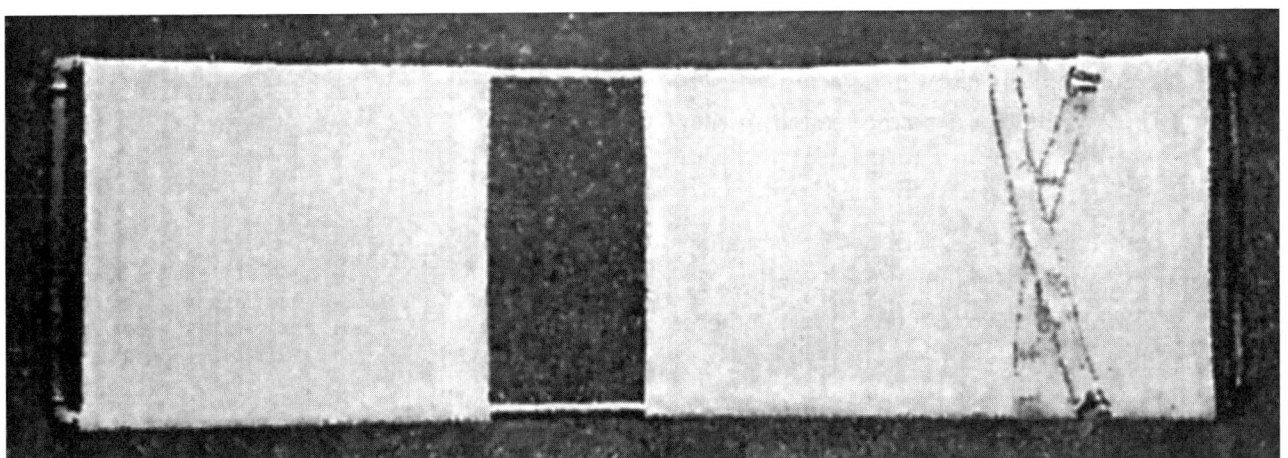

Bradford frame. Originally designed to treat patients with tuberculosis of the spine in recumbency. Bradford called it a gas-pipe frame. *Treatise on Orthopedic Surgery*, 2nd edition, by Bradford and Lovett. New York: William Wood and Company, 1899. Columbia University Libraries/Internet Archive.

ought to be done as well as any general surgeon can do it, and which operation can be supplemented by the judicious use of mechanical appliances, in order to bring about the best possible result.

Club Feet

In 1889, three months before his presidential address, Bradford reviewed his personal results of treating 99 cases of congenital club foot, from a few weeks of age to 18 years. He graded his results as perfect, good, satisfactory and imperfect within the following groups:

- cases treated without surgery
- infants treated with tenotomy
- children walking (2–5 years of age)
- resistant cases

Perfect results were obtained in 10 of 12 cases treated without surgery (no imperfect results); good or perfect results in 15 of 25 infants treated with tenotomy (2 imperfect results); good or perfect results in 12 of 25 children between ages two to five years (5 imperfect results); and 28 good or perfect results in cases over five years of age that he classified as resistant (6 imperfect results).

He concluded that in each of these categories, treatment can be successful but "relapses will invariably occur unless the distortion is completely corrected and in fact overcorrected" (E. H. Bradford 1889d). Bradford further stated in that famous paper that:

> Many resistant cases…where persistency and attention cannot be commanded…operations on the bone, radical in character, are sometimes demanded…Of these methods three serve careful consideration: (1) forcible correction, preceded by thorough division of the ligaments and tendons; (2) removal of the astragalus, an operation frequently performed on the European continent, and advocated lately by Dr. Morton, of Philadelphia; (3) osteotomy of the neck of the os calcis and of the astragalus, preceded by careful division of the soft parts of the inner side of the foot.

By this stage of his evolving care of club-foot deformity, Bradford had come to accept Phelps's medial ligament releases and/or bone correction for resistant cases. He summarized:

> It has been said by some writers that the treatment of clubfoot is one of the most unsatisfactory undertakings in surgery. The reverse has also been said…Both statements are true… explanation of the contradiction…that imperfect methods give extremely unsatisfactory results in club-foot…in no branch of surgery can a cure be more confidently promised than in the treatment of club-foot, and in few surgical undertakings do half measures occasion greater annoyance. (E. H. Bradford 1889d)

By 1893, Bradford had acquired extensive experience in the nonoperative treatment of congenital club-foot deformity as well as complex surgical interventions for resistant and relapsed cases (n=160 cases) (E. H. Bradford 1893). It was only 17 years after he had begun working with Buckminster Brown at the House of the Good

TREATMENT OF CLUB-FOOT.
BY E. H. BRADFORD, M.D., BOSTON.
JBJS, 1889, Volume s1-1, Issue 1

Title page of Bradford's article describing his personal experiences treating 99 cases of club feet. *Journal of Bone and Joint Surgery* 1889; 1: 89.

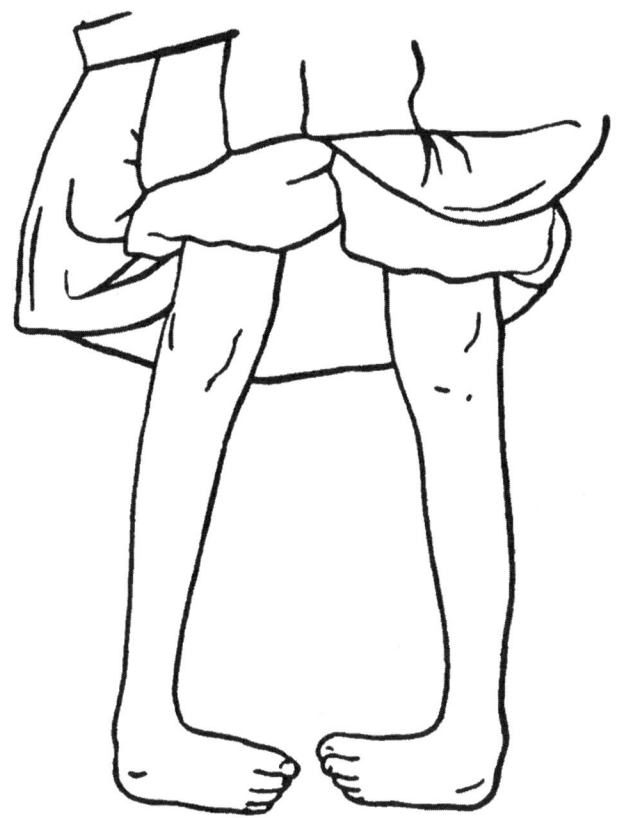

Bradford's sketch of a patient with bilateral club feet. *Journal of Bone and Joint Surgery* 1889; 1: 108.

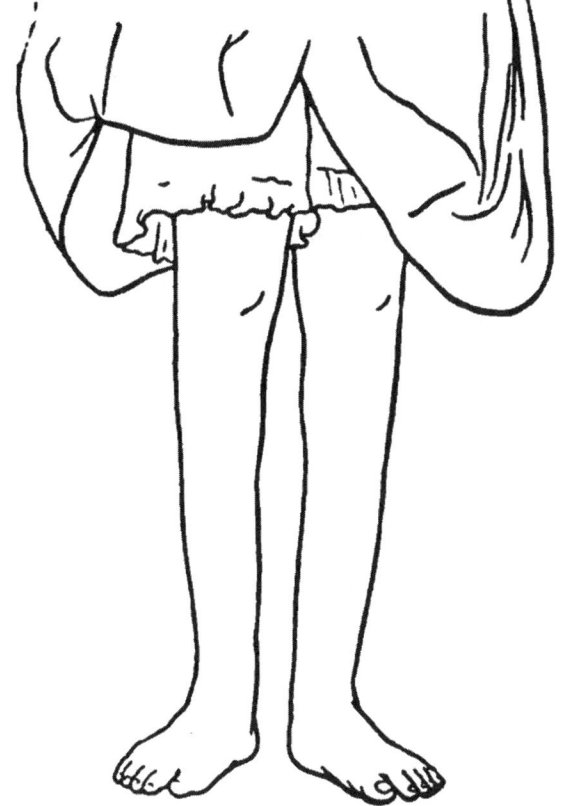

Bradford's sketch of the correction obtained in a patient with bilateral club feet. *Journal of Bone and Joint Surgery* 1889; 1: 108.

Samaritan, where the primary operation for clubfoot was a subcutaneous release of the Achilles tendon and possibly the toe flexors. That same year, he resigned from Boston City Hospital, where he had been employed for the past eight years, "and he dedicated his time to his work at Boston Children's Hospital, the House of the Good Samaritan, his own private practice, and to educating the next generation of physicians" ("F. C. S." [F. C. Shattuck], *Boston Medical and Surgical Journal* [*BSMJ*] 1926).

Bradford was now performing osteotomies in his practice at Boston Children's Hospital. Much like John Ball Brown and Buckminster Brown had illustrated their cases, Bradford illustrated his with drawings of casts made of the feet before and after correction, drawings of photographs and drawings of imprints of feet before and after correction. He wrote that in treating a resistant club foot with "osseous deformity of the neck of the astragalus and os calcis...perfect correction can be made with but little mutilation of the bone, by either a linear osteotomy of the neck of the os calcis and of the astragalus, or the removal from the neck of either or both a small wedge of bone, if this is preceded by a thorough division or stretching of the contracted soft parts" (E. H. Bradford 1889d).

Publication of the Seminal Text on Orthopaedic Surgery

Bradford was a highly productive writer, and a *Treatise on Orthopedic Surgery*—a textbook he coauthored with Robert Lovett in 1890—was the most significant of his works. The first five chapters focused on skeletal deformities from tuberculosis, and the textbook became a seminal work that most medical schools relied upon at the time.

It was eventually republished in five editions until 1915. The text consisted of 25 total chapters and was very large for a book of orthopaedic surgery at the time, 783 pages. In contrast to previous books on orthopaedics—with the exception of Dr. Lewis Sayre's excellent book—the authors stated in their preface that orthopaedic surgery includes "prevention as well as cure of deformity" (E. H. Bradford and R. W. Lovett 1890). It truly was a treatise at the time. They included a great deal of information on diseased joints, "nervous affections," and other related conditions. Not included were fractures, dislocations, or burns which were covered in surgery books.

A second edition was published in 1899 with only 22 chapters. Because of many advances in the field, they stated they had largely rewritten the book. The third edition appeared in 1905, with 21 chapters. Chapters were changed; new chapters were added on scoliosis, coxa vara, and non-tuberculous diseases of joints. New illustrations were included. The fourth edition was published in 1911 with 20 chapters. The authors wrote in their preface that because of the increasing interest in orthopaedic surgery, they produced: "a condensed handbook" (E. H. Bradford and R. W. Lovett 1911) focusing on surgery; the revised book was 410 pages and 20 chapters. They wanted the book to be used by both practitioners and students, and it emphasized surgical treatment, learned from work from the past 30 years at Boston Children's Hospital. References and bibliographical notes were reduced and discussion of different views eliminated. For the first time, they also dedicated the book "to our colleagues, the members of the AOA as a slight token of obligation and friendship" (E. H. Bradford and R. W. Lovett 1911). The final and fifth edition was published in 1915.

Bradford Frame

Tuberculosis of the spine and joints—with its subsequent skeletal deformities—was the most common serious disease that Bradford and other orthopaedic surgeons treated in the nineteenth century. Bradford designed the "Bradford Frame" to care for children with spinal deformities with the goal of achieving multiple purposes, including immobilizing pediatric patients who were being treated for diseases of the spine, hip, or knee from tuberculosis as well as from fractures. The frame was also intended to empower patients to use a bedpan while immobilized, reduce pressure on back wounds, and protect dressings and casts from becoming sullied. The Bradford frame was used for these conditions and in patients with paralysis well past the middle of the twentieth century.

The original description of the frame is described in the first edition of Bradford and Lovett's textbook:

> If the patient lies upon his back or upon his face on a hard surface, there is no superincumbent weight pressing upon any portion of the spine... If treatment by recumbency is to be adopted, it is not sufficient simply to place the child in bed. Sagging of the mattress, moving of the patient

Bradford and Lovett's *Treatise on Orthopedic Surgery*. First published in 1889. Columbia University Libraries/Internet Archive.

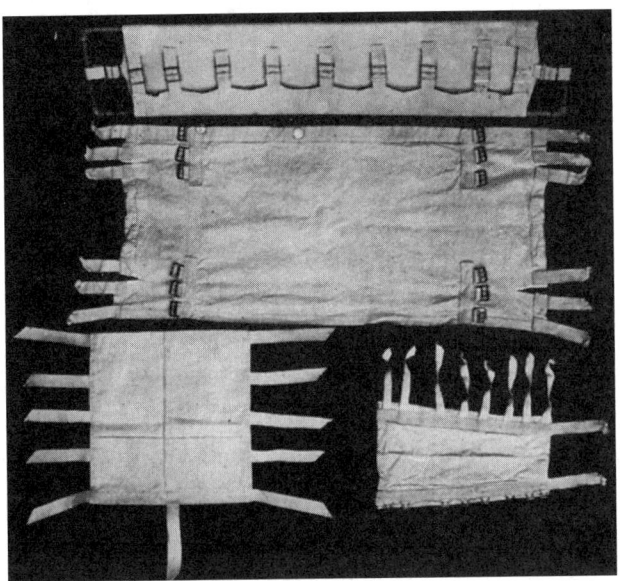

Bradford's frame with canvas covers. The frame was used for treating children with fractures and diseases of the spine, hip and knee. *Text Book of Orthopedic Surgery for Students of Medicine* by J. W. Sever. New York: Macmillan, 1925.

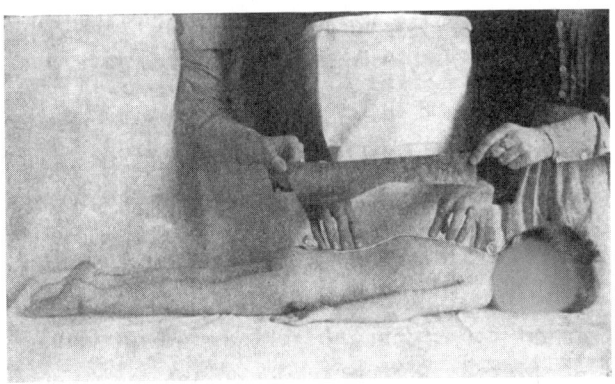

Method of measuring the gibbus deformity of the spine in Pott's disease. A cardboard model of the deformity is made and used to document any changes over time.
Treatise on Orthopedic Surgery, 2nd edition, by Bradford and Lovett. New York: William Wood and Company, 1899. Columbia University Libraries/Internet Archive.

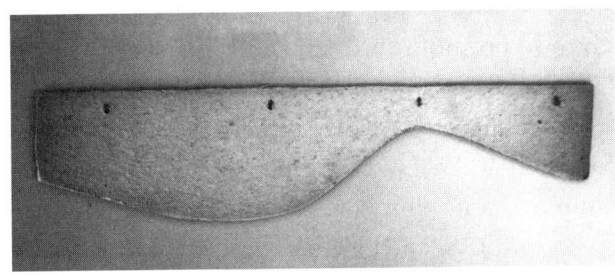

Example of the cardboard model of the spinal deformity.
The House of the Good Samaritan Records 1860–1966. Archival Collection—AC4. Archives of Children's Hospital Boston. Box 25, Volume 198. Orthopaedic patients. Taf-Z. Boston Children's Hospital Archives, Boston, Massachusetts.

from side to side, twisting and turning are all injurious, in that they cause motion between the vertebrae and change interarticular pressure, both of which are undesirable. It is necessary that the child should be fixed in a suitable position in bed. This can be done by securing the child in such a manner that the vertebral column at the seat of the disease is arched forward, diminishing the interarticular pressure. The simplest way of doing this is by means of a frame.

The rectangular bed frame…consists of a stretcher of heavy cloth attached to a rectangular gas-pipe frame. The child lying upon this frame can be secured by means of straps across the shoulders and pelvis and knees, and can be carried about without jar. When the frame is placed upon the bed, the cloth cover is no more uncomfortable than the surface of the bed. A child undergoing treatment on the frame should be turned once a day to have the back washed, rubbed with alcohol and powdered. (E. H. Bradford and R. W. Lovett 1890)

Julius Selva and others modified Bradford's frame. Selva wrote: "The Bradford frame, however, is very simple, practicable, and useful. It secures fixation and recumbency, and allows the patient to be moved about; but it does not bring about extension of the spine" (J. Selva 1896). He changed the frame by bending the side bars, "extending the spine in the dorsal decubitus" (J. Selva 1896). Dr. David Silver modified the frame by adding an extension to treat infants with fractured femurs (D. Silver 1909). Dr. Royal Whitman (R. Whitman 1901) also bent the frame (creating a curved Bradford frame) to overcorrect a kyphotic deformity in Pott's disease and cut an "oval hole in the canvas to admit the projecting kyphosis" (J. M. Berry 1907).

Others modified the frame for specific indications, even developing an adjustable frame (R. D. Maddox 1916).

Hip Disease

In 1894, Bradford and Lovett published a paper on the importance of distraction of the hip. They reached several conclusions after studying cadaver hip joints and treating a large number of patients. They wrote: "It is claimed that at a certain stage in hip disease traction force is desirable; that the amount of traction should be in proportion to the amount of muscular spasm and continued as long as the spasm persists...the separation of one inflamed bone from an adjacent inflamed bony surface, is desirable; that in this way every chance is given to promote cure and cicatrization of the previously inflamed bone...actual distraction, and that traction short of this is inefficient" (E. H. Bradford and R. W. Lovett 1894). Bradford designed a hip traction splint, a modification of the Thomas splint (A. R. Shands 1970).

Bradford and Lovett helped lead the way in the evolving treatment of tuberculosis toward the end of the nineteenth century. Working with Dr. Edward H. Nichols:

> the greatest impetus to the rational therapy of tuberculosis came from the pathological laboratory. Edward H. Nichols of Harvard, probably at the instigation of the Boston orthopaedic group [including Bradford and Lovett], studied 107 tuberculosis joints secured at the operating table or in the post-mortem room, and in 1898 reported his findings to the Association [American Orthopedic Association] in its longest communication (fifty-three pages). The occasion was dignified by the presence of Professor J. Collins Warren, head of the surgical department at Harvard, and of Professor William J. Councilman, head of the department of pathology. Both of them, as well as Gibney and Bradford representing the Association, expressed their appreciation of the significance of Nichol's study, which in reality laid the ground-work for our modern knowledge of the pathology of joint tuberculosis.
> (L. Mayer 1950)

After Nichols presented the results of his study, Bradford commented that "there was a need for the orthopedic surgeon to bestow a portion of his time on scientific investigation...this Association had done much good work in orthopedic surgery...but...tuberculosis in bone would need all the efforts of the pathologist...the bacteriologist and of the surgeon, and all the efforts of the experimenter, before it would be eradicated" (*Transactions of the American Orthopaedic Association* 1898, ["Discussion," pg 410]).

Congenital Dislocation of the Hip

Back in 1882, Buckminster Brown had reported his apparent successful treatment of a four-year-old girl with bilateral congenital dislocated hips by means of continuous traction for 13 months (see chapter 8, **Case 8.1**). Over the next 20 years, the "historical development [of congenital dislocation of the hip] is of particular interest because of swings of the pendulum, first toward the side of 'bloodless reduction,' then to open operation,

---

TREATMENT OF CONGENITAL DISLOCATION OF
THE HIP.

By E. H. BRADFORD, M.D.,

OF BOSTON.

Annals of Surgery
Volume 20 pgs. 1-
758 July/August/September/October/November/December 1894

Title page of Bradford's article in which he describes one of his first open reductions of a congenital dislocated hip.
Annals of Surgery, 1894; 20: 1.

then back to the closed method, then to open operation, finally to a combination of the two" (L. Mayer 1950). Bradford wrote several significant papers about congenital dislocated hips (CDH) during this period: its pathology, closed treatment by manipulative reduction, open reduction, femoral derotation osteotomy for anteversion, and the results of each of these treatments. He reported 21 cases treated at Children's between 1884 and 1896, seven by recumbent stretching and ambulatory traction, two manipulated under anesthesia, and 12 cases of open reduction and curetting a new acetabulum (all failed). For details on one of these cases, see **Case 15.1**. Included in one of the operative cases was a patient operated on by Professor Albert Hoffa (Berlin) who had visited Boston Children's Hospital. Earlier, Hoffa had been an advocate of closed manipulation. These were some of the first cases of open reductions performed at Children's Hospital by Bradford. One "famous contemporary surgeon [remarked], 'Before operation Hoffa's patients walk like ducks; after operation they walk like operated ducks'" (L. Mayer 1950). A duck's gait has been described as "waddling," and in humans a waddling gait is seen in patients who have a hip abductor weakness (called a Trendelenburg gait).

Bradford also reported his results on 34 patients with 44 congenital dislocated hips:

> The cases operated upon between 1890 and 1895 were not benefited by the operation... cases...between 1895 and 1898 show a small percentage of successful reduction, with one death from shock on a double operation, radical, on too young a child—one year old (an unjustifiable procedure and a preventable death)...In all...bloodless reduction was first performed, with a relapse...cases operated upon in the last year, 1899–1900, with improved technical experience...10 hips, all reduced first with bloodless operation, and all relapsed...2 relapsed after radical operation.
> (E. H. Bradford 1900)

Case 15.1. Surgical Treatment of a Congenital Dislocated Hip

> "Since the experiments were made upon cadaver, the writer has had an opportunity of performing the operation on a living subject, a child four years of age, with a congenital dislocation of the hip on the right side, the result confirming the conclusions reached by anatomical investigations. The operation was done...and reduction was made readily, the head of the femur slipping without difficulty into the acetabulum. It was found, after the attachment of the muscles to the trochanter had been divided, that on flexion of the limb, reduction by manipulation was readily made, but on attempting to straighten the limb, the head of the femur slipped instantly from the normal acetabulum. After, however, the anterior bands of the capsular ligament were freely divided, the head remained in its socket without difficulty in whatever position the limb was placed, without the use of traction. Some contraction of the adductor muscles was found on extreme abduction of the leg. The most resistant fibres of the adductor magnus were divided by open incision. The patient has recovered from the operation, the wound has healed, but, as only six weeks have elapsed since operation, the ultimate result cannot be reported as yet. The case can, however, stand as evidence of the readier method of successful reduction."
> —Unknown Case (E. H. Bradford 1894)

As Mayer stated, Bradford, was one among a few other orthopaedic surgeons who "must have been expert operators, some of them with a remarkable flair for originality" (L. Mayer 1950).

In 1899, Bradford, in arguing for early treatment of patients with CDH, reported a small series of adult patients with untreated CDH between the ages of 25 and 60 (E. H. Bradford 1899). All had moderate to severe disability, with pain, were often required to use crutches or cane, were unable to work, and walked with a limp. He then described the pathologic anatomy of a case of bilateral CDH in which closed manipulation followed by spica cast failed. Both hips re-dislocated in the cast after one month. He performed an open reduction on the right: "The ring of the cotyloid ligament [labrum] was found to be too small for the entrance of the head, being not more than a quarter of inch in diameter. This was dilated, the head passed through, the wound stitched, and the patient recovered" (E. H. Bradford 1899). Sadly, the patient died from whooping cough three months later before Bradford could operate on the patient's left hip. At autopsy, Bradford described the detailed anatomy of each hip, observing that the acetabulae in this case and others he operated on were of normal size. He recommended the following:

> [First,] stretching and overcoming all muscular contraction...by manual stretching or...use of a windless attachment...applied and a gradual stretching carried out under an anaesthetic... hamstring tendons can be divided subcutaneously and the ilio-tibial ligament cut some distance above the tibia...tensor vaginae femoris should also be divided subcutaneously, and... divide the insertion of the great adductor... The question then remains whether the capsule should be divided or not...a matter of judgment...where it is decided to cut down upon the capsule an oblique incision in front of the gluteus medius should be made, passing from the anterior-superior spine outward and downward, crossing the femur...between the tensor vaginae femoris and the gluteus medius...the capsule...should be cleared, opened and cut obliquely across...the head is put in through the cotyloid ring [labrum] into the acetabulum. If the ring is not large enough, it can be dilated...or cut by a herniotomy knife...the head...placed well in the acetabulum, remaining so in every position of the limb. (E. H. Bradford 1899)

In 1902, Dr. Adolf Lorenz, known for his expertise in closed manipulation and often referred to as "The Great Bloodless Surgeon," gave two demonstrations at Boston Children's Hospital to 300 guests at each one. He was well received and there was much mutual respect. He was known to have said, "[He] could teach them nothing" they did not already know (C. A. Smith 1983). Bradford later referred to Lorenz's visit, noting: "In 1902 there were twenty-two [CDH] cases treated; twenty reduced by forcible manipulation (including six operated upon by Professor Lorenz), with eight cures and two operated upon, open incision, with two cures" (E. H. Bradford 1909). Both Lorenz and Bradford had unsuccessful cases of closed manipulation of CDH (the bloodless method) as well as after open reductions; but less so. In fact, 24 years later, an *Evening Transcript* obituary described Bradford as "the Dr. Lorenz of Boston" because he was equally skilled, especially in pediatric cases (C. A. Smith 1983). Bradford used a device designed by Mr. Ralph W. Bartlett of Boston to reduce congenital dislocated hips, and he reviewed all cases treated at Boston Children's Hospital until 1909. He noted that "there has been a steady increase in the percentage of cures" (E. H. Bradford 1909) after both manipulative reduction and open reduction, especially in the last four years.

Occasionally Bradford performed a derotation osteotomy of the femur "owing to a twist of the neck of the femur, or an anterior obliquity of the plane of the acetabulum...at the middle or lower end of the femur" to avoid possible additional injury to the blood supply of the proximal femur (E. H. Bradford 1900). He did not want to keep the leg extremely internally rotated in order to maintain the hip stable in the acetabulum. Additional orthopaedic surgeons at Boston Children's Hospital, like Dr. D. R. Soutter who shared an office with Drs. Bradford, A. Thorndike, R. W. Lovett (1888) and E. G. Brackett (1889), probably also contributed some of the cases that Bradford reported to the American Orthopaedic Association in 1909.

Scoliosis

Bradford was also interested in lateral curvature of the spine. He designed two new techniques to evaluate and treat scoliosis. The first was a corrective device, in which he placed the patient (either standing or recumbent) in head/neck traction, stabilized the pelvis, and used wide straps attached to traction that applied lateral forces to the spine opposite to the deformity. Before applying the traction apparatus, he had the patients exercise and stretch to maximize their spines' flexibility. He then applied a plaster jacket after maximum correction was achieved, during the same period that Shulthess and Hoffa were doing similar work. With E. G. Brackett, he published two articles on this method in 1893 and 1895. In 1897, Bradford established a scoliosis clinic at Boston Children's

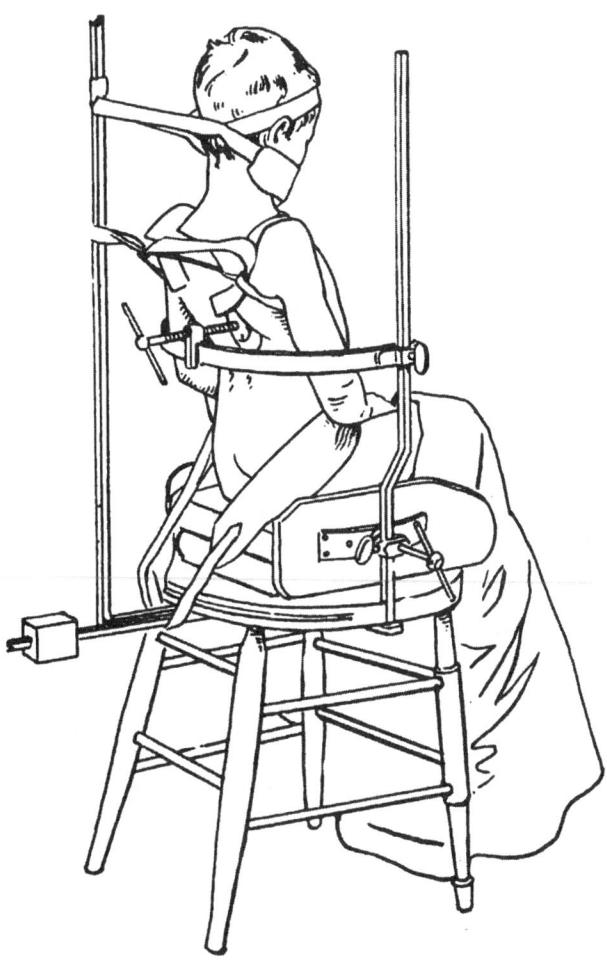

Example of a device used by Bradford to correct a scoliosis before applying a cast or jacket. In this case, the patient is standing with head traction and pressure pads applied to correct the lateral bend and rotation of the spine.

Bradford and Brackett, "Treatment of Lateral Curvature by Means of Pressure Correction," *Boston Medical and Surgical Journal* 1893; 128: 464.

Example of applying corrective forces to the spine with the patient sitting. Direct pressure pads are applied to the convex side of the curve and straps are used to decrease the rotational deformity.

Bradford and Brackett, "The Employment of Mechanical Force in Treatment of Lateral Curvature," *Boston Medical and Surgical Journal* 1895; 133: 357.

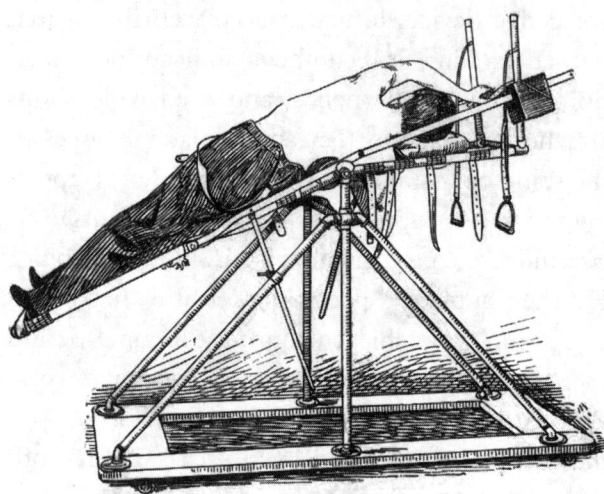

Example of applying corrective forces to reduce the scoliotic deformity with the patient supine and rotating the spine. No head traction is used.

Bradford and Brackett, "The Employment of Mechanical Force in Treatment of Lateral Curvature," *Boston Medical and Surgical Journal* 1895; 133: 357.

Hospital. He designed a second technique, a scoliosometer, which was described in 1906 as the "most accurate device for measuring the degree of the deformity due to rotation of the bodies of the vertebrae" (J. K. Young 1906).

ORTHOPAEDIC SURGERY AT THE BEGINNING OF THE TWENTIETH CENTURY

From almost 40 years after the earliest orthopaedic operation of a subcutaneous release of the Achilles tendon for club-foot deformity in 1838 by John Ball Brown until the beginning of the twentieth century, Bradford either contributed original procedures or advanced others in a wide array of surgical treatments available to orthopaedic surgeons. A brief list includes: drainage of abscesses, osteotomy of the femur, myotomy and tenotomy for deformity, amputation in advanced disease of the hip or knee, curetting infected sinuses, tenotomies in club foot, medial releases in club foot, cuneiform osteotomy, supramalleolar osteotomy, arthrodesis in paralytic club foot (tibio-tarsal), transplanting tendons/ muscles in limb paralysis from poliomyelitis or hemiplegia, tenotomy for torticollis and scoliosis, release of webbed fingers, tenotomies for hand deformities, surgical releases and open reduction of congenitally dislocated hips, and osteoclasis for bowlegs or knock-knees. This progress in surgery for musculoskeletal problems was remarkable and rapid and made possible by the birth of ether anesthesia.

Bradford also wrote about proper seating for school children, surgical treatment of spastic paralysis, use of tendon transfers (trapezius to deltoid insertion), the use of silk sutures, the treatment of bowlegs and knock-knees with an osteoclast he had designed, proper posture for children, recurrent patellar dislocation, and other orthopaedic treatments.

Schools for Disabled Children

Boston Industrial School for Crippled and Deformed Children

In 1893, Bradford opened the Boston Industrial School for Crippled and Deformed Children on Chambers Street with Drs. Augustus Thorndike and Elliott Brackett (see chapter 35). According to Thorndike, "Dr. Bradford was the founder and promoter of special training for cripples in America" (A. Thorndike 1926). Before opening the school, Bradford had often traveled to Europe in the summer, visiting the Pio Istituto Rachitici (1889) in Italy, which was a hospital devoted to children with rickets. It was there that "he first saw children gathered by an omnibus in the morning and returned at night; meanwhile they were bathed, fed, taught, exercised and allowed plenty of out-of-door play under the supervision of trained nurses and Sisters of Charity" (A. Thorndike 1926). He became convinced that children hospitalized for long periods of time in America needed the same attention and education.

Bradford, along with eight friends, including Thorndike and Brackett, led the planning for the industrial school for children in Boston. Initial efforts were unsuccessful. Bradford persisted, continuing to learn more about these special schools by visiting similar ones in London, Munich, and Copenhagen. Although meeting frequently and developing their plans, the group was unable to convince a newly opened New England Peabody Home for Cripples, which was designed "largely for the treatment of children with bone tuberculosis" (L. Snedeker 1969), to include a school to teach the hospitalized children. Undeterred, Bradford called a public meeting to hear about the successes of an industrial school in Christiania, Norway, from a visitor to Boston, whose two daughters, one disabled, ran the school:

He showed various articles made there—brushes, embroideries, cloth and linen handwoven by a one-armed girl, and by a boy who had impaired use of both hands. By slow, patient training, cripples, notwithstanding great handicaps, had learned to wash, to feed, and to dress themselves, and also to make things which could be sold toward self-support… Bradford said he believed that all that the cripples needed was to be shown and taught; and he instanced from history several distinguished hunchbacks…our American cripples, who really suffer mostly from the universal belief that no one who is a cripple can do anything.
(L. Snedeker 1969)

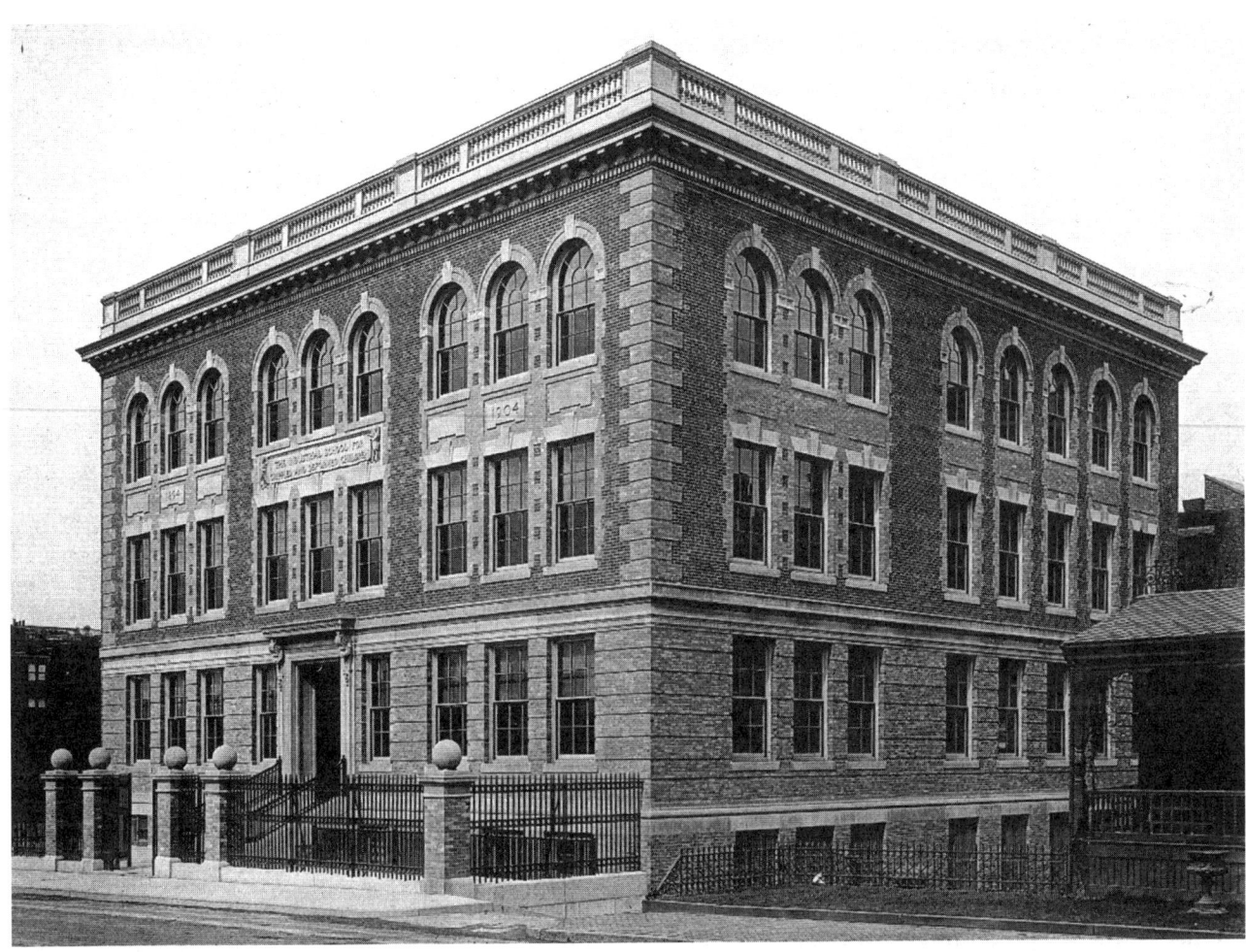

Industrial School for Crippled Children, 241 Botolph Street, Boston. Courtesy of Cotting School.

Bradford and his committee of friends immediately received donations ($28) and rent-free rooms for one year. After a few moves, the school was finally located in its own building on Botolph Street in Boston; it was renamed the Industrial School for Crippled Children. It was the first private, nonprofit day school for disabled children.

Bradford served as a trustee for many years. Thorndike commented on Bradford's personal qualities that led to his success in this role:

> There was a subtlety in the modest way in which Bradford advanced at the trustees' meetings, entirely new ideas and methods. He paid so much consideration and attention to the opinions of others, that his views were often followed without anyone at the close of the meeting being aware whose views they were...An example of his beneficent genius was shown in his selection of a crippled young man to be president of the Industrial School for Cripples in Boston. Frances J. Cotting, the second president, as a boy obliged to lie on a frame for some years for the treatment of disease of the spine, which left him with paralysis of both legs so that he could go about only in a wheel chair. This vital interest made a new man of him. (A. Thorndike 1926)

Bradford must have recalled Buckminster Brown's own personal history of years of bed rest for his spine disease.

The school later merged with the Kreb's School in 1986 and was renamed the Cotting School in 1974. Today, it is located on Concord Avenue in Lexington, Massachusetts. It consists of a "preschool, lower, middle and upper schools...[with] academic instruction focusing on a variety of skills and content areas, vocational assessment, and training...special education, assistive technology, art, music, library/media, dental, vision, nursing, occupational therapy, physical therapy, speech therapy, industrial

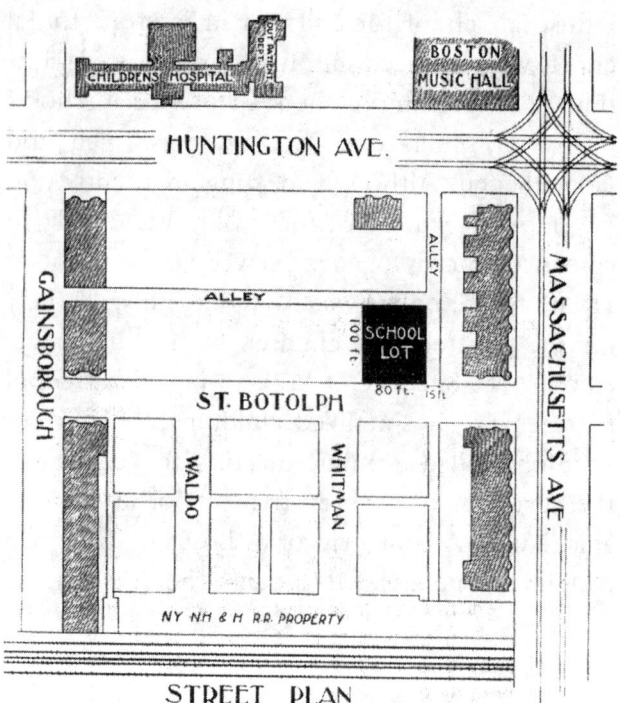

Street plan of Boston showing Children's Hospital (Huntington Avenue) and the future location of the Industrial School for Crippled Children (School lot on St. Botolph Street).
Courtesy of Cotting School.

arts, tutorial services, pre-vocational and vocational training" (*Wikipedia*, n.d., under "Cotting School").

Massachusetts Hospital School for Crippled Children

Bradford was not finished in his support, however, "of the right of handicapped children to special industrial training and general education [and] he persuaded Governor Bates and the Legislature of the State of Massachusetts of their duty to the State's crippled minor wards" (R. B. Osgood 1926a). A bill authorizing a Massachusetts Hospital School for Crippled Children was passed and signed by the governor in 1904. It was built in Canton, Massachusetts. Bradford was appointed chairman of the board of trustees, a position he retained until his death (A. R. Shands 1970). Opened in 1907, it admitted the first patients in

January of 1908. Patients were initially most commonly admitted with diagnoses of tuberculosis of the skeleton (first), polio (second), and cerebral palsy (third).

The building had a highly effective ventilation system, a plan of Bradford's own devising and one that limited upper respiratory diseases among the patients. Bradford was thoroughly "convinced of the value of an outdoor life for children, [and] he devised plans for the dormitories and other buildings to insure [*sic*] a maximum of constantly changing fresh air indoors" (F. C. Shattuck 1926). Along with the superintendent, he "made a careful…study of school-teaching methods [and] trained special teachers…[because] giving [the students] more play, less study, more fresh air produced healthier and brighter children" (F. C. Shattuck 1926). The attached infirmary was named in honor of Bradford, and one of his closest friends, Dr. Frederick C. Shattuck, wrote: "Perhaps his most conspicuous and lasting single service was his pioneer and continued work in connection with the education, mental and manual, of the pathetic child confined to bed on his back for months or years, or permanently crippled" (F. C. Shattuck 1926).

In 2016, Governor Charles Baker renamed the hospital the Pappas Rehabilitation Hospital for Children in honor of Dr. Arthur Pappas (see chapter 23).

Orthopaedic Surgeon-in-chief at Boston Children's Hospital

Bradford was a prominent figure in the early development of orthopaedic surgery in America, a mentor to the next generation and a leader among leaders. His vision led to Boston's role as an epicenter of orthopaedic practice and education in the United States, and he was described by Sir Arthur Keith as "the chief link between the old school and the new one" (A. Keith 1919). Boston Children's Hospital became an orthopaedic center as well as one of the most outstanding children's hospitals in the nation, largely due to his efforts and the outstanding orthopaedic surgeons he recruited.

As a member of the medical staff at Children's Hospital for 34 years (1878–1912), he started as a surgeon, later became surgeon-in-chief, and was recognized as the hospital's first orthopaedic surgeon. One of his more, if not the most, significant contributions to the emerging specialty of

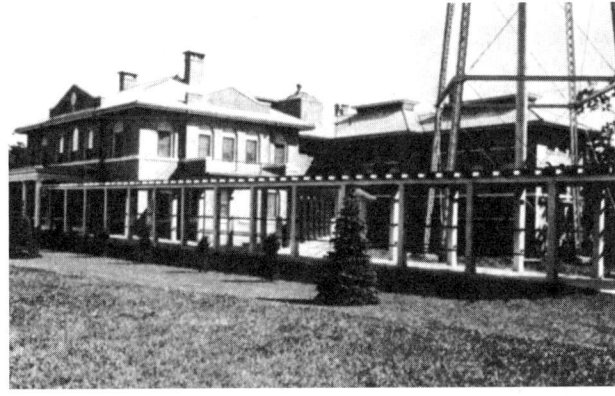

Bradford Infirmary or Wing of the Massachusetts Hospital School, Canton, Massachusetts. *The Early Orthopaedic Surgeons of America* by Alfred Rives Shands Jr., Saint Louis: Mosby, 1970.

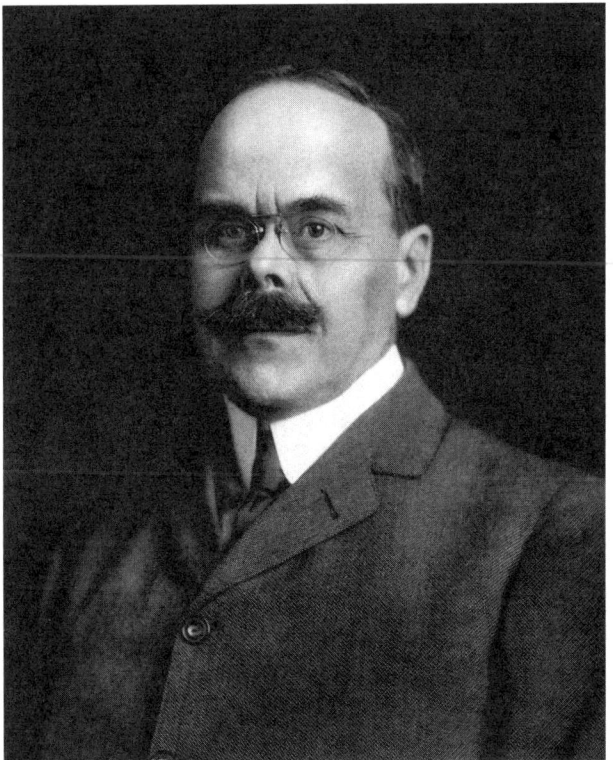

Edward H. Bradford. Boston Medical Library in the Francis A. Countway Library of Medicine.

orthopaedic surgery was his recruitment of other major future leaders of the specialty: Robert W. Lovett in 1888, Elliott G. Brackett in 1889, Augustus Thorndike in 1890, Joel E. Goldthwait in 1893, Robert B. Osgood in 1901, James W. Sever (his second cousin) in 1906, Arthur T. Legg in 1908, and others. Legg had been a medical intern there in 1900.

Under his leadership, the number of surgical admissions increased and remained at almost twice the number of yearly medical admissions from 1883 to 1913 (**Table 15.1**). Orthopaedics remained responsible for almost 50% of the total surgical admissions before it became an independent department in 1903.

Table 15.1. Orthopaedic Admissions at Boston Children's Hospital from 1883 to 1913

	1883–1885	1896–1898	1911–1913
TBC Spine (Pott's Disease)	66	201	234
TBC Hip	129	185	220
TBC Knee	19	56	66
Club Feet	37	73	163
CDH	3	28	145
Other	12	57	271
Total	266	600	900

(C. A. Smith 1983).

When orthopaedic surgery became an independent department at Children's Hospital in 1903—the first orthopaedic department in New England—Bradford was the Hospital's surgeon-in-chief. He remained at Children's as surgeon-in-chief and chief of the Department of Orthopaedic Surgery until his retirement, at age 65, in 1912. Harvard Medical School recognizes him as deserving of the "credit for establishing orthopaedics as a discipline separate from surgery" (*Harvard Medical School Perspectives* 1990).

Teacher and Dean at Harvard Medical School

Beginning with his first appointment to Harvard and throughout his career in the medical school, Bradford was "entrusted with the teaching of orthopedic surgery" (F. C. Shattuck 1926). At 41 years of age, eight years after his initial appointment to the surgical department, he received the first faculty appointment in orthopaedic surgery at Harvard as clinical instructor in surgery and orthopaedic surgery in 1889. In 1893, he was appointed assistant professor of orthopaedic surgery (at age 45). Simultaneously with his appointment as surgeon-in-chief in the orthopaedic department at Children's, he became the professor of orthopaedic surgery at HMS. He was the only professor of orthopaedic surgery, a position that would soon be endowed as the John B. and Buckminster Brown Professorship. Bradford was 55 years old. Throughout his tenure, he also served for years as a member of Harvard's Athletic Committee.

Bradford was an excellent teacher who was passionate about education and believed strongly in the use of models and illustrations to clarify learning. Osgood described him as methodically assembling over time:

> a unique and comprehensive collection of lantern slides of orthopaedic conditions, of primitive races and of gaits of ancient and modern footwear. With this collection he illustrated his talks. In the clinics he was determined that the students should do things themselves, that they should feel the lesion as well as hear of it, and in so far as possible should treat it. *"Morbi non eloquentia sed remediis curantur."* So, his teaching was profitable and popular, which is a not too common combination. (R. B. Osgood 1926a)

He later donated his extensive slide collection to the medical school. Bradford also started the first Harvard nose and throat clinic in the medical school (Countway Medical Library) in 1910.

The clinic gradually expanded to include all specialties as the patient demand increased. Treatment was free, and the clinic was used for teaching. It met daily, each afternoon 3:30–4:30. While dean, President Lowell asked him to support his efforts to establish an affiliation with a medical school in Shanghai. Bradford declined a position on its board of trustees, however, stating, it was "unwise for me to assume a position [with] increased responsibilities when it is difficult, if not impossible, for me to take an active part in the direction of the school in China" (Countway Medical Library).

Harvard's president, Abbott Lawrence Lowell, was so impressed by Bradford—as a teacher, leader, organizer, and a man with the highest principles and work ethic—that he asked him to become dean of the medical school at age 64. Bradford retired from Children's Hospital, became professor emeritus of orthopaedic surgery, and began a new career, dean of HMS. He remained dean for six years, from 1912 to 1918. Charles William Eliot, the previous president of Harvard, had reformed education, including medical education, at Harvard. Many improvements were in place when Bradford became dean. Some of the significant changes included new admission requirements, a new, more vigorous academic curriculum, and required written examinations. An optional fourth year was also added. Under Bradford's thoughtful eye, a new system of medical examinations was put in place to obtain the MD degree. Bradford was devoted to the medical students while further improving the medical school's organization and standards, and Lowell once commented that Bradford "gave a new birth to orthopaedic surgery in this country, and his administration as Dean prepared the way for the developments of the School that have since taken place" (G. H. Monks 1927). Osgood wrote that:

> Under [Bradford's] administration, the school grew and prospered and assumed leadership. He was elected to the Board of Overseers of Harvard College in 1919, and was made Chairman of its Medical Committee. He never lost touch with the students. He sought their point of view and valued their estimate of their teachers. He met them in large groups at his house and brought them in social as well as academic touch with their instructors. They could not fail to sense his purpose, his youth, and his unselfishness. (R. B. Osgood 1926a)

Although he did not intend to remain dean for more than five years, the complexity and breath of work of the deanship increased with each passing year (especially in light of the war), so he remained an additional year. Harvard medical students complained frequently about their curriculum, especially clinical courses in the third and fourth years. Bradford always made improvements, especially in his last several years as dean. Bradford was a member of the Committee on Education of the American Medical Association, and it was directly due to his guidance that medical students were able to continue their studies during World War I, graduate on time, and enter the military and aid the war effort. During World War I, he dealt with many of the students who requested draft exemptions, and

House Officer's Certificate, 1903. Signed by Bradford as surgeon-in-chief and Thomas M. Rotch as physician-in-chief.

Images of America. Children's Hospital Boston. Charleston, SC: Arcadia Publishing, 2005. Boston Children's Hospital Archives, Boston, Massachusetts.

he compiled a list of all first-year medical students in all US medical schools in an appeal to Washington to exempt all medical students from the draft. Washington was concerned, however, because the number of students entering medical school had been increasing each year. At the end of his term as dean, instruction in orthopaedic surgery began at HMS for military surgeons on May 1, 1918, under the direction of Dr. Robert Lovett. Dean Bradford had approval for this training by President Lowell on September 16, 1917. It was called the School for Health Officers (see chapter 16).

During the war, many faculty and hospital staff physicians and surgeons entered the military and were sent overseas, creating a shortage in each major hospital in Boston and elsewhere. There was a shortage of house officers as well. Such shortages created confusion and disorganization in the medical school and the hospitals. As adjustments were made, the American Medical Association requested that medical schools not lower their educational standards to avoid any deterioration in training. The senior staff at the Boston City Hospital requested that Dean Bradford modify the medical school's policy that "hospital time shall not count as school times" (Countway Medical Library). A memo from the executive committee at the Massachusetts General Hospital requested that HMS should "wave the rule forbidding the HMS students to accept house officer's positions at the MGH for the period of the war" (Countway Medical Library). Such changes approved by Bradford allowed the students to graduate sooner and enter the military service, which was something the majority of students wanted.

A list of the Harvard teachers of orthopaedic surgery for the military surgeons provided to the surgeon general included: Professor Lovett (age 59, major), Assistant Professor Brackett (age 58, colonel), Instructor Zabdiel B. Adams (age 43, captain), Arthur T. Legg (age 44, lieutenant colonel), Robert Soutter (age 48), Lloyd T. Brown (age 38), Henry J. FitzSimmons (age 37, contract surgeon, half-time), and Frank R. Ober (age 37, captain) (Countway Library Archives). A special list of essential teachers included Drs. Lovett, Legg, Soutter, and Brown.

Dean Bradford remained extremely busy during the war. His contributions included curriculum changes, a flexible and changing curriculum, an accelerated program to shorten time to graduation, a significant increase in the essential teaching of orthopaedic surgery to the HMS students and military surgeons, contributing to the needs of the Red Cross, leading operational issues of the draft, including exemptions and deferrals from the draft, as well as attention to local needs of the medical school, students, and the hospitals.

During his tenure, the Peter Bent Brigham Hospital was opened. He quietly hoped that, because of its closeness to the medical school, that it would become Harvard's teaching university hospital; Massachusetts General Hospital was across town, a distance of about five miles. Although extremely busy at Harvard, he volunteered to serve on the Board of Draft Appeal for Selective Service. Previously, he had volunteered during the Spanish American War of 1898, helping to organize and fund the return of the wounded from Cuba on the hospital relief ship, *Bay State*. He was eventually awarded an honorary degree, doctor of science, by the board of overseers.

Legacy

Dr. Bradford had married late in life, at age 52, to Edith Fiske in 1900. They had one daughter and three sons. Their daughter, Elizabeth Bradford, was a teacher. One of their sons, Charles Hickling Bradford, went on to become an orthopaedic surgeon. Charles' twin, Edward Hickling Bradford Jr., was a stockholder. Another son, Robert Fiske Bradford, would eventually serve as governor of Massachusetts. E. H. Bradford remained healthy for most of his life, never spending a day in bed except for "typhoid fever contracted from a casual glass of milk on a professional journey" (F. C. Shattuck 1926). But a bicycle accident in his early fifties left him blind in one eye with a deformed nose from a fracture (A. R. Shands 1970). This was particularly troublesome because he also had severe myopia. The injury occurred about the time he was named professor at Harvard and orthopaedics became an independent department at Boston Children's Hospital. After retirement at age 75, he lost the remaining sight of his functioning eye. A friend remembered him as saying, "I don't want any sympathy. Call me a damned fool if you like" (F. C. Shattuck 1926). Despite this personal challenge, he was tireless in his pursuits, studied Braille, and:

> learned to read with facility and with great pleasure...Speaking of his oncoming blindness, Dr. Bradford said that the first effect of this affliction was a sense of depression. "I was tempted to take a despondent view of life, but soon, however, on reflection I realized that all this was but incidental and superficial compared with the resources of life. I found that life was a very rich opportunity which I had only half explored. I found that life itself could be nothing more than a temporary aspect of that spiritual experience in which I might prepare myself for larger service. This reflection returned to me not only courage but enjoyment of life." (R. B. Osgood 1926a)

Bradford was a charter member of the American Orthopaedic Association, becoming its third president, 1888–1889; following Virgil P. Gibney, second surgeon-in-chief at the Hospital for the Ruptured and Crippled and first professor of orthopaedic surgery at Columbia University; and Newton M. Shaffer, surgeon-in-chief at the New York Orthopaedic Dispensary and first professor of orthopaedic surgery at Cornell University (A. R. Shands 1970). In 1915, he was elected an honorary member. In addition to his *Treatise on Orthopedic Surgery* (coauthored with Lovett), which remained the standard text in medical schools for 25 years (superseded in 1915), Bradford was founding editor of the series "Progress in Orthopaedic Surgery" published in the *Boston Medical and Surgical Journal* for 25 years (1878–1903). He was succeeded by Dr. Osgood. The scope of his knowledge was breathtaking; he wrote about almost every facet of orthopaedic surgery and, in addition to his textbook, published over 115 articles up to 1901. He was also a member of the American Surgical Association, as well as a number of other professional organizations. He volunteered in the Massachusetts Volunteer Aid Association, was a member of the Military Historical Society, served as president of the board of trustees of the Massachusetts Eye and Ear Infirmary, as a trustee of Simmons College, and as a trustee of the Boston Library Association. Two years before his death, he was appointed chairman of the Conservation Committee by Boston's mayor. He was the only American orthopaedic surgeon awarded honorary membership in the German Orthopaedic Association (*Harvard Crimson* 1912).

Dr. Bradford died on May 7, 1926. He passed suddenly of cerebral hemorrhage at 78. Comparing him to the famed knight Pierre Terrail, seigneur de Bayard, his obituary described him as "a man *sans peur et sans reproche*," or a man "without fear and beyond reproach" (Countway Medical Library). His son, Dr. Charles H. Bradford wrote, "[He] was a man of extraordinarily broad interests and tremendous intellectual power, and conversational association with him was extremely delightful and very informative; but his interests were so wide that we could talk together on many subjects and a person could know him well without realizing that he was even a doctor" (A. R. Shands 1970).

His friend Shattuck gave the following tribute:

> As self-critic he was merciless. As critic of others and their opinions he could be emphatic, but was always generous. His own intensity of conviction never dimmed the faith that those of opposing views might well be equally sincere and disinterested...His character did not greatly need the discipline of self-denial...[but] with the

saving grace of a sense of humor he was plentifully endowed. (F. C. Shattuck 1926)

Dr. J. W. Sever (1947), his second cousin and colleague, wrote:

[Bradford] was enthusiastic, generous to a fault, keen about progress of all kinds, a lover of art and music, and a truly religious man.

Dr. Osgood wrote two tributes about Dr. Bradford. In the *British Medical Journal*, he stated:

Professor Bradford was one of America's greatest surgeons and one of the most admirable of men. He will be remembered as a pioneer in the renaissance of orthopaedic surgery, as a public servant in many civic and military positions of responsibility, as a great teacher, and as former dean of the Harvard Medical School. His courage was as constant as his initiative was strong…Honored by his university and colleagues, beloved by students and patients, his spirit was yet most gentle and humble…Rarely has a man left a more stimulating record or presented the world an example more worthy of emulation. (R. B. Osgood 1926b)

In the *Journal of Bone and Joint Surgery*, Osgood wrote:

The world recognizes that important service given by a man to his fellowmen makes him great. If this man exhibits a constant and chivalrous courage while he serves, the world adjudges him still greater. To possess humility when both a man's service and his courage are honored is the epitome of greatness. Such greatness of mind, heart and soul shaped the life of Edward Hickling Bradford. (R. B. Osgood 1926a)

Before his death, some of Bradford's students convinced him to agree to have a portrait painted (R. B. Osgood 1926a). Painted by a friend and

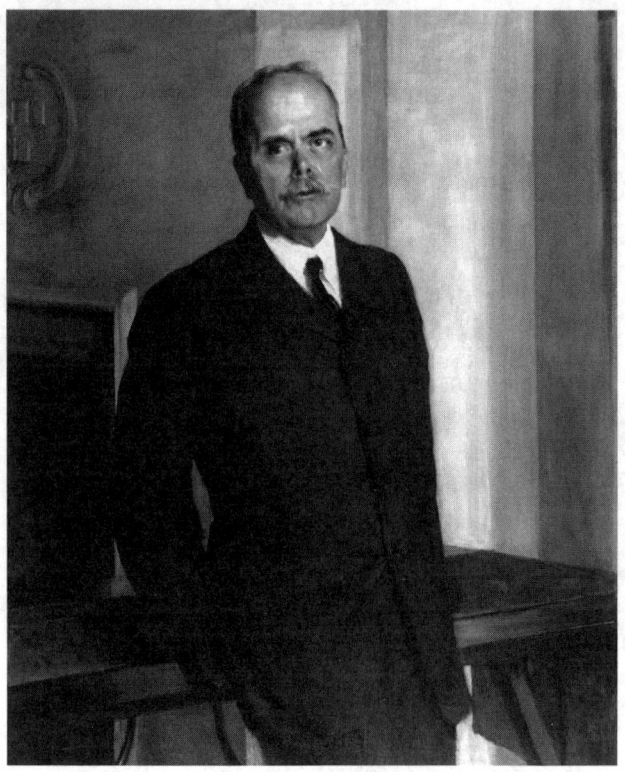

Portrait of Edward H. Bradford, ca. 1925.
Edward Hickling Bradford [1848-1926]; H345. Harvard University Portrait Collection, Gift of pupils and friends of Dr. Bradford "in recognition of his service, courage and humility" to the Medical School, 1924. Photo © President and Fellows of Harvard College.

well-known artist, it was hung in the faculty room of HMS. Shortly before his death, Bradford wrote these last words:

The doctor should be broadly human. He must deal with the vagaries of age, and the fancies of youth, the sports of boys and the appetites of men. In his profession he tests the aviator and rations the soldier, estimates the endurance of the laborer, cares for the worried mother and relieves the desk-ridden financier. His thought must reach to the ideals of the clergyman and interpret the flesh-prompted dreams of the man of the world. And in this service, neither the precision of science nor the efficiency of business methods will suffice, for above all else the practitioner must preserve and exercise the kindly indulgence of a considerate friend. In what academy can these lessons be taught? (F. C. Shattuck 1926)

CHAPTER 16

Robert W. Lovett
The First John Ball and Buckminster Brown Professor of Orthopaedic Surgery

Robert Williamson Lovett, the only son of John Dyson Lovett, a Boston merchant, and Mary Elizabeth (Williamson) Lovett, was born in Beverly, Massachusetts, on November 18, 1859. After attending Nobel's School, he graduated from Harvard College in 1881 and Harvard Medical School (HMS) in 1885 at age 26. Initially in his career, Lovett had expressed a broad interest in surgery and an early commitment to adding new knowledge to the fields of medicine and surgery. While a medical student, he had published a paper in 1884 in the *Boston Medical and Surgical Journal* [*BMSJ*] titled "Menstruation in Women and Animals." After graduation, he spent the next 18 months as a house officer on Dr. Bradford's service in surgery at the Boston City Hospital, interrupted by "a brief period at the New York Orthopedic Hospital" (*BMSJ* 1924).

EARLY TRAINING AND PRACTICE

In 1885, Lovett began his first year of practice as a house officer with an appointment as "Surgeon to Out Patients at the Boston City Hospital" (*BMSJ* 1924). He began a daily diary—each year beginning a new volume—in which he noted his activities, rounds, surgeries, social events, visits with friends and other people, and attendance at church. He worked as a surgeon in the outpatient clinic most days until just before or after lunch. He

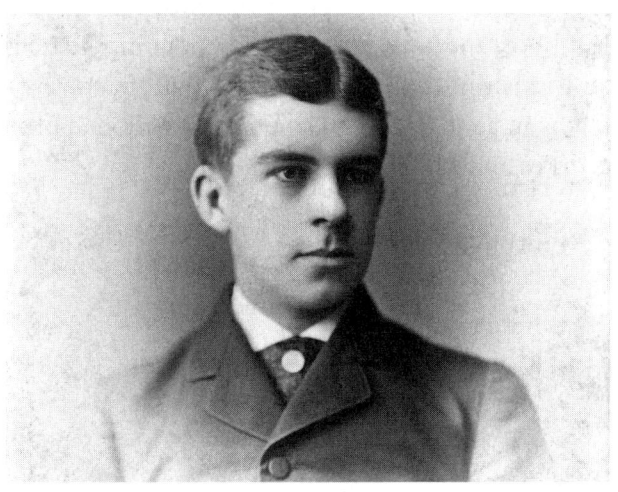

Robert W. Lovett, early in his career. Robert W. Lovett. [Senior Photograph]. HUP Lovett, Robert W. (1). Harvard University Archives.

Physician Snapshot

Robert W. Lovett

BORN: 1859

DIED: 1924

SIGNIFICANT CONTRIBUTIONS: The first John Ball and Buckminster Brown Professor of Orthopaedic Surgery at Harvard Medical School; accepted the first resident (Frank Ober) in a one-year orthopaedic residency at Children's Hospital; conservative orthopaedist whose major focus was on research and education; major contributor to the understanding of the pathomechanics of scoliosis; expert in poliomyelitis: developed the clinical use of the spring muscle test with Ernest G. Martin, diagnosed and treated Franklin Delano Roosevelt, member of the Massachusetts State Board of Health, founder and chairman of the Harvard Infantile Paralysis Commission, preferred and replaced the commonly used word "crippled" with "disabled" recorded his first handwritten note on surgery on January 1, 1885: "Slept until 7.30, got to breakfast, SOPD [surgery outpatient department] till 11...plastic for eyelid [accompanied by his small drawing of the procedure]...then after dinner casts on etherization...till 4.30. House calls until 6 this evening...went to Cambridge to evening party (dancing class)" (R. W. Lovett [Diaries] 1885). His diverse case load included treatments such as scraping of an old hip with necrosis, removing a necrosed phalanx, performing a tracheostomy, repairing a broken leg and two arms, removing a fish hook and foreign bodies, amputating fingers, and repairing an external epicondyle fracture of elbow in an infant. He also briefly mentioned procedures and surgeries that included:

- exploration of bladder
- rodent ulcer
- hernia
- aneurysm
- greenstick fracture (tibia)
- fractured ankle
- fractured clavicle
- fractured toe
- wrist injury
- nose polyps
- fractured femur
- depressed skull fracture
- ruptured cornea
- pistol wound of leg
- elbow sprain
- gunshot wounds
- burns
- both bone forearm fracture
- subcoracoid shoulder dislocation
- Pott's fracture
- Dupuytrens
- both bone fracture of leg
- Colles fracture
- urinary retention
- fractured patella
- humerus fracture
- ischial abscess

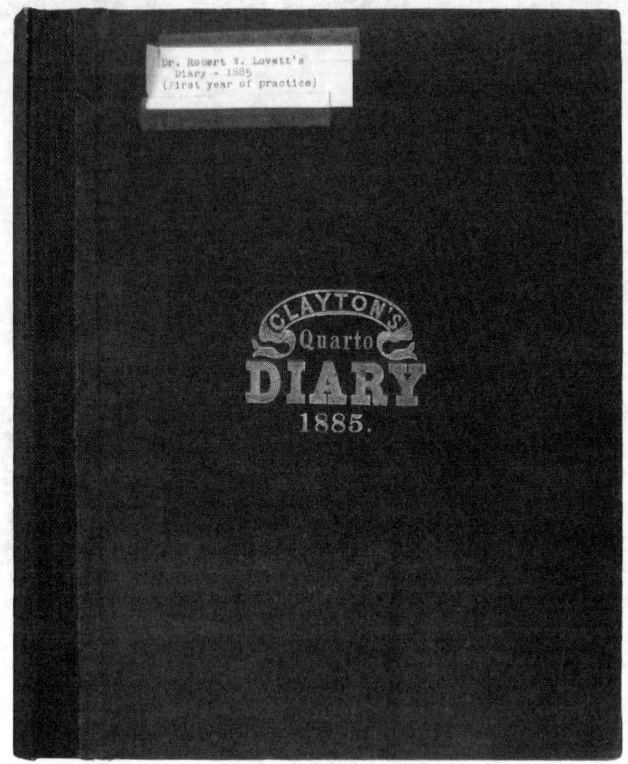

Lovett's diary in his first year as a house officer, 1885.
Harvard Medical Library in the Francis A. Countway Library of Medicine.

He stated, "probably 60% or more...[were] orthopedic cases [and this number] increased as the year went on" (R. W. Lovett [Diaries] 1885).

During his first year there, Lovett also published a paper on a "Case of Glanders." Common in horses, mules, and donkeys; glanders is rare in humans, and has not been reported in the US since 1945. Lovett reported a case of a stable groom who contacted the disease from a sick horse, developed extensive vesicles and pustules on his face and extremities, and died 20 days after contracting the disease. Lovett attended his autopsy and reported histologic findings of small micrococci and fine rods (*Burkholderia mallei*). By August, the service changed to Dr. Bradford. On September 5, Bradford wrote a letter to Dr. Rowe at Boston City Hospital stating, "The Senior [Lovett] of my service is decidedly run down from heavy work and needs a change of air[,] which I have recommended him to take for a week at least" (R. W. Lovett

[Diaries] 1885). The remainder of Lovett's first diary includes only a few brief entries about social events. He stated that on Monday, November 2, "[I] went back to work today" (R. W. Lovett [Diaries] 1885). It's possible Lovett had some form of illness that forced him to be away from work for almost two months. He had spent the majority of his first year working long hours in the hospital, operating, caring for patients, and performing autopsies. His last entry in volume 1 of his diary, dated Wednesday, December 2, 1885, states, "[I] did my first amputation tonight," which treated a forearm injury (R. W. Lovett [Diaries] 1885).

Lovett's diary of his second year in practice as a house officer begins on Friday, January 1, 1886. He described it as follows: "[I did a] hip and gland operation…went home late to lunch [and] put on a…plaster jacket with Paul's help ["Paul" was possibly an assistant on the surgical service or another house officer]…and had a very busy afternoon…after ten we took a death mask…went home…went to the Parkers which was a great crush and very much as all other parties…then I went to the club…[then] drove to the hospital and had one or two ward calls" (R. W. Lovett [Diaries] 1886). The next day, he wrote, "[I] rode to Lawrence, Cambridge and Brighton… return[ed and did] some casts and did a Colles fracture…went to bed early and had as usual some ward calls" (R. W. Lovett [Diaries] 1886). Lovett continued to work hard and for long hours. For example, just a few days later on Wednesday, January 6, he recorded that a "case came in at 8.30 [p.m.]…and [I] stayed up all night with brief intervals of sleep…got to bed at 6.30 [a.m.]." (R. W. Lovett [Diaries] 1886). By that Saturday, he wrote: "At 2 a.m. in my cutaway coat and black best trousers I appeared in the ward and asked who called me. The nurse quietly sent me back to bed" (R. W. Lovett [Diaries] 1886). He wrote frequently about how little sleep he had.

It was during this second year as a house officer that he discussed spending about four months with Drs. Charles Taylor and Newton M. Schaffer in New York at New York Orthopaedic Hospital, then known as the New York Orthopaedic Dispensary and Hospital. Shaffer, who followed Taylor as surgeon-in-chief and was in that role during Lovett's training there, had grown the hospital into an influential organization in the city. Shaffer had a forceful personality and taught his students well; his expertise lay in perfecting the design and fit of braces for his patients. Lovett had many strong characteristics that allowed him to identify with Shaffer. Both believed in gaining expertise in surgical technique through hours of careful and meticulous effort. Both also believed in the importance of learning through hands-on experience; they lobbied for laboratories in which students could practice the art of orthopaedics with the appropriate and necessary equipment, embodying

Handwritten note (diary) of Lovett with a sketch of a Smith's fracture he treated in 1885. Harvard Medical Library in the Francis A. Countway Library of Medicine.

the concept of a skills or simulation laboratory before its time. Furthermore, they both believed that instead of using a one-size-fits-all regimen, i.e., "this treatment for that injury," orthopaedic surgeons should evaluate and treat patients on the basis of their presenting pathology and circumstances—something that Lovett emphasized in his teachings and writings.

While in New York, Lovett also visited other hospitals, including Roosevelt, Polyclinic, Mt. Sinai, and Brooklyn's Foundling Hospital. At Roosevelt, he observed a surgery one afternoon with Taylor. He mentioned seeing: "Sands cut down on a Pott's sinus and...a tumor of neck...and an ostitis" (R. W. Lovett [Diaries] 1886). He "studied in the evening," and on Sunday, January 31, he "went to see an operation at Dr. Abbe's. Dupuytren's contracture—under cocaine began at 20–25 minutes after injection an incision made and the band dissected out and sewed up with continuous catgut suture" (R. W. Lovett [Diaries] 1886). He mentioned that he "visited Taylor frequently and [made] some [visits] to Shaffer" (R. W. Lovett [Diaries] 1886) and "did also have requests to see occasional patients in their home" (R. W. Lovett [Diaries] 1886). On one occasion, he attended an orthopaedic society meeting and heard a paper discussed by Drs. Sayre, Shaffer, Judson, and Gibney.

After returning to Boston, on Monday, May 3, he "went with Bradford to the Good Samaritan and went around there. Then to the Children's [Hospital] till 6" (R. W. Lovett [Diaries] 1886). He also described many personal meetings with friends and a variety of other acquaintances. He includes letters from some in which he was addressed more familiarly as "Bob" or often "Rob" by his friends. Interestingly, he never mentions giving any lectures or teaching. At the end of that year on Monday, December 6, he stated that he "did my first real operation at 9 a.m. Excision of [illegible]—Good Samaritan—Bradford and Thomas" (R. W. Lovett [Diaries] 1886). In addition to working with Bradford, Lovett also worked with Dr. Henry P. Bowditch in his laboratory on experimental pharmacology in the medical school on North Grove Street.

The notes in volume 3 of his diaries throughout 1887 (the last year of his diaries) are brief and similar to those in volumes 1 and 2. Chronically tired, he described that he often slept late on Saturday or Sunday mornings. He maintained contact with his mentors in New York, and on Thursday, January 27, he visited Roosevelt and St. Luke's Hospitals and saw Taylor in his dispensary. On Saturday, January 29, he had dinner at Shaffer's home with other surgeons, including Drs. Virgil P. Gibney, Charles F. Taylor, Samuel Ketch, Lewis A. Sayre, Hitchcock, Drovkin, W. B. DeGarmo, Brown, Arthur J. Gillette, H.W. Berg and John Ridlon. They "talked until 1 a.m." (R. W. Lovett [Diaries] 1887). He returned to Boston the following week, and that February Lovett received an invitation by a special committee of V. P. Gibney, N. M. Shaffer, and Lewis A. Sayre to attend an evening meeting (8:30 p.m. on February 24, 1887) to hear the committee's report on organizing a national orthopaedic association. He was invited to join the organization, which eventually became

> *New York, February 19th, 1887.*
>
> *Dear Doctor:*
> *You are requested to attend a meeting to be held at 285 Fifth Avenue, on Thursday, February 24th, 1887, at 8:30 P.M., to hear the report of the Committee on Organization of the Orthopedic Association.*
>
> *Very Respectfully,*
> **V. P. GIBNEY,**
> **N. M. SHAFFER,** } Committee.
> **LEWIS H. SAYRE,**

Lovett's invitation to attend a meeting to hear a report of a special committee organized to form a national orthopaedic association—eventually becoming the American Orthopaedic Association. The constitution and bylaws were written by the founding members, including three surgeons from Boston: Drs. E. H. Bradford, Buckminster Brown, and Robert W. Lovett. Harvard Medical Library in the Francis A. Countway Library of Medicine.

the American Orthopaedic Association. Lovett also mentioned seeing patients with Bradford at Children's Hospital and the House of the Good Samaritan. He was appointed district physician to the Boston Dispensary on April 14, but he resigned that same year in September, stating: "It will be impossible for me to continue" (R. W. Lovett [Diaries] 1887). He gave no concrete reasons, but he must have been too busy with his expanding practice at Children's Hospital and the House of the Good Samaritan. That same year, he published the results of 327 cases of tracheostomy. While working with Shaffer, Lovett also coauthored his first orthopaedic paper, "On the Ultimate Results of Mechanical Treatment of Hip-Joint Disease. An Analysis of 51 Cases Occurring in the Service of the New York Orthopaedic Dispensary and Hospital." It was the first of his many orthopaedic publications.

During these three years after graduating from medical school, Lovett mentioned numerous social events, parties, and weddings that he was invited to and attended. Obviously popular, he was elected into the Puritan Club in 1885, the Union Boat Club in 1886, and the St. Botolph Club in 1887. The Union Boat Club is a private social and athletic club and the longest continuing rowing club in Boston (UnionBoatClub.org, n.d.). He also went with Dr. Bradford to the Tavern Club, a private club whose members present plays and musicals, usually written and performed by the members (TavernClub.org, n.d.). Notables in the Tavern Club included Oliver W. Holmes, Alexander W. Longfellow, Henry P. Bowditch, and Henry Forbes Bigelow. The St. Botolph Club included prominent members of a variety of professions, including Charles W. Eliot, the president of Harvard. It was founded "for the purpose of promoting social intercourse among persons connected with, or interested in the arts, humanities and sciences" (info@stbotolphclub.org, n.d.).

Lovett was eventually appointed surgeon at the House of the Good Samaritan, where he came in contact with Buckminster Brown, surgeon-in-chief. Lovett continued to work with Edward Bradford, who succeeded Dr. Brown in 1888. Influenced by both of these mentors, he followed Bradford to Boston Children's Hospital at the Huntington Avenue location that same year, and he became Assistant Out Patient Surgeon. His office was located at 234 Marlborough Street with Dr. Ober. A few years later he resigned from Carney Hospital and "in 1901 from the City Hospital to devote his attentions exclusively to orthopedic surgery"; he continued his work at Boston Children's Hospital (*BMSJ* 1924, "Robert Williamson Lovett, M.D.," obituary, no author listed).

Lovett's first orthopaedic paper was coauthored with Dr. Newton W. Shaffer—presented at the New York Academy of Medicine. Harvard Medical Library in the Francis A. Countway Library of Medicine.

ORTHOPAEDIC CONTRIBUTIONS BEFORE WORLD WAR I

Two of Lovett's earliest publications—both published in 1888—included a study on strychnine poisoning and a study on the time and amount of ether required for anesthesia. In the last five decades of the nineteenth century, the discovery of ether anesthesia and antisepsis techniques led to the birth and rapid growth of the field of surgery. Appendectomies, oophorectomies, repairs of strangulated hernias, treatment of bowel obstructions, and treatment of emphysema opened a new era of surgery. These two major discoveries also allowed surgical specialties to make major advances. Dr. Bradford was busy during this period, and Lovett joined him and other orthopaedic surgeons in the last two decades, leading the way for the explosive development of orthopaedic surgical treatments that became available during the turn of the twentieth century.

One of his most notable contributions was the classic textbook on orthopaedic surgery, *A Treatise on Orthopedic Surgery*, which he coauthored with Bradford and published in 1890. The book's copyright contract with the publisher, William Wood and Company, called for a 500–700-page book on orthopaedic surgery to be published by October 1, 1889 (Countway Medical Library, "Robert Lovett's scrapbook"). Bradford was paid $250 upon publication. Also contained in Lovett's personal scrapbook are numerous letters; some to Bradford, some to Lovett. Many were complimentary and congratulatory in nature. But one particular series of letters was troubling.

On September 30, 1890, Bradford received a letter from Dr. Charles F. Stillman, a professor of orthopaedic surgery at Chicago Polyclinic. Essentially, he accused the authors of using photographs of his patients: "cuts and illustrations of mine that appear [in the book] without my consent and without credit from you" (C. F. Stillman 1889). He also accused the authors of using some of Dr. Lewis Sayre's photographs without permission. After commenting on each photograph, including a page number, Stillman wrote: "And now my dear Doctor, I don't wish to blame you publicly, if you can give me a satisfactory account of this proceeding, so I shall await your answer for a reasonable length of time... piracy among members of any profession should not be encouraged" (C. F. Stillman 1889). An anonymous editorial had appeared in the *Western Medical Reporter* (Chicago) in July 1890. Entitled "Eastern Gall," it essentially accused Bradford and Lovett of "downright literary piracy... there is hardly an original line in the work...the author in this instance prefers to crib everything and give no credit to anyone...In this work on 'orthopaedic surgery,' by Bradford and Lovett, there are more stolen plates than in any work of its size extant" (*Western Medical Reporter* 1890). Stillman denied writing the editorial.

Apparently, Stillman had had a previous agreement with William Wood and Company to write a textbook on orthopaedics, four years before Bradford and Lovett's book was published (W. Wood

Bradford and Lovett published a major textbook on orthopaedics, which was popular for over two decades.
Columbia University Libraries/Internet Archive.

1888). The publisher had already spent $400 on wood engravings for Stillman's book, but no draft of the book was available. The publisher decided against waiting longer and offered Stillman the opportunity to purchase all the woodcuts for $200. He refused, allowing the company "to use the woodcuts in any way we may please" (W. Wood 1890). Stillman, in response to the letter he received from the publisher in 1888 stated that "he had almost completed his manuscript, but I cannot see sufficient demand for such a work… With regards to the engravings, if you can use any of them [the woodcuts], you are perfectly at liberty to do so" (C. F. Stillman 1888).

As it turned out, Wood and Company offered Bradford and Lovett the engravings to use in their textbook (E. L. Bradford, n.d.). Some of Sayre's engravings, in the hands of the publisher, were included by mistake with Stillman's woodcuts that were given to Bradford and Lovett. Bradford wrote to Sayre, explaining the situation, which was totally acceptable to Sayre. In a later correspondence in 1890, Sayre wrote, "[Stillman] has been known as erratic in many of his actions…[and thinks Bradford's] explanation is perfectly satisfactory" (L. Sayre 1890). Stillman was criticized by others, including the American Orthopaedic Association (C. F. Stillman 1890). Bradford had been publicly forgiving of Stillman, because Stillman later thanked Bradford for defending him at the 1890 AOA meeting in Philadelphia. Bradford and Lovett's book went on sale on January 1, 1890. By May 12, 1891, Woods reported that 842 copies had been sold (W. Wood [sic] 1891)—more than had been expected. The book remained the major textbook on orthopaedics in the United States for over two decades.

In his first two years in practice in Boston, Lovett had published a large series of cases of cerebral palsy treated at Boston Children's Hospital and a paper on differentiating true from apparent leg-length discrepancy. He published numerous other studies, including one on intubation versus tracheostomy in 1892. Lovett also wrote about a wide variety of orthopaedic conditions and treatments, but he is recognized for his major contributions in understanding hip disease, the mechanics of scoliosis, flatfeet, and especially infantile paralyses and muscle testing (R. W. Lovett Collected Papers). Other topics he wrote about included:

- an article about Percival Pott
- the outdoor treatment of tuberculosis
- joint infections
- paralysis of the arm in newborn children
- issues of balance and posture influenced by corsets and high-heeled shoes
- chronic backaches
- Pott's disease
- The neurasthenic spine
- painful spines without organic disease
- round shoulders
- roentgenographic deformities in rickets
- the use of heliotherapy in chronic open bone infections (Thézac-Porsmeur method of sun treatment)

Lovett's devotion to research and establishing a scientific foundation for orthopaedic practice can best be summed up by his American Orthopaedic Association Presidential Address in 1898, entitled "Pathology and its Relation to Orthopedic Surgery." He stated: "American orthopedic surgery stands pre-eminent in its mechanical and practical side. My plea today is for working out a more exact scientific basis than we now have, which can only come from accurate etiological and pathological knowledge." However, according to Mayer (1950): "Even as thoughtful a student as Robert Lovett [was], in his presidential address in 1898… [he] does not mention the work of Röntgen, nor did he seem to envisage its meaning for the pathological knowledge he considered so important to orthopaedic advance."

In 1907, Lovett described the operative treatment of spina bifida (R. W. Lovett Collected Papers). Before his article, treatment of spina bifida consisted of tapping, ligation, or injection of irritant fluids. He described an operative technique that consisted of four stages: bilateral skin incisions through normal skin, closure of the sac like a hernia repair, use of flaps of muscle and fascia to close the opening, sealing the area to prevent spinal fluid leakage and skin closure. By 1910, he coauthored another book, *The Surgery of Joints*, with E. H. Nichols.

Hip Disease

Lovett had maintained an interest in hip disease after publishing his first paper with Newton Shaffer back in 1887. Two years after returning to Boston, he published three papers from Boston Children's Hospital on the treatment of tuberculosis of the hip, including the use of salicylic acid and the prevention and treatment of abscesses. Goldthwait coauthored the paper on treatment and prevention of hip abscesses in 1889 (R. W. Lovett and Goldthwait 1889). They stated:

> As a general rule, surgeons have advocated the early incision of these pus collections... Many of the leading orthopedic surgeons in America, on the other hand, advocate very strongly letting the abscesses break of their own accord unless their character is so acute as to render operative interference necessary. Their reasons for this are: first, the possibility that the abscess may disappear spontaneously; secondly, that the operation has no effect upon the original disease to which the abscess is only incidental; and third, that there is a risk of septic infection due to operation.

Lovett and Goldthwait reviewed the records of 360 patients treated at Boston Children's Hospital during the previous five years. They admitted and operated on 33% of patients with hip abscesses. Postoperatively, the patients were managed in traction or splints. They used Lister's antisepsis technique. In the "Discussion" following Lovett and Goldthwait's article (*Journal of Bone and Joint Surgery* 1889), Dr. Virgil P. Gibney of New York—the second surgeon-in-chief at the Hospital for the Ruptured and Crippled and known for treating over 2,000 cases of tuberculosis of the hip—commented: "From what I have seen of the institutions you have in Boston, it would seem that the children are treated antiseptically and treated well in the Children's Hospital." In the same "Discussion," Dr. Reginald H. Sayre also agreed: "I am in favor of thoroughly opening abscesses when they show signs of growing too rapidly."

For his research on hip disease, Lovett received the Fiske Prize in 1891 (G. F. Shrady 1891). The prize included $300. His essay was entitled "The Etiology, Pathology, and Treatment of Diseases of the Hip Joint." He followed this publication with the results of his use of traction to treat tuberculous hips in 1894 (R. W. Lovett 1894). He studied normal hip joints in seven children, diseased hip joints in 12 children, normal hips in a number of cadaver adults and children, and one child with a diseased hip of six months' duration who died of scarlet fever. Using a marking system over the anterior superior iliac spine, the greater trochanter and the lateral malleolus and with leg traction of either 10 pounds or 20 pounds, he measured the lengthening of the limb, i.e., distraction of the hip joint. In cadavers, he observed that "checks to

Lovett continued his interest in tuberculosis of the hip after this initial paper on hip abscesses that he coauthored with Dr. Goldthwait. *Journal of Bone and Joint Surgery* 1889; s2-1: 1.

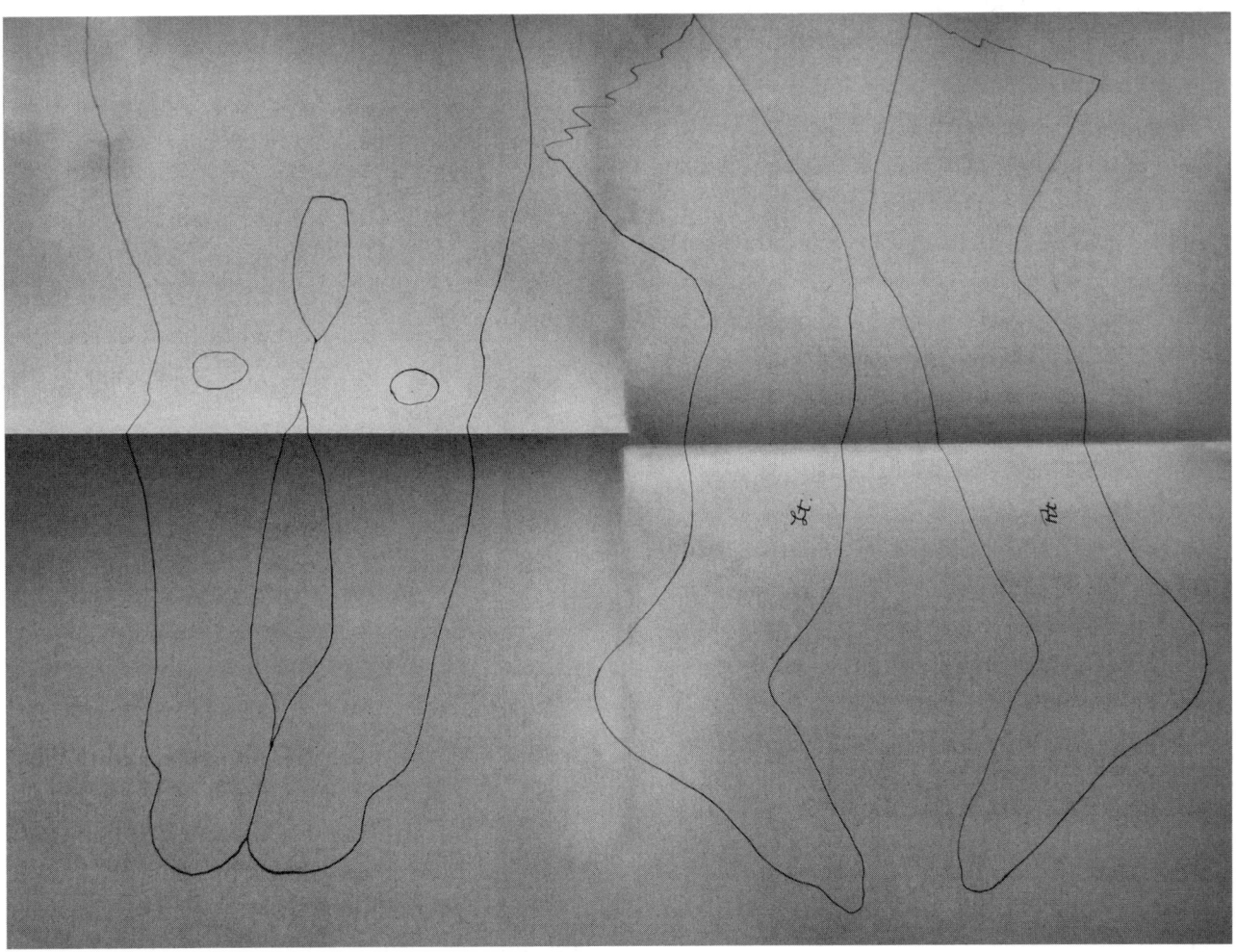

Before x-rays were available or commonly used, surgeons would trace a patient's deformities before and after treatment on paper and enter them into the medical record. In this example, there is an anterolateral bow of the left tibia (July 20, 1905).

The House of the Good Samaritan Records 1860-1966. Archival Collection—AC4. Box 13, Volume 29. Surgical Records, July 3, 1902–July 19, 1905. Boston Children's Hospital Archives, Boston, Massachusetts. Photo by the author.

distraction…lay in the resistance, first, of the capsular ligament, especially the anterior bands of the ilio-femoral ligament; second, in the resistance of the cotyloid ligament [acetabular labrum], and to a slight degree in atmospheric pressure" (R. W. Lovett 1894). In normal children, traction with 10 pounds did not lengthen the limb, but 20 pounds resulted in 0.25 inches in length. In children with diseased hips, he noted: "traction of ten pounds in children before puberty…produces lengthening of the leg in hip disease…due to separation of the joint surfaces…[but] in general less in older children than in young ones…that twenty pounds traction, as a rule, produces more separation than ten pounds" (R. W. Lovett 1894). He recommended the use of traction in patients with tuberculosis of the hip with a traction force sufficient to overcome any muscular spasm and to continue treatment until the spasms stopped. "In treating hip disease at a certain stage the object should not be simply rest, or fixation, or protection from jar, but actually distraction, and that traction short of this is insufficient" (R. W. Lovett 1894). An example of one of the severe cases he reported is described in **Case 16.1**.

In 1901, Lovett published the results of a study of incision and drainage of psoas abscesses (R. W. Lovett 1901). He reviewed all cases treated

Case 16.1. Tuberculosis of the Hip: Treatment by Prolonged Traction

> "Annie F. entered the out-patient department of the hospital in February, 1888, being at that time fifteen years old. The disease had been in progress for two years, one of which had been spent in bed. Pain had been severe and night cries frequent.
>
> "An abscess had formed, and the joint was flexed and fixed. Traction treatment was begun and continued for two years with traction splint and crutches. A protection splint was worn for four years more.
>
> "*Present Condition.* — Twenty-one years old; strong, healthy woman; weight, one hundred and twenty-one pounds. The sinus has been healed three years. There is motion in flexion of ten degrees at the hip joint. There is no motion in other directions. Patient walks well. There is a three-inch shortening, but the trochanter is not above Nélaton's line. There is no deformity."
>
> (R. W. Lovett 1894)

at Boston Children's Hospital over 10 years, from 1890 to 1900. Forty-nine of 54 cases were operated on during this period. Mortality rate was high (35%). In order for drainage to occur after incision, Lovett recommended that the patient be placed in a plaster jacket so that the patient could sit erect, allowing the abscess to drain.

Although roentgenograms were discovered in 1895, and used soon thereafter at Massachusetts General Hospital and at Boston Children's Hospital by Dr. Robert Osgood in 1900, Lovett did not report on the use of radiographs in hip disease until 1905, in a paper he coauthored with Dr. Percy Brown, radiologist to Children's and Carney Hospitals. To determine whether radiographs were accurate in determining early disease in the hip, the writers were blinded to the name of the patient, the clinical history, and the diagnosis in 100 consecutive cases taken from the files of Boston Children's Hospital Radiology Department. They wrote:

> Our conclusion as to the value of radiographs in the diagnosis of hip disease, and especially early disease, is that they are of great value in the hands of persons of average experience; that a radiograph free from abnormal appearances does not show that hip disease is absent or will not develop, but that in a case of doubtful clinical diagnosis a normal x-ray is a matter of weight and makes the likelihood of speedy recovery greater than will radiograph with abnormal appearances…
>
> In only two cases was hip disease diagnosticated where it was not present, and here the writers were misled by an extra-articular collection of pus. (R. W. Lovett and P. Brown 1905)

Foot

Sherk (2008) claims that Lovett authored the first article on conditions and injuries of the foot published in the orthopaedic literature in the USA. Lovett (1896) made numerous clinical observations by examining 250 nurses at Boston City Hospital. The most significant finding regarding prognosis, in his opinion, was a view of the sole of the patient's foot while standing on a glass table. He developed this technique at Boston Children's Hospital, a technique used for generations of orthopaedic surgeons and residents in training there (E. H. Bradford 1897). This view of the weight-bearing foot through glass allowed the observer to see the areas of the sole and heel that bore the weight of the individual to determine if the foot was pronated, in varus, and with a high or medium arch or no arch.

Lovett believed that patients experience more issues because of flat, pronated feet than feet "without breakdown of the arch" (H. Sherk 2008). He agreed with Bradford that "the shoe should be so designed that the toes are not crowded and free action be possible especially for the great toe" (E. H. Bradford 1897). Nurses' feet often hurt after working long hours; Lovett suggested soaking

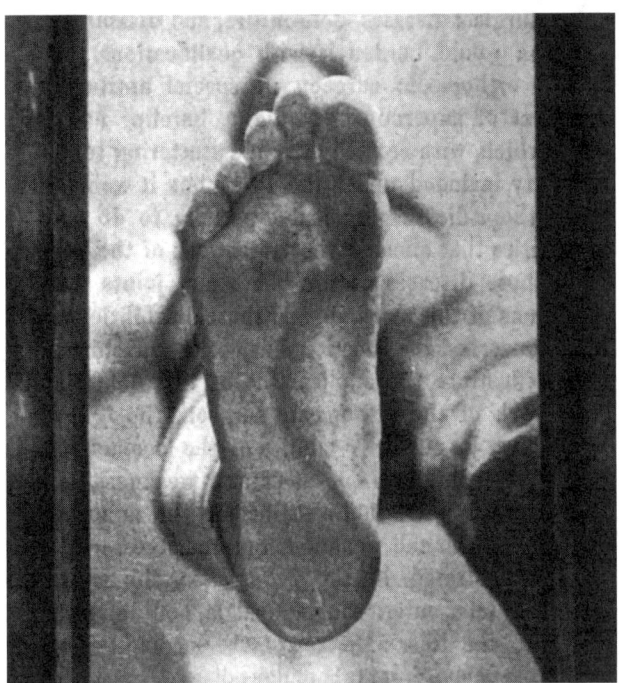

Photograph of the foot through glass with minimal weight-bearing. Lovett learned this technique from Dr. H. J. Hall, a former house officer at Children's Hospital. He preferred this method contrasted to the commonly used methods of smoked or wet tracing of the foot. As a resident in the late 1960s, I remember using this technique to demonstrate a foot deformity. Lovett, "The Mechanics and Treatment of the Broken-Down Foot," *New York Medical Journal* 1896; 63: 796.

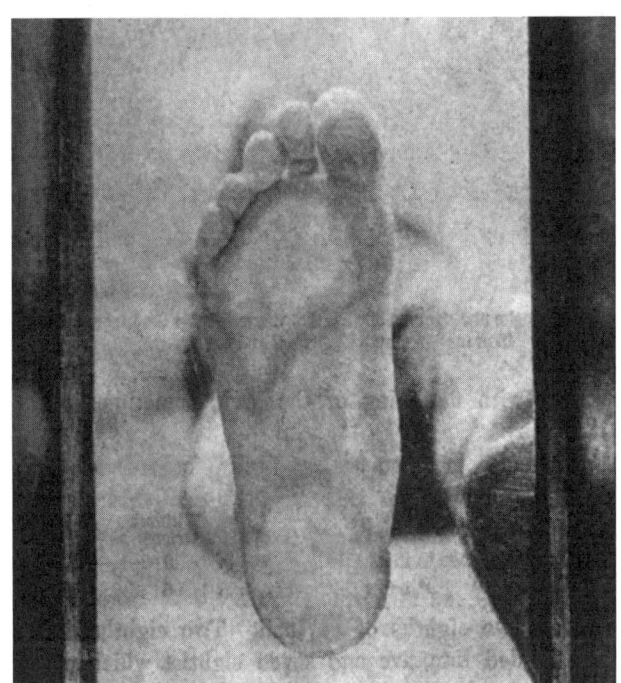

Photograph of the foot through glass with weight-bearing. The normal foot in this case assumes a pronated position. Lovett, "The Mechanics and Treatment of the Broken-Down Foot," *New York Medical Journal* 1896; 63: 797.

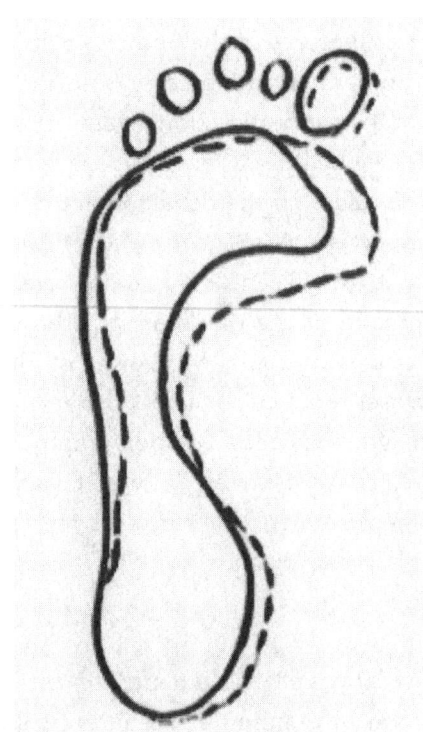

Tracing of the foot taken through glass. The black outline is the normal position and the broken line is the pronated position. Lovett, "The Mechanics and Treatment of the Broken-Down Foot," *New York Medical Journal* 1896; 63: 797.

in hot and cold water, wearing padding in the shoes, resting, and other treatments. Lovett even designed footwear that was "wide as the foot in front but [with a] straight inner edge [last] and high arched, stiff shanked and constructed on a slightly curved line so as to hold the foot in its position of strength" (H. Sherk 2008). Although he tried to make nurses wear them, they initially rejected the shoe because of its appearance and belief that it would not relieve their pain.

However, later that year—when Lovett presented his research in the article "The Prevention of Flat-Foot and Other Similar Affections of the Foot" (*Boston Medical and Surgical Journal* 1897)—Dr. Dewey is quoted in the "Discussion" of the paper at the meeting of the Boston Society for Medical Improvement that:

at the hospital we find that a large number of the nurses at first complain that their feet are tired, but at the end of the first fortnight, as a rule, they get the boot prescribed; and after that their troubles rapidly cease in the majority of cases. The nurses, as a rule, are satisfied with the regulation boots...The results to us at the hospital have been wonderful. Not a day has been lost by the nurses on account of their feet, whereas formerly a good many days were lost and some of the nurses had to leave the school. We are very grateful to Dr. Lovett for what he has done.

Lovett's research and design are all the more impressive because as late as 1900 he had not yet written about the use of x-ray:

The omission is all the more significant since Lovett was already thinking in terms of the x-ray in 1898, when with [Frederic J.] Cotton he employed roentgenology in his study of "The Anatomy of the Foot." No doubt the apparatus when available was so incapable of demonstrating fine bone detail that even the far-seeing Lovett failed to realize that the x-ray would help the development of orthopaedic surgery more than any other discovery of the next half-century. The only orthopaedic surgeon of the day that stressed its significance was Louis A. Weigel of Buffalo. He presented a paper in 1899 dealing with the diagnostic value of radiography. X-ray films were, he asserted, "not as fallacious as had been claimed." It is interesting to note that his paper did not elicit any discussion. (L. Mayer 1950)

Almost 20 years later, and after his experiences with Osgood in examining the feet of soldiers in World War I (see chapter 63), he published a paper on painful feet: "The Superstition of Flat Foot." He summarized his thoughts about flatfeet at the time (R. W. Lovett 1915b):

Feet vary in shape...some are naturally flat, others have a moderate arch, and some a very high arch.

Any foot may become painful from foot strain without any change in the height of the arch under unfavorable conditions, overuse, ill health, etc.

Boots are a predisposing factor to foot strain not only by cramping the foot, but especially by not supplying adequate support to the sole of the foot. For this reason persons with high arches are quite as liable to foot strain as persons with low arches, if not more so.

When foot strain occurs, it is desirable to rest the tired structures by support, most often a metal plate. Exercises in acute cases and the use of a flexible shoe generally do harm rather than good.

My final heresy consists of the belief that painful feet are more often helped by raising the heels than by lowering them.

Lovett didn't believe in the use of exercises for acute foot strain nor in the use of flexible shoes. In such acute cases, he treated patients with a supportive shoe with a metal arch support and often massage. After a short period of weeks or months, he would wean them from the metal arch support and return them to a more flexible shoe. During this transition period, he often prescribed exercises as well.

Scoliosis

It was in 1900 that Lovett began writing about lateral curvature of the spine. His early papers and a paper in 1905 were eloquent studies on the mechanics of scoliosis in cadavers and volunteer models. He studied normal movements of the spine in models: forward flexion, extension, lateral bending, and torsion (R. W. Lovett 1900). He acknowledged previous cadaver studies by Bradford and unpublished cadaver studies by Elliott G. Brackett. He also quoted from Henry

Title of Lovett's article in which he used living models to understand the normal flexion, extension, and rotation movements of the spine. *Boston Medical and Surgical Journal* 1900; 142: 622.

J. Bigelow's 1844 Boylston Prize Essay: "The principle of torsion is illustrated by bending a flat blade of grass on a flat, flexible stick in the direction of its width. The centre immediately rotates upon its longitudinal axis to bend flatwise in the direction of its thickness. In the same way the spine, laterally flexed, turns upon its vertical axis to yield in its shortest or antero-posterior diameter" (H. J. Bigelow 1845). As Leo Mayer (1950) stated, "our understanding of the mechanism of scoliosis was given a mighty forward surge in 1900 by the unusual research of Robert Lovett... Lovett's observations still hold good."

In his initial experiments, he fastened thin boards to the chest and pelvis and cardboard markers to the skin along the spine, and he observed the motions and positions of the spine. He then repeated these studies in cadavers with the boards and hat pins inserted into the spinous processes "of the first sacral, one of the lower dorsal, one of the upper dorsal, and one of the lower cervical vertebrae, to mark the antero-posterior axis of each vertebrae" (R. W. Lovett 1900). He concluded after his experiments:

> In flexed positions, bending is associated with torsion in one direction, in extended positions by torsion in the opposite direction. Torsion and side flexion of the spine are parts of one compound movement, and neither exists to any extent alone. Lateral deviation of any part of the spinal column is therefore necessarily associated with torsion (rotation) at the seat of the deviation...In this it follows simply the mechanical law governing flexible rods...the kind of torsion observed in scoliosis...originates in the flexed position of the spine...The immediate cause of lateral deviation is in some asymmetry of development or posture...causing the spine to deviate from the middle line. (R. W. Lovett 1900)

Lovett reported his research at the 14th Annual Meeting of the American Orthopaedic Association in Washington, DC, in 1900. In the discussion of his paper, Shaffer agreed with Dr. Lovett, but later in this discussion he "felt

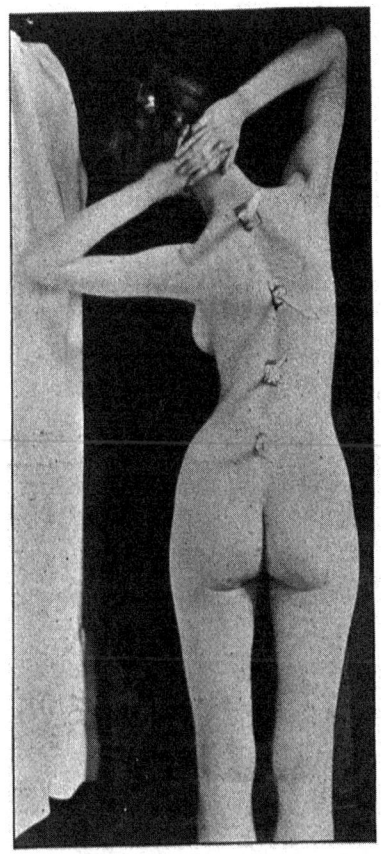

Example of a model bending her spine to the left in extension. Lovett placed cardboard markers on some of the spinous processes, which he states show that the spinous processes have turned to the right and the vertebral bodies to the left.
Boston Medical and Surgical Journal 1900; 142: 625.

Title of Lovett's article in which he used models as well as cadaver spines with pins inserted into the spinous processes to continue his research into normal and abnormal movements of the spine. *Boston Medical and Surgical Journal* 1905; 153: 349.

firmly convinced that lateral curvature of the spine is dependent primarily on changes in the muscles, though quite probably an underlying cause was to be found in the nervous system" (R. W. Lovett 1900). Bradford, in the discussion of a paper on the futility of correcting a scoliosis after bone changes had developed, "insisted that there were certainly some cases in growing children that were benefitted by treatment" (R. W. Lovett 1900).

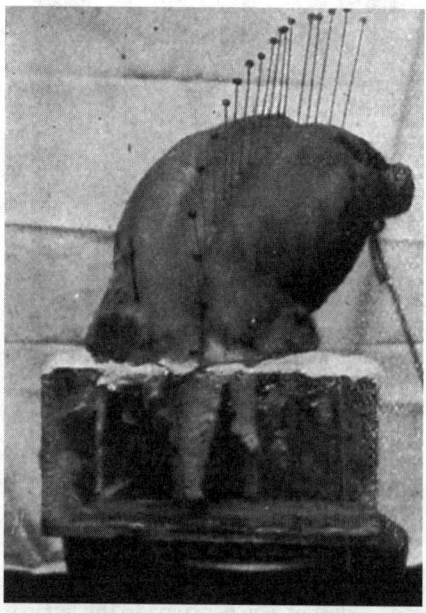

Side bending to the right, in flexion, in a cadaver spine. Lovett reported that a curve convex to the left was formed and that the vertebral bodies turned to the left. *Boston Medical and Surgical Journal* 1905; 153: 359.

By 1905, Lovett reported on additional experiments he conducted on spine mechanics in normal individuals and patients with scoliosis. In reviewing the literature from Europe and the United States, he wrote, "Nowhere can be found an accurate, concise, clean-cut description of spinal movements" (R. W. Lovett 1905). He did additional studies on cadavers, models, and children with scoliosis. In the cadavers, he inserted pins into each of the spinous processes of the entire spine. In models, "lead strip tracings and photographs were used, and tracings of side curves were taken on crinoline gauze laid over the back through which the spinous processes were felt and marked...[also] in the cadaver" (R. W. Lovett 1905). He concluded the following in the three regions of the spine:

1. In the lumbar region flexion diminishes mobility in the direction of side bending and rotation.
2. In the dorsal region hyperextension diminishes mobility in the direction of side bending and rotation.
3. In flexion the whole spine side bending is accompanied by rotation of the vertebral bodies to the convexity of the lateral curve, the characteristic of the dorsal region.
4. In the erect position and in hyperextension of the whole spine, side bending is accompanied by rotation of the vertebral bodies to the concavity of the lateral curve, the characteristic of the lumbar spine.
5. The dorsal region rotates more easily than it bends to the side...the lumbar region bends to the side more easily than it rotates.
6. Rotation in the dorsal region is accompanied by a lateral curve, the convexity of which is opposite to the side to which the bodies of the vertebrae rotate.
7. The column of vertebral bodies obeys in flexion, hyperextension, side bending and rotation and in the combinations of them the same rules which govern the intact spine. (R. W. Lovett 1905)

Lovett concluded his paper with observations of patients with scoliosis and commented on simple curves, double curves, the rotation of the shoulders and spine, and classified two distinct types of scoliosis: postural curves without bone changes and curves with structural changes in the vertebrae. He believed that the observations he made in normal spines could be used to treat flexible postural curves, but he remained doubtful about treating patients with structural scoliosis: "We are no longer dealing with a spine distorted by the normal mechanism, but by a malposition to which is added a distorting pathologic process. That a knowledge of spinal mechanics will make clearer the treatment of structural scoliosis I have no question, but…further study and careful investigation [are needed]" (R. W. Lovett 1905). It is very surprising that Lovett did not use or refer to x-rays in his early studies on scoliosis.

With Dr. James W. Sever, Lovett published a paper on the treatment of scoliosis (1911). They discussed treatment of both postural (functional) and structural (organic) curvatures. They stated: "We must recognize that bone is an adaptive structure, and we must remember also that we are dealing with a lateral bony deformity of the spine… it would seem as if our best chance of remedying the bony deformity was to force the spine into as normal a position as can be obtained, and to hold it in that position during part of the period of growth" (R. W. Lovett and J. W. Sever 1911). They described the use of exercises to gain flexibility and strength for mild curves. For more severe curves, they used removable or permanent jackets. They reported one interesting observation in 1911:

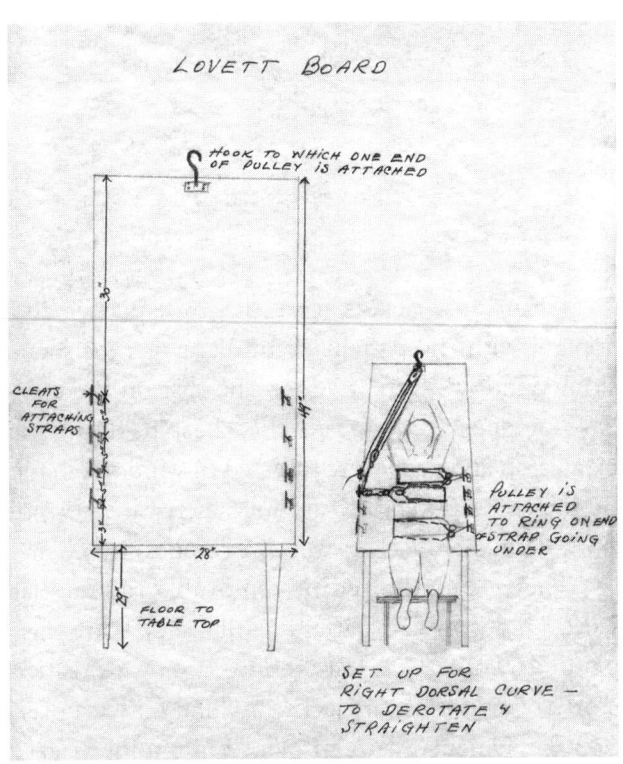

Lovett Board. Sketch of a prototype apparatus to derotate and straighten a scoliotic spine.

The House of the Good Samaritan Records 1860–1966. Archival Collection AC12. Box 2, Folder 22. Boston Children's Hospital Archives, Boston, Massachusetts.

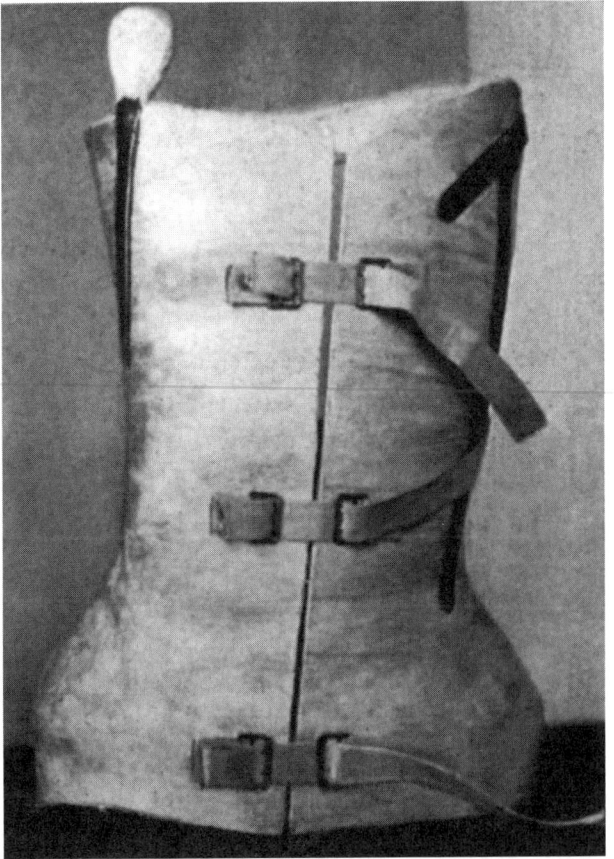

Removable jacket made from a plaster torso mold of the patient after initial correction. *Principles of Orthopedic Surgery* by J. W. Sever, New York: Macmillan, 1940.

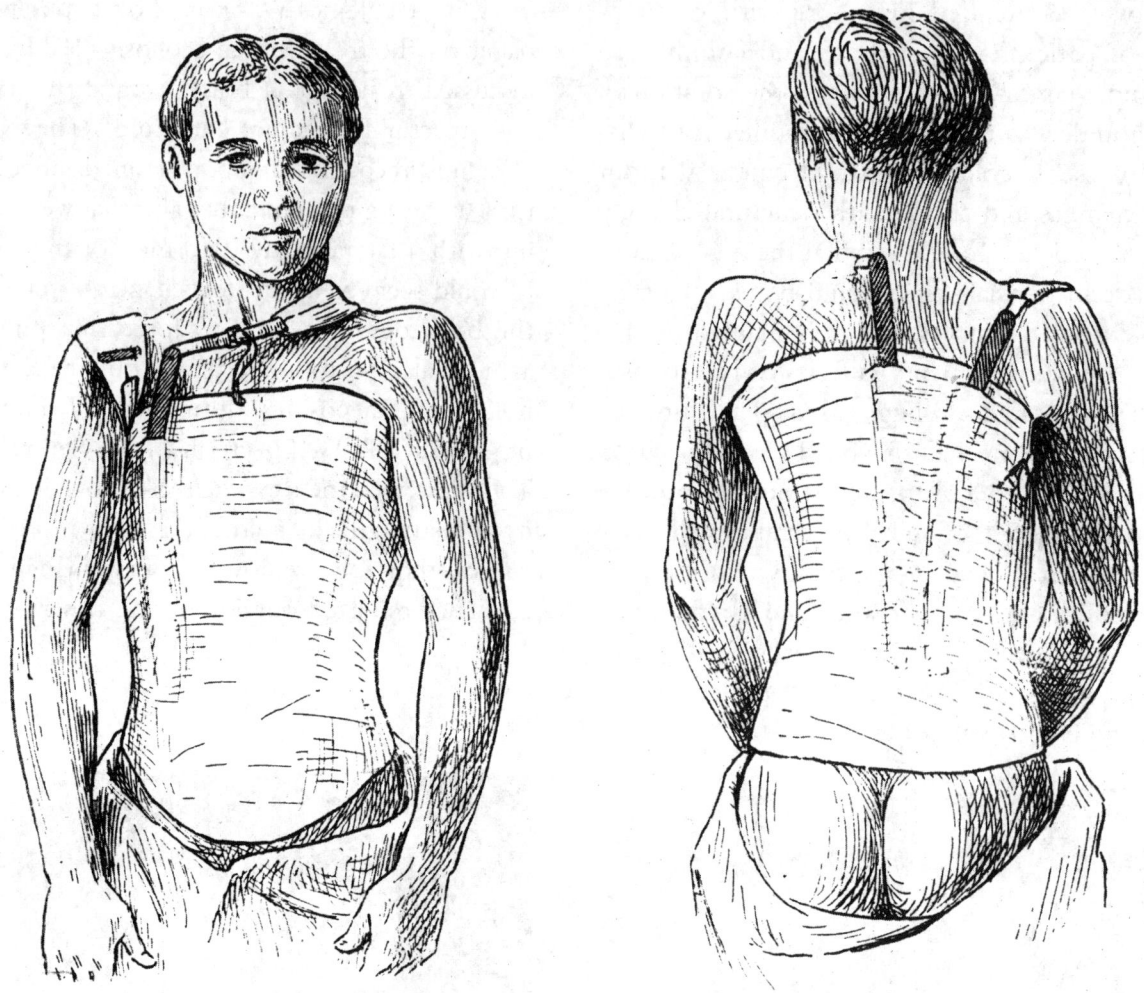

Sketch of a corrective plaster jacket used by Lovett and Bradford. *Treatise on Orthopedic Surgery*, 2nd edition, by Bradford and Lovett. New York: William Wood and Company, 1899. Columbia University Libraries/Internet Archive.

A curious experience directed our attention to the possibility of this [permanent cast or jacket during growth] method. A girl with a severe lateral curvature applied at the Children's Hospital for treatment. A forcible plaster jacket was applied and an x-ray of the spine in the corrected position taken through windows cut in the jacket. The girl was instructed to return in two weeks to have the jacket changed…she stayed away fourteen months and came back wearing the same jacket. The improvement in her position…was extraordinary, and an x-ray… showed an improvement in the bony curve. This suggested a treatment which has been followed…during the last three years. (R. W. Lovett and J. W. Sever 1911)

Permanent jackets were made of plaster and applied with the patient recumbent or in suspension. Windows were made in the cast on the concave or depressed side of the chest to allow for expansion and pads were inserted in windows made on the convex side for continued increasing correction. Permanent jackets were worn up to two years.

They were followed by removable jackets that were made on the patient while they were suspended. This jacket was removed and a positive (torso) made from the jacket by filling it with plaster. The patient was then placed in another jacket while the torso was remodeled, introducing further corrections into a future removable jacket. The torso remodeling included removing the prominent side and building up the opposite side "until it has become decidedly more symmetrical than the patient…On this corrected torso a plaster jacket is applied which is to be the removable jacket worn by the patient" (R. W. Lovett and J. W. Sever 1911). It was fitted with shoulder pads, straps and buckles on the open front of the jacket. The jacket was worn constantly, except for exercises. This same type of jacket, although later made of celastic, was made by the residents at Boston Children's Hospital until the arrival of Dr. John Hall in 1970. Lovett and Sever showed photographs of patients successfully treated with this method, but no x-rays.

Infantile Paralysis

The first major epidemic of infantile paralysis (poliomyelitis) in the United States had occurred in Vermont in 1894 (L. F. Peltier 1993). Between 1894 and 1916, multiple epidemics continued throughout New England; many experienced long-term effects or were paralyzed and in need of physical therapy (M. M. Plack and C. K. Wong 2002), and there was the pressing need for the development of new innovative orthopaedic surgical procedures to restore as much function as possible. Only basic facts about the disease were known: the virus was contracted most often by children and adolescents, and that infection occurred during only one season (summer). This widespread lack of knowledge of the disease inhibited the ability of hospitals and physicians to handle epidemics or to suggest and assess ideas for prevention and treatment (C. A. Smith 1983).

In 1907, Lovett was named by the governor to the Massachusetts State Board of Health because of his "work in orthopedic surgery, and particularly that which relates to the proper seating of school children and allied matters, should make him a particularly valuable member of the board" (*BMSJ* 1907b). This major appointment in public health, in addition to his early reports on infantile paralysis, led to another major appointment. In 1908 and 1909, Lovett, with others, published pamphlets and books on infantile paralysis in Massachusetts, its occurrence, and methods of treatment (*BMSJ* 1910). In 1910, he coauthored a major paper with Bradford, Brackett, Thorndike, Soutter, and Osgood entitled, "Methods of Treatment of Infantile Paralysis." As the authors stated: "The purpose of this paper is to furnish to the practitioner, as far as possible, a summarized guide in the treatment of poliomyelitis in its various stages of development" (E. H. Bradford et al. 1910). They emphasized the importance that the treating physicians needed to recognize the stages of the disease and the methods used in each. The stages were "stage of invasion; stage of recovery; stage of permanent paralysis and disability; stage of progressing deformity; stage of developed contraction and deformity" (E. H. Bradford et al. 1910).

In 1913, Lovett published a five-year review of the epidemiology and research of polio by the Massachusetts State Board of Health from 1907 through 1912 (R. W. Lovett 1913b). Surveys were sent to physicians to complete about each patient with polio. In 1907, there were 136 cases reported in Massachusetts; in 1909, there were 932 cases. From 1907 to 1910, 2,138 cases were reported. Polio was not made reportable in Massachusetts until 1909. Lovett mentioned that the disease was infectious and could be produced in monkeys. Seasonal occurrence was reliable: "the disease reaching its height in either July, August or September…but never quite disappearing even in winter" (R. W. Lovett 1913b). Not knowing whether insects such as the mosquito or stable fly were vectors, "we found what appeared to be evidences of transmission by direct personal contact in 13% of cases" (R. W. Lovett 1913b). With support from the legislature, the state board collaborated with the medical schools to continue active research to understand the etiology, epidemiology, contagiousness, pathophysiology, and treatment of this dreaded disease.

This report was followed by Lovett's paper on his study of the Vermont epidemic in 1914 (R. W. Lovett 1915c). There had been 293 cases of polio in Vermont that year. He visited the state

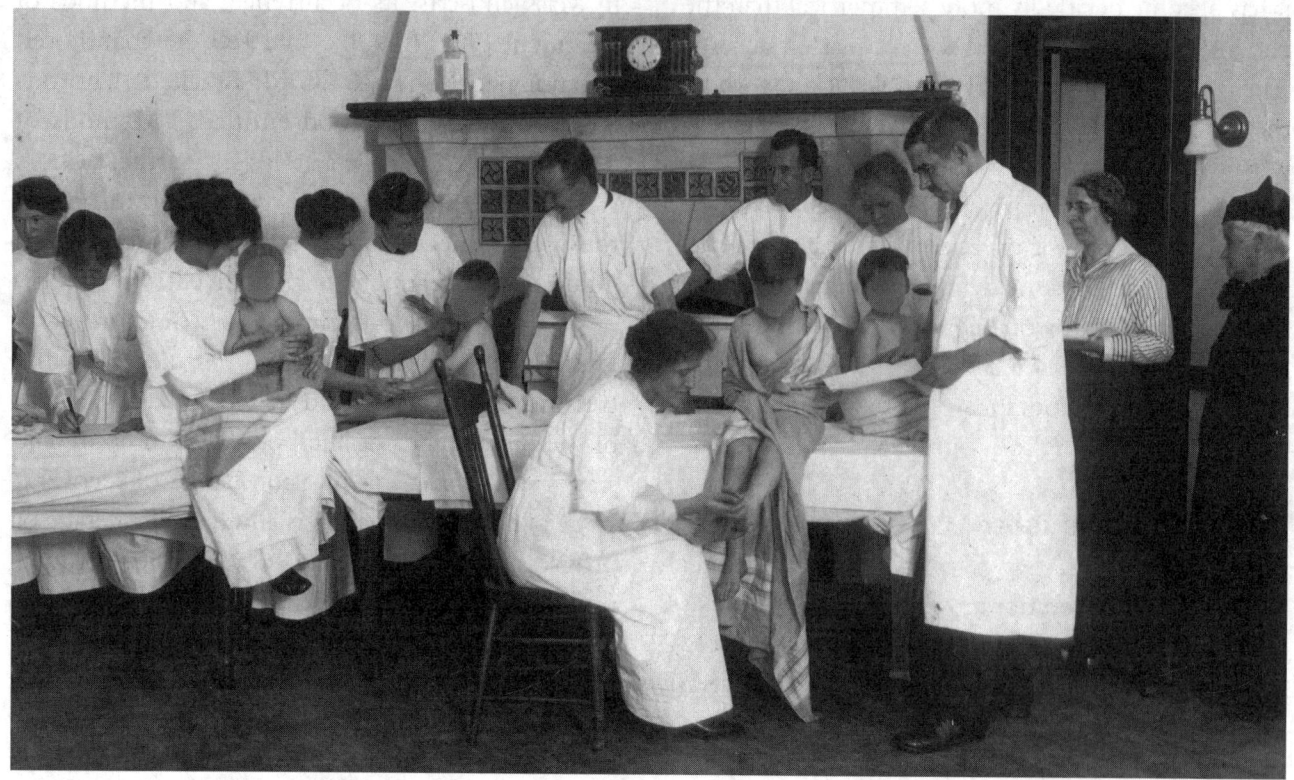

Dr. Lovett (standing in the foreground on the right) leading a clinic at BCH with nurses, doctors, and observers. Boston Children's Hospital Archives, Boston, Massachusetts.

many times and personally examined 149 patients, noting: "All patients were stripped, and the muscles were individually tested as to function…The muscles were classed as wholly paralyzed, partly paralyzed, and normal…The condition of each muscle was then marked on charts" (R. W. Lovett 1915c). He observed that partial paralysis was the most common finding: "Of 1452 muscles affected, 416 were totally paralyzed and 1036 partly, that is, the relation of partial to total paralysis was 2.5 to 1" (R. W. Lovett 1915c). He found that muscles of the lower extremity (quadriceps, gluteals, and gastrocnemius) were more frequently involved than those in the upper extremity. Abdominal muscles were affected in over 50% of the cases and spinal muscles more than 25%. Paralysis of muscles in the upper extremity was more common about the shoulder and decreased in frequency down the arm to the hands. He observed the same frequency in the lower extremity, i.e., more frequent paralysis about the hip and diminishing down the leg to the foot. Paralysis was more common in the left upper extremity, but it was similar in incidence in both lower extremities. He speculated that this pattern of muscle weakness could be because of the close association of certain centers in the spinal cord, the muscles responsible for walking, and the erect position that have large centers of motor cells, or it could be due to the predominance of certain muscles that are associated in function and not antagonists to the other. He offered no definitive answer.

He discussed three treatment programs for early cases: massage, electricity, and muscle training. He observed only local effects on circulation with massage. He completed a preliminary study in which cases were treated on one side with daily galvanic electricity and none on the opposite side, with no difference noted between the two sides. He noted that "muscle training, on the other hand, rests on a sound physiologic basis, works out empirically better than any other of the measures, and the large proportion of partial paralysis

> **THE TREATMENT OF INFANTILE PARALYSIS**
> PRELIMINARY REPORT, BASED ON A STUDY OF THE VERMONT EPIDEMIC OF 1914*
> R. W. LOVETT, M.D.
> BOSTON
>
> JOUR. A. M. A. VOLUME LXIV
> JUNE 26, 1915 NUMBER 26

Title of Lovett's report of the 1914 polio epidemic in Vermont.
Journal of the American Medical Association 1914; 164: 2118.

Case 16.2. Importance of Rest in Acute Poliomyelitis

> R. W. Lovett, March 4, 1916:
>
> "A man of 22 was referred in the fourth week after his onset. He had involvement of the right leg and arm, walked with a limp and could not raise his right arm. The left arm appeared to be slightly weakened. Examination by the usual method showed extensive weakness in the left arm, very little power in the right deltoid, and a general involvement of the right leg. His right arm was put in a sling, he was cautioned against much walking and the use of the arm, and weekly muscle tests were made, showing a general slow gain, but no therapeutic exercises were allowed at first. At a test, October 4, an increase of 50 per cent in the power of the right gastrocnemius muscle was observed, and on questioning it was found that he had been daily rising on his toes as a trial. This seemed to indicate that he was ready for therapeutic exercise, on which he then began with success. The test, October 26, showed a loss of 25 per cent of power in the wrist and finger flexors of the right hand, and it was found on questioning that he had been writing too much. This was stopped, and on the following week a return of the former power was found in these muscles, an instance of the information afforded by the test in directing routine and defining treatment."
>
> (R. W. Lovett and E. G. Martin 1916)

in the cases observed shows its reasonableness" (R. W. Lovett 1915c). The most important factor to Lovett, however, was early rest and the avoidance of fatiguing weak muscles (**Case 16.2**). He stated, "It must be an easy thing to overexercise them" (R. W. Lovett 1915c). When discussing patients in his private practice, he wrote, "Power might begin to return in a very faint degree to a muscle while under muscle training, and that with care this power would steadily increase, but if that muscle were exercised even very gently every day, that power would diminish or disappear, so that we exercise such muscles only once in three days at the outset, increasing the work most carefully" (R. W. Lovett 1915c). Lovett continued his work on infantile paralysis during and after World War I.

CHIEF AT CHILDREN'S HOSPITAL AND HARVARD EDUCATOR DURING CRISIS: WORLD WAR I

Lovett's initial appointment at Harvard Medical School had been as an assistant in clinical surgery. He was reappointed in 1899 and then appointed assistant in orthopaedics in 1902. From the beginning of his teaching career, he was well-known for his clinical and teaching skills, he routinely applied new knowledge from basic and clinical research to his patients. As described by Sir Robert Jones, Lovett had a "clearness of thought and simplicity of expression [that] made him a great teacher. Students appreciated his ability to give clearly the reasons for diagnosis and for treatment" (*BMSJ* 1924). He continued to be promoted until 1915, when he was named the first John Ball and Buckminster Brown Professor. This professorship was the first in orthopaedics at Harvard and the second in the United States, following Lewis A. Sayre's appointment as professor of orthopaedic surgery at Bellevue Medical College in 1853. It would be almost 50 years before the second orthopaedic professorship would arrive at Harvard Medical School.

Lovett would go on to lead curriculum changes at HMS during a critical and transformative time in the history of the United States: World War I.

Meanwhile, at Boston Children's Hospital, Lovett was involved with the move in 1914 from its current location on Huntington Ave. to its new location on Longwood Ave., and he eventually was appointed as visiting surgeon. By 1915, the same year he was promoted at HMS, he became the chief of the orthopaedic department (succeeding Dr. Bradford), a position he held for seven years.

The United States declared war on Germany (April 6, 1917) only two years after Lovett had succeeded Bradford as chief, and after he was named the first John Ball and Buckminster Brown Professor of Orthopaedic Surgery at HMS. During that two-year period, debate at Harvard, as well as across the nation, had focused on the possibility of entering the war and the question of whether to increase the military forces, debates that included pacifists opposing those who favored the United States entering the war. Gradually the tide shifted in favor of those who believed the United States should enter the war. Harvard President A. Lawrence Lowell also began changing admissions and the culture at Harvard at this time, expanding the types of students accepted to the college and introducing the ideal of public service as part of students' education (Shapley 1967). The class of 1917 had begun a trend of admitting a majority of students who had received a public education, although because so many entered the military, it was not a full class (Shapley 1967). Almost 90% of the class fought in the war; almost 30% of those who fought were included among the casualties (Shapley 1967).

The US declared war three years after the Allied Powers had already been fighting Germany and the other Central Powers. It would be the first time US troops were deployed in Europe. In anticipation, the American Orthopaedic Association (AOA), at its meeting in Washington, DC (May 1916), formed a committee "to consider the needs and equipment of orthopaedic hospitals" (US

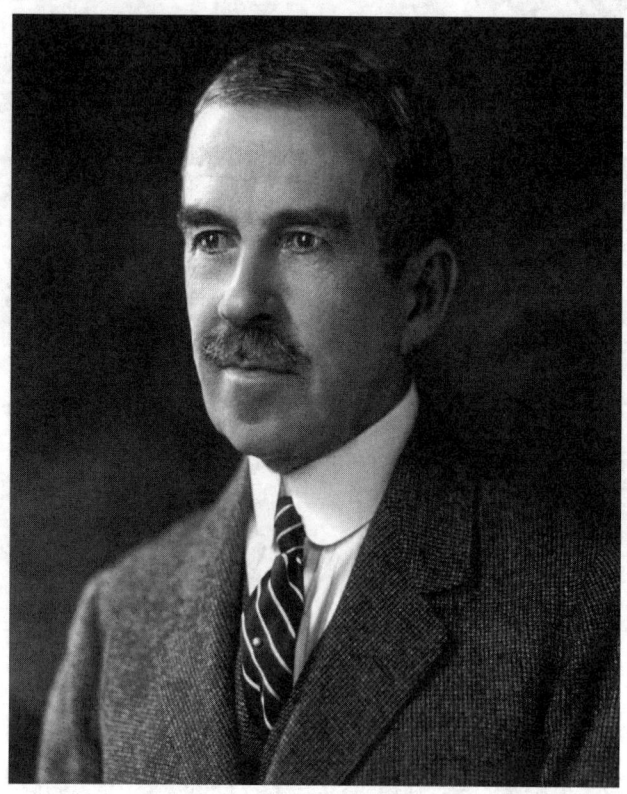

Robert W. Lovett as the John Ball and Buckminster Brown Professor of Orthopaedic Surgery. *The Evolution of Orthopedic Surgery* by R. B. Osgood. St. Louis: C. V. Mosby Co., 1925.

Surgeon General's Office 1921) (see chapter 63). The committee presented its recommendations the next year at its annual meeting in Pittsburgh (president was David Silver). Charles F. Painter was president of the AOA at the time of their review. He had graduated from Harvard, was house officer at the Massachusetts General Hospital, and worked at many hospitals in Boston: Robert Breck Brigham Hospital, Beth Israel Hospital, Carney Hospital, the Massachusetts Women's Hospital, and the House of the Good Samaritan. While in the military in World War I, he was stationed at the Chelsea Naval Hospital. He had become dean of Tufts Medical School in 1913.

After discussion, members of the American Orthopaedic Association adopted resolutions and presented them to the surgeon general. Briefly, they offered the services of all members of the AOA to the government, probably including active service, but especially in offering their services to provide orthopaedic education in "methods of examination, treatment, and instruction of conditions affecting the soldier in training" (US Surgeon General's Office 1921). Accepted by the surgeon general, the American Orthopaedic Association committee prepared a document to be used by surgeons in the military. It included instructions on conducting an orthopaedic examination, emphasizing the foot, footwear, the spine, etc. At the same time, the military was receiving reports from Europe about the large number of disabled wounded soldiers, raising concerns that the United States did not have the orthopaedic workforce to meet the demands in Europe after entering the war—nor at home when disabled soldiers would eventually return. In August 1917, an orthopaedic advisory council for the surgeon general was formed, consisting of many past AOA presidents and members of the orthopaedic section of the American Medical Association. The committee surveyed all orthopaedists who were available for service and recommended that special orthopaedic training be made available in the universities and hospitals.

As a result, a division of orthopaedic surgery was established for the first time in the United States Army. In addition to enlisting orthopaedic surgeons to active duty in France and England, additional personnel and hospital equipment were priorities of this new division. Recognizing that there were not enough orthopaedic surgeons to serve overseas nor to provide care for disabled soldiers returning home, plans were activated to train more orthopaedic surgeons by providing intensive periods of about three months for surgeons and for physicians as assistants to orthopaedic surgeons. Some Harvard orthopaedic surgeons were sent to England and France, including Robert Osgood, Joel Goldthwait, and others. Some were asked to remain at their teaching institutions to provide the intensive short training programs. Robert Lovett was in this latter group.

In the fall of 1917, Harvard and the New York College of Physicians and Surgeons were selected to begin an intensive six-week training program in orthopaedics for military surgeons. Within a few months, courses were also begun at Case Western Reserve, the University of Pennsylvania, Northwestern, and Washington University in St. Louis. The surgeon general expected that the medical schools would train the maximum number of surgeons in orthopaedics that was possible for each faculty, requesting that at least "one competent man" (F. F. Russell and R. L. Wilbur 1919) be retained in addition to the department chief who could assume the responsibilities of these intensive training programs.

On July 3, 1917, Dean Bradford wrote President Lowell requesting that Harvard Medical School be permitted to train military medical officers in orthopaedic surgery. Lowell approved his request on September 16, 1917, and the new school was named the School for Health Officers. The graduates of the class of 1917 received orthopaedic training at the Chelsea Naval Hospital (27 men) or in Portsmouth, New Hampshire (11 men). Harvard was selected as the first medical school to organize a course in orthopaedics for military officers, and Lovett was chosen by Dean Bradford to develop and teach the course.

The first course at Harvard began on October 1, 1917. Twenty men were enrolled, and a total of 35 men completed courses in the fall of 1917. Lovett wrote that the men were older, had practiced before, but had "a very imperfect knowledge of orthopaedic surgery" (R. W. Lovett, n.d.). He noted that the military leaders wanted men trained in orthopaedics for the "purpose of making them acceptable assistants in the camps, with a view to their later assuming greater responsibility as their experience increased" (R. W. Lovett, n.d.). Lovett was named a major in the army that year, and Bradford had him devote half of his teaching time to the new School for Health Officers (US Army) and the other half to the third- and fourth-year students. In a letter to Bradford dated March 16, 1918, Lovett expressed his desire to give all the lectures to the medical students himself in order "to improve the medical education in the orthopaedic department" (R. W. Lovett 1918c), and to fulfill a promise he had made to Bradford when assuming the chair at Children's Hospital: "Finally...I am accomplishing something in my present rather scattered activities...to hold up the standards of orthopedic surgery as I learned them from you" (R. W. Lovett 1918c).

Lovett enlisted in the US Army Medical Reserve Corps as a major. The next orthopaedic course for military surgeons at Harvard began on May 1, 1918. Over a two-year period, Lovett directed multiple six-week courses; each better than the previous one. Anatomy, which Lovett felt was fundamental for these military surgeons, was taught at the Harvard Medical School's anatomy department. The bulk of exercises were held in the orthopaedic outpatient department at MGH, usually in the morning with the afternoons in anatomy at the medical school or lectures in the Children's Hospital amphitheater. The officers spent about six hours each day (five days per week) in lectures, anatomy dissections and discussions of clinical cases. One day (Tuesday) was occasionally spent at the Peter Bent Brigham Hospital; some courses were also held at the City Hospital. Occasional lectures were held on Saturdays.

Most lectures were given by Lovett, including clinics in the foot at Canton, scoliosis in the Peabody Home, and an operative clinic at the Hospital School. He often lectured on neuromuscular mechanism, on pathology of joints, osteotomies and bone pathology. Other faculty and their lectures/demonstrations included:

- Major Pelters: foot splints
- Dr. Ehrenfried: plaster techniques; x-ray interpretation
- Dr. Legg: joint anatomy; operative clinic
- Dr. Soutter: operative surgery; joint incisions; gave first lecture on artificial leg
- Dr. Sever: spine fractures
- Dr. FitzSimmons: plaster application, joint anatomy

Lovett (n.d.) noted that he "gave frequent written examinations," and he and Rogers (who taught at the MGH) gave a final examination.

The first course was named a "Course in Orthopaedic Surgery." Lovett renamed it "A Course in the Principles of Orthopaedic Surgery" (R. W. Lovett, n.d.). Lovett's opinion about the course was that it became "perfectly evident soon that any attempt to teach these men orthopaedic surgery in 4, 6 or 8 weeks, was futile... most that we could hope to do was to ground them in the principles of orthopaedic surgery... which they might apply in practical work" (R. W. Lovett, n.d.). He then organized subsequent courses "around major topics: joints–structure and function, bones and pathologic disturbances, muscles...paralysis, tuberculosis, osteomyelitis, traumatic synovitis, etc." (see volume 5, "Military Orthopedic Surgery" July 9, 1918) (R. W. Lovett, 1918).

In July 1918, the surgeon general requested a list of all essential teachers of orthopaedic surgery because the "medical schools were disorganized" (R. W. Lovett 1918d). The list from Harvard included Professor Lovett and instructors Arthur T. Legg, Robert Soutter, and Lloyd T. Brown. Additional lectures on fractures and gunshot wounds were given to the military surgeons. Charles L. Scutter wrote to Bradford that he had "three separate squads of army surgeons assigned to him for instruction in fractures of bone" (C. L. Scutter 1918) and other topics. Numerous courses were held at medical schools from Boston to Los Angeles in the summer of 1918, and "in all 691 officers passed through the different schools" (US Surgeon General's Office 1921). Three courses were held at Harvard, "the shortest...some 130 hours of instruction, far more than any undergraduate would receive in that specialty in any year of his medical course" (R. W. Lovett 1918b).

Robert Lovett was honored by the University of Pittsburgh when he was chosen to deliver the fourth annual Mellon Lecture on May 10, 1918.

The title of his lecture was "The Problems of the Reconstruction and Re-education of the Disabled Soldier." David Silver was the professor and chair at the University of Pittsburgh at the time. In his lecture, Lovett discussed the problem of the severely injured soldier who returned home with a disability, the effects on the soldier's family, the importance of society's acceptance, and the government's responsibility to care for them and to re-educate them in some form of gainful employment. Based on the Canadian experience, Lovett speculated that about 20% of the injured soldiers would not be able to resume their previous job, and they would need re-education and training in another profession or trade. He was one of the first orthopaedic surgeons to use the word *disabled* instead of *crippled* in describing these soldiers, the latter of which he said was "so much in vogue in the newspapers" (R. W. Lovett 1918a). He described three steps in their reconstruction, or "the attempt to rehabilitate and, if necessary, re-educate the man who has been physically disabled" (R. W. Lovett 1918a). The first was to complete all medical and surgical care needed by the injured soldier. The second focused on their rehabilitation, including "treatment to loosen up joints, develop muscles, free tendons, improve resistance to fatigue…[although] partly accomplished by massage and similar measures, it has been found in this war that it is better brought about…by actual work either in bed, bedside occupations, or in shops equipped for the purpose known as curative workshops in which an occupation is pursued which is of itself curative." In the third step, "the disabled man must…be educated in a new trade or occupation [because] he may be unable to follow his original one on account of the nature of his injury…the third stage of reconstruction activity spoken of as 'vocational training' or 're-education'" (R. W. Lovett 1918a).

Lovett continued in his lecture with a comparison of the injured soldier to the previously crippled child who had been neglected in both Europe and the United States. It wasn't until 1832 that Germany started a school for disabled children and not until 1893—60 years later—that the first attempt at re-education for them was made in America, when "a private educational and industrial school for cripples was started in Boston" by Edward H. Bradford (R. W. Lovett 1918a). Lovett also compared the medical care and rehabilitation required for the man seriously injured in the workplace. Although many were uneducated, with "a surprisingly large proportion of cases being wholly illiterate…trades…were often closed to him in his uneducated position, but…in many instances by proper surgical attention, by general education and by special training, he could be made a wage earner and a useful citizen instead of being a burden on his family or becoming an almshouse charge" (R. W. Lovett 1918a).

> Of the returned men [American soldiers], 75 to 85 percent are to be classed orthopedic. The definition of orthopedic as established by the ruling of the Surgeon General of the United States, of August 1917, a ruling which is in general accord with the English and Canadian classification is as follows:
>
> a) derangements and disabilities of joints including ankylosis;
> b) deformities and disabilities of feet;
> c) malunited and un-united fractures;
> d) injuries to ligaments, muscles and tendons;
> e) cases requiring tendon transplantation or other treatment for irreparable destruction of nerves;
> f) nerve injuries accompanied by fractures or stiffness of joints;
> g) cases requiring surgical appliances
> (R. W. Lovett 1918a)

American orthopaedic surgeons learned from the European and British orthopaedic surgeons who had been in the war for over three years before the United States joined forces with them. One significant contribution was made by Colonel Sir Robert Jones, who emphasized the importance of the curative workshops. Lovett (1918a) credits him for "useful manual work has largely supplanted the older system of mechanotherapy." Jones emphasized the importance of active movements of the extremities and joints over the previously emphasized passive motion, especially in splints. "As soon as the patient is fit to get about, he should have some occupation for this mental, moral and physical welfare. Here the curative workshop is an invaluable aid to his gymnastic treatment" (R. W. Lovett 1918a). These rehabilitation techniques addressed the complex and debilitating condition of reflex sympathetic dystrophy (today called chronic regional pain syndrome or CRPS). The former director of the British Army Medical Service, Sir Alfred Keogh, stated, "Nothing has been more remarkable than the overthrow of the old-fashioned purposeless orthopedic exercises for the cure of muscle weakness, stiff joints, etc." (R. W. Lovett 1918a). Orthopaedic surgeons, by their experience and contributions to injured soldiers had now become responsible for the treatment of fractures, malunions, and non-unions, as well as for the field of rehabilitation.

After the war, Lovett continued with his busy practice and teaching at Children's Hospital and Harvard Medical School. Though his personality was reserved, Lovett's passion for the work was exemplified in, for example, his undaunted leadership of projects such as chairing the Infantile Paralysis Commission and leading training of medical officers during World War I, and his extensive private practice. Many other physicians sought his council and consultation (*BMSJ* 1925).

Based on his experiences teaching military surgeons the basics of orthopaedics, he advocated for a change in teaching the specialty to medical students. He wrote that by teaching the undergraduate, "giving didactic or clinical instruction... in those different affections...scoliosis, clubfoot, the deformities of poliomyelitis, tuberculosis of the spine, flat foot, torticollis, round shoulders, etc....is simply making the student...into a medical encyclopedia...Although this might pass, and has passed, unchallenged in the undergraduate curriculum, it did not stand the test of intensive instruction when instruction became an unusually serious and responsible business [as for military surgeons about to enter the war]" (R. W. Lovett 1918b). Lovett changed the teaching method for military surgeons and proposed that the new method should be used for teaching future medical

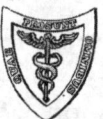

Cover of *Medical War Manual No. 4: Military Orthopaedic Surgery*. Orthopaedic Council: Major Elliott G. Brackett, Director of Department of Military Orthopaedic Surgery to the Surgeon-General; Major Joel E. Goldthwait, Director of Military Orthopaedic Surgery for the Expeditionary Forces; Major David Silver, Assistant Director of Military Orthopaedic Surgery to the Surgeon-General; Major Fred H. Albee; and Drs. G. Gwilym Davis, Albert H. Freiberg, Robert W. Lovett, and John L. Porter. Francis A. Countway Library of Medicine/Internet Archive.

students. "The plan was adopted of first taking up general principles, and then illustrating these clinically. It thus became the reverse of the so-called 'case system,' because the student first heard the principles stated, and after being grounded in them, was made familiar with their application... in this way he would, or should, be better able to approach a new and unusual condition which he had not met clinically" (R. W. Lovett 1918b). Lovett's list of general principles included: affections of the joints, diseases and affections of the bones, affections of the muscles and neuromuscular mechanisms, static affections (overweight, foot abnormalities), congenital affections, apparatus (bracing splints, casts), and reconstruction (rehabilitation, prostheses). His new pedagogy became "the principle of proceeding from the general to the special" (R. W. Lovett 1918b).

We can gain insight into Lovett's person and the vision he held for future leaders in his field from his speech as president of the Boston Surgical Society in 1921, when he introduced the first recipient of the Henry J. Bigelow Medal, Dr. W.J. Mayo. In his introduction, Lovett expressed his thoughts about leaders in medicine:

> Rising thus to leadership by their own attainment, and by that alone, it follows that no influence, no money, no power, no notoriety can make a man a leader in medicine, and no combination, no authority, and no clique can prevent him from becoming a leader, provided he has within himself the necessary requirements. The leader in medicine is essentially a self-made man, standing on his own feet, strong in his own convictions, relying on his own achievement. He must win and hold his place by honesty, strength, skill and ability...he must possess something more than mere professional skill and ability—call it what you will, character, spirituality, or vision, there must be something in the man that commands personal respect and confidence, or he cannot qualify.

(*BMSJ* 1921)

ORTHOPAEDIC CONTRIBUTIONS DURING AND AFTER WORLD WAR I

Lovett continued producing a tremendous number of contributions in orthopaedics during and after World War I, as did his mentor and chief, Dr. Bradford. In total, Lovett published over 173 papers and several textbooks. During the war, he was one of many authors of the military orthopaedic manual "Medical War Manual No. 4, Military Orthopedic Surgery," published in 1918. He also coauthored another textbook, *Orthopedic Surgery* with Sir Robert Jones in 1923. It was published in two volumes, replacing *Treatise on Orthopedic Surgery* as "the latest authority on the subject" (*BMSJ* 1924).

Title page of Jones and Lovett's textbook, *Orthopedic Surgery*.
University of California Libraries/Google Books.

Infantile Paralysis

In 1916, in the midst of World War I, the well-known Harvard Infantile Paralysis Commission (appointed by the University Corporation) named Robert Lovett (founder) as its chairman. According to Mayer: "It was not until the extensive epidemic of 1916 and its pathetic harvest of crippled bodies that orthopaedic surgeons began to note the numerical increase of paralyzed patients in their clinics and in their office practice" (1950).

Lovett's and Martin's Spring Test

With a generous gift from an anonymous donor to Vermont's State Board of Health, Lovett and Ernest Martin (assistant professor of physiology at Harvard Medical School) studied the treatment of polio victims in Vermont and at Boston Children's Hospital. They used a spring system of measuring muscle strength, originally developed by Martin, to study over 177 patients (13,000 observations) and a group of normal patients in the scoliosis clinic at Boston Children's Hospital. They classified partial paralysis as "severe (one third or less of normal power) or moderate (one third or more of normal power)" (R. W. Lovett and E. G. Martin 1916). Lovett wanted to accurately measure a muscle's strength and follow the change in strength over time and while the patient was being treated.

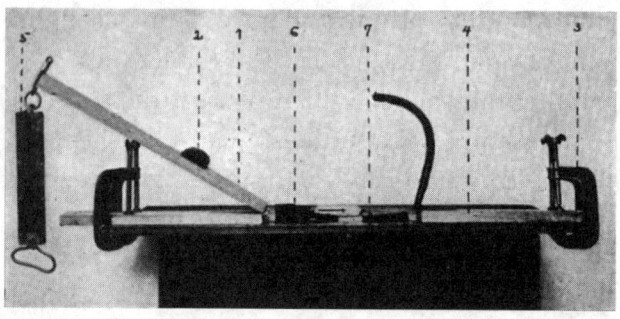

Apparatus designed and used by Martin and Lovett to measure muscle strength in polio patients.
Lovett, "The Spring Balance Muscle Test," *The American Journal of Orthopedic Surgery*, 1916; 14: 417.

The spring test worked in his hands. According to Mayer (1950), "Lovett's spring balance test for muscle strength...added considerably to the accuracy of our methods of examination. He developed a series of exercises for paralytic cases which, with the aid of his physical therapist, Miss Wilhelmine Wright, have found the basis of the system of so-called 'muscle education'" (L. Mayer 1950). Lovett and Wright used the spring test to treat a large number of patients with polio. (Wright later published the book *Muscle Function* in 1928 as a guide for physicians and physical therapists. In addition to describing actions of each individual muscle, normal muscle function, abnormal function in polio, she wrote about the need for re-education of muscle-tendon transfers in polio

CERTAIN ASPECTS OF INFANTILE
PARALYSIS

WITH A DESCRIPTION OF A METHOD OF
MUSCLE TESTING *

ROBERT W. LOVETT, M.D.
John B. and Buckminster Brown Professor of Orthopedic Surgery,
Medical School of Harvard University

AND

E. G. MARTIN, PH.D.
Assistant Professor of Physiology, Medical School of
Harvard University

BOSTON

Title of article by Lovett and Martin in which they described the spring muscle test. University of Toronto/Internet Archive.

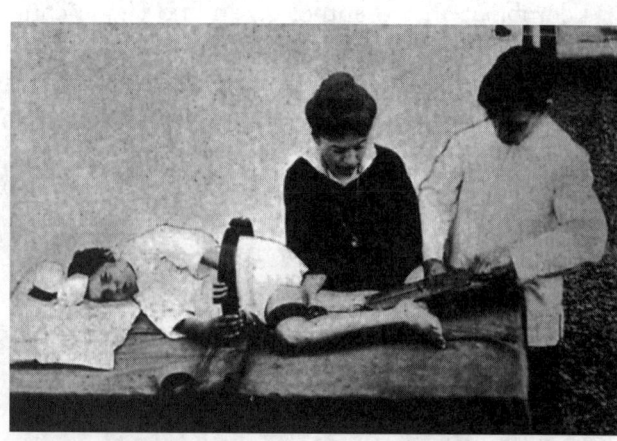

Photo of patient having her quadriceps muscle strength measured in the spring apparatus. Lovett, "The Spring Balance Muscle Test," *The American Journal of Orthopedic Surgery*, 1916; 14: 417.

patients.) However, not all patients could perform Lovett and Martin's spring balance muscle test. Patients who could not perform the test included those with extremely weak muscles or contractures. They were also unable to devise reliable methods for testing shoulder rotator cuff muscles, back muscles, and abdominal muscles. About 20 years later, the Nerve Injuries Committee of the Medical Research Council of Great Britain developed a simpler method that graded muscle strength on a 5-point scale. Clinicians could more easily apply this to patients with a larger variety of conditions, and it eventually became the gold standard.

The Treatment of Infantile Paralysis: An Early Classic

Not long thereafter, Lovett published the early classic on polio "The Treatment of Infantile Paralysis" in 1917. In it, he stated:

> The attack itself, apart from these characteristics, [referring to changes in the spinal fluid] may resemble an ordinary gastro-intestinal attack, a common cold, influenza, the beginning of one of the exanthemata or other of the common acute affections of childhood. The appearance of tenderness often masks the condition and leads to incorrect diagnosis; it must be remembered that tenderness is a routine symptom in the majority of cases.
>
> When the paralysis has occurred, the diagnosis as a rule presents but little difficulty. It is a motor paralysis, or weakening, of erratic distribution, most marked in the legs. Reflexes are diminished or lost, the reaction of degeneration is present in the most severely paralyzed muscles, atrophy, retarded growth, coldness, and sluggish circulation supervene in the latter stages in many cases. Atrophy of the thenar eminence is a frequent occurrence in infantile paralysis and at times throws light on the diagnosis of doubtful cases.

> But even when paralysis has developed the diagnosis is not always quite easy...The history is often misleading and one must at times be prepared to make the diagnosis on the physical signs which are left after the attack without regard to the history. The origin of the paralysis is at times attributed to trauma by the patients. (R. W. Lovett 1917a)

He summarized treatment during the acute phase: "Rest until the tenderness has disappeared, absence of meddlesome therapeutics, either medicinal or physical, the use of warm salt baths in the later part of this period, and possibly the early injection of immune blood serum...prevention of contractures [is important]" (R. W. Lovett 1917a).

PHYSICIAN TO FRANKLIN D. ROOSEVELT

Franklin Delano Roosevelt (1882–1945) was 39 years old when he became ill and met Dr. Robert Lovett for the first time. When they met, Lovett had already published his classic "The Treatment of Infantile Paralysis" and had responded to the Vermont polio epidemic. Roosevelt had already been a state senator in New York, assistant secretary of the navy, and in 1920 lost the election as vice-president. He had previously become ill during the 1918 flu pandemic and survived.

In the summer of 1921, Roosevelt left Washington, DC, for a vacation in his summer house on Campobello Island in New Brunswick, across the bay (Lubec Narrows) from both Eastport and Lubec, Maine (home of Charles Lowell; see chapter 3). At the time, Roosevelt was president of the Greater New York Boy Scouts Council and on July 7, 1921, he stopped to visit the Boy Scout Camp at Bear Mountain. He left a few days later, sailing to Campobello and arriving on August 9, 1921. Campobello was beloved by Roosevelt, having summered there since his childhood. The next day, after sailing with his children, Roosevelt became ill:

He complained of fatigue and a backache, which had been present for several days and had become more intense. He skipped dinner and went directly to bed. Later in the evening, he had chills and an elevation of temperature. On awakening on the morning of August 11, he noted that his left leg was weak. Within a few hours, both legs were weak, the back pain had become worse, a severe headache had developed, and his temperature had climbed to 102° F. (Z. B. Friedenberg 2009)

Dr. Eban E. Bennet, Roosevelt's family physician in Lubec, Maine, was called to see him. Visiting Campobello on August 12, 1921, Bennet was very concerned. He made a clinical diagnosis of a cold but "became uneasy with the diagnosis as his patient was having difficulty with urination, severe headaches, malaise and increasing weakness of his legs" (Z. B. Friedenberg 2009). Dr. W. W. Keen, a well-known surgeon and professor at Jefferson Medical School, was vacationing in Bar Harbor at the same time. Famous as a surgeon, both in the Civil War and World War I, he had secretly operated on President Grover Cleveland during his second term to remove a cancerous tumor from his upper jaw and palate. Bennet spent some time searching for another consultant to see Roosevelt, found Dr. Keen, and asked him to visit Campobello. Keen visited Roosevelt two days later (August 14) and "diagnosed a blood clot in the spinal artery in the lower spine. He was optimistic and predicted a full recovery, but the next day the paralysis had spread to the trunk muscles" (Z. B. Friedenberg 2009).

Eleanor Roosevelt was very concerned and communicated her concerns to James (called Rosy), Roosevelt's half-brother, and to her uncle, Frederick Delano. Frederick Delano went to Boston, recording that he "thought to consult the best man in Boston. The great Dr. Lovett" (F. A. Delano 1921/Papers of Eleanor Roosevelt). Lovett was out of town, but Keen (at Eleanor Roosevelt's request) eventually contacted Dr. Lovett. Lovett examined Roosevelt at Campobello on August 25, 1921 (on Friday, one of his regular operating days) with Keen. After examining him, Lovett wrote to Dr. George Draper, an expert on poliomyelitis at the Rockefeller Institute, stating:

> There was some uncertainty in their [Keen's and Bennet's] minds about the diagnosis, but I thought it perfectly clear so far as the physical findings were concerned and I never felt that the history is of much value anyway…There had been some hyperaesthesia of the legs preceding the bath for a day or two. He had, I thought, some facial involvement, apparently no respiratory, but a weakness in the arms, not very severe and not grouped at all. There was some atrophy of the left thenar eminence…His bladder was paralyzed…There was scattered weakness in the legs. (R. W. Lovett 1921a)

Lovett and other physicians never recommended a spinal tap, so confident were they in the diagnosis, although he and Draper often did one to help establish a diagnosis in other patients.

In several letters from 9, 20, and 21 September 1921, Lovett described his thoughts about the treatment of poliomyelitis. Initial treatment was "quarantine [for] three to four weeks…Mr. Roosevelt is not to be regarded as a source of danger from infection at the present time" (Countway Medical Library [Lovett's collected papers]). Writing to Dr. Bennet on September 20, he discussed the use of convalescent serum: "We used it in the epidemic in Massachusetts in 1916 [and] thought we got good results from it, especially in the preparalytic cases[, but Dr. Francis Peabody, in a controlled series,] conclu[ded] that cases without it did as well as the cases with it" (Countway Medical Library). The Harvard Infantile Paralysis Commission did not use intraspinal serum in the Boston epidemic of 1920 (about 1,600 cases). Writing to Keen in Philadelphia, in response to his letter one week before expressing Roosevelt's request that he needed more treatment, Lovett described his treatment philosophy: "In a good many cases…I allow no treatment of any kind

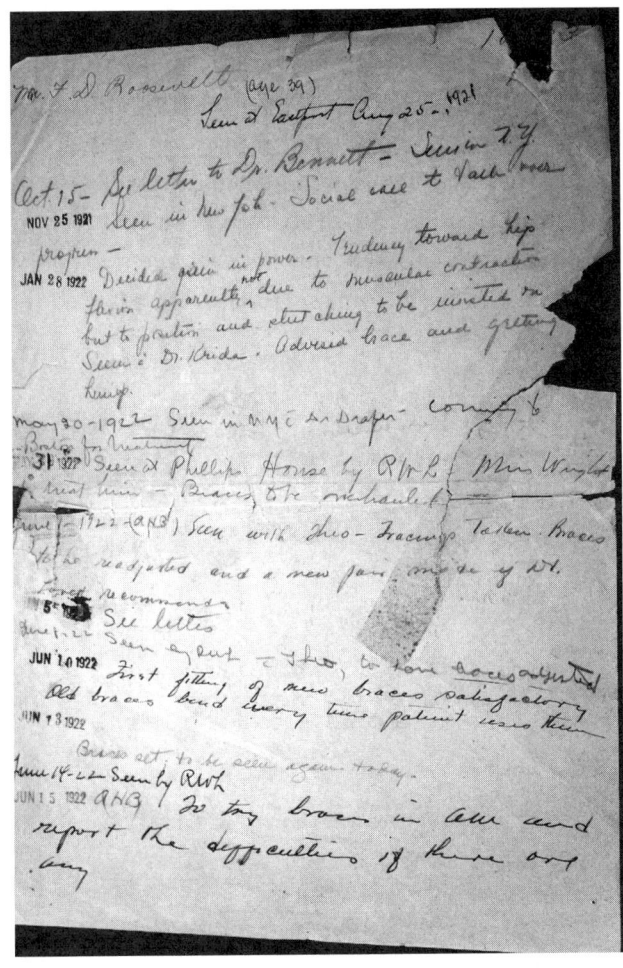

Lovett's handwritten notes about his visits with Franklin D. Roosevelt (1921–1922).

Case of Franklin Delano Roosevelt, 1921-1931 (inclusive), 1921-1925 (bulk). B MS c39. Boston Medical Library in the Francis A. Countway Library of Medicine.

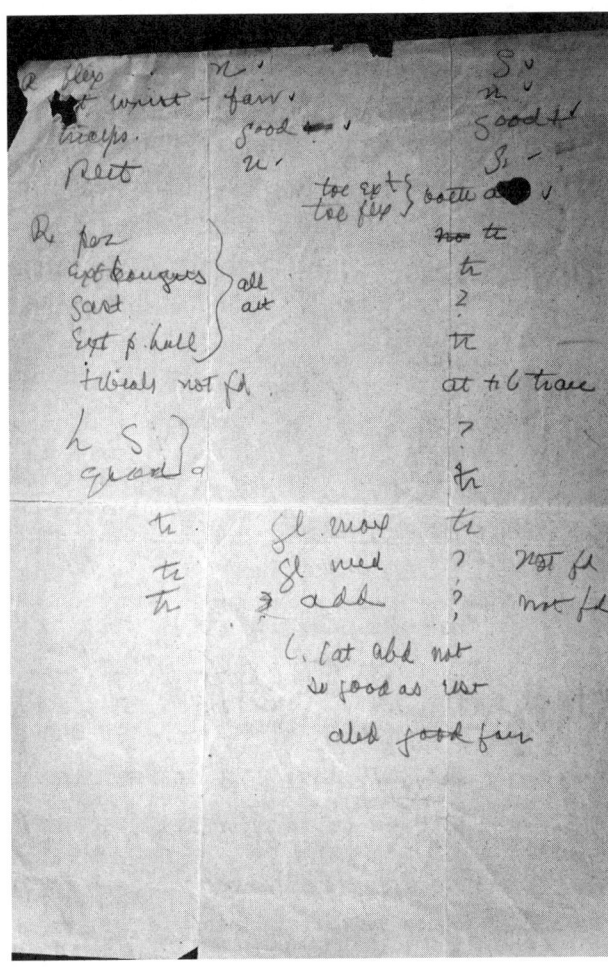

Lovett's handwritten note of his muscle exam of Franklin D. Roosevelt (date unknown).

Case of Franklin Delano Roosevelt, 1921-1931 (inclusive), 1921-1925 (bulk). B MS c39. Boston Medical Library in the Francis A. Countway Library of Medicine.

for months…my experience with it is this—I found that following massage, in early cases…the tenderness increased…giving massage in cases before the tenderness had absolutely disappeared nearly all of them were stirred up by the massage…I have seen massage frequently cause such severe pain that morphia had been required…seen massage keep up the tenderness five or six months in the hands of ignorant chiropractics and similar persons" (Countway Medical Library). In response to Draper's concern about Roosevelt's bladder paralysis, Lovett wrote on September 26, 1921, that "involvement of the bladder is almost always associated with abdominal weakness" (Countway Medical Library).

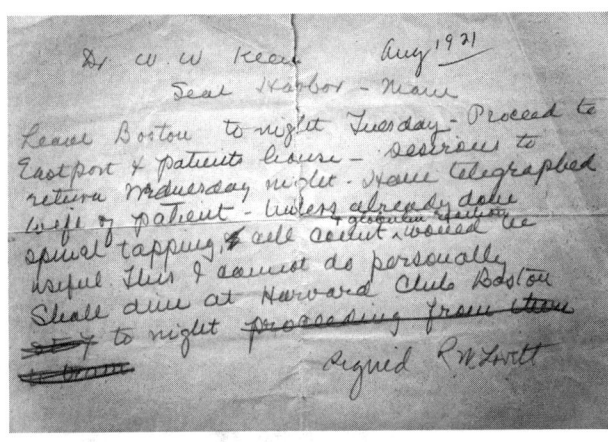

Lovett's handwritten letter to Dr. W. W. Keen (August 1921).

Case of Franklin Delano Roosevelt, 1921-1931 (inclusive), 1921-1925 (bulk). B MS c39. Boston Medical Library in the Francis A. Countway Library of Medicine.

Although Roosevelt's hospital records were destroyed, "Lovett decided that Roosevelt was sufficiently recovered from the acute phase of the disease [that] he allowed him to be moved. In a private railway car, he [Roosevelt] traveled from Eastport, Maine to Grand Central Station in New York City. He was admitted to the Presbyterian Hospital, where he received physical therapy and supportive treatment and remained until October 21" (Z. B. Friedenberg 2009). Before leaving Campobello, Dr. Bennet (who continued to treat Roosevelt) sent a telegram to Lovett on August 31, 1921, stating, "atrophy increasing, power lessening causing patient much anxiety…can you recommend anything to keep up his courage and make him feel the best is being done?" (E. H. Bennet

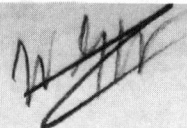

FRANKLIN D. ROOSEVELT
HYDE PARK, DUTCHESS COUNTY
NEW YORK

September 22, 1922.

Dear Dr. Lovett:

Many thanks for your letter which I should have answered long before this, but I am glad to be able to report that I have faithfully followed out the walking and am really getting so that both legs take it quite naturally, and I can stay on my feet for an hour without feeling tired. I think the balance is coming back also, and though I can negotiate stairs if I have a hand rail I cannot get up steps with only the crutches, and I doubt if this feat can be accomplished for a long time.

If it is convenient to you I will come on to Boston by motor getting there about 4 or 5 o'clock on Sunday, September 30th. Will you be good enough to ask them to reserve two room and bath at Philips House, as Miss Rockey will be with me as before. If they have a room on the 3rd floor where I was before it would be nice. If you would rather have me come later let me know.

I hope you had a delightful summer at Newport. Up here on the Hudson River we have had a good deal of rain but literally no really hot weather, and I am in fine condition.

Very sincerely yours,

Franklin D. Roosevelt

Franklin D. Roosevelt's letter to Dr. Lovett in which he describes his progress and asks Lovett to arrange a room for him in the MGH Philips House and visit him. Case of Franklin Delano Roosevelt, 1921–1931 (inclusive), 1921–1925 (bulk). B MS c39. Boston Medical Library in the Francis A. Countway Library of Medicine.

1921). Lovett continued to oversee the care of Roosevelt and answered other letters of concern and requests for advice by Dr. Bennet.

Lovett arranged that Roosevelt's care in New York be led by Dr. George Draper, and he made recommendations to Draper. While in Presbyterian Hospital, Draper sent a letter to Lovett on September 24, 1921. He was "concerned about [Roosevelt's] slow recovery" (G. Draper 1921a), noted Roosevelt's continued pain and severe weakness, atrophy of the spine [muscles], buttocks, posterior deltoid, and right triceps, and twitching of the forearm muscles. Describing Roosevelt's lower extremities as "most distressing…no motion in toe extensors…minimal motion right perinei…cannot extend the feet…little ability to twitch the bellies of the gastrocnemii…little power in the left vastus…both sides [have] similar voluntary twitches of the ham-string muscles" (G. Draper 1921a).

Draper expressed his concern that Roosevelt may not be able to sit because of the weakness of his back muscles and asked that Lovett "devise some kind of support…brace or corset…[but Roosevelt] believes them [upper extremities] to be untouched by the disease…biceps [are] pretty good" (G. Draper 1921a). Stating that Roosevelt "has such courage and ambition…[he] has made up his mind that he is going to go out of the hospital in the course of two or three weeks on crutches" (G. Draper 1921a), Draper asked Lovett to visit Roosevelt in the hospital as soon as he became pain free.

Lovett visited Roosevelt in Presbyterian Hospital on Sunday morning, October 12, 1921. A letter to Lovett from Draper on November 19, 1921, stated: "Roosevelt has been moved to his house…navigates successfully in a wheelchair…[and is] anxious to try crutches" (G. Draper 1921b). Roosevelt moved back to Hyde Park in June. On June

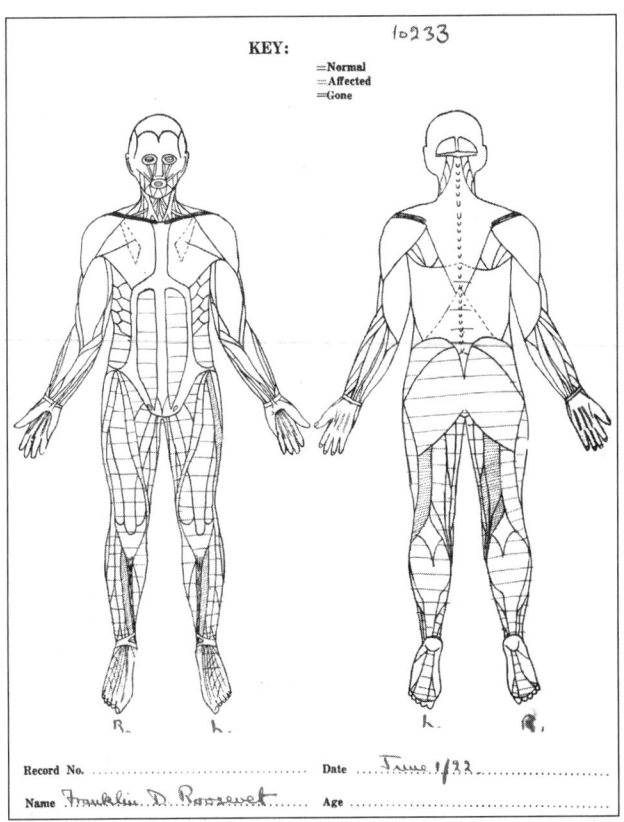

Lovett's diagram of Roosevelt's muscle exam on June 1, 1922.
Case of Franklin Delano Roosevelt, 1921–1931 (inclusive), 1921–1925 (bulk). B MS c39. Boston Medical Library in the Francis A. Countway Library of Medicine.

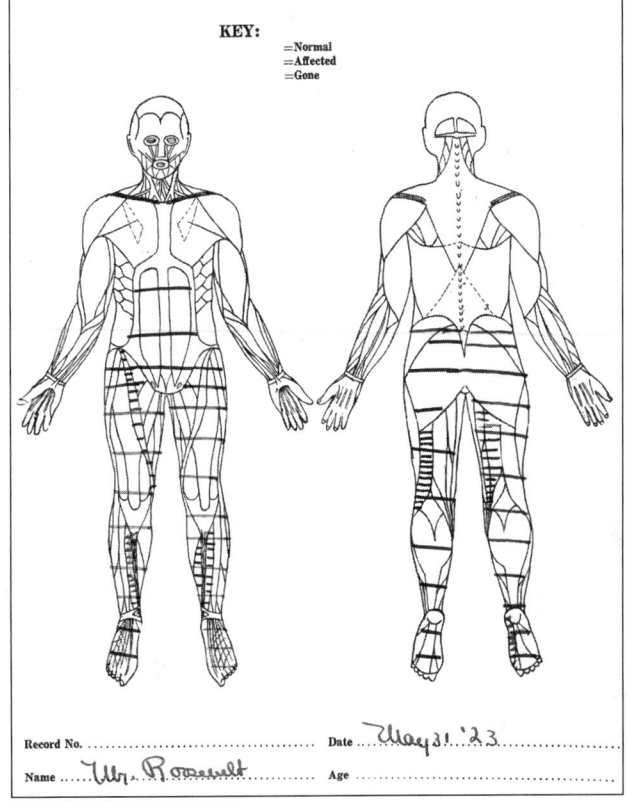

Lovett's diagram of Roosevelt's muscle exam on May 31, 1923.
Case of Franklin Delano Roosevelt, 1921–1931 (inclusive), 1921–1925 (bulk). B MS c39. Boston Medical Library in the Francis A. Countway Library of Medicine.

5, 1922, Roosevelt was admitted to the Philips House at Massachusetts General Hospital (R. W. Lovett 1921e). His braces had been made of soft metal and new, stronger braces were required. Lovett, in a letter to Draper after Roosevelt's discharge, stated that three things helped Roosevelt: (1) walking and activities of daily living education by Wright, (2) new braces made with a stronger metal, and (3) elastic straps to "substitute for hip flexors…hip abduction straps for him to try…with them on he got his legs forward better and handled himself better" (R. W. Lovett 1921f). About one year later at a follow-up exam, Lovett noted that:

> all muscles of the upper extremities were normal. The trunk and abdominal muscles were rated 2 to 3; the pelvic and femoral muscles were 1 to 3; the anterior and posterior tibial muscles were 0; and the right and left gastrocnemius muscles, peroneals, toe flexors and extensors were 2 to 3…This muscle rating remained unchanged throughout the rest of Roosevelt's life. (Z. B. Friedenberg 2009)

Roosevelt had many opinions about how he should be treated, often sharing his thoughts with physicians. In one memorandum to Lovett, he stated that "following my suggestions may prove of value in other cases as they proved useful on a small houseboat in Florida" (R. W. Lovett 1923).

Roosevelt had just returned from vacationing in Florida on a 60-foot boat and was seeking an appointment in Boston with Lovett (May 1923). He had five suggestions for Lovett to consider when treating other patients (F. D. Roosevelt, n.d.):

1) Getting up and down stairs: "I solved by sitting down on the third step from the bottom and by placing my hands on the steps lifting myself up (or down) one step at a time. A handrail on one side only was of great assistance."

2) Narrow passageway: "Extremely difficult to use crutches. I was able to get about without crutches by reaching up to the deck beams above, this gave me enough balance and support to move the legs forward in walking."

3) Getting into a small motor boat (deck 10 feet above water): "I had a section of the side rail cut out and hinged…From [the forward davit] I [was] suspended [on] a plain board…The davit was then swung out and I was lowered into the motor boat…or water [when going swimming]."

4) Exercising the quadriceps muscle: "I found that a small, light, low rocking chair without arms was of great value…I could rock back and forth by using only the knee and the lower leg and foot muscles."

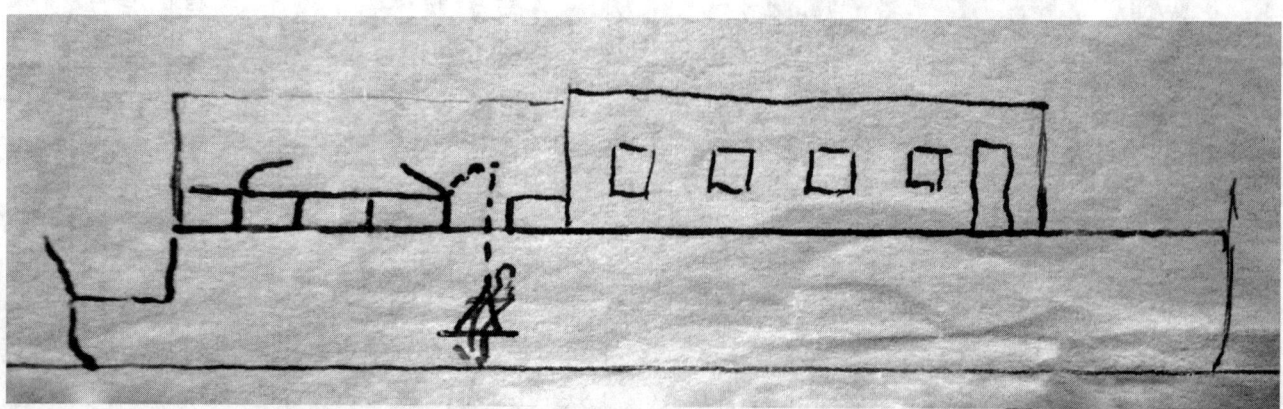

Roosevelt's sketch of the chair lift he designed to enable him to get on and off his yacht. Case of Franklin Delano Roosevelt, 1921–1931 (inclusive), 1921–1925 (bulk). B MS c39. Boston Medical Library in the Francis A. Countway Library of Medicine.

> 5) Fishing: "I managed to catch a number of large fish, some running as high as 40 pounds...I tied a strap around my chest and around the back of the revolving fishing chair."

Roosevelt also tried nonstandard treatments such as high-intensity lights and a "high-pressure atmospheric chamber to increase his oxygen intake" (Z. B. Friedenberg 2009). He studied polio extensively, learning not only the treatment methods of Lovett, but also those of Drs. Goldthwait, Hibbs, McDonald, and those referred to as the Chicago method, the St. Louis method, and others.

But his experiences of swimming and exercises at Warm Springs, Georgia, were his favorite. In "the pool...the water remained at a constant temperature of 88°F and was highly charged with limestone and other salts that provided buoyancy [after] exercising in the water, then exercising out of the water...he tested his muscles and was sure they had gained strength [in the pool]" (Z. B. Friedenberg 2009). At Warm Springs, Roosevelt helped finance the Georgia Warm Springs Foundation, a nonprofit organization to care for the poor. "He taught his patients exercises and examined them for improved muscle function...Roosevelt was known as Doctor" (Z. B. Friedenberg 2009). Roosevelt also recognized the importance of the need for a physician to supervise the patients arriving at Warm Springs. He located a physician six miles away in Manchester, Dr. J. A. Johnson, who "had tremendous interest in the polyo [sic] cases...a live wire" (F. D. Roosevelt 1925). In a letter to Dr. Frank Ober, Roosevelt described the progress of one of Ober's patients, another of Dr. Osgood's, himself, and four other cases, often describing in detail the patient's muscle weaknesses: "All in all, I consider this pool the best after-care treatment for polyo [sic]" (F. D. Roosevelt 1925). In the same letter, Roosevelt asked Ober to allow Dr. Johnson to visit him in Boston for two months of special training, to "work under your office and in the Children's Hospital, studying your methods" (F. D. Roosevelt 1925). Ober agreed.

As the polio program at Warm Springs grew, Roosevelt felt obliged to continue to raise money for the foundation. He wanted:

> a scientific stamp of approval on the project. At the Annual Meeting of the American Orthopaedic Association (AOA) in Atlanta, Georgia, in April 1926, Roosevelt had requested permission from the president of the association, Michael Hoke, to be in the program and address the membership. When this was refused, he then requested that the association form a committee to investigate the work of the Warm Springs Foundation and its rehabilitative successes. Hoke and most members of the executive committee were suspicious...that Roosevelt would use the name of the Association to advertise the virtues of the Foundation and profit from it.
> (Z. B. Friedenberg 2009)

No official committee was appointed by Dr. Hoke. But several prominent members supported Roosevelt, including Robert Osgood, Albert Freiberg, Fred Dickson, George Bennett, and LeRoy Abbott. They formed an ex officio committee chaired by Freiberg, with an orthopaedist and rehabilitation expert (Dr. Leroy W. Hubbard) from New York in charge of reviewing cases sent to Warm Springs over a six-month period. Hoke described these efforts:

> Bob Osgood was very insistent that Mr. Franklin Roosevelt, proprietor of Warm Springs, be given an opportunity to address the Association about Warm Springs in its relation to the treatment of infantile paralysis. Bob thought I was rather hardboiled because I refused to invite him to address the Association. Bob then decided a committee be appointed...to supervise the experiments that Mr. Roosevelt was to carry out. I was just as insistent and did all I could to keep the Executive Committee from making such an appointment.
> (M. Hoke, n.d.)

Dr. Hubbard evaluated 23 patients and reported his findings in December 1926. "No miracles occurred, but the majority of patients made more progress than they would if they had stayed at home" (Z. B. Friedenberg 2009). Dr. Hubbard became surgeon-in-chief and was assisted by Dr. Frank Brostrom who worked two years at Boston's Children's Hospital and Dr. Johnson who held clinics three days each week.

The board of consultants of the Georgia Warm Springs Foundation included Drs. LeRoy Abbott, Fred Warren Bailey, George Bennett, Frank D. Dickson, George Draper, Albert H. Freiberg, Bruce Gill, Ludvig Hektoen, Michael Hoke, Frederick C. Kidner, Arthur T. Legg, Belveridge H. Moore, Frank H. Ober, Robert B. Osgood, John Lincoln Porter, and DeForest Willard. Eventually, Roosevelt even persuaded Dr. Hoke to become the chief surgeon at Warm Springs.

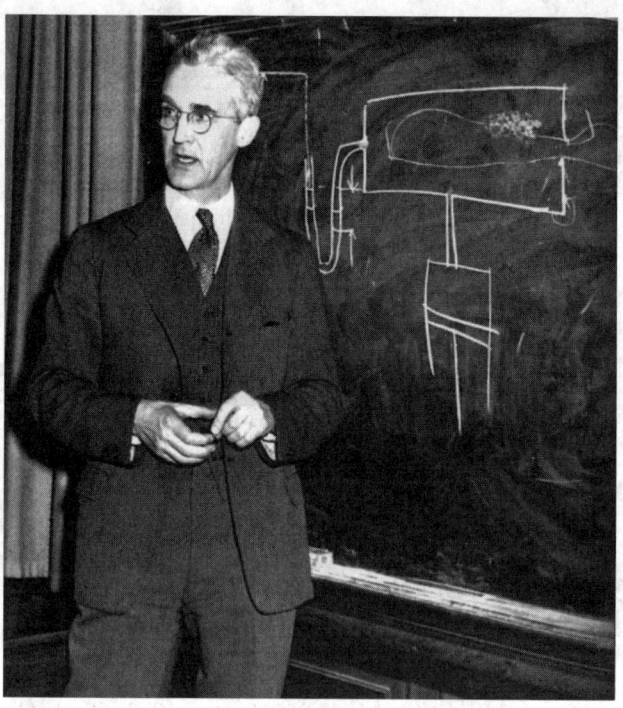

Dr. Philip Drinker, inventor of the iron lung, in 1928.
Images of America. Children's Hospital Boston. Charleston, SC: Arcadia Publishing, 2005. Boston Children's Hospital Archives, Boston, Massachusetts.

EVOLVING ORTHOPAEDIC TREATMENTS FOR POLIO

Orthopaedic treatment—immediately following diagnosis—became essential in a few years following the report of the Vermont epidemic and the publication of Lovett's classic work, as well as his other publications on polio. Diagnostic spinal taps had mixed results; treatment with convalescent serum had varying degrees of success. Lovett's regimen for preventing contractures—comprising rest, the avoidance of therapeutics, and warm salt baths —was commonly followed. However, Peltier (1993) described Lovett's approach as one in which the physician was fairly uninvolved. In 1916, Boston Children's Hospital had held polio clinics three times a week at 300 Longwood Avenue. After Lovett's death in 1924, orthopaedic surgeons began treating polio patients with muscle training after an initial period of rest for six to eight weeks. Following another six to eight weeks, any residual contractures were addressed by manipulation, soft tissue (tendon, fascia, capsule) releases, and tendon transfers; any frail or unstable joints were stabilized as well. By the 1930s, many clinicians also supplemented Lovett's method for preventing contractures with immobilization in plaster casts, which relieved patients' pain but precluded evaluation and caused muscles to atrophy.

As noted by Jones (1933), orthopaedic surgery had developed only through "repeated trial and error." Another significant contribution to the treatment of poliomyelitis occurred at Boston Children's Hospital in 1928, four years after the death of Dr. Lovett. Dr. Philip Drinker, at the Harvard School of Public Health, invented a mechanical respirator or iron lung, which initially was commonly used by only a single patient. Because of the often-sudden increase in patients, Dr. James L. Wilson (also at Boston Children's Hospital) created a large iron lung that could accommodate up to four beds, allowing clinicians to more easily care for multiple patients simultaneously. In 1928, President Edsall requested that each medical department describe their most important research during the past 20 years (Countway Medical Library). Dr. Edward H. Churchill responded from the Department of Surgery: "I do not feel that I have any investigative work to report which is important enough to be included in such a history." Dr. Robert Osgood, from the Department of Orthopaedic Surgery, responded, "I should list three." He then briefly mentioned the significant work of Dr. Legg, followed by that of Lovett, and third the research by Dr. Joseph Freiberg on experimental septic arthritis. When describing Lovett's research, he wrote: "Dr. Lovett's research into the physiotherapeutic treatment of infantile paralysis by means of rest and special training exercises…resulted in the restoration of very much larger amounts of function than by older method[s] of immediate attempt to regain function in deranged nerve muscle mechanism…[and] the elaboration of muscle function tests" (Countway Medical Library).

Boston Children's Hospital treated the orthopaedic problems of polio victims until the late 1960s. They were initially led by Lovett as the first director of the Infantile Paralysis Clinic (1916–1920); he was followed by Dr. Arthur T. Legg (1921–1939) and finally by Dr. William T. Green (1940–1960). In 1946, the Harvard Commission stopped providing care for patients with polio; Boston Children's Hospital took over and continued that care until there was no longer a need for it.

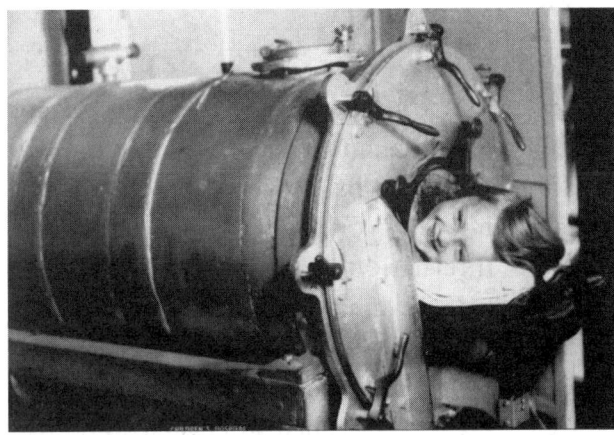

Iron lung respirator in the early 1930s.

Images of America. Children's Hospital Boston. Charleston, SC: Arcadia Publishing, 2005. Boston Children's Hospital Archives, Boston, Massachusetts.

SCOLIOSIS

Lovett also continued writing about lateral curvature of the spine throughout his career. In 1922, toward the end of his career, he provided a detailed account of the then current understanding of the pathophysiology and treatment of scoliosis in his monograph "Lateral Curvature of the Spine and Round Shoulders." It wasn't until 1924—the same year that he died—in a paper coauthored by Dr. A. H. Brewster, that Lovett reported on the outcomes of treatment of scoliosis using x-rays. In this paper, they also reported a new method of

Title page of Lovett's book, *Lateral Curvature of the Spine and Round Shoulders* (1922). Francis A. Countway Library of Medicine.

treatment: the use of a turnbuckle cast. (See chapter 23.) Made in the same fashion as the removable jacket described above, the turnbuckle jacket was made by "dividing [it] transversely at the level of the apex of the lateral curve and fastened together by a garden-gate hinge at the side of the trunk, which allows the jacket to be opened on that as an axis. On the other side a turnbuckle connects the two segments, fastened to the jacket by iron boxes" (R. W. Lovett and A. H. Brewster 1924). This allowed three-point pressure: "one at the maximum of the curve; two and three, as near both ends of the curve as possible" (R. W. Lovett and A. H. Brewster 1924). However, "the cure of scoliosis had to be handed down to future generations of orthopaedic surgeons…Lovett couldn't disprove Phelps's claim…'I have yet to see [by 1900] the first case of lateral curvature of the spine, in which bone changes had taken place, cured by any plan of treatment known to the scientific world'" (L. Mayer 1950).

LEGACY

Dr. Robert Lovett retired from his professorship in 1922 at age 63 with his health impaired by atherosclerotic heart disease. He became ill on one of his many trips to England. He was planning to visit his great friend, Sir Robert Jones. Seriously ill with pericarditis, he died in Sir Jones's home on July 2, 1924. Lovett left behind a wife and one daughter. He had married Elizabeth Moorfield Storey of Boston on October 5, 1895.

He had been active in organized medicine, both in Massachusetts and nationally (*BMSJ* 1924). In addition to the many important leadership positions he held (already listed in this chapter), Lovett was surgeon-in-chief to the Massachusetts Hospital School in Canton and the Peabody Home for Crippled Children. **Box 16.1** provides a partial list of his many other memberships. He was also elected into membership of the British, Italian, German Orthopaedic Associations, and the International Surgical Society. In 1920, Lovett was honored by the University of Cincinnati with an Honorary Degree of Doctor of Science.

Box 16.1. Lovett's Professional and Society Memberships

> Lovett was a member of the following organizations and clubs:
>
> - Advisory Board on Orthopedics of the United States Army
> - Boston Orthopedic Club
> - Puritan Club
> - Tavern Club
> - Somerset and Harvard Clubs
> - University Club of New York
> - Cosmos Club of Washington
>
> He also was active in other groups:
>
> - collaborating on the formation of the Orthopedic Section of the American Medical Association
> - acting as councilor of the Massachusetts Medical Society
> - member of the editorial staff of the *Boston Medical and Surgical Journal*
> - the first secretary of the Harvard Medical Alumni Association

In 1913, he had written to Professor Hans Spitzer, of Vienna, and Professor Vittorio Putti, of Bologna, with a proposal for a new international orthopaedic organization called SICOT (Société Internationale de Chirurgie Orthopédique et de Traumatologie). Lovett also suggested a new review journal, the *International Journal of Orthopaedic Surgery*, as a publication of SICOT. World War I had stopped any progress to forming this new organization despite support in the United States and Europe. After the war, in 1923, Putti and Sir Robert Jones met with Lovett in Boston to develop plans for the new international organization. Sir Robert Jones became the first president of SICOT when it eventually formed in 1929.

Sir Jones wrote the following tribute to Dr. Lovett (*BMSJ* 1924):

> The death of Professor R. W. Lovett will be deeply felt by our profession the world over. He sailed for this country with his family, intending to enjoy a much needed rest; he arrived in Liverpool desperately ill, and died in four days. No words can convey the pathos and tragedy of so overwhelming a catastrophe. He represented the highest ideals of our art, and brought to bear upon it the rich powers of a cultured mind. An indefatigable worker, a keen and critical observer, he sought and paid unswerving fidelity to truth. His thoughts were expressed in clear, incisive English—always the product of analytical study and logical acumen.
>
> He has enriched the literature of orthopaedic surgery by many classical contributions, and his work on scoliosis and infantile paralysis will have lasting value. As professor of orthopaedic surgery at Harvard he showed his great gifts in organization and teaching, and it was always an inspiration to accompany him round his wards. His demonstrations were models of lucid and judicious statement; whether in complete agreement with him or not, one never found his point of view obscure. He was a great teacher who, by the combination of character and ability secured the affection and respect of the student, and he was one of a small band of surgeons who formed a school of disciples. His reputation was international, and almost at any time distinguished foreign surgeons could be met at his hospitable board. Although 64 years of age, his mind was actively productive to the end and showed not the slightest trace of deterioration—even on his death-bed he wished to explain a new solution to the problem of scoliosis. It may be truly said of him that he died in harness.
>
> How difficult it is for a close friend and intimate colleague to strike a personal note under the bewilderment of so recent a remembrance and bereavement! I cannot attempt it. He had a heart of priceless gold, only fully revealed to those he loved. His end was peaceful, surrounded by his family in a country which he liked best next to his own, and all that skill and affection could suggest was done by his physicians. Our thoughts will be with his wife, who nursed him with tender devotion in the home of a friend.

After Lovett's death, money was "collected for an endowment for the medical school as a memorial for Dr. Lovett. Dr. Lovett's work was entirely in the medical school and had nothing to do with the school of public health" (D. L. Edsall 1931). So wrote Dean Edsall in a letter to Dr. C. K. Drinker, chair of the Lovett Fund Committee, in a response to a request to transfer the funds to the school of public health. A committee to oversee the use of the fund had been formed by Dean Edsall in December 1926. Dr. Drinker chaired the committee, and the two other members included Dr. Ober, who represented orthopaedic interests,

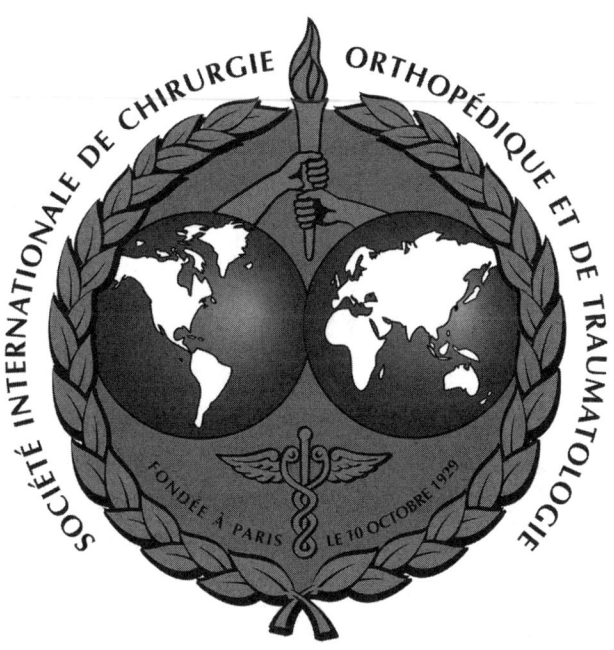

Logo of SICOT. Courtesy of SICOT.

and W. Lloyd Aycock, who represented preventive medicine (poliomyelitis).

Initially the fund was used to support research on arthritis by Dr. Walter Bauer at MGH. In a letter to Dr. Ober in 1929, Dr. Osgood acknowledged the use of the Lovett Fund to support arthritis research. Under Dr. Bauer's leadership, the arthritis research program at the MGH grew and was very productive. Dr. Bauer named his research unit the Robert W. Lovett Memorial Unit for the Study of Crippling Diseases. He served as director from 1929 to 1958. In 1951, he was named the chief of the medical services at MGH. An audit of the fund (June 30, 1930) sent to Dr. Ober stated that the Robert W. Lovett Fund had a value of $167,038.22 ($2,458,802.60 in 2019 dollars).

Dr. Ober was asked to chair the Lovett Fund Committee by Dean Edsall in 1931. In a letter to Mr. Archie S. Woods (vice president of the John and Mary R. Markle Foundation), dated August 24, 1936, Dr. Drinker wrote: "The Robert W. Lovett Memorial Fund was given to the Medical School some years ago and the University authorities placed the fund under the nominal direction of myself, Dr. Frank Ober and Dr. W. Lloyd Aycock... We reported to the authorities that we believed the total income from the fund...should be devoted to study upon arthritis" (C. K. Drinker 1936).

In 1999, after inactivity for several years, the Lovett Memorial Fund was activated by the dean as an endowed professorship in orthopaedics for Dr. Christopher Evans (first incumbent), an internationally known arthritis and cartilage investigator who led the first clinical trial on the use of gene therapy to treat rheumatoid arthritis. He was recruited by myself, then Partners Chairman of Orthopaedic Surgery, from the University of Pittsburgh. His new laboratory was in the Department of Orthopaedic Surgery at the Brigham and Women's Hospital.

CHAPTER 17

James W. Sever
Medical Director of the Industrial School for Crippled and Deformed Children

James Warren Sever was born in Kingston, Massachusetts, on July 4, 1878. Soon after, the family moved to Cambridge, where his father, Charles W. Sever, headed University Book Store and was "well-known to all Harvard men" (*Cambridge Chronicle* 1923); he was also president of Cambridge Savings Bank. James's mother, Mary Caroline (Webber) Sever, was a first cousin of Dr. Edward H. Bradford. Charles and Mary had five children. The Sever family lived on Friable Place in a scholarly, upper-class neighborhood just off Harvard Square, not far from the Mallinckrodt Chemistry Laboratory. Charles Sever's jobs were nearby and James received an early education at the Browne & Nichols School (then located on Garden Street). After high school, he immediately entered Harvard Medical School, graduating in 1901 at age 23. Sever was greatly influenced to practice orthopaedics by his second cousin Bradford.

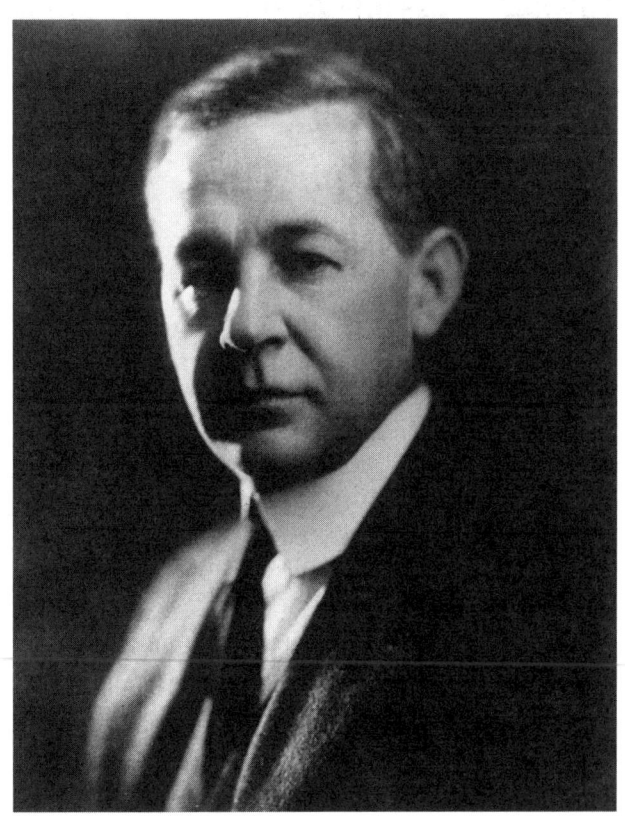

James W. Sever. MGH HCORP Archives.

EARLY CAREER AND RESEARCH

After completing an internship at Children's Hospital in 1901, Sever became a family doctor in Plymouth, Massachusetts, where his ancestor, William Bradford, had been the second governor of the Plymouth Bay Colony: "There he used a horse, Nancy, and shay [carriage] to get from one oil-lit home to another on the hill above Massachusetts

Physician Snapshot

James W. Sever
BORN: 1878
DIED: 1964
SIGNIFICANT CONTRIBUTIONS: Developed a surgical treatment for obstetrical paralysis; described calcaneal apophysitis or Sever's disease; codeveloped the Lovett-Sever method for treating scoliosis

83

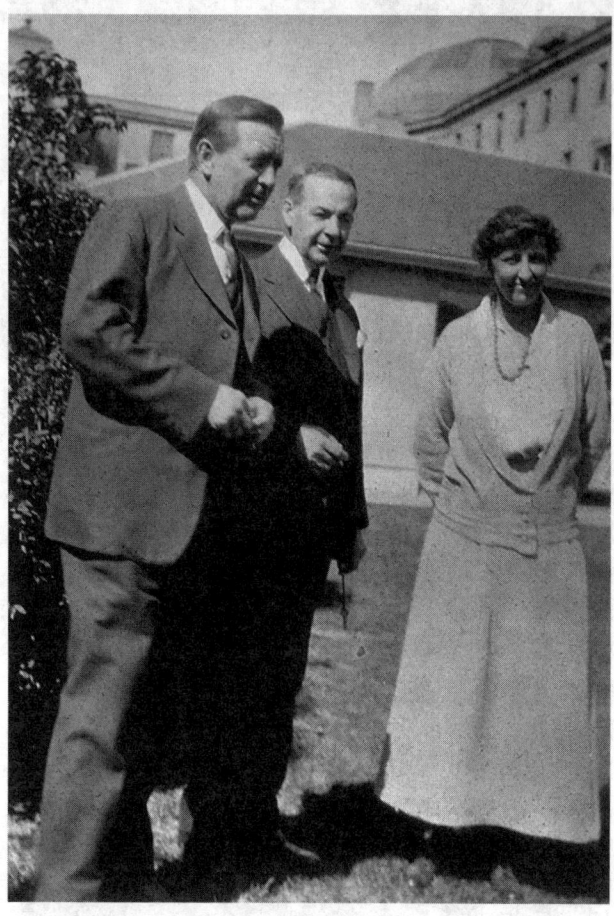

Photo of Drs. Arthur Legg (left) and James Sever (center). MGH HCORP Archives.

Bay and the country around" (Children's Hospital Archives [Annual Report 1963]). As a house officer at Children's Hospital, he would travel to the Children's Convalescent Home in Wellesley to change patients' dressings. The home was opposite the Town Hall and Poor Farm, where the Wellesley Country Club is currently located.

In 1906, he received his first appointment, as a junior assistant orthopaedic surgeon, at Children's Hospital, where he remained as a member of the orthopaedic staff for more than 40 years as assistant orthopaedic surgeon. (There are no further details available on the specifics of his later promotions.) During that time, he was also on staff at five other hospitals: Boston City Hospital, Mt. Auburn Hospital, Waltham Hospital, Quincy Hospital (all in the Boston area), and York Hospital in York, Maine. Sever was a prolific writer throughout his career, and he published his first paper in 1909, which was read at the Annual Meeting of the American Orthopaedic Association (1908). It was titled "Acetone: Its Occurrence in Orthopedic and Surgical Care." He would eventually concentrate his study on scoliosis, calcaneal apophysitis, obstetrical paralysis, and fractures, but he also wrote five papers on infection; three on tuberculosis of the knee, spine, and ankle; one on pneumococcal arthritis in the hip, knee, and shoulder; and one on epiphyseal changes after tuberculosis, syphilis, and osteomyelitis. After observing wide variation in white blood cell counts in healthy children, he also—much later in his career—penned a letter to the editor raising concern about using that cell count as an indication for surgery.

Scoliosis

As junior assistant surgeon at Children's Hospital, Sever worked four half days a week in the scoliosis clinic, which had been in operation since 1894 and was "under the direction of the senior out-patient surgeon…assisted by one of the junior assistant surgeons, who does the actual work of the clinic and sees all of the cases at regular intervals of not more than two weeks" (J. W. Sever 1910b). In 1910, he published a report of his experience treating those patients with scoliosis. At the initial visit, photographs (with the camera 70 inches from the patient) and x-rays were obtained under standardized conditions. At that time, other surgeons—including Walter Truslow, a surgeon from Brooklyn, New York, who published widely about scoliosis—were critical of the value of photographs. No accepted measurements were available for the curves on x-rays, though Bradford had been attempting to develop a method of obtaining such measurements. Sever, in his discussion of a 1913 paper by Dr. Z. B. Adams, emphasized the need for such measurements: "We are going through an experience meeting and talking about beliefs, and not facts. We are not keeping a sharp line of demarcation between what we think are facts and

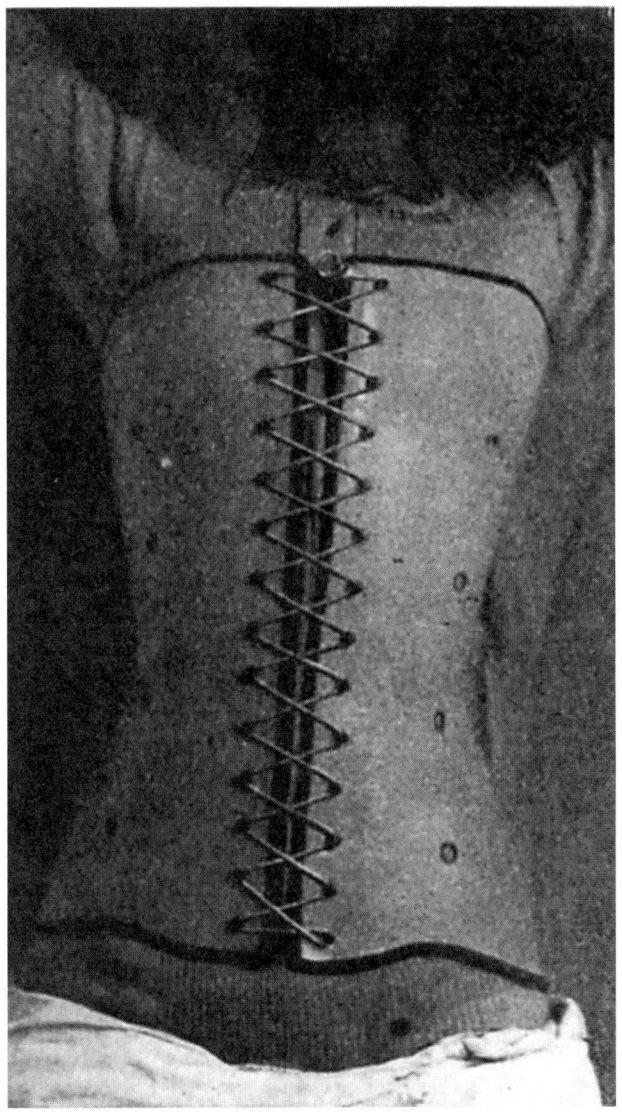 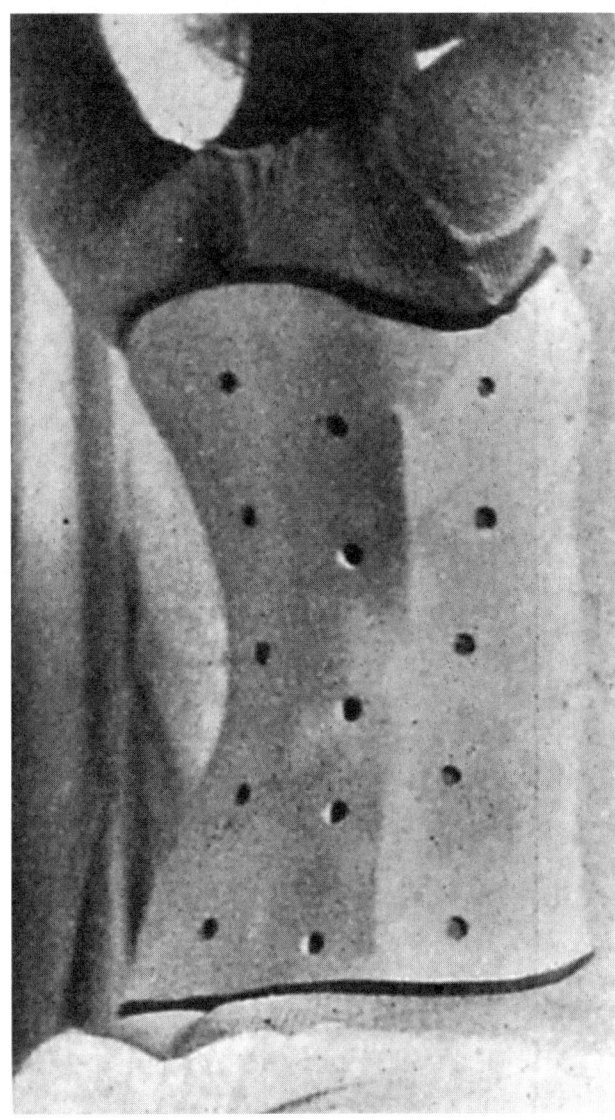

Celluloid jackets used by Sever and Lovett. *Handbuch der Orthopaedischen Chirurgie*, ed. Georg Joachimstahl. Berlin: Gustav Fischer Verlag. Francis A. Countway Library of Medicine/Internet Archive.

what we know are beliefs…I should like to suggest that we have a symposium next year on the same subject. Then let the men who have methods, such as Freiberg, Forbes, Abbott, Cook, and others, use them from now until that time, so as to be able to report to us next year facts, and not beliefs" (Sever 1913). During his discussion at the actual meeting, applause from the audience followed his remarks.

At the time, at Children's Hospital, patients with scoliosis were divided into three classes. Class I comprised cases of either functional scoliosis, which was treated with exercises (30 minutes to 1 hour, four times weekly), or, in patients with round shoulders who did not respond to exercises, a plaster jacket which the patient wore for 6 to 12 weeks. Class II represented structural scoliosis, which was treated with exercises or, in the case of moderate deformity, a patient wore a removable jacket "night and day, and removed [it] only for exercises, which are given for an hour daily…to increase…flexibility and…to develop holding power" (Lovett and Sever 1912). Class III included severe fixed curves that were treated with a permanent jacket, which the patient wore for one to two years. Such corrective permanent jackets were made of plaster and applied while the patient stood with the pelvis held with leather straps and the head held in a sling, and they were changed every two to three months.

Sever and others at Children's Hospital used two kinds of removable jackets:

> One is made of rather heavy leather, fitted wet over the corrected plaster torso [the mold made from a plaster jacket removed from the patient and corrected by shaving or skiving the mold over the prominent area to build in correction with the final jacket] and when dry is saturated with a solution of barbary [sic] wax...this soon dries and makes a hard and durable jacket [and] require[s] about ten days to two weeks to make. The other type is the so-called leather celluloid jacket, made of light weight leather, fitted to the torso as before and lined with several layers of celluloid...which is painted over several layers of gauze on the inside of the jacket. These jackets are more efficient when fitted with steel strips...are lighter than those made of Barbary wax...[and are] perforated for...ventilation. (J. W. Sever 1910b)

The jacket was "furnished with straps and buckles and shoulder pads" (Lovett and Sever 1912). These jackets were the precursors to the celastic jackets residents made during my training at Children's Hospital about 50 years later.

Lovett and Sever reported better results when using nonremovable (permanent) plaster jackets rather than removable plaster jackets to treat patients with a structural scoliosis. They made windows in the permanent jackets on the concave side of the deformity, which enabled them to increase the amount of padding on the convex side in an attempt to decrease the deformity. Other orthopaedists preferred to continually decrease the deformity by frequently changing the jacket.

Sever used additional apparatus to treat scoliosis, including Lovett's stretching board and Adams's machine. The stretching board allowed:

> correction of the lateral curve...by pressure on the spine through the medium of the ribs and... head traction...by having the patient lie prone. The corrective force[s] correct the rotation and...the side deviation...The patient lies face downward...on a board three feet wide by four feet long...[For] a right dorsal curve, a broad canvas strap is passed around the left upper thorax...and fastened to a cleat on the right side of the board...a point of pressure to the left... at the level of the axilla. A broad canvas strap is then passed around the pelvis...and is fastened to a cleat at the right side of the board...a point of pressure to the left at the level of the pelvis. A broad canvas strip is then passed around the thorax at the level of the greatest point of the curve...its upper end is fastened to a cleat at the left side of the board. Its lower end is fastened...into a compound pulley attached to a cleat at the left side of the board. By means of this pulley any reasonable degree of force may be exerted against the right side of the thorax, pulling it to the left, and at the same time... reduce the rotation...Head traction is applied in combination with this. Structural cases are treated with this apparatus from fifteen to twenty minutes daily. Dr. Lovett's board does not use head traction, but is an addition made by the writer [Sever]. (J. W. Sever 1910b)

Z. B. Adams at Children's Hospital devised Adam's machine, which was similar to Lovett's board except that the canvas straps were replaced with three circular rods supported by a gas pipe frame. Two pressure rods on each circular rod were applied directly to the trunk deformity allowing the spine to be derotated by moving each circular rod.

Sever (1910b) stated that he devised pelvic machines that were "used to fix the pelvis during exercises...these machines are made of gas pipe and are screwed to the floor. They consist of an upright made in two pieces, one sliding within the other, on top of which is a horizontal arm...to which is

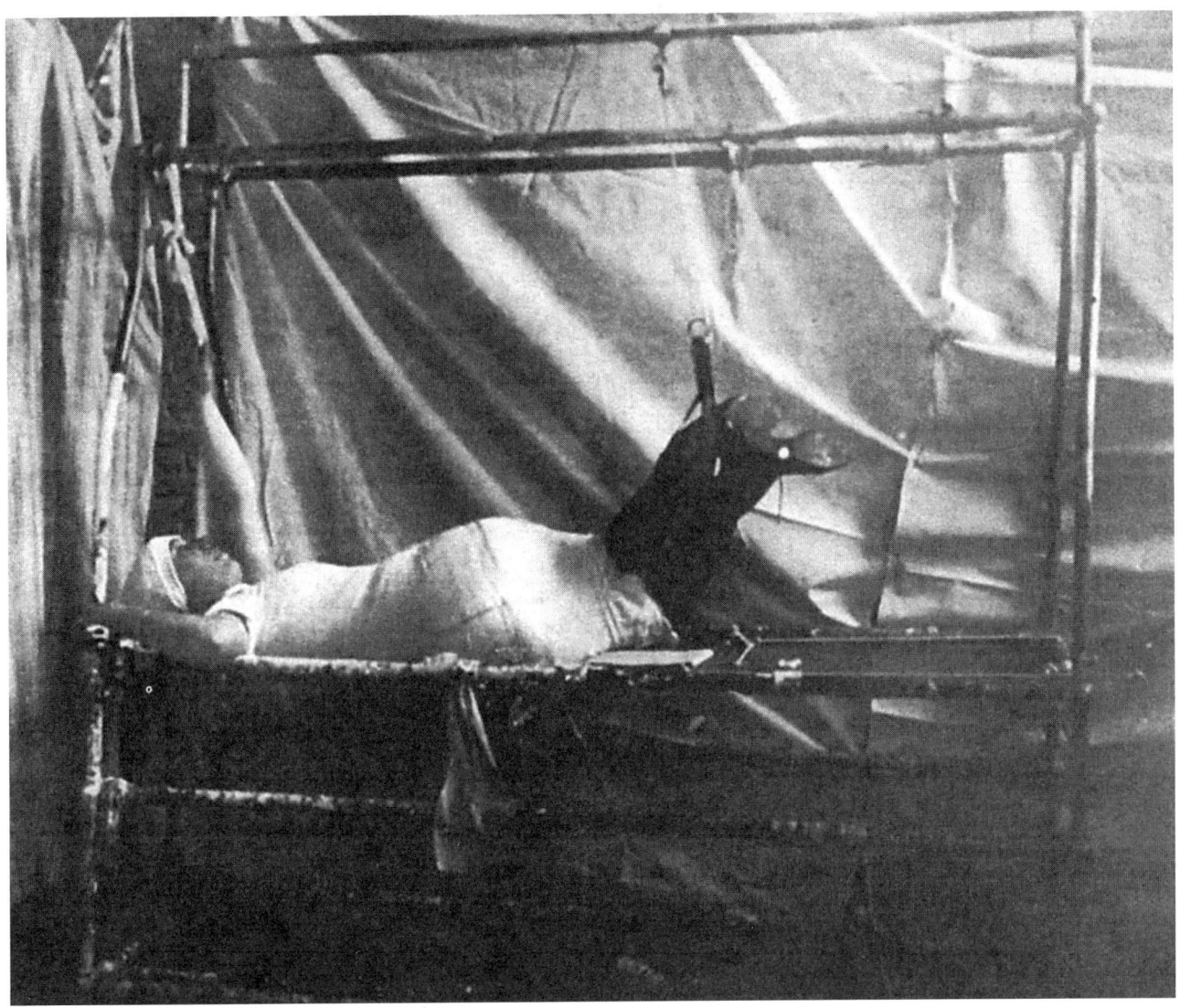

Forbes method of correction of a scoliosis and application of a body cast. A. Klein, "Subsequent Report on the Treatment of Structural Scoliosis at the MGH," *Journal of Bone and Joint Surgery* 1924; 6: 864.

fastened two sliding arms…to grasp a pelvis of any width. These arms are connected by a leather strap which passes firmly about the pelvis and holds the patient firmly."

In 1913, the American Orthopaedic Association formed a committee—Albert H. Freiberg, David Silver, and Robert B. Osgood—to evaluate three newer methods for treating structural scoliosis. Sever demonstrated for the committee what he called the Lovett-Sever method, in which he used an apparatus to apply pressure to the spinal deformity and rotate the spine with straps. This was an "intermediate between the older procedures by corrective jackets and the newer ones involving other theories of correction" (*American Journal of Orthopedic Surgery* 1914), and presented six cases of its application.

A. Mackenzie Forbes, from Montreal, demonstrated the Forbes method, in which corrective jackets were applied by rotating the arms to achieve flexion and rotation of the spine. E. G. Abbott, of Portland, Maine, applied corrective jackets while the spine was flexed and rotated, but pads were placed on the convex side of the chest to the anterolateral side of the chest below the shoulder.

The committee graded each of the three presentations, concluding that Abbot's method could overcorrect the deformity and achieves "better results in his [Abbot's] own hands than in others," that Forbes's method improved rotation in some cases but that correction was not maintained, and that "the method of Lovett and Sever shows no decided gain over older methods" (*American Journal of Orthopedic Surgery* 1914). With all three methods, the committee did not see "complete correction...at any stage, while in several, relapse has followed the removal of the retentive jackets" (*American Journal of Orthopedic Surgery* 1914). Each physician likely continued to use his own method, and newer ones evolved over time.

Calcaneal Apophysitis (Sever's Disease)

Sever became well-known for his study of calcaneal apophysitis, attaching his name to it so that it is now commonly referred to as Sever's disease, Sever's phenomenon, or Sever's syndrome (see **Case 17.1**). Sever originally described this condition in five cases in 1912, concluding that:

1. Apophysitis of the os calcis is not an unusual condition.
2. It may occur from muscle strain in rapidly growing children.
3. It may occur less frequently from direct trauma, but presents then the same clinical picture.
4. It never occurs after puberty.
5. The treatment is rest and protection.
6. The cure in all cases may be arrived at eventually. (J. W. Sever 1912b)

The original description he provided—first published in his initial article and then repeated almost verbatim in each of his three books—follows:

There is a painful condition of the heel often called to one's attention, which always occurs

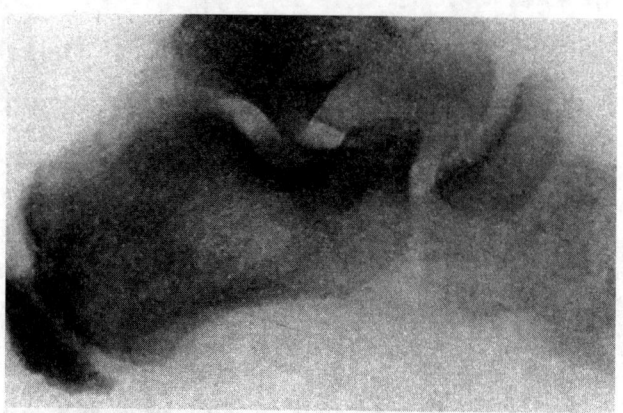

X-ray appearance of calcaneal apophysitis or Sever's disease.
J. W. Sever, "Apophysitis of the Os Calcis," *New York Medical Journal* 1912; 95: 1026.

in children, generally those who are overweight for their years, who are physically active and have strong muscles.

The picture is somewhat as follows: the child is usually seen on account of a slight persistent limp, with a marked disinclination to complete the full step in walking. There is also tenderness complained of about the posterior aspect of the heel, low down, which has persisted for several weeks or months without change. The child has usually worn a low shoe or sandal, with either a spring heel or none. There may or may not be a history of injury, but the child is generally overweight for its years, has been very active, and is strong physically. There also may be a slight amount of pronation of the foot. That the condition may also be secondary to undue shoe pressure on the heel from a tight or too close fitting counter, I believe, has not been determined.

An examination shows a moderately tender area on pressure over the posterior portion of the os calcis, deeply situated, and localized in front of the tendo achillis [*sic*] on either side. There is invariably moderate porky thickening about the whole posterior portion of the os calcis, with some tenderness, and with partial obliteration of the hollows on either side of the tendo achillis. The motions of the foot are all slightly limited, especially in full dorsal flexion, and any movement which tends to put a strain on the tendo achillis causes pain.

There is pain and tenderness on weight bearing when the heel is placed on the floor, but less so when walking on the toes with the heels elevated.

The disease resembles somewhat the condition of achillobursitis, an inflammation of the bursa between the tendo achillis and the os calcis, but is much more extensive and deep seated. One should also consider before making a diagnosis the condition of tenosynovitis of the tendo achillis, and calcaneal spurs on the under surface of the os calcis. These spurs, however, rarely if ever appear so early in life. Tenosynovitis is easily distinguished by the presence of the tendon crepitus and pain referred to the tendon itself on motion. There is also the condition where the bursa between the tendo achillis and the skin of the heel is irritated from shoe pressure, which has to be differentiated.

The x-ray will usually clear up the question at once, but even without this the condition is fairly characteristic. The x-ray findings are of interest, and are practically constant whenever the ossification of the epiphysis is sufficiently developed to show the characteristic changes… There is always to be seen in comparing the plates of the two feet, an enlargement of the epiphysis itself on the affected side, both in thickness in the anteroposterior plane, and also in length from top to bottom. There is also considerable cloudiness along the epiphyseal line between the epiphysis and the os calcis, suggesting a deposit of new bone, and often with a partial obliteration of this epiphyseal line. These findings are typical and constant, and never occur in any other condition. Often the condition suggests a slipping of the epiphysis, with the customary inflammatory reaction following such a condition, or epiphysitis. Similar conditions existing in the tibial tubercle have been spoken of as Osgood-Schlatter's disease.

In differentiating this condition from tuberculosis, it must be remembered that tuberculosis generally attacks the anterior portion of the os calcis, does not lead to bone hypertrophy, and is usually unilateral. (J. W. Sever 1912)

Sever had correctly identified the most common condition of heel pain in children: an inflammation of the calcaneal apophysis most likely caused by repetitive trauma.

Case 17.1. Calcaneal Apophysitis

> "Girl, aged seven years, weight seventy-two pounds. Had had trouble with both heels for six months. No cause known. Pain in heels and disinclination to walk, especially on first getting up in the morning. Heels, tender and limp. Some swelling about posterior portion of os calcis. Child well over weight for years and very active. She was relieved of this condition for a year by raising the heels of her shoes, removing the counters from them, and giving her an inside pad of sponge rubber. A year later, after a period of considerable activity, the left heel began to trouble her. At this time the examination showed considerable thickening about the region of the epiphysis of the os calcis, and the epiphysitis was demonstrated by an xray [sic] picture. Weight then eighty pounds.
>
> "The treatment at this time was as follows: A Thomas heel was applied with the whole heel of the shoe raised. Hot and cold soaking was ordered for a week, and later the heel was strapped with adhesive plaster, and rubber heels were ordered for the shoes. The recovery was then rapid under this protective regime."
>
> (James Warren Sever 1912b)

Obstetrical Paralysis

Sever wrote about numerous elements of orthopaedic surgery, but according to Green, his work on the causes and treatment of obstetrical paralysis was his "most outstanding" (Countway Medical

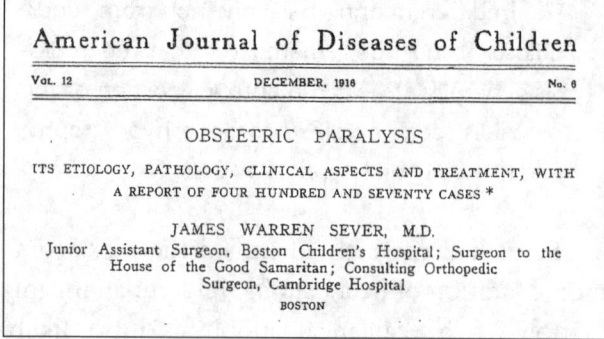

Title of Sever's article reviewing his experience treating 470 cases of obstetric paralysis. *American Journal of Diseases of Children*, 1916; 12: 541.

Title of Sever's article in which he argued that obstetrical palsies were an orthopaedic problem. *American Journal of Orthopedic Surgery*, 1916; 14: 456.

Library). Although he became well-known early on for his study of calcaneal apophysitis, his name also became attached to the procedure he developed for releasing muscles in obstetrical palsy. He developed the shoulder contracture release, or Sever procedure, which is still used today (but is now combined with tendon transfers, as described by James B. L'Episcopo, and is called the Sever-L'Episcopo procedure). In 1916, Sever published three papers on obstetrical paralysis in which he reviewed the etiology and pathology of, and his personal experiences treating, 471 cases, often repeating the data. The first was coauthored by the neurologist John Jenks Thomas, who had previously published a report of two cases of paralysis with rare involvement of only the lower cords of the plexus (Klumpke paralysis). Thomas had also reported on the importance of early massage and exercises that had been developed and used by clinicians in the Children's Hospital neurology department for more than 20 years. They published their abstract in May and the full article in October. Sever published two additional articles on these cases as sole author. In one of these—published in August—he discussed the role of the orthopaedist in treatment, and he stated that the condition was an orthopaedic problem. The *American Journal of Orthopedic Surgery* published it because "the Orthopedist has not taken a great deal of interest in this subject…[because] the possibilities of treatment are not generally known…and to emphasize the importance of orthopedic treatment" (J. W. Sever 1916c). In the other—published in December—he completed a major review of the cases and detailed the mechanism of injury to the brachial plexus during the birth process from his dissections in Nichol's lab at HMS.

Early in his career at Children's Hospital, Sever also worked in Harvard Medical School's Laboratory of Surgical Pathology, whose director then was Dr. Edward H. Nichols. There Sever focused his research on brachial plexus injuries during birth. He wrote:

> By numerous dissections on infantile cadavers, [I have] shown that traction and forcible separation of the head and shoulder puts the upper cords, the fifth and sixth cervical roots of the brachial plexus, under dangerous tension…This tension is so great that the two upper cords stand out like violin strings. Any sudden force applied with the head bent to the side and the shoulder held would without question injure these cords…forcible abduction and elevation of the arm and shoulder put the lower cords of the plexus, the eighth cervical and first thoracic on a stretch, and when much force is applied it may well lead to a tear rupture or other injury to these segments. This condition is seen in breech cases,

with arm extended…with the shoulder held and the head carried to one side…the suprascapular nerve always snapped first…with considerable force the fifth and sixth cervical nerves could not be completely torn across at Erb's point, but frayed…in some cases there could be produced an avulsion from the spinal cord of the fifth and sixth cervical roots…In no case, even with all the force I could apply with my hands, could I rupture the joint capsule, or even separate the humeral epiphysis. Neither could I dislocate the head of the humerus. The clavicle can be broken without great force, but fracture of the other bones… is practically impossible. (J. W. Sever 1916a)

He studied Lange's theory, which stated that just after a shoulder capsular tear, the infant would not move the arm because of pain, and stiffness resulted. In cadavers of infants, Sever injected the shoulder joints with methylene blue and then ruptured the anterior capsule. After placing the cadavers supine in a preserving solution and leaving them for several weeks, he dissected the shoulders, discovering that the methylene blue was present around the brachial plexus but not above the clavicle. On the basis of these results, Sever (1916a) argued that in living infants this would result in "paralysis of the whole arm below the joint, but would in no way affect the nerves above the clavicle…the typical picture of obstetric paralysis [that is, paralysis] of the fifth and sixth cervical nerves." This was a significant finding because he had ruled out other causes of obstetrical paralysis or the appearance of it, including:

1. fractures (because the joint is largely cartilaginous, fractures are rare).
2. soft tissue injury (although the infant would not move their arm in such cases of joint capsule rupture during delivery, the arm would not be held in the position of a birth palsy from an injury to the brachial plexus).

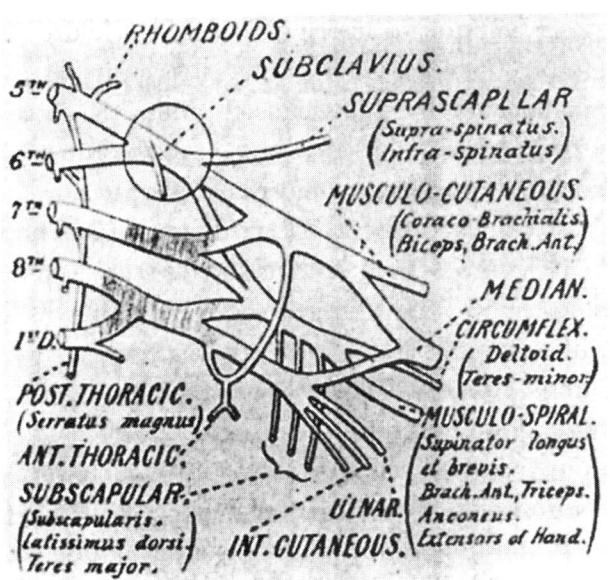

Sever's drawing of the brachial plexus with a circle at the site of injury in upper arm palsies and the shaded area indicating the site of injury in lower arm palsies.
J. W. Sever, "Obstetrical Paralysis—an Orthopedic Problem," *American Journal of Orthopedic Surgery*, 1916; 14: 456-475.

Fractures

In 1916, Sever also treated tibial tuberosity fractures nonoperatively in three patients and made the following observations: "It seems probable that two of these cases of mine, in view of their increased outward rotation and lateral mobility or abduction of the tibia, had torn anterior crucial ligaments. Possibly an operation to repair this damage might have given them a more stable joint" (J. W. Sever 1916b). By that time, only six cases of direct repair of the anterior cruciate ligament had been reported: one by A. W. Mayo Robson in England in 1903, and five by D. H. Goetjes in Germany in 1913. Note that this was 37 years after Paul Segond had associated avulsion fractures of the anterolateral margin of the tibial plateau with injuries to the ACL, one year before Ernest W. Hey Groves reported his reconstruction of a torn anterior cruciate ligament with a strip of fascia lata, and 20 years before W. Campbell in the United States first reported reconstruction of the torn anterior cruciate ligament with a patellar tendon graft.

In addition to his employment at Children's Hospital, Sever was for several years an impartial examiner for the Massachusetts Industrial Accident Board. In 1917, in a lecture to the International Association of Industrial Accident Boards and Commission, Sever reported of his experience as a medical examiner: "For several years now it has been my good fortune to have seen many cases with stiff and painful backs...It has been a great surprise to me to find that a large number of these cases showed fractures of one or more vertebrae... many [patients] had gone for periods of time varying from several weeks to even a year with no diagnosis and no treatment" (J. W. Sever 1917). He concluded, "first of all, [that the cases he presented demonstrated] the necessity and value of a diagnosis...and, second, that few cases get a careful and adequate examination" (J. W. Sever 1917).

Sever also lectured and wrote about other back disabilities caused by industrial accidents and emphasized the importance of physician participation. For Sever (1919a), physicians should "[first] assist in the recovery of the patient and to complete the operation of the law...[and second]... act as impartial examiners in disputed cases." He reported that the Industrial Accident Board in Massachusetts allowed "only $15 a week for the care of a patient who is receiving compensation... [but] allowed the Massachusetts General Hospital $17.50 a week...the standard rate charged by the hospital to all patients able to pay" (J. W. Sever 1919a).

LATER CAREER AND RESEARCH

Sever also dedicated time to teaching at Harvard Medical School and publishing multiple books throughout his career. He was initially appointed as instructor of orthopaedic surgery there in 1922 and promoted seven years later to assistant professor of orthopaedic surgery. He also published three books around this time: *Principles of Orthopedic Surgery* and *The Principles of Orthopedic Surgery for Nurses*, in 1924, and the *Textbook of Orthopedic Surgery for Students of Medicine*, in 1925. With few exceptions and additions, each book "was the result of many lectures on orthopedic surgery" (J. W. Sever 1924a), which were based on material from Boston Children's Hospital.

Principles of Orthopedic Surgery, his first book, was dedicated to "E.B.S.," whom I believe refers to his first wife, Elizabeth Bygrave Sever. His second book, written for nurses, was dedicated to Dr. Edward H. Bradford "in grateful recognition for many things" (J. W. Sever 1924b). Sever dedicated his third book, written for medical students, to Dr. Harvey Cushing, who "stimulated" Sever to write the book (J. W. Sever 1925a). The books were comprehensive and included chapters on fractures. Some chapters were similar—often identical—between books, including the same illustrations and photos. In the third book, however, he expanded and added some new chapters. A review of that textbook in the *Journal of Bone and Joint Surgery* (1926) stated, "[It] is a presentation of the subject to the student as a simple and easily digestible pabulum...the fundamental principles of orthopaedic surgery are enunciated and stressed as adequately as one would expect of an author who is conservative, temperate, and a well-balanced thinker on orthopaedic subjects."

Additional Interests in the Foot

Sever did not publish any other articles on calcaneal apophysitis later in his career, but he did write two on the foot. The most significant was a review of astragalectomy or Whitman's operation in 195 patients to resolve paralytic deformities of the feet or calcaneovalgus deformity, which he had published in *JAMA* in 1920. Early in the twentieth century, Naughton Dunn (1922) wrote that "Whitman's operation of astragalectomy with backward displacement of the foot, is, I think, generally recognized in America and perhaps in this country [England] as the standard operation

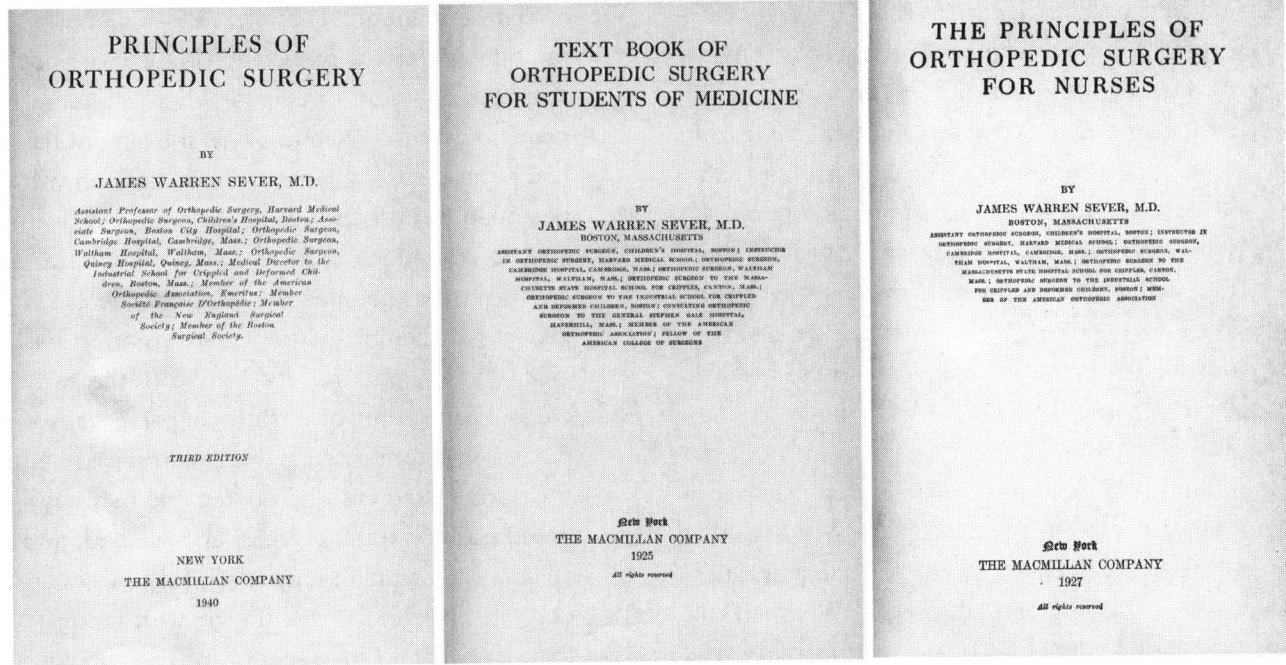

The three books published by Sever: *Text Book of Orthopedic Surgery for Students of Medicine* (1925), *The Principles of Orthopedic Surgery for Nurses* (1927), and *Principles of Orthopedic Surgery* (1940). Collected by the author.

for stabilization of the paralytic foot...originally devised for calcaneo-valgus deformity, but has in recent years largely been employed in securing stability in other types of paralytic deformity." With regard to astragalectomy, Sever (1920), after a thorough analysis, concluded that:

> astragalectomy is not an operation to be advised for any foot showing lateral instability as a result of the paralysis of one muscle group alone. The lateral instability at the ankle may be averted but more subsequent deformity may develop. It is as good an operation as any in feet which are flail or have only one muscle group left. In the presence of toe flexors varus is likely to develop later and lead to a bad weight-bearing position. The best results I have seen are in those feet in which there was good muscle power before operation and where after operation there was good motion between the tibia and os calcis and good weight-bearing position of the foot. In the latter cases I believe it should never have been performed. It is not an operation which will cure a limp or even improve one as a rule. It is not an operation to be advised lightly or invariably for foot deformities, but should be performed in older children on selected cases.

Based on these findings, Sever determined astragalectomy was not a preferred operation except in rare cases of paralyzed feet in older children.

Dunn, in his presentation before the Royal Society in 1922, mentioned Dr. Royal Whitman's criticism of Sever's paper: "[Whitman] ascribes the results of astragalectomy at the Children's Hospital, Boston, largely to improper selection of cases and failure in operative technique and after-care. These would explain failure in any branch of surgery, but probably the work at Children's Hospital, Boston, would not compare unfavorably with that of other hospitals where this class of case is treated." Dunn (1922) then quoted Robert Lovett's review of a large number of cases after astragalectomy:

> My [Lovett's] experience has never led me to feel that astragalectomy should be performed

in young children, except in cases of severe calcaneus for which the operation was originally devised by Whitman, or in connection with really serious and threatening deformities of other types. Performed after the age of 14 years it seems to me to be an admirable operation where operation is necessary. It gives a stable foot with little movement at the ankle-joint and in skillful hands a good ultimate result is easily obtained by proper technique, but this I believe is not generally the case in children.

Dunn (1922) admitted his limited experience with astragalectomy but agreed with Whitman that it is "the only effective remedy for paralytic calcaneus…[but] the operation devised by Whitman fails from its not controlling or correcting mid-tarsal deformity while it limits movements at the ankle, even in cases where this movement might be easily controlled by transplantation of the unparalysed [*sic*] muscle."

Obstetrical Paralysis

Sever continued his work and writing on obstetrical paralysis during this time. In a few of Sever's early cases, he noted, "where the joint has been opened [showed] a persistent loss of motion in the shoulder and the arm remained permanently abducted and outwardly rotated, with no motion in adduction…Too long fixation following operation with exercises and massage will also lead to slow recovery of motion in rotation and adduction" (Sever 1918). In the discussion of a paper on operative procedures of the shoulder written by Arthur Steindler in 1921, Sever stated:

> In regard to the stretching…for definite muscular contracture of the shoulder joint, secondary to obstetrical paralysis, I have not been successful with it because it depends on the fixation of the scapula so much that manipulation, forceful or otherwise, without that fixation, is apparently not very successful. I think that the after-treatment of any of these cases is of paramount importance, particularly in the cases not operated on—not, of course, where there has been an arthrodesis, but where the patient has had a muscle transplantation or a tenotomy. It has been our practice, when there have been cutting operations about the shoulder, to start an exercise as soon as the wound is healed… Prolonged fixation without early motion has given us very poor results. In two of the early cases in our series of obstetrical paralysis, we put the plaster casts on the children and had their arms fixed in the abducted and fully supinated position for six weeks, and we had, and still have, a beautiful arthrodesis [of] the shoulder joint…we found that the greatest factor in failure to obtain full function of the shoulder was lack of early motion. (Sever 1921)

His clinical experiences proved to him that early exercises after shoulder surgery—not including arthrodesis—were essential to restore function.

In 1925—around the same time as the publication of his third book—Sever published in the *Journal of the American Medical Association* an article providing "accurate data" for more than 1,000 infants with obstetric paralysis—the largest such cohort studied to that date (J. W. Sever 1925b). He reviewed the patients' demographics; their pathology, radiographs, and clinical findings; and the treatment they received. In both of these papers, the details and results of which he had also reported in 1918, Sever described his operation:

> An incision is made on the anterior aspect of the arm, beginning at the tip of the acromion and carried down to below the insertion of the pectoralis major. The cephalic vein is found generally in the outer edge of the wound and tied or retracted outward. The tendinous insertion of the pectoralis major is then defined, raised on an instrument, and divided all the way across. The pectoralis major muscle is then retracted inward, out of the way, bringing

into view at the bottom of the wound the inner edge of the coracobrachialis muscle. This muscle is then defined upward until the coracoid process is reached, the arm being outwardly rotated and abducted. The tip of the coracoid process, which is usually found elongated, is completely separated from its base, together with the insertion of the coracobrachialis, the short head of the biceps and the pectoralis minor. Not more than about one fourth or three eighths of the tip needs to be removed to accomplish this. This allows the coracobrachialis and the short head of the biceps to retract downward out of the way, and allows much freer outward rotation and abduction of the arm. The capsule of the shoulder joint is then seen in the bottom of the wound as well as the three horizontal circumflex veins. Just above the upper vein is the lower edge of the subscapularis tendon. This lower edge should be defined. A curved instrument is then inserted just underneath this tendon, which is fairly wide at this point, and the tendon completely divided on the instrument. This prevents any opening of the shoulder joint capsule; and, once this subscapularis tendon has been divided, outward rotation, abduction and elevation of the arm are perfectly free.

The only condition then that will block free outward rotation, abduction and elevation is a considerable degree of hooking of the acromion. If this condition exists, such portions of the acromion as block the restoration of the head of the humerus to the glenoid should be removed. The operation is then complete and the only stitches needed to close the wound are stitches to the fascia and skin. The arm is then put up on a splint in an abducted, elevated, outwardly rotated and supinated position.

Muscle reeducation, active and passive use of the arm, begins just as soon as the stitches are out, which is in about eight or ten days.

We have operated in about sixty or seventy cases. Our results have been satisfactory, that is, in the upper arm types, and while we cannot restore the arms to normal, we can improve them functionally, so that they are very useful.

There are one or two preoperative conditions that have bothered us a good deal: 1. For about a year after this operation, and sometimes even longer, there is considerable difficulty in inwardly rotating the upper arm, or in putting the hand on the opposite shoulders. 2. In almost all cases after operation there is a good deal of limitation of rotation in the joint itself, which, however, is eventually overcome. 3. With the arm hanging at the side, there persists almost always a considerable rotation of the scapula in a vertical plane, even when there is apparently free motion of the shoulder joint. Just why this is we have not been able to determine. It does not impair the function of the arm, but does not make for a cosmetic success.
(J. W. Sever 1925b)

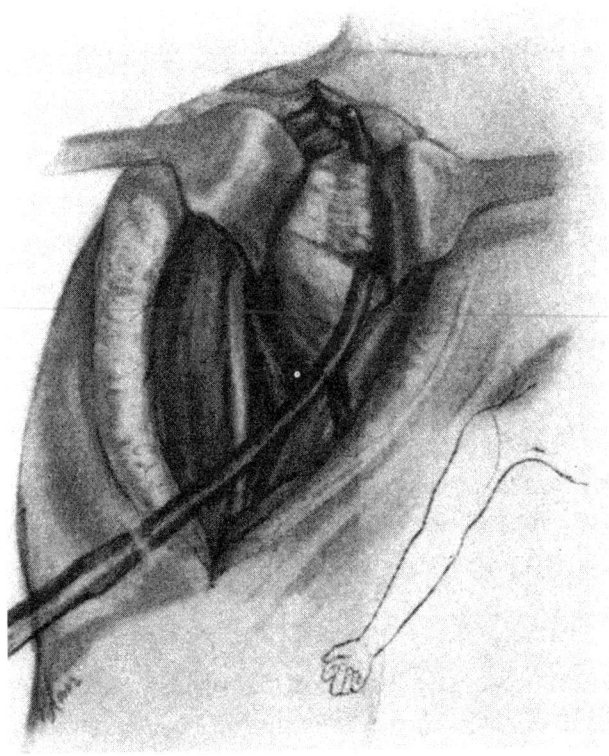

Drawing from Sever's article demonstrating the subscapularis tendon with a probe between the tendon and the shoulder capsule. J. W. Sever, "Obstetrical Paralysis—an Orthopedic Problem," *American Journal of Orthopedic Surgery*, 1916; 14: 456-475.

Sever's operation included an extensive anterior release of the shoulder—including the insertion of the pectoralis major, the origins of the coracobrachialis and the short head of the biceps, and the insertions of the pectoralis minor and the subscapularis—but did not include opening the joint capsule. In most cases, he found he was able to restore passive shoulder abduction and external rotation. It was an original and major contribution which at the time became the "accepted" procedure. It was only later supplemented or modified by L'Episcopo to include tendon transfers to provide the patient with active motion of abduction and external rotation.

Sever was not the only physician who studied brachial plexus injury through anatomical dissection of cadavers. Dr. J. H. Stevens (1871–1932), a surgeon who was seven years older than Sever, "had for a long time made a hobby of studying the brachial plexus" (J. H. Stevens 1934). Dr. E. Amory Codman was Stevens' neighbor and convinced Stevens to write a chapter for his upcoming book on brachial plexus paralysis; as Codman states in his introduction to the chapter, Stevens had not written about the subject (see chapter 34):

> [Stevens] had at the time dissected ninety-two plexuses through the courtesy of the Tufts Medical School; and since then, through the kindness of the anatomical department of the Harvard Medical School, he had been able to dissect a good many more...On March 24, 1932, Dr. Stevens died suddenly from heart disease, leaving his work in preliminary manuscript forms for me to use...I have used the portions of his manuscript which seemed to me original and enlightening. (E. A. Cadman)

Although Sever and Stevens probably knew each other, and knew of the other's investigations—maybe they even shared discussions of traction injuries to the brachial plexus—I was unable to find any references to such collaboration. Codman does not refer to Sever or his operation in his book on the shoulder.

Fractures

From 1916 to 1935, Sever had published six papers on fractures of the tibial tuberosities, neck of the femur, proximal humerus, head and neck of the radius, and elbow; and on nonunions of the humerus. Sever's last publication on fractures, published in 1935, reported five cases of nonunion of the humerus. He observed that nonunion was common for transverse fractures of the middle one-third of the humerus, though the etiology of the nonunion was generally unknown. He did, however, describe one case in which "the ends of the bone were found tapered off and lying in a thick fibrous capsule, filled with a material that resembled joint fluid [and stated that] massive or onlay graft, followed by a sufficiently long period of fixation to insure union and to carry one by the period of absorption and possible fracture of the graft," is worth doing despite being unpredictable (J. W. Sever 1935). Sever's interest in the topic led him

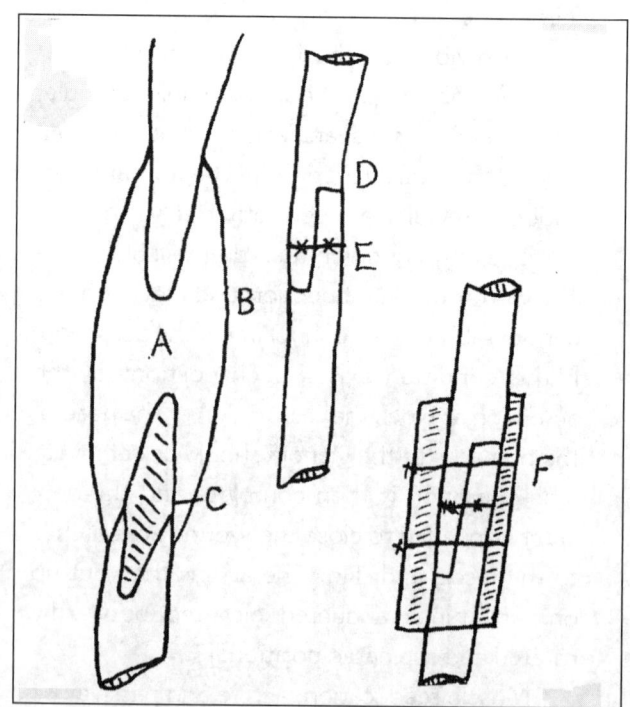

Sever's drawing of the large onlay bone graft technique he used to treat chronic nonunions of the humerus.

J. W. Sever, "Nonunion in Fracture of the Shaft of the Humerus: Report of Five Cases," *Journal of the American Medical Association* 1935; 104: 383.

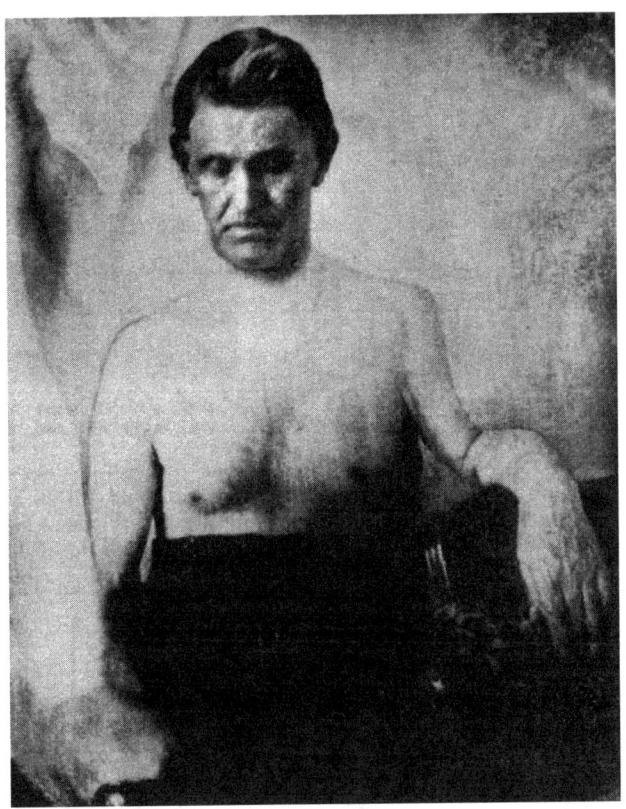

Photograph of a man with complete resorption of his left humerus following a fracture. The arm is preserved in the Warren Museum; prepared by Dr. Thomas Dwight.

J. W. Sever, "Nonunion in Fracture of the Shaft of the Humerus: Report of Five Cases," *Journal of the American Medical Association* 1935; 104: 383.

to study an 1819 case of complete resorption of the humerus in a patient with a history of three (re)fractures of the humerus over a two-month period. He found the patient's dissected arm preserved in the Warren Museum at Harvard Medical School.

WORK WITH DISABLED CHILDREN AND ADULTS

Sever was greatly interested in disabled children and adults, dedicating more than 50 years to the Industrial School for Crippled and Deformed Children in Boston's Back Bay where he served as medical director (*Boston Globe* 1964). Since 1894, the Industrial School had been providing a high school education/industrial training and therapy for over 1,000 disabled children—the majority of whom (~75%) had (or had recovered from) polio—(*Daily Boston Globe* 1939). In this role, Sever followed the values of Dr. Bradford, whom Sever quoted in his statement at the opening of the school: "We must have an institution in Boston for cripples, and I have come to believe that it ought to be a school where medical supervision, nursing, good food, and prescribed periods of rest can be given along with schooling" (Bradford quoted in J. W. Sever 1938). Sever (1938) accepted that children who could meet the physical demands of regular classes should be included there, but he thought it was ideal for children with disabilities to be taught separately so they could receive more attention from their doctors and have ample time available for therapy. We do not know when he was first appointed medical director, but most likely it was about 1906 and early in his career. He devoted time throughout his entire professional career to the school and its children.

AN ORTHOPAEDIC PERSONALITY WITH A MEMORABLE LEGACY

Sever had lived in Cambridge and in Cape Neddick, Maine, until his retirement in 1946, when he moved to his farm in Peacham, Vermont. His first wife, Elizabeth Clark Bygrave, had died in 1944. In that same year, he had married Josephine (Dormitzer) Abbott, who also had been previously married and who also died before him. Sever had remained in his post at Harvard Medical School until his retirement, having taught orthopaedic surgery for about 40 years in several faculty appointments.

Sever had also served as trustee of the Browne & Nichols School for many years. He was a member of the American Medical Association, and in 1932 had served as chairman of the Section on Orthopaedic Surgery. He was a fellow of the American Orthopaedic Association, the American Academy of Orthopaedic Surgeons, and the

American College of Surgeons; and a member of the New England Surgical Society, the Boston Surgical Society, the Société Francaise d'Orthopédie of France. He ended up participating as a member of the Massachusetts Medical Society for an astounding 63 years. An article about Dr. Sever appeared in the *Daily Boston Globe* in 1953. Written by F. Burne, it quoted Sever as he described his thoughts about the improving profession of medicine:

> It's extraordinary how much doctors have improved…The graduate of a good medical school and the house officer in a good hospital like ours today are so ahead of what we were that it isn't funny. When they begin to talk—my goodness I just want to crawl under the amphitheater…What they have to learn is the art and practice of medicine. But what they know is extraordinary—all this heart surgery, and blood work, it's just amazing…Have you ever noticed…how many people used to die in "languishment"…That just meant they didn't know what in the world they had. Today medicine is an expert profession…Today there is a much more intelligent treatment of infantile paralysis…We are doing more for spastic children. Practically a fracture treatment today is turned over to the orthopedist. For the last few years of my teaching life I couldn't find a case of bone and joint tuberculosis to show my students.

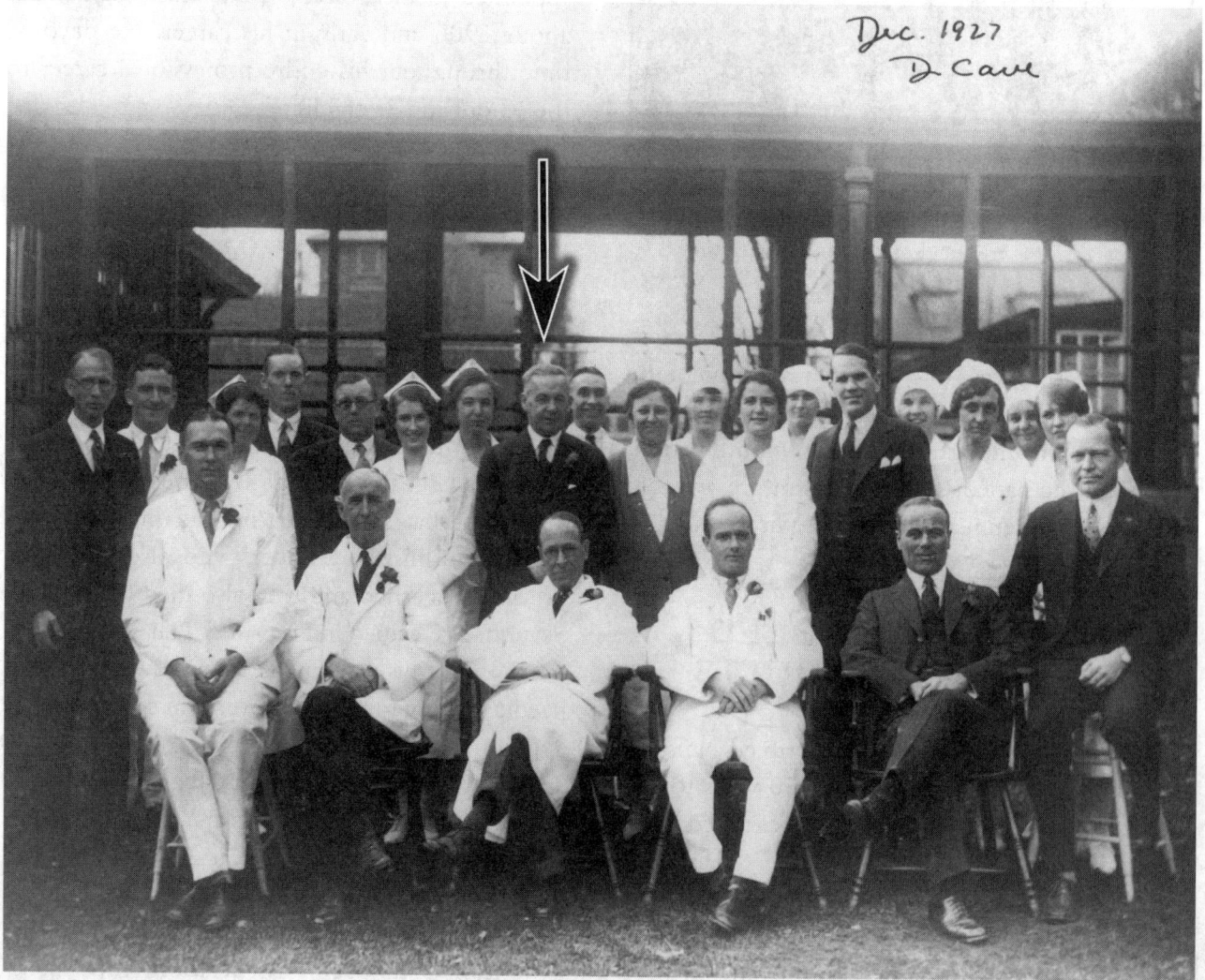

Orthopaedic Staff at BCH in December 1927. Sever is identified in the first standing row. MGH HCORP Archives.

The following year, at the Annual Meeting of the American Orthopaedic Association in 1954, Leo Mayer, a prominent orthopaedic surgeon, presented a paper about orthopaedic personalities in the first quarter of the twentieth century. He stated:

> I have been one of the few orthopaedic surgeons still living who have [sic] been privileged to witness...the evolution of orthopaedic surgery from the strap-and-buckle phase to its proud position as a major surgical specialty...First, let me undeceive those among you who may think that, because of the appellation "strap-and-buckle period," good surgery was non-existent during the late years of the nineteenth and the early years of the twentieth century. Bradford, in Boston, as early as 1895 operated successfully for recurrent dislocation of the patella...In contrast to...outstanding surgeons, there were many high-ranking orthopaedic specialists who never entered the operating room except to apply a plaster-of-Paris dressing or, occasionally, to perform a subcutaneous tenotomy. (L. Mayer 1955)

Mayer labeled Dr. Newton Shaffer of New York as one of these "rarely operating" orthopaedists who preferred mechanical therapy. Early in his career, Robert Lovett had studied under Shaffer. Mayer (1955) stated, "In Boston, Dr. Robert Lovett...was no surgeon, but his pathological studies, his research into the mechanics of scoliosis, his brilliant teaching and his organization of the Harvard Infantile Paralysis Commission have won him a high place in our society." Mayer reminded the audience that "orthopaedic surgery at the turn of the century did not demand surgical skill and knowledge as a prerequisite. The change in emphasis from mechanics to surgery has been one of the noteworthy advances of our specialty. Let no one gain the impression that this transition was easy and peaceful...[as] it precipitated a clash with the general surgeon, who disputed the new surgical claims of the young specialty" (L. Mayer 1955). Mayer (1955) quoted from A. M. Phelps's 1894 Presidential Address: "The orthopaedist was always at war with the general surgeon...There never was a time when they could lie peacefully together in the same bed, excepting like the lion and the lamb—one inside the other, and the poor orthopede was always inside." Mayer concluded by saying, "I am staggered by the changes which occurred...It is good for us today to realize our indebtedness to the past."

In a discussion of Dr. Mayer's speech, Sever made the following comments:

> Dr. Mayer's paper has been extraordinarily interesting to me. I've known all these men whom Dr. Mayer has talked about. When I read my first paper at The American Orthopaedic Association in Washington in 1907, the Association was small; we had perhaps thirty or thirty-five members. Dr. Bradford, under whom I trained, and Dr. Lovett, in whose office I worked for so many years, I knew well. Lovett was a hard task-master; he was a hold-over from the brace days and he was very much interested in and very insistent upon teaching the art of brace-making to his house officers and having his patients equipped with perfectly fitting braces. He knew nothing about surgery. I think that in thirteen years we did perhaps one tenotomy, as a private case, and one amputation of an arm for sarcoma of the elbow.
>
> When I started doing orthopaedic surgery, The American Orthopaedic Association was in its transition stage between the brace surgeons and the surgically trained orthopaedic men; and when I was asked about that time to take over the orthopaedic surgery at the Boston City Hospital, I was told by the surgeons that the only patients whom I could treat were those with flat feet, scoliosis, and rickets. Well, I didn't want to do that, because it didn't seem to me worth while [sic]. Dr. Brackett at that time was at the Massachusetts General Hospital and all of you knew Dr. Brackett and the wonderful work

he did, not only in surgery, but also as Editor of our "Journal" for many years. He developed it to the point from which Dr. Rogers has carried on. (from the "Discussion" in L. Mayer 1955)

Sever was honored by the states of Massachusetts and Maine for his long and distinguished service. He died at his farm in Vermont on July 19, 1964, at age 86, "survived by a daughter, two sons, four grand-children and five stepchildren" (*New England Journal of Medicine* 1964). He is buried in Mount Auburn Cemetery in Middlesex County, Massachusetts. He made an abiding impression on the field of orthopaedics—focusing on that specialty early in his career, and his knowledge and research led to many indelible contributions and a lasting influence. Dr. James Sever's name will always be associated with his signature contributions—developing the Sever operation for treating obstetrical palsy, and identifying calcaneal apophysitis (now often called Sever's disease).

CHAPTER 18

Arthur T. Legg
Dedicated to Disabled Children

Arthur Thornton Legg was born on April 19, 1874, to parents Charles Edmund and Emily (Harding) Legg in Chelsea, Massachusetts. He had one brother, Allen. After graduating from Chelsea High School in 1894 and spending two years at Harvard College, he entered Harvard Medical School, graduating in 1900. He completed an internship at Children's Hospital of Boston and then began his practice in 1902, limiting it to orthopaedic surgery.

GIFTED SCHOLAR AND SURGEON

Legg remained on the staff at Children's Hospital for his entire career, 39 years, but early on he also joined Joel Goldthwait at Carney Hospital. Goldthwait, who initially focused on pediatric orthopaedics, gradually increased his interest in adult orthopaedic problems. Legg assisted Goldthwait in establishing an adult orthopaedic clinic at Carney Hospital, which "was the first orthopaedic clinic for adults in the United States" (R. B. Osgood 1939). Legg was eventually placed in charge of a large foot clinic there during the same period that Osgood worked in the clinic at Massachusetts General Hospital.

In 1907, Osgood designed an apparatus to test the strength of foot adductor and abductor muscles in patients with flat feet. "Dr. Legg, always

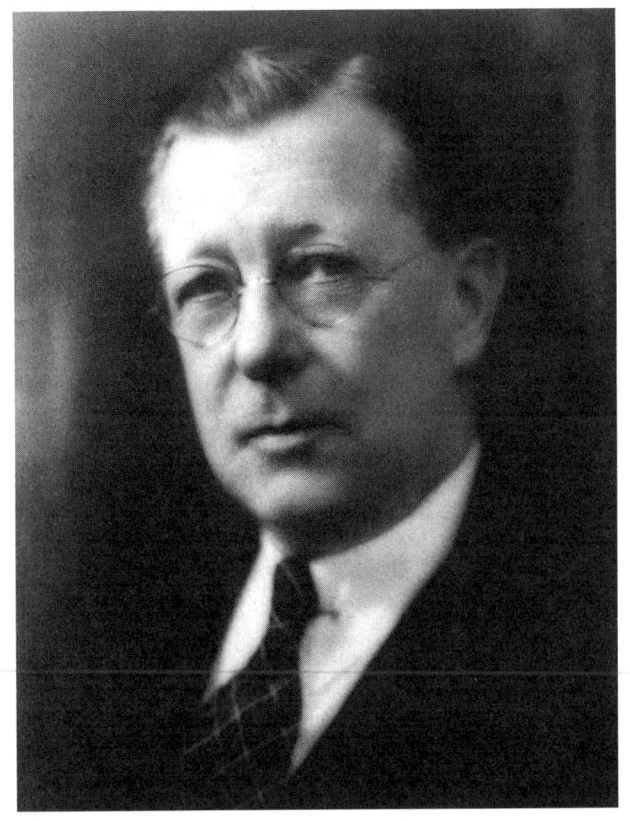

Arthur T. Legg. Boston Children's Hospital Archives, Boston, Massachusetts.

Physician Snapshot

Arthur T. Legg
BORN: 1874
DIED: 1939
SIGNIFICANT CONTRIBUTIONS: Pioneered work on coxa plana (Legg-Calvé-Perthes disease); founded first gait laboratory at Boston Children's Hospital

101

the kindest of men, did the testing at the Carney Hospital. [Osgood and Legg] agreed to test the comparative strength of these two groups of muscles in four different types of feet: symptomless feet; feet that were symptomless but [where] pronation was exhibited; feet that tired easily…and frequently exhibited…more exaggerated pronation; and painful feet [that were] covered by shoes that bulged on their inner sides [and which were] commonly called 'acute flat feet'" (R. B. Osgood 1942). Both Osgood and Legg agreed to do a clinical prospective trial with a control group—questionably unheard of at the time—and to an early attempt at a power analysis. Osgood noted that "Dr. Legg and I agreed not to discuss or compare our findings until we had tested a sufficient number of feet to give some reliability to our statistics. When a total of a hundred and twenty tests had been made…we compared our figures. To our surprise…the average ages…in the two different clinics were well-nigh identical" (R. B. Osgood 1942). They reported no change in muscle strength in the first two symptomless groups. However, in the third group "the pounds pull of the everters…was definitely stronger than that of the inverters [that were] in the fourth group [and] the ratio of the pounds pull of the inverters to that of the everters was approximately 4:5, [which was] the reverse of the ratio that existed in the test of normal symptomless feet" (R. B. Osgood 1942).

In 1908, he was appointed junior assistant surgeon at Children's Hospital. Legg also served as a consulting orthopaedic surgeon at the Massachusetts State Hospital in Canton, the Chelsea Memorial Hospital, and the Lakeville State Sanatorium, where he eventually became the senior orthopaedic surgeon.

Simultaneously during his research and work as a surgeon, Legg also fulfilled multiple teaching appointments. He started as an instructor in orthopaedic surgery at Harvard Medical School and eventually was promoted to assistant professor of orthopaedic surgery in 1929, an appointment which continued until his death. Legg was also appointed first assistant in orthopaedic surgery at Tufts University, where he was employed from 1903 until 1908. His students learned about musculoskeletal problems at Carney Hospital. He and Charles Painter, whom he assisted, were the only orthopaedic faculty at the university. During World War I, "he was kept in this country as an essential teacher and serv[ed] under Major Robert W. Lovett [at Children's Hospital and] did yeoman['s] work in fitting younger surgeons for service in army hospitals in Europe and America" (R. B. Osgood 1939).

LEGG'S DISEASE (COXA PLANA)

Legg contributed 22 publications throughout his career (detailed later in this chapter). He was a keen observer and a careful writer and "never wrote unless he had something worth while [sic] to put on paper" (R. B. Osgood). He was the first to identify the condition of coxa plana—a nutritional condition without infection—as separate and distinct from those cases previously grouped under a tuberculosis diagnosis. According to Osgood, Legg's seminal work on this unique condition addressed:

> a series of [five] cases of hip disease in children, published in February, 1910, [and] brought him international recognition. He was the first to recognize and demonstrate that the patients whose symptoms he described were not suffering from tuberculosis of the hip joint but from a deformity of a growth at the epiphyseal

AN OBSCURE AFFECTION OF THE HIP-JOINT.*

BY ARTHUR T. LEGG, M.D., BOSTON, MASS.,
Junior Assistant Surgeon, Children's Hospital.

Title of Legg's original article describing what would become known as Legg Calve Perthes Disease (1910). *Boston Medical and Surgical Journal*, 1910; 162: 202.

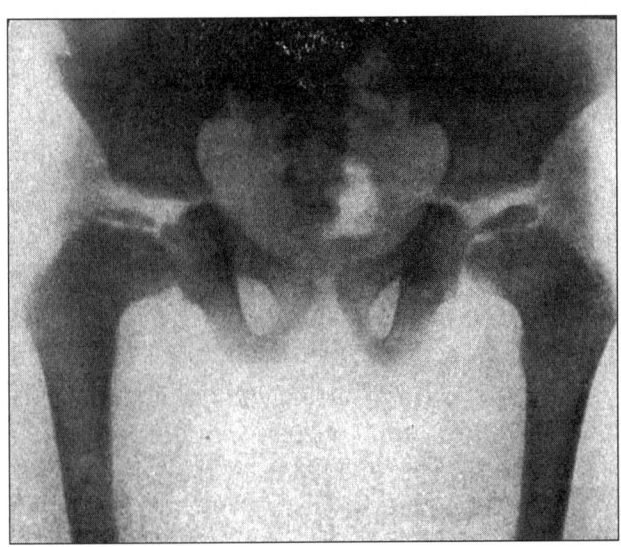

Case example with flattening of the right femoral head, and shortening and widening of the femoral neck.

A. T. Legg, "An Obscure Affection of the Hip-Joint," *Boston Medical and Surgical Journal* 1910; 162: 202-203.

line. Although farthest from his thought or wish, the osteochrondritis juvenilis or coxa plana which he first described became more generally known as Legg's disease in this country and brought him international recognition.

(R. B. Osgood 1939)

Smith-Petersen agreed that "a large per cent of the so-called cured cases of tuberculosis hip diseases are without doubt cases of Legg-Calvé-Perthes disease" (M. N. Smith-Petersen 1924). Legg had originally reported these observations in a paper he presented to the American Orthopaedic Association the summer of 1909, which were then recorded in the *Boston Medical and Surgical Journal* in early 1910. His first case is presented in **Case 18.1**. Similar cases (n=10) were reported the summer of 1910 by Jacques Calvé and in fall 1910 by Professor George Perthes (6 cases). The disease "is known by each of these names as well as by the names osteochondritis deformans juvenilis, coxa plana, pseudo-coxalgia, osteochondritis of the hip, osteochondral trophopathy, etc." (L. D. Smith 1935). Several of Legg's most noteworthy observations are recorded in **Box 18.1**.

Case 18.1. Legg's First Recorded Case of Coxa Plana

> "The first case, a well-developed girl of eight, was brought to the Children's Hospital in October, 1907, with a history of a fall nine months before, immediately followed by a limp on the right which had persisted. There had been no pain or constitutional symptoms.
>
> "Examination showed normal flexion of the right hip with all other motions much limited. There was very slight spasm, slight atrophy of the thigh and calf, but no shortening. There was a slight amount of thickening anterior to the neck. The motions of the left hip were normal.
>
> "A traction hip splint was applied, which she has worn since. She has had no acute symptoms, nor pain, and had remained in excellent general condition. The very slight spasm present at the first examination disappeared in about a month.
>
> "Examination of the right hip at the present time shows motion in flexion to 100°, abduction to 50°, adduction normal. Internal and external rotation is possible to about 45°. The thickening about the joint has remained the same, and the right leg now measures one quarter of an inch longer than the left.
>
> "There has been no pain or limp on the left, and the motions of this hip are normal. A slight amount of thickening, however, is felt about this hip.
>
> "The Von Pirquet test [tuberculin skin test] was negative. Roentgenological examination shows the head of the right femur to be flattened and apparently spread out. The neck appears thickened and shorter than normal. An area of increased radiability appears in the upper part of the head and neck. The left or apparently normal side shows the same condition with the exception of the area of increased radiability."
>
> (Arthur T. Legg 1910)

Between his initial seminal work and his second publication on the topic, Legg exhibited remarkable fortitude. He was a devoted son to a father who was "crippled by rheumatism for many years before his death in 1914...Although [Legg's] days in town were very full, he slept at night at his father's home in Chelsea in order that he might constantly minister to the needs of his widowed parent's body and spirits" (R. B. Osgood 1939). In 1918, not long after his father's passing and eight years after his seminal work, Legg published his second paper on coxa plana. He described 75 cases that he had personally followed.

Box 18.1. Legg's Observations in "An Obscure Affection of the Hip-Joint" (1910)

> **Identifying limp:** "In all cases for patients aged five-to-eight years, help was requested only because of a limp. Their patient history revealed injury and limp but no pain."
>
> **Roentgenogram results:** "[S]howed a flattened head and a distinct necrotic area just outside the epiphyseal line in the neck, with apparently some thickening of the neck."
>
> **Unknown Etiology:** "Is this condition the result of congenital deformity or faulty development[?] We see many cases of congenital dislocation of the hip [but] none of these shows a condition similar to the one described."
>
> **Analysis:** "In this group of cases, with a history of distinct injury in all of them[,] a possible explanation of the condition is that the injury may indirectly cause this condition by causing injury or displacement of the epiphyseal line, whereby the nutrition of the head, coming mostly through the neck, is impaired; and by the poorly nourished epiphysis bearing on the acetabulum, it becomes flattened...It does not seem probable to me that the change in the head...is secondary to...infection...for we see many cases of infection in the neck, and in none of these have I seen the condition described present in the head."
>
> **Conclusion:** "I am glad to have brought them to your attention in the hope that in so doing more cases of this type may come under observation and that by further study their true etiology may be determined."
>
> —Arthur T. Legg 1910

Called osteochondritis deformans juvenilis or coxa plana by many at the time, the etiology was still unknown. Some believed it was congenital; others believed infection caused the deformity. Legg noted that Calvé thought the condition "was due to an earlier rachitic condition" (A. T. Legg 1918). Still others agreed with Legg "that the affection is a circulatory disturbance" (A. T. Legg 1918). Legg reported that 25 cases had no history of trauma, 26 had "distinct trauma immediately preceding the limp[, and] twenty-four showed the condition after reduction of a congenital dislocation of the hip [and] in all these cases more than one attempt had been made before complete reduction was attained" (A. T. Legg 1918). He went on to note that:

> Any blocking of this [blood] supply (at the epiphyseal line) will cause atrophy of the epiphysis, and it is not hard to conceive that weight-bearing on an atrophied epiphysis would cause flattening of this structure [and] that a trauma about the hip may cause an injury at the epiphyseal line whereby the nutrient vessels to the epiphysis are blocked and atrophy and flattening follow...The writer [Legg] continues to believe, as he has previously stated, that the condition showing the flattening of the upper femoral epiphysis is due to a circulatory disturbance at the epiphyseal line, causing atrophy and flattening, and is generally due to trauma.
> (A. T. Legg 1918)

Johann H. Waldenström had simultaneously published his experience with Legg's disease in 1910. At the time, he incorrectly believed the disease to be caused by tuberculosis, but he also introduced the term "coxa plana." Waldenström concentrated on etiology, whereas Legg focused on the end results. In 1927, Legg published his last paper on coxa plana, a series of 40 cases that he had followed for 10 years or more and which included his original five cases from 1908. He observed that there was significant variation in femoral head involvement revealed via x-ray and in mobility limitations experienced by the patient. He noted imaging was necessary to identify the patient's prognosis, and he concluded that the final course of coxa plana showed either a "mushroom type" or a "cap type" on x-ray. Legg believed that treatment—including support during weight-bearing activities—did not ultimately affect the final resulting deformity or the patient's functional ability over time. In Perthes's earlier 1910 article, he agreed with Legg that treatment did not influence patient outcomes. In the discussion of Dr. Legg's paper on end results of coxa plana, Dr. Osgood stated: "We obtained permission from the parents [of one patient with a cap deformity] to explore the hip. Dr. Legg did so and found an almost normal looking head and acetabular cavity. He tunneled into the area of radiability which appears as a cavity in the x-ray, but obtained no pus and the culture was sterile on all media tried" (R. B. Osgood 1927). Dr. W. E. Ryerson disagreed and believed treatment with a Thomas caliper splint led to good results as long its use was continued until imaging showed complete ossification. He believed it important to not leave the condition untreated—which he observed led to a broad and short neck of the femur and flattening of the head—and that results from treatment could be expected within as little as a few months or as long as three years.

Legg never sought public praise. When Dr. Willis Campbell recommended giving him credit by naming the condition after Legg in his discussion, Legg responded by stating he would prefer to have the condition labeled coxa plana. Dr. Osgood described Legg's "most admirable [characteristics

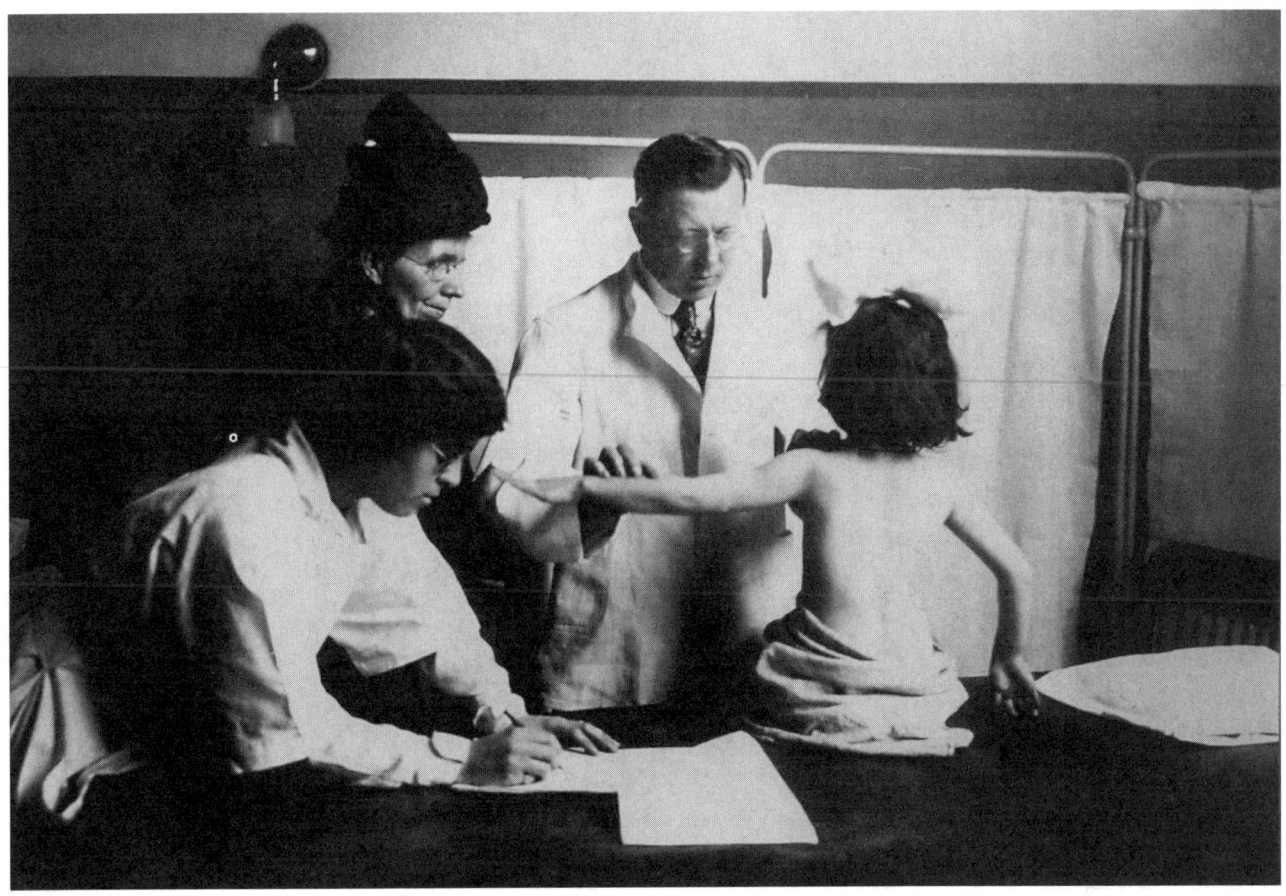

Legg examining a child in the orthopaedic clinic, ca. 1930. *Images of America. Children's Hospital Boston.* Charleston, SC: Arcadia Publishing, 2005. Boston Children's Hospital Archives, Boston, Massachusetts.

as] his devotion to the needs of the crippled child, his reserve and his modesty. [Legg's own] father complained of the necessity of 'pumping him' before he could learn either of his doings or his thinking" (R. B. Osgood 1939). Legg's work was one of three major research contributions from the orthopaedic department. In 1928, Dr. Osgood—the department chair at Boston Children's Hospital—in response to a report from Dean Edsall about the most important research in the past 20 years in orthopaedic surgery, wrote that Legg's research on coxa plana "has [had] far reaching effects on the treatment of these conditions and the original work has stood the test of time" (R. B. Osgood 1928).

I recall from my time as a resident at Boston Children's Hospital in the late 1960s that cases of coxa plana were called Legg-Perthes disease. Currently, only the name Perthes is used at Children's now. It's not clear when the name changed, but residents, fellows, and faculty at Harvard should give precedence to its first founder, Dr. Legg, who was on the staff at Boston Children's Hospital and on the faculty at Harvard for 39 years, by calling the disease Legg's disease or Legg-Perthes disease.

PEDIATRIC ORTHOPAEDICS

Legg will be forever remembered for his pioneering research on coxa plana. Nevertheless, he made many other significant contributions in the newly developing field of pediatric orthopaedics.

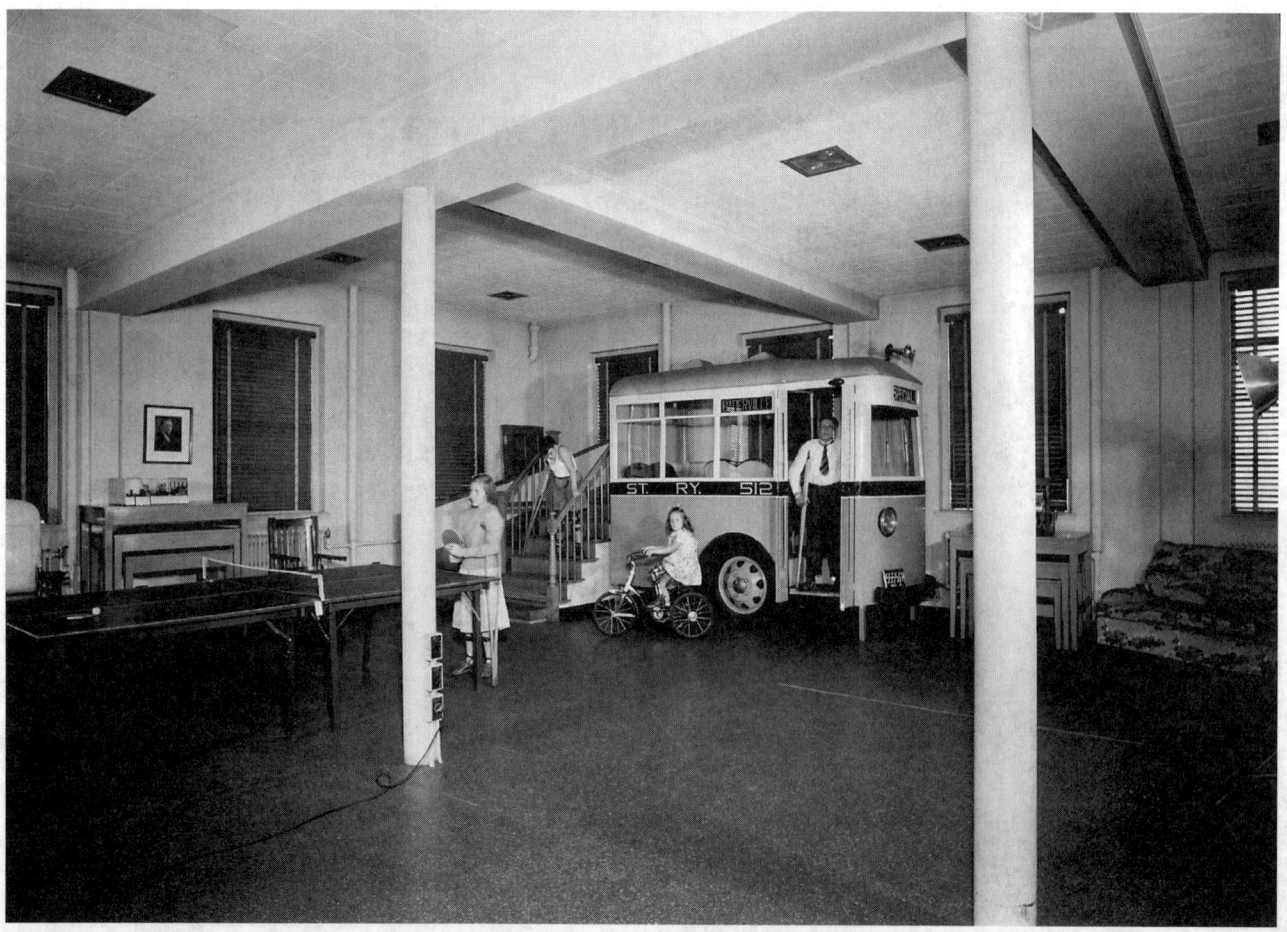

Bader Functional Room (Arthur T. Legg Memorial Room). *Images of America. Children's Hospital Boston.* Charleston, SC: Arcadia Publishing, 2005. Boston Children's Hospital Archives, Boston, Massachusetts.

He succeeded Dr. Lovett in 1921 as director of the Massachusetts Infantile Paralysis Clinics of the Boston Children's Hospital, and some of his most important contributions were his work with Dr. Lovett in treating patients with poliomyelitis. He remained as director for 18 years, serving under the department chairmen: Drs. Lovett, Osgood, and Ober.

Around 1923, Legg established the first attempt at a gait laboratory at the hospital. The Children's Hospital Annual Report noted that "Investigations are being conducted by Dr. Arthur T. Legg by means of moving pictures of the gaits caused by the weakness of the different muscles and muscle groups affected by infantile paralysis, [and] [t]he equipment and running expenses of this investigation are provided by the income of the Helen Hallett Thompson Fund." This grant was one of the first provided to an orthopaedist, and its procurement highlights Legg's innovative work and the greater significance of the gait lab at the time. Legg worked closely with the physical therapy department—especially its director, Janet Merrill. In 1932, Legg and Merrill published a book together, *Physical Therapy in Infantile Paralysis*. Legg provided the therapists with equipment of his own design for rehabilitation of paralyzed children. This rehabilitation work—including learning how to accommodate for and complete activities of daily living—was completed on the sixth floor of the Bader building, and the room was later renamed in his honor as the Arthur T. Legg Memorial Room. I was not able to locate the Arthur T. Legg Memorial Room during the time of writing this book.

When the state clinics for crippled children were established "under the provisions of the Social Security Act, Legg was placed in charge of the Haverhill Clinic" (R. B. Osgood 1939). He also served on the Advisory Council of the Georgia Warm Springs Foundation and was a consultant to the State Department of Public Health, where his "wise advice and counsel played a considerable part in maintaining the satisfactory relation between the profession and the Department of Public Health" (P. J. Jakmauh 1939). He attended monthly clinics each year in Haverhill. However, "his most important and far reaching influence was exerted as a member of the General Advisory Committee of Services for Crippled Children[,including] his aid during the summer of 1936, when the Department of Public Health was laying the foundation of Services for Crippled Children and was obtaining the good will of the medical profession as the cornerstone of the structure, [which] will never be forgotten by those who went to him for advice" (P. J. Jakmauh 1939).

CONTRIBUTIONS TO THE LITERATURE

Of Dr. Legg's 22 papers, Osgood identified almost half as Legg's most important contributions to orthopaedics. Three were about Legg's disease or coxa plana and four discussed polio.

Early Research

Legg wrote two papers discussing the foot early in his career. In 1907, he published his experience at Carney Hospital on the treatment of rigid flat-foot by excision of the scaphoid. He wrote that it was "probably first performed by Richard Davy and Golding Bird. The objects of their operation are to remove a wedge from the inner side of the foot, thus allowing correction of the arch and the relief of pain" (A. T. Legg 1907). Legg reported on 13 cases, which he followed for one to five years. He made the following conclusions: "The pain is relieved in all cases. The deformity in most cases can be corrected...The flexibility of the foot cannot be maintained [and] we cannot promise a cure [however] that this operation weakens the foot as some claim, the writer does not agree" (A. T. Legg 1907). Dr. James Warren Sever reported fewer positive results published later in 1920 from Children's Hospital.

In 1913, he reported on transferring the tibialis anterior from the first metatarsal/medial cuneiform to the plantar surface of the scaphoid. He reported successful results in 10 children under the age of four years. He also wrote several papers about infection in the hip joint, first reporting (with Dr. George) 10 cases of children with bacterial infections treated at Children's Hospital over 2.5 years 1905 to 1908. He operated on one patient, Lovett on three, Bradford and Brackett on two each, and Thorndike on one. Positive cultures were obtained in six cases, five with Staphylococcus infections and one with Pneumococcus. None were reported positive for tuberculosis. He stated: "We feel great harm has been done in the diagnosis, and especially in the treatment, by using the term 'hip-disease' to designate all conditions that attack the hip-joint and accepting the term hip-disease to mean tuberculosis [and] the writers hope that the term hip-disease will be discarded [so that] the exact pathological condition [can] be made" (Legg and George 1908). The authors acknowledged the importance of x-rays and the need for immediate surgical treatment, and Legg later wrote that "early incision and evacuation of the pus in the joint will in many cases save the femoral head" (A. T. Legg 1914).

Tendon Transplantation

In 1916, Legg had coauthored a paper with Ober on the results of tendon transplantation in 100 patients with polio. They set forth the basic principles of tendon transfers and described common causes of failure, identifying "the chief cause [as the] selection of a case in which there are no tendons of sufficient strength to assume new function" (Legg and Ober 1916). Besides poor selection of cases, they also reported failure because of faulty technique and insufficient postoperative treatment. In 1923, Legg reported a transfer of the tensor fascia femoris in 15 patients with a weak gluteus medius and a positive Trendelenburg sign. Transferring the insertion of the tensor fascia femoris posteriorly into a femoral periosteal flap 2½ inches below the greater trochanter, he reported that "so gratifying have been the results of this operation[that] the Trendelenburg sign has disappeared and the lateral swaying of the body [is] diminished, if not disappeared" (A. T. Legg 1923). Ten years

Title of the article in which Legg describes his results with transferring the origin of the tensor fascia femoris posteriorly to improve or correct a Trendelenburg limp. *New England Journal of Medicine* 1933; 209: 61.

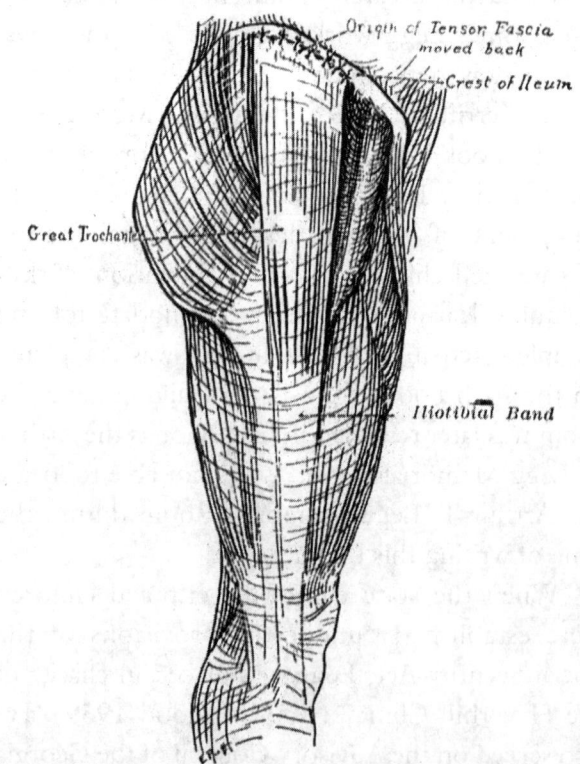

Drawing of the posterior transfer of the tensor fascia femoris origin.

A. T. Legg, "Tensor Fascia Femoris Transplantation in Cases of Weakened Gluteus Medius," *New England Journal of Medicine* 1933; 209: 62.

later, he reported two modifications of his original procedure in another paper. Because the initial transfer continued to have a flexion force, he had avoided this in 1926 by transferring the origin of the tensor fascia femoris posteriorly on the iliac crest, placing the muscle directly above the greater trochanter. Then, in 1928, he had stopped doing the second stage of inserting the iliotibial band into a periosteal flap of the femur, "since the iliotibial band…representing the tendon of the tensor fascia femoris, normally extends down the whole thigh to the outer condyle of the tibia, [and he] believed that a still better mechanical pull could be obtained" (A. T. Legg 1933). He reported excellent results in 25 cases.

Polio

In addition to reporting his technique for transferring the tensor fascia femoris, Legg published another four papers on polio. Legg also gave many talks about polio on the radio, to welfare workers specifically as well as the general public. In 1920, he reported his experience in treating over 1,000 cases during the 1916 epidemic. In summary, he stated:

- During the sensitive stage the patient should be at perfect rest.
- No active treatment should be started until tenderness has entirely disappeared.
- All beginning deformities should be corrected as soon as they appear.
- An accurate muscle examination of the entire body should be made before starting any treatment.
- Sitting and walking should be prohibited for two or three months at least, and then allowed only when the patient can be kept in a normal position.
- Braces should be applied, (1) to prevent deformity; (2) to allow locomotion.
- Fatigue must be constantly guarded against.
- Massage and muscle training is our best method to reestablish power. (A. T. Legg 1920b)

In 1924, he reported his six years' experience following the disabilities in 2,400 cases treated at the Harvard Infantile Paralysis Commission Clinic. He emphasized that "the evil results of over fatigue, general exercise treatment without regard for muscle balance, weight-bearing without mechanical support in positions which favor deformity, tendon transplants without regard for the bone mechanics of a foot, are not matters of theory, but are facts which have been proven to me by the personal examination of these twenty-four hundred cases, not only once, but many times" (A. T. Legg 1924). He also discussed tendon transfers in both upper and lower extremities; and in closing the discussion at the end of his presentation to the American Orthopaedic Association in 1923 stated: "The point of this paper I wish most to bring out is the fact that a great deal of bony deformity can be prevented if we have an opportunity to watch the cases from the beginning, and oftentimes in these cases we may prevent any bony deformity from occurring and we can do a transplantation which will re-establish balance in the limb" (A. T. Legg 1924, "Discussion").

In his personal writings, in 1931, Dr. Green recorded a successful operation by Dr. Legg on an 11-year-old polio patient who had a spine deformity secondary to polio. The patient "had a growth arrest of his trunk with back paralysis. [A] section of his shin bone [probably an osteoperiosteal graft] was grafted to the boy's spine thereby permitting the expansion of the chest and normal growth of the body" (Countway Medical Library). Legg's last paper on polio was published in 1937, two years before his death. He summarized his experience with the 1935 epidemic and compared it to the epidemics of 1916, 1927, and 1931. He wrote: "The distribution was greatest in the eastern part of the state. Seasonally, the peak was reached in August and September. The lower legs were more affected than the abdomen and upper legs…The severity of paralysis appeared to have no relation to the age of the individual. Both the frequency and severity of involvement corresponded…with the epidemic of 1927. The severity and extent of paralysis when compared with that of other years was less in 1935" (A. T. Legg 1937).

Leg Lengthening

Leg lengthening at Children's Hospital may have been led by Dr. Legg in 1929. Legg performed three cases after learning the technique from Dr. Frank Brostrom—his assistant whom he had sent to St. Louis to observe Dr. LeRoy Abbott, who had pioneered the method on 35 patients at Shriners Hospital. Legg gained two inches in four weeks in his first patient, a young girl who had contracted polio. He did a Z-lengthening of the tibia, "performing an osteotomy [of one half of the tibia] just above the ankle [and] another osteotomy just below the knee on the opposite side…the bone [was then] sawed lengthwise connecting the two previous osteotomies [where] the leg [was] fastened securely in a metal frame… grip[ped] near knee [and] grip[ped] near ankle [so that] the bones [were] pulled apart in traction" (Countway Medical Library). Next, a "lever in the frame [was] turned with the physician on one side, the patient on the other…each time together" (Countway Medical Library). After an extension process of four weeks, another "four to six weeks [was needed] for the bone to harden and for the child to begin walking and restore function (especially lost knee joint motion)" (Countway Medical Library). Two inches was the maximum length felt possible at the time.

PROFESSIONAL ORGANIZATIONS

He was elected into the American Orthopaedic Association at its twenty-second annual meeting in Chicago in 1908. His thesis was entitled, "The Cause of Atrophy in Joint Disease." He wrote: "Not until Brackett, in 1890…has anyone claimed that functional inactivity may alone account for atrophy seen in joint disease. His study is wholly from a clinical stand-point, but goes far to prove that functional inactivity plays a great, if not the entire, part in explaining atrophy from joint disease" (A. T. Legg 1908b). Legg demonstrated his interest in research, as he had done with Osgood on the strength of muscles in patients with flat feet (1907), by studying the effects of joint disease and inactivity in three groups of rabbits. He infected knee joints with human tubercle bacilli in two groups; one group was immobilized and the other was allowed to use the infected leg. In the third group, the joint was immobilized in a plaster cast, but it was not injected with the bacilli. After 42 days, the rabbits were euthanized, and he measured sections of the rectus femoris muscle, the femoral artery, and the femur's diameter and cortex thickness. His results allowed him to conclude that "the atrophy of muscle, artery and bone from disease alone was as great as when the joints were infected and immobilized…the atrophy produced by injection and immobilization and that from immobilization alone was greater than when the joint was infected and the animal allowed to use the leg…general atrophy from disease in no way [is] dissimilar from that caused by infection and immobilization" (A. T. Legg 1908b).

Legg then studied muscle atrophy in 50 children without joint disease who were placed on bed rest. He reported that "in all cases atrophy was seen in forty-eight hours…With an average of two weeks in bed, the thigh showed an atrophy of $^{11}/_{16}$ inch and the calf $^{3}/_{8}$ inch" (A. T. Legg 1908b). In his conclusion, he noted "from these experiments and clinically it is seen that atrophy from functional inactivity alone is as great as that which occurs when the joint is infected and immobilization [sic], while infected joints produce less atrophy than immobilization alone, if these joints are more or less active" (A. T. Legg 1908b). Legg was elected vice president of the American Orthopaedic Association in 1933.

Legg was highly dedicated to the Section for Orthopedic Surgery of the American Medical

Association, and he was eventually elected chairman. This new Section for Orthopedic Surgery formed in 1912 because many surgeons who had limited their practice to orthopaedics (and who lacked time or intent) were unable to become members of the American Orthopaedic Association. The purpose of the Section for Orthopedic Surgery was to allow them to make contributions to their specialty and further "the cause of orthopedic surgery in its broader relations with the medical profession at large [which] could be greatly aided and our own Association's aims more readily attained" (*American Journal of Orthopedic Surgery* 1912).

Legg was an active member of the Massachusetts Medical Association, the American College of Surgeons, the American Academy of Orthopaedic Surgeons, the Boston Orthopaedic Club, the Society of Sigma Xi, and the American Pediatric Society. He turned down an opportunity for membership in the International Society of Orthopaedic and Traumatological Surgery, but he also participated in the Interurban Orthopedic Club. The organization was founded in 1907, and included:

> some of the orthopedic men in the more eastern cities of New England, the Atlantic States and Canada. The cities represented in the membership are Montreal, Boston, Hartford, Rochester, NY, New York City, Baltimore, Pittsburg[h], and Washington, DC. The object of the club was to bring together the members twice each year, not for the purpose of listening to prepared papers, but to see in the orthopedic clinics the methods of treatment employed, any refinements of diagnosis which were being practiced, and to hear the results of investigations being carried on in whatever stage they might be. Inasmuch as the meetings are in different places each time, the members are obliged to break away twice each year from the ruts of their own clinics and mingle with others…the first in Boston…the meetings lasted two days. (*American Journal of Orthopedic Surgery* 1909)

Although very active in his professional associations, he was less involved in social organizations. Osgood mentioned that Legg was a member of the Harvard Club of Boston, the Star of Bethlehem Lodge of Masons in Chelsea, and the Vesper Country Club.

LATER YEARS

After moving from his office at 535 Beacon Street in 1929, Legg practiced from his new office in the Longwood Medical Building at 319 Longwood Avenue during his last 10 years. He lectured frequently at local medical societies, regional and national medical associations. His favorite topics were coxa plana and polio. Osgood described him as "an able, careful surgeon who often called attention to his mistakes but rarely to his many successes. His diagnostic skill was extraordinarily keen, and his therapeutic judgment wise and kindly… Though he held strong opinions, he consistently refused to be controversial. He belonged to that small group of useful men who are undemanding, pleasant in companionship and seemingly quite unaware of the sterling nature of their own admirable attributes" (P. J. Jakmauh 1939).

In addition to his many professional accomplishments, Legg was a kind and compassionate person who experienced personal tragedy. Although he seemed a "self-sufficient bachelor" for most of his life, he married Marie L. Robinson at age 62 on August 27, 1936 (R. B. Osgood 1939). They had met at Boston Children's Hospital, where Robinson worked as a nurse. After their marriage, they went to Grenfell Mission—where Robinson had previously served—to continue Legg's work. The mission—founded in the late-nineteenth century in St. Anthony, Newfoundland and Labrador—served the poor and included an association with St. Anthony Hospital. It was here that Dr. Legg—along with Dr. Arthur Krida, head of orthopaedics at New York Bellevue Hospital—treated patients experiencing orthopaedic complications from tuberculosis, infantile paralysis, or congenital conditions in 1937.

Legg and Robinson had been married less than two years when she sustained severe injuries and burns from a gas explosion in their apartment; she died two weeks later on May 24, 1938, at age 45, at 1950 Commonwealth Avenue. She had left an unsigned note and $120 in her purse. In her note, she expressed her love to Legg and a sense of melancholy responsibility for "ruining" his life. She indicated the money was intended to cover the cost of her wedding present. Osgood described her passing as leaving "a wound which those who knew [Legg] intimately realized would never heal, although he bravely and efficiently continued to meet his many medical responsibilities" (R. B. Osgood 1939). Not long thereafter, Legg died unexpectedly at age 65 on July 8, 1939, at the Harvard Club in Boston, where he had recently moved. His death "brought a sense of personal loss to a surprisingly large number of physicians and patients, and to many medical groups—surprising, because we have rarely known a medical servant endowed with a superior mental equipment and capacity of friendship who was so completely self-effacing" (R. B. Osgood 1939).

CHAPTER 19

Robert B. Osgood

Advocate for Orthopaedics as a Profession of Physicians and Surgeons Who Restore Function

Like his predecessors at Harvard, Robert Bayley Osgood made many unique and significant contributions to the progressive development of orthopaedic surgery in the United States. He was born on July 6, 1873, into "good New England stock" (P. D. Wilson 1957) to John Christopher Osgood and Martha Ellen Whipple in Salem, Massachusetts. His family was originally from Hampshire, England. John Osgood, whose ancestors were sailors, was the first Osgood to settle in America, and he arrived in Andover, Massachusetts, in 1638. Robert Osgood, after graduating from the Salem public school system, attended Amherst College and studied the classics in English, Latin, and Greek literature. He was known as Bob to his friends. He was an active member of the glee club (as a tenor) and in drama, both were interests that remained throughout his life. He was a "delightful companion. He loved poetry and could quote from it for hours. He also loved music and had a good musical understanding, although he played no instrument until in later years, when he learned to play the flute and fife for amusement" (P. D. Wilson 1957). He graduated from Amherst in 1895 at the age of 22 years.

Osgood entered Harvard Medical School (HMS) the same year that he graduated from Amherst. It is not known why or when this student of classics decided to become a physician. In his senior year, he was a house officer at the House of the Good Samaritan (1898–1899). He was one

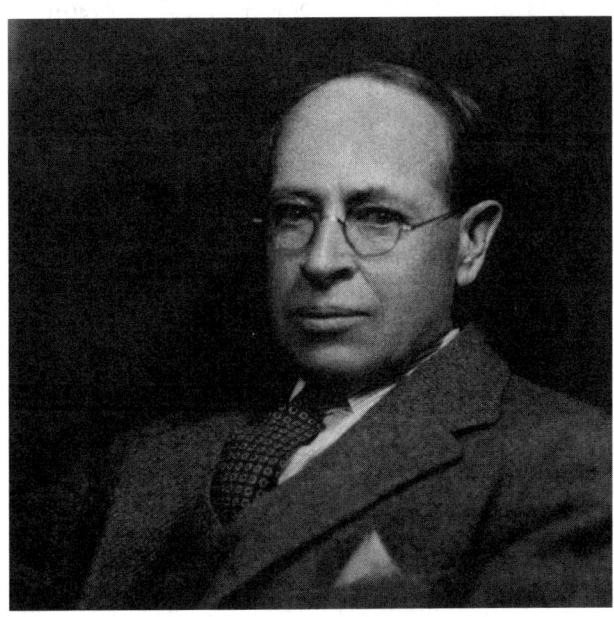

Robert B. Osgood. Boston Children's Hospital Archives, Boston, Massachusetts.

Physician Snapshot

Robert B. Osgood
BORN: 1873
DIED: 1956

SIGNIFICANT CONTRIBUTIONS: Clarified the role of the orthopaedic surgeon during World War I; made significant contributions to the standardization of splints and transportation of the wounded; served as assistant director American Expeditionary Forces to Sir Robert Jones and consultant to the Surgeon General; appointed only first-class surgeons; founder of the Harvard Combined Orthopaedic Residency Program (HCORP); initiated the tradition of weekly meetings of residents with the chief.

of 15 house officers who were listed at the House of the Good Samaritan between 1893 and 1899. Upon graduation in 1899, he completed a surgical internship at the Massachusetts General Hospital (MGH) and then entered private practice.

EARLY INFLUENCE OF ORTHOPAEDIC SURGEONS

The founder of the House of the Good Samaritan—Anne Smith Robbins—died while Osgood worked there as a house officer in 1899. Bradford had stepped down as chief of the surgical service, but he had remained as a consultant surgeon. The chief surgeon during Osgood's time was Augustus Thorndike. Lovett's practice was growing, both at the House of the Good Samaritan and at Boston Children's Hospital. Other orthopaedic surgeons at the House of the Good Samaritan, who Osgood most likely worked with, included Joel Goldthwait and possibly Elliott Brackett. "Undoubtedly, it was from assisting such orthopaedic surgeons… that he became interested in orthopaedic surgery" (P. D. Wilson 1957). Typical ward cases that Osgood would have taken care of included tuberculosis of the hip and spine, knock knees, bow legs, congenitally dislocated hips, coxa vara, club foot, hemiplegia, and polio. Examples of orthopaedic operations in 1905 at the House of the Good Samaritan included: knock knee: 8; coxa vara: 1; club foot: 1; bow legs: 2; and congenital dislocated hip: 1. Outcomes were documented at discharge as well: relieved, not relieved, died, or in hospital (a classification that was used by the MGH and Boston City Hospital at the time). Cases reportedly treated in the outpatient department included all the above, plus rickets.

The hospital records at the House of the Good Samaritan were all handwritten, brief, and unsigned in one large book. The left page contained information about a specific individual patient, including all data, the history, and physical exam. The opposite page contained daily notes about any patient (not only the one detailed on the left). Descriptions of the patient included the date along with the patient's name, age, address, birth location, father's occupation; health of the mother, father, and siblings; a list of any relatives with lung disease, rheumatism, joint disease or nervous disease; condition of the patient as a baby, bottle fed or nursed, previous illnesses, location of the present trouble (duration, cause, history of injury, if any, labor, first symptoms noted, pain and when worse, night cries, lameness, loss of flesh, other symptoms, previous treatment); and remarks. Additional pages in the patient's record included the date, subsequent history, and summary of treatment. Occasional drawings of the patient's deformity were included as well as tracings of the legs before and after surgery. No x-rays were available at the time there. See **Box 19.1** for examples of typical operations at the House of the Good Samaritan a few years before Osgood's arrival.

Radiologist at Boston Children's Hospital

After his internship at the MGH, Osgood's first hospital appointment was at Boston Children's Hospital as a radiologist from 1901 to 1903. He had been preceded by Dr. Ernest A. Codman, who had become the first skiagrapher (radiologist) there, which was a part-time appointment in 1899. They obviously knew each other, but they never collaborated or published papers together. Codman was an assistant in anatomy at HMS and began using the Crookes tube to produce x-rays with the help of Professor William Trowbridge of Harvard and Professor Elihu Thomson of the General Electric Company in Massachusetts.

Dr. Osgood, on the other hand, had formed a close relationship with Dr. Walter J. Dodd, a pharmacist at MGH, who in 1896 had begun experimenting with the first x-ray machine at the MGH. Osgood most likely learned about this new technology from Dodd during his internship. While serving as radiologist, Osgood "made the observations on

Box 19.1. Surgical Records from the House of the Good Samaritan

The following are the surgical records, found in the Children's Hospital Archives, of three operations at the House of the Good Samaritan not long before Dr. Robert Osgood's arrival:

1. Dr. Goldthwait Operation

   September 6, 1894: (patient with knock knees; age unknown).

   Ether operation. Dr. Goldthwait. Double osteotomy. Osteotome introduced on inside of each [leg] just above the adductor tubercle and bone nearly divided; axis of links then straightened by forcible manipulation, and correct position maintained by plaster bandages.

   On October 18 the "plasters [were] removed. Leg in much better position. Tracing taken. To be kept in bed."

   October 25. "to be allowed to play on ward."

   November 30. "Discharged." Almost three months after operation.

2. Dr. Thorndike Operation

   April 2, 1895: Patient with continued pain and draining sinuses. In traction since January 15, 1895.

   Operation: Dr. A Thorndike. Patient etherized for incision of the abscess. The sinuses were probed to make out the lay of the land. The upper sinus was curetted lightly. The first stroke of the curette was followed by a brisk hemorrhage. This…was so copious that the femoral artery was suspected. A cut was made down to the artery…and a small nick was found in the…side of the artery caused by the sharp edge of the curette. The abscess had worked its way under the vessels of the thigh and the finger in the upper sinus felt the femoral artery directly. The femoral artery was tied. An incision was made in the abscess…which several ounces…of foul pus was discharged. Irrigated with boiled water. Packed with sterilized gauze. Large dry dressing applied to whole thigh and pelvis. Three subcu of Brandy were given during the operation. Pulse was rapid—irregular of low tension. Child came out of ether pretty well. Given a subcu of Digitalis…Morph gr $^{1}/_{16}$ and Brandy. Orders left for Brandy ev. 15' during the night.

3. Dr. Thorndike Operation with Dr. Bradford Present

   May 2, 1895: (Second operation)

   Operation: Dr. A. Thorndike with Dr. Bradford present. Patient had not been doing well. Incisions [under ether] made in left hip – 3" long in exterior posterior part of thigh. Another incision on the anterior aspect. [Found] several ounces of thin tuberculosis pus… Capsule of his joint was eaten off so that femur was dislocated forward. Cavity extended all around end of femur. Cavity drained with boiled water. Dislocation corrected – dry dressing applied. Foot held corrected by plaster to cradle. Patient came out of ether well.

   Dr. Thorndike changed the patient's dressing daily. By May 18 the "child was in pretty poor condition…face puffy…has had profuse diarrhea…urine Sp Gr 1.012 [with] hyaline and granular casts." At one month (June 1st) after surgery the patient "has been failing gradually for past two or three weeks. This morning had three convulsions…unconscious at time of morning visit…Two more convulsions before 12 o'clock… Remained unconscious all day. Died at ten P.M."

the growth and traumatic disturbances of the tibial tubercle during adolescence which were published in a paper on January 29, 1903. These lesions have since become known as Osgood-Schlatter disease, Schlatter having at a later date also described the condition" (P. D. Wilson 1957). See **Case 19.1** for a description of one of the cases from that paper. In the paper, Osgood refers to Lovett's earlier description of the normal ossification of the tibial tubercle that he published in the *Philadelphia Medical Journal* on January 6, 1900, and recognizes the earlier observations of tibial tubercle fractures by Drs. Paul Vogt and De Morgan and A. Shaw. In addition to his radiologic observations, Osgood dissected the knees of fetuses (specimens prepared by Dr. E. B. Young at HMS) and two adult knees.

Osgood and Dodd eventually published a paper together "in 1906 on the technique and interpretation of roentgenograms as applied to surgery" (P. D. Wilson 1957). Dodd continued to be unprotected from exposure to x-rays, as did Osgood, until he resigned to focus on his busy private practice. Dodd "remained active in the field, and indeed was one of its great pioneers, [but he] incurred skin cancers in the hands which ultimately proved fatal" (P. D. Wilson 1957). Osgood recognized the early complications of the use of x-rays, noting that "in unskilled hands the therapeutic use of the x-ray includes the serious danger of burns" (R. B. Osgood 1905). He too developed many skin cancers of the hands, and he "underwent several operations and a cure resulted" (P. D. Wilson 1957). Codman, however, eventually died from melanoma (chapter 34). In 1903, for reasons that are unknown, though most likely to gain more knowledge about orthopaedics, "Osgood went to study in Germany, France and England; in England he made the acquaintance of Hugh Owen Thomas and his nephew Robert Jones, whose work made a deep impression on him" (P. D. Wilson 1957).

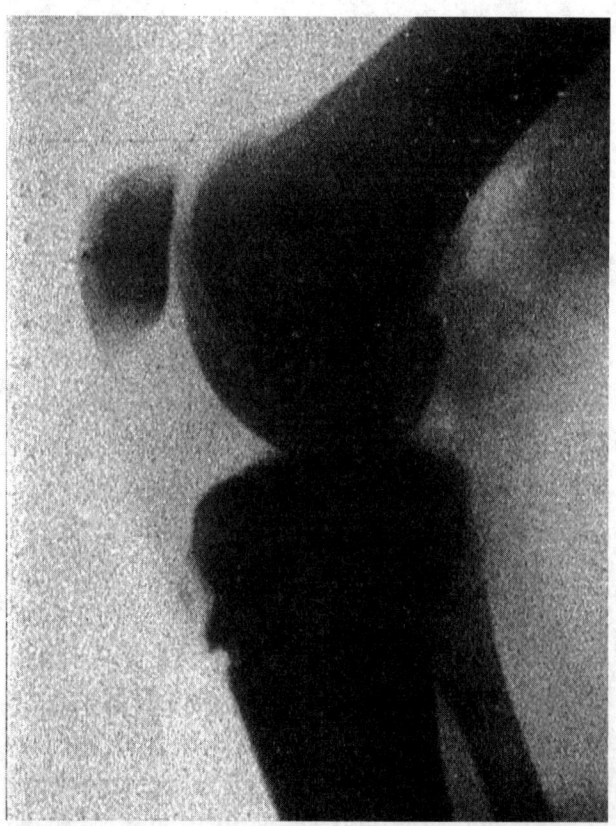

Title of Osgood's article describing the abnormal changes in the tibial tubercle named after him. *Boston Medical and Surgical Journal* 1903; 148: 114.

X-ray of one of Osgood's early cases demonstrating irregularities in the tibial tubercle.
R. B. Osgood, "Lesions of the Tibial Tubercle Occurring during Adolescence," *Boston Medical and Surgical Journal* 1903; 148: 114-115.

EARLY PRACTICE OF ORTHOPAEDICS

Upon his return to Boston, Osgood began his practice of orthopaedic surgery in association with Drs. Joel E. Goldthwait and Charles F. Painter in their office at 372 Marlborough Street. His first hospital appointment in orthopaedic surgery was at the Carney Hospital; his second was at the MGH, 1904–1907, as assistant orthopaedic surgeon in the Outpatient Department. Goldthwait was the first orthopaedic surgeon (a new specialty) at MGH, appointed in 1903 by the Medical Board and Trustees of MGH as consulting orthopaedic surgeon.

Osgood became very active clinically and demonstrated a strong interest in research and education. As a teacher, he became an instructor in surgery at HMS in 1906. Ward I, the first orthopaedic ward at MGH, opened in 1907, and "all orthopaedic surgical procedures were performed in a room in the basement of Ward I, across the hall from the conference room" (MGH HCORP Archives). Osgood was promoted to orthopaedic surgeon in the outpatient department at MGH

Case 19.1. Lesions of the Tubercle Occurring During Adolescence

> "A thin, muscular boy sixteen years old, exercising in the gymnasium, slipped from a jumping board and gave a sudden muscular jerk backward to prevent himself from falling. He felt immediate acute pain in the right knee, and could not step or move the leg forward. The physical examination showed a marked effusion of the joint. The right patella was drawn up higher than the left; and 6 cm. below its lower edge, in which no change could be felt, was a bony knob covered by tense skin, movable and resting 2 cm. from the tibial crest. On movement crepitus could be elicited. By strongly pushing downwards on the patella, this fragment could be made to approach the tibial crest. After the effusion had subsided under appropriate treatment, attempts to completely replace the fragment were still unsuccessful. Firm fibrous union finally occurred, and though slight lateral motion was still possible, a good functional result was obtained (Dr. Paul Vogt; 1869)...It is possible however, to have a partial separation of the tubercle and the interference with normal function be so slight that the condition is often unrecognized and the diagnosis made of a bursitis or periostitis, or even a joint fringe. The x-ray evidence of this is apparently indisputable and the clinical picture absolutely consistent with the true condition... These lesions occur in boys at or shortly after the age of puberty, when the epiphyseal growth is most rapid and a layer of cartilage intervenes between the epiphysis and the tibial shaft...there is felt acute pain in the knee referred to below the patella...often slight swelling...[and] distinct tenderness at this point. The ability to use the leg is only slightly diminished, and the acute pain is soon replaced by a feeling of weakness on strong exertion...a severe handicap to the active athletic life which this class of patients wish to lead...x-rays confirm [the diagnosis]...[and] complete immobilization may be necessary."
>
> —R. B. Osgood, January 29, 1903

that same year, a position he held until 1911. He served as assistant visiting orthopaedic surgeon from 1911 to 1917 and as visiting orthopaedic surgeon from 1917 until 1919. In his first 10 years of practice, Osgood published 20 papers and one book. The book, *Disease of the Bones and Joints*, was coauthored with Goldthwait and Painter and published in 1910. The book was divided into three sections: section 1 on tuberculosis of bones and joints; section 2 on non-tuberculous disease of the joints; section 3 on other conditions, including: lues, rachitis, osteogenesis imperfecta, osteitis deformans, gout, hemophiliac joints, flat feet, subdeltoid bursitis, round shoulder, and the use of plaster of Paris. His research papers ranged from metabolism in arthritis, to nerve grafting in polio, to transmission experiments with the polio virus in monkeys and humans, and to human carriers of polio. His clinical papers varied even more widely, focusing on traumatic lesions of the atlas and axis, prevention of foot strain, methods of distal femoral osteotomy for knee flexion contractures, mobilization of stiff joints, the posterior surgical approach to the knee, and the use of a frame to standardize photographs of scoliosis patients. "In 1910, in collaboration with Dr. Samuel J. Mixter, he reported the first open reduction of dislocation of the atlas on the axis, the reduction being maintained by a fixation with a strong suture. This operation forecast the pattern of the operation that has since been followed; only the silk suture has been replaced by stainless-steel wire and fusion has been combined with the fixation" (P. D. Wilson 1957).

WORLD WAR I

Two years before the United States entered World War I and Osgood enlisted in the US Army, he volunteered to care for the injured in France at the American Ambulance in Neuilly, France (see chapter 63). HMS, as well as other American medical schools, rotated some of their physicians and staff at this 190-bed unit set up in an empty school building (Lycée Pasteur) in the western suburbs of Paris. Neuilly-sur-Seine had been the location of the American hospital, a small hospital supported by the generosity of many Americans living in Paris. However, a larger facility was needed to care for the rapidly increasing number of injured French soldiers. A new school building under construction was converted to a field hospital, becoming the American Ambulance Hospital in Lycée Pasteur. Its organization succeeded thanks to the unflagging efforts of Dr. Joseph Blake, a retired surgeon from the College of Physicians and Surgeons living in France. The American Ambulance Hospital in Lycée Pasteur could eventually accommodate more than 600 wounded men, and Blake invited rotating surgeons from American medical schools for three-month periods to guide and oversee its efforts. These schools included HMS, Lakeside Medical School, and the University of Pennsylvania.

Blake, a keen observer, noted the frequent deformities and contractures developing in the injured while in the care of surgeons. He "began the organization of convalescent homes, where consistent and continued after-treatment of deformities could be carried out by means of mechanotherapy, massage, and apparatus, to the end of the reestablishment of the efficiency in the shortest possible time" (R. B. Osgood 1917c).

In addition to money and hospital supplies, "automobiles were given and lent; men and women of all sorts offered their services; and within a few weeks…a number of ambulances, rudely extemporized from touring cars, limousines and automobile chassis, were ready to bring in the wounded" (Andrew, Sleep, and Galatti 1920). Hundreds of young Americans volunteered to drive the ambulances "back and forth night and day between the western end of the Marne Vallue and Paris. This was the beginning of the American Ambulance Field Service" (Buswell 1916) and its associated hospitals (called American Ambulance). As a result, "an American volunteer formation function[ed] as an integral part of the armies of France" (Andrew, Sleep, and Galatti 1920). In the "steep mountain passes in Alsace which the French auto-ambulances are unable to cross…wounded soldiers were formerly carried on mule-pack" (Buswell 1916). By using small cars, the American volunteers were "able to reduce the duration of the journey of the wounded between dressing-stations and the hospitals from four or five hours to less than one" (Buswell 1916). Their primary role "was to get the wounded as rapidly and comfortably as possible from the battle-line to a field hospital, usually only a few miles back, where they could receive proper treatment under advantageous conditions" (Andrew, Sleep, and Galatti 1920).

Osgood volunteered to serve in the American Ambulance in Neuilly with other Harvard

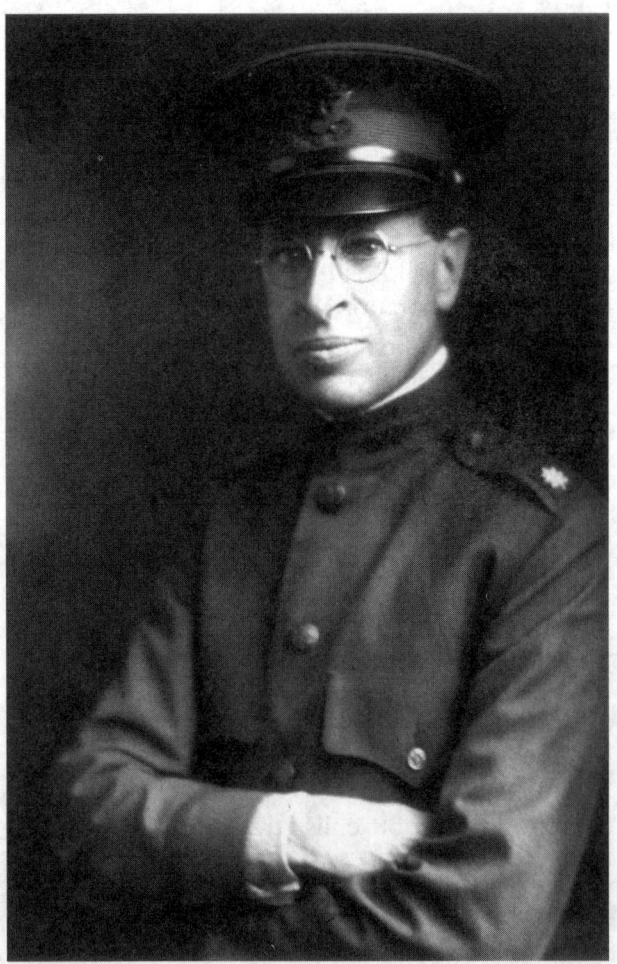

Osgood in his US Army uniform.
U.S. National Library of Medicine.

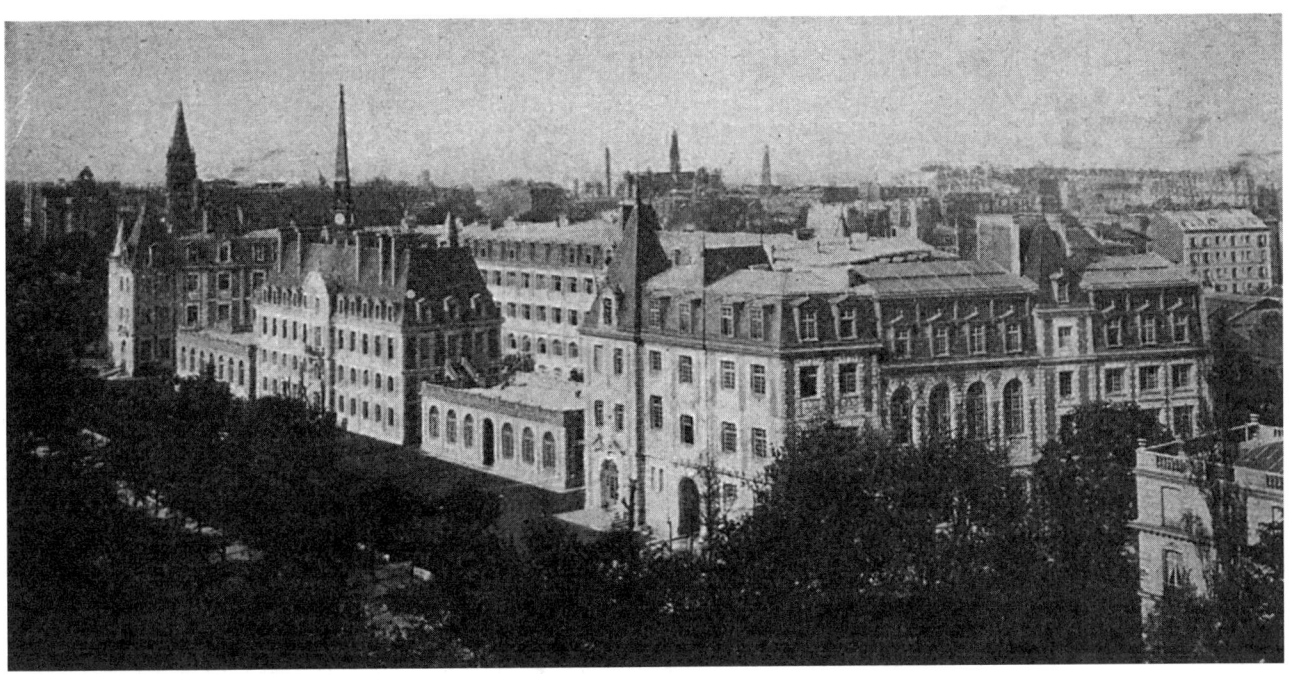

American Ambulance. Formerly the Lycée Pasteur. R. B. Osgood, "Orthopaedic Work in a War Hospital," *Boston Medical and Surgical Journal* 1916; 174: 110.

volunteers. He was the orthopaedic surgeon in April, May, and June of 1915 and was followed by Dr. Nathaniel Allison. The Harvard surgical unit was led by Dr. Harvey Cushing, the Moseley Professor of Surgery and Dr. Robert B. Greenough, his executive officer. Other future members of the Harvard Surgical Unit of the American Hospital in Neuilly following Cushing, Osgood, Greenough, and Allison included: Eliot Cutler, Fred Coller, Lyman Barton, George Bennett, Orvill Rogers, Philip Wilson, Marius Smith-Petersen, and Beth Vincent. The experience had a profound effect on Osgood and "was enough to convince [him] of the frequency and importance of wounds of the extremities involving skeletal structures caused by machine-gun fire and high-explosive shells and of the need for experienced orthopaedic surgeons to provide the necessary expert care" (P. D. Wilson 1957).

Osgood wrote that "the university division, of which the orthopaedic service was a part, represented one of the best examples of 'team play' we have ever seen, thanks to the organizer Dr. Greenough" (R. B. Osgood 1916a). Originally somewhat skeptical of this endeavor by an orthopaedic surgeon, he further stated: "We confess to some doubt at the beginning, as to whether an orthopaedic service at a war hospital would prove interesting to the orthopaedic surgeons or be useful to the other departments of the hospital. The doubt as to the interest of the orthopaedic problems presented disappeared at once and the work assigned to the orthopaedic surgeon, seemed to answer the other questions" (R. B. Osgood 1916a). He wrote at least four papers about his early experiences with the care of orthopaedic war injuries from this experience. In his first paper (1915), he stated:

> I have been somewhat uncertain since coming to the Ambulance as to just what an orthopaedic surgeon is supposed to be or to do. In a "sauf-conduit" I have been described as an "orthopédiste" which is apparently a chiropodist or corsetier. In France, orthopaedic surgery has been most closely associated with tuberculosis of the bones and joints in children…of late years, especially in America, we have been receiving some crumbs from the masters' tables of Medicine and Surgery among adults and like

to derive the words from orthos and the verb paideno, meaning to educate or train straight, quite without regard to whether children or adults are concerned. (R. B. Osgood 1915)

> **Original Articles.**
>
> ORTHOPAEDIC WORK IN A WAR HOSPITAL.
>
> By ROBERT B. OSGOOD, M.D., BOSTON,
>
> *Orthopaedic Surgeon to the Harvard Medical School Unit, Serving at the American Ambulance in Paris During April, May and June, 1915.*

Title of Osgood's article describing the treatments to severely injured soldiers provided by orthopaedic surgeons.
Boston Medical and Surgical Journal 1916; 174: 109.

After only a few weeks in the American Ambulance, Osgood described his initial observations of the difficulty of caring for infected open fractures and joints while immobilizing the involved limb "both for the promotion of union in a good position, and the prevention of osteomyelitis of a chronic type" (R. B. Osgood 1915) as well as the difficulty of maintaining joint motion and function; the difficulty of maintaining the best functional position for contracting joints; and the difficulty in "preventing overstretching of the paralyzed muscles [in wrist drop and foot drop] by allowing the malposition to be maintained" (R. B. Osgood 1915). He concluded:

> There can hardly be any question as to the value of the appreciation of the principles of the prevention of deformity to the cases under treatment...Later on, undoubtedly, surgeons will have the opportunity of acquiring a more perfect technic in operations for recovering motion in stiffened joints. Arthroplasty is still in its experimental stage...some of the apparatus which is being employed by the Harvard Unit; little of it is original, and it is of value only in so far as it makes war surgery more easy and aids in preventing and correcting deformity and adding to the comfort of the patients. (R. B. Osgood 1915)

Osgood grouped the orthopaedic patients into six categories: simple fractures, compound fractures, joint injuries, ankylosis of joints, tendon and/or muscle contractures, and nerve lesions resulting in paralysis. During his three months in Neuilly, he treated 19 simple fractures, 99 compound fractures (not including those in the hands and feet), numerous open joint injuries (with and without fractures), "some nine shoulders, six elbows, four knees, and two wrists received special attention [because of ankylosis]" (R. B. Osgood 1916a), 50 muscle tissue wounds resulting in contracture and tendon contractures of the hand/wrist and the foot/ankle, and many nerve injuries resulting in wrist drop or foot drop. He noted that:

> During the months of April, May, and June about 450 cases were under the observation of the Harvard Unit, and of these between 20 and 25 per cent presented some problem for the solution by which the help of the orthopaedic surgeon was sought. Touch with all the cases was kept by a combined visit with the surgeon to all the cases at least once a week and usually twice. The house surgeons were constantly on the watch for contracting tendons and muscles, and for joints which were in danger of becoming ankylosed or maintained in a position unfavorable for future function. Much after-treatment and deformity was undoubtedly spared by this attention. Careful records with a chronological, alphabetical, and diagnosis index were kept. (R. B. Osgood 1916a)

He described in detail the use of a variety of splints to correct or prevent deformity, the use of physical therapy and massage and the importance of an associated convalescent home "where the ambulatory cases may be watched and controlled and where massage and mechano-therapy can be had…[which] adds greatly to the value of the orthopaedic work" (R. B. Osgood 1916a). He concluded from his early experience with war injuries:

> [T]he essentials for efficient orthopaedic work are
>
> 1. a person with knowledge and interest in orthopaedic surgery, including the mechanical principles of bone and joint fixation and restoration of fractures;
> 2. availability of proper materials including plaster of Paris, a machine shop, splints, fracture table; and
> 3. sufficient time and assistants to care for the patients (in addition to performing surgery and the burden of administrative duties). (R. B. Osgood 1916a)

Almost immediately thereafter—with his exposure to extremity war injuries and his observations of the consequences of surgeons not experienced with the alignment of fractures, proper positioning of joints and limbs, and the concepts of rehabilitation and restoration of function—Osgood wrote:

> Finally, but perhaps most important of all in any long conflict, each must see to it that those large numbers who do not lose their lives, but who by reason of their mutilating wounds lose their fighting power, do not become a burden on the industrial community already depleted and vastly overburdened by the necessity of support of the armies in the field…Our thesis is to be that orthopedic surgery has a very large part to play in (1) assuring physical efficiency in the ranks; (2) in conserving and restoring the function of the locomotive apparatus of the wounded; (3) in providing the physical possibility

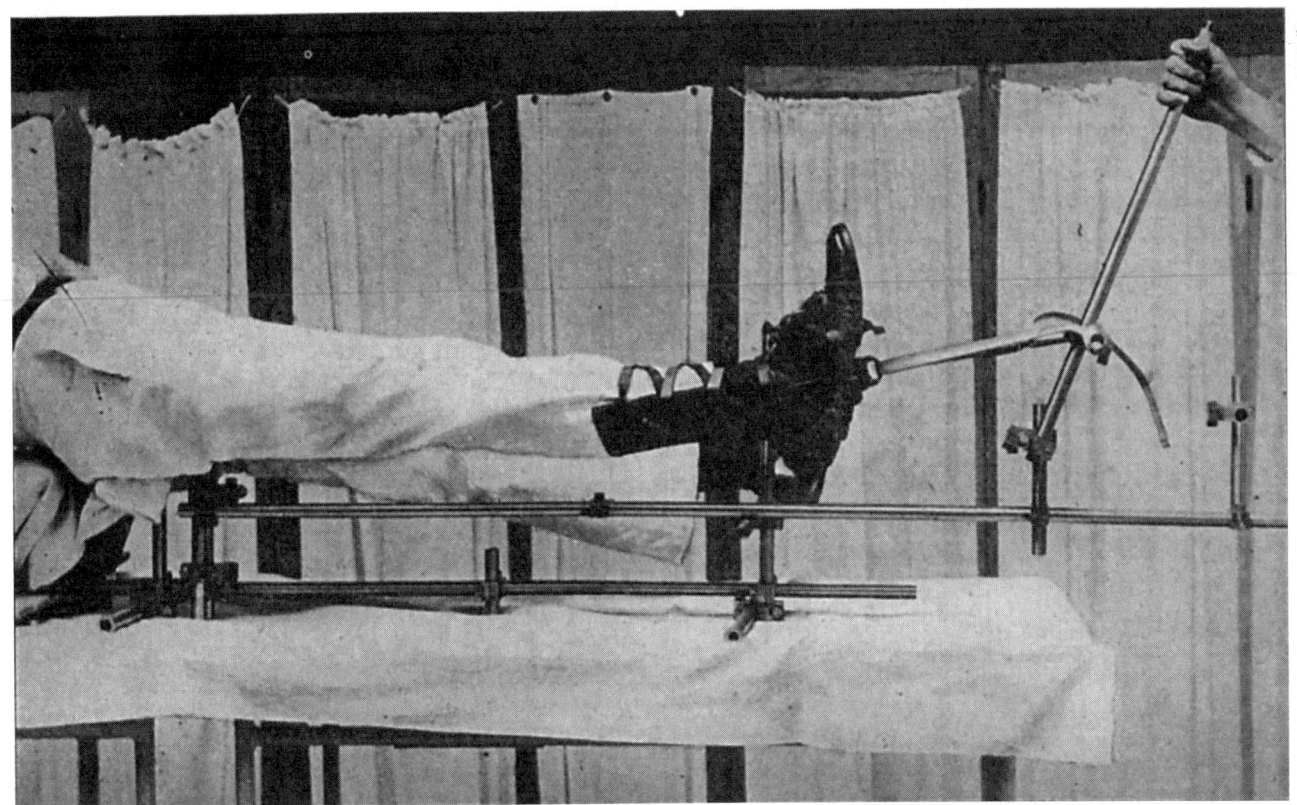

Fracture table designed by Dr. Robert Maddox (of Cincinnati) was available to the Harvard Unit. R. B. Osgood, "Orthopaedic Work in a War Hospital," *Boston Medical and Surgical Journal* 1916; 174: 111.

and perhaps reorganizing the means by which the war cripples may become happy, productive, wage-earning citizens, instead of boastful, consuming, idle derelicts. (R. B. Osgood 1916c)

Osgood had become a strong advocate for orthopaedic surgeons to have a major role in the care of extremity injuries, including fractures, which had been in the domain of the general surgeon. He began to use the term "preventive orthopedic surgery" and wrote:

I would remind you that no surgeon should be as well qualified to deal successfully with these problems as an orthopedic surgeon...Many limbs are saved now that formerly would have

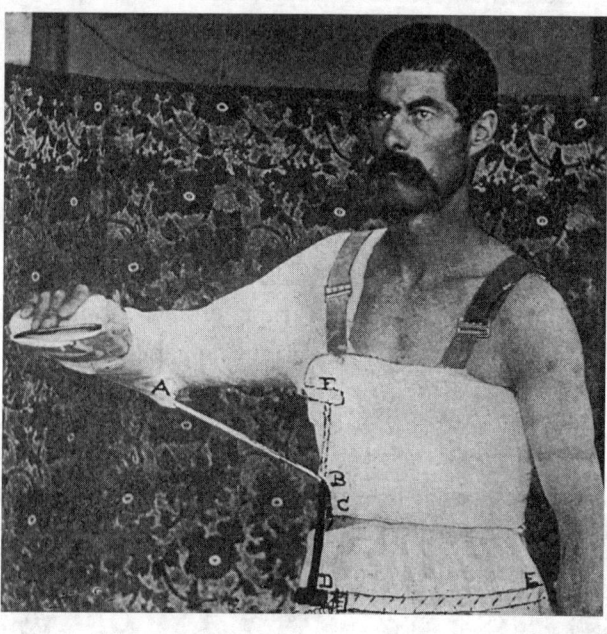

Fracture of the proximal humerus treated in a wire arm splint incorporated in a plaster swaithe and supported with a metal bar. R. B. Osgood, "Orthopaedic Work in a War Hospital," *Boston Medical and Surgical Journal* 1916; 174: 113.

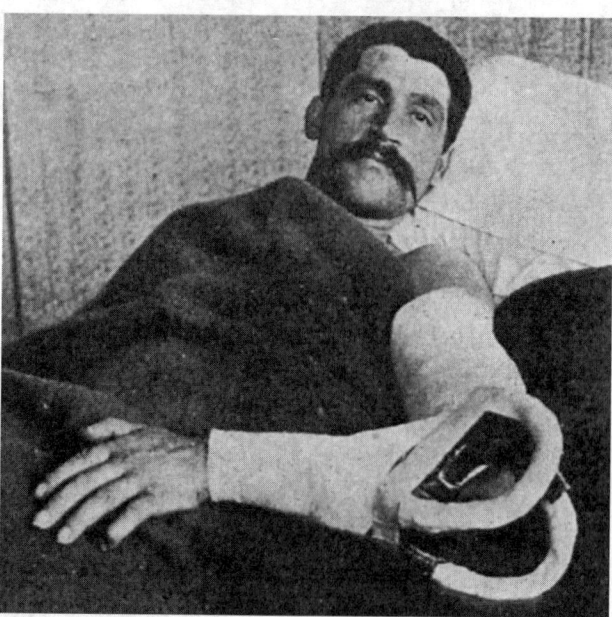

Treatment of an open fracture of the elbow in what Osgood called a basket plaster. R. B. Osgood, "Orthopaedic Work in a War Hospital," *Boston Medical and Surgical Journal* 1916; 174: 116.

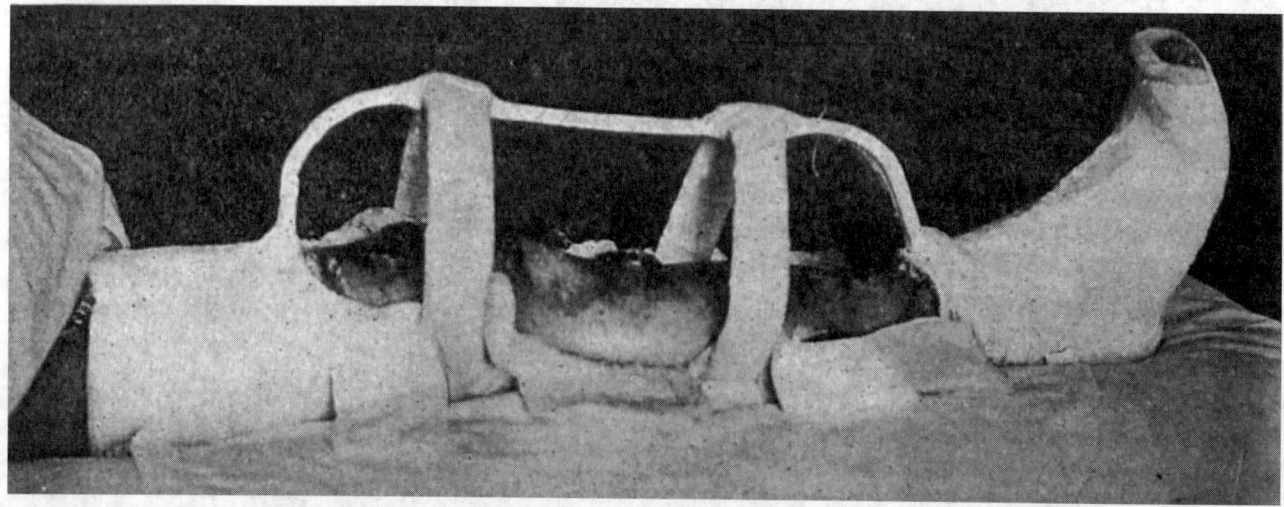

Use of a plaster cast with a long arch and supporting rings to treat a severe open fracture of the tibia and fibula with multiple anterior wounds. R. B. Osgood, "Orthopaedic Work in a War Hospital," *Boston Medical and Surgical Journal* 1916; 174: 117.

been amputated…A foot allowed to become fixed in equinus, a knee in extreme flexion, a hip in adduction, a wrist dropped, a straight elbow, a shoulder which is not abducted is a severe handicap and an entirely preventable one.

(R. B. Osgood 1916c)

Osgood had previously completed a study with Smith-Petersen in 1915 on their experience in the Harvard Unit at Neuilly with Philip Wilson; their study focused on feet sores with poorly fitting

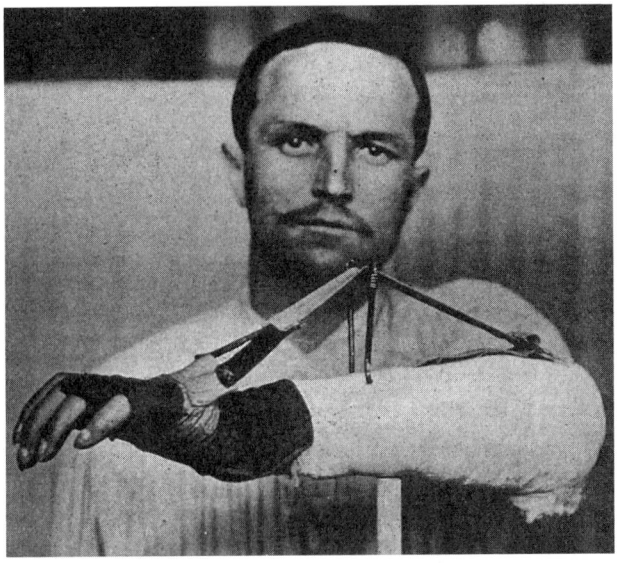

Patient with a wrist flexion contracture and radial nerve palsy treated in a removable long arm cast with an elastic outrigger to increase wrist extension and support the fingers.

R. B. Osgood, "Orthopaedic Work in a War Hospital," *Boston Medical and Surgical Journal* 1916; 174: 124.

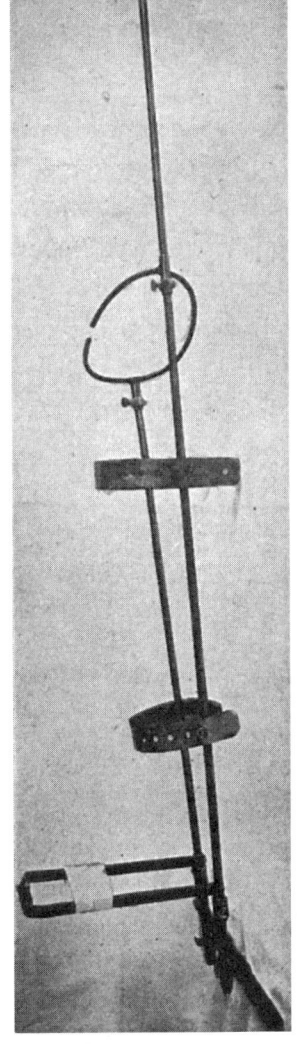

Early model of a Thomas splint with all parts adjustable to fit any size leg. R. B. Osgood, "Orthopaedic Work in a War Hospital," *Boston Medical and Surgical Journal* 1916; 174: 114.

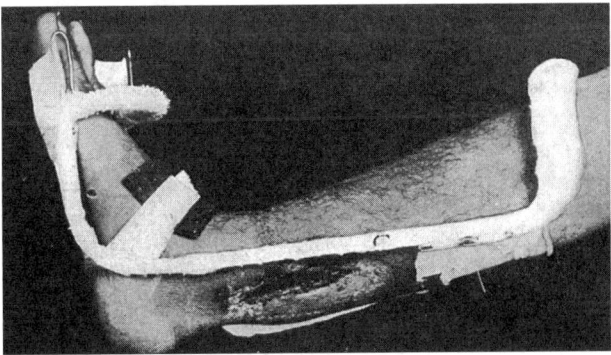

Example of a wire drop foot splint with a soft band across the ball of the foot to allow ambulation.

R. B. Osgood, "Orthopaedic Work in a War Hospital," *Boston Medical and Surgical Journal* 1916; 174: 126.

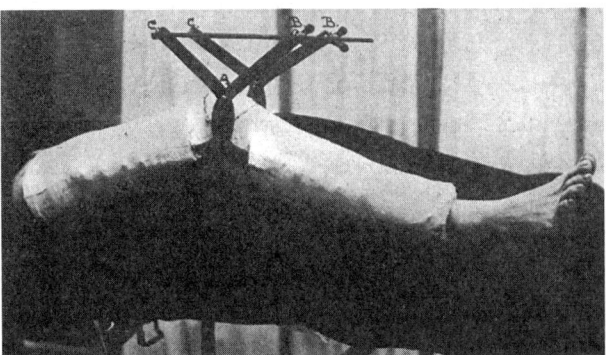

Use of an iron extension hinge (described by Dr. W. H. Turner of Montreal) to correct a knee flexion contracture.

R. B. Osgood, "Orthopaedic Work in a War Hospital," *Boston Medical and Surgical Journal* 1916; 174: 125.

shoes but it was not published. Together with Smith-Petersen, Osgood had:

> examined the feet and inspected the shoeing of a hundred soldiers and attempted to discover whether they had suffered from foot discomfort which had interfered with their efficiency. More than half of these men had had bad blisters from ill fitting and badly balanced shoes. Some of them had suffered from foot strain and weakened arches. A few had actually acquired foot deformities. Their efficiency had been… temporarily lessened…many cases seriously impaired for a considerable time…sometimes half a company [French troops] would be foot sore and laggards…the infantry wore boots thirty years old and had not enough of these.
> (R. B. Osgood 1917c)

Osgood must also have had some contact and discussions with Sir Robert Jones about the role of orthopaedic surgeons in the care of war-injured patients. He recorded in his diary in May of 1916 that he presented a paper to the research committee of the Red Cross at a meeting in Paris on the development of military orthopaedics under Sir Robert Jones. Not long after the publication of Osgood's paper, on April 6, 1917, the United States Congress declared war on Germany. Osgood volunteered almost immediately and received his commission as a major in the US Army Medical Corps on May 5, 1917. Before returning to France from the United States, he was appointed to the US Army Medical Board "to standardize splints, appliances, and surgical dressings for the American Expeditionary Forces" (P. D. Wilson 1957). About this same time, a British Commission arrived in Washington, DC, with a request from Sir Robert Jones for 20 orthopaedic surgeons to work in British hospitals and orthopaedic centers. Britain had a serious shortage of physicians, especially orthopaedic surgeons. In response, "Dr. Goldthwait immediately accepted a commission as Major and set about the organization of the first Goldthwait unit. This unit was organized at once from volunteers by telegraph" (W. H. Orr 1921).

The declaration of war by the United States had been discussed and anticipated for a couple of years. Orthopaedic leaders in both the American Orthopaedic Association (AOA) and the Orthopaedic Section of the American Medical Association appointed committees on preparedness with Goldthwait as chairman of each committee. Other members of the AOA Committee included:

> Drs. Allison, Henderson, Forbes and Irving… The committee…was appointed with the idea of trying to standardize, or decide what is the best equipment for an orthopedic base hospital, or what material should be used in any hospital unit which might be established, whether a general or special orthopedic unit. It was also thought possible to have all the men in the country who are interested in orthopedics get together, so as to be made available for service in case of need…to have collections of material stored…ready for use…doing something that will put us in a position very different from what most of the nations abroad were in when the war begun [sic]…It is the hope of the committee that any of the men…will communicate with the committee…[which will] have the names classified so that the government will have men fitted for different kinds of service. Some could go to the front; others could go to the base units. (J. E. Goldthwait 1916)

This preparation was begun about 18 months before Lovett taught his first Harvard course on orthopaedic surgery for surgeons and one year before the first unit of orthopaedic surgeons, led by Goldthwait, arrived in England.

Goldthwait's first unit of volunteer orthopaedic surgeons consisted of an additional 20 men. They set sail from New York in May 1917 to Liverpool, England, over the course of about one week. During the trip, Goldthwait gave talks and held discussions with the orthopaedic surgeons once or twice daily. Target practice with three- and six-inch guns was frequent. H. Winnett Orr, a member of Goldthwait's unit and later president of AOA and editor of the *Journal of Bone and Joint Surgery*, noted, "There was an obvious increase in nervous tension as we approached the European Side and the boat began to zig-zag instead of going straight ahead. Lookouts for submarines were increased in number and kept constantly on duty. The gun crews remained by the guns at all times" (W. H. Orr 1921).

Osgood, who was not a member of Goldthwait's unit, arrived in England on his way to Harvard's Unit Base Hospital No 5 in Boulogne, France. His unit had set sail on the *Saxonia* from New York on May 11, 1917, and landed in Falmouth, England on May 22, 1917. Osgood had two days of leave before departing England for France, and he took the opportunity to visit his friend in Liverpool:

> to sit at the feet of Sir Robert Jones to whom I always make a pilgrimage as a disciple whenever opportunity offers, whether that opportunity happens to find me on the western or the eastern shore of the Atlantic. We were together in the historic house at No. 11 Nelson Street, redolent still with the memories of that great master of orthopedic surgery, Hugh Owen Thomas. The telephone rang…at the other end…was Goldthwait's voice speaking for twenty earnest American orthopaedic surgeons who…had answered England's call…to help with the increasing problems of the war crippled when England had not that help to supply. (R. B. Osgood 1918a)

He was with Sir Robert Jones when he met with the Goldthwait unit. He wrote:

> It was a wonderful meeting almost too much for the tired nerves of the Director of Military Orthopaedics of Great Britain, who had been struggling with entirely inadequate help to care for the maimed and halt and palsied victims alike of the German war and of hasty, ill-considered surgery. His emotional gratitude was harder to express than his professional, for this man had come, not only to serve his nation, our ally, but to serve him, because to a man they trusted him and looked to him for leadership. He did it wonderfully, and it was a happy and contented group of men that met him on his lawn, at 11 Belvedere Road, that afternoon. (Osgood 1918a)

After seeing the American orthopaedic surgeons again in London the next day, Osgood sailed for France to lead the surgical department of Base Hospital No. 5. The director of the Harvard Unit was Major Harvey Cushing; the orthopaedic surgeon was Captain Frank Ober. Osgood wrote that

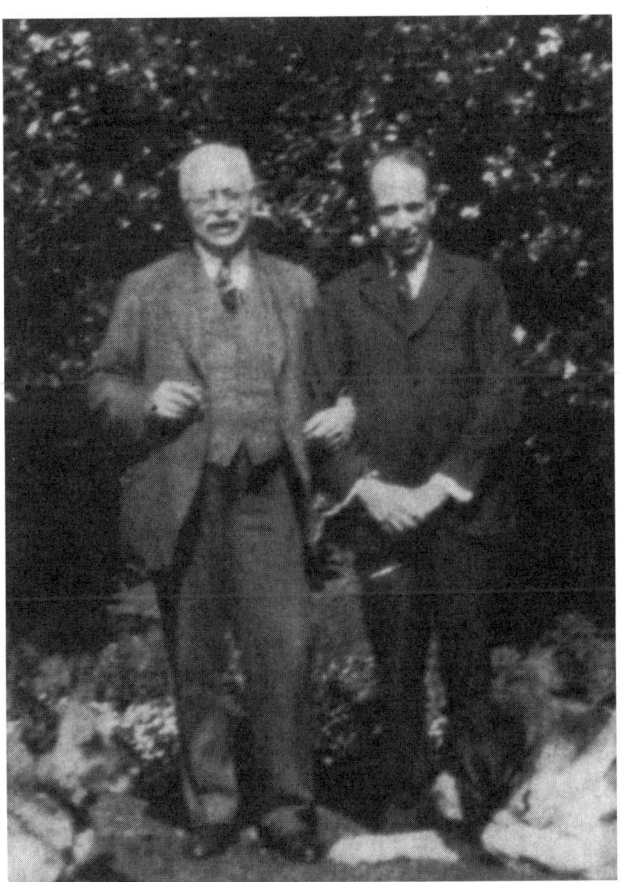

Photograph of Sir. Robert Jones (left) and Dr. Robert Osgood. MGH HCORP Archives.

it was upon "the broad back of kind Frank Ober [that the] brunt of the burden of orthopaedic surgery [and other surgical specialists was placed], I should have felt quite unequal to the task" (R. B. Osgood 1918a). Osgood worked there for four months and noted:

> I shall never cease to be grateful for these four months of hot, strenuous work—a hospital of 450 beds, expanding to 1800 when the pushes came. We were organized to care for 500, convoys of 1000 in 36 hours, dressing tents of 300 a day, night work, day work, rest and play, but always team work and a splendid spirit and close companionship. (R. B. Osgood 1918a)

Osgood kept a brief personal diary during his two years in England and France (1917 and 1918) in which he detailed descriptions of his travels, hotels, meals, operating expenses, and personal experiences. He occasionally played tennis with Cutler or Cushing. In July 1917, he acquired a dog from the adjutant, which he estimated to be about one year old. Originally named Jack, he called the dog Jock. Jock traveled everywhere with Osgood. But in September, he was called back to London to assist Sir Robert Jones. He wrote, "I had wished for the job, but it was harder than I thought to say goodbye to my comrades in active service and to my little dog Jock, especially after their very hard strafing from the bombs of the Hun war bird, which saddened us all" (R. B. Osgood 1918a). On July 4, 1917, he recorded the: "quietist and perhaps the somest [sic] Fourth most of us have spent, perhaps not the safest [German planes sighted]...I tooted a rather weak Star Spangled Banner on my little fife before breakfast" (R. B. Osgood, "Personal Diary"). On July 6, 1917, he met the Queen, who was touring the hospitals and visiting the troops. He said "her handshake was pleasant and her manner gracious and quite regal and simple" (R. B. Osgood, "Personal Diary").

A week later, he wrote about a soldier who died "from this terrible infection with gas producing bacillis [sic]...only saving treatment is not surgery but butchery, and when it doesn't save it seems quite too horrible" (R. B. Osgood, "Personal Diary"). A few brief notes about other cases included descriptions of back injuries from shell blasts causing compression fractures, removal of bullets from joints, the continuing need for transfusions that were often donated by the physicians or other patients, and an increasing number of cases of "delayed tetanus or lock jaw...immediately after being wounded men are given protective inoculation" (R. B. Osgood, "Personal Diary"). Osgood questioned why these inoculations were often not effective and why they were not given to soldiers before going overseas. He also mentioned that although the British preferred splints, the French commonly used plaster of Paris. He recorded that:

> A manual of splints and appliances for our army had to be written, and along with Nat Allison and Billy Baer, Major Joseph Black and Colonel Keller of hallux valgus fame, we had a hand in that, and while I was testing the bitter food of hell in front of the guns at Ypres to be sure our conclusions held water at the front, orders came for my detachment from the unit to serve as deputy to Sir Robert Jones in England. (R. B. Osgood 1918a)

During this period near the front, the hospital "frequently was attacked by enemy aircraft, and on the night of September 4, 1917, suffered several casualties...one nurse and twenty-two patients were wounded" (J. P. Hatch 1919). These were the first deaths of the American Expeditionary Forces in World War I. On September 21, 1917, Osgood was transferred to duty in London, as assistant director, section of orthopaedic surgery, in the American Expeditionary Forces and assistant to Sir Robert Jones. The central office for the organization of orthopaedic centers was located in the Medical War Office (Adastral House) along with the offices of the surgeon-general and the overall leader of medical services in Great Britain. Sir Robert Jones had already been responsible for establishing Orthopaedic Centers distinct from general military hospitals at 11 different locations (**Box 19.2**) At the time, "New centers [were] being started in Reading, Newcastle, Southampton, Birmingham and Manchester, and the cry for more orthopedic beds [went] up" (J. P. Hatch 1919).

Osgood's office was in Adastral House, and "he worked closely with Sir Robert Jones in the establishment and organization of orthopaedic hospitals in Great Britain" for six months (J. S. Barr et al. 1957). He noted several famous American orthopaedic surgeons working in these orthopaedic centers, always under the charge of a British military surgeon: Danforth (Rhode Island) at Edinburgh; MacAusland (Boston) at Alder Hey, near Liverpool; Orr (Nebraska) at Cardiff in Wales; Kidner (Detroit), and DeForest Willard (Philadelphia) at Shepherd's Bush in London. Osgood reported on some of their significant advances (see **Box 19.2**). The orthopaedic surgeons increasingly emphasized rehabilitation. In Aberdeen, soldiers with injured upper extremities exercised their hands and stiff fingers by making and repairing fishing nets. "Recent statistics from other centers have been dealing with this class of hopeless cases [serious lesions and bad surgery] have returned [to duty] on average 75%. Orthopedic surgery may be said to have come into its own, and this department of surgery, which is the specialty of a principle and not of a portion of anatomy, has vindicated itself at last on a conspicuous scale" (R. B. Osgood 1918a).

After six months in Great Britain, Osgood returned to France where Goldthwait was responsible for developing the orthopaedic service under the army's chief surgeon. Osgood described Goldthwait's momentous task:

> Major Goldthwait is preparing the way for the huge number of beds—35,000—which our government has directed him to make ready in France…We start—thanks to the far sight of General Gorgas and our Medical Department, based on a knowledge of the British and French experience—at a vantage point. We are to have charge of the cases from the time

Box 19.2. Significant Advances of the Orthopaedic Centers in Great Britain

> **Aberdeen (500 beds):** provided a well-equipped gymnasium, therapy room (hydro and electro), curative workshops (rehabilitation), and photographic studies
>
> **Belfast (200 beds):** center for treating hand and foot injuries
>
> **Bristol (300 beds):** contained a unique hydrotherapy plant and a large electro-therapeutic facility
>
> **Cardiff (500 beds):** Orr developed a system of medical records, focused on tendon transplants with the established rehabilitation program consisting of printing a weekly Welsh newsletter
>
> **Dublin (200 beds):** had none of the original American unit
>
> **Edinburgh (1000 beds):** Danforth studied end-results with detailed x-rays and photographs
>
> **Glasgow (500 beds):** focused on the treatment of osteomyelitis
>
> **Leeds (1800 beds):** had numerous hutments in which Osgood noted "every factor for efficiency is considered…light, heat, fresh air, cleanliness and comfort. As far as I know, the Children's Hospital in Boston has been the first to realize that this method of construction is not only the cheapest in the short run, but in the long run also. The cost per bed is enormously decreased" (R. B. Osgood 1918a).
>
> **Liverpool (1350 beds):** Cone (Baltimore) discovered a new nerve tissue stain
>
> **Shepherd's Bush in London (1100 beds):** housed a very large hydro-and electro-therapy facility in addition to rehabilitation workshops, which included a patient's orchestra
>
> **Oxford (400 beds):** one of the last centers; headed by Captain Gathorne Girdlestone

of the reception of the wound until the man is discharged from the base hospital back to the army or to civil life. As Matthew Arnold says in a sonnet: "Man must begin where Nature ends." The support of our Government has been most cordial and generous. The opportunity is a great one. There can be no excuse if we fail to meet it. (R. B. Osgood 1918a)

Osgood served as deputy to Goldthwait, first at Tours and then at Neufchâteau, in the American Expeditionary Forces. In his diary, he described his responsibilities as traveling city to city visiting hospitals including evacuation hospitals (15–20 km behind the line), "reviewing bone and joint cases" (including x-rays), examining the water supply to camps, attending conferences and lecturing on splints and methods of treatment as well as "to straighten out a few splint and dressing supply tangles" (R. B. Osgood, "Personal Diary"). He observed that the wounded were operated upon five–ten hours after injury. His days were long. He would have breakfast about 7:00 a.m. and turn into bed about 11:00 p.m. each night. On one occasion, he saw his dentist who told him his "incisors were smoked-stained" (R. B. Osgood, "Personal Diary"). The month following the German offensive in 1918—on Wednesday, April 17—after recently arriving in Tours, he wrote about an incident that portrayed the feelings of the French toward the American soldiers. He wrote, "While waiting in line for bread tickets [a long line of men and women] one man stepped out of line [and said] you are military, sir, and therefore take precedence; let me speak to the gendarme [and although Osgood begged him not to]…he did and this policeman admitted [him ahead of everyone]…not with accompanying scowls of the waiting crowd, but with smiles" (R. B. Osgood, "Personal Diary"). Inside the building, he recorded that he was pushed forward by the crowd to the desk where the lady in charge gave him four tickets for four days. He had asked for only three.

Osgood traveled by trains, sometimes accompanied by Allison to inspect different hospitals. He visited villages within a mile of the front "often with German planes flying over…with snipers in trees…[looking] directly on no man's land… often with guns firing" (R. B. Osgood, "Personal Diary"). Wounds were left open after debridement but some were closed "under twelve hours or in a few days…avoiding infections and painful future dressings" (R. B. Osgood, "Personal Diary"). Others described Osgood as possessing "gentleness and a kind of saintliness," and one of his colleagues reported that:

the hospital orderly went to Dr. Osgood's tent to waken him to see a very ill patient in his own ward. It took some shaking to rouse Dr. Osgood, but when he was only half awake he warmly thanked the orderly for calling him and added that he was sorry he was difficult to rouse. As one of his colleagues has recently said: "This convinced us that he was a saint by night as well as by day." (J. S. Barr et al. 1957)

On Tuesday, May 14, 1918, Osgood met with Goldthwait, who wanted him to return to the United States to do reconstructive surgery on veterans. Osgood returned as orthopaedic consultant to the surgeon general, where his work with splinting and methods to move the wounded had a significant impact. There he "did valuable work through periodic visits to the large base hospitals in the United States where he was able not only to examine the quality of the work being done but also because of his large experience, to help in the resolving of individual problems" (P. D. Wilson 1957). He was promoted and discharged as colonel from the Medical Reserve Corps in 1919.

During and shortly after the war, Osgood published 18 papers on war injuries, splinting, and transport of the injured. He also wrote 13 poems, which are contained in his private papers at the Countway Library. The theme of his poems was World War I. Their titles were: "Strife, The

Box 19.3. Examples of R. B. Osgood's Poetry

AMERICA.

(Impressions on Returning).

    You are real; My Country!
Not the rich and boasting thing that
    patient France and England seem to see
You are strong, My Country!
    And you struggle hard to break the bonds
Of sons who would not have you free.

    You are true, My Country!
The dross will clear and leave you, The
    fire is lit, the melting pot is hot
You are pure, My Country!
    And your molten spirit shall cleanse wounds,
and make the ancient grudge forgot.

    You must mourn, My Country!
While you suffer and the gates of Death
    Close round you and the Peril looms,
You must fight, My Country!
    You shall show that Heroes may be rich
and great men bred in clerks and grooms.

    We are yours, My Country!
Take us, break us, shape us to your ends
    And weld us in a glowing mass.
We are yours, My Country!
    Hurl us, glowing, conquering; then by
Mercy cool us when the grief shall pass.

TO GENERAL SIR ROBERT JONES (On the presentation of a gold chain from the first group of American Orthopaedic Surgeons who were sent to help him in June 1917)

As King you called across the sea
We came to serve your cause and you,
Not homage on the bended knee,
But tribute paid to leadership.

To withered arm and crooked bone
To heart distressed and crippled mind
You brought the healing from your throne
And gave your life to Britain's need.

From out the travail of the earth
By stress of war an art is born
The times of Peace shall bless that birth
Your skill and vision gave to men.

With gladness by your spirit driven
We serve and strive to learn this Art
Your friendship ever freely given
Begets expression from your friends.

A token to a master kind
A pledge of faith from Peers to King
A slender chain but strong to bind
Our common Purpose to the end.

—R. B. Osgood, "Personal Diary"

Voyage," "To Sir Robert Jones," "Peace, America (Impressions on Returning)," "Home Coming," "Beautemps (The Song of the French Women Working in the Fields)," "The Song of the French Calvary Man in Training," "Mallow (The Dream of the Irish Tommy)," "The Half Built Wall (Between Portiere's and Bordeaux)," "Ypres 1917," "The Battle Song and Tears August, 1918," and "Camp Sherman March 12, 1919." Examples of two of his poems are included in **Box 19.3**.

CHIEF AT MASSACHUSETTS GENERAL HOSPITAL

Following his discharge from the army, Osgood rejoined the medical staff at MGH in the role of orthopaedic surgeon from 1919 until 1922. Shortly after Osgood's return, Brackett also returned to MGH, assuming his position as chief of the orthopaedic service. He retired as chief later that year in 1919 and Dr. Osgood was promoted as his replacement. Brackett remained in practice, and, in 1921, he became the third editor of the *Journal of Bone and Joint Surgery*. Osgood easily settled back into practice. He had just published an important paper in the *Journal of Orthopaedic Surgery* entitled "The Orthopaedic Outlook," in which he asked the questions: "What is our position at present with the other branches of the medical profession and what is our attitude toward them...what is our position at present with relation to the other branches of the medical profession... are we in contact with them or are we really isolated?" (R. B. Osgood 1919a). He then described the transition that had occurred for orthopaedic surgeons, their chosen profession, and the reasons for the transition (see **Box 19.4**).

In 1917—prior to enlisting in the US Army Medical Corps—Osgood and Dr. Charles Scudder, a general surgeon, established the first fracture clinic in the United States at the Massachusetts

Box 19.4. Osgood's Analysis of the Transformation of the Orthopaedic Surgeon's Profession

"We have been a small specialty. Our early masters were pioneers...In the early days, and in what we may, at present, call pioneer medical communities, orthopaedic surgeons were, and are, looked upon with askance. There is a reason for this and, to some extent, a just reason. It is because our artist [physician/surgeon] abhors a mechanician [orthopaedist]. The early orthopaedic surgeons were brace makers and we, their descendants, are brace makers still. A man may be respected if he is a surgeon by ability and intent and a brace maker by necessity. He will not be respected if he is a brace maker first and a surgeon afterwards, nor will he be respected if he is a surgeon only by necessity.

"From the barber surgeon developed the Royal College, but not because they became better barbers as the years went on...We like to derive the polyglot work...to educate straight. A specialty of function and not of anatomy...Does not all medicine and surgery attempt to make it straight? What right does a small body of men to claim it as their special task? The only right is because a few surgeons and few internists have considered it their task. The derelict no one wanted. When the wound made by nature or by art was healed, too often the task has been considered done. The foot fixed equino valgus after a Pott's fracture, the flexed knees of an arthritis whose fire has long died out, these are bad surgical and medical results which have excused the existence of the orthopaedic surgeon and given him his daily bread. Of late years they have helped to give him his hospital and teaching positions also...the lay public are discovering what the rank and file of the medical profession have failed to appreciate, that lesions of the joint mechanism of the body, bones, muscles, nerves, must be treated physiological quite as much as anatomical methods...the end result must be judged by the amount of useful function and not by the beauty of the scar. This conception which was gradually taking shape, has become much more definite since 1914. Cases began to stream back from the war... whose wounds were healed, whose fractures were united, whose joint sepsis was over, but whose contracted muscles and badly aligned bones and joint deformities represented crippling problems demanding longer and more specialized treatment than the original lesions...for which no one surgeon was to blame, but...half of them might have been prevented...It is true that many orthopaedic surgeons have the respect and confidence of many general surgeons, but the specialty as a whole, has not...The lack of confidence has been caused by the general impression which exists in the profession that orthopaedic surgeons are surgeons only in name. The feeling approaches a benign contempt. As long as we stay as a class, basically mechanicians, we shall deserve this contempt and not deserve its benignity... No living surgeon...combines...technique...perfect asepsis...absence of faddism...manual dexterity...anatomical knowledge...power of diagnosis and such ability to obtain functionally good end-results as Sir Robert Jones...a general surgeon of wide practice and unusual success long before he determined to devote his life to functional surgery of the extremities and the spine. He is an orthopaedic surgeon, not because he cannot be a general surgeon, but because the cripple appeals to his great heart as it did to

General Hospital. Upon his return after the war, the fracture clinic became an independent unit, under the combined purview of general surgery and orthopaedic surgery. The first conference on fracture treatment was organized by Osgood in 1921. It was a two-day meeting that included both general surgeons and orthopaedic surgeons. About 50 surgeons attended the meeting in Boston; proceedings were published in a special bulletin of the American College of Surgeons ("A Primer of Fracture Treatment"); and they resulted in the formation of the Fracture Committee of the American College of Surgeons, which is now called the Committee on Trauma. As chief of the Orthopaedic Service, Osgood's:

> weekly orthopaedic rounds were stellar performances, not so much because of what he said, but because of the opportunity he offered for all staff members for full discussion. Ultimately he

---

his uncle, Hugh Owen Thomas, before him…The complicated fresh joint fracture, especially if it be compound, is usually safer still as an emergency in the hands of the eminent general surgeon than the eminent orthopaedic surgeon…Later, after the acute surgery is done, the orthopaedic surgeon may be trusted to think of the end result in terms of function…which chiefly concerns the patient; but ought we to be obliged to divide the authority? There is no excuse for failure to acquire good surgical technique… an orthopaedic surgeon…[who] thinks too much operating is being done. This does not excuse him…[from] keep[ing] his 'hands in,' he had much better keep both his hands out and turn his operative work to another. Surgical judgment is a real thing. It is born in few men and is usually acquired only by experience. We have far too small a proportion of operating surgeons whose judgment is good, whose anatomic knowledge is accurate and whose aseptic technique is faultless. We must have a larger portion if we are to talk about conserving function and have our peers as well as our patients listen…We must progress beyond the ultimate wish of the German surgeon, 'I pray that they do not die on my hands' and cherishing the dictum of Ambrose Paré that the first duty of a surgeon is to do no harm, we must contend that his last duty is to give back to the patient his fullest degree of function…The war has suddenly brought into prominence a small specialty. It is fair to say that many honest surgeons believe into too great prominence. Will it remain a specialty? Probably yes.

"We believe that the specialty has rendered a great service to the soldier and to the nation by insisting that locomotive, wage-earning function, conserved and increased, is the chief end of life-saving surgery…that a small group of surgeons were specially fitted to direct this conservation and repair. We believe it was right to do so. It was not being done without them; it is being done with them…

"The name is nothing; the principle is everything, and the principle has been demonstrated to be valid and enormously important in war surgery. The war is over and war surgery will finally disappear. Shall we swing back to rest on our braces or can we apply the principle more widely than we have done to the lesions of civil life? There is a field in which are produced crops of injuries [similar to] war injuries…The field is Industrial Surgery…We believe that industrial surgery opens a wide door to orthopaedic principle and practice…We must still teach human mechanics and even braces. We must track the conservation of function in chronic bone and joint disease…in paralytic conditions…we must learn also…[to] teach how to apply these principles…in traumatic lesions of adults in which chronicity and loss of function are threatened. We must measure up to surgical standards of general surgeons…Our desire is to attract them to the work so as to furnish the best possible treatment to soldiers and civilians and to incorporate these principles of treatment into the education of the general surgeon."

—R. B. Osgood, "The Orthopaedic Outlook." *Journal of Orthopaedic Surgery*, Jan. 1919

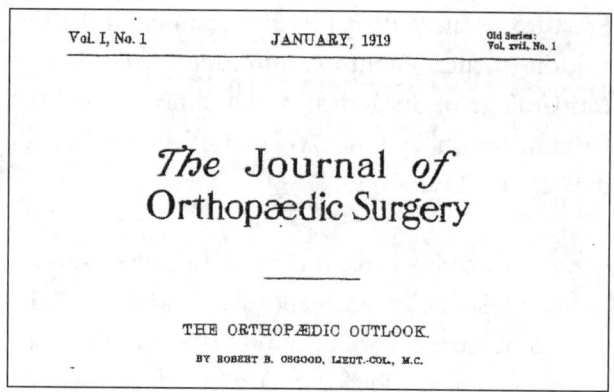

Title of Osgood's article in which he describes the transition of orthopaedists into orthopaedic surgeons and the importance of the specialty. *Journal of Orthopaedic Surgery*, 1919; 1: 1.

summarized the discussion which clearly guided the final decisions as to treatment. He operated only often enough to maintain his technical skill; feeling always that the surgical opportunities should be given to the junior staff surgeons. He devoted himself to his residents, learning to know them and their families personally, so that he was familiar with all their problems. When a man did not come up to the standards required, he redoubled his efforts in the hope that he would find a way to stimulate him and set him on the right path. (P. D. Wilson 1957)

When honorary president of the Robert Jones Orthopaedic Society, Osgood hosted the spring meeting in Boston, April 21 and 22, 1919. The society consisted of practicing orthopaedic surgeons along the east coast of the United States and Canada.

CHIEF AT BOSTON CHILDREN'S HOSPITAL

In June 1921, two-and-one-half years after Osgood published his provocative paper, "The Orthopaedic Outlook," Osgood published his presidential address to the American Orthopaedic Association, "Backgrounds of Orthopaedic Surgery." The themes of both papers were similar: the development of a new specialty in surgery, one that emphasized end results and function. He listed six basic characteristics of orthopaedic surgery (R. B. Osgood 1921b), as contrasted to general surgery:

1. The prevention of deformity;
2. The importance of "rest as a curative agent in diseases and injuries of the bones and joints";
3. The "rational mechanics of rest and protection" by the use of "simple and mechanically perfect splints";
4. The importance of "research and the physiology of surgery...extremities and spinal column," as being essential for the specialty;
5. The essential requirements for an orthopaedic surgeon include "anatomical knowledge, general [surgery] training, and technical skill in surgery"; and
6. Orthopaedic patients (adults and children) should be segregated in specialty departments in hospitals and "hospitals for crippled and deformed children" be developed under the direction of orthopaedic surgeons specializing in the care of the disabled.

Interestingly, he emphasized that this latter new specialty group of surgeons "must be ready to delegate to others...the operative procedure necessary to the fulfillment of our purpose...or else train ourselves to the accuracy of operative technique which the case requires" (R. B. Osgood 1921b). Osgood believed that this was a "temporary limitation, a passing phase" and that with the achievement of the six main characteristics that he listed for his colleagues "universal training of Orthopaedic Surgeons [will lead] to the recognition by great institutions and...State and Federal governments that the segregated care of the handicapped under the direction of specially trained surgeons is not only a humanitarian measure, but of advantage to the body politic" (R. B. Osgood 1921b).

> The first duty of a surgeon is to do no harm; his last duty is to give back to the patient his fullest degree of function.
>
> —R. B. Osgood

In 1922, Osgood left the Massachusetts General Hospital to assume the position of chief of the orthopaedic department at Boston Children's Hospital, the position of leadership in postgraduate training in orthopaedic surgery, and the professor of orthopaedic surgery at HMS. In 1924, he was named the second John Ball and Buckminster Brown Professor of Orthopaedic Surgery, succeeding Robert Lovett. The chair was originally designated for the professor and head of orthopaedics at HMS—a position that traditionally had been located at Boston Children's Hospital—and Osgood persuaded the dean at HMS to extend eligibility for the position to both the chief of Boston Children's Hospital and the chief of MGH.

In his early career, Osgood had demonstrated an interest in poliomyelitis, specifically its transmission route. However, at Boston Children's Hospital, Dr. Arthur Legg managed the infantile paralysis clinics. In addition to his clinical practice, organizational responsibilities, and administrative duties, Osgood emphasized the importance of education and teaching the next generation of orthopaedic surgeons. He met with all the orthopaedic students weekly for a one-hour conference. As recalled by some of his residents:

> one of the most pleasant memories of our Children's training was of tea at five o'clock once a week with Dr. Robert Osgood in his office. It was known as "Bobby Osgood's tea." We seldom missed it…It was a delightful and stimulating hour for us, as Dr. Osgood in his conversation took us out of the hospital to many parts of the United States and the world. In this way, we were introduced to many orthopaedic leaders and personalities, and to current orthopaedic and medical problems and their suggested solutions. (C. L. Rowe 1996)

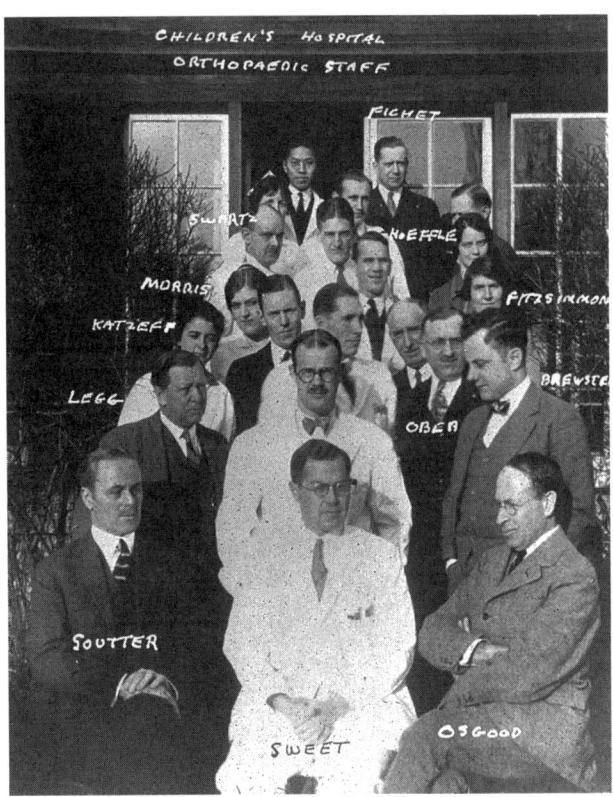

Orthopaedic staff at BCH. Osgood, seated in the front right, is chief of orthopaedics, ca. mid-to-late 1920s.
MGH HCORP Archives.

For years, he held meetings on Sunday mornings at Children's Hospital at which the outcomes of all patients treated at least one year previously were discussed in detail. All residents and staff participated.

In late 1923, the year following Osgood's move to Boston Children's Hospital, Dr. Nathaniel Allison was recruited as the next chief of orthopaedics at MGH. Allison was the chair of orthopaedic surgery and dean of the Washington University School of Medicine. Osgood and Allison had known each other for years, both attended HMS together, graduating two years apart, and had served together in France during World War I. Both were very interested in education. In 1921, Allison had written a thoughtful paper on "The Teaching of Orthopaedic Surgery." (see chapter 36) The educational requirements for training orthopaedic surgeons had become a national topic of discussion, and a special committee of the American Medical Association (N. Allison 1921) reported that:

The minimum requirements to become an orthopaedic surgeon are:

1. Standard medical school course, Class A school, four years
2. Surgical internship at least one year
3. Graduate course, one year as interne on service devoted entirely to orthopaedic surgery
4. Six months in allied studies, physical therapy, shop work, and schools for cripples.

These were not ideal requirements according to Allison. He was of the opinion that "from us, as orthopaedic surgeons, must come the definition of our field of teaching and training for the future orthopaedic surgeons; and in us must be the ability and power, as teachers, to hand on 'to him our knowledge and skill, and to stimulate him to constant advancement'" (N. Allison 1921). Just as Osgood had emphasized the importance of an orthopaedic surgeon to be a surgeon first and a user of splints and braces second, so did Allison, who wrote, "He must always be a surgeon plus considerable of special qualifications. He must never be a specialist with low-grade ability as a surgeon. Much harsh criticism has come upon us from this, one of our faults in the past. Future developments must correct it" (N. Allison 1921). This latter opinion struck a strong chord with Osgood, both firmly believed this.

Both Osgood and Allison were also outstanding teachers and extremely committed to education, specifically orthopaedics to medical students and orthopaedic surgery to medical school graduates who wanted to become orthopaedic surgeons. An opportunity arose for them together, as chief of orthopaedics at Boston Children's Hospital and Harvard and chief of orthopaedics at MGH, to improve postgraduate training in orthopaedic surgery in the Harvard teaching hospitals. In addition, Osgood was a friend to many at MGH, had been a successful chief of the orthopaedic service and also had a strong relationship with the general surgeons, having served as assistant director of the fracture service. He was also a strong leader and excelled in diplomacy. This diplomacy served him well as students across North America were attracted to their program between 1922 and 1930:

The orthopaedic program had been a one-year program at Boston Children's Hospital. It expanded under the leadership of Osgood and Allison to include a second year of adult orthopaedics—especially fracture management—at MGH and six months of basic sciences at HMS.

It was the most advanced and comprehensive program of orthopaedic training in the United States and served as a model for many other medical schools. (P. D. Wilson 1957)

As the professor of orthopaedic surgery at HMS, Osgood also had great influence on the orthopaedic education of medical students. In 1925, he described problems associated with orthopaedic lectures and the changes he and the faculty made in the third-year curriculum:

The subjects to be considered in the twelve lectures have been chosen, not because of their prime importance in the practice of orthopaedic surgery as a specialty, but rather because of their important relationship to the practice of general medical and general surgery...[each lecture was] written out...to stress the fundamentals of etiology and diagnosis, and...the broad general principles of a rational therapy...a few references...given...the lecture was given to each man...about a week before...the date set for the delivery of the lecture [for] the students...to read...The lecture hour [was] divided into three twenty-minute periods...first twenty minutes the students...ask[ed] the lecturer questions...the second twenty minutes...were devoted...to illustrative cases and the third and last twenty minutes the lecturer quizzed the students. (R. B. Osgood 1925b)

Osgood concluded that "the results of this lecture system seem to us to justify its continuance... the students...liked it...their interest in the subject stimulated...the students [had a] greater grasp of the subject...We are...hopeful that some of these fundamentals will be acquired permanently and be found useful in the practice of medicine" (R. B. Osgood 1925b).

Osgood also gave two major named lectures in 1925. He gave the First Detroit Orthopaedic Lecture to the Wayne County Medical Society. In addition to tracing important discoveries in orthopaedics, he closed by stressing the need for future changes in the profession: specifically, more focus on investigation and less on therapy as a means to continue the evolution and transformation of the orthopaedics specialty. Before the Medical Institution of Liverpool, on June 2, 1925, he gave the Hugh Owen Thomas Lecture entitled "The Orthopaedic Aspects of Chronic Arthritis."

Other Achievements

In 1930, Osgood "retired voluntarily, earlier than necessary, in order to make room for a younger man" (P. D. Wilson 1957). Mr. H. J. Seddon said:

> the most outstanding quality of Dr. Robert Osgood's, greater even than his reputation as a surgeon, was his beneficence; it embraces causes and individuals alike. His command of orthopaedics was profound...what mattered far more to him was that orthopaedics in America should be done well...I visited two Shriners' hospitals... [and asked] an American friend how it was that all the Shriners' hospitals I had ever visited were staffed by such excellent men. His answer was that from the first the policy had been to appoint only first-class surgeons. 'Bob Osgood used to do it, you know.' (*British Medical Journal* 1957)

He had served as the first chairman of the Advisory Board of Orthopaedic Surgeons to the Trustees of the Shriner's Hospitals for Crippled Children and a member—and later chairman—of the Advisory Committee of the Services for Crippled Children of the Children's Bureau in Washington (Department of Labor). "He was [also] a member of the Advisory Board of the Alfred I. DuPont Institute and helped in planning its hospital" (P. D. Wilson 1957). Even after retiring, Osgood remained active in his vision to improve the caliber of orthopaedic practice and medicine. Dr. Osgood was influenced by Codman's end-result idea, and he was ever driven in his goal to see continued excellence in the field.

Osgood published over 30 papers during his time at Boston Children's Hospital and four books during his career in orthopaedics. In 1931, he and Allison published *Fundamentals of Orthopaedic Surgery in General Medicine and Surgery*, lectures given to the Harvard medical students. They dedicated their book to John Ball and Buckminster Brown, pioneers in orthopaedics, and to Edward Hickling Bradford. These were the same 12 lectures that were given to the third-year students each week before the scheduled lecture. Students were to read and be prepared to ask questions of the lecturer, observe cases, review illustrations, and answer questions asked by the lecturer. The topics (chapters) were:

1. Introduction, General Joint Phenomena
2. The Reactions of Developmental and Adult Bone; Its Response to Infection
3. Nutritional and Growth Disturbances Resulting in Changes in Bones and Joints.
4. Congenital deformities
5. Cerebral and Spastic Palsy; Obstetrical Paralysis; Volkmann's Deformity; Dupuytren's Contracture
6. Scoliosis
7. Tuberculosis
8. Anterior Poliomyelitis (Infantile Paralysis)
9. Chronic Rheumatic Arthritis (Arthritis Deformans)

10. Traumatic Affections of Joints and Bursae
11. The Relation of Orthopaedic Surgery to Industry
12. Body Mechanics and Statics

The purpose of the lectures and the book was to teach medical students enough of orthopaedics "to meet the demand of a general practice with intelligence and safety...to make reasonably accurate diagnoses and recognize certain conditions which demand immediate appropriate treatment" (*Naval Medical Bulletin* 1932).

Osgood, along with coauthors Allison, Wilson, Bucholz, Soutter, Low, Danforth, Brown, Smith-Petersen, and occasionally others, published 31 reports on the progress in orthopaedic surgery from 1912 through 1927. Originally, the "Report of Progress in Orthopaedic Surgery" was published in the *Boston Medical and Surgical Journal* (now the *New England Journal of Medicine*). Thirteen reports, consisting of one-to-four parts were published in different issues of the *Boston Medical and Surgical Journal* until 1919, a period of eight years. Osgood was the first author on all the papers, except for 1917 (one part) and 1919 (two parts). Hermann Bucholz was first author in 1919, and Murray Danforth was first author in 1917. Osgood, a coauthor, was listed as lieutenant colonel in these reports during World War I. No progress report was published in 1918. There was no report published in 1920, but they resumed in 1921 in the *Archives of Surgery*. Over the next seven years, Osgood and his coauthors published another 18 reports, consisting of one or two parts in different issues of the journal. Osgood remained first author on all reports, except for number 26 (one part) and number 27 (two parts) in 1925. Allison was first author on reports numbers 26 and 27. He had joined the group as coauthor in 1924. In 1923, Smith-Petersen joined the group as a coauthor. Occasionally an additional one-time coauthor participated, such as Arman Klein and Loring T. Swaim. Over a total of 25 years, the group published 31 progress reports, 25 parts in the *Boston Medical and Surgical Journal*, 23 parts in the *Archives of Surgery*. The last progress report was published in 1931. Philip Wilson was first author. Osgood published an additional 22 papers after retiring as chief at Boston Children's Hospital in 1930, covering a wide variety of topics.

In New England, Osgood was president of the New England Surgical Society in 1928, a member of the Physician's Committee for the Improvement of Medical Care, a trustee of the Massachusetts Hospital School at Canton, and a member of the Massachusetts Medical Society. "In 1931, on his retirement from the Medical School, the *New England Journal of Medicine* devoted an issue to honoring his career and his contributions" (J. S. Barr et al. 1957). "This journal contains several articles which are contributions from the Orthopedic Department of the Children's Hospital...most of the work set down in the individual papers went on while he was chief of the Orthopedic Department" (*New England Journal of Medicine* 1933). Included was a brief tribute to Osgood and nine original articles from his colleagues and staff at Boston Children's Hospital, including Ober, Souter, Legg, Sever, FitzSimmons, Brewster, Fitchet, Morris, and Katzeff. In 1943, the *Archives of Surgery* dedicated an issue to Dr. Osgood, which was organized "by his former associates on the

---

SPECIAL NUMBER

DEDICATED TO

DR. ROBERT BAYLEY OSGOOD
Emeritus Professor of Orthopedic Surgery,
Harvard Medical School

BY

HIS FORMER ASSOCIATES ON THE OCCASION
OF HIS SEVENTIETH BIRTHDAY

Title of the special issue of *Archives of Surgery* dedicated to Dr. Osgood on his 70th birthday. *Archives of Surgery* 1943; 46: 589-590.

occasion of his seventieth birthday" (Kuhns 1943). There were 33 publications on a wide range of orthopaedic topics: five on fractures, one on rehabilitation after the war in Great Britain, a biography of the contributions of Henry Jacob Bigelow, and 12 articles of surgical treatments. Two unusual papers were about an operation for recurrent dislocation of the jaw and dysmenorrhea as a result of a postural defect. Two articles became well-known and frequently read: treatment of slipped capital femoral epiphysis at the MGH by Klein, Joplin and Reidy; and a review of surgical operations of the upper extremity in rheumatoid arthritis by Smith-Petersen, Aufranc, and Larson.

Osgood's efforts and personal friendships influenced the formation of several major orthopaedic national and international organizations, especially the British Orthopaedic Association. Osgood was a "specially invited guest" at the first meeting of the British Orthopaedic Association, which was held February 2, 1918. His diplomacy and tireless efforts had played a significant role in its founding. Others included the Canadian Orthopaedic Association and the International Society of Orthopaedic Surgery and Traumatology (SICOT). He became a member of SICOT, an honorary member of the British Orthopaedic Association, as well as an honorary member of the Australian Orthopaedic Association, the Italian and the Scandinavian Orthopaedic Associations, an honorary fellow of the Royal College of Surgeons and the Royal Society of Medicine. He was also an active member of the American Academy of Orthopaedic Surgeons and the American College of Surgeons.

Additional honors he received included, "the degree of Doctor of Science, honoris causa, from Amherst College in 1935" (P. D. Wilson 1957). He was also a corresponding member of the Belgian Orthopaedic Association (J. G. Kuhns 1943). He was president of the American Orthopaedic Association in 1920. The American Orthopaedic Association's meeting in June 1921, with Osgood as president, met in Boston. It was the largest meeting in the history of the organization; Lovett, Bradford, Ober, Sever, Lloyd T. Brown, Painter, Mark H. Rogers, Brackett, FitzSimmons, Smith-Petersen, Goldthwait, Loring T. Swain, Z. B. Adams, Philip Wilson, Augustus Thorndike, John Dane, and Soutter participated in the operational functions of the meeting. Osgood's guests included Sir Robert Jones and Professor Putti. Dr. Nathaniel Allison was elected president to follow Dr. Osgood, and "as a member of the American Committee on Rheumatism, [Osgood] helped to organize the American Rheumatism Association (President, 1944)" (P. D. Wilson 1957). In 1944, a "group of [his former] pupils and associates united to arrange for the painting of his portrait by Mr. Samuel Hopkinson. This excellent work now hangs in the Massachusetts General Hospital" (P. D. Wilson 1957).

On December 18, 1939, Osgood read a paper before the New York Medical Society entitled "The National Health Act of 1939." It was later published in the *New England Journal of Medicine*. The occasion was a symposium on the Wagner Health Bill, Senate Bill 1620, which would mandate use of federal funds for healthcare. Osgood was a member of the Committee of Physicians for the Improvement of Medical Care, "which expressed its sympathy with the general purpose of the Wagner Bill, and agrees with the American Medical Association that a functional co-ordination of all federal and medical activities is almost a necessity…there should be an allotment of such funds as Congress may make available to any state in actual need for…prevention of disease…promotion of health and the care of the sick…should be an extension of medical care for the indigent and medically indigent" (R. B. Osgood 1940a). After a detailed review of the issues, Osgood stated: "I subscribe to the belief, which I think is rather generally held, that no nationwide system of compulsory health insurance should be imposed, and that the non-profit voluntary systems which are spreading so fast should be given a fair and sympathetic trial" (R. B. Osgood 1940a). In the same year, in an obvious toast before an unknown alumni group

(R. B. Osgood 1939a), Osgood raised similar issues being debated today: the role of government in healthcare, national health insurance, the care of the indigent, and the need for financial support of medical education and medical research. His speech appears in **Box 19.5**.

LEGACY

Dr. Robert Osgood had married Margaret Louisa on April 29, 1902. They had one daughter, Ellen Osgood Jennings, and four grandchildren. P. D. Wilson described Osgood as conveying a "strong

Box 19.5. Osgood's Speech: "The Nation and the Hospital" (Before an Unknown Alumni Group)

"Mr. Osborne, Guests and Gentlemen of the Alumni: I think I am reasonably sober, but if I were not I am sure that I should become so in attempting to reply to the toast, 'The Nation and the Hospital.' The future relation of the nation to such a splendid philanthropic private hospital [Massachusetts General Hospital] as this is a very sobering matter. A recent thoughtful book is entitled, "Medicine at the Cross Road" [by Bertram M. Bernheim, 1939]. It is of the utmost importance that medicine and the great privately endowed hospitals take that road of progress which will give them the fullest opportunity to serve their fellow men.

"The evolution of medicine and its application in the form of medical care has progressed more rapidly than the evolution of economics and sociology. The majority of the medical profession believe that medicine, if left alone, can be trusted to improve steadily the quality of medical care without governmental interference either Federal, State or Local. However certain portents have appeared in the medical skies of the United States which strongly suggest that the medical profession is not to be allowed to thus proceed without interference to improve the quality and if necessary, to increase the quantity of medical care.

"Perhaps the most significant of these portentous signs is the amount of space now given in the daily press and in the popular magazines to medical matters. The lay appetite for medical articles is becoming increasingly avid. Medicine has outgrown the days of charms and secret formulae and of 'wizard men.' It is being 'exposed' and the curtain is being raised by the physicians themselves. This is as it should be. If the illumination is fair and complete, not discovered by tricky lighting or distorted by prejudice, the foundations of medicine will be discovered to be as firm as ever and the superstructure architecturally sound. Neither need we fear that the spirit which today activates the vast majority of physicians will appear less noble than the spirit which dictated the oath of Hippocrates.

"The Public is the great consumer of medical care. If it becomes convinced that the quality of medical care is inferior, or the quantity insufficient, public opinion will demand that existing conditions be bettered.

"This 'consumer demand' has become audible.

"If the Federal surveys are reliable, there are some 40 million people living in families whose total annual income is less than nine hundred dollars. These people are not indigent, but it is quite evident that in case of need they cannot, even by the most careful budgeting, purchase the best that medicine is now to provide in the way of prevention and treatment of disease and injury. If we accept the premise that health is not a commodity, and that every citizen and his dependents have as inalienable a right to health as they have to 'life, liberty and the pursuit of happiness,' then some organization either medical, philanthropic, or governmental must endeavor to do something about it. The consumers of medical care demand that it shall be done. The members of the medical profession are the experts who should plan this 'something-to-be-done' and being experts, are most likely to plan wisely. They cannot pin a sign on themselves, 'Noli me tangere' and then bury their heads in the sand in false security. The votes of our one hundred and forty thousand physicians will not bulk large against the many million votes of laymen.

"Unless the medical profession is ready to be the star actor in the drama and win over its public audience, the Federal and State governments may feel, in duty bound, to steal the role although they are likely to play the part somewhat awkwardly.

"The Wagner Health bill now before the Senate is a case in point. It seems to many of us to be an honest attempt to make available to the indigent and the low income groups tradition of elegance," including "elegance of appearance, of behavior, and of professional work. Those who took his Second Year Course in Bandaging will remember his insistence on form and appearance as well as effective function in surgical dressings, and they will never forget his final demonstration. Dressed in impeccable morning clothes, he applied a plaster cast (a body spica), making a beautiful cast and ending up without a spot on his elegant and unprotected garments" (P. D. Wilson 1957). It was of the utmost importance that everything was impeccable, from

> a higher grade of medical care than it is now possible for them to command. It recognizes the rights of the individual states to work out their own programs and the outstanding contributions to the improvement of medical care which privately endowed institutions like your own have made and are continuing to make. It proposed to make the fullest possible use of these independent institutions. Nevertheless, as physicians, we believe the bill to be seriously defective in many respects. One of the most glaring defects of the bill is that no provision is made for Federal grants-in-aid for medical education or research. Upon the brains, the bill calls for large appropriations of federal money, perhaps not enough, perhaps too much.
>
> "You are all aware that the Federal Treasury is dangerously ill. Perhaps another serious defect in the bill is that there is no provision for a special hospital consecrated to the recovery of the U.S. Treasury.
>
> "The last portent we shall mention is the increasing participation of the Government in the practice of medicine. Over 50% of all the hospital beds in the United States are today supported by Federal or State or Civic governments. We have already become accustomed, for example, to think of hospitals for the insane and sanatoria for tuberculosis as public institutions. It is no longer possible for the Federal or State departments of public health to confine their activities to sanitation and the control of epidemics. Preventive and curative medicine have grown to be not only close relatives but insuperable Siamese twins. Practitioners of medicine are finding that departments of public health [i.e. governmental] and their laboratories and hospitals are already essential to the practice of medicine.
>
> "Where will this so called 'socialized' or 'state medicine' stop? We do not know the answer. Many of us do not fear continuing socializing of medicine if philanthropy is unable to provide the facilities which the private practitioner and his patients require for efficient treatment. What nearly all of us do fear (and will resist) is the socialization or regimentation of physicians and of the great privately endowed hospitals and clinics. I am an optimist and I believe we shall find an American way out. If hospitals are placed under direct governmental control there is grave danger that their hearts will become sclerotic. The hospital with a sclerotic heart is moribund. You may remember one of Santyana's early sonnets:
>
> > 'It is not wisdom to be only wise.
> > But it is wisdom to believe the heart —
> > Columbus found a world and had no chart
> > Save the one faith deciphered in the skies.
> > To trust the soul's invincible surmise
> > Was all his science and his only art.'
>
> "This hospital has never hardened its heart and in my opinion, at thirty years of observation, the multiple heart of the trustees and the staff is beating today more strongly and efficiently and sympathetically than ever before and I offer it my warmest congratulations.
>
> "I hope it is fitting for me to express my conviction that since the advent of the present director not only has this splendid old hospital taken on a new lease of life, but the whole spirit of orthopaedic surgery in this great city has become more effective and cooperative than ever before. I will not try to commend him in detail for our warm friendship and our former intimate colleagual [sic] relations in war and in peace would make my testimony partial and prejudiced. My feeling for him is in the same place as that of the little girl, etc."
>
> —R. B. Osgood, "The Nation and the Hospital," 1939

research to character. He had been a driving force in orthopaedic practice and education, and Herbert Seddon—internationally famous for his classification of nerve injuries still used today—gave the following tribute remembering his first visit to Boston Children's Hospital:

> I met Dr. Osgood [about 1930] and, having listened to him in the course of a ward round, I realized that here was a great man…when we finished he asked me if I could sing…[and] asked me to have dinner with him that evening and then go with him to a carol practice… Dr. Osgood was a respectable tenor…(Dr. Philip Wilson in an adjoining group was, I think, a magnificent basso profundo). On Christmas Eve we were let loose on Beacon Hill, and finished up in the snow-covered courtyard of the Massachusetts General Hospital for our last performance. Then we went back to Beacon Hill…in no house was the welcome warmer than in Dr. and Mrs. Osgood's; there was supper for everyone and presents from the Christmas tree…I was one of scores of young men who Robert Osgood guided with good advice, always given greatly and humbly. This cultivated Bostonian, one of the small band of outstanding men who gave their city its unique place in orthopaedics…all that is best in American orthopaedic surgery owes something to Robert Osgood. (*British Medical Journal* 1957)

Dr. Osgood continued to write poems during his lifetime. He had published anonymously in the Amherst Graduates Quarterly, *The News*. In 1943, he published a poem entitled, "The Unforgiven Sin," stating that men and women struggle and fight to shape the world. For Osgood the unforgiven sin was lethargy. Dr. Osgood died at the age of 84 on October 2, 1956. Dr. Rodney F. Atsatt (MGH orthopaedics, 1926) wrote: "Robert B. Osgood was an individual [who] has inspired his students and colleagues" (MGH HCORP

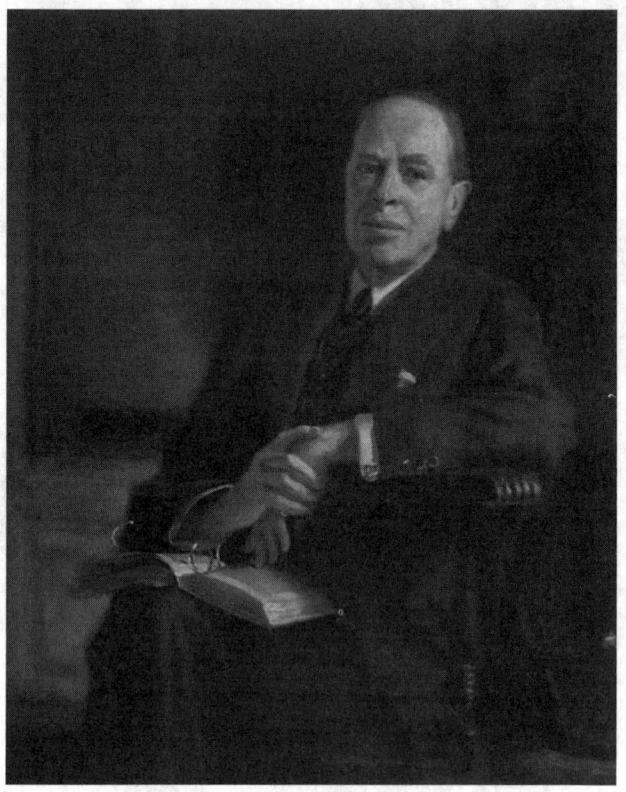

Portrait of Dr. Osgood. Massachusetts General Hospital, Archives and Special Collections.

Archives). Dr. George H. Jackson Jr. (MGH orthopaedics, 1919) wrote: "All who have been privileged to serve under Dr. Osgood know how truly this expression of regard to their own former chief, whose kind sympathy and ready understanding will never be forgotten (MGH HCORP Archives). On November 4, 1956, the medical advisory board of the Alfred I. DuPont Institute of Nemours Foundation wrote the following resolution (MGH HCORP Archives): an expression of "deepest appreciation for what Dr. Osgood did for the Foundation and the Institute and gave it to his wife and daughter [Mrs. Ellen Osgood Jennings]." Thirteen members of the board signed the resolution included Joseph S. Barr, Philip D. Wilson, Alfred R. Shands Jr., and Mrs. Alfred I. DuPont. The Osgood Visiting Professor was later established in his honor, with the first lecture given in the 1980s (**Box 19.6**).

Box 19.6. The Osgood Visiting Professor

Early 1980s
    Thornton Brown, M.D. "Orthopaedics at Harvard: The First 200 Years"
1983
    Henry H. Banks, M.D. "Osgood Lecture"
1999
    Joseph A. Buckwalter, M.D. "Surgical Methods of Restoring Articular Cartilage"
2000
    Robert B. Bourne, M.D. "An Experiment with Electronic Point-of-Care Data Collection: The Southwestern Ontario Joint Replacement Pilot Project"
2001
    Vernon T. Tolo, M.D. "The Evolution of Pediatric Fracture Care"
2002
    James D. Heckman, M.D. "Subtle Injuries of the Ankle and Foot"
2003
    Scott Boden, M.D. "Bone Graft Substitutes: Update 2003"
2004
    James E. Nunley, M.D. "Achilles Tendon Disorders: Non-insertional and Insertional Disease"
2005
    Frank Eismont, M.D. "Infections of the Spine"
2006
    Russell F. Warren, M.D. "Progress in treating Rotator Cuff Disease"
2007
    James Kellam, M.D. "Orthopaedic Trauma: Our Evolution and Future"
2008
    Vincent D. Pellegrini, Jr., M.D. "Prevention of Pulmonary Embolism after Total Joint Arthroplasty: Who Knows Best?"
2009
    James H. Herndon, M.D., MBA "The Birth of a Specialty"
2010
    James N. Weinstein, D.O. "Where's the Wisdom in Healthcare"
2011
    James Heckman, M.D. "Pursuing Research Throughout Your Orthopaedic Career"
2012
    Ken Yamaguchi, M.D. "Risk and Clinical Significance of Rotator Cuff Deterioration: Implications for Treatment"
2013
    Tony Herring, M.D. "No Limits: Stories of Human Adaptability"
2014
    James H. Herndon, M.D., MBA "Significant Historic Events in Boston's Orthopaedic History"
2015
    Peter J. Stern, M.D. "Man's Inhumanity to Man"
2016
    Daniel J. Berry, M.D. "Introduction of New Technology in Orthopaedic Surgery: Lessons from Joint Arthroplasty"
2017
    Robert V. O'Toole, M.D. "Do We Know Who Has Compartment Syndrome?"
2018
    William N. Levine, M.D. "Education in Orthopaedic Surgery—It's Not as Easy as It Used to Be!"
2019
    Scott H. Kozin, M.D. "Touching Hands Project: Inception to Implementation"
2020
Canceled due to COVID-19

CHAPTER 20

Frank R. Ober
Caring Clinician and Skilled Educator

Frank Roberts Ober, "of Down-East Yankee stock" (Joseph S. Barr 1962), was born on June 1, 1881, to Otis Meriam Ober and Melita Josephine Roberts. He was born in Mount Desert, Maine, on Mount Desert Island, which encompasses a large swath of Acadia National Park. This small town, incorporated in 1789, had a census of only 2,109 people (962 households) in 2000. During Ober's youth, Mount Desert became increasingly popular as a location for summer residences of wealthy families—the Rockefellers, Fords, Vanderbilts, Carnegies, and others. He chose to attend college at Westbrook Seminary, a coeducational institution near Portland, Maine, about 170 miles from Mount Desert. (Note that in the nineteenth century, the terms "college," "seminary," and "institute" were used interchangeably.) Established in 1831 by the Kennebec Association of Universalists, Westbrook's purpose—like that of any college—was to educate. The seminary also taught piety and morality. In the early 1930s, it was renamed Westbrook Junior College. In 1996, it merged with the University of New England, becoming the Westbrook College Campus or the Portland campus.

Ober left Westbrook after two years and entered Tufts University Medical School. He graduated from Tufts in 1905. After receiving his medical degree, Ober completed a one-year rotating internship at Carney Hospital. He then returned home to Mount Desert Island and opened a general practice in Northeast Harbor, where his only

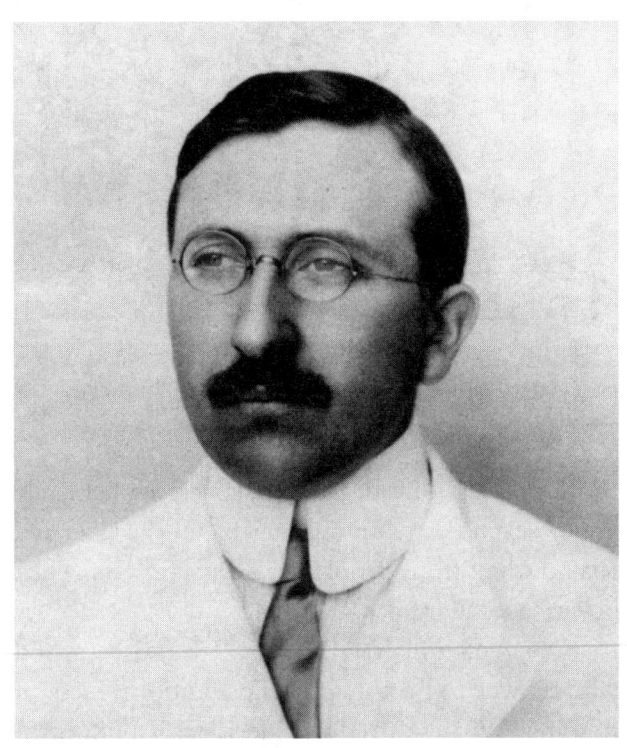

Dr. Frank R. Ober as an orthopaedic resident at BCH in 1914.
Boston Children's Hospital Archives, Boston, Massachusetts.

Physician Snapshot

Frank R. Ober
BORN: 1881
DIED: 1960
SIGNIFICANT CONTRIBUTIONS: Developed and perfected many muscle transfer procedures; developed a test to determine *tensor fascia lata* contracture (the Ober test); provided care to hundreds of children with polio and other disabilities; substantially influenced the development of graduate and postgraduate medical education

143

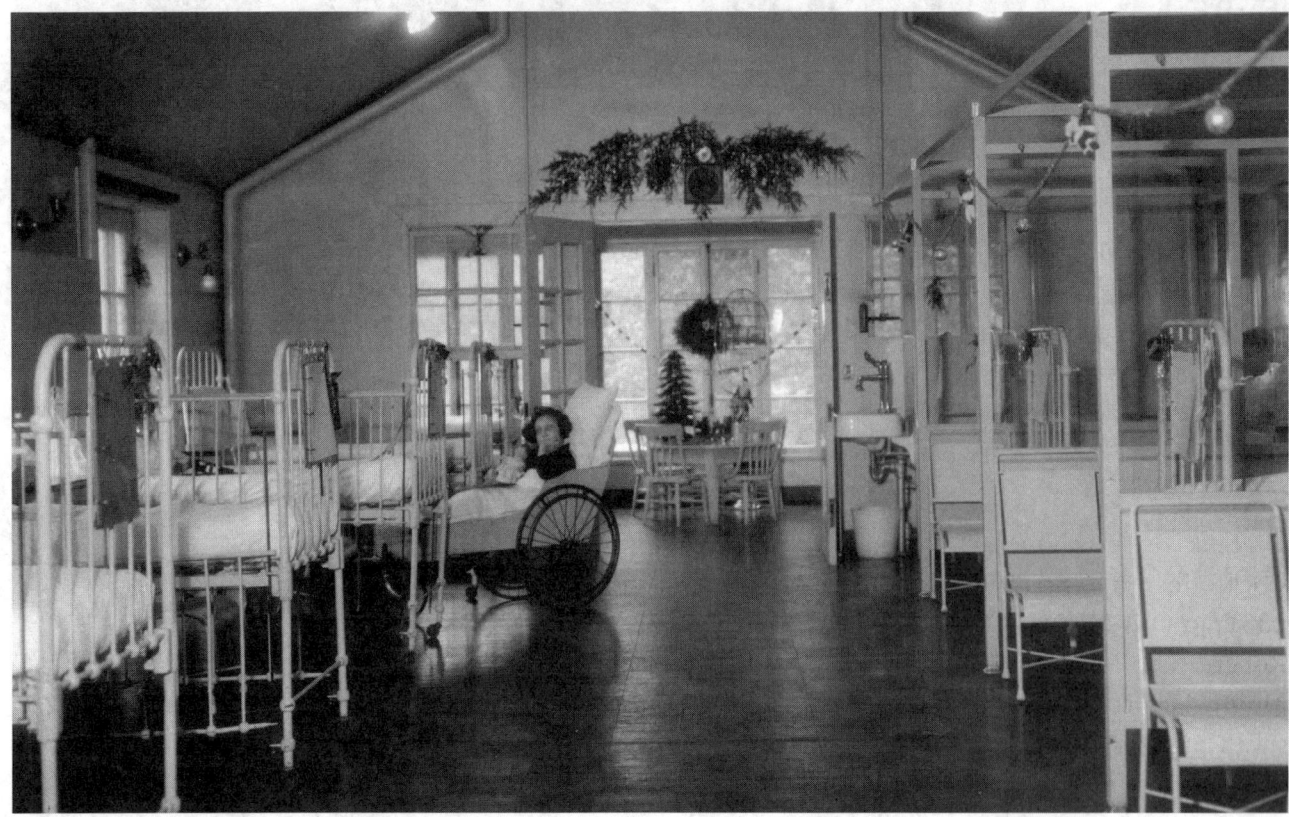

Standard ward in Children's Hospital in 1914. *The Children's Hospital of Boston: Built Better Than They Knew* by Clement A. Smith. Boston: Little, Brown and Co., 1983. Boston Children's Hospital Archives, Boston, Massachusetts.

brother, Ernest, lived. Ober practiced medicine for about seven years, during which time he married Ina Spurling from Brookline, Massachusetts. They never had children.

Ober left his practice in 1913 and returned with his wife to Boston to obtain additional medical training. What spurred this decision is unknown. He began a second internship at Children's Hospital, after which he became "the first resident in orthopaedics [there] under the late Dr. Robert W. Lovett, who had originally inspired Dr. Ober to enter this field" (*New England Journal of Medicine* 1961). Ober's one year of specialized training (residency) in orthopaedic surgery began the evolution of the residency program at Massachusetts General Hospital and Children's Hospital—what would, about 65 years later, become the Harvard Combined Orthopaedic Residency Program. Ober completed his orthopaedic residency in September 1915, becoming the second house officer on the orthopaedic service. (Around 1910, several years before Ober became an orthopaedic resident, Henry J. FitzSimmons had completed a six-month internship in orthopaedics under Dr. Lovett. Chapter 23 provides more details about FitzSimmons's education and career.) In 1915, Ober joined the staff at Children's Hospital and the faculty at Harvard Medical School, "where he continued for the rest of his life" (R. B. Osgood 1935).

EARLY LIFE AND CLINICAL CONTRIBUTIONS

Ober's mastery of anatomy and his surgical planning and skill resulted in excellent outcomes for his patients. His brusque attitude often intimidated nervous residents and nurses—"even Dr. [William] Green was afraid of him" (H. Yett, pers comm. 2013)—but he was always kind and generous toward his patients, whatever their circumstances. "One of Dr. Ober's great contributions to life was his gentle and loving care of his patients. Beneath his calm exterior, he had a great human sympathy, with a keen and kindly appreciation of the personal as well as the physical needs of his patients" (Massachusetts Medical Society 1961). This care for his patients was one reason he had been able to build a large and successful practice at Children's Hospital just as he had in Maine. His practice kept him busy, and he frequently (often monthly) consulted for patients in New York and occasionally in Philadelphia. Ober returned to Maine every August, where he provided care to both seasonal residents and locals in Northeast Harbor.

OPERATIVE CORRECTION OF CLUB FEET

Ober made quick work of original contributions to the field while completing his residency program; "he also made an important contribution to the operative correction of club feet by his procedure… in which he divided the deltoid ligament and any other restraining bands on the medial side of the foot" (L. Mayer 1950). In 1915, Ober reported his experience in treating club feet:

> After studying several hundred cases before and after several methods of treatment, and eight specimens in various stages of dissection, certain conclusions were drawn…First the equinus is due principally to a contracted Achilles tendon and a short posterior calcaneofibular ligament… The varus is due to contraction of the posterior and anterior tibial tendons, an outward rotation of the anterior end of the astragalus and the os calcis and to an adduction of the forefoot [with] subluxations and dislocations of the mid-tarsal joint and the posterior tarsal joint…The inversion of the whole foot is due to contraction of the two tibial tendons and of the deltoid ligament. (F. R. Ober 1915)

In that paper Ober described his operation in 10 children aged three to 13 years. Through a medial approach, he dissected:

> both layers of the deltoid ligament…as a flap dissected off the bone [distal tibia]…the superior calcaneo-scaphoid ligament is divided transversely…these ligaments are actually boned off of the inferior surface of the sustentaculum tali and well down on the internal surface of the os calcis. It is not often necessary to cut the posterior tibial tendon…and… not necessary to cut the Achilles tendon except in older children. The plantar fascia may be divided if there is considerable cavus… The foot is manipulated into an overcorrected position…The deltoid ligament is sutured at either corner, low down on the malleolus, so that this important structure will be preserved intact…A plaster is applied from the toes to mid-thigh, maintaining the foot in the overcorrected position and the knee flexed to a right angle. (F. R. Ober 1915)

His report was one of the earliest to illustrate the importance of releasing the medial deltoid ligament to correct resistant inversion of the hindfoot.

WORLD WAR I AND RESUMING CLINICAL PRACTICE

After a few years at Children's Hospital, Ober joined other orthopaedic surgeons from Harvard in volunteering for duty in the US Army in May 1917, just after the United States entered World War I. He was assigned to work in France at Army Base Hospital No. 5, where he headed up the orthopaedic department until April 7, 1919. He was honorably discharged in 1919 with the rank of lieutenant colonel.

Returning to Boston, Ober resumed his practice at Children's Hospital in association with

Lovett. That year, at Harvard Medical School, Ober was appointed an instructor in orthopaedic surgery. After only a few years on the staff at Children's Hospital, Ober demonstrated his vision and inclusiveness of the future of medical education. He joined Dr. James S. Stone from Children's Hospital and Harvard, along with other noted faculty from medical schools throughout the United States, to speak at the "First Post-Graduate Course in Medicine and Surgery for Negros in the South" at the John A. Andrew Memorial Hospital (Tuskegee Institute) in Alabama. Its successful conclusion advanced the "belie[f] that this coming together of the white and colored physicians in the launching of this post-graduate course means that a distinctly new epoch is established in negro medical education" (*New England Journal of Medicine* 1921).

Initially, his practice had been associated with Lovett's at 234 Marlborough Street in Boston. Albert H. Brewster later joined Lovett and Ober's practice there (chapter 23). After Lovett's death in 1924, Ober and Brewster remained together, along with Nathaniel Allison and Ralph Ghormley, in private practice. Joseph S. Barr became an associate in 1929. Their group became Marlborough Medical Associates and continued to expand. Over the next 30 years, numerous other physicians joined the practice, including: Eugene E. Record, Dr. Thomas I. DeLorme, Paul W. Hugenberger, and Charles L. Sturdevant. In 1960, Record and DeLorme resigned from the group, leaving Ober, Brewster, Hugenberger, and Sturdevant together at 234 Marlborough Street.

APPROACH TO THE HIP AND THE SHELF PROCEDURE

Another of Ober's early innovative approaches to clinical practice included modifying the posterior approach to the hip joint, described by Jones and Lovett, by making an incision:

in line with the neck of the femur directly over the center...fibers of the gluteus maximus are in line with the skin wound. These fibers are separated...The fatty layer is now separated by blunt dissection...the short rotators are divided in the direction of the neck...The capsule is split throughout its entire length...the ascetabulum [sic] and neck are freely exposed.
(F. R. Ober 1924)

He preferred his method over the standard approaches developed by Langenbock and Kocher, which were widely used at the time. He believed his approach was "a more direct muscle splitting approach to the joint than those above" (F. R. Ober 1924). His concern with Langenbock's and Kocher's approaches was that "there is considerable hemorrhage to be controlled...a distinct disadvantage on account of the depth of the wound [, and] the communication to the joint is not so direct... making drainage in septic cases more difficult" (F. R. Ober 1924). After describing in detail one patient treated with his modified surgical approach, Ober concluded that "rapid and free drainage was obtained with a minimum of bleeding" (F. R. Ober 1924). Indications for the operation included "1) Septic arthritis of the hip joint; 2) Osteomyelitis of the neck of the femur; 3) Excision of the head of the femur; 4) Osteotomy of the neck of the femur; 5) Removal of foreign bodies" (F. R. Ober 1924).

MODIFICATION OF THE USE OF THE SACROSPINALIS

In the lower extremity, he described a modification of the use of the sacrospinalis (erector spinae) muscles in treating paralysis of the gluteus maximus, which Lange and Kreuscher had each previously described separately. Lange used heavy silk sutures to attach the muscles to the greater trochanter. Kreuscher modified the operation by placing a piece of fascia lata between the muscle

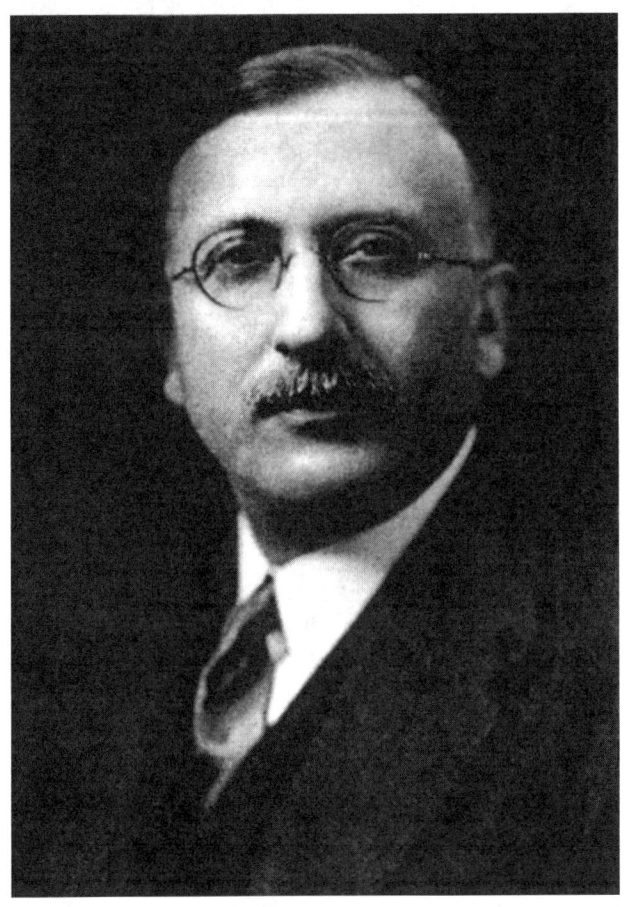

Dr. Ober when he was chief of the orthopaedic department at BCH. *Journal of Bone and Joint Surgery*, 1962; 44:787.

VOLUME 88 JOUR. A. M. A.
NUMBER 14 APRIL 2, 1927

AN OPERATION FOR THE RELIEF OF PARALYSIS OF THE GLUTEUS MAXIMUS MUSCLE

FRANK R. OBER, M.D.
BOSTON

Title of Ober's article on the use of erector spinae muscles transfer for a weak gluteus maximus muscle.
Journal of the American Medical Association 1927; 88: 1063.

and the crest of the ilium to prevent adhesions. Ober modified the transfer by replacing large silk sutures with a long, thin piece of fascia lata and iliotibial band to connect the freed erector spinae muscles:

A free flap of muscle about 5 inches long, 1 inch wide and three-fourths inch thick...a long flap of fascia 1 inch wide...[was] drawn through the hole [made at the level of the gluteus maximus tendon insertion on the femur] from before, backward...The free end of the fascial flap was drawn up under the gluteal fascia...care being taken to keep the gliding surface of the fascia next to the iliac bone...the edges of the fascial flap and the aponeurosis of the erector spinae muscle [overlapped 2 or 3 inches] were sutured under moderate tension.
(F. R. Ober 1927)

After describing a successful case, Ober reported that he had done the operation on 14 other patients; he implied that these were also successful.

SURGEON-IN-CHIEF AND IMPORTANT CLINICAL CONTRIBUTIONS

In 1930, Dr. Ober was promoted to assistant professor of orthopaedic surgery at Harvard Medical School. After Robert Osgood's retirement the following year, Ober, now 50 years old, was named surgeon-in-chief of the Orthopedic Department at Children's Hospital and a clinical professor of orthopedic surgery at HMS. He became the John Ball and Buckminster Brown Clinical Professor of Orthopedic Surgery by 1937, an appointment he held until 1946 (*New England Journal of Medicine* 1961).

Transfers to Supplement Weakened or Paralyzed Muscles

In 1931, Ober reported to the Vermont State Medical Society his and Lovett's experiences operating on patients with polio and their rehabilitation. He named five "general rules in tendon transplantation" (F. R. Ober 1931):

1. To remove fixed deformities.
2. To be sure that there are muscles enough of good function present so that the transplant will function in its new position.
3. To see that the tendon is inserted so that sufficient leverage will be obtained to make the transplant function.
4. To have the tendon go as nearly in line with the one it replaces as is possible.
5. To transplant the tendon under fascial compartments and not through tunnels in the fat. Fat tunnels make for adhesions.

Ober then described the stabilization procedures he preferred for the ankle and foot, as well as various tendons at the hip, knee, shoulder, and hand that could be transferred to substitute for weakened or paralyzed muscles. He had developed these transfers on the basis of his extensive experience treating polio patients in Vermont. Ober's name is attached to other transfers as well. In one, the fascia lata is attached to the erector spinae muscles to help strengthen a weakened gluteus maximus. In another, in the upper extremity, the biceps and triceps are proximally transferred in order to restore shoulder abduction in cases of paralysis of the deltoid muscle. He transferred the proximal long head of the triceps (with a small piece of bone attached) to a bone flap on the posterior aspect of the acromion, and transferred the short head of the biceps so it was attached to the anterior aspect of a split acromion. Both transfers were then sutured together one inch from the tip of the acromion. He preferred this transfer over shoulder arthrodesis because "in children arthrodesis is not particularly satisfactory because the weight of the arm causes the humerus to bend downward either at the joint or at the epiphyseal line" (F. R. Ober 1932b). One patient "was able to raise the arm voluntarily against gravity and hold it in either the forward or lateral position. She could also elevate her arm above her head" (F. R. Ober 1932b).

> JOUR. A. M. A.
> DEC. 24, 1932
>
> AN OPERATION TO RELIEVE PARALYSIS OF THE DELTOID MUSCLE
>
> FRANK R. OBER, M.D., BOSTON

Title of Ober's article on tendon transfers for paralysis of the deltoid muscle. *Journal of the American Medical Association* 1932; 99: 2182.

In a tribute to Dr. Robert Osgood, Ober published a paper titled "Tendon Transplantation in the Lower Extremity" in the *New England Journal of Medicine* in 1933. Following his own requirements for a successful outcome after tendon transfers, Ober described the transfers he commonly used in polio victims. In transfers about the ankle joint:

> tendon transplants...must be combined with an arthrodesis for two reasons. First, because removing a tendon from the lateral aspect of the ankle joint and conveying it to another position increases the instability of the joint and, secondly, because stabilizing the joint permits the tendon to divorce itself from its former function of stabilization and speeds up its new function.
> (F. R. Ober 1933)

He then described in detail tendon transfers about the foot and ankle, transfers about the knee for weak quadriceps or hamstring muscles, and transfers about the hip for weak abductors or extensors. He summarized his thoughts at the time (F. R. Ober 1933):

1. Tendon transplantations at the ankle improve function if the cases are well selected and the operative technique is carefully followed out.
2. Tendon transplants combined with stabilizing questions are more useful because

better stability results in better muscular control.

3. Many transplants may be done now which were formily [sic] thought to be valueless.
4. Tendon transplants at the knee result in improved function and better security and stability of the knee.
5. The sartorius and tensor fasciae are the more ideal muscles to use; first, because of their anatomical situation, and secondly, the function of these two muscles is not so opposite as that of the hamstrings.
6. Transplants at the hip result in improved function and minimize an unsightly and troublesome gait.

Author Recollections

During my residency in the late 1960s and more recently, however, a common rumor circulated about Dr. Ober and a triple arthrodesis. On at least one occasion, Ober had driven the osteotome through the patient's foot and into the sandbag supporting it. Dr. Henry H. Banks (1999), who as a resident had assisted Ober in the operating room, described Ober as a quick and efficient surgeon and an excellent teacher with a strong and commanding personality.

Vermont's Poliomyelitis Rehabilitation Program

Upon Ober's return to Children's Hospital in 1919 after serving in World War I, Lovett had turned over to him the responsibilities of Vermont's poliomyelitis rehabilitation program, which Ober led until 1944. Traveling around Vermont in 1933, Ober "conducted clinics in ten towns of the state, with an attendance of 485 patients" (*New England Journal of Medicine* 1933). He would perform operations free of charge. Ober gained a tremendous amount of clinical experience in these polio clinics and developed joint stabilization procedures and muscle/tendon transfers to replace muscles in the shoulder, elbow, hip, knee, and ankle that had been weakened by polio. His techniques gained traction throughout the field and were used by both his resident-trainees and his peers.

Treatment for Hip Abductor Paralysis

In cases of hip abductor paralysis, Ober achieved excellent results with the use of the Legg technique of transferring the origin of the tensor fascia lata posteriorly in line with the femur and inserting the *fascia lata* into the lateral femur below the trochanter. He modified the procedure by mobilizing the anterior border of the tensor:

> The origin is divided along the crest of the ilium…The belly of the muscle is next freed from the deep structures and the whole muscle is turned backward on itself so that the anterior edge is sutured to the fascia behind the trochanter. In this way there will be a straight pull from the crest of the insertion of the iliotibial band. (F. R. Ober 1933)

During his time examining and treating patients with polio in Vermont, Ober observed that:

> the quadriceps muscle is more frequently paralyzed in the thigh than any other. The two muscles most often spared are the sartorius and the tensor fasciae latae, and their use as knee extensors is fairly satisfactory and causes less disability than transplanting the hamstrings. There is a danger of the knee hyperextending when one or more of the hamstring muscles are used. The tensor through its gluteal attachment helps to extend the knee and the anatomical situation of this muscle and the sartorius gives a

better physiological action [in phase transfer] on the patella and is in better anatomical relation to the anterior structures of the knee than is a hamstring. (F. R. Ober 1933)

To replace a paralyzed quadriceps muscle in order to gain some knee extension power, Ober freed the iliotibial band from the fibula and maintained it as a three-quarter-inch wide flap. He then freed the tensor muscle and with a tendon passer redirected the freed strip of iliotibial band and sutured its distal end to the patella tendon. With the knee:

> flexed to a right ankle, the belly of the sartorius is exposed and freed from its surrounding structures, and the tendon is severed at its insertion...The muscular septum between the sartorius and the quadriceps is next perforated, and, by means of a tendon carrier, the sartorius is also drawn out of the wound over the quadriceps tendon...[and] firmly sutured to the patellar tendon. (F. R. Ober 1933)

He sutured the sartorius tendon to the patellar tendon first, and then the iliotibial band, running over the sartorius tendon, was sutured to the patella tendon: "Each edge of this band is sewed to the reflected edges of the aponeurosis of the patella and to the edge of the sartorius muscle... the transplants are placed under the fascia lata and not subcutaneously, as is so often done" (F. R. Ober 1933).

Treating Patients with Weakness or Paralysis of the Foot and Ankle Muscles

Ober had certain preferences for treating patients with weakness or paralysis of foot and ankle muscles. For isolated paralysis of the anterior tibial muscle, he transplanted the peroneus longus through a hole in the lateral septum into the anterior compartment, suturing its distal end into "an osteoperiosteal bone bridge...in the base of the first metatarsal near the insertion of the anterior tibial" (F. R. Ober 1933). With an additional posterior tibial paralysis, he transferred the "extensor proprius hallucis muscle...[which was] implanted into the neck of the first metatarsal bone [by] passing the cut end of the tendon through a drill hole made from above downward. The tendon entering the hole at the inferior medial aspect is withdrawn and the end sutured to the capsule and bone at its exit" (F. R. Ober 1933). To avoid a hammer toe deformity, he sutured the distal portion of the extensor hallucis longus tendon to the extensor digitorum brevis. "In paralysis of the peroneals, the anterior tibial tendon with some attached bone is passed through the sheath of the common extensor and sutured to the base of the third metatarsal" (F. R. Ober 1933).

Ober preferred to transfer the peroneus longus and posterior tibial tendons for gastrocnemius paralysis. After freeing the ends of the tendons, he "passed [them] down through the tendo-Achilles compartment, crossing behind the tendon, and passed through a drill hole in the os calcis, the posterior tibial from without inward, and the peroneal from within outward. The cut ends are sutured to the os calcis and the tendo-Achilles" (F. R. Ober 1933). He agreed with Dr. Naughton Dunn that the flexor digitorum communis can be added to increase the strength of the transfer. He also preferred performing a triple arthrodesis (as described by Michael Hoke) in addition to these transfers because "the function of plantar flexion will be increased a great deal [, though one must be] careful to displace the foot backward in order to obtain more leverage" (F. R. Ober 1933). In cases of severe weakness of the calf muscles, including the posterior tibial and the peroneals, he transferred the anterior tibial tendon posteriorly and did a triple arthrodesis; that "operation was first done by Ralph Ghormley, who was formerly associated with me" (F. R. Ober 1933). With anterior tibial and peroneal muscle paralysis and intact calf muscles, the foot becomes fixed in equinovarus. Ober mentioned that:

there has been a good deal of adverse discussion about transplanting the posterior tendon forward...Tenotomy of the posterior tibial and correction of the varus deformity relieve the situation in part, but it is difficult to prevent the recurrence of equinus and it seems an unwarranted waste to throw away the power of a good muscle. (F. R. Ober 1933)

In these cases, he successfully transferred the posterior tibial tendon through the interosseous membrane, attaching the distal end of the tendon in a groove at the base of the third metatarsal. To prevent recurrent deformity and lateral stability, he combined the transfer with a triple arthrodesis.

Use of the Shelf Procedure for Congenitally Dislocated Hips

As mentioned in chapter 15, Bradford reported his early results of open reduction for congenitally dislocated hips. In 1934, Ober reported his own results with the shelf procedure to treat persistent dislocation of the hip in 26 cases over 11 years; in 20 cases that procedure was performed for congenital dislocation, the other six because of infection. The shelf procedure was becoming increasingly popular at that time, and many orthopaedic surgeons were reporting its use.

Although early in his experience Ober usually did not open the capsule, he noted that between 1930 and 1934 "we have opened the capsule in practically every case" (F. R. Ober 1935c). This allowed him to remove contracted or dense fibrous tissue, thereby preventing reduction. He observed in these patients that:

> where the shelf was constructed without pulling the head down, there were a Trendelenburg sign and an abductor limp which are distressing to the patient, the parents and the surgeon...In an effort to combat this limp, we have lately been transplanting the trochanter...down the shaft of the femur...In one-half of the cases treated, the shelf partially or wholly disappeared leaving the head in its original position. (F. R. Ober 1935c)

Ober concluded that:

1. ...the Trendelenburg sign persists even though a suitable shelf is apparent...with the hip in situ.
2. The shelf should be made of acetabular tissue when possible...the roof turned down...cartilage intact [; the] roof should be nearly horizontal.
3. The head...must be pulled down...to construct such a shelf.
4. all obstructing tissue should be removed but [it is] unwise to remove much fibrous tissue from the acetabular cavity.
5. If...two failures [occur while] secur[ing] manual reduction...do an open reduction before the acetabular roof disappears.
6. In spite...that the shelf has melted away in many of these cases, the hips are more stable than when there is no good false acetabulum or no acetabular roof present. (F. R. Ober 1935c)

His work demonstrated the importance of reducing the hip before completing the shelf procedure as well as the need to advance the greater trochanter to improve gait.

The Ober Test

Ober first described one of his most significant contributions in his 1935 paper entitled "Back Strains and Sciatica." The Ober test, sometimes called the Ober sign or the Ober abduction sign, determines the tightness of the iliotibial band, the tensor fascia lata, or both. The patient lies on one side, with the lower hip and knee flexed to reduce lumbar lordosis, and the examiner holds the upper leg with the knee flexed. The examiner then flexes and abducts the upper hip and then extends it, bringing both structures over the greater trochanter.

> THE RÔLE OF THE ILIOTIBIAL BAND AND FASCIA LATA AS A FACTOR IN THE CAUSATION OF LOW-BACK DISABILITIES AND SCIATICA*
>
> BY FRANK R. OBER, M.D., BOSTON, MASSACHUSETTS
>
> VOL. XVIII, NO. 1, JANUARY 1936

Title of Ober's article describing his procedure releasing a contracted iliotibial band. *Journal of Bone and Joint Surgery* 1936; 18: 105.

The examiner then attempts to place the upper leg, with the knee still flexed, parallel to the lower leg. An inability to do so indicates that the iliotibial band, the tensor fascia lata, or both are tight. Ober syndrome is a contracture of these structures. Ober knew that a contracted iliotibial band or tensor fascia lata caused poor posture.

He followed up his first paper with a second article in 1936, entitled "The Role of the Iliotibial Band and Fascia Lata as a Factor in the Causation of Low-Back Disabilities and Sciatica." At the time, the etiology of low-back pain and sciatica was unknown, even though Mixter and Barr had just published (in 1934) their observations on herniated intervertebral discs. Ober reported his results of the release of a contracted iliotibial band: 33 of 42 patients were well or improved, whereas nine patients experienced no relief (see **Case 20.1**). He concluded that:

1) The simple surgical procedure described relieves sciatic pain in spines which show no bone pathology by x-ray.

2) Contracted iliotibial bands and fasciae exert pulls on the pelvic bones, resulting in bad posture.

3) One more diagnostic sign has been added to our present knowledge of low-back disabilities, which should be helpful in clearing up another group of lame backs that have not responded well to other treatment.

(F. R. Ober 1936)

Case 20.1. "Back Pain and Sciatica"

"F. K., a white women [sic], aged 33, married, seen July 16, 1934, complained of a lame back of twenty-one years' duration. She had been worse since the birth of a boy ten years before. She had been in constant pain and more or less uncomfortable with attacks of sciatica down the right leg. One year before she had a bad attack and was confined to bed from November to July. For six weeks she had been very uncomfortable. During that time she was up once but had severe pain in the left leg going down to the heel and the side of the foot. Sometimes she had pain over the outer side of the thigh, which kept her awake. She was uncomfortable in any position except the semiprone position with the left thigh flexed.

"Physician examination, July 16, showed that when she was standing all motions of the spine were limited, with moderate muscle spasm. Straight leg raising was markedly limited on both sides but more on the left. There was marked shortening of the iliotibial bands, more marked on the left. Other reflexes were normal. There was weakness in the dorsal flexion of the left foot.

"On July 18, under general anesthesia, both iliotibial bands were divided. July 26, straight leg raising was possible to 50 degrees on the left side and 60 degrees on the right. The power of dorsal flexion had increased. She was taking no sedatives after having taken them for nearly a year. Pain was decreasing. By August 11 the conditions had improved markedly. She walked better, with less sciatica. There was no weakness in dorsal flexion of the foot. September 16 she still had a moderate amount of sciatica in the posterior aspect of the thigh, but none down the leg. The patient could put on shoes without difficulty, which she could not do before the operation. Straight leg raising was 80 degrees on the left side and to a right angle on the right. There was still slight limitation of the back motions, with a list to the left. The patient felt better than she had for years.

"A pathological report of the specimen removed at the time of operation was acute and chronic inflammation. Muscle fibers showed loss of striations."

(Frank R. Ober 1935)

Ober Operation

Fixed contractures at the hip and knee, often with a tilted pelvis, can occur secondary to contracture of the tensor fascia lata, the iliotibial band, and the intermuscular septum. Ober described a proximal release of these tissues primarily in the region of the hip. Yount described a distal release of the iliotibial band and the intermuscular septum just above the knee. In severe cases both procedures (an Ober-Yount fasciotomy) may be required to correct the contracture deformities.

Ober described his operation for an abduction contracture of the hip that had increased stress on the lower spine and pelvis and thereby caused low-back pain:

> Operation...The incision is oblique and begins at a point a little lateral to the anterior iliac spine, attending downward and backward to a point about one inch posterior to and one inch above the greater trochanter and exposing the fascia lata. The iliotibial band and fascia lata are incised posteriorly well over the anterior portion of the gluteus maximus muscle. The incision is now carried forward to a point just below the anterior-superior spine and includes the fascia surrounding the tensor fascia latae. All intermuscular septa in this region are divided. As soon as the section is completed, there is a marked separation of the cut surfaces. The fascia is further separated by blunt dissection until there is a gap of two inches. In some instances, pathologic examination of the iliotibial band has shown chronic inflammation.
> (F. R. Ober 1936)

This procedure was done to relieve sciatica as well as to improve posture and gait. It was successful in relieving back and leg pain in some patients, and it also improved posture and gait with better alignment of the lower extremity and increased motion at the hip and knee.

Brachioradialis Transfer

In 1938, Ober described the brachioradialis transfer for triceps weakness. He gave examples of arm movements that require sufficient power (at least fair) from the triceps, including fully extending the elbow and pushing movements. Importantly, brachioradialis muscle transfer achieves high-quality outcomes only when the muscle's original function is good or normal. This transfer procedure can incorporate the extensor carpi radialis longus if additional strength is required. Ober identified the anterior margins of the muscle and indicated that the anterior margin should be rolled laterally and then secured to the periosteum of the ulna and to the triceps tendon. He noted that the surgeon must preserve the nerve and the blood supply during the procedure. This transposition allows the brachioradialis to now extend, rather than flex, the elbow. Ober reported that he had performed this operation successfully on five patients; the first was in 1934. He stated that function of the out-of-phase

Drawing from Ober's article demonstrating the separation of the contracted tensor fascia lata after release.
F. R. Ober, "Back Pain and Sciatica," *Journal of the American Medical Association* 1935; 104: 1582.

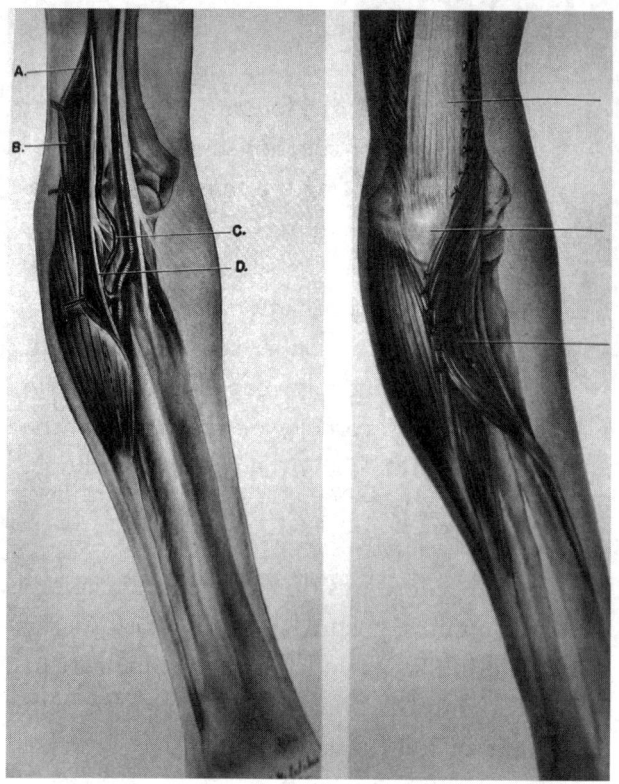

Drawing from Ober's article demonstrating the brachioradialis transfer for triceps weakness.

F. R. Ober and J. S. Barr, "Brachioradialis muscle transposition for triceps weakness," *Surgery, Gynecology and Obstetrics* 1938; 67: 106.

transfer occurred easily in all five patients after the procedure, achieving at least fair muscle strength in each.

Shoulder Arthrodesis Versus Muscle Transfers

In 1942, Joseph Barr reported the findings of the American Orthopaedic Association's Research Committee on outcomes of shoulder arthrodesis in 90 children with poliomyelitis, almost half of whom had had a previous muscle transplantation. "Satisfactory muscle transplantations were found only in those cases possessing fair power in the deltoid preoperatively" (J. S. Barr et al. 1942). The committee concluded that a fusion was indicated for patients six years or older; younger patients developed better motion than older patients, but their fusion rates were lower. Optimal position of the fused shoulder was "45 to 55 degrees of abduction, 15 to 25 degrees of flexion and 15 to 25 degrees of internal rotation" (J. S. Barr et al. 1942). The committee agreed "that arthrodesis of the shoulder joint is the operation of choice in all cases of infantile paralysis with complete paralysis of the shoulder" (J. S. Barr et al. 1942).

Ober noted that a biceps-triceps transplant won't effectively resolve a paralyzed supraspinatus muscle in cases with a poor deltoid:

> When there is an avulsion of the shoulder cuff and the supraspinatus tendon...The insertion of the trapezius muscle is freed as is done in the Mayer transplant...a piece of fascia is attached to the free end of the trapezius...passed underneath the acromion and attached to the head of the humerus, just distal to the insertion of the supraspinatus. (F. R. Ober 1944)

Ober also described two other transfers for weakness about the shoulder. First, in cases with an intact posterior deltoid but a paralyzed anterior and middle deltoid, he detached the posterior deltoid from the spine of the scapula, "turned [the muscle] over on itself and sutured [it] to a slit in the periosteum or the posterior superior surface of the clavicle" (F. R. Ober 1944). Second, for cases with painful subluxation and no muscular power in the extremity other than in the upper trapezius muscle:

> the insertion of the trapezius [is] cleared...the tendon of the long head of the biceps is severed from the muscle belly...a hole is drilled from before backward through the surgical neck of the humerus...the free end of the tendon is passed from before backward through this hole and the distal end of the tendon is snugly sutured with No.4 braided silk to the free end of the trapezius. (F. R. Ober 1944)

For paralysis of the serratus anterior, a rare problem in polio, Ober wrote:

It is very unsightly and results in the so-called angel wing deformity [with] loss of power in reaching forward and also difficulty in elevating the arm above the horizontal level…because the serratus anticus function is to carry the scapula forward thus allowing complete elevation of the arm. Several years ago, I did a transplant of fascia lata to elongate the tendon of the sternal portion of the pectoralis major. The fascia was trapezoid in shape. The narrow portion was sutured to the vertebral border of the scapula subperiostally [sic]. This operation was not published as it was discovered that [Alfred] Tubby had performed a similar operation in 1909. The results in the two cases have been excellent and have lasted. (F. R. Ober 1944)

OBER AS EDUCATOR

In addition to his role as a clinician, Frank Ober was a leader in medical education, especially postgraduate education (residency), throughout most of his career. He challenged students by using the case method during grand rounds, and they could observe his technical skill during surgeries; both approaches made him a compelling teacher. He served as "Assistant Dean of the courses for graduates, serving with distinction from 1928 to 1946" (*New England Journal of Medicine* 1961). He may have been the first to hold that position.

The Art of Diagnosis

Early in his career (1926), he had published a paper on "Diagnosis in Orthopedic Surgery." Obviously recalling his experiences in World War I, he stated that despite thorough training, orthopaedic surgeons of the time confronted numerous deformities that either had no cure or were relieved only after inducing serious injury, and he believed that an accurate initial diagnosis could avoid such problems. He suggested that all necessary efforts should be made to arrive at a correct diagnosis and that:

> most weaknesses in solving problems in diagnosis are due to:
>
> 1. Bad elementary training.
> 2. Insufficient knowledge of the fundamental subjects in medicine.
> 3. Lack of proper hospital training.
> 4. Incomplete physical examinations.
> 5. Failure to make a thorough search for a cause of the ailment.
> 6. Premature selection of a specialty.
> 7. Dependence on the roentgen ray alone.
> (F. R. Ober 1926)

Ober mentioned two worrisome deficiencies in some students as they begin their career: a lack of both (1) solid observational skills and (2) the ability for logical thinking. For Ober, both of these derived from poor training. He believed that interns and residents need solid knowledge of anatomy/physiology and pathology, as issues with structure and function cause most orthopaedic conditions. Students and trainees should also receive extensive training in patient examination and diagnosis to ensure they dig deep enough to identify the true underlying issue. Ober also derided the dependence on roentgen studies to actually make diagnoses; instead, he insisted, the roentgen ray should aid a clinician in making a diagnosis, not be in itself the basis for a diagnosis.

Ober believed that treating physicians should focus on an accurate and an early diagnosis as their goals. He condemned diagnoses of hysteria and snap diagnoses, concluding that a poor examination or only a cursory one by the clinician wrongly labels patients or could endanger them. Late diagnoses, for Ober, are also a problem, resulting from a physician's lack of knowledge or preparation, their reliance on usual methods, uncooperative patients, or too few data.

Ober reflected on how to enhance clinicians' ability to provide a proper diagnosis—mainly through higher quality education and training, thorough physical and laboratory testing in order to establish early diagnosis.

When Ober was the assistant dean at Harvard Medical School and a clinical professor of Orthopaedic Surgery, he gave a thoughtful and provocative presentation to Tufts Medical School alumni. The speech was entitled "Your Brain is Your Invested Capital," and it provided some insight into his values. Ober's use of the word "capital" referred to a physician's brainpower: those physicians who share knowledge or develop a useful practice or procedure that benefits patients will leave a lasting legacy. His advice to the physician audience of the elements necessary for being successful included:

- a comprehensive education in school and extensive training afterward,
- constant study, through attendance at meetings and conferences, discussion with colleagues, and reading medical and surgical journals,
- hard work, emphasizing the need for extensive knowledge and the cost of mistakes,
- cleanliness and a congenial attitude—both of which benefit relationships with patients and colleagues.

"To be successful," he said, "is to be more useful, and in general these are three good rules for success: To be on time, do our job better today

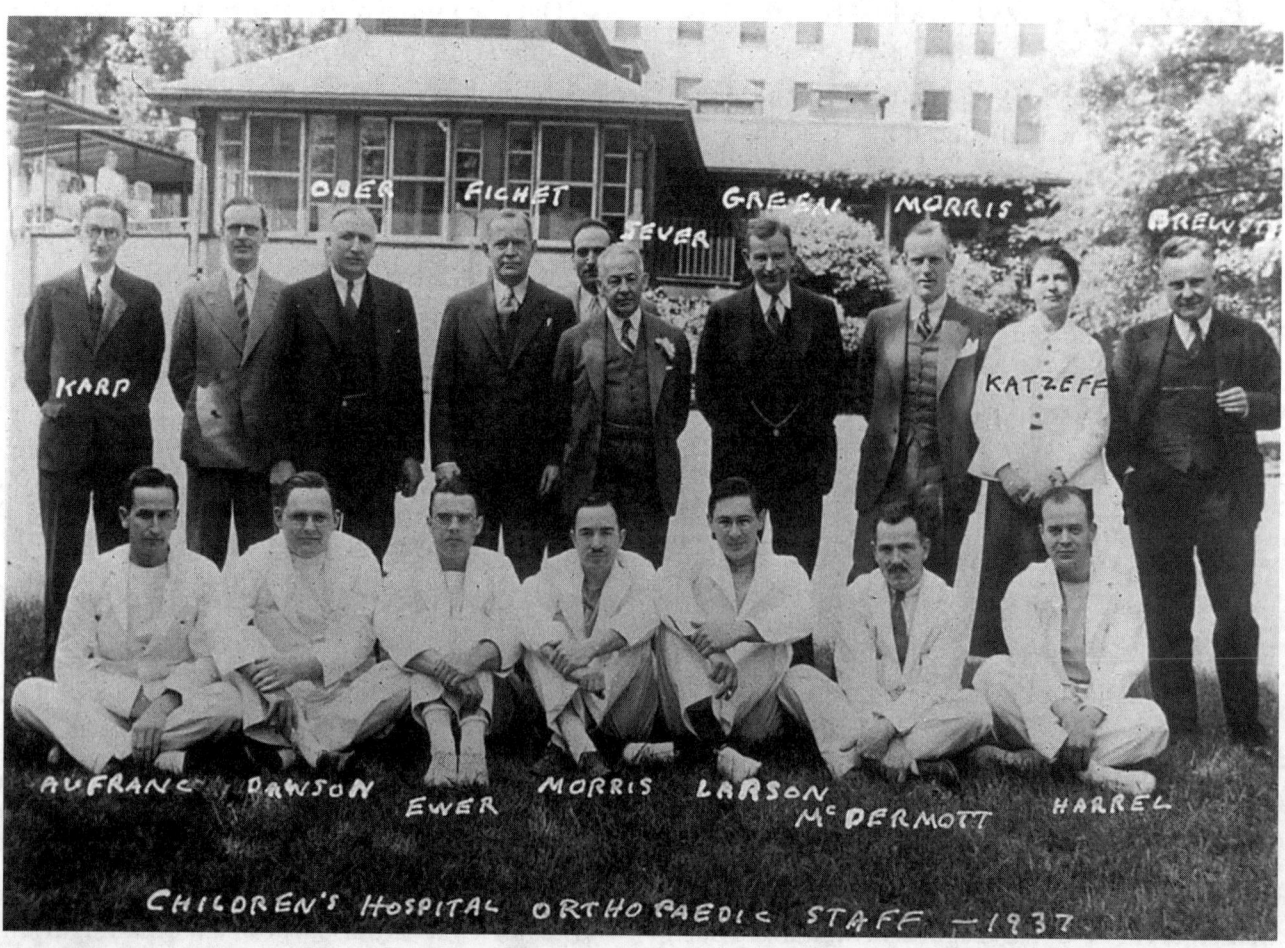

Orthopaedic staff at BCH in 1937. MGH HCORP Archives.

than yesterday and above all, be human" (Ober 1939b). He emphasized that because of all the effort the aforementioned elements require, "no one should go into the study of medicine unless he wants to do that more than anything else in the world" (F. R. Ober 1939b). A larger extract from Ober's speech is provided in **Box 20.1**.

Postgraduate Education

By 1930, Ober had already been recognized as a leader in orthopaedic education for students and residents. That year—just one year before Ober was promoted to the John Ball and Buckminster Brown Professorship at Harvard Medical School—Dr. R. B. Greenough, the president of the Massachusetts Medical Society, asked Ober to present a paper on postgraduate teaching at Harvard Medical School. The occasion was a meeting of the New England Medical Council, a group of "five members from each state…representing the State Medical societies" (*New England Journal of Medicine* 1930) to address the topic of "The Relation of Clinics and Health Associations to the Medical Profession." Five papers were read and discussed in the Aesculapian Room of the Harvard Club.

Ober addressed two main postgraduate initiatives at Harvard. The first was a series of "short courses whereby general practitioners may have opportunities to improve themselves in diagnosis" (F. R. Ober 1930b). Today these courses fall under the category of continuing medical education. Recognizing that it was difficult for busy clinicians to leave their practices to attend courses, Harvard Medical School offered "some extension courses which are carried out in different cities in the state, the doctors clubbing together and each one paying a small fee…the Medical School send[s] men who are interested in a special line of work so that they may have a clinic once a week…we hope in this way to carry graduate teaching to more practitioners" (F. R. Ober 1930b). The second initiative focused on specialty training—that is, residencies. In 1930, specialty training at Harvard included 6- to 24-month programs in orthopaedics, neurology, ophthalmology, and pediatrics; future programs were being planned in urology, gynecology, obstetrics, dermatology, and laryngology. Ober described the orthopaedic program as:

> a two-year course, eight months of which are given at the Massachusetts General Hospital, eight months at the Children's Hospital and their third eight months are spent in some of the chronic hospitals and in the laboratories [and basic science] at the Medical School. Along with these courses the men are given clinical instruction by the members of the Visiting Staff, and they are allowed to do operations assisted by members of the Staff on service in the wards of the hospitals. These men have the care of the patients in the wards under the direction of the visiting surgeon and are held responsible for their care. (F. R. Ober 1930b)

The orthopaedic residency Ober described had changed from its predecessor. A few years earlier, Robert Osgood and Nathaniel Allison had added one year of adult orthopaedics at the Massachusetts General Hospital and six months of basic sciences at Harvard Medical School to the one-year orthopaedic residency program at Children's Hospital. Now, in 1930, upon Osgood's retirement, the program was reduced from 30 to 24 months, as described by Ober. The residents continued to receive instruction in the sciences and in adult

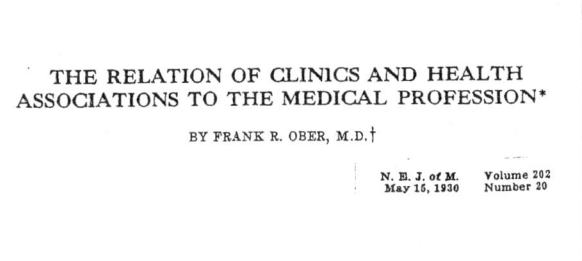

Title of Ober's article in which he described the two-year residency in orthopaedic surgery at HMS. *New England Journal of Medicine* 1930; 262: 953.

Box 20.1. Your Brain is Your Invested Capital

"The undergraduate must realize from the start that the study of medicine is a life job in which there are great and often grave responsibilities. To meet them, one must have a versatile education in order to deal with the varied problems of humanity. Hard work must be your slogan. Those who do not know how to study will have the most difficult time and the poorest grades, so it behooves this group to acquire the art of study…It is impossible in four short years to learn all there is to know about medicine…The education received in the medical school serves only as a meager foundation for a life, which must to its end be devoted to constant study of all the problems that relate to disease in every-day practice and research.

"How do you propose to practice medicine? Are you going to settle down to a humdrum life, having made up your mind you know all there is to be known…he who ceases to learn is already on the side of the down grade. Nothing ever stands still. It either dies or it lives.

"Take your choice. Anything that lives must progress. If you choose the self-indulgent road, your competitors and the cults will win. You will lose and life will be full of disappointments and bitterness and the blame will be at your own door…The human machine in no way resembles the motor car, but the human is too often treated as if he were a machine. The human patient has a personality and his illness may or may not be affected or altered by his personality.

"The secret of success in practice is hard work. No person ought to devote his life to such a calling unless he is prepared to undertake the responsibility…Mistakes are too often costly, so it behooves us to know and to learn as much as is humanly possible…we must be untiring in the devotion to our calling.

"There are many things which help to contribute to success in medicine. First, clean habits in persons; i.e., make the best of your personal appearance. It is a little thing for the doctor to wash his hands before he examines a patient, but it means a lot to the patient. Second…An agreeable personality is a real asset…[it] means more than being agreeable. It means poise, radiating energy, stimulating confidence in others, giving people honest assurance and not being under-or over-enthusiastic. Having a good voice…is a distinct asset.

"The world is full of specialists today. Some think we are overspecialized…The very best preparation for a specialty

and pediatric orthopaedics, along with training in chronic orthopaedic conditions. Osgood was likely the one to implement these changes, as Ober had not become a full professor and head of orthopaedics at Harvard Medical School until 1931, after Osgood had retired.

In the discussion after Ober's presentation, Dr. Greenough stated that he and Dr. George Blumer had been asked by the New England Medical Council to urge the deans of medical schools in Boston and New Haven to develop graduate programs that would adequately prepare students to practice their chosen specialty. The issue of whether the graduates of these specialty residency programs should receive a graduate degree was also discussed. Greenough's opinion was that the New England Medical Council should cooperate with the American College of Surgeons to establish and develop the college's fellowship, because the public already recognized the high standards of the American College of Surgeons. The council did not agree with awarding graduate degrees; the general consensus was that such degrees were unethical, serving only to advance the name of the institution awarding them.

At the 45th Annual Meeting of the Association of American Medical Colleges (AAMC), a major symposium on graduate medical education held in Nashville, Tennessee, in October 1934, Dr. Ober spoke about the "Value of the Short Course in Graduate Teaching." He commented that longer short courses lasting one or two months are considered a burden on clinicians, and those lasting only half-days were attended only at the clinician's convenience—and other distractions always existed. Ober referred to these as the "doldrums."

> after adequate hospital training [rotating internships] is a general practice for three or four years…[during which] what is far more important, one learns how to deal with people…
>
> "The lone wolf in general medicine is apt to have a hard time. It is wise to mix with your fellows, attend the meetings of your medical societies regularly and above all, when you have something to say in these meetings, get on your feet and say it. Cultivate the area of speaking by speaking… If you have anything worth saying then it is worth saying well…
>
> "'Your capital is your brain.' Did you ever know anyone who was satisfied for very long with the amount of money he happened to acquire?…If we all applied the money-getters' dissatisfied ambition to our own capital, brains, we would go on acquiring knowledge from reading books and journals, attending hospital clinics and medical meetings, and taking graduate and postgraduate courses.
>
> "Subscribe to a few well selected medical and surgical journals and read them…
>
> "One of the great weaknesses in medicine today is the failure of the doctor to go to school after he has been graduated. There are probably many reasons for this; but most of them boil down to inertia, disinclination to spend the necessary money, or self-satisfaction. Inertia may be overcome.
>
> "The money can be saved for postgraduate courses out of income…self satisfaction is an unrealized sin and no amount of praying will cure such a disease; it must be plucked out.
>
> "Increasing your capital can be done only by education, because that which the brain receives, it stores, and there is no limit to the capacity of that storehouse. Remember then, — there is no short cut to knowledge, any more than there is to permanent wealth. Wildcat schemes have no place in medicine and will catch up with you as they do in finance. To be successful is to be more useful, and in general these are three good rules for success: To be on time, do our job better today than yesterday and above all, be human.
>
> "Finally, no one should go into the study of medicine unless he wants to do that more than anything else in the world."
>
> —F. R. Ober, "Your Brain is Your Invested Capital," 1939

He recommended major changes, including limiting the number of clinicians in order to more closely engage those who attend, and providing to attendees a syllabus and easy-to-access references.

Ober reported on one such successful course, lasting a full day, wherein a notable physician led rounds; facilitated a discussion of cases, problems, and procedures; and taught an evening session on a topic of interest to the attendees. He also briefly described the successful annual course on fractures at Massachusetts General Hospital, which had been popular with clinicians for almost a decade (see chapter 31). In 1934, more than 100 physicians had attended from across the United States and Canada. The course lasted almost 10 hours each day for one week. Attendees learned about and discussed the diagnosis, treatment, and outcomes of fractures, and they attended demonstrations and participated in question-and-answer sessions. Ober suggested other topics for one-week-long review courses:

- Endocrine disturbances
- Arthritis
- Cancer
- Diagnostic problems in surgery
- Vaccine therapy
- Poliomyelitis
- Diabetes
- Diseases of the blood
- Circulatory disturbances
- Fractures
- Brain and cord lesions

In the discussion following Dr. Ober's presentation, Dr. Leroy Perkins of Harvard University told the audience that he had met with the governor of Massachusetts about postgraduate medical education. The governor was supportive and requested that Perkins and Ober name a group of five physicians and five prominent laymen to organize financing for physicians' postgraduate education. Ober and Perkins, along with Harvard Medical School Dean David Edsall, declined to do so in order to maintain control over such education by physicians only and to ensure costs remained reasonable. (L. D. Perkins 1935)

In his closing remarks, Ober stated:

there are a few things which have to do with the weakness of graduate teaching. In the first place, undergraduate teaching is usually of prime importance and graduate teaching is of secondary importance…The graduate student [is] too willing to ride along with the knowledge he gets in undergraduate days. Many of them rarely read their medical journals and, I fear, too few keep up with modern medical literature. If the man is successful in a financial way, there is no incentive to encourage him to search for more knowledge, and too few realize that when a man stops studying in medicine, he belongs to the past. The best way for the graduate to combat the cults is…to keep in touch with all the modern programs in medicine. (F. R. Ober 1935e)

Ober then recommended that the AAMC evaluate the curricula of "all the graduate medical programs throughout the United States and set standards that would sufficiently reflect the importance of graduate education" (F. R. Ober 1935e).

Graduate Education in Orthopaedic Surgery

In 1933, the American Orthopaedic Association appointed a committee to report on the status of residency programs in orthopaedic surgery. The committee comprised five members: Ober as chairperson, LeRoy Abbott, of San Francisco; William E. Gallie, of Toronto; Edwin W. Ryerson, of Chicago; and DeForest P. Willard, of Philadelphia. Ober represented the committee and presented its findings at the 1934 American Orthopaedic Association Annual Meeting in Philadelphia; the final report was published in 1935 in the *Journal of Bone and Joint Surgery*.

```
GRADUATE INSTRUCTION IN ORTHOPAEDIC SURGERY
REPORT OF COMMITTEE APPOINTED BY THE AMERICAN ORTHOPAEDIC ASSOCIATION *
    WILLIAM E. GALLIE, M.D., Toronto, Canada
    DeFOREST P. WILLARD, M.D., Philadelphia, Pennsylvania
    EDWIN W. RYERSON, M.D., Chicago, Illinois
    LeROY C. ABBOTT, M.D., San Francisco, California
    FRANK R. OBER, M.D., Chairman, Boston, Massachusetts
VOL. XVII, NO. 4, OCTOBER 1935          VOL. XVII, NO. 4, OCTOBER 1935
```

Title of the report of a committee appointed by the American Orthopaedic Association to study the status of orthopaedic residency programs in the United States. *Journal of Bone and Joint Surgery* 1935; 17: 1072.

Seventy-six institutions completed the questionnaire, including 62 medical schools, 11 Shriners Hospitals for Children, and 3 other hospitals. Findings revealed that:

- Fifteen were medical schools with teaching hospitals that had an orthopaedic department, which included interns who averaged about two months on an orthopaedic rotation. Nine of these 15 schools/hospitals offered short courses (two weeks long) for practitioners and long courses (up to two years long) for interns, but only five of these nine offered internships in orthopaedic surgery.
- Thirteen were medical schools that had no orthopaedic departments, but six of these had hospital affiliations that offered short (28 days to 2 months) orthopaedic rotations to house officers.
- Twenty-five offered no graduate courses in orthopaedic surgery.

- Eleven had hospital affiliations and made available short orthopaedic internships (three to six months long).
- One offered an orthopaedic residency (one or two years long).
- Seven were Shriners Hospitals that had orthopaedic rotations for residents that varied from one to two years. Most of these programs gave no certificate or degree upon completion of the program.
- Data is unavailable or unknown for four of the institutions surveyed.

By contrast, at Harvard, "the course in Orthopaedic Surgery…now consists of eight months of pathology, an interneship [sic] of eight months at the Children's Hospital, and eight months at the Massachusetts General Hospital, making a total of twenty-four months. Both hospitals have a Chief Resident on each service, part of whose time is spent in teaching" (Gallie et al. 1935). Harvard required its house officers to have graduated from an accredited medical school, and they "must have served a rotating internship of at least two years or a one-year surgical interneship [sic]" (Gallie et al. 1935). Harvard also offered short courses (one or two months long) in orthopaedic surgery.

The committee commented only briefly on intern's compensation in their report: "At the New York Orthopaedic Hospital, the interns received $50.00 per month and maintainance [sic]. The Fellows [residents] on full time work from 8:00 a.m. to 6:00 p.m. and receive…adequate salary" (Gallie et al. 1935). What was $50.00 per month, or $600 per year, in 1935 equates to ~$945.00 per month, or $11,337, in 2019. In 1965, when I was an intern at the Hospital of the University of Pennsylvania, I received a salary of $1,200 per year (plus a night call bed, meals, and three sets of white pants and shirts)—a salary that in 2019 would have been valued at $9,739.31.

Dr. Ober was president of the American Orthopaedic Association in 1943. As might be expected on the basis of his devotion and commitment to graduate medical education, the title of his presidential address was "The Future of Graduate Medical Education." Drawing on his experience during World War I, he began by stating that:

Many of the wounds of that war [World War I] and WWII were of the organs of locomotion. There were then too few trained and experienced men in England or America to meet a great situation involving thousands of wounded men in the early days of the first war. It was not until 1917 [before it was] realized that the fractured femur due to gunshot wounds was one of the great disasters of the war. Many of these men died in shock and none up to that time were rehabilitated…in the spring of 1917…it was at his [Sir Robert Jones]… [suggestion] that the fractured femur was splinted on the field…the mortality rate was greatly diminished. Such results stimulated a widespread interest among surgeons and a greater respect in the care of bones and joints. It became apparent that the general surgeon needed to know more about surgery of the extremities, and it also became apparent that the orthopaedic surgeon of insufficient training needed to know more about general surgery. (F. R. Ober 1943c)

After briefly reviewing wartime efforts to provide short intensive orthopaedic training to surgeons, Ober noted young physicians' increased interest in and desire to train in orthopaedic surgery (others such as Osgood and Dr. Alfred B. Shands Jr. had recognized this trend as well). Ober recognized the problems caused by the lack of both minimal requirements for certification and of the teaching of basic sciences at some medical schools. He also described issues with:

the sharp line drawn between the preclinical and the clinical years…[and the effects of war which] has disrupted the teaching of graduates in the great foreign clinics…has also disrupted undergraduate and postgraduate medical education in this country; first because the armed forces have called into service all physically fit medical students who are limited to one year of hospital training which practically nullifies the pools from which doctors...wish to go into special fields; second, physically fit physicians...for postgraduate courses have been called to active duty; and third, the teaching school faculties have been so depleted that there are scarcely enough teachers to maintain the teaching of the undergraduate. (F. R. Ober 1943c)

Ober called on his colleagues to engage in providing sufficient graduate education to students:

If we are to keep up our standing in the medical world that preparations be started now to organize a program of graduate education which will meet the demands that must surely come when the war is over...It should be our duty to supply adequate additional educational advantages for all those young doctors who have had a one-year internship, and also for older doctors who wish to improve their education before returning to their practices...thousands of both...will desire more hospital experience...One great fault...of graduate medical education is that for the most part...the student pays all the fees...It is obvious that the great medical centers...should be endowed on a permanent basis. (F. R. Ober 1943c)

Ober provided several recommendations for this education (**Box 20.2**). He then ended his speech with the following:

The orthopaedic surgeon has a large stake in graduate medical education. It is up to us as members of this, the oldest association of orthopaedic surgeons, to do our part in promulgating plans for the future of graduate medical education...Let us put our shoulders to the wheel now...Let us hope that our successors have

Box 20.2. Ober's Recommendations for the Future of Graduate Medical Education

Establish centers of graduate instruction

- Include centralized graduate instruction in basic and clinical sciences at specified medical schools
- Teach clinical subjects in approved hospitals and medical schools
- Establish standardized minimum requirements before students are eligible to begin courses
- Seek and create endowments to maintain these graduate centers

Specialty departments

- Appoint a director for each special department to manage undergraduate, graduate, postgraduate, and research divisions
- Establish specialty research laboratories

Faculty

- Create a process and "pedagogical group" for instructing junior faculty and establishing research laboratories

Publication

- Set up a clear process to publish scientific articles

Residencies and Fellowships

- Determine a consistent method of instruction and supervision for interns and residents
- Organize fellowships for candidates following a specified selection process

learned from us all we have to give, will go on exploring new fields and new opportunities, realizing that where one starts out in life to be educated, a diploma is not the period or end, but education is a continuing affair until life has ceased. (F. R. Ober 1943c)

OBER THE MAN AND HIS MANY ACHIEVEMENTS

In 1961, Dr. William T. Green described Ober, one of his own teachers, as an extremely accomplished individual who was full of life. Green emphasized Ober's skill at teaching residents:

> Dr. Ober was first a surgeon, and he brought as chief of service an emphasis on surgical skills. His productions and interests varied from a new operation for recurrent dislocation of the patella to low back pain…He was particularly interested in the methods of surgical rehabilitation…applicable to poliomyelitis and congenital deformities.

In 1999, Dr. Douglas Brown presented his presidential address to the American Orthopaedic Society for Sports Medicine. In it he described Dr. Ober and the care that he gave Dr. Brown's father:

> If you will indulge me, I want to share a personal story with you that illustrates how the practice of medicine is unique. My father somehow contracted polio as an infant, at age 6 months to be exact, in 1911. He was living in a small paper mill town of Waterville, Maine. Shortly after he became ill with a high fever, he seemed to lose the function of his left arm and his right leg. There were no local options for his treatment in Waterville, Maine, but Boston's Children's Hospital was 150 miles to the south so my grandparents took my father to Boston by train, carrying him on a pillow. After examining him and confirming their worst fears, Dr. Robert Lovett, a renowned Boston orthopaedic surgeon, arranged for my father to be immediately hospitalized and for my grandparents to take up residence in an apartment he owned adjacent to the hospital, an arrangement that lasted many weeks and without any cost to my grandparents.

> That was my father's first trip to Boston, but there were dozens and dozens of other trips over the next 20 years. During that time, those Boston Children's Hospital doctors, nurses, bracemakers, and many others were like saints to my father and my grandparents. Through years of repeat visits for check-ups, new exercises and braces, and multiple surgeries, often accompanied by month-long stays in the hospital, they gave my father encouragement, his mobility, and helped nurture his determination.

> There came a time when—as an awkward 15-year old boy with a full-leg brace on one leg, a weak and withered opposite arm, and a heavy plaster-of-paris body brace to control his scoliosis—my father paid a visit to Boston to his then-orthopaedic surgeon, Dr. Frank Ober. According to my father, Dr. Ober was a stern man, but kind in his own way. "Young man," Dr. Ober began after he had finished examining my father, "I want you to pay close attention to what I'm about to say to you. We both know that you've got problems with that leg and that arm of yours that are never going to go away. But the day you make up your mind that you're no different than anyone else, is the day you'll realize that you can do anything you set your mind to.

> It has now been 73 years since Dr. Ober said that and, although my father passed away 16 years ago at the age of 73, everyone in my family still proudly quotes Dr. Ober, just as my father did all his life. I am very proud of how my father dealt with his handicaps and how he lived his life, exactly, as I see it, as Dr. Ober recommended. The year I was born, in 1945, my father started one of the first radio stations in Maine, and for the next 30 years he was a successful radio and television broadcaster. When he decided to use a motorized wheelchair when he was in his 70s, it was simply a way to increase his mobility and his independence! Throughout his life there was no place my father would not try to go and nothing he

would not try to do, much to the terror of his parents when he was young, and to my mother when he was older. (D. W. Brown 1999)

Ober wrote and spoke about many other orthopaedic problems in children: osteomyelitis, septic knee joints, fractures and dislocations of the patella, neuritis, proper shoe wear, the lame back, use of corsets for backache, rheumatoid arthritis pain, and others. He used the Hibbs spinal fusion procedure to treat scoliosis that developed quickly. A superb clinician, Ober was frequently asked to speak at local, regional, and national meetings. He often presented and discussed cases or presented papers at meetings of the Boston Orthopaedic Club, the New England Pediatric Society, the Suffolk District Medical Society, and the Tufts Alumni Association, and at numerous conferences of the Massachusetts Medical Society. As a member (and later chairman) of the Committee on Postgraduate Medical Instruction, he initiated a series of postgraduate courses for the Massachusetts Medical Society. He also conducted, weekly, a long-standing series of combined medical, pediatric, surgical, and orthopaedic surgical clinics with staff, faculty, and residents from Children's Hospital and the Peter Bent Brigham Hospital, where they were held. Dr. Ober was very active in the Massachusetts Medical Society and served as president in 1940. At the time, he was 59 years old. He served as chairman of the Committee on Post-Graduate Instructions, the Central Professional Committee, the Committee on Society Headquarters, and the Committee on Expert Testimony, and he presented many reports at the society's meetings. He even published a paper about the society's meeting places over its almost 200-year history.

Ober was a leader of and had great influence in the Massachusetts Medical Society. As president, he presided over a debate on proposed changes to the bylaws on April 15, 1942. The meeting lasted seven hours, during which time Ober demonstrated his effective leadership skills—he moderated the debate, obtained timely votes on issues, got members to collaborate, achieved results, appointed members to appropriate committees, and allowed full discussion of issues without being directly involved. On another occasion, he supported a requirement that new members of the Massachusetts Medical Society be required to have a license and to have practiced for at least two years, contradicting the proposed draft requiring only one year of practice; his motion to amend was defeated, a decision he accepted. In 1944, as chairman of the Committee on Expert Testimony, he reported the committee's recommendations (after two years of meetings): "1. That a standing committee of five or more, to be called the committee on Medicolegal Problems, be appointed by the president. 2. That the by-laws of the Massachusetts Medical Society be amended to provide for such a body" (*New England Journal of Medicine* 1944). The report was accepted, and, in the discussion, Ober made the following observations:

> There are a great many matters that have to be considered with this thing. First, there is the bad medical witness, and there is the court testifier who goes around testifying as an expert in all sorts of things…the question of subpoenas, having a constable come into your office and serve you with a subpoena as an ordinary witness, and you get down there to the court and find you are going to be qualified as an expert witness…that does not seem to be quite fair to some of us. Then there is the question of one doctor testifying against another…The Committee on Ethics and Discipline is a court, as I see it, to settle many problems of this nature… Every doctor should be informed concerning what constitutes malpractice and concerning proper conduct toward his patient, so that he does not interfere with the code of ethics of the American Medical Association…so that he will not tell some patient, "Well, so-and-so just treated you rottenly." We should like to stop all that…Under the prevailing system of trial by jury…the conduct of a lawsuit is a bilateral

contest to see which side will win…Too often the debate is emotionalized and dramatized by one side or the other in order to influence the jury. Therefore, it would seem in the interests of justice that some other method of considering expert testimony might be worked out which would be superior to our present system…

The functions of a standing committee on medical expert testimony should be twofold; first, punitive and, second, educational. It should set up a program of education for the physicians. (*New England Journal of Medicine* 1944)

In addition to the numerous organizations in which Ober actively participated, he was engaged with organizations that supported the care of patients with polio: he was a trustee of the International Poliomyelitis Congress, chairperson of the Advisory Committee of the National Foundation for Infantile Paralysis, and a member of the Board of Consultants of the Warm Springs Foundation. (Franklin D. Roosevelt was president of the Warm Springs Foundation trustees, others of whom included Osgood and Legg, both from Children's Hospital.) Ober served on the Board of Associate Editors of the *Journal of Bone and Joint Surgery* along with A. R. Shands Jr., Leo Mayer, and G. E. Haggart. (William Rogers was editor.) In 1948, Ober served as president of the Tufts Alumni Association and was a trustee of Tufts University.

Ober was surgeon-in-chief of the New England Peabody Home for Crippled Children for almost two decades, and one of the trustees for 14 years before his death. During his tenure as chief, he and the staff provided care to hundreds of ill children, most of whom had skeletal tuberculosis. Ober encouraged open discussion among the staff and visitors in order to achieve the best treatment for each patient, most of whom recovered fully from their illness. Ober also supervised the care of children at the Perkins Institution and the Massachusetts School for the Blind.

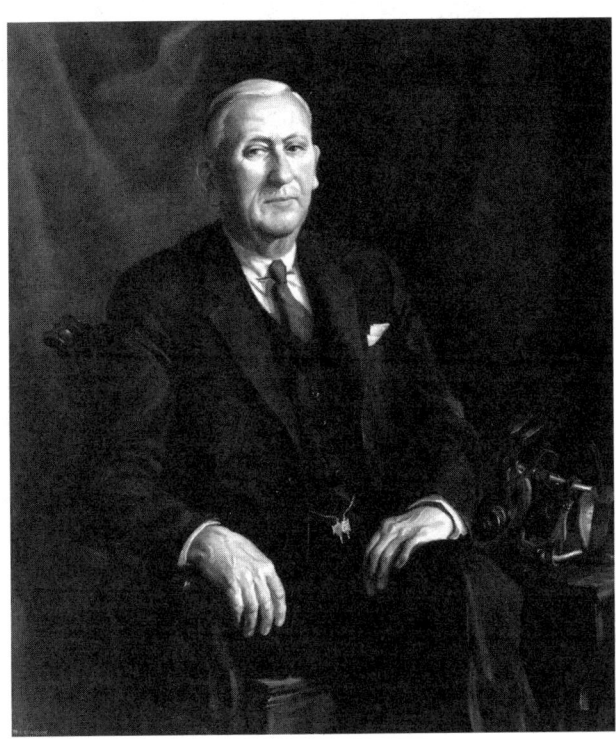

Portrait of Dr. Ober. Boston Children's Hospital Archives, Boston, Massachusetts.

Although Dr. Ober had no children, he had an intense interest in them, especially those who were crippled or handicapped in any way. To improve their lot, as well as that of adults, he established the Frank R. Ober Research Fund at the Children's Hospital Medical Center, by obtaining gifts and contributions from his patients. This fund with additions, will serve as lasting memorial to his vision. (*New England Journal of Medicine* 1961)

Ober was recognized by his alma mater in 1943 when the Tufts University School of Medicine awarded him an honorary doctorate of science. He also received an honorary degree from the University of Vermont, likely in recognition of his many years spent caring for patients with polio in that state:

His philanthropic interest in all handicapped people is exemplified in his being largely responsible for establishing "The Robert W.

Lovett Memorial Foundation" at Harvard Medical School...created 'for the study of diseases causing deformity.' It sponsored the arthritis clinic at Massachusetts General Hospital where active research in the study of this disease has continued from 1928. (*New England Journal of Medicine* 1961)

In 2000, the Robert W. Lovett Professorship was activated from this Lovett memorial fund. Christopher Evans, PhD, was named as the first recipient.

Ober was not only a caring clinician and skilled educator. He enjoyed writing and undertook the work of revising the first edition of Jones and Lovett's textbook *Orthopedic Surgery*. He was an avid hunter and fisherman, vacationing each year in the Adirondacks, and he liked to play cards with friends. Ober continued practicing until he was hospitalized after an operation. Hugenberger, who had been in practice with Ober and had visited him in the hospital on Christmas Day 1960, reported Ober's eagerness to be discharged so he could be available to perform upcoming surgeries. Ober had also been working on the third edition of *Orthopedic Surgery*. Ober's plans were cut short on December 26, 1960, when he died from a pulmonary embolism. He was survived by his wife, Ina Spurling, in Brookline, and his brother, Ernest, in Maine.

CHAPTER 21

William T. Green
Master in Pediatric Orthopaedics

William Thomas Green, known to his friends as "Bill" and to colleagues and staff as "WTG," was born in Waucoma, Iowa, but grew up in southern Indiana. His father, an 1898 medical school graduate who became a general practitioner in a small town in Indiana, married a nurse and had two children: "Willie" (as Green was called as a boy) and his sister, Jean, who remained her entire life in Indiana (spending a brief period as a journalist with the *Washington Post*). William Green attended the University of Indiana—becoming a "crusty Hoosier" (H. Banks, pers. comm., 2009). He graduated with an AB degree in 1921 and an AM degree in anatomy in 1922. While he was pursuing his master's degree, he was an instructor of anatomy at the Indiana University School of Medicine, from which he later graduated, in 1925.

TRAINING AND EARLY PRACTICE

Green spent the following five years training in general surgery and orthopaedic surgery, eventually choosing orthopaedics as his specialty. In 1926, he interned at Indiana University Hospital and was an assistant resident in general surgery at Henry Ford Hospital. He returned home and practiced with his father from 1927 to 1928. Green's motivations for leaving his father's practice are unknown, but, in 1928, he returned to Henry Ford Hospital for

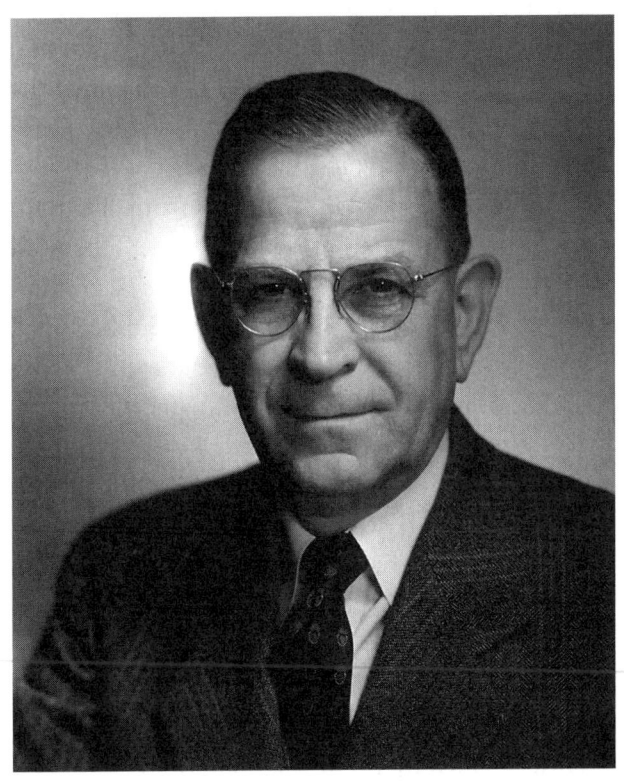

William T. Green. *Clinical Orthopaedics and Related Research*, 1968; 61: 3.

Physician Snapshot

William T. Green
BORN: 1901
DIED: 1986
SIGNIFICANT CONTRIBUTIONS: Leader in orthopaedic education for medical students and residents; expert in the diagnosis and treatment of numerous pediatric conditions, especially in polio, cerebral palsy, and congenital abnormalities

a one-year residency in orthopaedic surgery. After that, Green moved to Boston, residing in the Longwood area. He spent one year (1929–1930) as an assistant resident in general surgery under Harvey Cushing at the Peter Bent Brigham Hospital. From 1930 to 1931, he was a resident in orthopaedic surgery at Children's Hospital under Dr. Frank Ober—he was Ober's first orthopaedic resident, in fact. His residency occurred during the transition from Dr. Robert Osgood's leadership as chair of the orthopaedic department to that of Ober. After all that—an internship, work in his father's practice, two years of a general surgery residency, two years of an orthopaedic residency, and then a stint as chief resident—Green joined the staff at Boston Children's Hospital and the Peter Bent Brigham Hospital.

Green met Gladys Griffith, from Detroit, during his residency at Henry Ford Hospital, where she was the superintendent's secretary. They wanted to marry. Gladys had asked her boss, Henry Graham, for advice about the man she was thinking of marrying. Graham "advised her not to marry [him because] his mistress was orthopaedics" (W. Green Jr., pers. comm., 2009). Gladys didn't take her boss's advice, and in 1930 she married Green and they moved to Belmont at 126 Prospect Street. At the time, under Cushing at Peter Bent Brigham Hospital, residents were not allowed to marry, and William and Gladys "kept it quiet" (W. Green Jr., pers. comm., 2009). They eventually moved to Brookline, where they had three children: William T. Green Jr., who also grew up to become an orthopaedic surgeon, and two daughters, Janet and Elizabeth. Janet later became a specialist in Soviet affairs, serving as a writer and administrator of the Russian Research Center at Harvard. (No additional information was found for Elizabeth.) The family had a summer home for years in Duxbury, Massachusetts, about 35 miles southeast of Boston.

As Ober began his tenure as chair of orthopaedics at Children's, he wanted someone working full time to help accomplish the orthopaedic department's goals, which included upgrading the level of teaching and expanding efforts for both clinical practice and research. After Green completed his training, Ober invited him to join the staff there and Ober's practice on Marlborough Street.

EARLY CONTRIBUTIONS TO ORTHOPAEDICS

Over the next the 15 years, Green rose through the ranks at Children's Hospital, from junior assistant orthopaedic surgeon to visiting orthopaedic surgeon to orthopaedic surgeon. During that time, he also advanced at Harvard Medical School: he was an assistant in orthopaedic surgery for three years, becoming an instructor in orthopaedic surgery in 1934 and assistant professor in 1940.

Green would make many original contributions in various areas of the growing field of pediatric orthopaedics, but he never published some "experimental and clinical investigations of major significance" (H. H. Banks 1968). According to Banks:

> [Green's] first endeavor was a striking demonstration of the concept that wire, nail, or tendon implants through the center of the epiphysis do not arrest growth in the epiphysis, while compression and screw fixation in the same area causes fusion of the epiphysis. These observations were readily applicable to the problem of tendon transplantation and epiphysiolysis and to the treatment of injuries of the growth zones of the skeleton. In addition, Dr. Green investigated the circulation of the head of the femur in children and described the blood vessels in the retinacula of Weitbrecht. Using investigations of the blood vessels of the hip joint, Green devised a set of principles of closed treatment of congenital dislocation of the hip and open reduction of slipped capital femoral epiphysis.
> (H. H. Banks 1968)

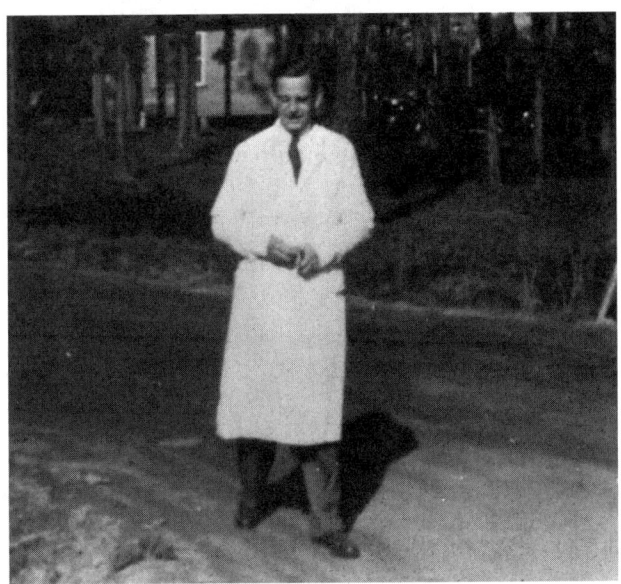

William T. Green as a young man. MGH HCORP Archives.

> **Author Recollections**
>
> Although Green published numerous papers and gave many presentations at regional and national meetings, those who knew him personally and worked with him—myself included—know that he never published many of his ideas and original surgical procedures. For many years early in my practice, I kept an archive of my surgical dictations of Green's operations from Children's Hospital; before undertaking a specific operation that Green or others had developed, I would refer to those dictations to help me recall the important details of the procedure.

The works that he did publish included contributions to bone and joint infections, skeletal growth (normal and abnormal), polio, cerebral palsy, Volkmann contracture, Legg-Calvé-Perthes disease, congenital dislocation of the hip, slipped capital femoral epiphysis, bone diseases (neurofibromatosis, eosinophilic granuloma, and osteochondritis dissecans), Sprengel deformity, and tendon transfers. He also often emphasized the importance of rehabilitation.

Osteomyelitis

Early in his career as a visiting orthopaedic surgeon at Children's Hospital in 1932, Green spoke frequently and published several papers on osteomyelitis and septic joints in infants (aged two years or younger). He presented his experience and treatment concepts to both pediatricians and orthopaedic surgeons. He differentiated osteomyelitis in infants from that occurring in children over the age of two years: In infants, the duration is shorter, wound healing occurs more quickly, and sequestration and recurrences occur less often. *Staphylococcus* is the most common pathogenic organism in osteomyelitis among older children, whereas both *Staphylococcus* (63%) and *Streptococcus* (30%) have been identified in those younger than two years. Also, lesions often fully heal in younger children, whereas sclerosis of the bone remains in those older than two years.

Ober, in discussing one of Green's presentations to the American Medical Association, stated that in the early 1900s infants with osteomyelitis required an immediate operation with "removal of a piece of bone, tunneling the shaft" (F. R. Ober 1925), and afterward, frequent dressing changes. The resulting mortality was ~50%. Ober stated that "it was not until Dr. Green began his study of osteomyelitis, however, that any of us became aware of the fact that, no matter what was done in the way of surgery, the reaction of the bone was practically the same. Of these ninety-five cases… only six show[ed] sequestration" (F. R. Ober 1925). Green reported a mortality of 21% among these infants, i.e., all children under 2 years old. Mortality was 44% in patients under six months of age and 13.4% in patients between six months and two years of age.

He advocated limiting invasive treatments to the extent possible and endorsed supportive treatment, with immobilization of the limb with a splint while waiting for an abscess to form, which could then be drained. If no abscess formed, he recommended that the surgeon make a small window in the bone to allow drainage. In one paper Green stated that "by allowing an osteomyelitic process in infancy to localize, a minimal amount of surgery may be done with very good results" (W. T. Green 1934a).

Bone Growth and Leg Length Discrepancy

Green also developed an early and avid interest in normal bone growth and correction of leg length discrepancies, which he maintained throughout his career. According to Anderson, Green, and Messner (1963): "In planning the surgical control of unequal extremity lengths during the growing years, knowledge of the amount of growth which may occur in the long bones after various ages is fundamental." Dr. Thomas Morgan Rotch had performed the first studies of bone age at Children's Hospital, and in 1907 he published the first book in the field, titled *The Roentgen Method in Pediatrics*. In 1933, Phemister published a now classic paper on his technique of epiphyseal arrest and his study of leg length measured by using teleroentgenography in six children (**Table 21.1**).

Table 21.1. Leg Lengths Measured from Teleroentgenograms

	Femur		Tibia	
	Entire Bone	Diaphysis	Entire Bone	Diaphysis
Female				
8 years	37.0 (14.500)	33.0 (13.000)	31.0 (12.125)	28.8 (11.125)
13 years	42.8 (16.875)	39.5 (15.375)	36.5 (14.375)	33.5 (13.250)
13 years [sic]	44.5 (17.500)	39.7 (15.625)	35.5 (13.875)	32.6 (12.875)
Male				
12 years	40.0 (16.000)	36.8 (14.25)	31.7 (12.500)	29.0 (11.375)
14 years	44.5 (17.500)	39.6 (15.625)	35.0 (13.250)	32.4 (12.750)
16 years	48.0 (19.125)	43.2 (17.000)	39.0 (15.500)	36.5 (14.375)

Data are in centimeters (inches) (D. B. Phemister 1933).

Phemister based the timing of epiphyseal arrests upon his study of leg length in healthy growing children. Fifty years earlier, Toldt had reported similar measurements taken from skeletons of children of various ages and adults (**Table 21.2**).

Table 21.2. Total and Diaphyseal Lengths of the Femur and Tibia as Measured by Toldt

	Femur		Tibia	
	Entire Bone	Diaphysis	Entire Bone	Diaphysis
Female				
4 years	21.3	18.2	17.8	15.3
Adult	41.1	—	33.5	—
Male				
6.5 years	25.6	22.2	20.3	17.6
12 years	38.3	34.5	30.8	28.0
15 years	42.2	38.3	35.3	32.1
Adult (mean of 9)	46.7	—	37.4	—

Data are in centimeters (D. B. Phemister 1933).

Phemister stated that the method used by Kenelm H. Digby to calculate the longitudinal growth of the long bones that occurred from each of the proximal and distal epiphyses in the upper and lower extremities was probably the most accurate (**Table 21.3**).

Table 21.3. Longitudinal Growth of Long Bones as Measured by Digby

Bone	Growth from the Epiphyses (inches)	
	Upper End	Lower End
Femur	5.000	11.000
Tibia	7.500	5.000
Fibula	7.500	5.000
Humerus	9.500	2.500
Radius	2.000	6.000
Ulna	1.750	5.625

(D. B. Phemister 1933).

Green would go on to make significant contributions to this field as well. His first paper on the normal development of the foot was published in 1938. Like Phemister, he also studied and published on the use of orthoroentgenograms and his early experiences with epiphyseal arrest.

Arthritis

About two years later, in 1940, Green presented a paper entitled "Mono-Articular and Pauciarticular Arthritis in Children" at the seventh Annual Meeting of the American Rheumatism Association. Only a brief abstract was published in the *Journal of the American Medical Association*. He reviewed 43 cases of arthritis of the knee and 35 cases of pauciarticular arthritis. Then, as today, "pauciarticular arthritis" referred to cases involving four or fewer joints. Today the term is applied to juvenile idiopathic arthritis or juvenile rheumatoid arthritis. Green summarized that, at least in Boston and its surrounds, the "mono-articular and pauciarticular type [of arthritis] in children is more commonly nonspecific than [that] due to syphilis or tuberculosis" (W. T. Green 1940). He noted that rheumatic fever was often the cause of pauciarticular arthritis. Dr. J. Albert Key, in discussing Green's presentation, agreed, noting that cases could be caused by Still's disease or rheumatic fever, though Key noted, "Long ago I heard Dr. Osgood say, 'when confronted with chronic progressive mono-articular arthritis in a child, the diagnosis is tuberculosis until proved otherwise'" (W. T. Green 1940, in "Discussion"). Dr. Walter Bauer of Boston also agreed: similar to adult patients, children with this type of arthritis often have "an atypical form of rheumatic fever or rheumatoid arthritis" (W. T. Green 1940, in "Discussion"). No patients in Green's series had antistreptolysin titers measured. Regarding orthopaedic treatment, Green emphasized rest and "local treatment [, which] in the chronic group involves the active correction of the deformity. Traction applied to the joints allows correction of the deformity and active painless motion" (W. T. Green 1940, in "Discussion"). He also noted that the involved extremity often lengthened in both groups: "In twelve of the cases in which the knee was involved, there was an average lengthening of 1.3 cm. with squaring of the epiphysis" (W. T. Green 1940).

Bone Granuloma

The following year, in 1941, Green and Dr. Sidney Farber presented a paper entitled "A Recently Defined Destructive Lesion of Bone" at a meeting of the Boston Orthopedic Club. They stated, "A new disease under the name 'solitary granuloma' and 'eosinophilic granuloma'…has been described in the recent literature" (Green and Farber 1941), specifically in two papers, one by Lichtenstein and Jaffee, the other by Otani and Ehrlich. Green and Farber reported on ten patients under the age of 12 years who had bone lesions similar to solitary bone cysts, as seen on radiographs. The pathologic tissue "was essentially a granulomatous process in which eosinophilic infiltration was frequently a prominent feature" (Green and Farber 1942), as in tissue from patients with Hand-Schüller-Christian disease or Litterer-Siewe disease. They concluded that eosinophilic granuloma was not "a new or a separate disease entity" (Green and Farber 1942).

At the annual meeting of the AAOS in 1942, they reported 13 cases followed at Children's Hospital since 1930. That paper was published later the same year in the *Journal of Bone and Joint Surgery* and reported outcomes from 10 (of the original 13) patients with significant follow-up 10 years after diagnosis. Green and Farber (1942) noted, "Ordinarily, the lesions have healed quite promptly after roentgen radiation, and, on occasion, after curettage."

Cerebral Palsy

Green's first publication on cerebral palsy, cowritten with Leo McDermott, was also published in 1942. Bronson Crothers (1884–1959), a pediatrician, had been assigned to a new neurology service at Children's Hospital in 1920. Two types of patients were usually treated on that service: the most common were those with a birth palsy of the upper extremity, followed by those with cerebral palsy. By 1930, a neurological ward (Ward Nine) was opened for treating these patients (commonly through physical therapy, pool exercises, carbon-arc and ultraviolet light treatments) and for performing clinical research. (Before his retirement in 1942, Crothers, with coauthor R. S. Paine, began writing a book on cerebral palsy, which they published 15 years later as *The Natural History of Cerebral Palsy*.) It was during this early and active program for patients with cerebral palsy—specifically sometime soon after Green became a visiting orthopaedic surgeon—that he developed an interest in cerebral palsy and began treating patients with the disorder. Green and McDermott's first publication reviewed their experiences in treating 160 patients at Children's Hospital and the Peter Bent Brigham Hospital from 1925 to 1940. A total of 421 operations were done during that 15-year period. The paper is important because they reported outcomes of treatment, after a mean follow-up of six years, with three different methods of result analysis. They concluded that only some patients with spastic paralysis, and not many with extrapyramidal cerebral palsy, would benefit from operative orthopaedic procedures, and thus these surgeries should not be the main form of treatment in such patients.

Green and McDermott reported procedures they used for the foot, knee, hip, and wrist, as well as the results obtained after those procedures. For the foot, they reported that heel-cord lengthening was beneficial; patients who also had a triple arthrodesis (Hoke type) showed the best results. For the knee, hamstring lengthening was the most common procedure, and patients with lengthening of both the hamstrings and the proximal gastrocnemius achieved the best results. They reported disappointing results with adductor myotomy and obturator neurectomy in the hip. Other less common hip procedures included Ober fasciotomy and a release described by Soutter and Legg. Green and McDermott reported excellent results with flexor carpi ulnaris transfer to the extensor carpi radialis longus for wrist flexion/forearm pronation contractures; neurectomy of the pronator teres was not as successful. In general, their results were not favorable in quadriplegic patients, those with very weak muscles, and patients with mental retardation. Green expressed strong support for lower extremity surgery in those who were unable to walk, but only if their prognosis for walking was favorable.

Green's early experience in treating cerebral palsy influenced his thinking about the importance of treatment and rehabilitation of patients after they undergo an orthopaedic procedure—something he would underscore his entire teaching career. Green and McDermott emphasized the use of physical therapy postoperatively, particularly for the muscles that work against the deformity. They noted that insufficient care provided postoperatively and poor patient and caregiver training mainly contributed to unsatisfactory results. A lack of extensive immobilization was their most common mistake, and to avoid this they suggested applying corrective casts to be worn overnight.

Later that same year—this time as sole author—Green reported his early surgical experience with tendon transfer for the treatment of flexion and pronation deformity of the wrist. It would be many years before Green published any further work on cerebral palsy.

Congenital Pseudoarthrosis of the Tibia

The so-called birth fracture, or congenital pseudarthrosis of the tibia, was first described by Sir James Paget in 1891. Barber associated this condition with neurofibromatosis in 1939; Moore did the same in 1941, followed by Green in 1942. Green and Rudo reported the case of a young girl with anterolateral bowing of the tibia who developed a pseudarthrosis of the tibia and fibula (see **Case 21.1**). They reported, for the first time, the histology of tissue at the fracture site, which consisted of neurofibromatous tissue, most likely from nerves in the bone itself. This information

Case 21.1. Tibial Pseudarthrosis in Neurofibromatosis

Part 1

"I.D., a girl aged 6 years 11 months, was admitted to the Children's Hospital on May 14, 1940, complaining of a tender swelling in the right arm and a deformity of the right leg. A lump in the right arm was noted eight months prior to admission. It had increased slightly in size since original observation, and although it did not interfere with the use of the arm, it was quite sensitive to pressure.

"The bowing of the right leg had been present since birth and, except for the deformity, had caused no symptoms. The mother was of the opinion that the degree of deformity had not changed over the years. There was no history of trauma, and at no time had there been any complaint of discomfort. The other details of the history obtained were not considered pertinent to this presentation except that the father had small café au lait spots on his skin.

"Physical Examination. — The child was rather undersized and undernourished. Her skin showed multiple areas of pigmentation, so-called café au lait spots. Her head was markedly dolichocephalic in type and her jaw was prognathic. Her posture was poor, with increased lordosis, protruding abdomen and round shoulders. There was no beading of the ribs or Harrison's groove. Otherwise the examination was not significant except for findings in the right arm and the right lower extremity.

"Palpation of the lateral aspect of the right arm at the junction of the lower and the middle third revealed a tender firm nodular mass beneath the subcutaneous tissue, the main portion of which was about 3 cm. long and 0.6 cm in diameter.

"The right leg showed increased knock knee with anterolateral bowing of the tibia. The left leg was entirely normal, and the lower extremities were equal in length.

"Roentgenograms of the right leg taken at the time of admission revealed an ununited oblique fracture in the distal portion of the fibula, which had evidently been present for some time, and a sinuous bowing of the tibia, most marked in an anterolateral direction. The tibia showed an irregular thickening of the cortex, which was maximal at the level of bowing, but no localized defects could be seen in the bone at this time. Roentgenograms of the remainder of the skeleton showed no significant abnormalities. However, a review of roentgenograms which had been made elsewhere two years previously revealed that the facture of the fibula was not present then, although the appearance of the tibia and the fibula was otherwise similar to that seen in the more recent films.

"Laboratory examinations on admission showed no particular abnormalities. The values of blood calcium and phosphorus were 9.9 mg. and 5 mg. per hundred centimeters, and the value of phosphatase was 9.3 Bodansky units. An intradermal test with tuberculin in the dilution of 1:1,000 was negative, as was the Hinton test for syphilis. The blood cell counts were normal, as were the findings in the urine.

"First Operative Procedure: — On May 27 the mass in the right arm was exposed and found to be a wormlike nodular whitish tumor, which was attached to the radial nerve and in part had to be dissected from it. There were many continuations from the main mass into the fascia and muscles, although bone and periosteum were not involved. All recognizable tumor tissue was excised.

"An incision was then made over the distal third of the right leg so as to expose the tibia at the site of maximal cortical thickening and the fibula in the area of the defect which was visible in the roentgenograms. About 5 cm. above the lateral malleolus, the periosteum over the fibula was found thickened and the underlying bone was bulbous. Incision of the periosteum exposed a definite area of nonunion, from which a rectangular block of bone was removed so as to give a representative longitudinal section of the area. Following this, a section of bone for microscopic examination was removed from the tibia at the site of the greatest cortical thickening. The leg was immobilized in a plaster splint from the toes to the groin, with the knee flexed at about 45 degrees.

"Pathologic Examination of the Tissues Obtained at the First Operation. — The material excised from the right arm was a serpentine mass of thickened nerves. Microscopic examination showed the nerve bundles to be thickened by a proliferation of loosely arranged elongated spindle-shaped cells, a picture typical of plexiform neuroma.

"The block of bone and attached periosteum removed from the region of the ununited fracture of the fibula displayed a freely movable line of dense soft tissue 2 to 3 mm. wide. This zone corresponded to the fracture line seen in the roentgenograms.

"On microscopic examination the fracture fragments were seen to be separated by a vascular cellular tissue composed of streaming bundles to elongated cells with little or no intervening collagen. The nuclei in some areas showed a tendency to form parallel rows or 'palisades.' Osteoblastic activity and osteoid formation were evident along the margins of the fracture fragments and in this region there was an intermingling of the described cellular tissue with fibrous and osteoid tissues. This intermingling of the soft cellular tissue with the osteoid material produced a defective type of osteoid, poorly calcified.

"There were areas of a more cartilaginous type of callus in which there was a tendency for the tissues to disintegrate with formation of eosinophilic debris. In these areas osteoclastic giant cells were numerous.

"The bone at a little distance from the fracture line was entirely normal. The periosteum did not contain any cellular tissue of the type that was found between the fracture fragments. The pathologic diagnosis was intraosseous neurofibroma of the fibula with pathologic fracture and pseudarthrosis.

"The specimen taken from the right tibia was found on microscopic examination to consist of cortical bone which was not unusual except for slight enlargement of the haversian canals. The connective tissue within the canals was quite vascular and showed no neoplastic change or other abnormality. The overlying periosteum was not abnormal. The diagnosis was cortical thickening of the tibia with enlarged haversian canals."

Part 2

"Course in the Interval Before the Second Admission. — When the splint which had been applied at the first operation was removed, Sept. 5, 1940, fourteen and one-half weeks after the operation, there was still no roentgenographic evidence of union of the fibula, although the defect in the tibia created by the removal of the block for microscopic examination had healed.

"Roentgenograms taken on September 19 showed a new rounded defect in the tibia, distal to the site of the previous removal of a section of bone and opposite the site of nonunion in the fibula. This was interpreted as probably a neurofibroma of bone. It was decided that no intervention should be made at this time, but that the defect should be observed.

"Second Admission to the Hospital. — On December 14, seven months after the previous admission to the hospital, the patient was readmitted, with the story that eight days before, while playing the in snow, she fell and injured her right leg. She was taken to a nearby hospital, where an unsuccessful attempt was made to reduce a fracture of the right tibia and fibula. She was then transferred to this hospital with her leg immobilized in a plaster splint. Roentgenographic examination showed a transverse fracture of the tibia at the juncture of the distal two thirds and proximal one third, with a new fracture of the fibula at this same level. The tibia had been fractured approximately through the area of previous removal of bone for biopsy, although no gross defect from this procedure was visible in the roentgenograms. The line of fracture did not involve the defect in the tibia which had been recognized at the last roentgenographic examination and interpreted as a neurofibroma of bone. Attempts at closed reduction of this fracture were unsuccessful in that, although the fracture could be reduced, the surfaces seemed to be smooth and could not be locked in position.

"Second Operation. — Open reduction of the fracture with biopsy of the defect of the tibia was performed on December 23. There seemed to be a small amount of fresh subperiosteal callus at the site of fracture and some similar tissue between the fragments. This was resected down to healthy-appearing bone, and the fracture was fixed with a four screw vitallium plate. Following this, the defect in the tibia distal to the fracture was exposed. The tissue in this area in its gross aspect resembled granulation tissue in many particulars and was separated from the periosteum by a thin layer of cortical bone. It was resected for histologic examination.

"Pathologic Examination of Tissues Obtained at the Second Operation. — The soft tissue nodule removed at the site of roentgenographic defect and the material from the site of the nonunion both showed a histologic picture entirely similar to that seen in the tissue from the area of nonunion in the fibula previously described. The diagnosis was (1) neurofibroma of bone and (2) pathologic fracture of the tibia with neurofibroma of bone."

Part 3

"Course in the Interval Before the Third Admission. — The extremity was immobilized in a plaster splint, which was not removed until April 9, 1941, approximately three and one-half months after the operation. At this time union was solid and there was definite callus with obliteration of the fracture line.

"Third Admission to the Hospital. — The girl was again admitted on June 5, 1941 with the story that ten days before this she had stumbled over a cobblestone, with immediate pain in her right leg. The trauma was minimal. She was able to walk, but the leg became swollen and painful.

"Examination showed tenderness in the distal portion of the tibia, below the site of the former fracture. Roentgenographic examination showed a transverse fracture of the tibia, distal to the previous fracture, at the site of the most recent removal of tissue for biopsy, although the defect created at that time had almost completely healed. There were, however, a few new defects anteriorly just below the fracture line. There was no displacement, and the extremity was immobilized in a plaster splint for several weeks. Since at the end of this time there was no evidence of union, and definite defects in the bone adjacent to the line of fracture existed, an open procedure was performed.

"Third Operation. — On July 29 an incision was made in a longitudinal direction over the distal third of the tibia, excising the scar of the previous operation in this area. The vitallium plate which was used in the immobilization of the previous fracture was removed. Union was solid in this area, and no abnormal tissue was noted. The site of the recent fracture was then exposed. There was no evidence of union. The bone adjacent to the line of fracture in the tibia was resected, as was the area of nonunion in the fibula. The resected portion of the tibia contained certain defects occupied by tissue of fibrous type. The surfaces of the tibia were coapted and plated in position. The distal fragment of the tibia was very atrophic and friable. The use of a large bone graft was considered, but deferred at this time; small osteoperiosteal grafts were placed across the line of fracture. The extremity was immobilized by means of a circular plaster splint extending from the toes to the groin.

"Pathologic Examination of the Tissue Removed at the Third Operation. — The tissue was similar to that seen in previous sections. The histopathologic diagnosis was recurrent neurofibroma of bone with pathologic fracture.

"Fourth Admission to the Hospital. — Roentgenograms of December 15 showed the bone plate to be holding the fragments in good position, but there was no evidence of union: in fact there was absorption of bone from the adjacent surfaces. The patient was then allowed partial weight bearing, a modified Boehler walking iron being used. The absorption of bone from the adjacent fragments which was in evidence in the roentgenograms of December 15 increased markedly, and the patient was readmitted to the hospital on May 16, 1942. The roentgen picture at this time was typical of pseudarthrosis of the tibia.

"Fourth Operation. — On June 25 the vitallium plate, which had broken, was removed, the tissue occupying the fracture line, which was of gray glistening character, was widely excised, and two large bone grafts removed from the opposite tibia were inserted in onlay fashion with fixation by vitallium screws after the technic used by Boyd.

"Pathologic Examination of the Tissue Removed at the Fourth Operation: — Again, histologic examination of tissue from the site of nonunion led to the diagnosis of recurrent neurofibroma of bone.

"On October 15 roentgenograms of the tibia showed solid union."

(William T. Green and Nathan Rudo, 1943)

contributed to our current understanding of the pathophysiology of this rare problem. Green and Rudo suggested that complete excision was necessary, as any of this tissue retained in the bone could allow recurrence and cause the union to fail. After failing to achieve union in three operations, Green and Rudo used large dual onlay bone grafts fixed by screws, as described by Boyd, and reported a successful outcome.

Slipped Capital Femoral Epiphysis

In 1944, at the Section on Orthopedic Surgery at the 49th Annual Session of the American Medical Association, Green discussed 26 patients with a slipped capital femoral epiphysis (SCFE) who had been treated at Children's Hospital and the Peter Bent Brigham Hospital. He published the series the next year in the *Archives of Surgery*. His initial findings on examination included muscle spasm about the hip and loss of range of motion, especially flexion, abduction, and internal rotation. Hip, thigh, or knee pain in an adolescent, especially one who is obese, may be indicative of the condition. He also noted early changes visible on x-ray (lateral view), including resorption in the proximal metaphysis of the femur and subluxation of the femoral head on the neck of the femur. He concluded that the condition must be diagnosed before the epiphysis becomes extensively displaced in order to achieve acceptable outcomes.

Green made four recommendations for achieving good results in hips with a slipped capital femoral epiphysis:

1. Minimal displacement: Internal fixation in situ
2. Minimal to moderate displacement: Initial traction followed by hip-spica cast
3. Severe displacement: Use open reduction and internal fixation
4. Overall, avoid closed reduction (W. T. Green 1945a)

During my residency, Green preferred to fix the head with a single large wood screw. He also stressed the importance of maintaining circulation to the head of the femur.

In discussing Green's paper on slipped capital femoral epiphysis, both Dr. Fremont Chandler and Dr. Walter Blount emphasized how controversial the treatment was at the time, highlighting quick transitions between "conservative" and "radical" therapies. Blount commented on reports of poor results using a flanged nail, sharing his belief that using more small nails or screws achieves a better result than one large nail. Such comments may have influenced Green to favor using a single large wood screw. Green treated patients with spasm accompanying the SCFE using skeletal traction. To avoid further bone trauma, he used internal fixation but not the flanged nail once the spasm was relieved. He also believed in the use of assistive devices, e.g., crutches, that allow partial weight bearing after internal stabilization of the femoral head would help achieve good outcomes.

CHIEF AT CHILDREN'S HOSPITAL AND LEADER IN ORTHOPAEDIC EDUCATION AND RESEARCH

After numerous distinguished contributions to the field, Green was appointed chief of orthopaedics at Children's Hospital in 1946 at 45 years of age. The following year, he was appointed clinical professor and co-head of the orthopaedic department at Harvard Medical School, where he led undergraduate and residency education. During this time, Green held other orthopaedic leadership positions as well, including director of the Harvard Infantile Paralysis Clinic, president of the American Academy for Cerebral Palsy, and president of the American Academy of Orthopaedic Surgeons (AAOS).

As a surgeon, Green designed many new and innovative procedures. He was a "slow, meticulous

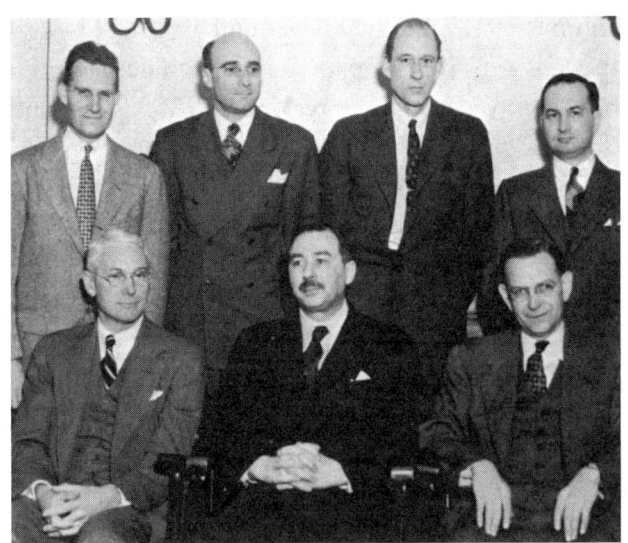

Department chiefs at Boston Children's Hospital, 1949. Dr. Green is seated on the right in the first row.
Boston Children's Hospital Archives, Boston, Massachusetts.

surgeon[,] often assisted by Dr. Grice" (H. Banks, pers. comm., 2009), and later by Dr. Trott. However, "He wasn't a good technician and residents used to make fun of him" (McCarthy and Cassella, pers. comm., 2012). During one epiphyseal arrest, the procedure took so long that resident Eric Radin commented to Green that another growth study would be needed in order to accurately determine the additional bone growth that had occurred during the procedure. Dr. Robert M. Smith, the chief of anesthesia at Children's, recalled both Green and Ober in the operating room:

> Dr. Green was a very good surgeon, but extremely slow. Dr. Ober was working on a case, and he was pretty rough. He would break a bone to set it and push it together again. [Someone would ask,] "Are you going to take an x-ray?" "I don't need an x-ray; I know it's all right," he'd say. He was operating on one of his late cases, and Dr. Green put…his nose in and said, "Dr. Ober, when are you going to quit?" Dr. Ober says, "When I get to be as slow as you are, then I'll quit." (D. Dyer 1993, "Interview with Robert M. Smith")

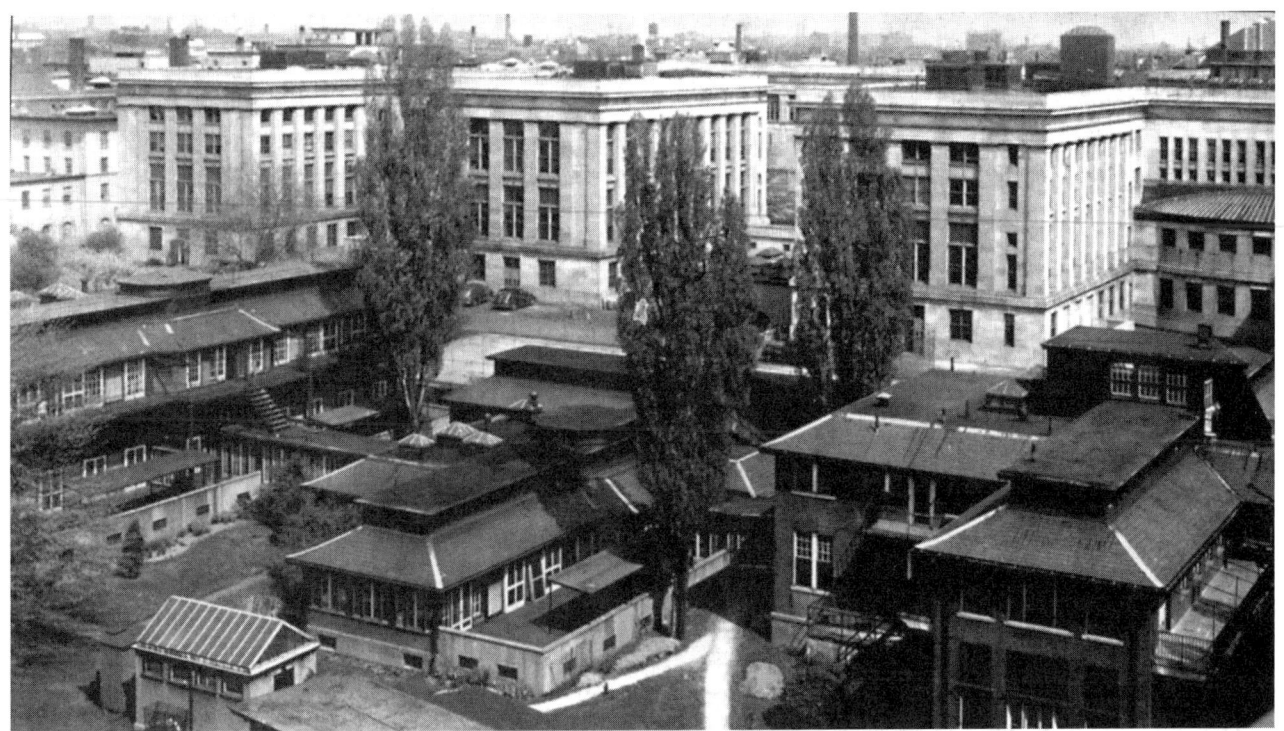

Boston Children's Hospital (foreground) in 1953. *Images of America. Children's Hospital Boston.* Charleston, SC: Arcadia Publishing, 2005. Boston Children's Hospital Archives, Boston, Massachusetts.

Clare McCarthy and Mickey Cassella, physical therapists who worked for decades at Children's Hospital from 1953 and 1954, respectively, referred to Green as "a great teacher...a task master"; they remembered that "Dr. Green always taught and took time to explain" (McCarthy and Cassella, pers. comm., 2012). Jack McGinty recalled that Green was a "good, but always a tough teacher...You liked him or hated him" (J. McGinty, pers. comm., 2009). "He [Green] crucified us and the residents" at Grand Rounds (McCarthy and Cassella, pers. comm., 2012), but he "never embarrassed physical therapists in front of patients and families [though he] often did so to the residents" (McCarthy and Cassella, pers. comm., 2012).

Green saw his patients daily, including Sundays. He led grand rounds, which lasted about one hour on Tuesday mornings: "It was a rigorous teaching experience. All residents were groomed in freshly laundered uniforms and clean white shoes. Dr. Green demanded precise presentations" (H. Banks, pers. comm., 2009). During grand

Author Recollections

I remember attending grand rounds with Green during my residency. On one occasion, the presenting resident could not answer Green's questions about the patient's family history. Green became angry; he stood, told the resident to prepare better for grand rounds, and walked away. On another occasion, when I was a pup and was required to present radiographs in chronological order on the viewing box at the front of the auditorium, Green whispered to me, asking me to retrieve the x-rays on two babies with congenitally dislocated hips who had recently been treated in the hospital by one of the attending physicians. These two patients had not been originally scheduled to be presented on that day. Each had undergone a closed reduction and application of a spica cast under general anesthesia in the operating room the previous day. Green favored preliminary traction and adductor massage which neither child had received before the reductions; and somehow, he knew it. After presenting the x-rays of these two patients, Green lectured the audience about treating congenital dislocation of the hip and criticized the attending physician. It was an embarrassing incident for me, for the audience, and especially for the unprepared surgeon, who was caught unaware when Green began discussing his patients during grand rounds.

I also recall an occasion when Green saw my partner, a senior resident, studying in the library. Green told the resident that he would teach him all he needed to know about orthopaedics and to resume his clinical duties on the floor or he would give him some casts to make. I also remember having to remake casts that Green found to be unacceptable when he examined them during inpatient rounds. Green would mark an "X" on the cast with a green marker and expected the cast to be remade before rounds the next morning—including spicas and body casts.

During Green's tenure as chief, residents had to make celastic body jackets—rigid, form-fitting jackets made for patients to wear for six months postoperatively after a Risser cast had been removed. They were made through a stepwise process that took approximately 14 hours to complete: first, a plaster mold of the body was made while the patient stood upright, suspended in traction. Plaster was then poured into the mold. Once hardened the plaster form was carved and shaved with linoleum knives in order to build additional correction into the final product. Residents sculpted these replica forms during off-hours at night and on the weekends. Once completed, celastic fabric was wrapped around the replica form, allowed to harden, and rounds, senior residents presented the patients, providing a detailed description of the patient's history and physical examination, and a review of the x-rays and appropriate studies; pups and junior residents insured that the x-rays were labeled and presented chronologically. After each case had been presented, Green would call on other residents for their opinion, then he would critique those opinions and comments. "Everyone was terrified about being called on" (H. Banks, pers. comm., 2009). Following grand rounds, all residents and staff accompanied Green on bedside rounds, when they saw all inpatients.

To prepare for Tuesday's grand rounds, on Mondays physical therapists performed muscle examinations on the patients to be presented at rounds. During the grand rounds, physical therapists sat in seats at the back of the auditorium, behind the residents and staff physicians. Green sat in the front seat to the left of the center aisle. (When Green was away, no one would sit in his empty seat.) McCarthy and Cassella recall one

then removed. Technicians in the brace shop would add straps, buckles, and a cloth lining, removing rough edges. The completed jacket was fitted to the patient, and Green or another attending physician would do a final inspection. If the inspector found the jacket to be unsatisfactory, a new one had to be made. Obviously, each resident attempted to make the best jacket possible—not only for the benefit of the patient, but to avoid having to repeat the entire process.

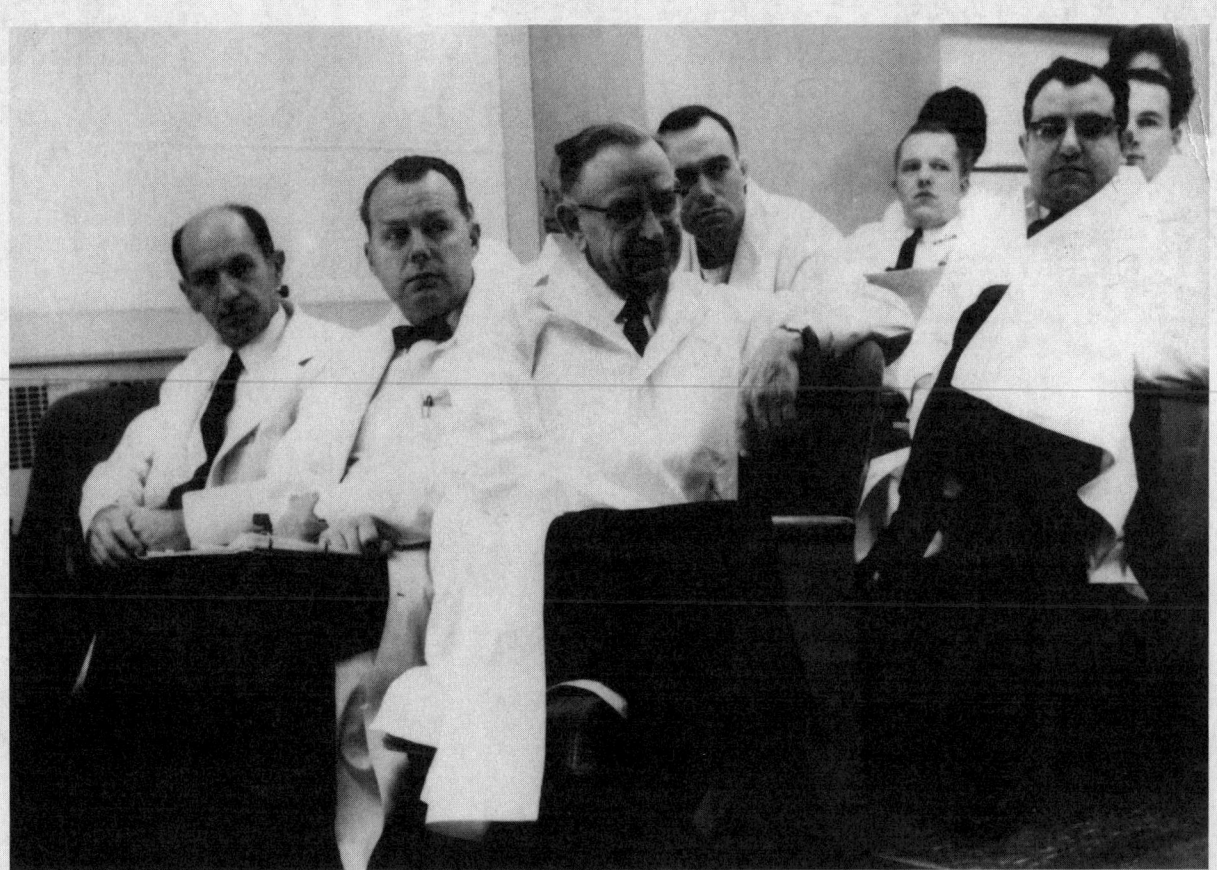

Orthopaedic Grand Rounds. Dr. Green is in the front row on the right. To his right is Dr. Trott and next to Trott is Dr. Cohen. MGH HCORP Archives.

particular incident during McCarthy's presentation of a patient who had been partially paralyzed by polio. McCarthy had reported that the patient's gluteus muscle had fair-minus strength, but the resident had rated the muscle strength as good. Green asked McCarthy to come up and examine the patient in front of the large audience. Green himself also evaluated the patient's muscle strength, rating it fair-minus and supporting McCarthy's finding. McCarthy, obviously upset, stated, "I have never recovered from that" (McCarthy and Cassella, pers. comm., 2012). It has been rumored that Green could tell the grade of a muscle by its appearance.

McCarthy and Cassella also recalled a physical therapy student named Beryl Dunn, who had been visiting from London. After another physician presented a case that centered on the indications for triple arthrodesis versus pantalar fusion in a patient with a complex foot and ankle problem, the audience made no comments. Dunn—who "was dressed up and had only been at Children's Hospital a few months" (McCarthy and Cassella, pers. comm., 2012), and who on this occasion was seated in the last row at the back of the auditorium—eventually raised her hand. Green immediately asked her, "Would you like to come down and lecture us?" (McCarthy and Cassella, pers. comm., 2012). She did. She named the bones seen on the x-rays, described a unique modification of the triple arthrodesis, and recommended it for the

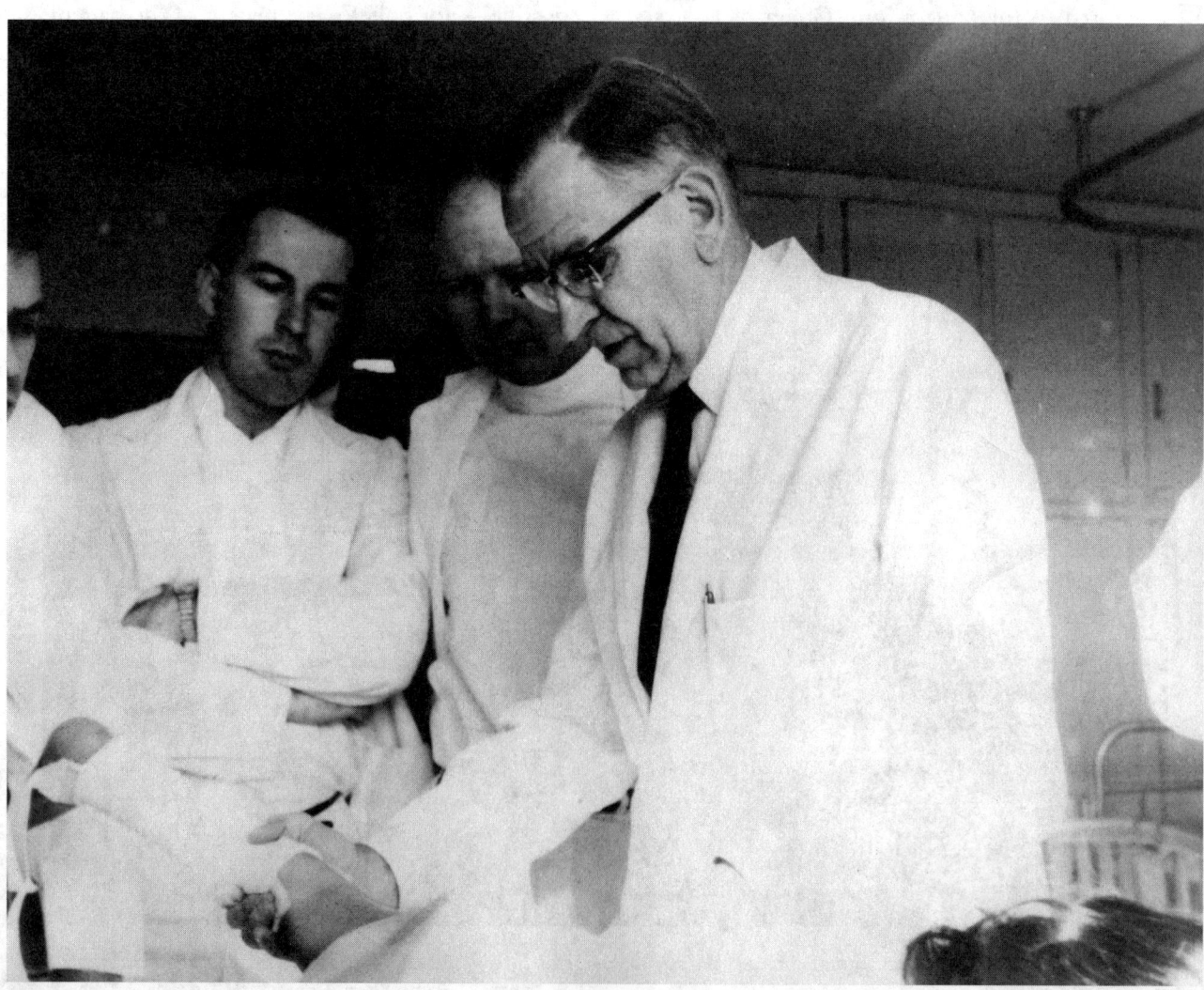

Dr. Green teaching residents on ward rounds. MGH HCORP Archives.

patient. Both the audience and Green were taken aback. Dr. Green asked her, "Where did you find out this information?" (McCarthy and Cassella, pers. comm., 2012). To everyone's surprise, she said her father was Naughton Dunn, an orthopaedic surgeon at the Royal Orthopaedic Hospital in Birmingham, England, who in 1922 described his own modification of a triple arthrodesis in which he completely removed the navicular bone, fusing the head of the talus to the cuneiform bones, the os calcis to the cuboid, and the talus to the os calcis; Beryl Dunn had described her father's modified procedure. By all accounts she stayed on at Children's Hospital for a couple of years. I do not know whether Green personally knew Naughton Dunn, but he most likely was aware of Dunn's operation and publication. (Dunn had trained under Sir Robert Jones, cared for wounded soldiers in World War I, and was well-known throughout Europe and the United States for his operations on paralyzed feet.)

In addition to rounds, Green led other conferences with staff, including a weekly meeting with all residents in his office at Children's Hospital. The chief would express his views about problematic issues in the department and allowed residents to gripe or complain. This weekly meeting had originally been held on Sunday mornings and thus was referred to as the "prayer meeting"; the name stuck, although the day of the meeting changed from Sunday to Saturday and then to Wednesday.

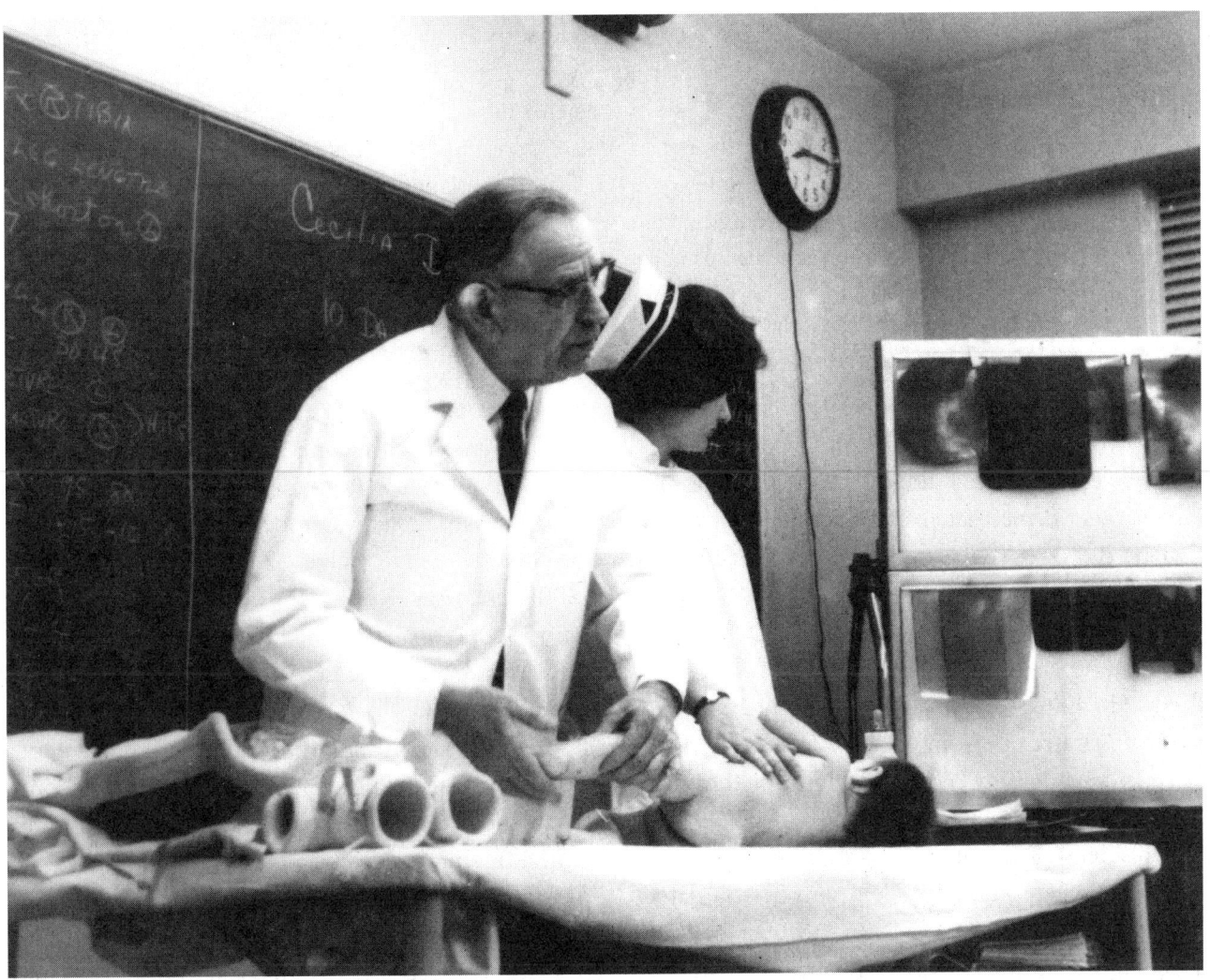

Dr. Green examining an infant at Grand Rounds. Notice the bivalve casts in the left foreground. MGH HCORP Archives.

After these Sunday meetings, Green, accompanied by staff and the residents, would visit all inpatients at the Children's Hospital and the Peter Bent Brigham Hospital. Sometimes these rounds lasted most of the day. He also held a monthly chief's consultation clinic, in which residents presented complex patients, especially those for whom treatment decisions had to be made, and Green gave his advice; often complex issues related to growth disturbance, such as in the foot, were discussed. Although Green "knew only his chief residents by name, he did not know anything personal about the residents or their families…[but] he did learn about those in trouble, who were poor performers or didn't do orthopaedics right" (Z. Zimbler, pers. comm., 2009). According to McCarthy and Cassella, "His patients and families adored him, but he thought a lot of himself…he had a big ego… he terrified us. He got the best out of us by fear" (pers. comm., 2012).

Green was a hard worker, "seemingly inexhaustible [, working] long into the evening hours" (H. H. Banks 1968). I can remember being on call at Children's Hospital and Green sometimes calling around 8 or 9 p.m., telling me to take him on rounds of the inpatients. He routinely ate dinner in the hospital cafeteria, continuing to work, and then leaving the hospital around 9 or 10 p.m., taking two full briefcases with him. According to his son, however, he often didn't open them at home. Green Jr. told me that his father always "felt bad that he didn't have enough time for research; he was continually pulled into education and patient care" (W. Green Jr., pers. comm., 2009). Green also held others to his own high and exacting standards. He didn't treat his staff as colleagues; he had an authoritative persona (A. L. Zaoussis 2001). His residents greatly respected him, but they also feared him. "I was afraid of him" reflected a former resident (Z. Zimbler, pers. comm. 2009). He "polarized everyone…you liked him or you hated him" (J. McGinty, pers. comm., 2009). He had a demanding teaching style, an obvious irritation when residents answered questions incorrectly, and expectations that residents work long hours (sometimes more than 14 hours in a shift), which overtaxed the residents but also taught them all they needed for a solid foundation for a career in pediatric orthopaedics.

At a recent ceremony honoring Dr. Amory Codman, Dr. Hardy Hendren told me a brief story about a nurse who worked with him and Green at Children's Hospital. Hendren had met the nurse for the first time when she was crying in a hallway. When Hendren began to console her, she told him that Green had said she was a horrible nurse because she wouldn't hold the plate while a patient received x-rays; she hadn't wanted to be exposed to the radiation and refused. Hendren was upset at Green because of his behavior and hired her as his own nurse. She worked for him at the Massachusetts General Hospital and then for another 20 years after he moved to working almost exclusively at Children's Hospital.

Not only residents and staff, but also attendings feared the chief. Neither the chief resident nor the attendings would leave the hospital until Green had left. Green would park his car (a Thunderbird) in front of the Jimmy Fund Building, and attendings would check frequently to see whether his car was still in its spot. On one occasion Green had parked his car at Children's Hospital while he was out of town to attend a meeting. The chief resident at the time stayed at the hospital for a couple of days—until the chief's car was gone. This was not unusual, as Green "was away a lot" (Z. Zimbler, pers comm. 2009), serving as president of the American Academy of Orthopaedic Surgeons, the American Board of Orthopaedic Surgery, and the Academy for Cerebral Palsy.

Nevertheless, Green would often take residents to Harvard football games, and he always encouraged them to develop practices in other hospitals and academic medical centers. And as tough as he was on residents, he "never fired anyone" (Z. Zimbler, pers. comm., 2009). Dr. Zeke Zimbler remembers Green being angry at Drs. Lupien and Weinfeld because they had improperly positioned and draped a patient in the operating room. He told them both that they were fired. After receiving assistance from others to reposition and redrape the patient, Green—now satisfied—ordered Lupien and Weinfeld back into the operating room to assist him. Both graduated from the residency program.

In 1962, Dean George P. Berry named Green the first Harriet M. Peabody Professor. The previous department chiefs had been essentially in private practice. Green, however, "became the head of the first department of orthopaedic surgery to be established on a full-time basis in the history of the Harvard Medical School," all of which was made feasible by a 1961 donation from the trustees of the New England Peabody Home for Crippled Children (*News of the Children's Hospital Medical Center* 1962 [Children's Hospital Archives]). According to the stipulations of the donation at the time, "William T. Green's activities will be centered at Children's Hospital and Peter Bent Brigham Hospital...the influence of his Department will extend throughout the entire orthopedic program of the Medical School's Associated Teaching Hospitals" (*News of the Children's Hospital Medical Center* 1962 [Children's Hospital Archives]).

LEADER IN UNDERGRADUATE AND RESIDENCY EDUCATION AT HARVARD

A conference on teaching orthopaedics to medical students was held in June 1948—about one year after his appointment as clinical professor and co-head of the orthopaedic department—at a joint meeting of the American Orthopaedic Association and the Canadian Orthopaedic Association in Quebec, Canada. Dr. A. Bruce Gill of Philadelphia organized this meeting in response to a 1947 report from the Committee of Undergraduate Training of the American Orthopaedic Association that uncovered problems in undergraduate orthopaedic education. In addition to Gill, the committee members were Leroy C. Abbott, Joseph S. Barr, Guy A. Caldwell, Fremont A. Chandler, Paul C. Colonna, John L. McDonald, and Alfred R. Shands Jr. The committee hoped to produce transactions that would serve "as a guide to the deans of the medical schools and the teachers of orthopaedic surgery in the planning for the curriculum of undergraduate orthopaedic education" (*Journal of Bone and Joint Surgery* 1949). A total of 155 orthopaedic educators were invited to attend; they hailed from 55 of the 70 medical schools in the United States, from eight of the nine medical schools in Canada; and from Great Britain.

Attendees discussed four main topics: "(1) Objectives of Teaching, (2) The Curriculum, (3) The Use of Audio-Visual Aids, and (4) The Relationship of the Division of Orthopaedic Surgery with the Other Divisions in the Medical School" (*Journal of Bone and Joint Surgery* 1949). Five speakers focused on undergraduate education; one addressed the issue of the relationship between a division of orthopaedic surgery and other surgical divisions. Attendees from the Alfred I. DuPont Institute, and from the medical schools of the University of Michigan, Johns Hopkins University, Stanford University, and Harvard University, also presented. Shands Jr. summarized the committee's findings, stating that they identified four important objectives for teaching orthopaedic surgery to medical students:

THE WELL-BALANCED CURRICULUM IN ORTHOPAEDIC SURGERY
By WILLIAM T. GREEN, M.D., BOSTON, MASSACHUSETTS
Harvard University
THE JOURNAL OF BONE AND JOINT SURGERY
VOL. 31-A, NO. 1, JANUARY 1949

Title page of Green's article in which he describes his views about orthopaedics in a medical school's curriculum.
Journal of Bone and Joint Surgery 1949; 31: 207.

The first objective should be to give an accurate knowledge of the scope of orthopaedic surgery...that branch of surgery especially concerned with the preservation and restoration of the functions of the skeletal system, its articulations and associated structures. The second objective should be the instruction in how to take a satisfactory orthopaedic history and how to perform an adequate orthopaedic examination...The third objective should be a description of the more common bone and joint disorders, presented in such a way that these can be recognized and differentiated from conditions...in other fields of medicine [—] the differential diagnosis of the specialty. The fourth objective should be the teaching of the fundamental principles of therapy. (A. R. Shands 1949)

At the meeting Green presented "a well thought-out and detailed program" (W. T. Green

Box 21.1. Green's Sample Orthopaedic Curriculum

First Year

Emphasis
- Anatomy and physiology: general (musculoskeletal system, body mechanics); the trunk, neck, and back; upper extremities; lower extremities and gait; and bone growth and abnormalities in embryological development.

Tools
- Well-illustrated lectures emphasizing normal musculoskeletal mechanisms that offset by illustrations of abnormal states
- Dissection with supervision by an orthopaedic surgeon

Second Year

Emphasis
- Pathology (first semester) and orthopaedic exercises (second semester) to highlight abnormalities of the musculoskeletal system and illustrate patients with such abnormalities

Tools
- Illustrated lectures (1 hour each):
  1. Problems arising in the musculoskeletal system; examination of a patient
  2. Trauma of bones
  3. Infections of bones
  4. Joint phenomena, infection, trauma; tendons, bursae, and tendon sheaths
  5. Abnormalities of growth, tumors
  6. Paralysis
  7. Developmental and congenital diseases and abnormalities
  8. Mechanical abnormalities
  9. Metabolic disease (probably by division of medicine)
  10. Therapeutic measure, general, in relation to pathological processes; traction, casts, exercises, etc.

  - Sections (18 hours total):
    - Physical diagnosis of the musculoskeletal system, taught by an orthopaedic surgeon (sections limited to only six students, though demonstrations could accommodate larger groups)
    - Four exercises (total of twelve hours) comprising a 2- or 3-hour visit of each section to the orthopaedic out-patient department to illustrate the problems that arise (supervised by an instructor)
    - Ward rounds by each section to see the problems that are represented and the techniques of treatment
    - Instruction in basic first-aid and bandaging (if not covered elsewhere)

1949c, in "Discussion"). He believed "that somewhere between 20 and 25 percent of the teaching time in surgery should be to orthopaedic surgery…[and that] one of the main difficulties, other than that too little time is allotted to orthopaedic surgery, is that it is frequently worked into the curriculum in haphazard fashion…The Department of Orthopaedic Surgery should itself take part in first-year and second-year teaching [that is] correlated with the instruction given… in basic science" (W. T. Green 1949c). He noted that orthopaedic surgeons rarely served on the curriculum committees, and, even if they did, they had little influence on the amount of time that students were exposed to orthopaedic surgery. Green then presented "a sample curriculum" (W. T. Green 1949c) meant to guide discussion (**Box 21.1**). Green believed that instruction in orthopaedics should begin immediately, in the first year, and be incorporated throughout the

---

Third Year

Emphasis

- Focus on patients, orthopaedic surgery, and problems of the musculoskeletal system, with a goal of giving an understanding of the musculoskeletal system in its relation to the patient as a whole

- Emphasize work with patients, some teaching in large groups, particularly with visual aids. Sections would be of moderate size: a fifth or a sixth of the class for lectures and demonstrations, and smaller groups (approximately six students) assigned to each instructor for work with patients

Tools

- Approximately 20 lectures or exercises:

    1. The patient and the musculoskeletal system
    2. and 3. Congenital anomalies (specific problems, congenital hip disorders, club-foot, other anomalies)
    4., 5. and 6. Neuromuscular abnormalities, including poliomyelitis, obstetrical paralysis, cerebral palsy, etc
    7. and 8. The joints: arthritis, trauma, other conditions
    9. Specific infection of bone (osteomyelitis, tuberculosis)
    10. and 11. The back (the spine, including cervical spine, mechanical difficulties, back pain, sciatica, scoliosis)
    12. Tumors and related abnormalities
    13. Upper extremity, general
    14. Lower extremity, hips to knees inclusive
    15. Leg and foot
    16. Fractures (general management, simple, compound)
    17. Fractures, upper extremity
    18. Fractures, spine
    19. and 20. Fractures, lower extremity

- Sections spending time on the wards and in the outpatient department; students (in small groups) work with patients (with adequate supervision, assistance, and independence); approximately four weeks

Fourth Year

Emphasis

- Four months in surgery, including at least 2 weeks in orthopaedic surgery (including fractures), during which time students assigned to the orthopaedic department, still make the major teaching rounds on the general surgical service during this period, if possible; students in the large surgical section should make regular teaching rounds with the orthopaedic service (e.g., once a week).

Tools

- Patient workups

- "Scrub[bing] up" for operations on their assigned cases

- Participation in all the activities affecting their assigned patients

- One month of elective orthopaedic surgery, during which a student can work with the department, performing many of the duties of a junior house officer.

(Adapted from W. T. Green 1949c)

curriculum, "not merely to teach the facts in orthopaedic surgery, but to give the student a thoughtful approach to the problem of the musculoskeletal system and to medicine in general" (W. T. Green 1949c).

Green intended for this sample curriculum to provide an instructional framework, stressing the importance of gradually integrating instruction on orthopaedic surgery and the importance of beginning this instruction in the first year. He believed:

> The object should not be merely to teach the facts in orthopaedic surgery, but to give the student a though approach to the problems of the musculoskeletal system and to medicine in general. It should be mentioned that the allotment of sufficient time does not of itself assure good teaching in orthopaedic surgery. The more efficient the teaching, the less time is needed. The student's time must be well occupied. (W. T. Green 1949c)

His thoughts on pedagogy—and how to achieve this "efficient" teaching—extended to an analysis of lectures as a method of teaching. He highlighted the pros and cons of lectures:

> There is much to be said for and against the lecture including whole classes at this time. Such a lecture is likely to be delivered by a stimulating, capable individual, whereas, if all the teaching is done in small sectional groups, there is constant repetition, requiring a great extravagance of instructors' time. The result is that the teachers for such groups are not so stimulating or effective as those who might give a lecture to a larger group. A good portion of the work must be sectional, but part can be well covered in lectures. The difficulty of lectures to a large group is that they are likely to be entirely independent of the sectional work as to time. This is not good. The ideal would be to present the subjects, well illustrated and in lecture form, to the whole group and to correlate the sectional work with it; this is usually impossible. (W. T. Green 1949c)

In the same year that Green presented his thoughts on an undergraduate curriculum, he wrote an article on the ideal pediatric orthopaedic curriculum for residents (**Box 21.2**). He listed two "essentials" of a program providing training in pediatric orthopaedic surgery: "1. Sufficient diversified representative clinical material; 2. Capable orthopaedic surgeons in the children's field to spend sufficient time in teaching the men who are in training" (W. T. Green 1949d).

Green maintained the development of an "ideal" curriculum is complex, and not applicable to every training program. He wrote that he believed:

> the best type of training represents an evolution from the apprentice system, in which, in effect, the apprenticeship is to a hospital service with all its attendant diversification rather than to one individual. Essentially the institution should be centered about the problems as they arise on the service. Ordinarily, the problems presented by the patients, singularly and in the aggregate, serve as the axes about which training revolves. Progressive responsibilities and experiences should be given the trainee, as he is ready to receive them. Didactic lectures should be minimal, although, when judiciously used, they may have a place. On the other hand, conferences

---

THE IDEAL CURRICULUM IN CHILDREN'S ORTHOPAEDIC SURGERY

BY WILLIAM T. GREEN, M.D., BOSTON, MASSACHUSETTS

Children's Hospital

THE JOURNAL OF BONE AND JOINT SURGERY
VOL. 31-A, NO. 4, OCTOBER 1949

Title page of Green's article in which he describes the importance of pediatric orthopaedics in residency training programs. *Journal of Bone and Joint Surgery* 1949; 31: 889.

Box 21.2. Important Elements of a Graduate Orthopaedic Training Program

Appropriate Hospitals
- Sufficient patients representing all orthopaedic problems and all ages (growth periods)
- Large outpatient clinics
- Allow follow-up/observation of discharged patients
- Autonomous orthopaedic service
- Participate in undergraduate and graduate teaching in specialities [sic] other than orthopaedics, allowing trainees to grasp the breadth of approaches to childhood problems

Residency Assignments and Rotations
- At least two residents on a junior-senior relationship, both in time of service and experience, as trainees received much effective training by residents who are senior to him in the rotation
  - A larger number of residents is better because duties succeed through a "staggered system" of appointments and provide for a better discussion
- Organize the rotation through children's orthopaedic surgery at the start of the clinical training
  - Must have a senior resident(s) on the children's service who have completed at least two years of training; these residents have a teaching function and are prepared for senior surgical experience
  - Must have a chief resident who has completed three years of training and is prepared for great responsibility

Organization

Staff
- Orthopaedic surgeon-in-chief provides continuity in the program
- Resident staff perform the main activities of the clinics
  - Progress through positions, with increasing responsibility
  - Do the work, rather than simply observe others
- Several visiting physicians who spend time on and off service diversify the teaching program
  - Consult and advise in the outpatient clinics

Clinics
- Organized by condition, staffed by visiting physician with that particular interest
- Provide continuity of care and an excellent teaching element
- Teaching of Surgery
- Must be well supervised
- Evolution from assisting in procedures, to performing them with the assistance of the teacher, to performing them independently (senior residents)

Rounds and Conferences
- Formal rounds: conducted weekly by the chief of the service, with all visiting and house staff present; house staff present cases, giving their ideas; visiting and house staff then discuss the problem
- Resident rounds: conducted daily, with all residents present for the duration, during which visiting staff see the patients, discuss their problems, and consider new admissions
- Chief-of-service resident meeting: held weekly with residents to discuss administrative issues and residents' questions
- Seminars (organized by the chief resident): house staff present papers they've prepared or journal reports; visiting orthopaedic staff or physicians from other fields give talks; x-ray conferences
- Orthopaedic pathological conferences or basic science activities: include content related to pathological physiology and biochemistry; integrates basic science with clinical problems as they arise
- A special orthopaedic laboratory to allow free interchange between the laboratory and clinical groups
- Combined conferences: held weekly; attended by all pediatric services, each of which presents a case for discussion
- Follow-up clinics: all visiting physicians and residents attend; discuss patient outcomes and the results of various procedures

(Adapted from W. T. Green 1949d)

and exercises in which the trainees participate are valuable, and form an essential part of any program. (W. T. Green 1949d)

He understood that despite their best efforts, no curriculum could be used as a template without adjustment to the unique circumstances of each program.

LATER CONTRIBUTIONS TO ORTHOPAEDICS

Despite his unflagging commitment to orthopaedic education, his clinical work, and the large volume of work that remained unpublished, Green did continue to publish extensively as well. Green never published a textbook on pediatric orthopaedics, but two of his former residents, who eventually became colleagues, did: Dr. Albert B. Ferguson Jr., who became a professor and chairperson of the Department of Orthopaedic Surgery at the University of Pittsburgh after leaving his staff position at the Peter Bent Brigham Hospital, and Dr. Mihran Tachdjian, who left his staff position at Children's Hospital in Boston to become the chief of orthopaedics at the Children's Memorial Hospital (now the Ann & Robert H. Lurie Children's Hospital) in Chicago. Ferguson's book was entitled *Orthopaedic Surgery in Infancy and Childhood* and was first published in 1957; Tachdjian's book was entitled *Pediatric Orthopedics*. The patients described and the x-rays published in those books reportedly came from Children's Hospital in Boston. Green supposedly was furious at both "for using his cases without telling him, not asking for his permission or including him as a coauthor" (Z. Zimbler, pers comm., 2009).

Ferguson's book listed four contributors; Green was not one of them. Ferguson states that the cases presented in the text were his own experiences but had roots in the past, and he gave credit in the preface to Dr. Joseph Barr, Green, and his own father (Albert Ferguson Sr.). Yet Ferguson's text included drawings of the flexor carpi ulnaris transfer in cerebral palsy from one of Green's articles but did not credit Green with creating the images (except for listing Green's published article in the references at the end of the chapter). One photograph showed an illustration of a patient in a cast with a spring attached to his scapula after a procedure to correct a Sprengel deformity; that illustration had originally been included in an article by Green, but again, Ferguson did not note that Green's publication was the original source. Eventually Ferguson did credit Green with that procedure to correct a Sprengel deformity—but not until the fifth edition of the text, published in 1981. In that same edition he also credited Dr. Henry Banks and Green for the flexor carpi ulnaris transfer procedure.

Leader in Poliomyelitis Treatment and Research

Green had followed Dr. Arthur T. Legg as director of the Harvard Infantile Paralysis Clinic in 1940, a position he held until 1960. In 1946—the same year Green was appointed chief of orthopaedics at Children's Hospital—Harvard stopped providing patient care and transferred their polio programs to Children's. Green was responsible for this transition and remained in charge of the newly named Massachusetts Infantile Paralysis Clinics there. The Massachusetts chapters of the National Foundation for Infantile Paralysis paid the costs for patients in these clinics, which were adjusted annually. The clinic at Children's Hospital comprised the main center and external centers were scattered throughout nearby locations. Patients could receive physical therapy regularly at the external centers, but any new cases or problem cases were seen at the main clinic.

At the time of this transfer of the polio clinics to Children's Hospital, Green was also leading the Unit for Epidemic Aid in Infantile Paralysis of the National Foundation for Poliomyelitis, a national group that provided consultations regarding patient care and methods for organizing programs to dealing with polio epidemics throughout the United States. Personnel from Children's Hospital staffed the unit. Green led this group during many polio epidemics over seven years, from 1944 to 1951. During his time as director of the polio clinics and leader of the Unit for Epidemic Aid in Infantile Paralysis, Green published widely on poliomyelitis and its treatment: ~13 articles and abstracts, 3 book chapters, and 3 instructional course lectures (with Dr. David Grice) for the American Academy of Orthopaedic Surgeons (AAOS). He also compared the Kenney method for treating polio with that used by the Harvard Infantile Poliomyelitis Commission (1945) and reported no substantial difference in the results of either method.

In 1948, Green wrote the "Present-Day Status of Poliomyelitis" for the *New England Journal of Medicine*. For him, it was an important topic to review because he knew "of no other disease in which the public has such a great interest and… apprehension out of proportion to its incidence, morbidity and mortality. Many sensational statements regarding new developments are reported in the lay press…without scientific confirmation. The public is more likely to be aware of exaggerated, false claims then [*sic*] of actual scientific evidence" (W. T. Green 1948a). He recognized the great support for research provided by the National Foundation for Infantile Paralysis, but he also knew that research progressed slowly. He noted, the means of transmission remained unknown, that tonsillectomy was known to be associated with bulbar poliomyelitis and therefore should be avoided during an epidemic, and importantly, that "we are still without a method of increasing either passive or active immunity to the virus" (W. T. Green 1948a). After considering clinical issues, pathology, and treatment as they relate to polio, Green concluded that "treatment…may be very simple in patients with mild involvement [but] in a small percentage of cases, it is a long, arduous task requiring highly skilled, patient, physical therapists and careful medical supervision…All patients, from the onset of the disease, are best cared for in the hospital" (W. T. Green 1948a). The following year, he recommended that patients take 20-minute hot baths in a Hubbard tub before receiving physical therapy to correct deformities and increase joint motion. The hot baths relieved the patient's pain and relaxed tight muscles.

In his "Present-Day Status of Poliomyelitis," Green had written that "the real advance will come when infantile paralysis can be prevented" (W. T. Green 1948a). In 1949, Dr. John Enders and colleagues successfully created a tissue culture of the poliomyelitis virus; however, a vaccine was not yet ready. During this time and his final years leading the Unit for Epidemic Aid, Green helped found the Mary MacArthur Memorial Respiratory Unit at Wellesley Hospital; he served as director of that unit in 1950. He also organized polio-related courses at Children's Hospital; two courses were offered annually to health care providers—mainly doctors, nurses, and physical therapists, who traveled from around the country to attend.

Just a few years later, in 1952, Dr. Jonas Salk first tested his polio vaccine. In 1954, Green served on the Advisory Committee to the Poliomyelitis Vaccine Evaluation Center, which evaluated Salk's testing of his vaccine. The following year, the committee recognized the role the vaccine would play in curtailing the prevalence of the disease—and eventually ending its ubiquity. The polio vaccine became available to the public in 1955.

Green continued to research polio-related conditions, and, in 1956, he and Grice reported a series of 152 children with polio who developed a calcaneus deformity, a severe condition that is difficult to treat in older children. Green reported that the foot could be stabilized through an early (within 18 to 24 months after paralysis) tendon transfer in these children, avoiding severe deformity. He used any available muscles in the front of the foot, transferring them to the os calcis apophysis. Early in the series, he used supplemental arthrodesis, but later he found that the transfers alone, if strong enough, were sufficient. If arthrodesis was needed, he advocated for an extra-articular (subtalar) technique. Among 58 patients with a strong anterior tibial muscle and in whom the peroneus longus was transferred to the os calcis, 30 patients developed dorsal bunions. These bunions did not develop in patients with a weak or absent anterior tibial muscle. To avoid the bunions, Green recommended suturing the distal end of the peroneus longus to the peroneus brevis muscle tendon unit.

Dr. Arthur Trott, collaborating with Green and others, wrote two papers on circulatory changes in the lower extremities in patients with polio, noting that in those who had been paralyzed for a long time, poor circulation often causes "cold, clammy and often cyanotic extremities" (Trott, Hellstrom, and Green 1956). They measured skin and muscle temperatures at various sites on both the normal and the paralyzed (opposite) legs in 153 patients. They also measured temperatures at the same sites in 98 healthy people. They found that in healthy participants, simple bed rest reduced circulation to the same extent as the circulation measured in the patients with polio. They found no substantial

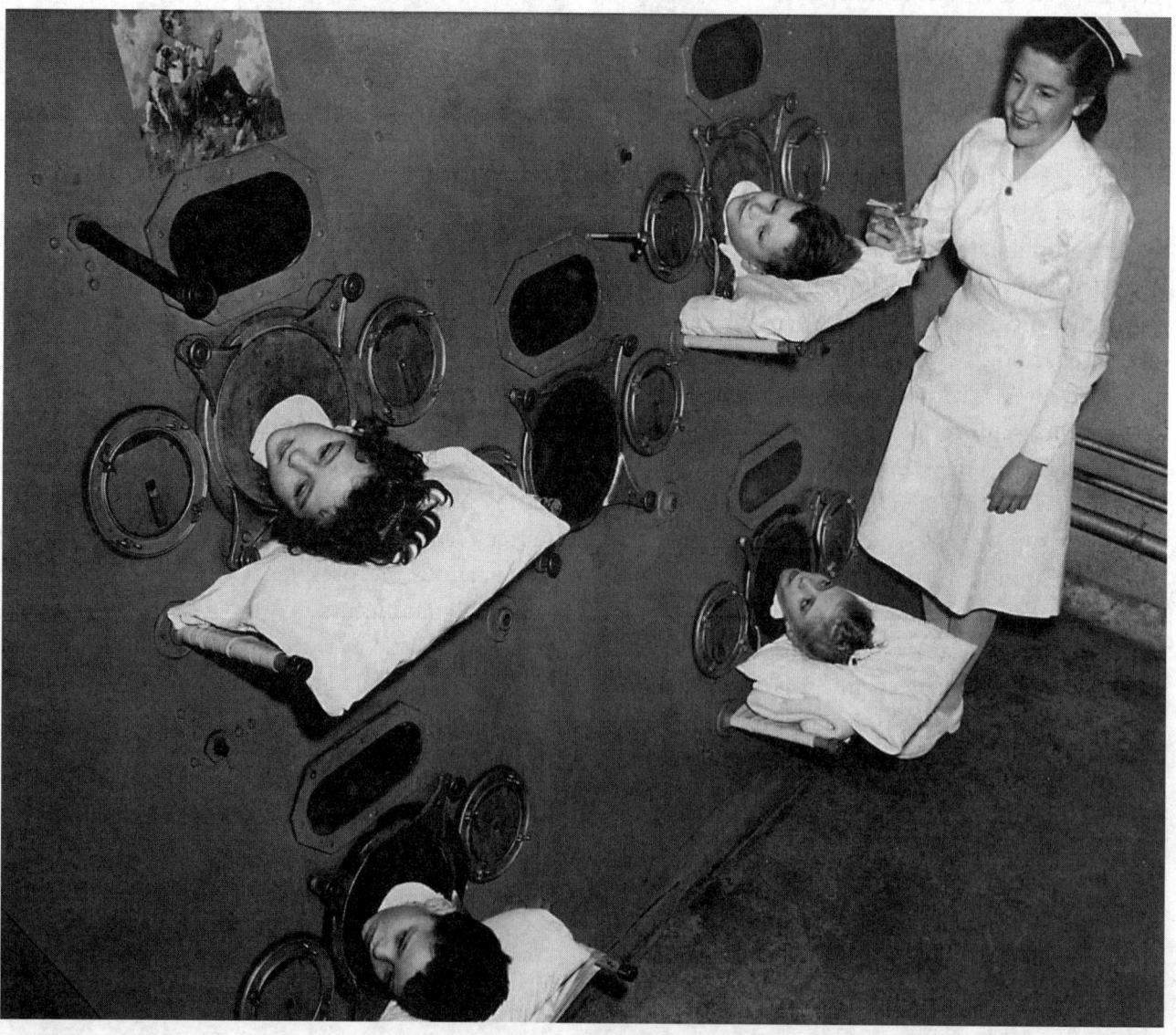

An iron lung designed to accommodate four children in a single room functioning as a respirator. Boston Children's Hospital Archives, Boston, Massachusetts.

vasoconstriction during the acute phase, but they did find colder limbs in patients with weaker muscles in the fair and poor range of muscle strength but not those with mild paralysis. These temperature changes occurred five–six months after the acute onset of polio.

Vaccine innovations and developments continued, and Albert Sabin first tested his oral vaccine in 1957, which was made available in 1962. The effect of these vaccines was enormous. The number of cases of acute poliomyelitis declined rapidly. Two institutions affiliated with Children's Hospital, the Wellesley Convalescent Home and the New England Peabody Home for Crippled Children, emptied of patients with poliomyelitis—as they had years before emptied of patients with tuberculosis and the hospital board of trustees realized that it could no longer economically support either home. The Wellesley Convalescent Home closed in 1958; the New England Peabody Home for Crippled Children closed in 1964, and its trustees donated funds originally designated for a Peabody Clinic at Children's Hospital to supporting a full-time Harvard Department of Orthopedic Surgery at Children's Hospital.

After Harvard had withdrawn financial support from and discontinued the activities of the Harvard Infantile Poliomyelitis Commission and transferred care, the Massachusetts Infantile Paralysis Clinic at Children's Hospital served the entire state of Massachusetts, though its activities had slowed as the polio vaccine was disseminated and the number of cases declined. The National Foundation for Infantile Paralysis assumed the operating costs of this clinic until 1960, when it required the hospital and patients to begin paying. The foundation did, however, continue providing funding—at that time almost $55,000—for the clinic's respiratory unit. In the late 1960s, while I was a resident at Children's Hospital, I remember seeing children disabled by polio at weekly clinics and performing numerous operative procedures such as tendon transfers, osteotomies, fusions, and epiphysiodeses to correct or improve their deformities.

In 1969, Lendon Snedeker paid tribute to Green's leadership (along with that of Trott and Grice) in sustaining the collaboration between Children's Hospital and the National Foundation for Poliomyelitis, and for helping it to succeed. During polio epidemics, Children's Hospital and its orthopaedic staff (surgeons, researchers, and physical therapists) played important leadership roles in combating this devastating disease. In addition to providing acute and chronic care and developing new methods of treatment for both, they organized and led initiatives to control epidemics in Massachusetts, Vermont, and New York (see chapter 16). Dr. Philip Drinker of the Harvard School of Public Health would go on to invent a mechanical respirator, widely known as "the iron lung," which saved the lives of innumerable patients with respiratory paralysis. Because of increasing demand, Dr. James L. Wilson later devised a "room-sized four-bed respirator...in which nurses and doctors...could minister to the bodies of patients whose heads were outside."

Continuing Bone Growth and Leg Length Discrepancy Research

In 1946 and 1947—at a time when Green was determining what kind of department he wanted to lead as chief of orthopaedics, beginning to innovate changes to the undergraduate and residency education at Harvard, and was simultaneously leading the transfer of the polio program to Children's—Green continued his earlier research on bone growth and leg length discrepancy. He reported on normal growth of the femur and tibia in children from the age of five years until their epiphyses closed. He wrote these papers in collaboration with Margaret Anderson, his long-time research associate. Green and Anderson were later assisted by research assistant Marie Blais Messner.

In 1947, Green and Anderson published their preliminary chart of corrections made possible by arresting the growth of the distal femur and the

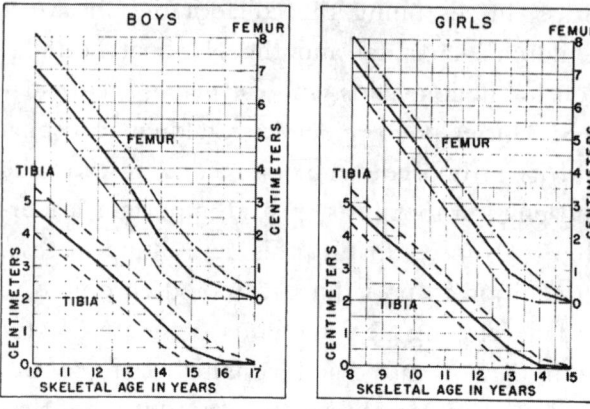

Figure 21.1. Example of Green and Anderson's preliminary growth chart, 1947.

W. T. Green and M. Anderson, "Experiences with Epiphyseal Arrest in Correcting Discrepancies in Length of the Lower Extremities in Infantile Paralysis: A Method of Predicting the Effect," *Journal of Bone and Joint Surgery* 1947; 29: 663.

Table 21.4. Percent of Cases that Achieved the Predicted Outcomes After Epiphyseal Arrest by Green and Anderson

Results	Arrests (n = 61)
• Within 0.5 in of the predicted value	54 (88.5)
• ≥0.5 inches above the mean predicted value	1 (1.7)
• ≥0.5 inches below the mean predicted value	6 (9.8)
• Delayed operative effect	4 (6.6)
• Other (one case)	2 (3.3)

Data are in (%) (adapted from Green and Anderson 1947).

proximal tibia (**Fig. 21.1**). They had followed "700 children, 87 per cent of whom have residual paralysis in one lower extremity on the other side; and it also includes observations on 158 normal children" (Green and Anderson 1947). They used orthoroentgenograms taken at 3- or 12-month intervals, a technique they had described in 1946. Their final measurements "were derived from three to six annual orthoroentgenograms of the normal lower extremity...of seventy-one boys and fifty-one girls with anterior poliomyelitis and from eight to ten consecutive yearly roentgenographic measurements of twenty boys and eighteen girls who are normal individuals" (Green and Anderson 1947). The values were only predictions, not actual measurements, because none of the children had yet achieved skeletal maturity. They reported 77 cases, 61 of which yielded adequate measurements (Green and Anderson 1947) (**Table 21.4**).

They later emphasized the importance of skeletal age in determining growth predictions, though they recognized that relative maturity may not remain the same as a child ages (Anderson and Green 1960). Although just over half of their participants (58%) maintained a particular skeletal maturity as they grew, the rest (42%) showed changes as they moved into adolescence.

Even though the surgeons involved used various methods to arrest growth, Green advocated the technique of epiphyseal arrest previously reported by Phemister, indicating that if done correctly, it should have an immediate effect and leave little deformity (**Fig. 21.2**). Complications included four valgus deformities and one varus deformity (with genu recurvatum); three received a corrective osteotomy, one was recommended, and the last had

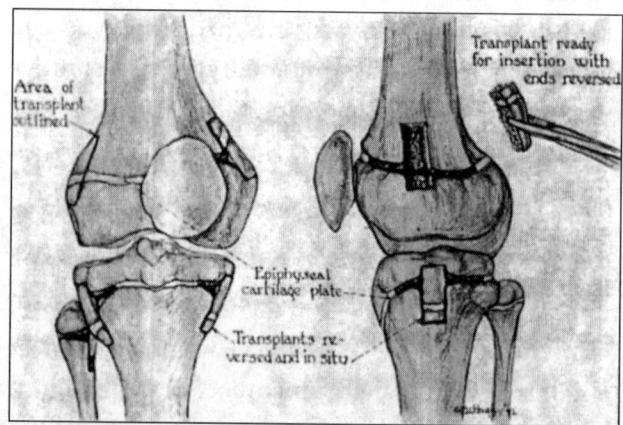

Figure 21.2. Drawing of an epiphyseal arrest as described by Phemister, 1933.

"Operative Arrestment of Longitudinal Growth of Bones in the Treatment of Deformities," *Journal of Bone and Joint Surgery* 1933; 15: 11.

a secondary arrest. Others included a case of osteomyelitis, one temporary peroneal palsy, and three overcorrections (two of which received distal femoral arrests in the paralyzed leg). The methods Green and Anderson used to predict bone growth and correct leg length discrepancies eventually came to be considered standard techniques and were used worldwide.

Meanwhile, Green established a center for what he referred to as his "Growth Study" at Children's Hospital. In his chief's report in the hospital's 1962 annual report, he wrote that "the Growth Study is a particular interest of mine. Particular areas of activity…include analytical studies of the growth of bone in children and the growth modified by surgery, further refinements of the tables of predictions of growth, study of the effects of trauma to the epiphysis on growth, a longitudinal study of the stimulation of growth arising from fractures of the shaft of long bones in the lower extremities, and a study of the abnormalities of growth which produce deformity of the hip and upper end of the femur. The Growth Study represents a major activity not only in research but in the care of patients as well" (Children's Hospital Archives, Annual Report 1962). The study was funded by a US Public Health Grant, by a Noemi chapter of the United Order of True Sisters, and in part by grants from the National Foundation for Infantile Paralysis and the National Institute of Arthritis and Metabolic Diseases.

In 1963, Anderson, Green, and Messner reported the final results of their earlier growth studies that included 100 children (50 girls and 50 boys) who had been followed annually until they reached maturity. All underwent orthoroentgenography of both lower extremities at least yearly, and the researchers determined each child's skeletal age by using the Greulich and Pyle atlas. Between the ages of 10 and 15 years, "71 percent of total femoral increment occurred at the distal metaphysis whereas 57 percent of the total tibial growth arose at the proximal metaphysis during this age interval" (Anderson, Green, and Messner 1963). The authors used these data to calculate new growth charts (**Fig. 21.3**), which were very similar to those published 16 years earlier, except they included both one and two standard deviations from the mean (rather than only one), and an additional two years of age on both ends (younger and older) for both boys and girls.

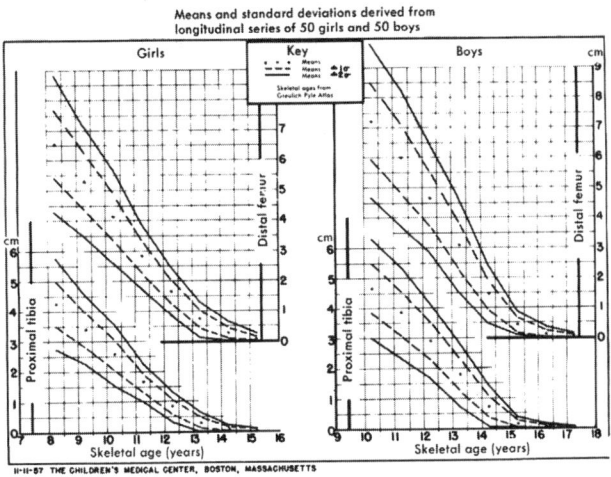

Figure 21.3. Example of Green and Anderson's final growth chart, 1963.

Anderson et al., "Growth and Predictions of Growth in the Lower Extremities," *Journal of Bone and Joint Surgery* 1963; 45: 10.

By my estimation, the main changes in the growth charts Green et al. published in 1963 versus that of 1947 was the amount of bone growth that occurs after the age of 12 years: in boys the femur will grow only another ~8% and the tibia, only ~5%; in girls, growth slows by ~8% in the femur and by 10–17% in the tibia. The revised growth chart of 1963 was meant to serve only as "a guide in estimating the effects of epiphyseal arrest at the distal end of the femur and proximal end of the tibia. Certain factors which may influence the amount of correction of discrepancy…included factors producing the discrepancy and its rate of increase, the child's maturity relative to his age in years, his/her pattern of growth, and his/her relative size for age" (Anderson, Green, and Messner 1963).

Green et al. published the last of the results from their Growth Study in 1964, 26 years after Green published his first paper on growth of the normal foot. During that time Green and colleagues had published at least 13 papers on bone growth and leg length discrepancies. Overall, Green and Anderson, along with Messner, made the following contributions regarding skeletal growth:

- Expected normal bone growth of both lower extremities and the foot until maturity
- The importance of skeletal age versus longitudinal age in predicting future growth
- Orthoroentgenography technique
- Patterns of growth in girls versus boys, showing that girls have a growth spurt at a younger age than boys
- The importance of bilateral serial longitudinal radiography in calculating growth and the percentage limitation of growth (including in the opposite, apparently normal limb)
- The effect of diseases such as polio on skeletal growth
- The discovery that implanting wires, nails, or tendons through the center of an epiphysis does not arrest growth, whereas growth may be partially arrested if such an implant is passed through the periphery of the epiphysis
- The discovery that passing a screw across an epiphyseal plate or compressing the epiphyseal plate often results in closure of the plate

Green's methods and the Green-Andersen growth charts for estimating future growth of the femur and tibia have been replaced by Moseley's straight-line graph method, which is widely used today. Moseley's method makes measurements easier to both visualize and employ by fitting data graphically along a straight line (**Fig. 21.4**), and allows procedural outcomes; e.g., of epiphysiodesis, lengthening, and shortening; and growth inhibition to be predicted. Neither Moseley's nor Green and Andersen's method, however, could estimate foot height (though Green had previously developed a radiographic technique to measure foot *length* in a standing position).

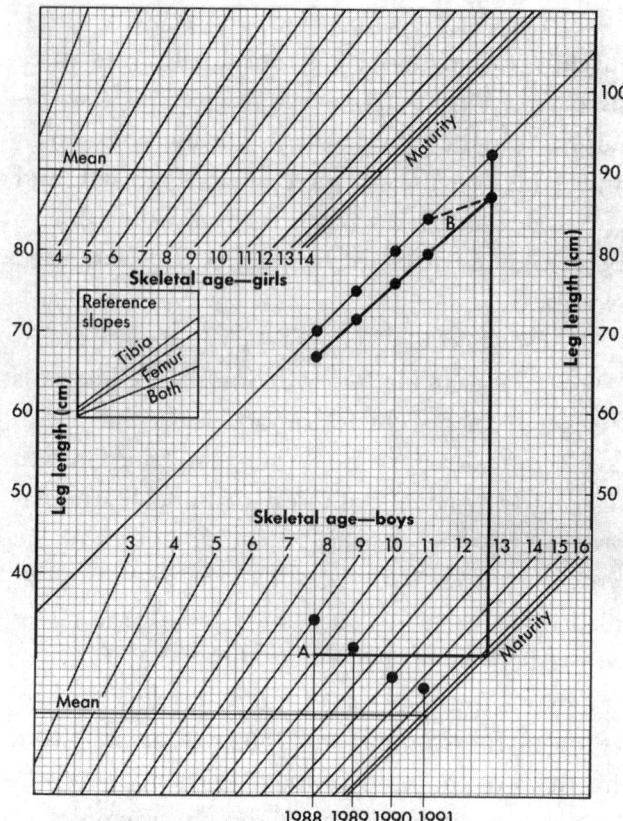

Figure 21.4. Example of Moseley's Straight-Line Graph.
Campbell's Operative Orthopaedics, 8th ed., by W. C. Campbell, S. T. Canale, and J. H. Beaty. Philadelphia: Mosby/Elsevier, 2008.

Other methods for estimating growth include that proposed by Menelaus and the Paley multiplier method. In 2013, Lee et al. compared the original Green-Anderson method, a modified version of it, Moseley's straight-line graph method, and the Paley multiplier method. They reported that although all of these techniques can predict leg length discrepancy, none of the predictions are accurate; they do, however, note that of the four methods, Green and Anderson's original provides the most accurate values.

Publications on Osteochondritis Dissecans

Quiet necrosis, the name Sir James Paget had given to osteochondritis dissecans in 1870, had been reported infrequently in children: only nine cases had been published by 1952, when, at the

AAOS meeting, Green and Banks reported 27 cases in patients under the age of 15 at Children's Hospital; they published the paper in 1953. They stated, "osteochondritis dissecans is not uncommon in children and…when the lesion is protected, the process can heal quite promptly…even in the patients in whom there is apparent sequestral formation within the confines of the cavity" (Green and Banks 1953). They studied the histology of some specimens obtained at surgery, confirming "that the basic process…is an aseptic necrosis involving the subchondral bone and that all the other changes are secondary" (Green and Banks 1953). They also concluded that "the etiology… remains in doubt[;] osteochondritis dissecans has a significant incidence [during] childhood[, and] in the majority of instances surgical intervention is not indicated" (Green and Banks 1953). Dr. Charles Herndon, in his discussion of Green and Bank's paper, stated:

> We are indebted to Dr. Green and Dr. Banks for bringing to our attention the facts that osteochondritis dissecans is not uncommon in children…I have been under the impression, as I believe most orthopaedic surgeons have, that osteochondritis dissecans is a disease which occurs in adults and which is distinctly uncommon in children…I believe that this paper is a real contribution and, if we keep this condition in mind when we examine children, we should recognize more cases during childhood and would begin treatment before permanent damage could occur. (Green and Banks 1953, in "Discussion")

Dr. Don King commented: "After hearing Dr. Green's paper, one wonders if some of the children who have growing pains, muscle cramps, and transitory limps might actually have osteochondritis dissecans…As far as I know, Dr. Green is the first to demonstrate this with a satisfactory series of proved cases" (Green and Banks 1953, in "Discussion").

Publications on Sprengel Deformity

Green also developed a procedure that was successful in treating Sprengel deformity, a rare congenital elevation of the scapula. In 1957, he reported the results of 16 cases at the Annual Meeting of the American Orthopaedic Association in Hot Springs, Virginia. Most patients had less than 120° of combined abduction before surgery. Postoperatively, they had gained a mean of 49° to 167° of combined abduction, and the mean change in the inferior position of the scapula was 4 centimeters. All patients achieved cosmetic improvements.

At Children's Hospital, Ober had previously developed a two-stage procedure to treat Sprengel deformity (**Fig. 21.5**). Green's procedure, completed in just one stage, "was extensive and one that required the attention to small details…as he [Green] stated 'it is precise, effective, and gives a most satisfying result'" (W. T. Green 1957a). The procedure:

> was entirely an extraperiosteal dissection of those muscles which attach the scapula to the spine and the trunk…completely freed in anatomical layers and…reattached after the scapula was brought down into its new position. If there was an omovertebral bone present, it was completely dissected out extraperiosteal [and removed, and] the supraclavicular portion of the scapula was excised along with the periosteum. The scapula was held down in place by wire traction applied to the spine of the scapula and attached to a small spring scale with three pounds of traction. This traction was maintained for three weeks [with] the child immobilized in a plaster spica…In some instances, the scapula had been osteotomized by a greenstick fracture to decrease its marked convexity. In all cases the lower pole of the scapula was very carefully placed beneath a pocket formed beneath the latissimus dorsi. Considerable care was taken to attach the…muscle groups so that they produced the desired downward displacement of the scapula. (W. T. Green 1957a)

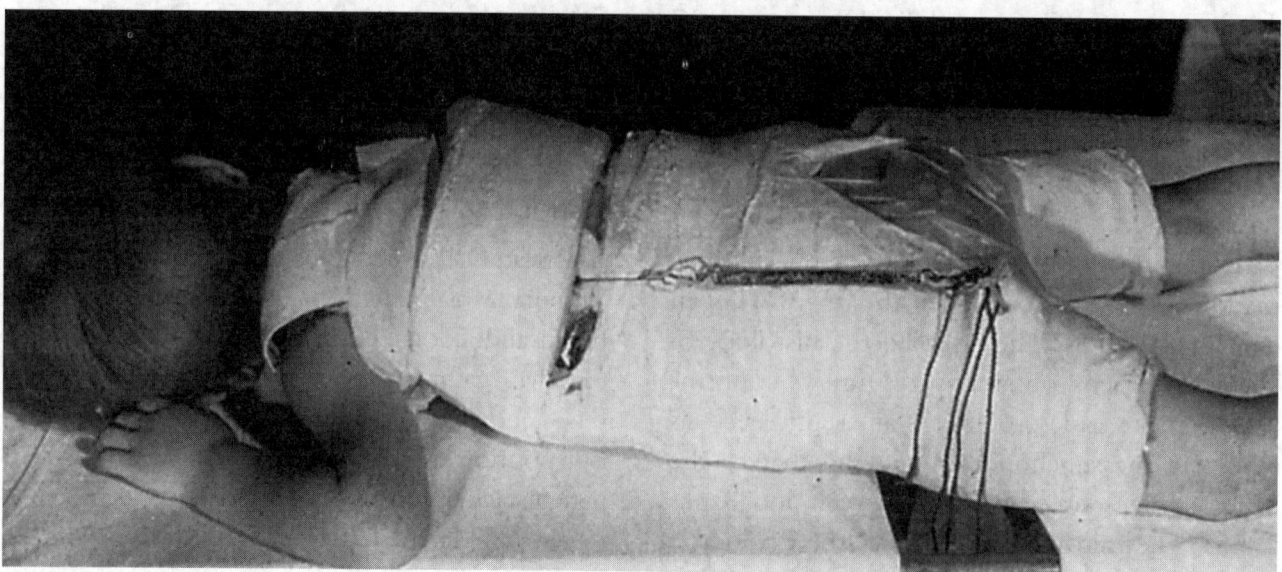

Figure 21.5. Photograph of a child in a plaster spica cast with wire traction in place after surgical correction of a sprengel deformity. *Orthopaedic Surgery in Infancy and Childhood* by Albert Barnett Ferguson. Williams and Wilkins, 1957.

His single-staged procedure followed by skeletal traction was successful in achieving very good cosmetic results and improved shoulder function in this rare deformity.

Leader in Cerebral Palsy Treatment and Research

Green also led the fight against another disabling disease: cerebral palsy. Between 1946 and 1952, Children's Hospital had successfully completed three fundraising campaigns, raising $7.8 million—more than twice the expected amount—enabling the hospital to add new programs and facilities, including a cerebral palsy clinic led by Dr. William Berenberg and incorporating the efforts of a multidisciplinary team. Fifteen years after his two previous publications, Green published another paper on cerebral palsy in 1957. Green had continued his research in the interim, and during this period:

> when the value of surgical procedures in cerebral palsy was in question, Dr. Green undertook a series of studies as to their effectiveness. He concluded that, in a large percentage of cases with spastic paralysis, properly chosen surgical procedures were of great benefit and may be dramatic in their effect. He pointed out, however, that the surgical procedure was only a step in the treatment and must be integrated into a general training and rehabilitation program. The surgical procedure enabled the other measures to be effective. He pointed out that a fundamental factor was the selection of cases in which the motor and mental capabilities of the child permitted him to achieve the benefits from surgery. Many operations which he developed in this field are now standard. (W. T. Green, n.d., "Unpublished Curriculum Vitae")

In 1956, at the Annual Meeting of the American Academy for Cerebral Palsy, Banks and Green presented a series of 78 patients with hip adduction contractures who they had followed since 1940 (in continuation of the larger series of studies). With the additional experience they had gained by that time, and with likely improved patient selection, they reported better results in their 1957 paper than Green did in 1942—now achieving good to excellent results in 69 patients (89%). Their preferred procedure included myotomy of the adductor longus, the adductor brevis, the gracilis, and the anterior portion of the adductor magus and a "neurectomy of the anterior branch of the obturator nerve" (Banks and Green 1957a).

Over the next few years Banks and Green studied another 11 cases and in 1960 published their results in the *Journal of Bone and Joint Surgery*. Almost half of the patients had been followed for more than 5 years—and some up to 17 years—after their surgery. Noting that "spasticity of the adductor muscles of the hip is a common disability in cerebral palsy…the most common hip deformity… second only to equinus deformity of the foot" (Banks and Green 1960b), the authors concluded that most patients improved after receiving the procedures. It was important to ensure "that the patient's mental and motor status [during the preoperative evaluation] meet[s] certain requirements. Adequate postoperative management and attention to certain minimum rules of care are major factors in the results. These patients must be followed over a long period of time for a maximum result to be obtained" (Banks and Green 1960b).

The next year, in 1958, Green was elected president of the American Academy for Cerebral Palsy. In his presidential address, he stressed, "the chaotic condition of the treatment of cerebral palsy in this country which led in the following year to a continuing 'Evaluation Study of the Treatment of Cerebral Palsy' fostered by the American Academy for Cerebral Palsy and supported by multiple foundations" (W. T. Green, n.d., "Unpublished Curriculum Vitae"). His efforts in that role led the Academy to support continuing studies of the outcomes and effectiveness of numerous surgical treatments in patients with cerebral palsy. At the time, those studies provided some clarity about the indications for and expected results when treating this complex disabling condition. During Green's year as president, he and Banks published their results on the treatment of equinus deformities and presented a paper on hamstring contractures at the Annual Meeting of the American Academy for Cerebral Palsy. These two studies were part of their 15-year (1940–1954) review of all patients with cerebral palsy who had been treated at Children's Hospital. End results were reported for 132 of 153 patients who had undergone surgery to treat equinus deformity and who had received a mean follow-up of seven years. Green had for years used a sliding type of heel-cord lengthening that had been described by J. Warren White. Green emphasized once again that in order "to obtain a good result the postoperative care of these patients must be very carefully and patiently supervised" (Banks and Green 1958b).

Occasionally a patient would undergo fractional lengthening of the gastrocnemius origin, which Green had described in his 1942 paper on the operative treatment of cerebral palsy; this was his preferred procedure. Associated foot deformities such as valgus, varus, or cavus were treated with a triple arthrodesis in which "the cuts in the bone were patterned so as to correct equinus deformity" (Banks and Green 1958b). In their discussion, Banks and Green drew attention to the negativity at that time regarding surgery for patients with cerebral palsy—both among surgeons and being reported in the literature: "It is stated time and again that there is no point in operating on patients with cerebral palsy because all or nearly all, of the deformities recur anyway…Contrary to this point of view, it has been our experience over the years that orthopaedic surgical procedures have a major role in the management of patients with cerebral palsy" (Banks and Green 1958b). They reported only a 5.5% recurrence of equinus deformity after a heel-cord lengthening; in their experience, recurrence was "usually associated with poor and inadequate follow-up, poor cooperation on the part of the patient and family, a motor status in the lower classification, and severe mental retardation" (Banks and Green 1958b). They did not recommend a triple arthrodesis for a severe equinus deformity because the height of the foot would be reduced after a sufficient amount of bone had been removed. In children over the age of five years with valgus deformity of the foot, they recommended

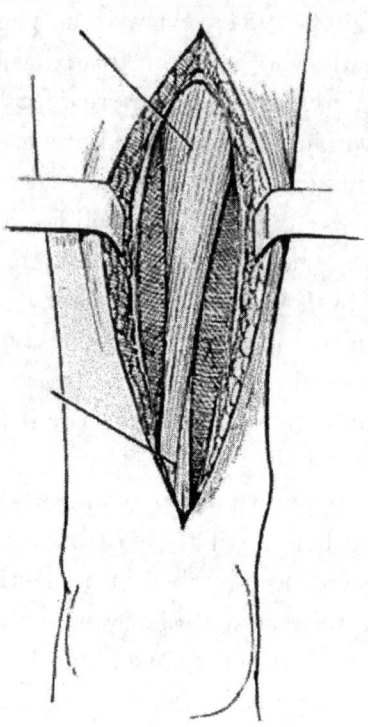

Drawing of the Achilles tendon with two pins in place, identifying the rotation of the tendon bundles proximally and distally, before the sliding procedure.
H. H. Banks and W. T. Green, "The Correction of Equinus Deformity in Cerebral Palsy," *Journal of Bone and Joint Surgery* 1958; 6: 1360.

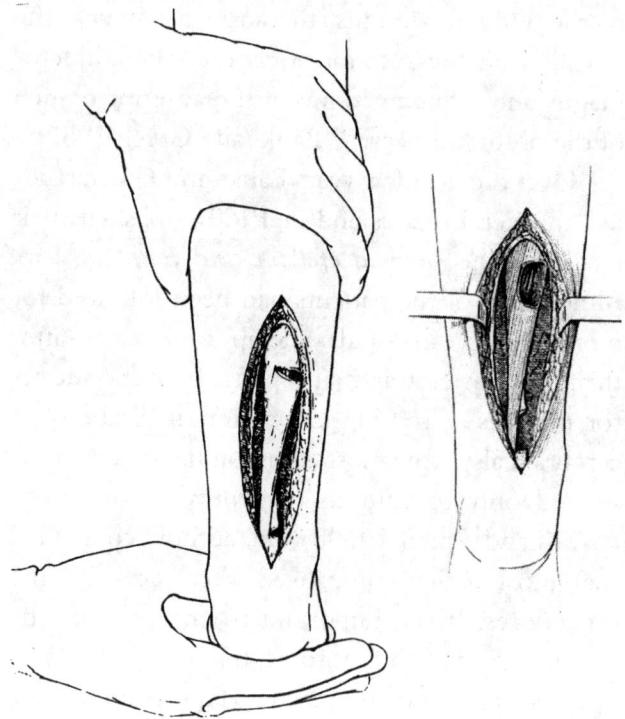

Drawings of the Achilles tendon sliding procedure after the appropriate cuts in the tendon and the final result with the selected gaps in the correct bundles proximally and distally. Contact is maintained with the bundles between the cuts.
H. H. Banks and W. T. Green, "The Correction of Equinus Deformity in Cerebral Palsy," *Journal of Bone and Joint Surgery* 1958; 6: 1362.

heel-cord lengthening and subtalar extra-articular arthrodesis, as described by Dr. David Grice.

Green's other contribution to the field of cerebral palsy during his presidency was the surgical correction of hamstring contractures. He and Banks presented the outcomes of 54 procedures in 29 patients with hamstring contracture—again from among those included in Green and Banks's general review of patients treated at Children's Hospital between 1940 and 1954—at the Annual Meeting of the American Academy for Cerebral Palsy in New Orleans in 1957. Twenty-one patients had been followed for 5 years or more, 12 for more than 10 years. The operation consisted of "a sliding or fractional lengthening of the hamstrings with an additional fractional lengthening of the tendinous origin of both heads of the gastrocnemius" (Banks and Green 1958a), and they reported good results in correcting flexion deformities of the knee. Once again, they "emphasized the importance of postoperative care, including physical therapy, bivalved night casts and supervised walking" (Banks and Green 1958a). Green and Banks published an abstract in the *Journal of Bone and Joint Surgery* in 1958, but they never published a completed article on the topic.

Four years later—and 20 years after his first description of the flexor carpi ulnaris transfer to the extensor carpi radialis longus or brevis—Green, again with Banks, published his last paper on cerebral palsy. Green believed that wrist fusion, advocated by some orthopaedic surgeons for flexion-pronation deformities, "often decreases rather than aids the functional capacity of the hand. Wrist motion and the ability to supinate and pronate the forearm are important complements to the function of the fingers and hand" (Green and Banks 1962). Green and Banks published their long-term results of this transfer in 47 patients at Children's Hospital and the Peter Bent Brigham Hospital from 1941 through 1960. Green's technique transferred the flexor carpi ulnaris:

> around the medial side of the ulna into the dorsal compartment of the forearm where it is attached to the tendon of the extensor carpi radialis brevis or longus. The tendon is detached from the pisiform. The muscle is then freed further until it will pass in a straight line from its origin to the border of the ulna and thence to the extensor compartment of the wrist. The nerve supply…is a delimiting factor in the proximal dissection. The intermuscular septum…is excised. A buttonhole is made in the extensor carpus radialis tendon through which the ulnaris tendon is passed and sutured under good tension with the wrist in full supination and the hand in at least 45 degrees of dorsiflexion. [The patient is placed in a long arm cast, including the fingers,] with the wrist extended, the forearm in supination, the fingers in the functional position just short of full extension, and the thumb in a position of abduction and opposition…The cast is bivalved and the exercises are ordinarily started on the fourth or fifth day after operation…maintained in a bivalved cast…for a least six weeks and often longer…The long night cast is usually used for many months and in some instances… for several years. (Green and Banks 1962)

Green chose the extensor carpi radialis brevis as the point of attachment if more dorsiflexion was

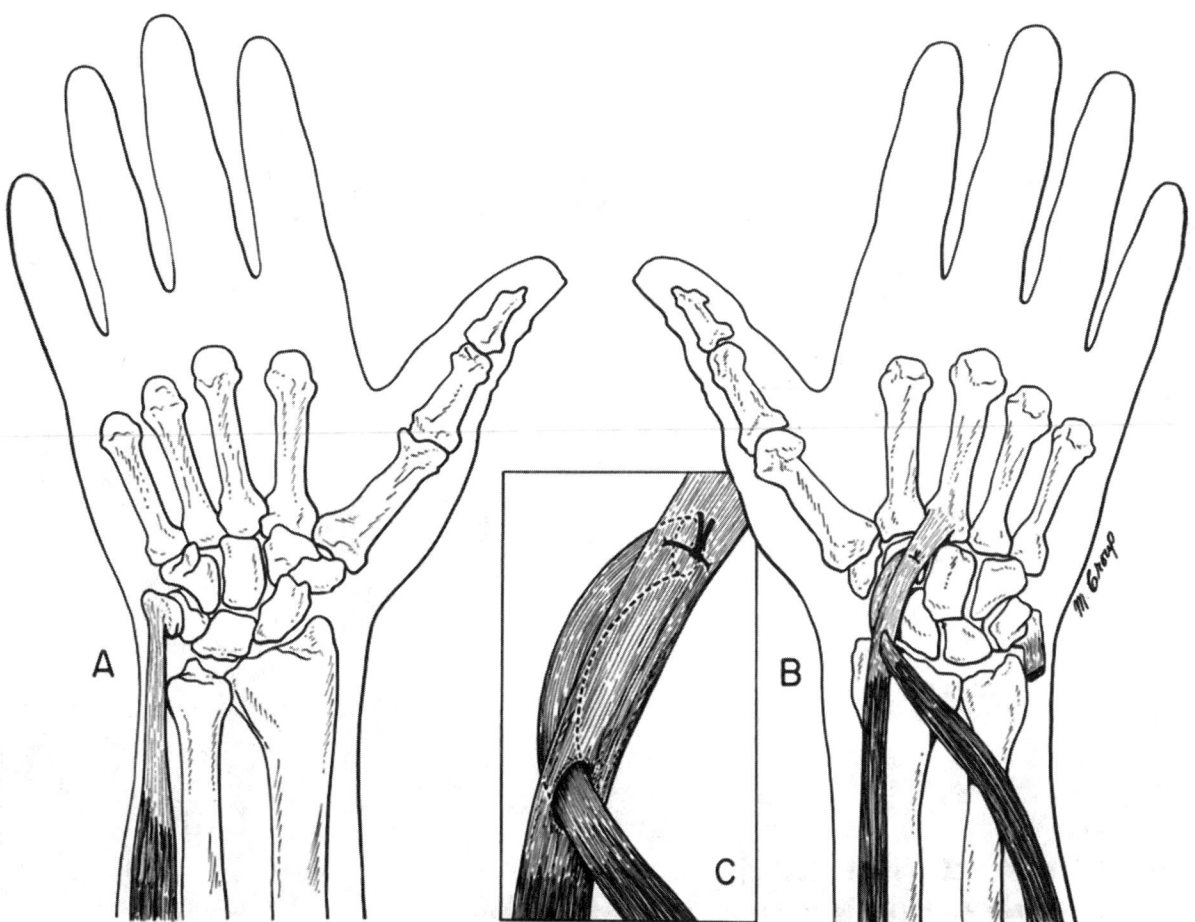

Drawings of the flexor carpi ulnaris transfer to the extensor carpi radialis or brevis. Green WT (1942). Albert B. Ferguson Jr., *Orthopaedic Surgery in Infancy and Childhood*, 5th edition, Baltimore: Williams and Wilkins, 1981: 702 [fig. 16.51.]

required, and the extensor carpi radialis longus if more correction of ulnar deviation was necessary. They advocated correcting any fixed deformities before the transfer, and although not contraindicated in cases of astereognosis, they noted that condition "does handicap the use of the hand" (Green and Banks 1962).

They reported good to excellent results in 24 patients (51%) and poor results in only 2 patients (4.3%). During his discussion of the paper in a presentation at the AAOS meeting in Chicago in 1962, Banks stated, "we have not found it necessary to do a wrist fusion in cerebral palsy in the last twenty years" (Green and Banks 1962).

Publications on Volkmann Ischemic Contracture

At the annual meeting of the AAOS in New York City in 1965, Dr. Richard Eaton, in collaboration with Green and Dr. Herbert Stark, presented a small series of patients with Volkmann contracture of the forearm. They had treated 14 patients over 25 years at Children's Hospital, and their work made two contributions: (1) a model of the pathophysiology of the development of an ischemic contracture and (2) the importance of epimysiotomy in preserving muscle integrity and function. In 1972, Eaton and Green reported their model of an ischemia-edema cycle (**Fig. 21.7**), where, after various types of trauma:

> arterial flow into a specific region is reduced by occlusion, compression or spasm [which] creates a proportionate degree of ischemia in the individual muscles…anoxia develops, with formation of histamine-like substances which increase capillary permeability…promoting a transudation of plasma into the muscle. The summation of this effect is increasing intramuscular edema…[a] progressive increase in the pressure of muscle enclosed in fascia and

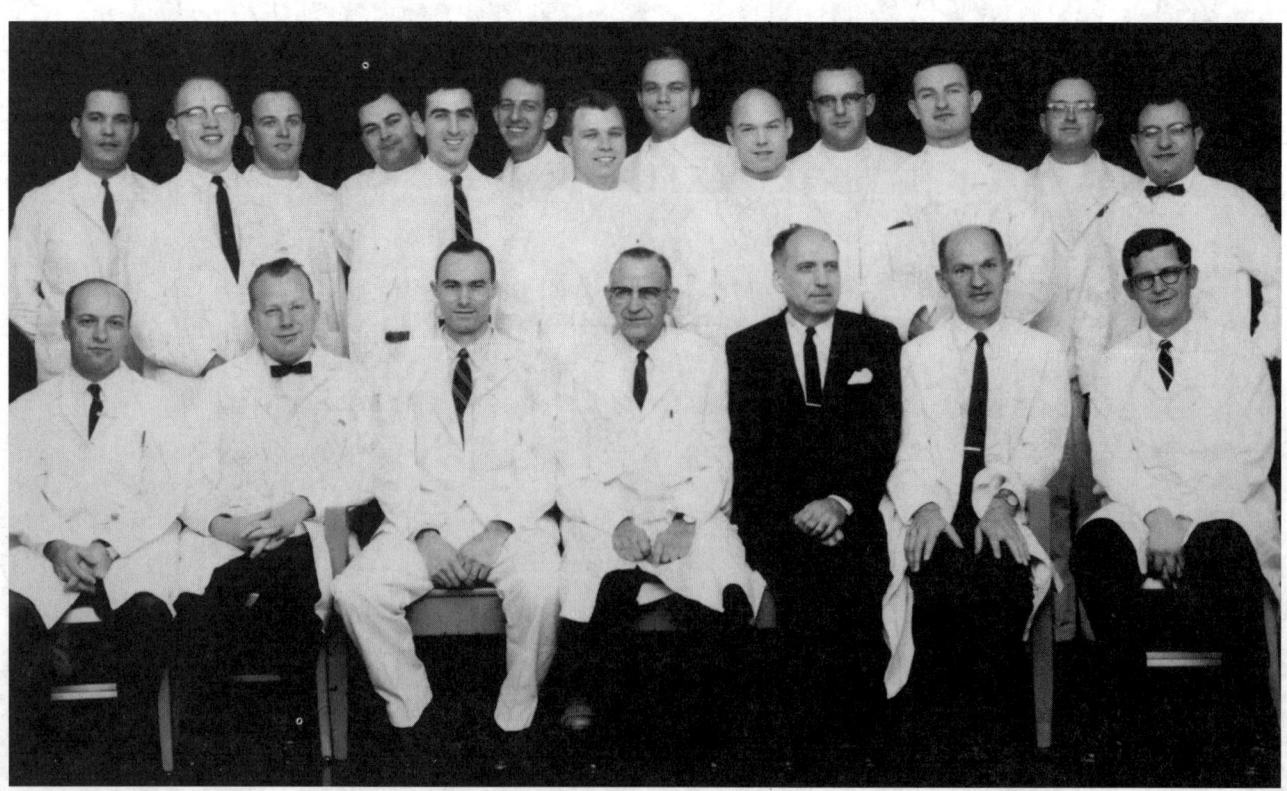

Orthopaedic staff at BCH, 1965. Front row (left to right): Drs. Banks, Trott, Eaton, Green, Hugenberger, Cohen, and Griffin.
MGH HCORP Archives.

epimysium. This pressure is compounded by any unyielding dressings encircling the arm…add to various compression [causing an] increase in intrinsic tissue pressure…set off a proximal reflex vasospasm…reinforces and perpetuates the initial vascular compromise, and a destructive ischemia-edema cycle develops. (Eaton, Green, and Stark 1972)

In 1975, they reported their experiences with 19 cases (including five additional cases since their 1965 article). Emphasizing the main physical findings of palpable induration of the volar compartment, sensory deficit, and pain upon passive finger extension, they advocated immediate surgical decompression, including "the superficial and deep portion of the volar compartment[;] division of the epimysium of the deeper muscles and, in particular, of the fascia of the flexor digitorum profundus and flexor pollicis longus should be decompressed by longitudinal incision" (Eaton, Green, and Stark 1975). "Despite a vigorous exercise program, dynamic splinting, and at least one reconstructive procedure, [three patients treated without fasciotomies] had poor results" (Eaton, Green, and Stark 1975). They recommended "decompression, not only of the compartment but of each individual muscle which shows evidence of vascular compromise" (Eaton, Green, and Stark 1975).

PRESIDENT OF THE AAOS: A LASTING INFLUENCE ON ORTHOPAEDIC SURGERY AND EDUCATION

Green was president of the AAOS in 1957. His remarks on education in his presidential address, titled "Orthopaedic Surgery, Yesterday and Tomorrow," were informed by a study of the state of medical education he had performed in preparation for it. To study students' exposure to orthopaedics, Green surveyed the deans of 65 medical schools; 49 of them responded. Over four years, students spent from 56 hours to 232 hours on orthopaedics—a huge difference. The mean time was 126 hours. Only an average of 14% of the total time for teaching surgery was dedicated to orthopaedics; among the schools, this ranged from 7% to 27%. Most orthopaedics—an average of 25 hours—was taught in the third year; only a mean of 3 hours of orthopaedics were taught in the first two years. In most schools:

> the students were receiving too little teaching to allow any reasonable approach to the subject…Furthermore, many areas in basic science which are important to understanding in this field were slighted…Orthopaedic surgery, by all measurements that we can make, is a major field of medicine. In this age of wars and accidents all physicians need to develop a better understanding of the musculoskeletal system and its problems. Teaching in orthopaedic surgery must recognize this and it should receive the emphasis which its position in the total medical picture warrants. (W. T. Green 1957b)

In his address, he reported these findings and made a few comments on orthopaedic education:

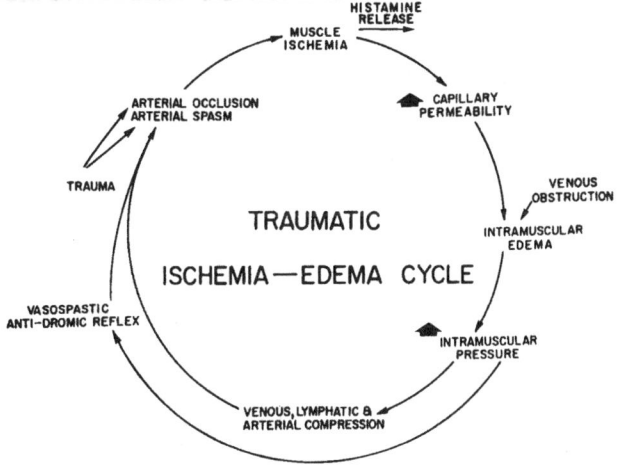

Figure 21.7. Eaton and Green's model of an ischemia-edema cycle.

"Epimysiotomy and fasciotomy in the treatment of Volkmann's ischemic contracture," *Orthopedic Clinics of North America*, 1972; 3: 177.

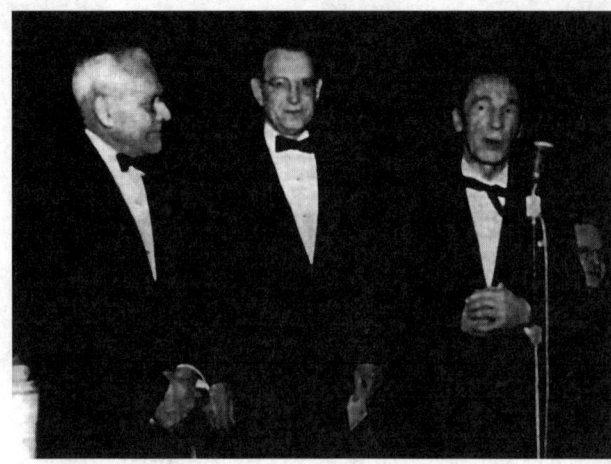

Dr. Green (center) at the annual AAOS banquet during his presidency. MGH HCORP Archives.

Orthopaedic surgery should attract its share of men…yet I do not believe that we do get our fair share of medical graduates off the top of the heap…interest in orthopaedic surgery is rarely generated in medical school, but rather in graduate training, often late in graduate training…[T]his arises, in large part, from the limited exposure of the student to orthopaedic surgery in medical school. (W. T. Green 1957b)

In his "American Academy of Orthopaedic Surgeons Committee on Undergraduate Teaching Report," Green recommended 220 hours of orthopaedic instruction for medical students over four years. "A good part of the practice in orthopaedics is medical…orthopaedic surgery is made up of both medical and surgical components. The percentage of teaching time assigned to orthopaedics should not be related just to surgery" (W. T. Green 1957b). In his presidential address, he further emphasized that, "as we consider the future of orthopaedic surgery and its responsibilities, increased research has a top priority. I would list three needs above the rest: (1) the need for more research and experimental investigation, (2) we need more men and more top-flight men in orthopaedic surgery, and (3) we need to improve undergraduate teaching and the position of orthopaedic surgery in our medical schools" (W. T. Green 1957b).

Green's concluding remarks during his presidential address focused on the gradual erosion of the influence of orthopaedics in the community and the increasing concentration of orthopaedists on only surgery, highlighting the need for such specialists to remain interested and to be active in providing continuing care:

Is this relative inactivity of orthopaedic surgery [in hospital and community activities] a natural evolution or is it the product of our own lethargy and a ducking of our responsibilities…We should be the leaders in community projects affecting our field. We should participate in organizations and in programs which represent the interest of orthopaedic surgery whether medical organizations or lay organizations. It does not look good to sit back and sneer. So, too, must we ask ourselves about our part in the total field of neuromusculoskeletal disease. Many of us seem to concentrate on the actual performance of surgical procedures and show little interest in other than surgical aspects of our specialty. If the particular province of orthopaedic surgery is the skeletal system and the organs of movements, our specialty is, in reality, more medical than surgical. Is it a natural evolution…[to] confine ourselves only to the surgical aspects? Is this sound? Many of us who are older look upon the surgical procedure itself as but a step of a continuous program in an individual's care and rehabilitation. [Are we] to be the technicians who come into a case when someone else decides it's time for surgery and someone else gives postoperative care, will we in fact come to know less and less about less and less. We must be careful not to sit in a self-satisfied reactionary state; yet we must always discriminate between progress and change. (W. T. Green 1957b)

Highlighting the need for orthopaedic specialists to remain interested and active in providing care, Green pushed others to strive for a level of commitment and action similar to his own.

He not only spoke to the AAOS about his ideas on education; he was also an active educator in the Academy: He was a frequent instructional course lecturer and a member of the Committee on Instructional Courses, among numerous others. He chaired the AAOS Committee on Education, Committee on Undergraduate Teaching, Committee on Graduate Education, and Subcommittee on Graduate Education in Children's Orthopaedics. In 1961, Green expressed some of his other thoughts on teaching, in addition to those he had previously included in the report:

> Teaching is the obligation of every department of orthopaedic surgery no matter what its circumstance. At what level the teaching is done depends upon the features peculiar to the center, but for all departments there is teaching to be done. If the center is related to a medical school, undergraduate teaching assumes a major position. Orthopaedic surgery must assume responsibility for instruction in the area of the neuromusculoskeletal system. To do this teaching in the most effective way should be the objective of every department. In every medical school the department of orthopaedic surgery should strive to obtain the necessary hours in the curriculum but, beyond all else, it should make the best possible use of the hours which it has. Adequate instruction in this field is essential to the well rounded experiences of a medical student. Teaching of the undergraduate is not only a responsibility but a privilege as well. Much of the judgment of orthopaedic surgery by our confreres in medicine arises from the impressions that they obtain in their undergraduate years. At this time, too, there is the opportunity to interest the students in orthopaedic surgery itself and to develop in him as appreciation of its importance in the total picture of medicine. It is up to each orthopaedic department to flavor its impressions well.
>
> Teaching of our residents and graduate students is a particular obligation since they are the orthopaedists of the future and will be responsible for carrying orthopaedics to new levels. Each department should have the best possible resident-training program that it can provide. Every endeavor must be made to create an atmosphere which will attract men into orthopaedic surgery and which will provide for their healthy growth. We need to entice more men into orthopaedic surgery. Included in our plans should be the provision of better financial support for our residents and for the young man who is starting his career in academic orthopaedics. (W. T. Green 1961b)

The previous year, in 1960, Green received an honorary doctorate of science from the University of Indiana. The citation summarized his efforts to enhance and advance medical education; it read, in part, "You have manifested a striking interest in the work of the medical student at every level, and a great talent for teaching so that former students of yours are now in positions of great responsibility and trust as a result of your inspiration and example" (W. T. Green, "Chairman's Archives").

LEGACY

Dr. William Green retired from Harvard on August 30, 1968, becoming the Harriet M. Peabody Professor Emeritus, a position announced by Dean Robert H. Ebert. At the same time, he also retired from Children's Hospital, where he was orthopaedic surgeon-in-chief, and from the Peter Bent Brigham Hospital, where he was chief of the Division of Orthopaedics.

Green's accomplishments are too numerous to recount in full in this chapter. From 1954 to 1956, Green served as president of the American Board of Orthopaedic Surgery. He was a founding member of the Orthopaedic Research Society, and he was a governor and member of the Orthopaedic Advisory Committee of the American College of Surgeons from 1960 to 1963. He chaired

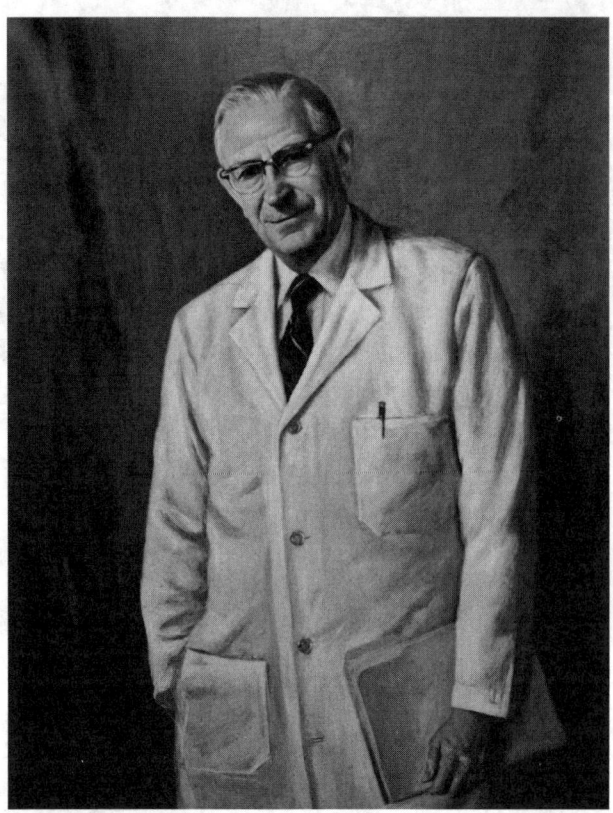

Portrait of William T. Green. Melvin Robbins/Boston Children's Hospital Archives, Boston, Massachusetts.

the Orthopaedic Section of the American Medical Association; in his address to the Section in the summer of 1956, he opened his speech on tendon transplantation in rehabilitation with a joke: "Up in Vermont they have a definition of a specialist...a specialist is an 'illigitimate [sic] fellow' from Boston with a box of lantern slides" (W. T. Green, "Chairman's Archives"). Green was also active in the American Orthopaedic Association, the American Academy of Pediatrics, the International Society of Orthopaedic Surgery and Traumatology, the Society for Pediatric Research, and the Society for Research in Child Development.

He received various honors, including membership in Phi Beta Kappa, Sigma Xi, and Alpha Omega Alpha, and in the following international orthopaedic organizations: the British Orthopaedic Association; La Sociedad Colombiana de Circugia Ortopédica y Traumatologia (Bogota, Columbia); La Sociedad Colombiana de Circugia Ortopédica y Traumatologia, Seccional-Antioquia (Bogota, Colombia); the Sociedad - de Pediatriade Antioquena (Medellín, Columbia); the Sociedade Brasilieira de Ortopedia e Traumatologia (São Paolo, Brazil); the Societa Italiana di Ortopedia e Traumatologia (Rome, Italy); and the Sociedad Latinoamericana de Ortopedia y Traumatologia (a multi-country organization).

In "A Tribute to W. T. Green" in 1968, Dr. Henry Banks wrote, "In the ability to put a sick baby at ease, to communicate the warmth and kindness of a father, and to introduce a strong sense of discipline with a keen sense of humor into a serious clinical situation, Dr. Green has no peer" (H. H. Banks 1968). As a clinician he was the best, very analytical, but at the same time controversial. He was "very committed to his patients [while treating them; he] wanted everything right [and] would even make casts for swimming if the patient wanted to continue swimming" (W. Green Jr., pers. comm., 2009). William T. Green Jr. recalls that his father received many letters from grateful patients who loved him. "The patient was always number one" (W. Green Jr., pers. comm., 2009).

Green was "uniquely disciplined and demanded perfection, nothing less in this regard [stressing] the importance of details of a patient's assessment and the importance of postoperative care" (H. Banks, pers. comm., 2009). He emphasized "the importance of maintaining correction of a deformity 24 hours a day by exercises or specially prepared supportive measures [e.g., bivalve casts]. He made the patients and/or parents learn how to do exercises at home...He has the patience to teach mothers to perform as nurses and physical therapists [in order] to care for their children at home" (H. H. Banks 1968). Clare McCarthy, a physical therapist who worked with Green for years, recalled the story of a wealthy Japanese family whose child Green had cared for. Apparently, the patient's mother did not work and wanted one of her helpers at home to manage the child's exercise program. Green refused to discharge the child unless the mother learned how to do the exercises

> ### Editorial Comment
> Academic Orthopedics—A Tribute to W. T. Green
>
> Clinical Orthopaedics and Related Research
> Number 61
> Nov.-Dec., 1968

Title of a tribute to Dr. Green published in CORR. *Clinical Orthopaedics and Related Research* 1968; 61: 3.

(McCarthy and Cassella, pers. comm., 2012). In his tribute to Green, Banks wrote, "His ability to examine a child and see much more than any other physician in a community filled with many other capable physicians, including a large number of his own pupils at Harvard Medical Center, is truly remarkable" (H. H. Banks 1968).

Banks wrote, "Dr. Green's greatest contribution has been in the field of education of medical students and residents in orthopaedic surgery and at the bedside and in the operating theater, and in the course of this work he performed experimental and clinical investigations of major significance" (H. H. Banks 1968). In recognition of Green's impact as a teacher, some of his former pupils and residents honored him on his sixty-seventh birthday by contributing papers to a special section of *Clinical Orthopaedics and Related Research*, published in 1968. In his editorial comment preceding the section, Banks stated, "Perhaps Dr. Green's most noteworthy accomplishment is his bedside teaching of the fundamentals of bracing, tendon transplantation, prevention [of rigid scoliosis by use of casts or braces], and correction of paralytic scoliosis, and bony stabilization of joints in patients with residual poliomyelitis…these teachings are now being applied with even greater diligence to the treatment of traumatic and other paralytic disorders" (H. H. Banks 1968).

Green was a long-time smoker, though Jack McGinty, a resident and clinical staff member at Children's Hospital in the 1960s, "never saw him smoke" (J. McGinty, pers. comm., 2009). William Green Jr. remembers his father quitting cold turkey. Despite this, Green eventually developed chronic emphysema. Also, "dementia later in life… was a major problem" for Green as well (W. Green Jr., pers. comm., 2009). After struggling with a long illness, he died on a Wednesday in July 1986 at Newfield House in Plymouth, Massachusetts (*Boston Globe* 1986).

CHAPTER 22

David S. Grice
Advocate for Polio Treatment

David Stephen Grice was born to John Grice and Elizabeth Fry Grice in Chicago on July 9, 1914. He graduated from Nicholas Senn High School, where he excelled and showed an early dedication to leadership and service as the commanding officer of the high school reserve corps. He went on to obtain:

> his A.B. degree from the University of Rochester in 1935, where he was an outstanding athlete in football, track, and baseball. He was captain of the football team in his junior year… [H]e went on to medical school at the University of Rochester, receiving his M.D. in 1938. His decision to go into medicine came early… [with] football…a major factor in his choosing to become an orthopaedic surgeon. He had a football injury to his knee which required an operative procedure. Certain complications following this greatly prolonged his convalescence and, in fact, caused him to have intermittent difficulty with the knee from that time on. This experience stimulated his interest. After graduating in medicine…he served an internship [1938–1940], followed by an assistant residency in surgery [1940–1941] at the Strong Memorial Hospital in Rochester. He had his resident training in orthopaedic surgery in Boston at the Children's Hospital [1941–1942, under chief Frank Ober] and the Massachusetts General Hospital [1942–1943, under chief Marius Smith-Petersen],

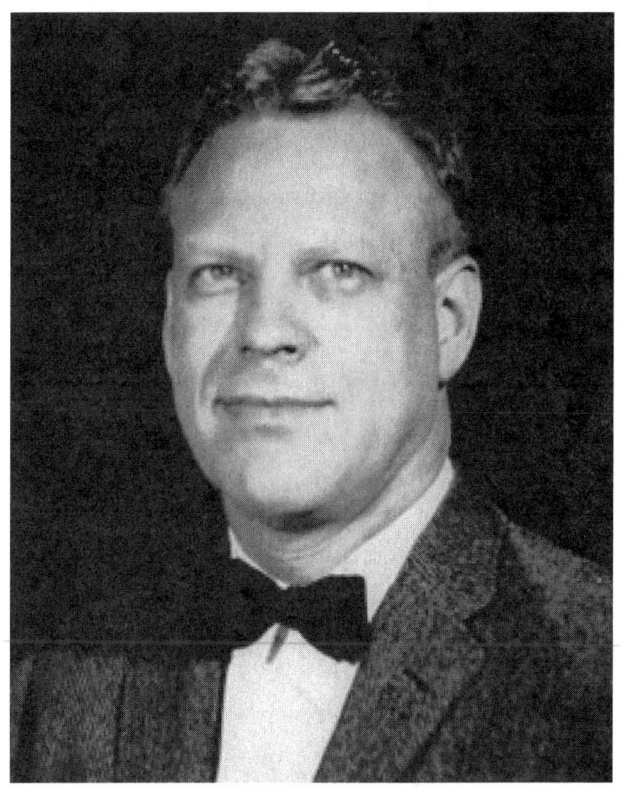

David S. Grice. W. T. Green, "David S. Grice 1914–1960," *Journal of Bone and Joint Surgery* 1961; 43: 319.

Physician Snapshot

David S. Grice
BORN: 1914
DIED: 1960
SIGNIFICANT CONTRIBUTIONS: First described subtalar extra-articular arthrodesis (the Grice procedure); expert in polio

finishing his last year of training in 1943–1944 as chief resident in orthopaedic surgery at Children's Hospital. In 1944 he became a member of the staff at the Children's Hospital and an assistant in orthopaedic surgery at Harvard Medical School. This began an association with Harvard Medical School, the Children's Hospital, and the Peter Bent Brigham Hospital which lasted until 1958. During this period…he was an immediate associate of Dr. William T. Green, with his offices at the Children's Hospital Medical Center, and was intimately concerned with the teaching program at Harvard…the resident training program at the Children's Hospital, and the general activities of the Department.
(W. T. Green 1961)

With his initial appointment at Children's Hospital, Grice was also named assistant director of the Massachusetts Infantile Paralysis Clinics at Children's Hospital.

Grice's "writings were not extensive in number but they were important in their significance" (W. T. Green 1961). He published six peer-reviewed articles, four American Academy of Orthopaedic Surgeons Instructional Course Lectures (presented at the AAOS annual meeting and later published), three book reviews, and one book chapter. His first paper, published in 1944 and cowritten with John F. Bell, described the treatment of club feet with the Denis Browne splint. Grice and Bell were both house officers at Children's Hospital, but after a brief period as assistant in orthopaedic surgery at Children's Hospital, Bell moved to Vermont, where he became an associate professor of orthopaedic surgery at the University of Vermont and director of the Crippled Children's Service for the state's Department of Health. Grice had previously succeeded Bell as chief resident at Children's Hospital in March 1943.

Grice had been appointed assistant director in 1944, and then "Associate Director of the Massachusetts Infantile Paralysis Clinic, [and] Orthopaedic Consultant to the Mary MacArthur Respirator Unit" (W. T. Green 1961). In 1945, Grice became an orthopaedic consultant for the Massachusetts Services for Crippled Children, and, in 1946, a junior associate in orthopaedic surgery at the Peter Bent Brigham Hospital. "[Grice] wrote on many phases of poliomyelitis, its therapy and surgical treatment. His particular interest over most of his medical career was in pediatric orthopaedics" (W. T. Green 1961). After becoming a member of the Massachusetts Medical Society, he presented in 1947 the first of his many papers on poliomyelitis, this one entitled "The Treatment of Infantile Paralysis During Convalescence." He also presented a second paper, "The Roentgenologist and the Orthopaedic Surgeon." That same year—a pivotal one—he advanced to associate orthopaedic surgeon in 1947 at Boston Children's Hospital and was promoted to instructor at HMS after five years as an assistant in orthopaedic surgery. Shortly thereafter, he was appointed orthopaedic surgeon at Boston Children's Hospital, in 1949, and clinical associate at HMS, in 1951. Over those next 12 years, Grice presented seven papers on poliomyelitis, and his four AAOS Instructional Course Lectures (three of which were done with Green) were also about that time. He published another five papers on other aspects of pediatric orthopaedics.

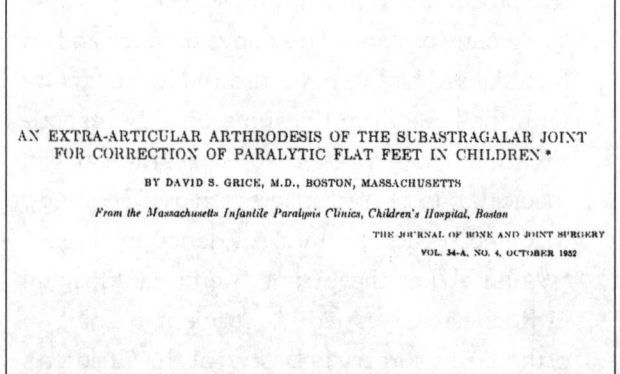

Title of Grice's article, "An Extra-Articular Arthrodesis of the Subastragalar Joint for Correction of Paralytic Flat Feet in Children." *Journal of Bone and Joint Surgery* 1952; 34: 927.

THE GRICE PROCEDURE: SUBTALAR EXTRA-ARTICULAR ARTHRODESIS

In 1952, Grice published his classic article, "An Extra-Articular Arthrodesis of the Subastragalar Joint for Correction of Paralytic Flat Feet in Children" (see the **Case 22.1**). It 2013, it was ranked forty-second among the 100 classic papers most cited in pediatric orthopaedics, and Dr. Robert B. Salter cited it as one of the "most significant advances in pediatric orthopaedics during the thirty-three-year period from 1954–1987" (R. B. Salter 1987). Grice wrote:

> It is the purpose of this paper to discuss the severe valgus deformity which has developed in children who have had paralysis of the anterior and posterior tibial muscles…Initially the deformity is similar…to that of a mildly pronated foot…Unlike the pronated foot with good musculature, the paralytic valgus foot usually becomes progressively worse. It is difficult to prevent the development of this deformity by the use of supportive apparatus, such as arch supports, braces, or casts…In the foot with paralysis of the posterior tibial alone or in conjunction with the anterior tibial muscle, the heel is displaced into eversion by the unopposed action of the peroneal muscles and the gastrocnemius. As the calcaneus is everted, its anterior portion is displaced laterally and posteriorly. As a consequence, there is loss of the normal support beneath the head of the astragalus, which drops into equinus and projects further anteriorly…The backward displacement of the calcaneus and the forward movement of the astragalus results in abduction of the metatarsus…If the deformity has persisted for a long period, secondary adaptive changes have occurred…the most significant…are contractures of the tibio-astragalar joint capsule, shortening of the tendo-achilles, contractures of the mid-tarsal joints, and adaptive changes in osseous structure associated with growth. The surgical correction of this deformity is for the purpose of obtaining several major objectives. The calcaneus must be replaced beneath the astragalus…[which] must be brought up out of equinus. Muscle balance should be restored by tendon transplantation to avoid recurrence. The deforming everting power of the peroneal muscles should be removed and active inversion and dorsiflexion should be restored to the astragaloscaphoid (talonavicular) area. Since it is desirable to correct this deformity in the young child before it has become fixed, the operative technique should not interfere with subsequent growth of the foot…This technique of using bone grafts placed in the

Case 22.1. Subtalar Extra-articular Arthrodesis

> "The first patient in this series was five years old when the operation was performed. The boy was born in 1940 and had onset of poliomyelitis in 1941. Residual involvement of the left leg was moderately severe. There was complete paralysis of the anterior and posterior tibialis, long toe flexors were fair, gastrocnemius was fair plus, and the other muscles were good. A severe valgus deformity of the left foot developed, with marked plantar flexion of the astragalus…The astragalus was in so much equinus that the foot was wedged up in plaster casts before operation. In August 1945, a subastragalar [extra-articular] arthrodesis was performed, with the use of bone grafts from the diaphysis of the tibia. At the same time the peroneus longus was transplanted beneath the calcaneoscaphoid ligament and inserted into the scaphoid. An excellent result was obtained and correction of the deformity has been maintained…The x-rays taken four years postoperatively revealed that the height of the tarsus has been maintained, and growth has occurred."
>
> (David S. Grice 1952)

sinus tarsi to obtain an extra-articular arthrodesis...was first used at the Children's Hospital in 1945 at the suggestion of Dr. William T. Green. (D. S. Grice 1952)

OPERATIVE TECHNIQUE

Grice, at the suggestion of Dr. Green, developed an operation to treat paralytic flat foot deformities in children with polio. To preserve bone stock and avoid injury to the potential of the talus and calcaneus, he inserted bone grafts into the sinus tarsi, which corrected the flat foot deformity without injuring the joint surfaces:

> A short curvilinear incision is made on the lateral aspect of the foot directly over the subastragalar joint...The cruciate ligament...is split in the direction of its fibers and the sinus tarsi is dissected free of adipose tissue...If the foot is placed down into equinus, the calcaneus can usually be replaced beneath the astragalus by inverting the foot. If the deformity is severe... it may be necessary to divide the posterior capsule of the subastragalar joint or remove a slight amount of bone laterally beneath the anterior superior articular surface in order to restore proper alignment. An osteotome...is inserted into the sinus tarsi as a block to demonstrate the stability which might be obtained with the grafts...[and] to determine the size of the grafts and the optimum position in which they may be placed...The sinus tarsi is prepared for the grafts by removal of a thin layer of cortical bone from the under surface of the astragalas and the superior aspect of the calcaneus...[Bone is taken from] the upper portion of the tibia...to provide cancellous as well as cortical bone... about 3.5 to 4.5 centimeters long and about 1.5 centimeters wide. The grafts are cut to size and are trapezoid in shape. The corners of the broad base are removed with a rongeur, so the grafts will countersink into the calcaneus bone and prevent lateral displacement...The grafts are placed in the sinus tarsi with the foot held in the slightly overcorrected position...as the foot is everted, the grafts are locked in the desired position...A cast is applied from toe to groin with the knee flexed and the foot in maximum dorsiflexion. If there is no residual equinus and tendon transplantation is indicated, it is preferable to do this at the same operation. Exercises for the transplant may be started at six weeks... and weight-bearing has been allowed when healing of the grafts is observed in the roentgenograms...usually about ten to twelve weeks after operation. (D. S. Grice 1952)

Earlier, in 1950, at the Annual Meeting of the American Orthopaedic Association (AOA), Grice had reported on nine cases of paralytic flat feet. In 1952, he published the results of 22 cases:

> Seventeen patients have been followed at least one year...fifteen have been classified as having a good result and two as having a poor result due to recurrence of the deformity. In all cases, the arthrodesis has been successful, and the grafts have become solidly incorporated into the adjacent bones...one patient has been followed for six years with no evidence of recurrence... Since the grafts are...essentially extra-articular [they] should interfere with growth in a minimal degree. (D. S. Grice 1952)

Grice was promoted to assistant clinical professor of orthopaedic surgery at HMS in 1954 and elected as an AOA member at the annual meeting that same year. There he presented his further experience with extra-articular arthrodesis of the subtalar joint:

> Based on his experience with fifty-two paralytic flat feet resulting from poliomyelitis...Thirty of the children were between four and eight years of age [and] growth of the foot is not interfered with...The two grafts are so placed that they lie

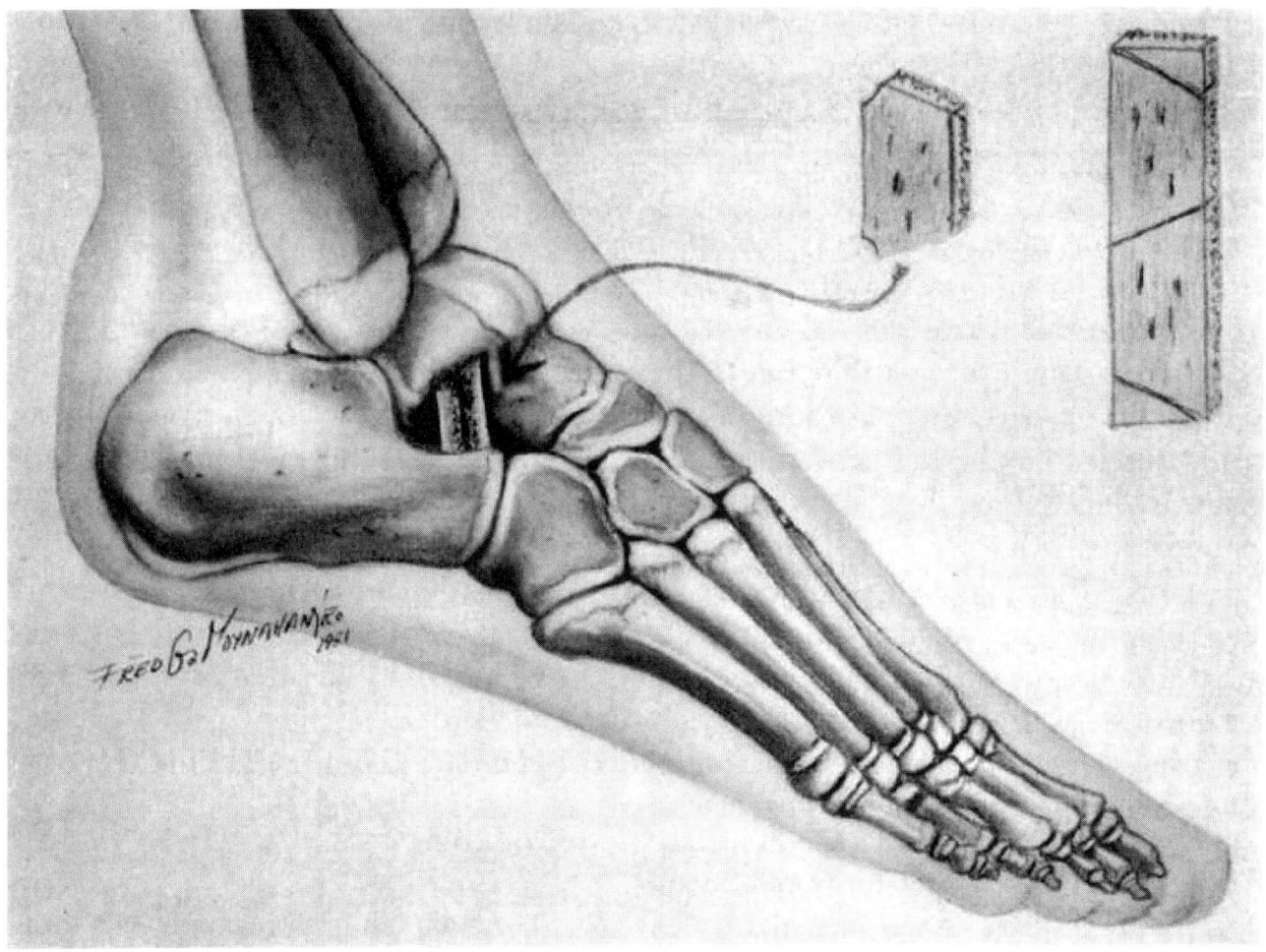

Drawing of the placement of the two cortico-cancellous grafts in the sinus tarsi (subtalar). D. S. Grice, "An Extra-Articular Arthrodesis of the Subastragalar Joint for Correction of Paralytic Flat Feet in Children," *Journal of Bone and Joint Surgery* 1952; 34: 933.

in a plane at right angles to the axis of motion of the subtalar joint, with cancellous surfaces apposed. The longest period of follow-up was nine years[, with] forty-one good results. In seven patients, there was insufficient correction; in four, there was overcorrection. In only three patients was there any difficulty in obtaining union" (*"Proceedings," Journal of Bone and Joint Surgery,* 1955. [Though not listed in the section, Dr. Grice was the author of this paper.])

In the discussion of that presentation, Grice commented, "We have lengthened the heel cords in several patients who had cerebral palsy, but discussion of that group of patients was not included in the presentation" (D. S. Grice 1955a). By the late 1960s, however, surgeons were expanding the indications for different types of patients who might benefit from the Grice procedure, including those with cerebral palsy. Seymour and Evans mention this in their 1968 article on the "Grice subtalar arthrodesis" published in the *Journal of Bone and Joint Surgery*:

> Extra-articular arthrodesis of the subtalar joint...is a satisfactory method of stabilizing mobile pes valgus in children. The established procedure is technically difficult, and this may explain a proportion of failures...This paper describes a method...devised by Batchelor [fibular graft] and used by him since 1955. It is technically easier and failures of fusion are rare...

As poliomyelitis has become less common the operation is performed less often. With increasing interest in the surgery of myelomeningocele and cerebral palsy, however, the operation is likely to be indicated more often...In the standard Grice procedure, difficulties in seating and retaining the graft in the sinus tarsi may result in failure to maintain correction of valgus of the heel and the need to place the graft under some compression may lead to overcorrection. (Seymour and Evans 1968)

The success rate of the Green-Grice procedure was reported at only 74–79% in other surgeons' hands (Grice and Green themselves had 79% success), and the indications to operate were broadening to include patients with cerebral palsy, myelomeningocele, progressive neuropathy, arthrogryposis multiplex congenita, Ehlers-Danlos syndrome, club foot, and congenital vertical talus. Thus, the use of the Green-Grice procedure combined with the Batchelor technique increased throughout the 1950s and 1960s, but with mixed results.

A large series of 149 Green-Grice procedures for valgus deformities in a variety of conditions were performed at the Shriners Hospital for Crippled Children in Louisiana and were reported in 1985. Almost half of these achieved poor outcomes because of graft failure or incompletely corrected deformity. McCall et al. (1985) suggested performing the Grice procedure with tendon balancing only for patients with cerebral palsy or polio, and avoiding it in those with myelodysplasia or flexible flatfoot because unrecognized ankle valgus could exist.

Scott et al. (1988) noted that the Grice procedure cannot offset ankle valgus, and that it should be combined with a balancing procedure or osteotomy in order to resolve a calcaneus deformity. Overcorrection of the hindfoot into varus led to poor results. An unrecognized valgus ankle can often be differentiated from hindfoot valgus only on radiographs of the feet and ankles during weight-bearing. They reported poor results in 61% of cases, mainly because of the aforementioned problems, and failure in 32%, including orientation of the graft in an anterior direction.

Alman et al. (1993) performed the Grice procedure on 53 feet of patients with cerebral palsy. They modified Grice's technique by lengthening the heel cord, placing the graft distally in order to minimize its height, and immobilizing the talocalcaneal joint with two threaded wires. To maximize results, they emphasize the importance of selecting appropriate patients who will most benefit from the procedure; muscle balance and normal neurological function are crucial. Those with neurological instability, valgus alignment of the tibial plafond, or extreme deformity may experience negative results.

OTHER CONTRIBUTIONS

Polio Expert

As assistant director of the Massachusetts Infantile Paralysis Clinic, Grice became recognized as a national expert in poliomyelitis. He, along with colleagues, nurses, and physical therapists—all of whom were specially trained in poliomyelitis—had volunteered as consultants to help communities deal with sporadic epidemics, as in Miami in 1946 and in three cities in Missouri in 1949. That year, they had also provided training courses in poliomyelitis and coordinated the delivery of equipment such as iron lungs and hydrocollators to hospitals and communities in Boston and throughout Massachusetts.

Grice continued to study polio and advance its treatment as the new decade began. **Box 22.1** provides a timeline of events of Grice's contributions to the study of polio through the mid-1950s. From the mid-fifties through the end of the decade, Grice spoke numerous times about extra-articular subtalar arthrodesis in patients stricken with poliomyelitis.

Box 22.1. Grice's Contributions to the Study of Polio between 1949 and 1955

- 1949. Grice participates in a roundtable discussion, "Respiratory Problems in Acute Poliomyelitis," at Boston University School of Medicine with Drs. Robert M. Smith and William Berenberg and others.
- 1952. Grice participates in a postgraduate course for the Massachusetts Medical Society, "Medical Aids for the Physically Handicapped," with Drs. Thorndike and Record.
- 1954. Grice presents a lecture, "Practical Considerations in Treatment of Poliomyelitis," to the Pentucket Association of Physicians.
- 1955. Grice takes part in a panel discussion, "Management of the Poliomyelitis Patient," at the Annual Meeting of the American Society of Anesthesiologists in Boston Demonstrates, with Green, Dr. Charles Janeway, and others, patients from the polio clinic at Children's Hospital through closed-circuit television to the Clinical Meeting of the American Medical Association, which was being held in Boston.

During an interview with the *Daily Boston Globe* about rehabilitation, Grice stated:

> Perhaps we have a patient who has had a cerebral accident...he's getting along all right. He has an offer of his job back as soon as he's well enough. But he finds himself being "rehabilitated" with all the resources of the community. "I don't need 'em," he tells them. "You gotta have 'em," he's told...rehabilitation should be saved for those who[se] lives have been changed by poliomyelitis, blindness, by heart crippling or psychiatric trouble and may need temporary adjustment or longer aid. But, he warned, "today everybody wants to jump on the bandwagon and help those who don't need it. To[o] often we work, not for the patient, but for the agency...Are you interested in your patient or in your press clippings? We are too prone to talk about the wonderful work we're doing. But we don't know where we're going." (F. Burns 1958)

A major polio epidemic hit the Boston area in 1955, causing mass hysteria. Dr. William Berenberg described days when 150 to 200 sick children were brought to the hospital by their parents—a long line of cars blocking the street—making the extent of the outbreak obvious. Berenberg described how he and Grice attempted to manage the rush of patients. They would walk from car to car in the dark of the night, quickly visually assessing the children in each. Those who were noted as experiencing respiratory distress or immobility were moved to the front of the line; the rest waited their turn.

A Difficult but Effective Educator

Grice was an accomplished orthopaedist and was known as a tough but effective teacher who pushed his students to excel. In addition to teaching at HMS, he was also a lecturer in anatomy at Simmons College. In 1958 he left Harvard to become a professor of orthopaedic surgery and the fifth chief (following Dr. Paul Colonna) of the Department of Orthopaedic Surgery at the University of Pennsylvania, which had been the first such department in the country, established in 1889.

> At the time of his resignation to accept this position he was assistant professor at Harvard Medical School, Orthopaedic Surgeon at the Children's Hospital Medical Center, Associate in Surgery at Peter Bent Brigham Hospital, Associate Director of the Massachusetts Infantile Paralysis Clinic, orthopaedic consultant to the Mary MacArthur Respiratory Unit, a consultant to the Massachusetts Crippled Service [Fall River Clinic] and a lecturer in anatomy at Simmons College...Dr. Grice was blessed with many attributes—brilliant of mind, original in his ideas, discerning, and critical. He carried in all his activities an enthusiasm which was boundless and exceeded only by his determination and persistence in striving to get the job done in the best possible way. There was no compromise

with expediency. He was a stimulating teacher who loved to teach and gave of himself to the full...He strove for the clear thinking mind in his students, and the easy, sloppy was intolerable to him. Many a resident burned under his searing criticism of the moment only to appreciate it the next day and to cherish and respect his teaching forever after. (W. T. Green 1961)

Grice was mainly interested in facts and truth, and some remember him as being confrontational with residents—tougher even than Dr. Green—often embarrassing them (and sometimes staff as well). Such confrontations with residents occurred frequently during evening rounds, sometimes in front of patients' families. Residents often had a difficult time returning after rounds to care for those patients and their families.

This method of teaching by fear had a downside for residents with type A personalities, as they didn't like to admit that they had done something incorrectly, missed some detail, or didn't know an answer. Grice made the situation much worse by publicly demonstrating their shortcomings. Dr. Z. Friedenberg (2002), in his historical summary of the orthopaedic department at the University of Pennsylvania, remembered Grice in a similar way—many disliked him because he would shame and deride the residents. According to Friedenberg, Grice acted in this way to cover his own lack of confidence and experience in treating adult patients.

A LASTING LEGACY DESPITE AN UNTIMELY DEATH

Grice was chairman of the Department of Orthopaedic Surgery at Penn for just two years. On October 5, 1960, at age 46, he died when a plane he was on—an Eastern Airlines Electra—crashed shortly after takeoff from Boston's Logan Airport because a large flock of starlings had been drawn into the engines.

Dr. Arthur Trott recalled that fateful day:

Dave and I had been on a court case in Worcester, involving a patient he had originally treated. Then when he went to Philadelphia to Penn Hospital, I took over his practice. They got to me first as far as giving testimony in court. He followed. He was supposed to catch that plane and get on it. We used to have a monthly meeting of people on the staff of Children's [Hospital]. They used to have a dinner and a talk at the Medical School once a month. So that was the night of the meeting. I went over to the meeting, got back to the hospital, walked into the office and the phone was ringing. It was Dr. Guy Brugler, who was the administrator at the time. Guy said, "Did you hear about Dave?" I said "No, what?" He told me about the plane crash, which had occurred while I was at the meeting. I spent the night checking to see if he had been on the plane. I finally got Mary Grice at 6:00 in the morning. She had just got the word. That was a rough night. (D. Dyer 1993, "Trott interview")

The board of editors and staff of the *Journal of Bone and Joint Surgery* announced their "sense of great loss—loss of a bright and rising star on the orthopaedic horizon, loss of one of our ablest and most faithful associate editors, and a loss of a dear and devoted friend...[we] extend to Mrs. Grice and the three children...[our] deepest sympathy" (*Journal of Bone and Joint Surgery* 1960b).

"Mrs. Grice" was Mary Burns of Rochester, New York, who married David Grice "on March 30, 1940, while [he was] an assistant resident in surgery at Strong Memorial Hospital" (W. T. Green 1961). They had three daughters. "One of the family's choicest times and spots was a cottage on a Massachusetts lake where they spent their summers. As might be expected, it was within a relatively short driving distance of the hospital and his work" (W. T. Green 1961). While Grice was a resident at Children's Hospital, the family lived at 108 Holden Green in Cambridge; they later moved to Dedham, Massachusetts. When he became chief at the University of Pennsylvania they lived in Wynnewood, about six miles northeast of the university.

Grice had been elected as a fellow of the American Academy of Orthopaedic Surgeons (AAOS) in 1950 (Otto E. Aufranc, Charles H. Herndon, and Eugene E. Record were also elected as fellows at that same meeting, and Dr. Joseph Barr became president-elect of the AAOS); he was appointed chairperson of the AAOS Program Committee the year of his death. In addition to his membership in the American Orthopaedic Association (AOA), he was also a member of the Orthopaedic Research Society and a representative to the American Board of Orthopaedic Surgery by the American Medical Association. He was also a member of the Forum Club and a trustee of the University of Rochester.

At the time of his death—in fact, only two days later—Grice had planned to participate in a conference of orthopaedic department chairpersons sponsored by the Committee on the Skeletal System convened by the National Research Council of the National Academy of Sciences. The purpose was to discuss "common problems relating to department-sponsored research programs...an outline of the more favorable factors affecting the conduct of interdepartmental research and some suggestions for the solutions of these problems" (*Journal of Bone and Joint Surgery* 1961).

As Green described so eloquently, Grice had a definite influence on his patients and the field of orthopaedics:

> He was an excellent clinician and a keen investigator...The procedure of subtalar extra-articular arthrodesis, which he first described, was well conceived...and should remain as one of our classic procedures in surgery. His judgments were good, and his counsel was much sought and appreciated. He had the happy faculty of going directly to the crux of the problem, analyzing the factors involved, and quickly coming to a decision. He was an individual of strong convictions and deep emotions...He had a great feeling of responsibility for orthopaedic surgery and for his duty as an orthopaedic surgeon. His patients meant much to him, and they, in turn, had great affection for him. He was a disciplinarian with his patients, with himself, and with those who trained under him...It was particularly gratifying to see the morale and enthusiasm which he instilled in the patients of this [Massachusetts Infantile Paralysis] Clinic. (W. T. Green 1961)

Upon Grice's death, his colleagues (and former patients) at both Children's Hospital and the University of Pennsylvania created memorial funds in his name:

> How much he was appreciated by his patients and by his associates in Boston was demonstrated by the fact that as a spontaneous expression of their feelings a memorial fund was established for him at the Children's Hospital Medical Center...the respect which he had already engendered amongst his confreres at the University of Pennsylvania is shown by the fact that an official memorial fund was established at the Orthopaedic Department there, where he had been for such a short time. (W. T. Green 1961)

At Children's Hospital, the fund was founded by the seven service chiefs:

- Dr. Sidney Farber, pathology
- Dr. George E. Gardner, psychiatry
- Dr. William T. Green, orthopedic surgery
- Dr. Robert E. Gross, surgery
- Dr. Frank Ingraham, neurosurgery
- Dr. Charles A. Janeway, medicine
- Dr. E. B. D. Newhauser, radiology

Grice's memory lives on at Children's Hospital today through the annual David S. Grice Annual

Lecture, which was started in 1984. **Table 22.1** lists the lecturers over the past 35 years.

The National Research Council—whose conference Grice had been scheduled to attend—best captured the feeling of the orthopaedic community upon hearing the news of his death: "The conference was saddened by the tragic and untimely death of Dr. David S. Grice…who died two days before the meeting…a relatively young man, [who] had achieved prominence in the field of academic orthopaedics[,] and his loss to the orthopaedic world will be keenly felt by all" (*Journal of Bone and Joint Surgery* 1961).

Table 22.1. David S. Grice Lecturers Since Its Inception in 1984

1984	G. Wilbur Westin, MD
1985	David Sutherland, MD
1986	Eugene Bleck, MD
1987	Jean Dubousset, MD
1988	G. Dean MacEwen, MD
1989	John A. Herring, MD
1990	Robert Hensinger, MD
1992	Timothy M. O'Brien, MD
1993	John Wedge, MD
1995	Vernon T. Tolo, MD
1996	John Hall, MD Symposium
1997	Klaus Parsch, MD
1998	Mervyn Letts, MD
1999	Hamlet A. Petersen, MD
2000	Mercer C. Rang, MBBS
2002	Charles T. Price, MD
2003	James G. Wright, MD, MPH
2004	Professor Reinhold Ganz
2005	James H. Beaty, MD
2006	Marc A. Asher, MD
2007	Perry L. Schoenecker, MD
2008	Professor H. Kerr Graham
2009	Charles E. Johnston, MD
2010	Alain Dimeglio, MD
2011	James Kasser, MD
2012	Marybeth Ezaki, MD
2013	Stuart Weinstein, MD
2014	Dennis R. Wenger, MD
2015	Steven L. Frick, MD
2016	Peter Newton, MD
2017	John Flynn, MD
2018	Deborah Eastwood, MD
2019	Lyle Micheli, MD

CHAPTER 23

BCH
Other Surgeon-Scholars (1900–1970)

In 1934, during his tenure as surgeon-in-chief of the orthopaedic department at Children's Hospital, Frank Ober, in the department's annual report, gave high praise to the surgeons who have cared for the hospital's young patients over the years:

> The men [and women] who have occupied staff positions through the period of the hospital's existence have given freely of their time and energy to aid the sick and crippled child. Each succeeding staff member has endeavored to do more than his part in mentoring the standards of the hospital at the same time in building up the standards of medicine and in keeping the Hospital a preeminent institution in the country.
>
> As a result of the efforts of these men, the productive results at the Children's Hospital have been valuable and worthwhile. We sometimes wonder if the general public is aware of what the Children's Hospital, or any hospital in the community, means in protecting the health of the people of that community.

The orthopaedic surgeons described in this chapter are some of the surgeons who practiced at Children's Hospital from 1900 to 1970. Harvard calls these and other clinicians "surgeon-scholars." The surgeon scholars covered in this chapter include:

Frank D. Bates	218
John F. Bell	219
Albert H. Brewster	221
Jonathan Cohen	231
John H. Dane	241
Richard G. Eaton	248
Seth M. Fitchet	251
Henry J. FitzSimmons	254
Thomas Gucker III	259
Llewellyn Hall	267
Paul W. Hugenberger	268
Miriam G. Katzeff	273
James G. Manson	275
John B. McGinty	277
Robert H. Morris	282
Arthur M. Pappas	285
Robert C. Runyon	289
Robert Soutter	292
Charles L. Sturdevant	299
Mihran O. Tachdjian	300
Augustus Thorndike	305
Arthur W. Trott	313

FRANK D. BATES

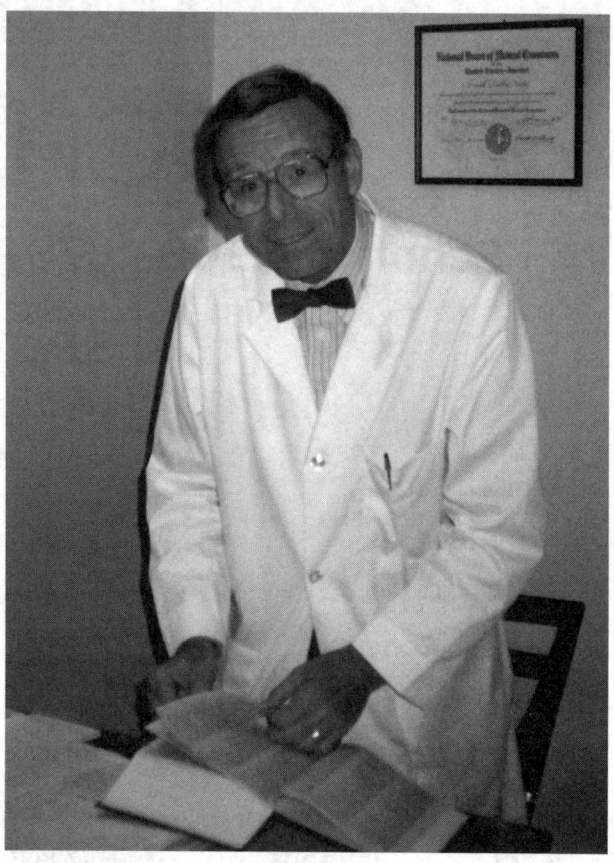

Frank D. Bates. Courtesy of Sarah Bates.

Physician Snapshot

Frank D. Bates
BORN: 1925
DIED: 2011
SIGNIFICANT CONTRIBUTIONS: Volunteer teacher and environmentalist

Frank Dudley Bates was born in Delmar, New York, outside Albany, in 1925. His family eventually moved to Snyder, New York, near Buffalo, where Frank attended Amherst Central High School. He spent his undergraduate years at the Massachusetts Institute of Technology (MIT) and then graduated from Harvard Medical School in 1948.

Few details are known about Frank Bates. He apparently trained in orthopaedic surgery at Veterans Association hospitals in Arkansas and Tennessee and at Children's Hospital in Boston. During the Korean War (1953–55), he served as a physician, with the rank of captain in the US Army, stationed at the 25th Station in Korea. To acknowledge his meritorious service, he was presented with a Bronze Star.

After being discharged from the army, Bates joined the clinical staff at Children's Hospital. He became a member of the Massachusetts Medical Society in 1957. In his private practice, he held appointments at several hospitals in the Boston area, but he lived in Winchester, and he performed most of his clinical and operative care at Winchester Hospital, where he eventually served as chief of orthopaedics (1970–75). Beginning in 1957, Bates served as an assistant in orthopaedic surgery at Harvard Medical School (a position he held until 1982) and as a junior assistant orthopedic surgeon at Children's Hospital. He became an associate surgeon in orthopaedics there in 1965 and a visiting surgeon in 1975. I recall Bates occasionally participating in teaching rounds at Children's Hospital while I was a resident. Despite extensive searches of the literature and various archives, I could not find any publications by Bates.

After leaving Harvard, in 1983, Bates, then 58 years old, began practicing at Huggins Hospital in Wolfeboro, New Hampshire. He retired from active practice in 1987 at age 62, but he remained on the hospital's board of trustees, serving on the finance and executive committees and as chairman of the board.

Bates remained very active in retirement; he loved being outdoors and was an avid mountain climber. He also volunteered clearing trails, and in doing so he injured his hip in 1993 and had to undergo surgery. While retired, he also served in various other roles in the community of Sandwich, New Hampshire: as a member of the Conservation Commission, the board of deacons and the choir at the Federated Church, as a member of the Benz Center Board of Trustees, and as the Bearcamp Valley Garden Club treasurer.

Bates had chronic lung disease, which led to his death at his home on May 23, 2011. He was

85 years old. In the "Guest Book" section accompanying his online obituary, Joseph Davis, one of Bates's former patients—in 1982, he had undergone spinal fusion at Winchester Hospital—praised Bates for enhancing his quality of life and said Bates had a "quiet but stern manner" (Mayhew Funeral Home 2011).

JOHN F. BELL

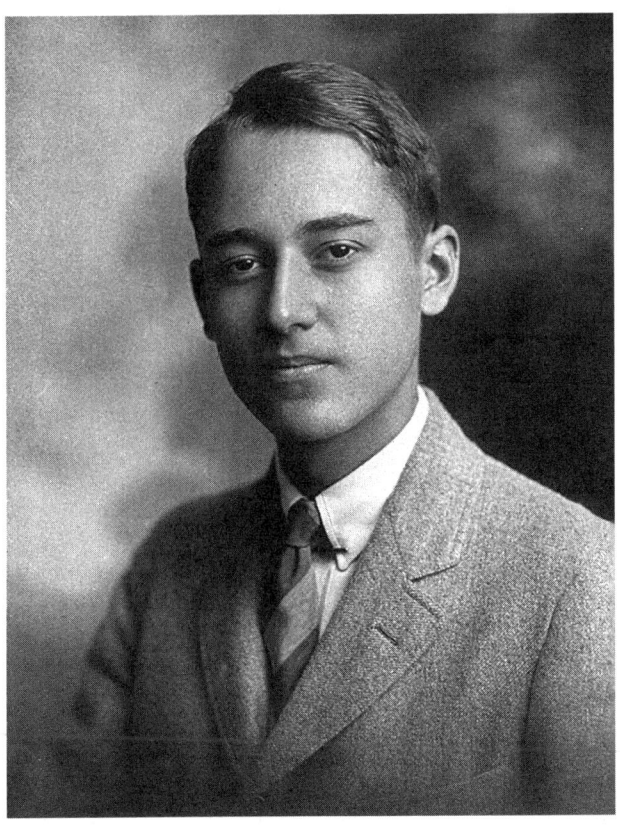

John F. Bell. Courtesy of Enoch F. Bell.

Physician Snapshot

John F. Bell
BORN: 1909
DIED: 1989
SIGNIFICANT CONTRIBUTIONS: Director of Vermont's Handicapped Children's Division of Child Health Services' Orthopaedic Program; established the Crippled Children's Clinic at the Mary Fletcher Hospital (Burlington, Vermont); chief of the division of orthopaedic surgery at the University of Vermont

John Frye Bell was born July 29, 1909. At the time, his family—father Enoch, a minister in a Congregational church; and mother, Anna Elizabeth (née Bowman)—lived in Newton, Massachusetts, but when John was three they moved to Sharon, Massachusetts. John had tuberculosis, prompting subsequent moves to Wellesley and then to Newton Center, in 1918.

John completed high school in Newton in 1926, and then, a year later, graduated from Philips Exeter Academy. He then matriculated at Yale. During his time there, he played baseball on the Phi Beta Kappa team; his roommate later noted that through his pitching John carried the team in a win against Harvard their senior year. In 1931, he received a bachelor of arts degree from Yale and went straight to Harvard Medical School. He received an MD degree in June 1935, and he stayed in Boston, where he immediately began an internship (July 1–December 31, 1935) at the Palmer Memorial Hospital.

The Palmer Memorial Hospital originally opened in 1920 on Blue Hill Avenue (see chapter 56). It had 39 beds and was used for housing patients with incurable conditions; staff there administered no treatments. In 1927, Palmer Memorial was revamped by the New England Deaconess Association: it now cared for patients with cancer, providing both surgical and radiation

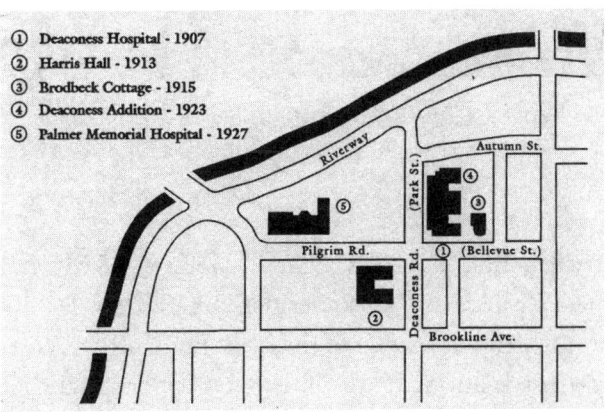

Map of hospital locations. Palmer Memorial Hospital (#5). The Ruth and David Freiman Archives at Beth Israel Deaconess Medical Center.

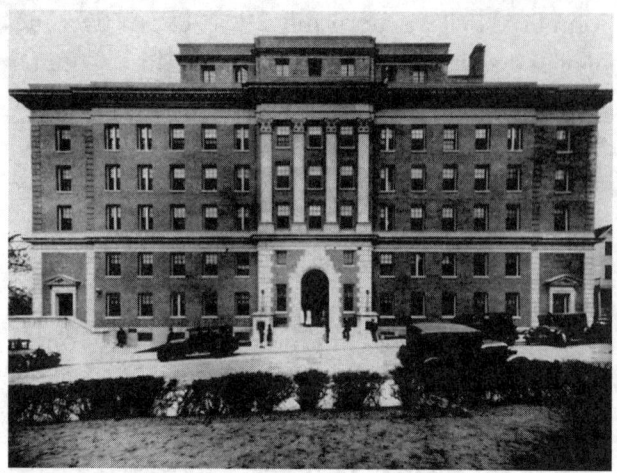

Palmer Memorial Hospital, 1927. George Brayton/The Ruth and David Freiman Archives at Beth Israel Deaconess Medical Center.

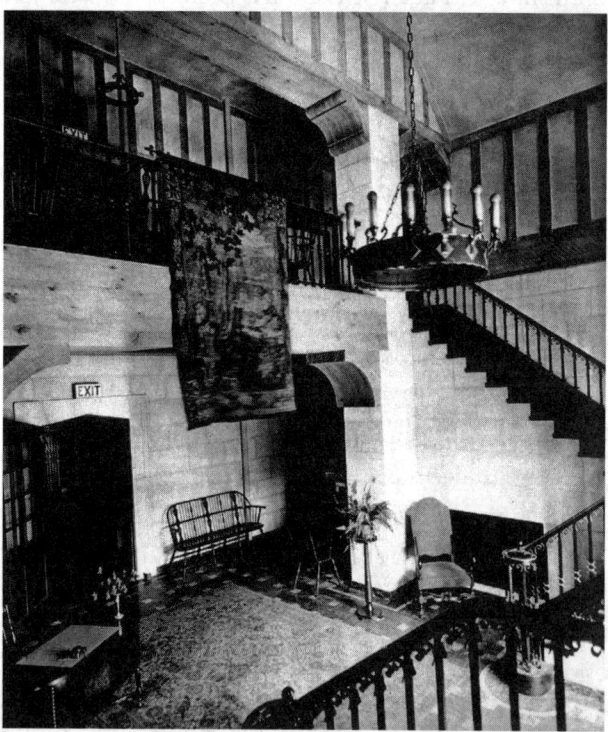

Lobby of the Palmer Memorial Hospital, ca. 1927. The Ruth and David Freiman Archives at Beth Israel Deaconess Medical Center.

treatments. The new Palmer Memorial Hospital had 75 beds and was considered a modern facility among the buildings of the New England Deaconess Association. It was in this cancer hospital that Bell interned in 1935.

Bell married Emily Jane Buck, a nurse, just after the new year in 1936. About five weeks later, Bell began a 15-month surgical internship at the Peter Bent Brigham Hospital, which he completed October 31, 1937. He continued his training through various residencies and fellowships, which are listed in **Box 23.1**.

Box 23.1. John Frye Bell's Training

- Arthur Tracy Cabot Fellow in Surgery, Harvard Medical School (November 1, 1937—October 31, 1938)
- Assistant resident, Peter Bent Brigham Hospital (November 1, 1938—February 29, 1940)
- Intern for orthopedic surgery (under Dr. Frank Ober), Children's Hospital/Massachusetts General Hospital (March 1, 1940—February 2, 1942)
- Resident for orthopedic surgery (under Dr. William Green), Children's Hospital (March 1, 1942—February 1943)
- Assistant in orthopedic surgery, Harvard Medical School (March 1, 1943—March 1, 1944)

During his training, Bell published two papers. The first, written with Thomas B. Quigley, J. Englebert Dunphy, and John L. Keely while Bell was a surgical resident at the Peter Bent Brigham Hospital, was entitled "Successful Autotransplantation of the Adrenal Gland in the Dog." The second, written with David S. Grice while Bell was an assistant in orthopaedic surgery at Harvard, was entitled "Treatment of Congenital Talipes Equinovarus with the Modified Denis Browne Splint."

In the summer of 1943, Bell was an assistant to Dr. Frank Ober at Ober's Crippled Children's Clinics in Vermont. Bell seemingly enjoyed his time in Vermont, and so he planned a move to the University of Vermont, but the United States was more deeply involved in World War II, and so he joined the army and served in the US Army Medical Corps in Europe.

After his army service, he picked up where he had left off: on New Year's Day 1947 he began at the University of Vermont as an associate professor of orthopaedic surgery and as chair of the division of orthopaedic surgery at the university's college of medicine (he held the latter position for almost 20 years, until he resigned on June 30, 1964). He also acted as a consultant to the state's Crippled Children's Division (he became its director at the end of 1950). In the early 1950s, he also established the Crippled Children's Clinic, which operated within the Durfee Clinic at the Mary Fletcher Hospital. His work with physically disabled children won him the Governor's Award in October 1953.

Throughout his career he focused his efforts on teaching, clinics, and private practice; he initially set up the latter out of his home in Burlington. Bell had faith in knowledge and education as the foundation for an orthopaedic surgeon's practice: "An orthopedic surgeon can do a lot with a piece of felt and a roll of adhesive tape and his knowledge of the pathology of musculo-skeletal disease" (E. Bell, n.d.). He returned to Harvard briefly to obtain a master's degree in public health (1951–52); afterward, back in Vermont, he became too busy and so began to care only for pediatric patients. He closed his practice in April 1958 after taking on a larger role in the Vermont Department of Health: he was named director of the Orthopedic Program for the Handicapped Children's Division of Child Health Services. During that time Bell spent two years (1963–65) as an associate editor for the *Journal of Bone and Joint Surgery*.

He stayed with the Vermont Department of Health for more than 10 years, becoming its director of medical care programs in 1970. He moved on in 1971 when he took the position of president of the Crotched Mountain Foundation in New Hampshire.

He published three additional papers on orthopaedic problems in children: one evaluating lower-extremity tendon transplantations in patients with polio, one evaluating operative procedures for congenital talipes equinovarus, and the last describing congenital defects in the shoulder, sternum, spine, and pelvis. Bell remained an active member of the Vermont Medical Association throughout his career and even after he retired; in 1982, he received the Association's Distinguished Service Award.

In 1989, he became ill and September 20 he died at the hospital he had labored at for so long. His son recalled Bell's devotion to his patients and the care he gave to his young patients: "He loved people and devoted his life to helping others, particularly crippled children. His private practice seldom paid much because he helped many who could not pay…Dad always spoke of duty as a driving force in his life and he always strove to do his duty, even if it meant significant sacrifice on his part. As a doctor he was always serving others" (quoted in E. Bell, n.d.).

ALBERT H. BREWSTER

Physician Snapshot

Albert H. Brewster
BORN: 1892
DIED: 1988
SIGNIFICANT CONTRIBUTIONS: Developed (with Lovett) the turnbuckle jacket; developed a modification of the triple arthrodesis—the Brewster countersinking procedure

Albert Howell Brewster was born in 1892 in Georgia and attended the Georgia Military Academy, an all-male school that opened in College Park in 1900 (it's now coeducational and known as the Woodward Academy). In 1914, he graduated from the University of Virginia with a bachelor of arts degree, and he then entered medical school at Johns Hopkins University.

In 1917, Brewster had just completed his third year at Johns Hopkins. Medical students entering their senior year enlisted in the US Army, and thus Brewster was 1 of 32 third-year medical students who volunteered to be part of the Johns Hopkins Hospital Unit that was mobilized to staff Base Hospital No. 18 of the American Expeditionary Forces in Bazoilles-sur-Meuse, France, in May 1917:

These men had been enlisted as privates in the Medical Reserve Corps with the understanding that they should be given practical training in a hospital in France, as well as organized teaching by the members of the Staff, and upon the completion of the course, would be granted a degree in medicine by the University and a commission in the army as medical officers. The possibility that some of these men who were in the St. Nazaire detachment would be unable to complete the projected course of study, and hence that the plan under which they had been enlisted would become impossible to carry out, was a source of a great deal of worry. ("History of Base Hospital No. 18" 1919)

Making its way through areas patrolled by German submarines, their ship landed at St. Nazaire, France, after 18 days at sea. Then traveling by train, they reached Bazoilles-sur-Meuse, the farthest advanced hospital at the time, though still well back from the front lines. While at Base Hospital No. 18, their training included:

Clinical work on the wards of the hospital, and in the operating room and laboratory…The staff of the hospital made every effort to give the students the training they considered essential for medical officers. Ward rounds were given by the chiefs of the various services and included cases from the general surgical wards, orthopedic wards, genito-urinary wards, infectious and general medical wards, and wards caring for eye, ear, nose and throat cases. ("History of Base Hospital No. 18" 1919)

In addition, the students attended lectures covering such things as "The practice of general medicine and surgery…[t]he organization and administration of the Medical Corps of the Army… [and t]he special problems pertaining to troop sanitation in and out of the line, evacuation of the wounded and, in general, the duties of battalion medical officers" ("History of Base Hospital No.

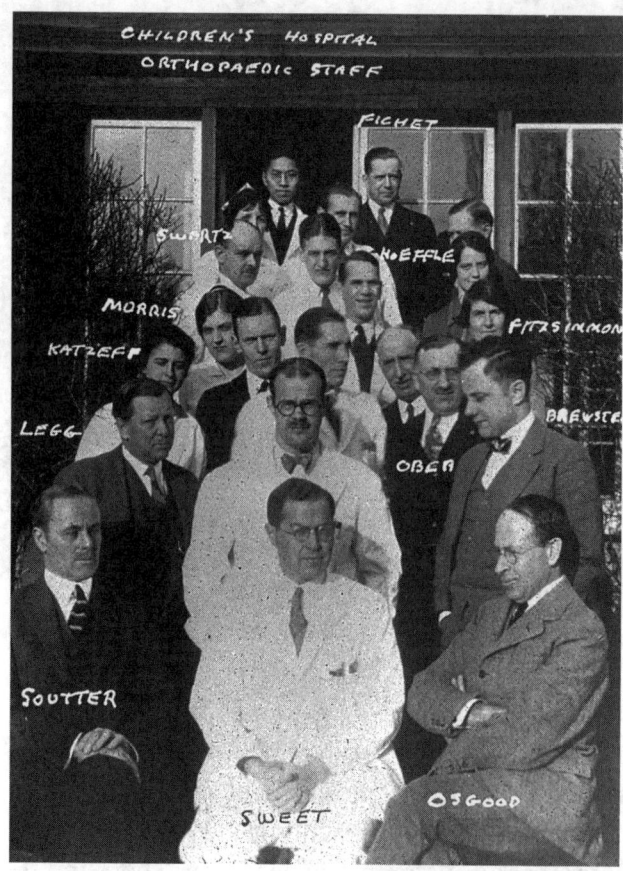

Orthopaedic staff at BCH. Dr. Brewster is standing on the right, just behind Dr. Osgood, who is seated. MGH HCORP Archives.

18" 1919). After almost 18 months, the staff of the base hospital had treated 14,179 patients.

Thirty members of the fourth-year class, including Brewster, graduated with a medical degree from Johns Hopkins in April 1918 and were commissioned as first lieutenants in the army. As a first lieutenant in the US Army Medical Corps, Brewster became an intern at the Peter Bent Brigham Hospital in 1919, after which he spent two years as a surgical house officer there (through June 1921). In 1922, he was appointed junior assistant surgeon at Children's Hospital. In 1926, he was an assistant surgeon, along with Seth M. Fitchet and Robert H. Morris, and he also worked with the junior assistant surgeon Miriam Katzeff and an assistant surgeon in the outpatient department, John G. Kuhns. He began as an instructor in orthopaedic surgery at Harvard Medical School in 1921, and he remained in this position throughout his career. Some of Brewster's instructor colleagues at Harvard in the early 1920s included Lloyd T. Brown, Henry J. FitzSimmons, Robert Soutter, and Loring T. Swaim; assistants included Joseph S. Barr, Edwin F. Cave, William T. Green, John G. Kuhns, Robert H. Morris, Sumner N. Roberts, and William A. Rogers.

Clinical Interests

Scoliosis

Brewster worked closely with Kuhns in the clinic for lateral curvature of the spine at Children's Hospital in 1928. Brewster became interested in scoliosis early during his career at Children's Hospital, and, in 1924, he and Dr. Robert Lovett published a preliminary report on a new method for treating scoliosis. Lovett had previously published (11 years earlier) with James Sever their experience in treating scoliosis with forcible permanent plaster jackets followed by removable jackets. Lovett and Brewster modified this earlier method. They first explained why most treatment for moderate or severe scoliosis was, in their word, "ineffectual" (or nonexistent):

> There are two reasons for this:
>
> 1. The problem is assumed to be largely a muscular one.
> 2. [T]he basic principles of general surgery are not sufficiently borne in mind, and fantastic notions derived more from tradition than from the knowledge of true surgical principles – are evidently the dominating factors.
>
> This failure to obtain results cannot be wholly attributed to the inefficiency of treatment by medical men, because for centuries this affection has in large part been treated by, or referred for treatment to, those who practice treatment by physical means without medical qualifications; but with this division of responsibility understood, the fact remains that the treatment of structural scoliosis has written for itself in general a record of failure, if one may judge from results. One has only to read the literature of orthopedic surgery for the last twenty years or more, or the literature of physical therapeutics in its relation to scoliosis, to see what a contradictory, unsurgical, confused mass of theories, notions and traditions it is, and how far much of it is removed from good surgical literature on other subjects. (Lovett and Brewster 1924a)

Title of Lovett and Brewster's article describing the turnbuckle cast. "The Treatment of Scoliosis by a Different Method from That Usually Employed," *Journal of Bone and Joint Surgery* 1924; 6: 847.

They then described the goals for their "method of attack that meets the principles of general surgery" (Lovett and Brewster 1924a):

> [W]e are trying to make straight a spinal column that has curved to one side and has become stiff in the curved position. There is contraction of the soft parts on the concave side of the curve; the vertebral bodies have become twisted and wedge-shaped, and partially or wholly ankylosed in the curved position, so that the patient is unable to assume a better position in standing and the curves do not disappear in recumbency. The rib circle of the thorax is unilaterally distorted… given so serious a distortion of the spine…the

influence of growth under the continuance of the malposition will tend to increase and aggravate the existing deformity. In our outlook…our sheet anchor must be found in the adaptability of growing bone to change its shape in consequence of changes in pressure, according to Wolff's Law…There is every prospect of a permanent straightening…the methods most commonly used in the past and at present seem to us to have failed to yield satisfactory results, largely because they did not take cognizance of a well-known mechanical law. The strongest structure known to the engineer is our arch and the strong part of an arch is the apex or its keystone. Most methods for the correction of structural scoliosis expend their force in pressing directly against the apex…the keystone of the arch. Such methods are known to be inefficient…because cases of structural scoliosis are so rigid and resistant that force enough to correct the curve…cannot be endured by the patient. (Lovett and Brewster 1924a)

Lovett and Brewster then described their modifications of the forcible jacket, the first of which they applied at the end of 1923 and into early 1924:

In the jacket…as now used by us, the mechanics are such that the ends of the arch are spread, using the apex of the curve as a point of resistance…a very marked degree of distraction or pulling apart at the point of greatest curve is exercised on the spine. This is because…an

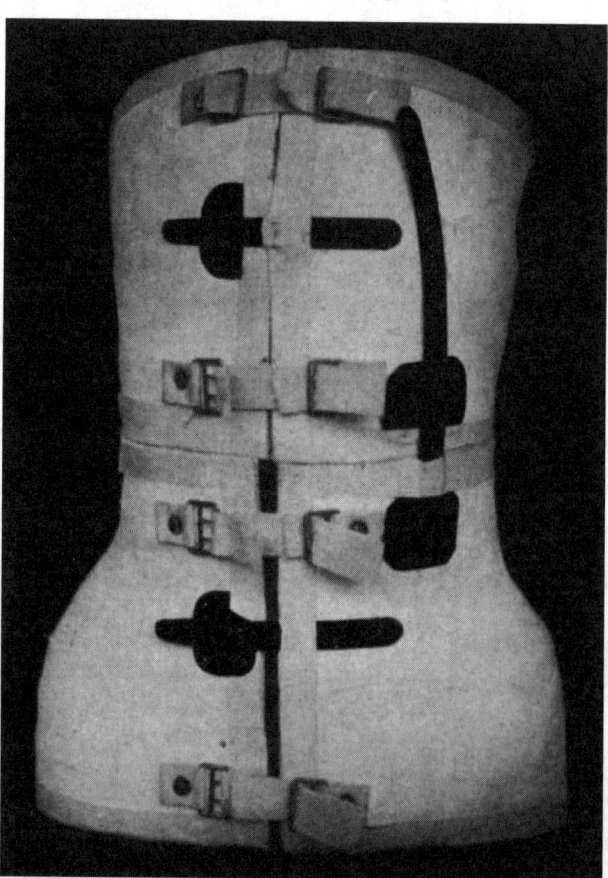

Photo of one of the original turnbuckle casts before applying the turnbuckle.
R. W. Lovett and A. H. Brewster, "The Treatment of Scoliosis by a Different Method from That Usually Employed," *Journal of Bone and Joint Surgery* 1924; 6: 848.

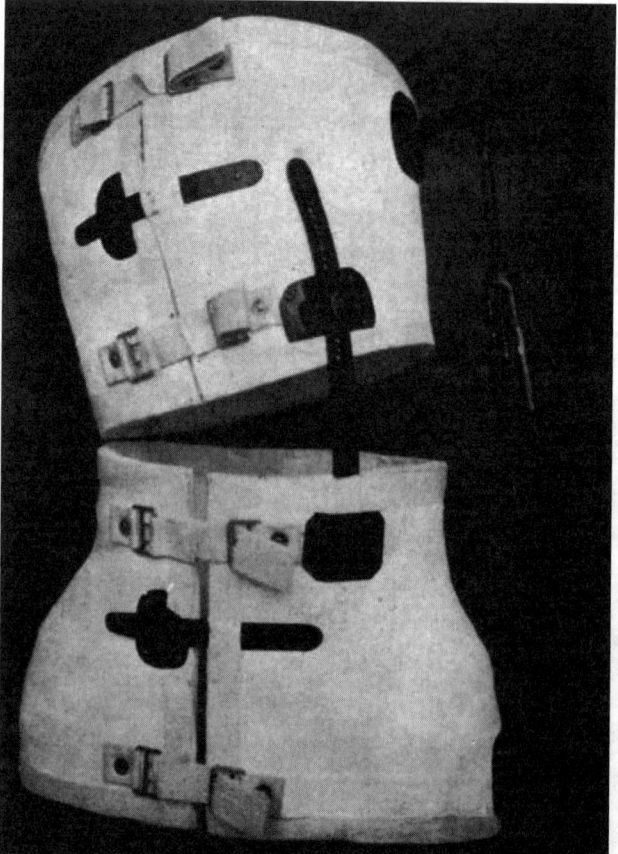

Photo of the turnbuckle cast after applying the turnbuckle and beginning correction of the scoliosis.
R. W. Lovett and A. H. Brewster, "The Treatment of Scoliosis by a Different Method from That Usually Employed," *Journal of Bone and Joint Surgery* 1924; 6: 849.

eccentric hinge on its [jacket's] periphery, while the center of motion, being in the spine, is in the middle line of the body; so that when the jacket is opened by the turnbuckle, enormous force on the spine may be exerted to straighten it and pull the thorax away from the pelvis.

This is done by...extending [the plaster jacket] from the axillae to the trochanters. The jacket is then divided into two parts by a transverse cut opposite the convexity of the lateral curve. This jacket is then provided with a hinge on the convex side of the lateral curve opposite its apex, and by means of a turnbuckle on the opposite side of the jacket at the same level the jacket can be opened on the concave side of the lateral curve. The thorax is held as a whole, and with the jackets firm grip on the pelvis, a great straightening force is exerted on the spine. The jacket must fit very accurately. (Lovett and Brewster 1924a)

They concluded by providing 10 points in support of this new method of treatment for structural scoliosis:

1. It effects [sic] mobilization of the spine.
2. The force applied spreads the ends of the arch and does not disregard the mechanical law that the keystone is the strongest part of the arch.
3. It permits of gradual correction.
4. It will produce an immediate correction in moderate curves, as described above.
5. It tends at the same time to decrease rotation as seen clinically and in the roentgenograms.
6. It stretches out the shortened structures on the concave side of the curve.
7. It allows the stretched structures of the convex side to retain their tone.
8. It furnishes a means of securing an adjustable overcorrection retention jacket.
9. It increases the patient's height.
10. It is not uncomfortable.

We...look forward to a permanent alteration in the bones of the spine. (Lovett and Brewster 1924a)

In Brewster's last paper on scoliosis, published in 1929, he referred to this new jacket as the turnbuckle jacket (it was often referred to as the Brewster turnbuckle jacket) (**Box 23.2**). In 1968, P. D. Wilson wrote an obituary for John Cobb—an orthopaedic surgeon who began the first scoliosis clinic at the Hospital for the Ruptured and

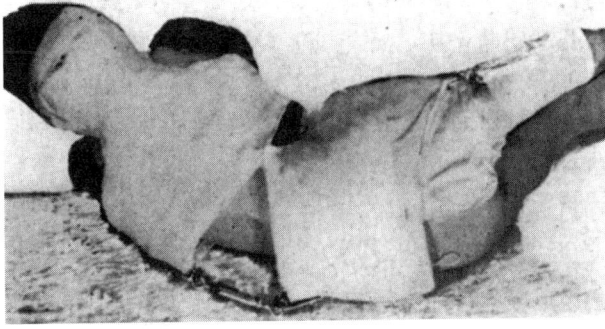

Photo of patient in a turnbuckle during process of wedging.
A. D. Smith, F. L. Butte, and A. B. Ferguson, "Treatment of Scoliosis by Wedging Jacket and Spine Fusion," *Journal of Bone and Joint Surgery* 1938; 20: 827.

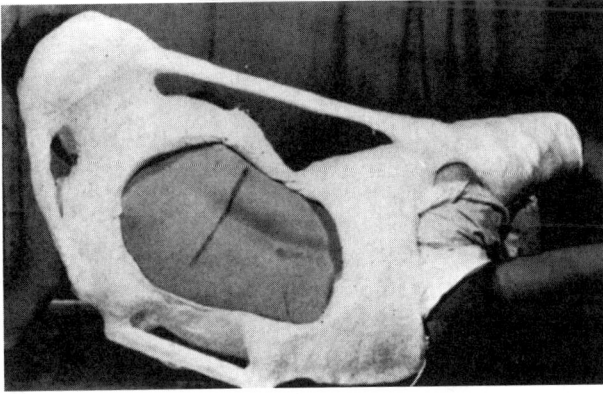

Photo of patient in turnbuckle after completion of the correction. A large posterior window has been made in preparation for surgery.
A. D. Smith, F. L. Butte, and A. B. Ferguson, "Treatment of Scoliosis by Wedging Jacket and Spine Fusion," *Journal of Bone and Joint Surgery* 1938; 20: 827.

Box 23.2. Application Technique for the Turnbuckle Jacket

"Construction. – A patient with a right dorsolumbar curve, with the apex of the curve at the twelfth dorsal vertebra, is suspended in a Sayer head sling until his toes are just touching the floor. He holds on to the bars above his head with his hands. This position hyperextends the spine and elevates the scapulae as well as making them prominent laterally. Both of these points are important in the construction of the jacket. A plaster jacket is then applied from high up in the axillae down over the greater trochanters, taking particular care to mark out the anterior superior spines and inguinal regions. This is immediately removed by a front midline incision and a few more plasters wound around to hold it in shape. A wooden box...[has] a hole... made through its center. A steel rod is passed through this hole in the box... [and placed] perpendicular to the floor. The jacket is so placed on the box that the steel rod passes directly through its center and is then filled with plaster mud and allowed to set. The jacket is removed and the torso is ready for hewing. The steel is placed in a vice and the torso is hewed. The prominence on the torso caused by the elevated scapulae is cut away...It is most important not to lower or change the contour of the iliac crest because such a change makes the final jacket very uncomfortable from pressure on these bones, particularly the anterior superior spines.

"With the squaring of the torso finished...correction of the torso is begun...the right prominence is shaved with a draw knife as much as it is evident the patient can stand. The left hip is then lowered and the part of the torso at the top, left posterior is hewed away. This decreases the left concave side of the body making it approach a straight line. By the foregoing procedure, it is readily seen that pressure is exerted at points [the apex of the curve on the right side and points above and below the curve on the left side]...

"After the torso is cut as described, a new plaster jacket is put on and immediately cut off...This jacket ought not to be more than three-eighths of an inch thick...Seven plasters will as a rule, give just about the right thickness.

"Application. – After the jacket is dry, about 4 or 5 inches are cut off at the top in order that the patient may be comfortable with the arms hanging at the sides...enough...so that the circulation will not be impaired. At the bottom, the jacket is cut off about 1 inch below the anterior superior spines tapering downward posteriorly. This allows the patient to sit comfortably.

"The jacket is put on...temporary straps are tightened... The jacket is worn for a day or so to be sure that it exerts pressure over the rotation being attacked...shown by a slight redness of the skin. The jacket must be comfortable...a string is tied about him [patient] at the level of...[the apex] vertebra. The jacket...is [again] applied. At a point in front at the level of the string, the jacket is marked...A line is then drawn around the jacket about one-half inch below the front mark. A cross is put in the left midaxillary line at

Crippled and who developed a simple and reliable method of measuring spine deformity (the Cobb angle). Wilson (1968) noted that Cobb believed this jacket "seemed to offer hope of correcting the deformity of the spine" and that he had "gradually became convinced that the best method of correction was the use of the turnbuckle plaster jacket combined with spine fusion." A 1998 publication called it a "breakthrough" in scoliosis treatment.

The turnbuckle jacket was used at Children's Hospital during my residency there in the late 1960s. At that time, however, the turnbuckle cast had been modified yet again to include the proximal hip and thigh on the same side of the convexity of the curve in order to better immobilize the pelvis. Patients would be placed in a turnbuckle cast and the curve gradually straightened to maximal correction; a rectangular opening posteriorly exposed a space to allow for posterior spine fusion while the patient remained in maximal correction in the turnbuckle cast. An osteoperiosteal graft would be taken from the tibia and placed along the corrected spinal segments. The patient stayed recumbent in the cast for three months. After the

the level of the circular mark to indicate where the hinge is to be placed. On the right side is the midaxillary line, at the top and bottom, crosses are made indicating the position of the boxings for the removable turnbuckle. Lines are drawn around the jacket indicating where it is to be steeled. In front, marks are made indicating where the boxes for the top and bottom stays are to be placed. The jacket is then sent to the appliance shop, and the hinge, boxings and steels are put on before the circular incision, separating the jacket into two parts is made…

"The mechanical principles of the turnbuckle jacket and shell are exactly the same…A laterally curved spine represents one or more arcs. The problem is to straighten the spine…[with] a method which entails no harm to the patient…three forces are necessary: (1) a resisting force on the convex side of the keystone at its center; (2-3) an active force at each end exerting pressure on the concave side. Such forces if strong enough will snap the arc… The turnbuckle jacket and shell furnish the forces used to straighten an arc. Another mechanical principal of the turnbuckle and shell is that they are eccentric. The hinge on either does not correspond to the center of motion in the spine and when they are opened they are elongated, which produces a distraction of the spine above and below the part opposite the hinge."

—A. H. Brewster 1929

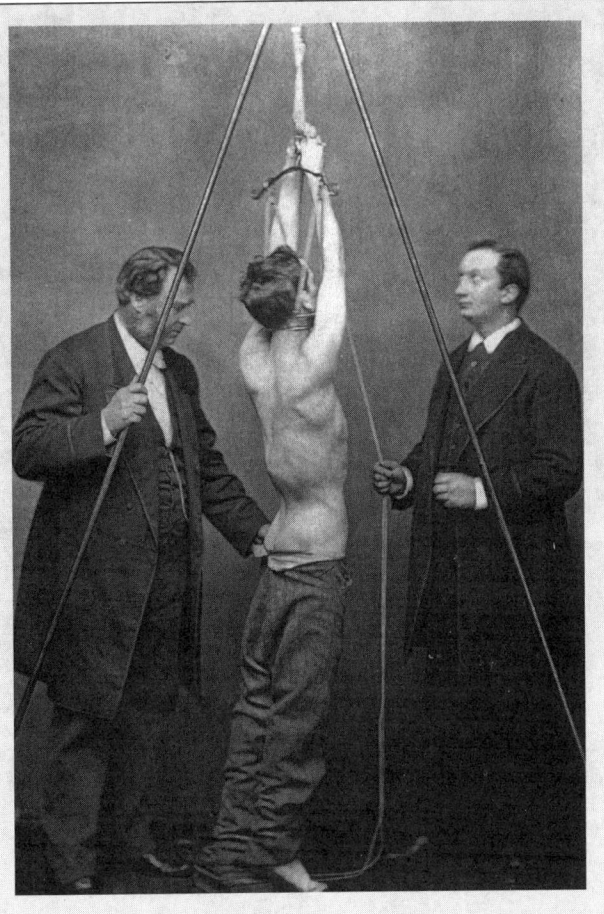

Dr. Sayre (left) with a patient in suspension-traction in preparation for application of a corrective body cast.

Spinal disease and spinal curvature: their treatment by suspension and the use of the plaster of Paris bandage by L. A. Sayre. London: Smith, Elder & Co, 1877. Francis A. Countway Library of Medicine/Internet Archive.

fusion had healed, the patient could ambulate in a plaster jacket, and then in a corrective celastic jacket for another 6 to 12 months.

In 1931, Brewster and Frank Ober revised the fifth edition of Lovett's *Lateral Curvature of the Spine and Round Shoulders*. Both surgeons had worked with and took over for Lovett in practice, and their goal with the text:

> was to keep alive the fundamental contributions of their renowned teacher…The editors added some valuable material, which includes the Galeazzi method of treatment and detailed descriptions of the turnbuckle jacket and the turnbuckle-shell treatment. The book contains an excellent history of scoliosis…The chapter on pathology includes the living and dissecting room subjects. The relation of scoliosis to school life is given in detail. The chapter on exercises has been practically rewritten with the assistance of Miss Wright. It is to be regretted that the chapter on the operative treatment has been given so little space. This book remains the best book on the subject at present and is

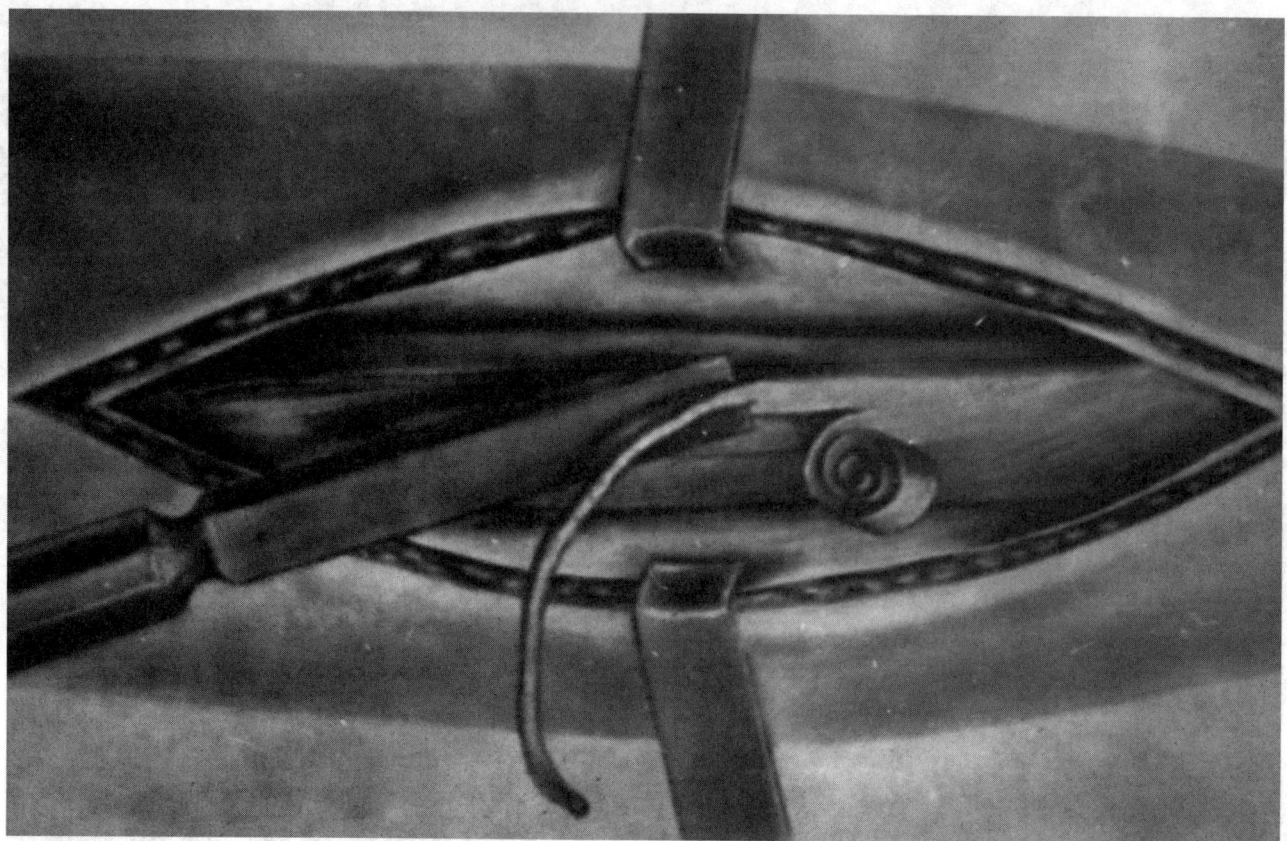

Drawing of Dr. Green's technique of obtaining a tibial osteoperiosteal graft. Unpublished; archives of Dr. William T. Green, Harvard Medical Library in the Frances A. Countway Library of Medicine.

recommended to medical students, interns, general practitioners, physical education students, physical therapists, pediatricians and orthopedic surgeons. (*Journal of the American Medical Association* 1931)

Deformities of the Foot

Another interest of Brewster's was deformities of the foot. He wrote two papers on the topic: an early one on an original type of triple arthrodesis in which he countersunk the astragalus, and another, seven years later, in which he reported his modified triple arthrodesis in cavus feet using a slightly different technique of countersinking the talus. He delineated four reasons for countersinking the talus into the calcaneus in paralytic feet: "First – Lateral stability of the foot. Secondly – Limitation of dorsiflexion. Thirdly – Limitation of plantar flexion. Fourthly – After the above is accomplished, the foot appears normal and is functionally good" (A. H. Brewster 1933). He then described his technique:

[A]t the junction of the neck and body of the astragalus, its inferior surface is removed in a plane parallel to the sole of the foot...a chisel is driven through the os calcis at right angles to the sole of the foot, and just posterior to the cartilage of the calcaneocuboid joint, from the lateral side to the medial. At right angles to this, the superior surface of the os calcis is removed parallel to the sole of the foot anteroposteriorly, until all the cartilage...in the joint between the astragalus and os calcis is removed. The head and neck of the astragalus are next removed at right angles to the sole of the foot...The posterior part of the astragalus is removed at right angles to the sole of the foot...Next, as much of the bony prominence on the posterior superior surface of the os calcis is removed at right angles to the sole of the foot…[allowing countersinking of the astragalus, after which]…the cartilage of the scaphoid…is removed. (A. H. Brewster 1933)

Brewster first performed the procedure in 1927, and he operated on more than 50 cases by the time of his publication in 1933.

In 1940, Brewster and Carroll B. Larson published a review of 200 cases of cavus feet—or "claw feet," as then called—treated at Children's Hospital. They noted "a cavus tendency in a high proportion of children who had been continuously in bed for six months or longer, even when the weight of the bedclothes had been removed. It would seem reasonable that gravity might play a role by allowing the forefoot to approximate the hindfoot" (Brewster and Larson 1940). In their opinion:

> The triple arthrodesis, when done to relieve the deformities of a claw foot, must accomplish several things: 1. The astragalus must be reshaped in order to elevate the forefoot, so as to flatten the long arch. 2. The os calcis must be relieved of its calcaneus position and set back, in order to reduce contracture and to increase leverage of the tendo-achilles. 3. The foot must be shortened, in order to relax the tightness of the plantar fascia and also lessen the cocked-up position of the toes by relaxing the contracted tendons. The triple arthrodesis has been modified in order to better accomplish these objectives…to date the results have been very gratifying. (Brewster and Larson 1940)

In 1942, William Green and Leo McDermott published a paper on surgical treatment of the foot in spastic cerebral palsy. They reported seven cases of Brewster's countersinking operation, some of which had been accompanied by tendon transplantation (most often transplanting the posterior tibial tendon into a metatarsal). In their experience, the two procedures together gave "the best results" (Green and McDermott 1942).

Contrary to these previous articles praising Brewster's countersinking procedure, in 1950—almost 20 years after Brewster's initial publication of his technique—Patterson, Parrish, and Hathaway reported their results with various types of bony stabilization procedures in the foot—including 10 cases of Brewster's countersinking procedure—at the Hospital for Special Surgery. They had not achieved much success with Brewster's procedure. For them, "the Brewster countersinking procedure…is difficult to carry out. There appears to be a tendency for displacement of the talus from the countersunk position and, unless adequate muscle power is available for transplantation to the dorsum of the foot, the operation cannot be relied upon to correct drop foot" (Patterson, Parrish, and Hathaway 1950). Their experience with four types of triple arthrodesis revealed "the percentage of failures to be quite similar (Hoke stabilization 12.5 per cent., Brewster countersinking operation 20.0 per cent., Lambrinudi stabilization 14.5 per cent., and triple arthrodesis 15.9 per cent.)" (Patterson, Parrish, and Hathaway 1950).

Supracondylar Fractures

Brewster cowrote his last published article, in 1940, with Meier Karp. Theirs was an end-result study of supracondylar fractures of the humerus in children. They examined eight cases of cubitus varus deformity and measured the length of the lateral side of the arm against the length of the medial side. In six patients, the lateral side of the arm was longer by one-quarter to three-quarters of an inch. "They concluded that this had been caused by stimulation of the external epicondylar and capitellar epiphyses" (L. Smith 1960). Lyman Smith (1960) considered "this explanation…most unlikely," because his own study showed "that simple medial tilt of the distal fragment gives the same appearance…it is difficult to explain the deformity on the basis of a pure growth disturbance in view of the overwhelming predominance (ten or more to one) of varus deformities."

Clinical Practice and Professional Involvement

Brewster's office was located at 234 Marlborough Street, where Lovett and his wife (Elizabeth Moorfield Storey) had lived and where Lovett practiced shortly after their marriage. Elizabeth Lovett owned the building, and although the couple moved from the house in 1901, her husband maintained his medical office there up until his death in 1924. Upon the Lovetts' move, James S. Stone moved into the house and had his office there, but in 1908 he and wife also moved to Framingham. Thereafter, the building remained occupied exclusively by medical practices. Ober had also established his medical office at 234 Marlborough Street, and in 1935 he purchased the buildings at 234 from Elizabeth Lovett and next door at 232, converting both to medical offices. It seems that Ober sold both buildings separately in 1961: 232 Marlborough Street was converted back into 10 apartments, and 234 Marlborough Street was purchased by Brewster; he continued to practice there. The hallways crossing between the buildings were closed.

Active in the Massachusetts Medical Society, Brewster participated in the postgraduate instruction series organized by Ober. He was also active in the Boston Orthopaedic Club and the Interurban Orthopaedic Club; in 1934, he presented to the latter club a paper on biceps and triceps transfers for deltoid muscle paralysis. Brewster was also a member of the American Orthopaedic Association and the American Academy of Orthopaedic Surgeons. A longtime participant in the Clinics for Crippled Children in Massachusetts, Brewster covered the clinic in Lowell. Other volunteer-physicians at the same time included Arthur T. Legg in Haverhill, Harold C. Bean in Salem, Mark H. Rogers in Gardner, George W. Van Gorder in Brockton, John W. O'Meara in Worcester, Garry de N. Hough Jr. in Springfield, Francis A. Slowick in Pittsfield, Paul L. Norton in Hyannis, and E. A. McCarthy in Fall River.

Clare McCarthy, a physical therapist at Children's Hospital, recalled that Brewster would come to grand rounds once every three months. He would sit in the first row, opposite William Green. She remembered one occasion when a physician presented a baby with increasing weakness. Someone mentioned polio as a possible diagnosis, and a large debate ensued. Brewster, however, commented that he thought the baby had scurvy—which proved to be the correct diagnosis.

Brewster was an orthopaedic surgeon at the New England Peabody Home for Crippled Children. The home opened in 1895 on 40 acres of what had once been part of Harvard surgeon Henry Jacob Bigelow's estate. Clinicians there treated the children who had what were then incurable diseases, such as tuberculosis and polio. Toward the mid-1900s, the facility had an operating and recovery rooms as well as a radiography suite, and ~100 patients lived at the home. The physicians limited visits by family in order to keep the children focused on healing—being away from their parents was tough for all of the them—but

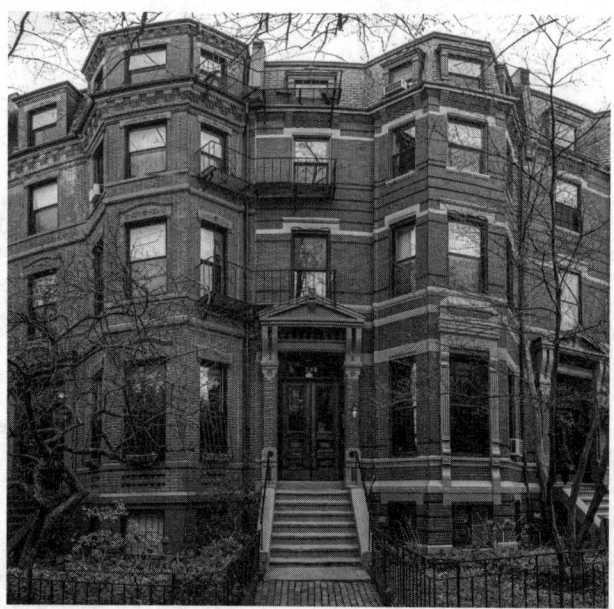

Brewster's office: 234 Marlborough Street. Kael E. Randall/Kael Randall Images.

the doctors did allow teachers in to educate the children, who ranged across first through twelfth grades, and sometimes special guests, like Ted Williams, would visit. The Peabody Home operated for almost 70 years; it closed in 1961 and Brewster became an emeritus surgeon.

In 1960, Brewster and Robert Morris, both of whom were at the time senior members of the orthopaedic staff at Children's Hospital, were named emeritus orthopaedic surgeons. Brewster was 68 years old. Also, in 1960, Brewster gave to the Boston Medical Library a letter written to Lovett by President Franklin D. Roosevelt in which Roosevelt explains to Lovett how he was able to get around on his houseboat. (I don't know how Brewster obtained this letter.) Brewster died on August 8, 1988, at age 95. He was survived by his wife, Elsie Estelle (née Carter), his daughter Nancy, and his grandchildren. His son Albert Howell Brewster Jr. may have predeceased him.

JONATHAN COHEN

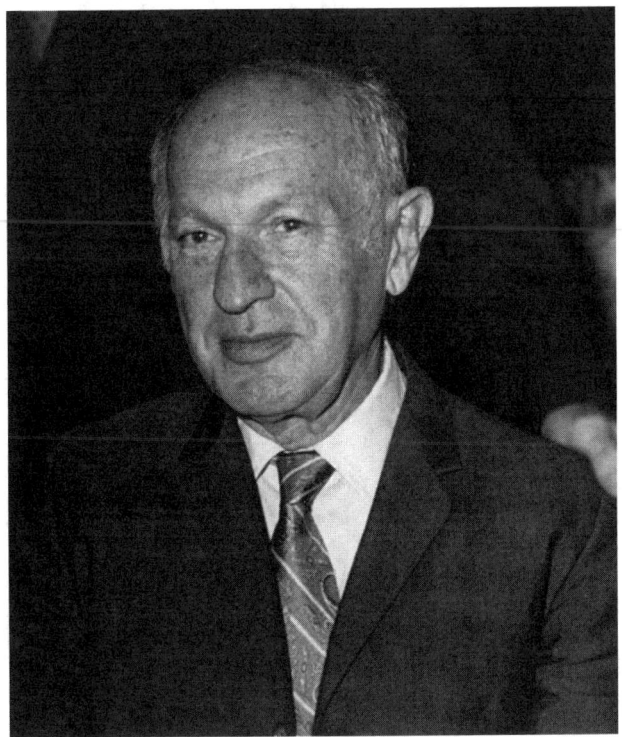

Jonathan Cohen. "Jonathan Cohen, MD, 1915-2003," *Journal of Bone & Joint Surgery* 2004; 86: 662.

Physician Snapshot

Jonathan Cohen
BORN: 1915
DIED: 2003
SIGNIFICANT CONTRIBUTIONS: Helped to develop the mobile army surgical hospital (MASH) units during his time in the military; established (with Wolbach, Farber, and Green) the Orthopaedic Research Laboratory at Children's Hospital; was the first to observe that a Ewing tumor of the talus appears similar to avascular necrosis; served as president of the Orthopaedic Research Society

Jonathan Cohen was born in New York City on February 26, 1915. His father, as a teenager, had immigrated to the United States from a small village on the Sea of Galilee. Jonathan "attended public schools and graduated from New York University in 1933" (M.H.McG., R.E.B, and H.J.M 2004) when he was 18 years old. In the early 1930s, "a quota existed for Jewish students who were seeking medical degrees in the schools of New York City. However, the Jesuit priests accepted Jonathan into St. Louis University School of Medicine where he was awarded his medical degree in 1938" (M.H. McG., R.E.B, and H.J.M 2004). After graduating from medical school, Cohen interned at the Jewish Hospital in St. Louis (1938–39) and then was a surgical resident in Georgia (1939–40) and in Montreal (1940–41). In 1941, during World War II, he joined the US Army. He served five years, "the first two years in teaching and administrative roles at the Infantry School in Fort Benning, Georgia...[and then] three years as an army surgeon" in the 105th General Hospital (M.H.McG., R.E.B., and H.J.M. 2004).

While in the army, Cohen was instrumental in developing mobile army surgical hospitals (MASHs), one of the benefits of which was how quickly they could be taken down and then reassembled elsewhere. According to Eliza Alden, Cohen's stepdaughter, "He was very passionate about his time during the war...It didn't matter if [his patients] were five-star generals or everyday soldiers. He treated them all the same" (M. Bartle

2003). Two of Cohen's more well-known patients were General Douglas MacArthur, who was treated for a leg wound, and Charles Lindbergh, who was treated for a shoulder injury.

Much later Cohen (n.d.) wrote *The Fourth Portable Surgical Hospital's Service in the War against Japan*, which was "a history of that hospital unit…for the archives of the Army and Air Force. The unit provided front-line surgical care for the wounded who were stationed along the western edges of the Philippines, New Guinea, and the Dutch West Indies" (M.H. McG., R.E.B., and H.J.M. 2004). Cohen's (n.d.) goal was "to provide historical documentation on one such hospital [a small portable hospital] activated (only six saw combat service)" in the Buna campaign. The Fourth Portable Surgical Hospital (4PSH) operated as a functional unit in New Guinea from September 20, 1942, until September 12, 1945 (see chapter 64). It was used in both the Buna and Mindoro campaigns. The hospital was a satellite of the 105th General Hospital at Gatton, Australia, 50 miles west of Brisbane. All physicians at the 105th General Hospital were from Harvard Medical School; their commanding officer was Dr. Augustus Thorndike. In a letter to Thorndike, Dr. Neil Swinton (commanding officer of the 4PSH) stated, "The rigors of the Buna campaign, consisted mainly of working long hours in jungle conditions that included lack of sanitation and inadequate prophylaxis against malaria, took their toll on the personnel of the 4PSH" (J. Cohen,

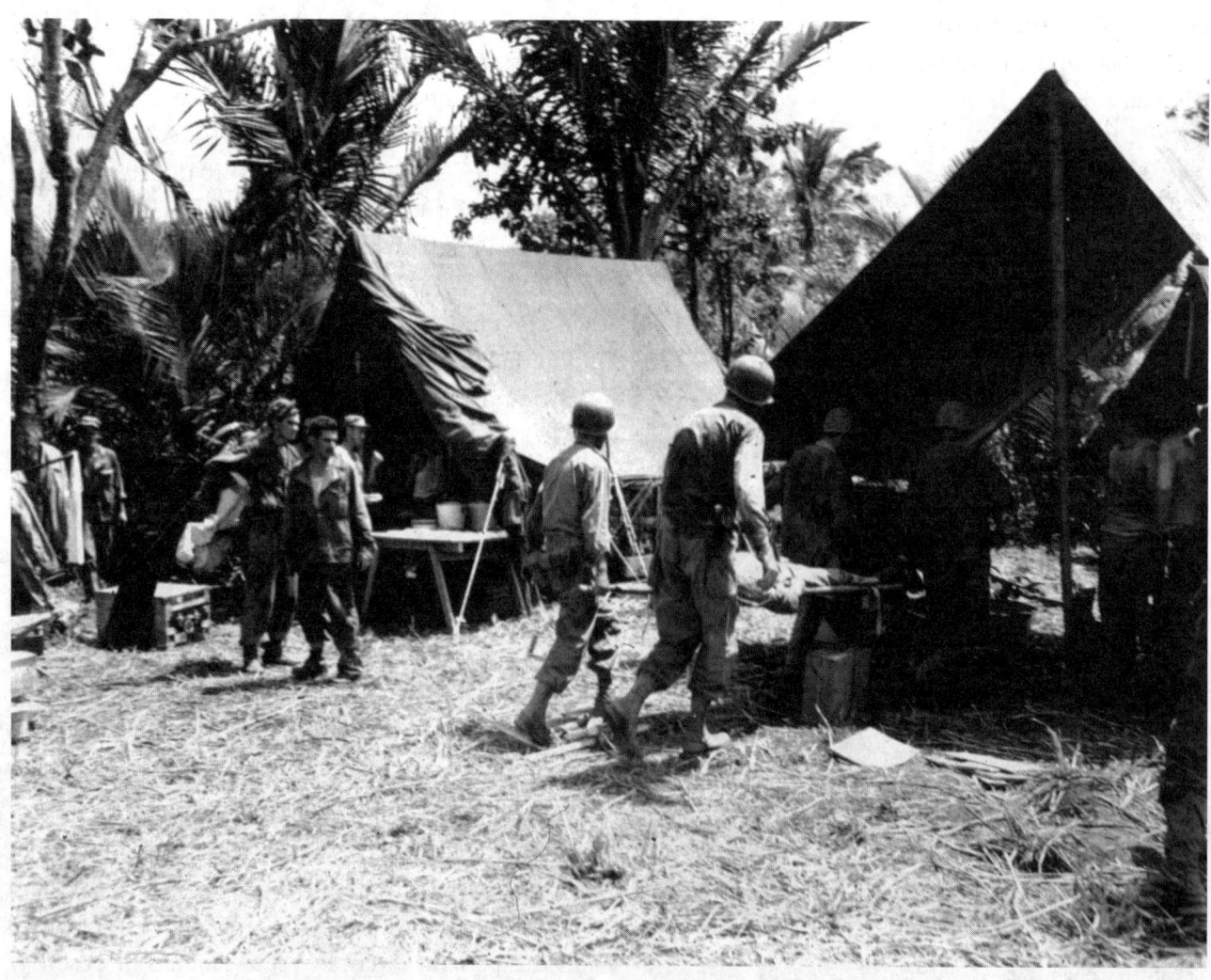

MASH Unit, 12th Portable Surgical Hospital, New Guinea (April 1944). U.S. National Library of Medicine.

n.d.). Cohen described the difficulties with travel and sanitation (the latter "was never satisfactory" [J. Cohen, n.d.]). At one time, the entire unit had dysentery; each man lost an average of 10–15 pounds.

Each portable hospital unit was staffed by four doctors and 33 enlisted men. The 4PSH was located 250–500 yards behind the battalion. The 4PSH had no refrigeration and initially no x-ray facilities. Intravenous pentothal was used as anesthesia for everything except laparotomies; then, open-drop ether was used. Superficial wounds were debrided after local administration of 1% or 2% novocaine.

The physicians initially treated wounded or sick soldiers at the 4PSH—this included performing amputations—but those who were more seriously ill or wounded were evacuated. Because the 4PSH did not have any vehicles, litter bearers carried these soldiers three miles to an evacuation hospital at the rear. Dysentery was endemic, 80% of the medically ill had malaria, and hundreds of soldiers had infected epidermophytosis. In *The Fourth Portable Surgical Hospital's Service*, Cohen recalled treating 20 Japanese prisoners at the 4PHS: "All were diseased and debilitated to the point of emaciation. All had malaria, malnutrition, anemia and intestinal parasites."

Cohen also described the wounds of injured Allied soldiers—many of which had been caused by gunshots and grenade explosions:

> Because of the high velocity of the Japanese rifle (3300 feet per second) and its small caliber (25 mm) the bullet wound often resembled a drill hole, even when the bullet passed through bone. The exit-hole would not be much larger than the entry-hole. Also the Japanese grenade was small and low-powered and our soldiers learned that they could sit on the grenade and accept a wound in the buttock in preference to the multiple and possibly more serious wounds from the grenade's unfettered explosion.
>
> (J. Cohen, n.d.)

Cohen described only one patient he treated, a second lieutenant who had a grenade explode in his right hand 30 minutes earlier. His hand was gone, and he had severely open, comminuted fractures of both bones of the forearm and extensive soft-tissue damage, a collapsed left eyeball, and multiple fragment wounds. Cohen performed an open guillotine amputation of the forearm six inches below the elbow, applied skin traction to the open amputation, excised the remains of the left eyeball, and debrided all the fragment wounds.

During the last few weeks of the 4PSH's service, two orthopaedic surgeons, Cohen and Dr. Eugene Suzedell (also from Boston), replaced the commanding officer and alternated their command. The hospital was officially disbanded on November 15, 1945. Cohen was discharged from the army in 1946. He was 31 years old.

Cohen moved to Boston after being discharged, and he spent the next two years as a resident in pathology at Children's Hospital, then as a resident in orthopaedic surgery at Children's Hospital and the Massachusetts General Hospital.

After completing both residencies, Cohen was appointed to the staff at Children's Hospital and Harvard Medical School, "where he taught and practiced for 17 years" (M.H.McG., R.E.B., and H.J.M. 2004). He was promoted to assistant professor at Harvard Medical School in 1959. The 1966 Children's Hospital Department of Orthopaedics annual report lists Cohen as an orthopedic pathologist in the Department of Pathology and a senior associate in orthopedic surgery (along with Drs. Henry Banks, Paul Hugenberger, and Arthur Trott) in the Department of Orthopedic Surgery.

Research

Cohen published papers on both bone pathology (including the effects of irradiation) and metallic implants throughout his career. He also wrote five papers on bone anatomy, physiology, and repair. He was a thorough and meticulous writer, which

I can attest to personally. In one publication we wrote together, I had to rewrite the paper six times before it was acceptable to Cohen.

One of his first papers, titled "Progressive Diaphyseal Dysplasia," was published in 1948 while he was still a resident. He was focused on research from the beginning:

> [His] research career began in 1950 and was focused on three topics. In two areas he and researchers from Massachusetts General Hospital and the Massachusetts Institute of Technology (M.I.T.) made notable contributions. One was the effect of radioisotopes that concentrate in bone (radium, thorium, radon, plutonium, and uranium)...The other was the development of metals (mainly alloys of cobalt, chromium, steel, or titanium) that are used in devices (e.g. total joint prostheses, screws and plates) for orthopaedic surgical treatment. He and the M.I.T. team contributed to the development of metals that are well tolerated by tissue...His third area, less immediate in its application, was a clarification of the physiology and morphology of bone growth and the depiction of various abnormalities, such as bone cysts. (M.H. McG., R.E.B., and H.J.M. 2004)

Cohen encouraged collaboration in research. For several years, he and Dr. Thomas Weller organized a beer and cheese club; this club began to meet in 1954 when Weller moved his lab from Children's Hospital to Harvard Medical School. The members met monthly in one of their homes. It allowed faculty who had labs at Children's Hospital and faculty who had labs at Harvard to discuss their current research activities, providing opportunities for collaboration. Members represented many fields including John Craig in pathology, Robert Smith in anesthesiology, Dick Wittenborg in radiology, David Nathan in oncology, Alex Nadas in cardiology, Shervin Kevy in hematology, and Park Gerald in genetics.

Orthopaedic Research Laboratory

Cohen, in collaboration with Burt Wolbach, Sidney Farber, and William Green (with whom he cowrote numerous research papers), developed a plan for and established an orthopaedic research laboratory at Children's Hospital. He requested 1,400 square feet of separate space with dedicated areas for electromyography, histology, and mechanical (a workshop providing equipment and space for working with bones and metal implants); a library/seminar room; offices for the laboratory director and a secretary; and a laboratory with two technicians, one for the bone histology and one for analytical chemistry. He initially requested an annual budget of $25,000 for research in the areas of epiphyseal growth and motor mechanisms. He envisioned an orthopaedic surgeon as lab director; three other orthopaedic surgeons who would be involved in research; and two–four residents who were aspiring to a career in academics, each of whom would spend one year in the lab. By 1963, Cohen and Green had successfully obtained a research training grant. Two or three fellows completed research projects in the lab each year, including Dr. Mohinder Mital, who studied metal toxicity on cells in tissue culture. Cohen's "investigations in the orthopaedic laboratory...[evolved to become] largely concerned with biologic reactions to metals...The causes of failure of metals which have been implanted in the human body are a particular interest. Dr. Cohen and his work are largely supported by a grant from the National Institutes of Health" (W. T. Green 1960). At that time the orthopaedic research laboratory facilities were located on the sixth floor of the Bader Building (Growth Study), the Jimmy Fund building (provided by Dr. Farber and the Cancer Research Foundation), and a small laboratory in the Saltonstall Laboratory on the second floor of the Farley Building.

Cohen had dual appointments at Children's Hospital: as assistant pathologist in the Division of Laboratories and Research, and as an assistant orthopedic surgeon in the Department of Orthopedic Surgery. In a letter to Sidney Farber on March 3, 1954, Cohen stated that his dual appointments "have given rise to several conflicts of administrative responsibilities during the past few years" (J. Cohen 1954a). According to Cohen's letter, from July 1950 through June 1953 (his initial years on staff at Children's Hospital), Farber funded his work through a grant from the Playtex Park Research Institute of Medicine Advisory Board. After the grant ended, he applied for a grant from the Muscular Dystrophy Foundation. That grant was delayed, and Cohen met with Green (then the orthopaedic surgeon-in-chief at Children's) about finances on two occasions (March 4 and 10, 1954). Cohen summarized the discussions in a written report:

> 1. Dr. Green expressed dissatisfaction with my relationship with his department…he did not wish to mention specific examples…he had the feeling I was not integrated into the service as much as he would like…I did not come to him frequently enough for consultations and reports of progress…I admitted differences of orientation…my own being along the lines of tissue reactions and pathology…his…was more clinical…no…financial…or laboratory facilities could be attributed directly to the Orthopedic Department since they were obtained through Dr. Farber…[therefore] disinclination for close integration and the Orthopedic Department was understandable…
>
> 3. Dr. Green stated that one of the principles which applied generally to members of his department was that financially each one would pay his way and his plan in my regard was to foster for me a limited private practice in the hospital with minimal expense, to afford me a measure of financial independence…I pointed out that if research work were to be my primary function, I could not be expected to earn my way by private patient care and still maintain the proper orientation for laboratory work as well as afford the necessary time…
>
> 4. Dr. Green stated that he had tried in allways [sic] to secure continuing financial support of my program and had figured the Muscular Dystrophy funds to become available a year before they did; and that was the reason for the lapse in financial support available to me. He said that future financial arrangements were still indefinite, depending on the decisions reached and the funds available.
>
> 5. Dr. Green stated that he considered it a great insult to him for a member of his department to make a request for funds from outside sources…such as the foreign body reaction assay project without his knowledge or approval…The matter of the application for a grant to study reactions to foreign bodies was not properly pertinent to the orthopedic department, but, I stated that if he could show me that it was pertinent, and that it was in the interest of all to withdraw the application, I would do so, but that otherwise I would prefer to allow it to proceed…
> (J. Cohen 1954b)

Cohen mentioned his "cooperative attitude [which] could be attested to by the fact of seven years of service to the Children's Medical Center under financial handicaps" and shared with Green his "continuing desire to build up interest and constructive work in research pertaining to Orthopedics" (J. Cohen 1954b). In the end, however, Green told Cohen he'd be unable to support Cohen's work.

In a second letter to Farber dated March 11, 1954, Cohen wrote that he had applied for a National Institutes of Health grant to evaluate a foreign body assay through Farber's department, but he preferred not to work in the Saltonstall Laboratory, though he would continue "my moral obligation to the Muscular Dystrophy program in running the clinic…and to a limited degree in the laboratory" (J. Cohen 1954a). He said he would, however, "be forced to reduce my other clinical duties in the Department of Orthopedic Surgery to a volume similar to that of other members of the Department" but would continue his teaching responsibilities and, he hoped, be "allowed a small private practice" (J. Cohen 1954a). Such matters he left to "be worked out between Dr. Green and Dr. Farber" (J. Cohen 1954a).

Bone Lesions and Tumors

Cohen published at least 15 papers on a variety of bone lesions and tumors. In 1960, he published a paper on simple bone cysts and in 1970 a paper on their etiology. His commonly known theory was that "the principal etiological factor is blockage of the drainage of interstitial fluid in a rapidly growing and rapidly remodeling area of cancellous bone" (J. Cohen 1960). Cohen had studied the fluid in the cysts in six cases and found that the protein and electrolyte content were similar to plasma in four cases and similar to blood in two cases. Later, his injections of contrast medium into the cysts of two patients demonstrated "the absence of drainage from the proximal part of the cyst wall—a sign of obstruction" (J. Cohen 1970). Today, "the cause of a unicameral bone cyst remains unknown. Theories have been proposed but none have definitely been definitively proven. [In addition to Cohen's theory, one] of these theories is that the cysts result from a disorder of the growth plate…[Others] speculate that repeated trauma puts the bone at risk for developing a bone cyst" ("Unicameral Bone Cyst" 2020).

During his retirement, Cohen remained interested in bone cysts. In 1997, when he was 82 years old, Cohen wrote a letter to the editor of the *Journal of Bone and Joint Surgery* (British volume) commenting on the publication by Lokiec et al., who had injected their study participants with autologous bone marrow; they had reported successful treatment of bone cysts as a result of the alleged osteogenesis of the injected cells. Cohen questioned their success, suggesting that their method may injure the cyst wall and that that injury—rather than the formation of new bone by injected cells—caused the cyst to reduce.

Cohen had a broad depth of experience with a variety of bone lesions, and he generously provided cases for others to include in their published series (**Box 23.3**).

Box 23.3. Published Series for Which Cohen Provided Cases

- "Dysplasia Epiphysealis Hemimelica," by Kettlecamp, Campbell, and Bonfiglio (1966)
- "Rickets Following Ureterosigmoidostomy and Chronic Hyperchloremia" by Specht (1967)
- "Osteoid-Osteoma with Multicentric Nidus. A Report of Two Cases," by Glynn and Lichtenstein (1973)
- "Multicentric Giant-Cell Tumor of Bone," by Peimer et al. (1980)
- "Subdural Abscess Associated with Halo-Pin Traction," by Garfin et al. (1988)
- "Aseptic Necrosis of the Femoral Head with a Forty-Year Follow-up. An Unusual Case," by Daley et al. (1991)

Cohen and his associates were the first to observe that Ewing's tumor of the talus appeared like avascular necrosis on x-ray, and he and Clement Sledge stated that diastematomyelia refers to the split in the spinal cord and not to a septum or bone spike in the split area.

Bone Irradiation

Another main interest of Cohen's was the effects of irradiation on bone. As early as 1952, he had cowritten a paper on the "Irradiation Effects of Roentgen Therapy on the Growing Spine." Cohen and his colleagues demonstrated that doses <1000 r did not cause vertebral deformities but doses >2000 r might (mainly vertebral contour), no matter the subject's age. Radiation exposure rarely causes scoliosis, but radiation of the epiphyses may cause exostoses to develop.

Working with colleagues at the Massachusetts Institute of Technology in 1955, Cohen demonstrated that high-energy cathode-ray sterilization of bone grafts provided results similar to those achieved with homologous bone grafts without such sterilization. His studies of radioactive calcium tracers in bone grafts in animals showed:

> a few intense hot spots [of activity] and often a ring of increased activity in or near the endosteum or periosteum. The hot spots corresponded to individual Haversian systems...up to thirty-five times that of the diffuse component...the distribution of Ca^{45} from radioactive grafts were systemic and [not]...preferential...to callus or nearby bone...in dogs which received non-radioactive grafts and injections of Ca^{45}, the specific activity of the callus was the highest observed anywhere in bone, up to 100 times that of the different component of the host's cortical bone...the time of calcification of callus occurred predominantly at about the third week after grafting. (Cohen et al. 1957)

In a later paper, Cohen and D'Angio (1961) reported two tumors (an osteoblastoma and a chondrosarcoma) that developed in children after irradiation with ≥1000 r. Six years later, he and his colleagues reported a mesenchymal chondrosarcoma that had arisen in a 12-year-old patient in whom a malignant intra-abdominal tumor had been irradiated.

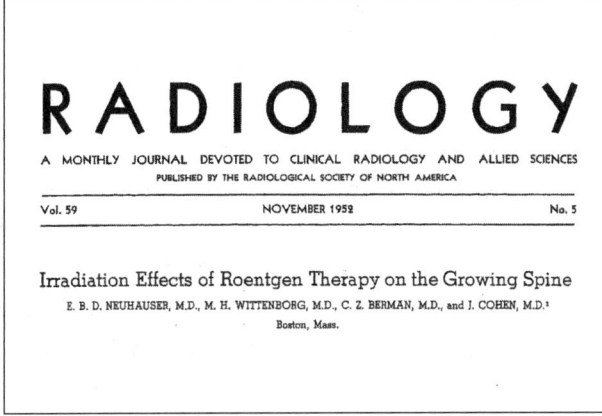

Title of Cohen's article on the effects of irradiation on bone. *Radiology* 1952; 59: 637.

Metals

Most of Cohen's published papers were about metal implants, the tolerance of tissues to metals, corrosion, and metal implant failure. As of 2003, he apparently held patents on upward of 300 prostheses. Across a 10-year period, beginning in 1959, he wrote more than 10 articles on metal implants, foreign body reactions, corrosion, the influence of surface finish, fretting corrosion, and the toxicity of metal particles. In 1960, he and W. S. Foultz reported a case of a painful rust granuloma in a patient whose fibular fracture had been stabilized with a Steinmann pin (see **Case 23.1**). They stated that the "Steinmann pin...showed marked pitting corrosion...the composition of the steel was the principal factor in promoting corrosion" (Cohen and Foultz 1960).

In 1961, Cohen "demonstrated that the surface finish on screws greatly affected the torque force required to extract them from bone. A rough surface finish afforded much greater resistance to extraction than a smoothly finished one. Most important of all, it was noted that the tissue reaction to rough and smooth-finished materials was the same in each instance" (Welsh, Pilliar, and

Case 23.1. Corrosion of a Steinmann Pin Used in Intramedullary Fixation

> "A woman, fifty-two years old, was seen for non-union of a fracture of the lateral malleolus of the right fibula. One year previously the patient had a trimalleolar fracture treated by closed reduction and plaster-cast immobilization. On September 18, 1956, the fibular fragments were cleared of intervening fibrocartilaginous tissue and the talotibial subluxation was reduced. A large lag screw of 18-8 SMO stainless steel inserted obliquely through the fibula into the tibia was used to narrow the widened ankle mortise and a Steinmann pin was drilled proximally through the lateral malleolus into the fibular medullary cavity to maintain alignment of the fracture fragments. An iliac-bone graft was applied across the fracture gap.
>
> "About two months later the patient began to complain of pain over the lateral aspect of the fibula. Two weeks after the pain began, roentgenograms revealed signs of healing of the fracture, but on the medial side of the fibula at the junction of its middle and distal one-thirds, there was some rarefaction and associated subperiosteal new-bone formation. This new bone did not extend to the area of fracture. Since the patient had had a questionably malignant lesion excised from the breast two years before, this area raised a considerable problem in differential diagnosis. Therefore, the area of periosteal reaction was biopsied at the same time the screw and pin were removed. The pin was withdrawn through the distal end of the fibula. The tissue removed from the region of the subperiosteal reaction in the fibula consisted of viable and necrotic granulation tissue, containing many foreign-body giant cells filled with brown pigment and large numbers of lymphocytes, plasma cells, and occasional polymorphonuclear leukocytes. An iron stain revealed large amounts of blue material in the macrophages and in the areas of brown pigmentation. The histologic diagnosis was rust granuloma.
>
> "The screw revealed no defects on careful gross examination. The Steinmann pin showed several defects. The bend visible on the postoperative roentgenogram was maintained. Areas of tarnish were evident all along the shaft and tip of the pin. At the middle of the shaft, extending nearly to the pointed tip, there was a series of pits in the metal. These were oriented longitudinally and measured from less than one millimeter to one centimeter in length and about one-half millimeter in width. They were filled with black granules of a crumbly material which, when removed, was [sic] shown by chemical analysis to be principally iron salts. The depth of the pits varied up to three over the rest of the surface...as determined by probing. The pits were most conspicuous on the convex side of the pin, but a smaller number of small pits was also evident on the concave side and scattered."
>
> (Cohen and Foultz 1960)

Macnab 1971). Cohen (1967) wrote that surgical implants made from biomaterials are very important in orthopaedic surgical procedures, as the better-quality components equate to better response and tolerance once the materials are implanted. He also recognized the various issues that were arising as the use of metal implants increased, citing the need for stronger metals that won't corrode once implanted.

Cohen was an active participant in the Committee on Surgical Implants (F4) of the American Society for Testing and Materials (A.S.T.M.).

Editor of the *Journal of Bone and Joint Surgery*

The *Journal of Bone and Joint Surgery* made Cohen a deputy editor in 1968, a position he held for 27 years, until 1995, when he was named emeritus deputy editor. Paul Curtis, a physician who worked with Cohen, praised Cohen's work as deputy editor: "When it comes to describing what he did for the journal, well he did a little bit of everything. He was an invaluable editor" (M. Bartle 2003). Another colleague, Dr. Henry

> **Biomaterials in orthopedic surgery.**
>
> Authors: Cohen J
>
> Source: American journal of surgery [Am J Surg] 1967 Jul; Vol. 114 (1), pp. 31-41.

Title of Cohen's article on the use of biomaterials in orthopaedics. *American Journal of Surgery* 1967; 114: 31.

Cowell, who had worked with Cohen for more than a decade, remarked that Cohen was "painstakingly accurate" and mentioned that Cohen called himself "resident curmudgeon" at the journal (M. Bartle 2003).

As deputy editor, Cohen wrote four editorials for the journal. His later ones focused on accurate data and measurements in research. He put much of the responsibility for such accuracy on the authors: "Readers and authors should be aware of the *Journal*'s policy to try to publish only meaningful data and analysis…[If] the attempt fails…the staff…takes some responsibility, but the ultimate responsibility rests with the author" (J. Cohen 1991). He also encouraged readers themselves to evaluate the publications they read: "The Editors… try to prevent authors from egregious departures from…appropriate and proper methodology… [but] readers have to decide these matters for themselves as applied to every so-called scientific article" (Burstein and Cohen 1993).

Beginning in 1955 and continuing throughout his tenure with the journal, Cohen wrote approximately 114 book reviews, usually 2–5 each year; in 1970 he wrote 12. Some of the famous books and authors he reviewed are listed in **Box 23.4**.

An example of Cohen's thoroughness can be seen in an excerpt from his 1968 review of Dr. Albert Ferguson's book *Orthopaedic Surgery in Infancy and Childhood*:

> In spite of its obvious defects as a text this book continues to be popular…the only book that serves the…needs of pediatricians, residents, students and…orthopaedic surgeons whose experience does not include much children's work…the book is not directed at those who actually are doing the surgery but more at those who are not…the book is well organized…the experience orthopaedist will…cringe at some of the author's lapses, grammatical or substantive. The index and bibliography are poor since they will not serve principal reader group…[but] there is an easy conversational style.

In another review, this one of Sir John Charnley's book on bone cement, Cohen (1971a) concluded: "This book will best serve the wary sophisticated orthopaedist who recognizes that there is much to recommend the ideas behind the procedure of total hip replacement, using acrylic, and the experience with it to the present, however fragmentary the evidence. Nevertheless waiting for all the evidence is hard, especially after ten years."

In his review of the reprint of Ernest Codman's 1934 book *The Shoulder*, Cohen (1966a) stated:

> It is a moot point whether Codman's *The Shoulder* has become a classic because of its delineation of the bursitis problem or because of the author's personal idiosyncrasies. The author's character, style, opinions, and autobiography find expression on every page and make the book a unique personal statement…it is astonishing how modern the book is, despite the thirty years…since its first appearance… the anatomy, pathology and clinical descriptions are quite to the point…unaffected by the recent great advances of science…only two operations are given—the repair of supraspinatus tears and the excision of calcareous deposits…[The book] teaches, it entertains, and it brings you face to face with Codman—his personality, his strong opinions about everything, and his medical career…The famous table in the Preface is the

Box 23.4. Books Reviewed by Jonathan Cohen

- *To Work in the Vineyard of Surgery: The Reminiscences of J. Collins Warren (1842–1927)* by Edward D. Churchill
- *Bone Tumors. General Aspects and an Analysis of 2276 Cases* by David C. Dahlin
- *Tumors and Tumorous Conditions of the Bones and Joints* by Henry L. Jaffee
- *Metals and Engineering in Bone and Joint Surgery* by Charles O. Bechtol, Albert B. Ferguson, and Patrick G. Laing
- *Bone Tumors* by Louis Lichtenstein
- *Tumors of Bone and Cartilage* by Lauren V. Ackerman and Harlan J. Spjut
- *Surgical Pathology* by Lauren V. Ackerman
- *The Shoulder* by E. A. Codman (reprint of the 1934 edition)
- *Orthopaedic Surgery in Infancy and Childhood* by Albert B. Ferguson
- *Nerves and Nerve Injuries* by Sydney Sunderland
- *The Biology of Degenerative Joint Disease* by Leon Sokoloff
- *Orthopaedic Biomechanics* by Victor H. Frankel and Albert H. Burnstein
- *Acrylic Cement in Orthopaedic Surgery* by John Charnley
- *Campbell's Operative Orthopaedics*, 5th ed., by A. H. Crenshaw
- *Heritable Disorders of Connective Tissue* by Victor A. McKusick
- *Heritable Disorders in Orthopaedic Practice* by Ruth Wynne-Davies
- *Adult Articular Cartilage* by M. A. R. Freeman
- *Orthopaedic Aspects of Cerebral Palsy* by Robert L. Samilson
- *Diseases of the Knee Joint* by I. S. Smillie
- *Fundamental and Clinical Bone Physiology* by Marshall R. Urist
- *The Musculoskeletal System. Embryology, Biochemistry, and Physiology* by R. L. Cruess
- *The Law of Bone Remodeling* by Julius Wolff
- *Limb Salvage in Musculoskeletal Oncology* by William F. Enneking

key to the book. It contains…personal history, the graph of his earnings, his diversions, logs and domestic minutiae and…the list of his publications (listed as advertisements).

Cohen continued to be active with the journal after his retirement; he participated in his last quarterly editor's workshop in 2003—the year of the 100th anniversary of the *Journal of Bone and Joint Surgery*. The editor at the time, Dr. James Heckman, announced in an editorial that "Because so many important events have been documented in the *Journal*, we asked Jonathan Cohen, MD, Deputy Editor Emeritus, to write a history. This elegant 100-page story is now available" (Cohen and Heckman 2003).

Professional Memberships and Service

In 1958, Cohen was elected as a member of the American Academy of Orthopaedic Surgeons. He was very active in the Orthopaedic Research Society, presenting papers on such topics as irradiated bone as a grafting material, studies on the fate of bone grafts and the distribution of the radioactive tracer (radioactive calcium), reaction of cells to metal particles in tissue culture, in vitro toxicity of metals. He was president of the Orthopaedic Research Society in 1964, when he presided over the 10th annual meeting in Boston.

In addition, Cohen was active in the AAOS and also often presented papers at the academy's meetings. He served as chairman of both the Committee on Scientific Investigation (which awarded the Kappa Delta Award) and the Committee on Pathology. In 1956, Cohen received a grant from the Orthopaedic Research and Education Foundation to study the three-dimensional anatomy of the Haversian systems in bone; Dr. William H. Harris presented their research at the AAOS annual meeting that year (see chapter 39).

The First Annual Review Course in Orthopaedics was held at Colby College in the summer of 1967. Cohen and other Harvard faculty participated in this popular course. Cohen also was active in the Gordon Research Conferences on Bone and Teeth and for many years was an examiner for the American Board of Orthopaedic Surgery.

Cohen was a member of the American Orthopaedic Association as well, along with some other professional societies. He was certified by the American Board of Orthopaedic Surgery in 1952.

Later Life and Career

Cohen spent 20 years at Harvard. In 1973, "he transferred his teaching activities to Tufts University School of Medicine" (McG.M.H., R.E.B., and H.J.M. 2004). He began to work with Mital at the Kennedy Hospital (now the Franciscan Children's Hospital and Rehabilitation Center), where his bone and joint research progressed. While teaching at Tufts, Cohen also lectured at the yearly pathology course for Boston-area orthopaedic residents. Achieving the role of professor in 1973, he was given the title of emeritus in 1988.

Cohen was a musician; he played the viola. In 1971, he had married Louise Alden, who had three daughters and had worked in admissions at Radcliffe College and Harvard University. The couple left Cambridge in 1988 and moved to Spruce Head, Maine. Fifteen years later, on November 13, 2003, Cohen died in a nursing home. He was 88 years old.

In 2005, Bryn Mawr College announced a gift of $3.3 million from him and Louise, who was a Bryn Mawr graduate and had been an active member of the college's alumni council.

JOHN H. DANE

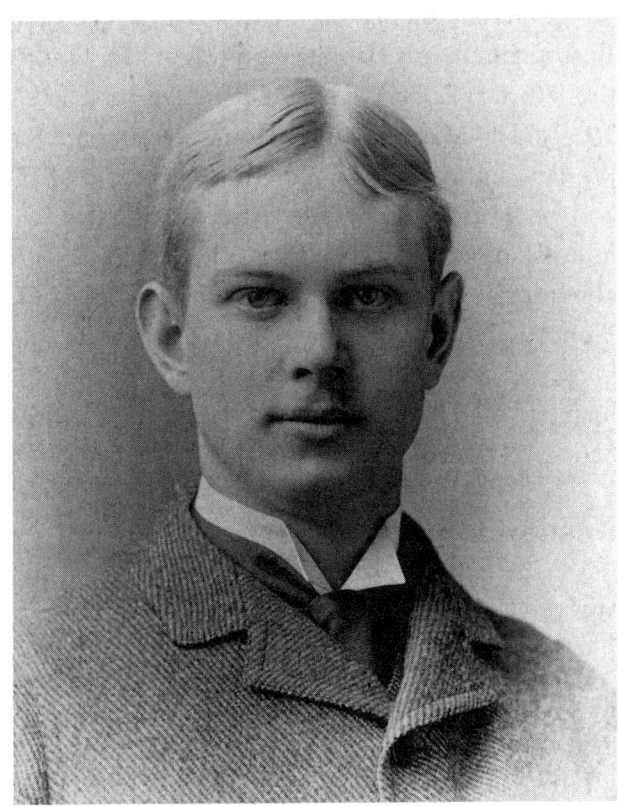

John H. Dane. Courtesy of Tamar Dane Dor-Ner.

Physician Snapshot

John H. Dane
BORN: 1865
DIED: 1939

SIGNIFICANT CONTRIBUTIONS: Modified the Whitman plate for patients with flat feet; designed modifications for the Thomas splint, the Taylor back brace (for patients with Pott's disease), and a splint for knock knees and bow legs; developed the Dane splint; put forth a new method for marking spinal curvature (by marking the apices of the spinous process with a tracing)

John Huntington Dane was born in Brookline, Massachusetts, on August 31, 1866. He attended Nobles Preparatory School in Dedham, which had been founded in 1866 as an all boys' preparatory school for Harvard College; in 1892 it was named

Noble and Greenough. Dane "graduated from Harvard University and received his medical degree from Harvard Medical School in 1892. After serving an internship at the Massachusetts General Hospital, he became connected with the Marcella Street Home, the Boston Infant's Hospital and the Boston Children's Hospital and was an assistant to the late Dr. Robert W. Lovett" ("Death. Dane" 1939). The Marcella Street Home was a home for orphans and homeless children; it opened in 1877 and operated for 21 years. After completing his internship, Dane apparently "made numerous trips abroad, visiting nearly all the hospitals in England, France, Germany and Italy where orthopedic surgery was a specialty. For several years he was an instructor in orthopedics at Harvard Medical School" ("Death. Dane" 1939).

Research on Flat Feet

We also know that Dane was a house surgeon at the House of the Good Samaritan in 1891. That year he published his first paper, "An Apparatus for the Correction of Talipes Equino Varus." Dane had an obvious interest in orthopaedics as a medical student, and at Harvard Medical School he wrote his senior thesis on the foot. It was entitled "A Study of Flat-Foot with Special Attention to the Development of the Arch of the Foot" and was published in four parts in the *Boston Medical and Surgical Journal* in 1892—the year he both graduated and was serving as a house officer at the MGH. In part one, "The Normal Foot," Dane goes into great detail about the three arches in the foot as described in the 10th edition of *Quain's Anatomy* (by Jones Quain, George D. Thane, and Edward A. Sharpey-Schafer) and by Adolph Lorenz. In part two, "The Pathological Foot," he notes that 89% of flat feet were static, that is, of "the form that is commonly understood by the term 'flat-foot,' and over which so much difference of opinion, both as to cause and treatment, has found its way into literature" (J. Dane 1892). Under the section on causation, he quotes Lorenz:

Title of Dane's thesis on flat feet and the development of the arch of the foot. *Boston Medical and Surgical Journal* 1892; 127: 430.

"'Valgus acquisition is that deformity of the foot which is caused by pressure [from the weight of body] and consists of a sinking of the external portion of the arch of the foot, together with a sliding off of the internal from the external arch of the foot'" (J. Dane 1892), going on to say that this definition, put forth by Lorenz in Austria, also holds sway in the US:

> Bradford and Lovett, in their "Orthopedic Surgery," say, "There can be now no question that the deformity results from the superincumbent weight falling upon an ankle and foot unable to sustain it. It is the result of a disproportion between the body weight and the apparatus for sustaining it"…This brings us back again to the question of which arch gives way first, and the answer seems clear. It is the internal arch. The weight of the body is normally transmitted through the astragalus upon the os calcis… [which] will, therefore, tend constantly to roll over…to tip the astragalus off its back in a direction inwards and forwards. This tendency is as constantly counteracted by ligamentous and muscular action…[and] the scaphoid is in its turn thrust so far upwards that in severe cases it may lie like a bridge upon the neck of the astragalus…If the foot is dipped in water and the patient allowed to stand upon a dry sheet of paper, an exact tracing of the sole is easily

obtained. Normally the outer margin is nearly straight, while the inner shows a sharp curve with the convexity outwards...When looked at from behind, the normal axis of the foot is seen to be parallel to that of the leg. As flat-foot advances, the foot assumes more and more the position of pronation; that is, the axis of the leg if prolonged falls to the inner side of the axis of the foot, the sole is turned outwards...In the pronated foot the external maleolus appears to have been lost...One peculiarity among the symptoms of the flat-foot needs special emphasis. It is that the amount of pain stands in no direct relation to the amount of deformity... This fact of painless flat-foot has led the Germans to make a separate class for them, calling it "Platte Fuss." (J. Dane 1892)

Dane (1892) also describes in the second part the pain that attends flat feet:

> The earliest symptoms of developing flat-foot are usually an undefined sense of fatigue upon long standing, which gradually increases to the degree of pain...Locality of the pain. 1) the first of these [localities] will be found over the head of the astragalus on the inner margin of the foot, and corrections to the over-stretched calcaneo-scaphoid ligament. 2) Usually second in appearance...is localized pain...through the heel just under and behind the malleolus... 3) Next comes pain at the calcaneo-cuboid joint, due to stretching of that ligament. 4) And, finally, more diffused pain all along the dorsal aspect of the tarso-metatarsal articulation.

Dane mentions that he treated three cases of flat feet at the MGH, but in part three of his thesis, he describes his research on the topic of arch development:

> With a view to finding out what the condition of the arch was in infancy and childhood, a series of tracings were taken under the immediate supervision of the writer, of the feet of nearly four hundred children, whose ages ranged from nine days to fourteen years. The method employed was...a modification of that of König. The child was allowed to dip its feet in water, and then stood for a moment upon a flat-sheet of brown paper. Wherever the feet touched, the paper would be moistened. The edge of this moist area was quickly marked with pencil, and the paper carefully dried. The writer

Tracings of feet obtained by the imprint of the wet sole standing on a piece of paper or on the floor. The bottom tracings are of two patients with severe, painful flat feet.

"A Study of Flat-Foot, with Special Attention to the Development of the Arch of the Foot," *Boston Medical and Surgical Journal* 1892; 127: 404.

here wishes to thank the officials of the following institutions for the uniform kindness...The deductions from the drawings are not in accord with the accepted authorities...Briefly stated... [f]rom one to eighteen months, arch distinct; sexes alike; one foot better than the other. From eighteen months to three years, arch mostly lost; exceptions are females. From three to four years arch building up; unequal in the two feet; females tending to form earlier. From four years upwards, arch established; sexes alike; both feet. (J. Dane 1892)

In his third part, in the midst of his description of arch development, Dane effusively thanked the institutions and organizations who helped him in his research, including "The Massachusetts General Hospital; the Boston City Hospital; the West End Nursery; House of the Good Samaritan; Church Home of Orphans and Destitute Children, Marcella Street Home and St. Mary's Orphan Asylum; and also to thank most heartily Mr. S.E. Bullard and Mr. Lyman Hodgkins of the Harvard Medical School for their cooperation in taking the tracings and making the experiments upon plates" (J. Dane 1892).

Section four of his thesis focused on treatment. He briefly describes nonmechanical treatment of gait training, emphasizing that the toes should point forward, and use of exercises. Dane writes in detail, however, about mechanical treatment, particularly elastic pads and plates, as well as manipulation under ether and operative treatment. Dane (1892) considered plates to be the "the best form of flat-foot apparatus." He described these as "consist[ing] of a thin sheet of metal fitted accurately to the sole of the foot and worn inside the shoe, generally outside the stocking" (Dane 1892). He went on to describe the types of plates used and some of their benefits and disadvantages:

For all kinds of plates a mould or a pattern of the foot must be taken. Whitman has a most elaborate method for this...A much simpler method is to flow plaster-of-Paris into a shallow trough, and when it is about to harden to have the patient step in it. In this negative a positive of the sole of the foot can easily be seen...The method used by the author...[incorporates] sheet wax, when put into hot water becomes perfectly supple, and can be moulded to the foot and cut to the desired shape. As it cools, it grows harder again, and can be greased and backed with plaster...Bradford and Lovett...plate[s] fitted at the Children's Hospital...have little tendency to slip and are quite comfortable; but they give only a limited support...Whitman has urged that [this type of plate] is unnecessarily heavy, and that it interferes considerably with the free flexion of the foot while walking...[whereas] as weight is put upon [Whitman's] plate [while standing or walking it] it...forces the body of the plate up against the calcaneo-scaphoid joint, and so preserves the damaged internal arch. The objection of this [Whitman's] plate is its unstable bearing, and the great difficulty of keeping it in its proper place. (Dane 1892)

He went on to explain in detail his experiments in modifying Whitman's original plate, elaborating their differences and describing how his modified plate it fitted and created:

During the summer of 1891 experiments were made by the writer in the Out-Patient Department of the Massachusetts General Hospital, and a shape of plate very similar to [Whitman's original] plate...was adopted. The points of difference would seem to be but two. (1) The flange on the outside...[was] made a little higher, and carried a little farther towards the heel...to pronate the foot...[2] bringing the plate up sharply on the inside...gives an inside bearing over the whole span of the internal arch...[T]he material used by Whitman is hammered steel...but the plating soon wears off...[and] such plates are quite expensive...An attempt has been made by the writer to get a flat-foot plate of hard rubber…It is exceedingly light…is uninjured in water…and does not tarnish or soil the stocking…A shell of the desired shape is made of wax…it is then greased and filled…with plaster…[The] cast…is sent to the Davidson Rubber Company, who fill the cast with a thin layers of sheet rubber, and vulcanize it at a temperature of 300° C. The price is one dollar and a half [at the time, the cost for similar plates made of steel ranged from three to six dollars apiece].

Dane noted that as of September 1892 he had applied more than 30 of his modified plates. He described his success as only "partial," noting that "For light women and for children the plate has answered most admirably…Further experiments are now being carried on in the hope of making the rubber plate still stronger" (J. Dane 1892).

In concluding his thesis, Dane discussed manipulation under ether and operative treatment. With regard to manipulation under ether, he stated:

The usual procedure in such cases [not easily cured] is to anaesthetize the patient and forcibly break down the adhesions, crowd the bones back into place, and at once restore the foot to its normal shape…the foot is put up in a plaster bandage in an over-corrected position, that is, forced adduction and flexion. After four weeks' rest this plaster is taken off and active treatment begun…the foot should be soaked in hot water and thoroughly massaged before any 'twisting' is begun…While the foot is…held…[in a corrected position], the patient is directed to flex and extend the toes, and to make voluntary efforts at abduction and adduction. This should be done once a day for at least two weeks…[and] the patient should be taught how to walk with his plate and should be directed to go through his gymnastic exercises by himself several times daily. (J. Dane 1892)

About operative treatment, Dane mentions just three procedures that have been "met with such favor":

[The] first…aims at forming an anchylosis between the astragalus and scaphoid bones…by removing their articular surfaces and fastening the bones together by means of ivory pegs in a correct position [first described by Alexander Ogston in 1884]. Second, a less severe operation has been advised by Mr. [William] Stokes…a wedge-shaped piece of bone from the enlarged head and neck of the astragalus is removed with an osteotome, and the foot is then put up in plaster in the corrected position. [A third option] which is rapidly gaining favor both in Germany and in this country is that advised by Von Trendelenburg…the operation of the future. It is nothing more than the artificial production of bow leg. The tibia and fibular are respectively chiseled through subcutaneously a short distance above the ankle joint. The ankle is then taken under the arm and the foot forcibly placed in the normal position. The ankle and foot are then put up in a plaster bandage, in which they remain for from ten to twelve days, after which time the bandage may be taken off and the position still further corrected if it is found necessary…After four or five weeks, the patient can be allowed to walk about with some form of light apparatus. Trendelenburg claims…it not only returns the foot to its normal position but restores its arch as well. (J. Dane 1892)

In a January 1893 meeting of the Boston Society for Medical Improvement, "Dr. F. B. Harrington made some remarks upon the value of Whitman's foot plate in paralytic valgus" ("Value of Whitman's Foot-Plate" 1893). During the ensuing discussion, Dr. H. W. Cushing commented on Dane's foot plate: "The Dane hard-rubber plate was devised in order to furnish a plate as light as possible, and also one which would not be injured by rust. I understand from

Dr. Dane that it fulfils three requirements when made of proper material, but that at present the quality of rubber furnished is often unsatisfactory. Those that I have seen have worn well" ("Value of Whitman's Foot-Plate" 1893).

In 1895 Dr. Robert Lovett and Dane presented a paper on flat foot at the Ninth Annual Meeting of the American Orthopaedic Association in Chicago. The shared six conclusions:

> (1) That feet of the infant at birth are not flat... tracing at the time resembles the adult normal foot...[2] That a body of fat develops under the arch, which gives the appearance of flat-foot for some years...(3) That the smoke tracing is not a perfect method of studying abnormalities of the arch of the foot...(4) That the element of pronation is more constant than breaking down of the arch of the foot...(5) That the condition of pronated foot without breaking down of the arch...should be recognized and not confused with flat-foot; [and] (6) That the treatment of pronated-and-flat-foot is the same...proper boots, the application of a pad or plate, the stretching of the gastrocnemius muscle where it is shortened. (Lovett and Dane 1895)

They published their findings in 1896 in two almost identical articles, one in *Transactions of the American Orthopaedic Association* and the other in the *New York Medical Journal*.

In 1898 Dane presented another paper on "Further Studies upon the Arch of the Foot in Infancy and Childhood," which was published the same year in the *Transactions of the American Orthopaedic Association*. In it, he revisited his 1892 study and his subsequent findings:

> [In a 1892] study of wet tracings of the feet, that the arch of the foot seemed to be present at birth...then broke down when the child began to walk, but at the age of three or four years... appeared again...However, further investigation, made by means of measurements and the study of hardened sections of the feet, had proved these first observations to be erroneous...A study of the hardened sections (mostly frozen) of intact feet, showed that the space is filled up with a pad of fat, and this was the reason for the erroneous impression given in the wet tracings. Each section showed plainly that the bones are in the normal position found in later life, and that the arch of the foot is perfectly formed in the vast majority of cases at birth. (J. Dane 1898)

In correcting his original 1892 findings, Dane performed two additional studies: "first, a series of measurements relative to the height of the tuberosity of the scaphoid above the level of the sole of the foot; and, second, an examination of hardened sections of such infants' feet as could be obtained for that purpose" (J. Dane 1898). He obtained a few of his specimens from the Warren Museum, but Dane doesn't state the source of the majority of them. He does note that "some of them were frozen and then the sections cut. A few were hardened in formalin before being cut" (J. Dane 1898).

Later Career and Research

Over the next 15 to 20 years, Dane continued to actively publish clinical papers, usually after presenting on the topic at meetings of the American Orthopaedic Association, the Boston Society for Medical Improvement, or the Suffolk District Medical Society. Dane was active for many years in the latter society, serving on the committees for social meetings and on system of records for patients of the hospital ship *Bay State*, "the first aid association ship that has ever been equipped under the Geneva Conference, Article XIII" (H. Burrell 1899). It was used during the War of 1898. Also, for at least three years (1897–99), he was secretary of the Suffolk District Medical Society. He also enjoyed membership in the Massachusetts Medical Society and the American Medical Association.

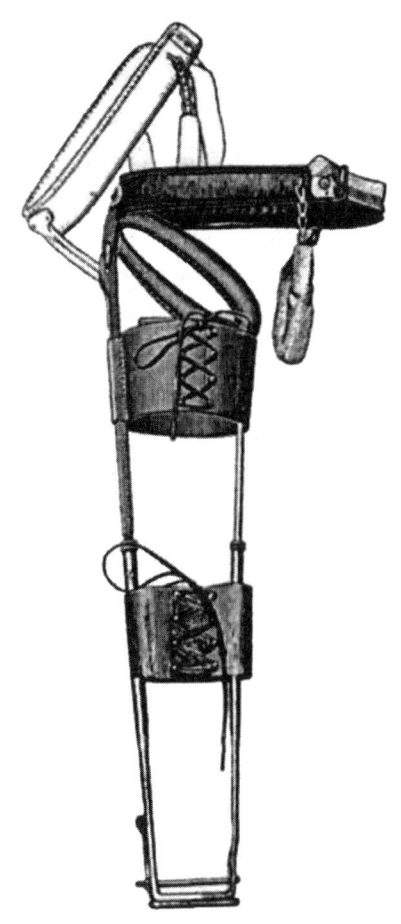

Dane's modification of the Thomas splint. With an added pelvic band and a perineal strap, the splint could not be applied incorrectly or migrate proximally. J. Dane, "A New Modification of the Hip Splint," *Boston Medical and Surgical Journal* 1892; 137: 60.

Dane published several articles about the skeletal anatomy of the foot (in collaboration with Professor Thomas Dwight of the anatomy department at Harvard Medical School), effects of pronation of the foot, and surgical procedures of the foot and ankle in patients with polio. He designed modifications for three splints: the Thomas hip splint, a splint for knock knees and bow legs, and the Taylor back brace for Pott's disease. Dane also "studied the amount of motion allowed by hip splints, and points to the value of grasping the pelvis in order to obtain good fixation…[and developed] the Dane splint" (Bradford and Soutter 1903).

During an in-person meeting with the Committee on Recording Lateral Curvature in 1899, Dane:

described a new method [of recording a spinal curvature]…by marking the apices of the spinous processes with an oil and lampblack cosmetic pencil. A sheet of blotting paper… was then pressed lightly against the marked back, thus obtaining a tracing of the position and relations of all the processes. A thin form of paper…bound up in letter files was the most convenient for use. Several tracings can be taken…in different positions…[and] after an interval of time, are superimposed and examined by transmitted light, a very suggestive and graphic picture is obtained. (J. Dane 1899)

During that same discussion, Dane reported that Edward Bradford (who did not attend the meeting) felt that photographs had proved to be the best method of recording scoliosis deformations at Children's Hospital.

In 1893, Dane was appointed as district physician at the Boston Dispensary; two years later, along with Dr. Joel E. Goldthwait, he was appointed visiting surgeon at the Marcella Street Home. The dates of Dane's appointments at Children's Hospital, however, are not fully known. He was appointed as junior assistant there in 1897 and was an instructor at Harvard Medical School in 1906. Robert Lovett, in his 1914 *History of the Orthopedic Department at Children's Hospital*, noted that some brilliant orthopaedic surgeons had been appointed, one of whom was Dane, along with Elliott Brackett, Joel Goldthwait, Edward Nichols, Robert Osgood, and Zabdiel Adams. We also know that Dane served as a lieutenant in the US Army during World War I. He was a member of the orthopaedic staff at the US General Hospital No. 2 at Fort McHenry, Maryland, in 1918 and 1919.

Dane, "of 33 Woodland Road, Jamaica Plain, died March 27 [1939]. He was in his seventy-fourth year" ("Death. Dane" 1939). He was survived by his wife, Eunice Cooksey, and his son, John Dane Jr.

RICHARD G. EATON

Physician Snapshot

Richard G. Eaton
BORN: 1929
DIED: —
SIGNIFICANT CONTRIBUTIONS: Named "a pioneer in hand surgery"; published *Joint Injuries of the Hand*, which contained descriptions of some of his original operations; developed a curriculum for the hand surgery fellowship at Roosevelt Hospital in New York City; director of the Hand Service at Roosevelt Hospital in New York City

Richard G. Eaton was born December 3, 1929. After attending Franklin and Marshall College, he graduated from the University of Pennsylvania School of Medicine in 1955. He stayed in Philadelphia, interning at the Graduate Hospital. He then moved to Boston for a year-long residency in general surgery at the Peter Bent Brigham Hospital (1956–57). From 1957 to 1959, Eaton was on active duty in the US Army at Ford Hood in Texas. Following his discharge from the army, he was a resident in orthopaedic surgery (1959–62) in the combined program of the Massachusetts General Hospital and Boston Children's Hospital. He briefly left Boston for New York City for a year-long fellowship with Dr. J. William Littler at the Roosevelt Hospital, but in 1963 he returned to Children's Hospital, where he was recruited by Dr. William Green to be on the geographic full-time staff. In 1964, he received a fellowship from the National Institutes of Health to develop an animal model of compartment syndromes. After two years as an assistant in orthopaedic surgery at both Children's Hospital and Harvard Medical School, Eaton rejoined Littler at Roosevelt Hospital as an attending orthopaedic and hand surgeon; he also became an instructor in orthopaedic surgery at Cornell University Medical College. In 1988, he was named director of the Hand Surgery Service at Roosevelt, a position he held until 1999.

Publications and Presentations

Eaton was a major force in orthopaedic hand surgery education, a surgical innovator, and a prolific writer. Among his more than 60 publications, 16 were about instability and reconstruction of the thumb basal joint; 9 about reconstruction procedures for wrist arthritis; 6 about proximal interphalangeal joint ligamentous injuries, contractures, and volar plate arthroplasty (see **Case 23.2**); 2 about each of a treatment for chronic paronychia and a fascial sling for ulnar transposition of the ulnar nerve; and 1 about a popular technique for managing painful neuromas in the hand. His early interest in compartment syndrome, which started during his fellowship with the National Institutes of Health, continued throughout his career.

Case 23.2. Volar Plate Arthroplasty of the Proximal Interphalangeal Joint

1. "A 24-year old patient suffered a fracture dislocation of the right index finger in [a] basketball game. Primary treatment consisted of splinting the PIP joint for 2 weeks, then encouraging active motion. Because of increasing pain and stiffness, volar plate arthroplasty was carried out 1 year following injury…Marked degenerative changes were present and involved the entire base of the middle phalanx with considerable cartilage erosion of the condyles of the proximal phalanx. Radiographs 14 months following arthroplasty showed a smooth contour at the base of the middle phalanx…Active range of motion was 100°."

(R. G. Eaton and M. M. Malerich 1980)

Eaton presented at multiple annual meetings of the American Academy of Orthopaedic Surgeons (AAOS). First, in 1962, he presented with Dr. William R. MacAusland Jr. an exhibit entitled "The Management of Sepsis Following Intramedullary Fixation for Fractures of the Femur." They subsequently published this paper in the *Journal of Bone*

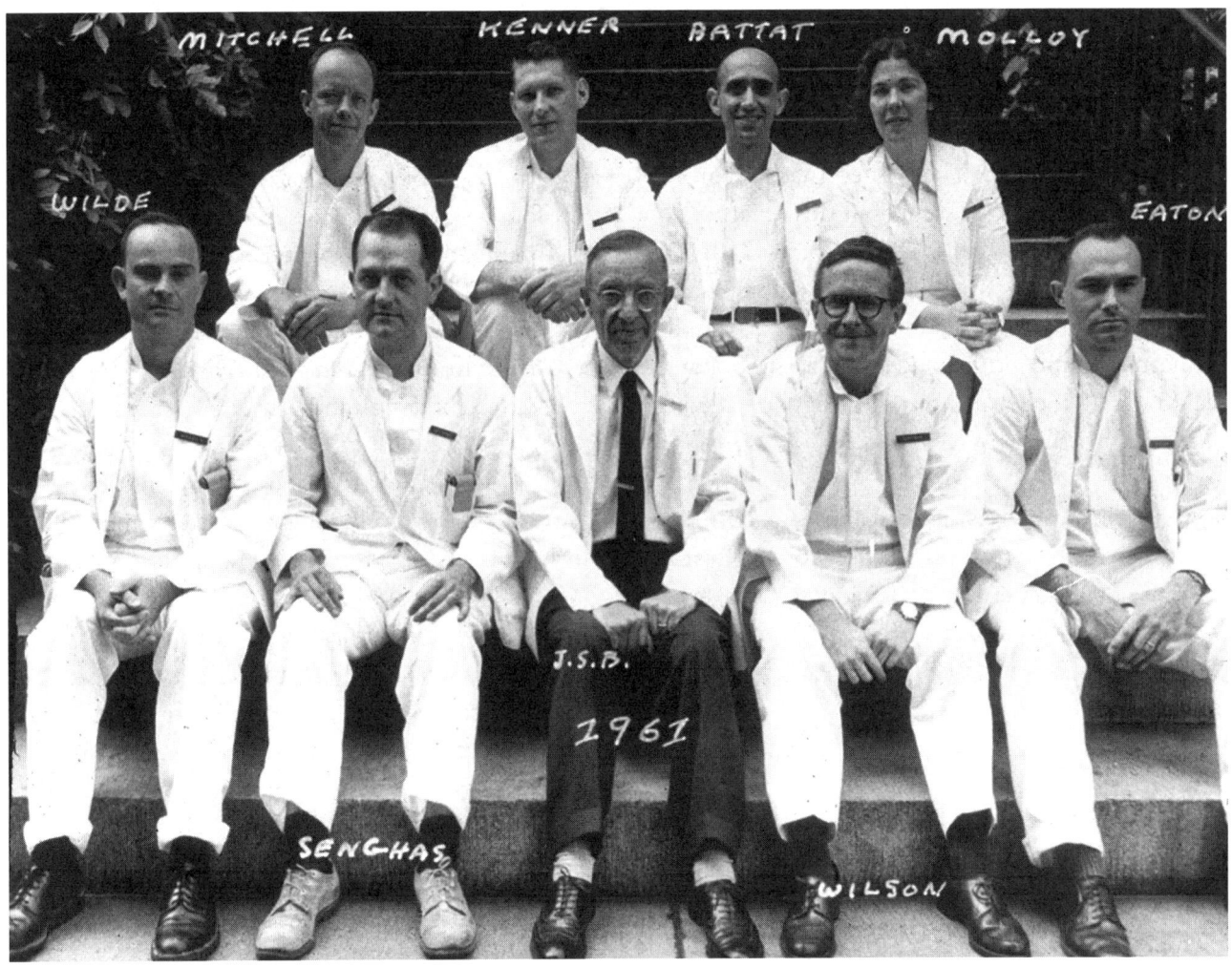

Dr. Barr and the orthopaedic residents at MGH. Dr. Eaton is seated in the first row, on the far right. MGH HCORP Archives.

and Joint Surgery in 1963. At that time there was no consensus in the field about "the management of these infections," in particular regarding "retention of the device…[or] removal of intramedullary fixation and curettage of the medullary canal" (MacAusland and Eaton 1962). After reviewing 14 patients with osteomyelitis following intramedullary nailing of femoral shaft fractures at Massachusetts General Hospital, they made "a plea…for the maintenance of rigid internal fixation, even in the face of seemingly disastrous infection, in order to achieve union of the fracture" (MacAusland and Eaton 1962).

Eaton presented again, in collaboration with Green and Dr. Herbert Stack, at the 1965 AAOS annual meeting in New York City. They reviewed 14 patients with Volkmann ischemic contracture of the forearm who had been treated at Children's Hospital over a 25-year period. In addition to proposing a pathophysiologic model for this unique and catastrophic event, they reported on the importance of (preferably early) fasciotomy and epimysiotomy, although they showed that these procedures were also beneficial for up to four months after the injury (see chapter 21).

Eaton published three other papers on compartment syndrome of the forearm, one in 1972, the second in 1975, and a third with Dr. Alan Sarokhan in 1983. In the last paper, the authors concluded that treating surgeons must have a strong understanding of forearm anatomy and the process of surgical decompression in order to successfully treat a compartment syndrome, as well as appreciating the underlying pathophysiology in Volkmann's ischemia. They noted that fasciotomy and epimysiotomy are essential in this regard.

He also published a case report with Dr. Joseph Barr. The patient, aged 31 years, had a painful, comminuted nonunion fracture of the distal humerus and both condyles. Barr and Eaton (1965) described the unique design of a distal humerus prosthesis:

> A stem-type prosthesis was designed...[by using] a plaster-of-Paris replica of the distal end of the humerus of an adult male cadaver[;] a stem was added...the Austenal Company...made a vitallium replica...of this...plaster-of-Paris model...the prosthesis was cast hollow to minimize its weight...two holes were made in the stem so that screws [could be] passed through both humeral cortices and the stem of the prosthesis...Elbow function four years after...was surprisingly good...[with] roentgenographic evidence of bone resorption and [a] broken distal screw...We believe that elbow prostheses of this general design are worthy of further trial in carefully selected patients with painful, unstable elbows.

"In 1971, he published a book entitled, *Joint Injuries of the Hand*, which was the seminal work in his career-long interest in small joint injuries" (C. C. Thomas 1971). In his review of Eaton's book, Dr. John Byrne (1971) wrote: "Dr. Eaton has taken a small field of hand surgery and brought it into clear focus...He stresses the need for an accurate immediate diagnosis of these injuries, which may require digital block anesthesia for final assessment."

Efforts in Education and Teaching

Eaton left the staff at Children's Hospital after less than two years to rejoin Dr. Littler in practicing hand and upper extremity surgery at Roosevelt Hospital in New York City. There he developed a curriculum for a hand surgery fellowship, through which he helped train more than 70 surgeons. In the early 1970s, Eaton offered Tufts residents from Boston a rotation on the Roosevelt hand service. I was a hand fellow with Littler and Eaton in 1973–74; it was a very educational and rewarding experience. Eaton conscientiously covered the fellows in the clinic and the emergency department. He always provided thoughtful and diligent care to his patients and performed innovative surgical procedures. Once Drs. Edward Nalebuff and Leonard Ruby provided such a fellowship in Boston (through Tufts University and the New England Baptist Hospital), students no longer needed to go to New York for that rotation.

Cover of Eaton's book, Joint Injuries of the Hand.
From Richard G. Eaton, *Joint Injuries of the Hand*, January 1, 1971. Courtesy of Charles C. Thomas Publisher, Ltd., Springfield, Illinois.

While at Roosevelt Hospital, Eaton also taught at Cornell and then Columbia, where, in 1986, he obtained the position of professor of clinical orthopaedic surgery. In that same year, the leadership at Roosevelt Hospital named him director of the Hand Surgery Service.

Recognition

Eaton was active in the American Society for Surgery of the Hand, which recognized him in 1995 by naming him the Founders Lecturer, which is given in order to honor the extensive influence of Dr. Robert Carroll on hand surgery education. Eaton's lecture was entitled "The Narrowest Hinge of My Hand," which was about the proximal interphalangeal joint and its supporting ligaments.

In 2010, in recognition of his enormous contributions to hand surgery, Eaton was named a "pioneer of hand surgery" by the International Federation of Societies for Surgery of the Hand. He was a founding member of the New York Society for Surgery of the Hand, of which he served as president in 1973. He was also president of the Hand Division of the Pan American Medical Association from 1982 to 1989.

After retiring in 2001 from his position as chief of the hand service at Roosevelt Hospital, Eaton continued to see patients in Brewster on Cape Cod in Massachusetts, where he has a summer home.

SETH M. FITCHET

Physician Snapshot

Seth M. Fitchet
BORN: 1887
DIED: 1939
SIGNIFICANT CONTRIBUTIONS: Published in 1929 an "extraordinary" paper on cleidocranial dysostosis in the *Journal of Bone and Joint Surgery*; interested in public health

Seth Marshall Fitchet was born in 1887. Little is known about his early life. Unhappy in school, he enlisted in the US Navy at age 18 and served for four years as a seaman in the Pacific Fleet. After being discharged with the rank of chief petty officer, he returned to school. "Failing any financial backing, his academic pursuits were necessarily carried out entirely on his own resources with the help of occasional scholarships" (A. T. Jr. 1939). Nevertheless, Fitchet completed a bachelor of arts degree at Clark University (Worcester, MA) in 1915 before entering Harvard Medical School, from which he expected to graduate in 1919. After only two years of medical school, however:

> as soon as the United States entered the World War…he enlisted [again] and after a preliminary period of training at Plattsburgh was commissioned a captain in Battery E of the 301st Field Artillery. During his training at Plattsburg, he sustained a severe injury when a camouflaged gun pit caved in, fracturing several cervical vertebrae and leaving him after a long convalescence with a slight residual paralysis. It was characteristic of the man that minor incidents such as this could not be allowed to interfere with duty, and with no complaints or incriminations, he carried on, went with his battery to the French front and was cited for bravery in action at Verdun and at Chateau Thierry. When the war was over, he returned home as a Major and maintained his commission in the Reserve Corps until 1934, finally resigning as a lieutenant colonel. (A. T. Jr. 1939)

After the war, Fitchet reentered Harvard Medical School, graduating with the class of 1921, along with Augustus Thorndike Jr. He was 34 years old. Later that same year, he was admitted into the Massachusetts Medical Society. He eventually also became a fellow of the American College of Surgeons, but I couldn't find out whether he was ever a member of the American Orthopaedic Association.

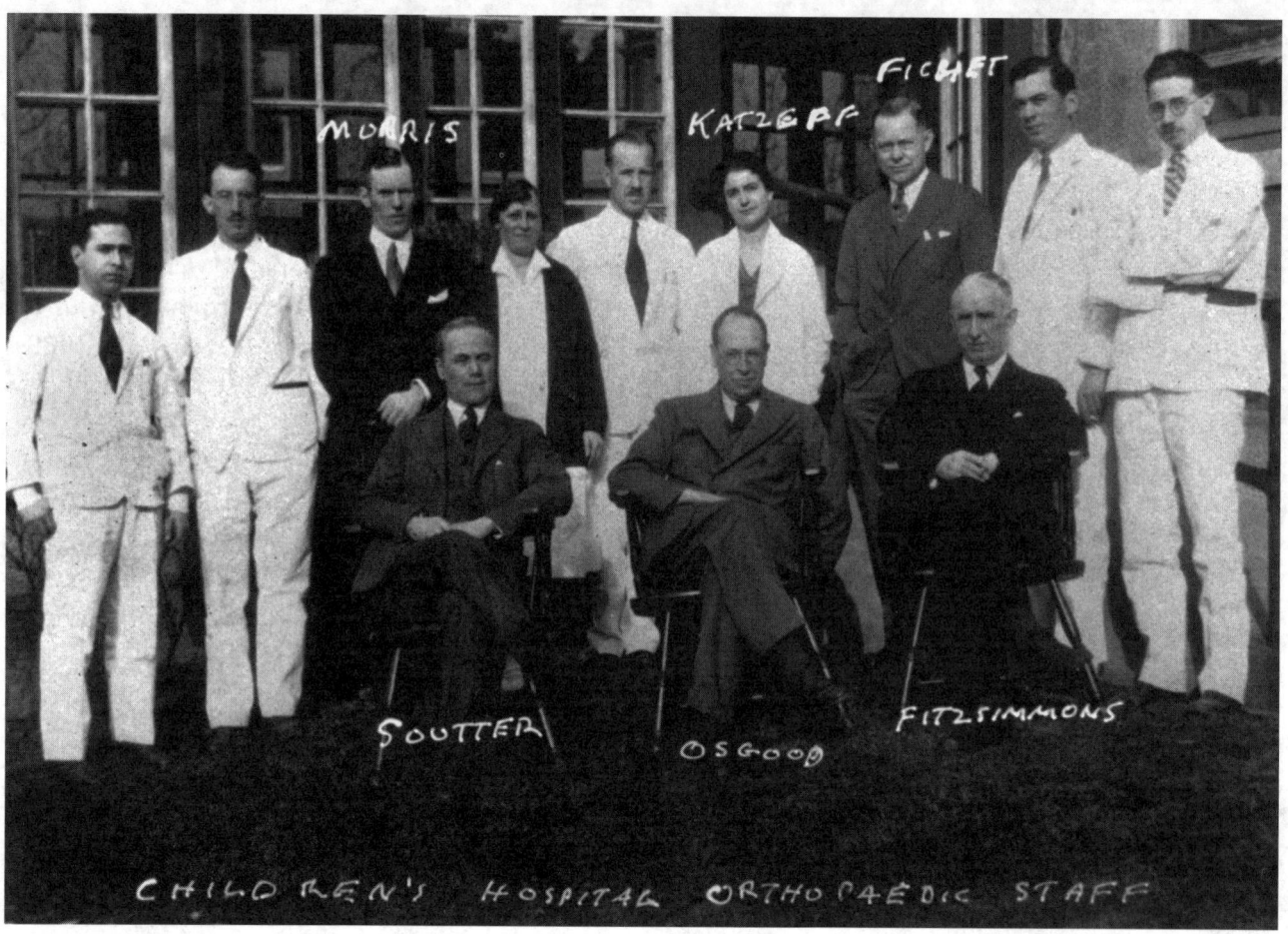

Orthopaedic staff at BCH. Dr. Fitchet is standing in the back row, third from the right. MGH HCORP Archives.

Fitchet became a surgical house officer at MGH, on the East Surgical Service (Thorndike was on the West Surgical Service), where he served for a full year, from October 16, 1922, to October 16, 1923. He worked for six months in the surgical outpatient department at Children's Hospital. In 1923, at age 36, he opened a private practice at 270 Commonwealth Avenue. He practiced there for six years until 1929, when he moved his office to the Longwood Medical Building at 319 Longwood Avenue.

Fitchet maintained staff appointments at both Children's Hospital and MGH. At Children's Hospital, he was a junior assistant surgeon in the orthopaedic department from 1924 until 1929, when he was promoted to assistant surgeon. His junior assistant and assistant colleagues at that time were Miriam Katzeff, Robert H. Morris, Albert H. Brewster, and Joseph H. Shortell. The associate surgeons at the time included Arthur T. Legg, James T. Sever, Henry J. FitzSimmons, and Frank R. Ober. In 1930, Fitchet was listed as an assistant visiting surgeon and, in 1931, as a visiting surgeon.

At MGH, Fitchet was appointed assistant in surgery, a position he kept during his entire career. In 1926, he was an assistant in orthopedic surgery at Harvard Medical School, where he would later be appointed assistant in orthopaedic courses for graduates. He was also an instructor in surgery at Tufts College Medical School, though I could not identify which particular years he spent there. His other hospital affiliations included consulting surgeon at the Massachusetts Eye and Ear Infirmary and associate surgeon at the New England Baptist Hospital. "In 1938 he became surgical director and chief-of-staff of the Josiah B. Thomas Hospital in Peabody" (A. T. Jr. 1939).

Fitchet seemed to develop an interest in public health, and he received a bachelor of public health degree (first and only recipient) from the Harvard School of Public Health in 1924, two years after its opening. In 1935, he was one of seven physicians to join the Harvard Department of Hygiene as assistant to Dr. Arbie V. Bock, then head of the department and the Stillman Infirmary and the Henry K. Oliver Professor of Hygiene. Thorndike Jr. was the head team physician in Harvard's Department of Hygiene. Fitchet was the assistant surgical advisor to the Stillman Infirmary. The Stillman Infirmary had been endowed by James Stillman of New York in 1902 for undergraduates at Harvard College. It functioned like a small private hospital, with inpatient beds (about 10) for overnight stays, one operating room, a dispensary, and a dining room. Care was provided 24/7. On occasion, up to 3000 patients were seen in the clinic each year. The students enjoyed having this resource available in a convenient location near the campus. Seriously ill students were sent to local hospitals. The infirmary remained fully operational for 113 years, but on June 1, 2015, it began caring for urgent cases only from only 8 a.m. to 10 p.m. each day. Although phone consultations were available overnight, the clinic no longer provided overnight services. Students who needed such medical care had to be seen in a local hospital's emergency department—the closest of which is Mt. Auburn Hospital.

Fitchet's publications throughout his surgical career reflect his interests in general surgery and orthopaedic surgery. He published 13 papers in all: one on public health in his first year in practice—a 1923 publication on the use of electric current to precipitate particles of dust, smoke, or fumes from the air—five papers on general surgery, and seven papers on orthopaedic surgery. The 1923 paper was the only one of his articles related to public health that I could find.

In addition to his contributions on ruptures of the serratus anterior (see **Case 23.3**), he also

Case 23.3. Injury of the Serratus Magnus (Anterior) Muscle

> "A boy of seventeen years had been in a football scrimmage. As he was leaving the field, he noted increasing pain in his shoulders and in testing out his motions…he discovered he could not raise his arm above the level of his shoulder. He was cared for by a masseur connected with the team, with subjective improvement. Three days after the scrimmage, I saw this man in a routine college physical examination. He had no complaint except an inability to elevate the right arm above the shoulder, and moderate lameness, with pain in his shoulder.
>
> "Physical examination…showed a moderate drooping of the right should…As viewed laterally with the arms at his sides, the inferior angle of the right scapula projected more than the left. When the arms were elevated, this projection became marked on the right. As viewed from the rear, as the arms were raised, the right vertebral border of the scapula remained almost vertical, parallel to the spine, and the scapula assumed the characteristic winged position…On palpation there was marked tendencies along with lower two-thirds of the vertebral border of the right scapula. There was an indurated area made out between the scapula and the chest wall…thought to be a hematoma…Pressure over the digitations on the right produced pain referred indefinitely to the region under the body of the scapula—his 'back'…
>
> "The diagnosis of rupture of the serratus magnus was made in this case because of the known trauma…he had a classical winged scapula…he was tender along the vertebral border of the scapula; and because he had an indurated area, probably hematoma, consistent with a rupture. There was no convenient way to have an electrical examination made…
>
> "The right arm was put in an aeroplane type of splint… kept for a period of six weeks. In three weeks, the indurated area had entirely disappeared. In five weeks, baking, gentle massage, and passive motion was started. In six weeks, the splint was removed…In twelve weeks he had entirely recovered the use of the serratus magnus."
>
> (Seth M. Fitchet 1930)

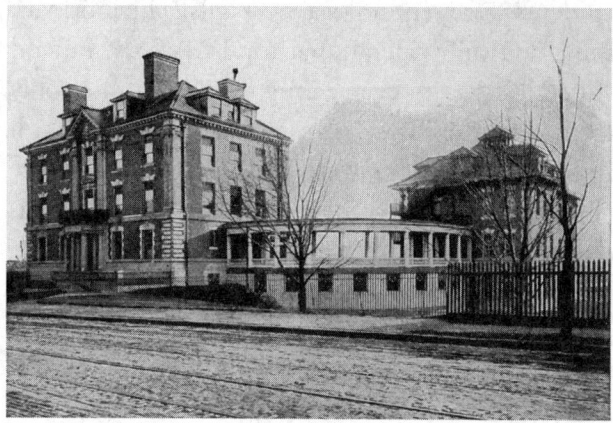

Stillman Infirmary. *The Harvard Book*. Boston: H. B. Humphrey Company, 1913. Library of Congress/Internet Archive.

described various other conditions, from congenital deformities, scoliosis and hip deformities, to epiphyseal fractures of the lesser trochanter. In 1929, after six years in practice, he published a paper on cleidocranial dysostosis in the *Journal of Bone and Joint Surgery*. Eighty-five years later, in their 2013 paper about "Rare Genetic Disorders That Affect the Skeleton," Mankin and Mankin described Fitchet's 1929 paper as "extraordinary" in that Fitchet both described the condition *and* cited 113 references from the literature. Four years before he died, he published his last papers: three in orthopaedics and one concerning a patient he treated surgically, which he presented at a clinical pathological conference and then cowrote with Joe V. Meigs and Tracy B. Mallory for publication in the *New England Journal of Medicine*.

Fitchet died on September 26, 1939, at age 52. About a year-and-a-half earlier, he had "consulted one of his closest medical friends for what seemed to be a minor ailment. It was apparent, however, that the malignant disease from which he actually was suffering was already far advanced and no possibility of cure existed. In spite of this, Seth Fitchet, the soldier, returned to his work and remained at his post as long as he could—courageous and simple and victorious to the end" (A. T. Jr. 1939).

HENRY J. FITZSIMMONS

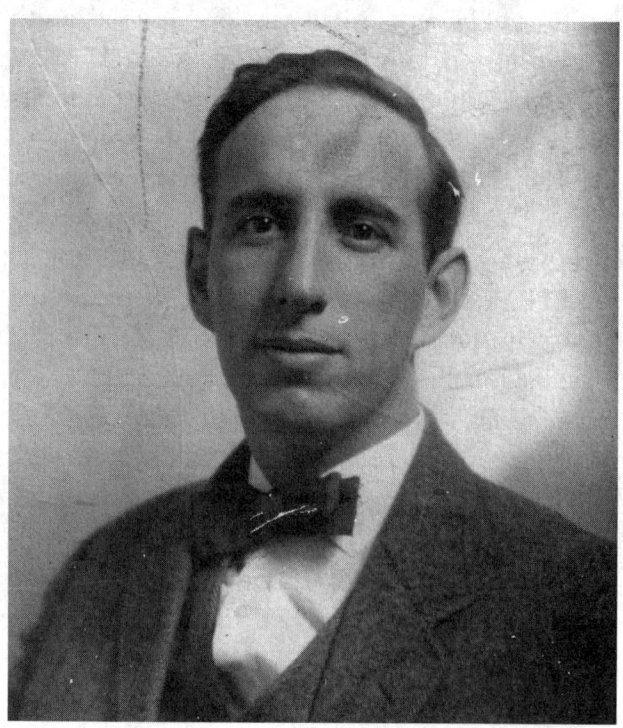

Henry J. FitzSimmons. He preferred to spell his name with a capital S after Fitz. Courtesy of Henry J. FitzSimmons Scannell.

Physician Snapshot

Henry J. FitzSimmons
BORN: 1880
DIED: 1935
SIGNIFICANT CONTRIBUTIONS: Introduced the implantation of silk artificial ligaments and tendons to the US (from Germany); reported long-term outcomes of patients with congenital torticollis; served some time during World War I at Camp Devens as the orthopaedic surgeon in charge

Henry Joseph FitzSimmons was born on February 21, 1880. He graduated from Harvard College in 1903 and from Harvard Medical School in 1908. Afterwards, he spent an 18-month surgical internship at the Boston City Hospital, and some time as a resident surgeon at the East Boston Relief Station (a branch of the Boston City Hospital that opened in 1908 and functioned as an emergency facility for injured and sick patients in the area). As a resident surgeon there, FitzSimmons would have treated outpatients, operating on those in need, admitting some for short stays, or transferring patients, if necessary, to Boston City Hospital. He then completed a six-month internship with Dr. Edward Bradford on the Orthopaedic Service of the Department of Surgery at Boston Children's Hospital.

FitzSimmons was well-liked at Children's Hospital. While there, he demonstrated a keen interest in orthopaedics:

> he determined to make orthopaedic surgery his chief concern, and was awarded a traveling fellowship for two years by the Boston Children's Hospital. These two years...were profitable ones spent under masters of orthopedic surgery. Six months with Sir Robert Jones, during part of which he was Resident Surgeon at the Liverpool Royal Southern Infirmary; work in the clinics of Calvé and Mennard at Berck Plage; work under Lamy in Paris, Putti in Bologna, Schanz in Dresden, Bielsalski in Berlin, Lange in Munich, and in the orthopedic clinics of Rome and Vienna. While [FitzSimmons was] in Munich, Lange perfected his original technique for the implantation of silk artificial ligaments and tendons. The young American orthopaedic surgeon became one of his [Lange's] favorite pupils. FitzSimmons may be said to have introduced the method into this country. Upon his return from Europe, he familiarized himself with the type of work being done in the orthopedic clinics of Baltimore, Philadelphia, New York, Chicago and Rochester, Minnesota. (R. B. Osgood 1935)

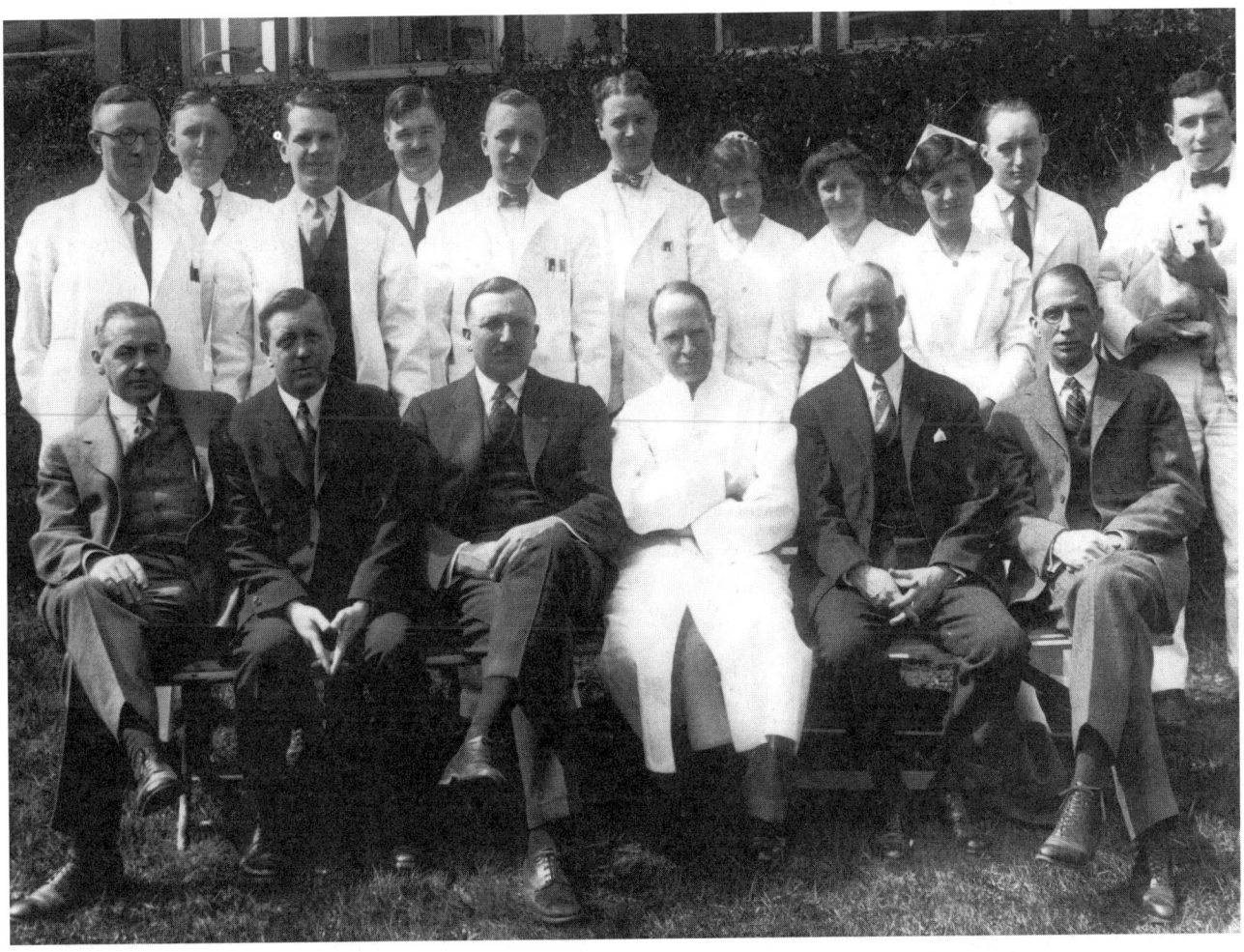

Orthopaedic staff at BCH. Front row, left to right: Drs. Sever, Legg, Ober, Osgood, and FitzSimmons. MGH HCORP Archives.

After his travels, he returned to Boston; he lived in Jamaica Plain, at 857 Centre Street, and his office was located at 370 Commonwealth Avenue in the city. He initially took a position as a junior surgeon at Children's Hospital, but he advanced during his career there, eventually achieving "the position of full Visiting Surgeon and Instructor in Orthopaedic Surgery at the Harvard Medical School" (R. B. Osgood 1935). In the 1935 Orthopaedic Department annual report, Dr. Frank Ober stated that FitzSimmons "was the first chief resident at the Children's Hospital and he served in the capacity for two years and demonstrated very well the need for the position." FitzSimmons remained clinically active at Children's Hospital throughout his career. He was also an orthopaedic consultant to Quincy City Hospital, Choate Hospital in Woburn, the House of Providence in Holyoke, and St. Margaret's and Mary's Infant Asylum. He held an orthopaedic clinic for years at the Day Nursery in Holyoke.

Research and Publications

Although FitzSimmons was heavily involved in clinical work, "he managed to carry out over a series of years important research studies as to the causes and treatment of Congenital Torticollis or 'wry-neck.'" (F. Ober 1935). After reviewing the literature as to the cause and types of torticollis, FitzSimmons stated three conclusions:

1. In all cases congenital torticollis results from fibrosis in the sternomastoid muscle consequent upon the development and absorption of the so-called "sternomastoid tumor" of infancy.
2. Sternomastoid tumor, and therefore torticollis, results from a temporary acute venous constriction in the muscle, this obstruction taking place during labour.
3. It is probable that such a temporary venous obstruction has been rendered permanent by patchy intravascular clotting in the obstructed venous tree. (F. Ober 1935)

Ober (1935) noted that FitzSimmons's "conclusions were made authoritative by a large true end-result study…a noteworthy contribution."

This end-result paper was published 18 years after FitzSimmons's first publication on torticollis. In his first paper, FitzSimmons mentioned the "dangers" inherent in the surgical procedure to resolve this condition, in which the sternoclavicular part of the muscle is most often "severed" (FitzSimmons noted that at Children's Hospital, among 100 patients, 97 had a sternoclavicular incision, whereas only three had a mastoid incision during the procedure). He went on to describe the "routine" procedure done at Children's:

Under ether the child is placed dorsally recumbent on the operating table, with the head twisted and the shoulder elevated so as to bring the offending muscle sharply into relief. The form of incision having been decided on and used, the dissection is carried down to the muscle at its tendinous portion, and all obstructing tissues are excised. The wound is closed in layers as tightly as possible, the skin approximation being as nearly perfect as can be. A collodion dressing is then applied over the skin wound, and the head held in an overcorrected position, while a plaster helmet is applied, which firmly holds this position. This helmet is then worn for two months, after which time the child wears a steel support, with a chin piece which maintains an overcorrected position of the head in its relation to the past deformity. The steel apparatus is worn for a year, being removed for purposes of massage and exercise. (H. J. FitzSimmons 1933)

He noted in his results that "the atrophy, facial asymmetry and compensatory scoliosis seem to depend on the duration of the torticollis…In all cases analyzed positively cured cases were 64 per cent.; 14 per cent. of cases were lost from the clinic; in 16 per cent…it was impossible…to classify the result" (H. J. FitzSimmons 1933). Thus, he concluded that the procedure "definitely offers

Case 23.4. Atypical Multiple Bone Tuberculosis

"This patient J.R., a boy of sixteen months came to the Out Patient clinic of the Boston Children's Hospital May 3rd, 1913.

"Four months before entrance the mother noticed a lump in the child's abdomen…[and] lumps upon the head.

"On entrance the child appeared well developed and well nourished…Over the right parietal portion of the skull were three tumor masses, each about ¾ inch in diameter. Two appeared hard and…connected with the bone, the other was fluctuant…The posterior cervical and…auricular glands were…enlarged. At the outer canthus of each eye there was a small fluctuant reddened area…The examination of the chest revealed good development with no signs of rickets…The lungs showed no areas of dullness, no rales nor adventitious sounds…On the surface of the right thigh are a few small areas…covered with dark crusts and surrounded…[by] induration… In the region of the upper third of the right tibia…anterior…one could feel an area of thickening about 2 inches long by 1 inch wide. Beneath the external nucleolus and extending towards the cuboid…over the region of the astragalus is a large tense area of swelling. The right upper arm appears normal save for some thickness of the lower end of the humerus…Over the right radial epiphysis is a swelling…which is slightly tender. This tumor is connected with the bones beneath. The right hand shows at the end of the fourth metacarpal a pustular lesion covered with a dry scab…surrounded with an area of induration ¼ inch in thickness. The left upper leg…[has] two inches below the trochanter…a small indurated dark colored lesion…about 1/4 inch in diameter. Just below the knee… is a similar lesion…which appeared to be fluctuant. The left lower leg presented nothing abnormal except a few scattered skin lesions. Over the first metatarsal of the left foot on the inner side was an area of swelling somewhat reddened but free of fluctuation. This swelling extended from the toes to the ankle joint…On the exterior surface of the upper third of the left ulnar was a tumor mass… connected to the bone, but did not involve the skin…not tender, reddened nor fluctuant. The left hand presented a fusiform enlargement of the first two phalanges of the first finger, upon which are dark crusts…There was motion in all joints…

"The Wasserman reaction…was negative. The Luctin test was negative. The Von Pirquet reaction was strongly positive. His blood examination showed leucocytosis 15,600; polynuclear forms 60%…

"October 3, 1913. While the child was under ether a section containing skin and cavity of the two superficial lesions in the left thigh was removed…Both contained… thick yellowish pus similar to that removed from tubercular cavities.

"October 21, 1913. Under ether…a three inch incision was made over the crest of the right tibia immediately below the tibial tubercle…a piece of cortex one inch long and ¼ inch wide was removed with a chisel…some yellow thick purulent material…[escaped from] a well defined abscess cavity…lined with a definite membrane.

"November 11, 1913. A small incision about ¼ inch long was made in…each tumor mass…under the eyelids…The abscess located over the external maleolus of the right foot was incised.

"November 18, 1913. The right arm…under ether an incision was made over the cavity…outlined by the x-ray, two inches below the elbow joint…The cortex was… chiseled through and the cavity opened. From this cavity a large amount of yellow caseous material was removed. This cavity was lined with a definite membrane…[measuring] 1 inch in length by one half inch in width.

"December 10, 1913. The general condition of the child to-day is much worse than it was one month ago, notwithstanding the fact that the child has had the benefit of outdoor treatment at the Convalescent Home at Wellesley…

"The child on December 19th had a positive Von Pirquet skin reaction…The bacteriologists have been unable to grow the material sent to them from the numerous operations. The pathologist reports…the specimen from the ulnar shows typical tubercles…A section through the fragment of bone [tibia]…shows…typical tubercles."

(Henry J. FitzSimmons 1914)

a cure for the deformity of congenital torticollis and the results are uniformly satisfactory" (H. J. FitzSimmons 1933).

Although he gave lectures at Children's Hospital and at orthopaedic meetings, FitzSimmons published only eight articles: two on torticollis, three on tuberculosis of bones and joints (see **Case 23.4**), one on rotary displacement of the cervical spine, one on orthostatic albuminuria, and one on the design of a traction table to aid in the reduction of difficult congenitally dislocated hips. The latter he had reported at a meeting of the Interurban Orthopedic Club in Boston on December 31, 1915.

Military Service and Later Career

As World War I began, before he entered active duty, FitzSimmons gave lectures in Lovett's course on orthopaedic surgery at Children's Hospital to army surgeons before they left for Europe. He enlisted in 1918 and served as a captain in the Medical Officer's Reserve Corps. He "saw service at Camps Greenleaf, Fort Oglethorpe, McPherson, Devens, and finally at Base Hospital No. 10, Parker Hill, Roxbury, Massachusetts" (R. B. Osgood 1935). While at Camp Devens, he was the orthopaedic surgeon in charge and had a staff of six other orthopaedic surgeons. In one month, they cared for 576 wounded soldiers. FitzSimmons was honorably discharged toward the end of June 1919.

FitzSimmons remained an instructor in orthopaedic surgery at Harvard Medical School until he resigned the position on September 1, 1935. He was also an assistant in orthopaedic surgery at Boston University. He was a member of various societies, mainly professional associations; some of these are listed in **Box 23.5**. Ober, in the 1935 department report, described FitzSimmons's retirement: "[He] was always willing to step in any emergency and gave freely of his time to the hospital. We are sorry to lose such a valuable member of the staff."

Box 23.5. FitzSimmons's Organizational Memberships

- Massachusetts Medical Society (joined in 1910)
- American Medical Association
- American College of Surgeons (from 1919)
- American Academy of Orthopaedic Surgeons
- Eastern States Orthopedic Club
- Boston Orthopedic Club
- Aesculapian Club
- Military Order of the World War
- Charitable Irish Society

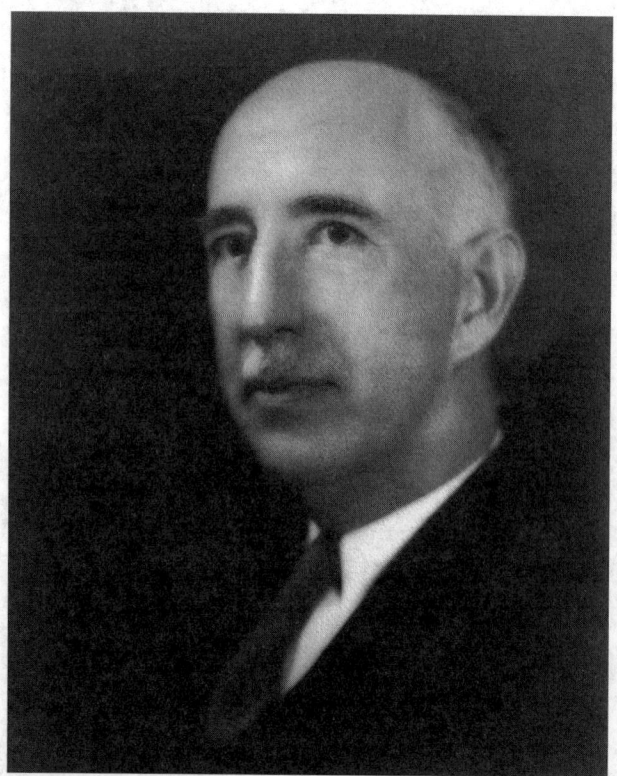

Henry FitzSimmons. Courtesy of Henry J. FitzSimmons Scannell.

On October 5, 1935, at age 55, FitzSimmons died in his home, just one month after he resigned his faculty appointment at Harvard Medical School. He was survived by his wife, Elizabeth Grace Rogers, whom he married in 1914, and their four daughters. Dr. Robert Osgood wrote an obituary for FitzSimmons, which was published in the *Journal of Bone and Joint Surgery*. Osgood noted that:

One of Dr. FitzSimmons' close medical associates is unable to remember ever hearing him speak in derogatory terms of any of his professional associates and all of us were conscious of his infinite kindness. His medical opinion was honestly given and valuable. He was a most generous consultant whose mind was open. His devotion to his private, industrial and hospital patients was complete. His monument will be the abiding memory of a 'talented, honest, generous, serviceable' gentleman…Gentleness also was his in attitude and actions. (R. B. Osgood 1935)

THOMAS GUCKER III

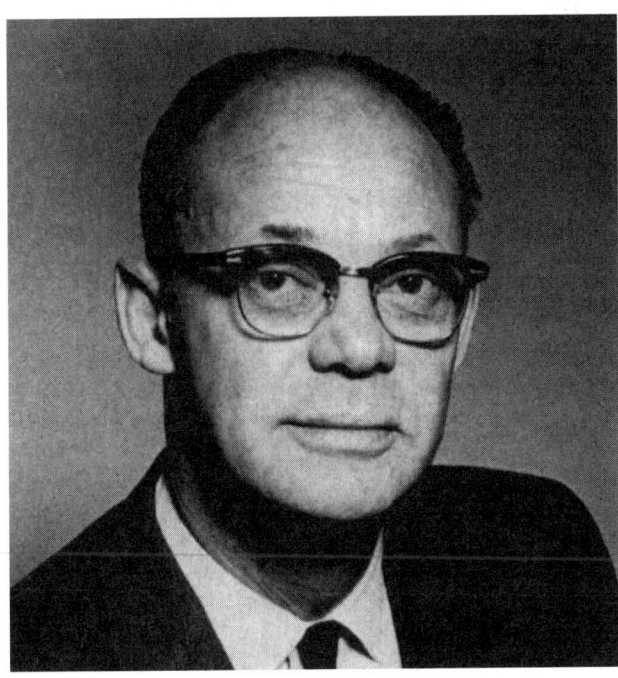

Thomas Gucker III. J.D.H., "Thomas Gucker, III, M.D. 1915–1986," *Journal of Bone and Joint Surgery* 1987; 69: 312.

Physician Snapshot

Thomas Gucker III
BORN: 1915
DIED: 1986
SIGNIFICANT CONTRIBUTIONS: An expert in poliomyelitis (and was afflicted with the disease); pioneer in orthopaedic rehabilitation; helped treat patients in Berlin during the city's 1947 polio epidemic; medical director of rehabilitation at the Orthopaedic Hospital of Los Angeles

Thomas Gucker III "was born in Philadelphia, Pennsylvania, on April 13, 1915. At the age of five years, he contracted poliomyelitis that left him with weakness and deformities of the lower extremities. He had to wear braces throughout his life" (J. D. H. 1987). After graduating from the Chestnut Hill Academy, Gucker attended Princeton University. He was an outstanding student and participated in athletics: "He was a member of the Princeton Gymnastic Team [all Eastern], intercollegiate champion on the sidehorse, and a world-record holder (1936 to 1940) of the twenty-foot (6.1 meter) rope-climb" (J. D. H. 1987). He also served in leadership roles in many organizations: student government, the Undergraduate Council and Student Faculty Association, the St. Paul's Society, and the University Council on Athletics. Studying psychology and taking a premed course—already he was planning to become an orthopaedic surgeon—"In 1937 he graduated summa cum laude…with a Bachelor of Arts degree, earned highest honors in psychology, and was elected to the Phi Beta Kappa Honor Society. At graduation he was selected as the Lyman Biddle Senior Scholar and received the M. Taylor Pyne [Honor Prize]" (J. D. H. 1987). The Pyne Prize has been given each year since 1921 to a senior who "has most clearly manifested…excellent scholarship, manly qualities and effective support of the best interests of Princeton University" (quoted in "Princeton Honors Leading Student" 1937). It is "one of the most prestigious awards [given at Princeton] that [exemplifies] excellence in academic and extracurricular activities" (J. B. H. 1987).

After Princeton, Thomas:

attended the University of Pennsylvania School of Medicine…received a Doctor of Medicine degree in 1941, and was elected to the Alpha Omega Alpha Honor Society. He also received the Spencer Morris Prize, the highest award that was given on the basis of academic standing and best performance on a special examination.

[His] postgraduate training was at the Hospital of the University of Pennsylvania…and Children's Hospital in Boston [where he was] Chief Resident in orthopaedic surgery from 1945 to 1946. At the time of his residency in Boston, 500 new patients who had poliomyelitis were treated on his service each year. After training, [he] was associated with the Harvard Infantile Paralysis Clinics and was leader of the Epidemic Aid Team at Harvard. (J. D. H. 1987)

Service during the Berlin Polio Epidemic

In 1947, Dr. William Green selected a team of three polio experts from Children's Hospital—Gucker, then an assistant in orthopedic surgery and leader of the Epidemic Aid Team at Harvard Medical School; Anne Fallon, the chief orthopedic nurse; and Elizabeth Zausmer, a physiotherapist—at the request of the National Foundation for Infantile Paralysis in response to an appeal by General Lucius D. Clay, the American commander in Berlin. The team from Children's Hospital traveled to Berlin to help treat the more than 1,500 cases of infantile paralysis that had been recorded (**Box 23.6**). The team took various equipment, including six iron lungs, which would not operate correctly because of the difference in voltage (110 volts in the US vs. 220 volts in Germany). To save some patients, they had to pump the iron lung manually. When asked by a Boston Globe reporter whether he would train the German and Russian physicians in Berlin, Gucker responded, "Medicine is above political boundaries" (quoted in "Polio Experts Return" 1947). Anne Fallon noted that the training would emphasize prevention through "education against mosquitoes, unwashed fruits and vegetables, overuse of fatigued muscles and sudden chilling after exercise" (quoted in "Polio Experts Return" 1947).

Upon returning to Boston, Gucker was interviewed by Frances Burns of the *Daily Boston Globe*. Gucker was very frank in his comments, stating the dirty conditions were "ghastly"; flies were everywhere; hospital supplies (such as hot water, bedpans, masks, gowns, penicillin, and respirators) and food were in short supply (what food was available was from gardens fertilized with human feces); and the physicians were young and inexperienced, lacking "fundamental training" and the critical thinking skills needed to appropriately treat patients (quoted in F. Burnes 1947). In addition to these issues, Gucker mentioned "lethargy" and "a fatalism, an indifference to the value of a single human life" (quoted in F. Burnes 1947) as factors in the extensiveness of the polio epidemic in Berlin. He went on: "The Germans have no feeling of repentance—they jolly well lost a fight, but they weren't wrong, is their attitude. But there is a sort of resignation—when 800 people were killed in an air raid, what is one more death from polio" (quoted in F. Burnes 1947).

Burns wrote that the German physicians could not provide even basic care to those with polio, such as administering fluids to dehydrated patients with fever, treating intestinal problems, or

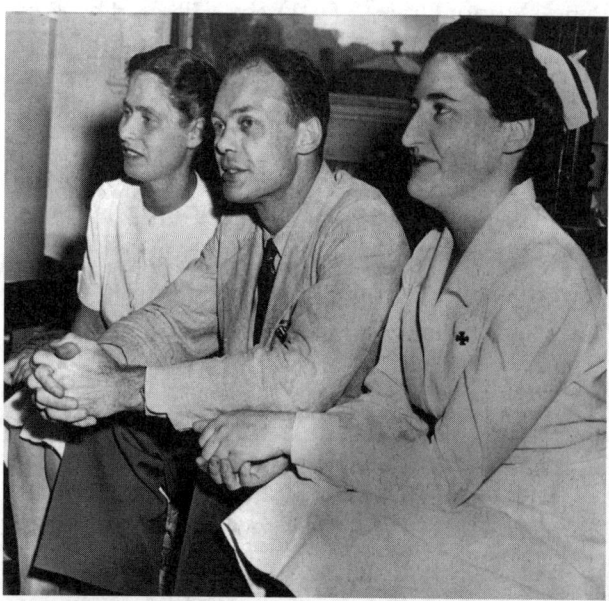

Thomas Gucker; Elizabeth Zausmer, PT; and Anne Fallon, RN; as they prepared to travel to Berlin to assist in the polio epidemic in September 1947. Boston Children's Hospital Archives, Boston, Massachusetts.

Box 23.6. Infantile Paralysis—What Does it Mean to the Patient?

"'Mrs. Brown, your son has infantile paralysis.' Suppose the doctor said this to you, what questions would race through your mind? Wouldn't you ask yourself whether your child would live? Would he have to be put in an 'iron lung'? Will his hands and arms be paralyzed? Could he ever walk again? Would he be a cripple for life? This fearful experience is occurring to more and more parents each year as poliomyelitis continues in unrelenting epidemics. Furthermore, because of greater publicity, even adolescents and older children are beginning to know of this dread disease. Consequently, not only their parents, but more and more patients are asking themselves the same frightening questions when they learn they have polio. And once an outbreak occurs, near panic may grip an entire community. There must be an answer to this demanding problem, and the answer must ultimately include all aspects of poliomyelitis. The picture is still incomplete. Just how a person contracts the disease is unknown. There is no reliable method of prevention. Even when the infection has reached the central nervous system, the amount and severity of paralysis cannot be predicted at once. But much is known today, and upon these facts we must build our defense.

"It is now recognized that actual infection with a virus of poliomyelitis is much more widespread than was realized previously. In any family when one member is diagnosed to have poliomyelitis, there is good evidence that the virus may well be present in practically every member of that family.

"Our next consideration is the patient himself; his psychologic make-up, and something of his immediate environment and relationships with others. In 1840 Jacob Heine reported the first sizable outbreak of poliomyelitis. Among his keen observations he noted that the paralytic patients were usually of a healthy and stronger constitution, and this conclusion has been substantiated throughout the years. The paradox remains that individuals who are generally more resistant to other infections are more vulnerable to the paralytic form of poliomyelitis. Fascinated by this aspect of the problem, Draper and later others have attempted to ascertain what are the inherent characteristics of the individual which make him susceptible. For a time certain constitutional traits including anthropometric and morphologic characteristics appeared important...At the present time the exact characteristics are not clearly evaluated. Yet it is well to remember that in general the patient is fundamentally of sound stuff, and that he is otherwise well constituted to hurdle the polio barrier. There is inadequate evidence that any one psychological type is more susceptible to paralytic poliomyelitis than another..."

Patients Reaction to the Disease

"We turn now to the reactions of the individual from the time that poliomyelitis is diagnosed. Excluding infants and very young children, it is well to assume that the patient knows more about his illness than we think he does. Frequently an overheard remark by the professional staff is misinterpreted by the patient resulting in an exaggerated concept of his difficulties. In response to direct questioning, one should remember the wise counsel of Montaigne that it is not always necessary to tell the whole truth, but, what one says must be true. Since the reactions of children are quite different from those of adolescents and adults, a separate analysis is necessary. Consider the child who has infantile paralysis and is taken to the hospital for the first time. Assuming that the child is conscious, the first difficulty is the fear of being left with a strange group of people away from the parents and home. This fear is aggravated by the general irritability and discomfort so characteristic of the disease in the acute stage. When paralysis occurs the child usually takes it much more in his stride than the adult does. In fact since the child is generally being treated by complete bed rest at this time, the seriousness of paralysis of an extremity is often not realized. Moreover the group in which the child finds himself is on restricted activity, and unless the upper extremities are severely paralyzed, the child is not hampered in keeping up with his mates. When he is allowed more freedom, the child finds out that he has certain limitations, and it is generally unnecessary to volunteer any detailed information about the paralysis. As the patient reaches the stage of recovery when walking can be undertaken, the difficulties assume greater proportions.

The child then attempts to do what he has always done to play and keep up with others, and finds that he cannot. Yet he will generally stick it out, and if uncontrolled he will use whatever muscles and means he can to do what he wants. A common complication is the tendency of adults to project themselves into the child and then expect the child to react to the situation as they themselves would.

"How then do the older children and adults react? First we must remember that poliomyelitis is known to most of these patients and usually their knowledge is distorted and exaggerated. Consequently as soon as they suspect the diagnosis, fears and misgivings begin. At times they believe they will die and conjure up memories of an iron lung which often signifies to them a desperate lifesaving measure or at least a machine which will hold them captive indefinitely. If that crisis is passed, the patient may wait fearfully for the onset of paralysis which, he assumes, occurs in all cases of poliomyelitis. Once he realizes that any part of his body is paralyzed, he may begin to speculate on what precious former activities will be denied him for the remainder of his life. Usually his prospect tends to be pessimistic, and it is no wonder that studies of such patients in the early convalescent stage have indicated a reaction of anxiety and depression. Some patients may even contemplate suicide. At one time or another most patients will show resentment toward their affliction and may query why they rather than some one [sic] else had to be stricken. This is most likely to occur when they are forced back into competition with others who appear to be unhandicapped. Yet the drive to survive and compete is strong.

"The outcome of the dilemma depends on many factors. If the patient had previously been introspective and had been babyed [sic] by his parents, the family may tend to be overindulgent. This is to be condemned for it can really force the patient to become a psychologic cripple dependent upon others even for things he could do for himself. If the former psychologic type was extrovertive, and he had been adequately adjusted to the usual situations of his age group, there is a strong possibility that the patient will overcompensate and overreact to the demands put on him. This may result in an aggressive, dominating response which may o'er leap itself. All variations between these two are found.

"Even the patients who come through with no significant residual paralysis must be considered. Pathologically it has been shown that the virus invades parts of the cerebral cortex even though there are no obvious signs or symptoms of involvement of his portion of the central nervous system. By electroencephalography abnormal tracings have been demonstrated in a high percentage of patients under 14 years age during the early convalescent state. These abnormalities generally tend to improve by the end of the first year after onset, but occasionally they may persist for years. The evidence is only suggestive, but it fits in well with the clinical observations that emotional disturbances and irritability are very common during the first year after onset even when no paralysis has been recognized. In one study 38% of the patients presented sufficient behavior problems to cause the parents to seek assistance. Again one must consider the over-all picture and not ascribe such abnormalities entirely to the effect of the virus upon the central nervous system of the host. Undoubtedly the nature of the patient's own reaction to his illness and the way he is treated by all who are with him during convalescence are of the utmost importance. A common example is the child who has limitations put on his activities because of the need to avoid fatigue during convalescence. The child meanwhile is resuming his usual activities with his playmates. He feels well and sees no reason why he can't try to do everything others do. He rebels against curtailed activities, enforced rest periods, and other parts of his treatment program. Many behavior problems can easily result from improper management of the patient during this period."

Comments on the Specific Approach to Treatment

"It is not the purpose of this paper to describe the details of treatment of poliomyelitis, and the reader is referred elsewhere for this information. Rather the emphasis is placed upon the 'man in the disease' (Draper), and his reactions to the various stages of his recovery. In no other branch of medicine is it more important to consider the patient as a whole which must also include the interaction of the patient and all who assume the great responsibility of his care and treatment. To treat Peter Brown who has paralysis, not simply a polio, requires a careful analysis of medical, orthopaedic, and psychological factors as they apply to Peter Brown specifically. To accomplish adequate overall treatment there must be co-ordinated teamwork. Ideally this encompasses the doctors, the nurses, the physical therapists, the occupational therapists, the school teachers, the social workers, and except for Peter himself, most important of all, his parents and immediate family. At least all of these aspects of treatment must be included and co-ordinated. It is essential that each one participating in the treatment program understand the basic problems and the particular steps in attaining the desired goal, namely, a well-adjusted, adequate member of society who may well have limitations, but should not be a handicapped cripple.

"In the acute stage while fever persists, the principal objectives are medical; to save life and to give supportive treatment as in any systemic febrile illness. But the patient must be treated as an individual, and especially if he is a child, the fears of separation from home and parents must be allayed. Remembering Montaigne's comment, it pays to be honest and whenever necessary to prepare the child for every unexpected or unfamiliar procedure. Rapport must be established as soon as possible, and a few extra moments spent in gaining the patient's trust and co-operation will be repaid a thousand fold in subsequent progress. Explanations of what is to happen should be direct, easily understood, and should prevent undue anxiety. As the therapist becomes more familiar with the patient as an individual, the complexity and tenor of explanations can be adjusted to suit the case.

"It is wiser to let the patient find out many of the implications of his paralysis, than to attempt to anticipate subsequent deficiencies upon which he can brood. Improvement is to be expected even though the paralysis is extensive. It is seldom advisable to make absolute statements that he cannot do this or will never to able to do that. This is particularly important during the early convalescent stage. However, as soon as muscle and functional tests allow a reasonable prognosis of future disabilities, and limitations, the emphasis should be shifted. Recovery takes time, but that in itself is fortunate because insight into the real meaning of paralysis comes gradually not as a sudden blow. By this time the patient himself may sense that he will never be able to walk without apparatus, and if the question is asked specifically an honest answer should be given. But as soon as possible the emphasis should be placed on what he can do, and not on what he cannot do. While the painstaking and lengthy period of muscle re-education is progressing, attention should also be directed toward the active use of the mind and unaffected extremities. Interest must be developed to take the patient out of himself and to direct his attention toward other people and things. He must be carefully evaluated as to his intellectual, temperamental, physical and functional capabilities. Then only can reasonable goals of attainment be set, and he must be stimulated to attain these goals, often by competition with others similarly afflicted. One should not expect the impossible, but when one is sure that a certain performance is within the patient's potentiality, he must be made to want to succeed in that undertaking and not give up until he has. Motivation is of prime importance, and the therapist will often require considerable imagination and ingenuity to satisfy the need. Above all the goal must be worthwhile and attainable within a reasonable time. It is pointless to encourage a youngster to be a second Babe Ruth when it is obvious that he will never walk without braces and crutches. It is, however, commendable to encourage him to make model airplanes, collect stamps, take up radio; in other words to pursue natural bents, and develop skills which are appealing to his own age group so as to make him one of the gang. Likewise the adult must have vocational guidance and purposeful activity geared to his future occupational needs. Successes in such undertakings even if they are initially small, must be assured. Bolstered by these, the patient can later successfully face the disappointments which are imposed on him by irremediable paralysis. As he matures and finally reaches a plateau of functional activity, he will then be ready to set further goals for himself, goals that are within his grasp because they are founded upon the positive aspects of his capabilities mental and physical, and not upon the negative. With this approach the patient can face life with confidence, unflinchingly, and life will respond."

—Thomas Gucker, "Infantile Paralysis – What does it mean to the patient?" *American Journal of Occupational Therapy*, 1949 administering antibiotics. The lack of iron lungs required patients to be rotated in and out. Thus, orthopaedic care for those patients was delayed by at least one year in Germany, whereas the orthopaedic team at Children's Hospital provides such care immediately and throughout the first years of follow-up to help diminish the paralysis. According to Burns (1947), "General Clay told the Boston staff that the work they did, not only was important in saving German lives…but that it was a practical demonstration of Democracy functioning through voluntary contributions of many people for the benefit of men everywhere."

Career and Research

Gucker was a student of polio, a patient himself, and a clinical researcher who treated patients with polio throughout his career. During his chief residency at Children's Hospital (1945–46), he treated 500 new patients with polio on his service. He became a lifelong friend of Dr. Albert Sabin, the researcher who developed the oral polio vaccine. He was eventually promoted to instructor of orthopaedic surgery at Harvard Medical School and associate orthopaedic surgeon at Children's Hospital, where he remained until 1950. That same year, he was certified by the American Board of Orthopaedic Surgery.

While at Children's Hospital, Gucker published four articles about the general care of patients with poliomyelitis. With Green, he wrote a paper in 1949 on the use of moist heat. They described the evolution of the therapy, noting that hot packs were first mentioned by another team of Children's Hospital physicians (including Edward Bradford, Robert Lovett, Robert Osgood, Elliott Brackett, Augustus Thorndike, and Robert Soutter) and were subsequently used in therapy to enhance muscle function and joint mobility, and later in aquatherapy throughout the phases of polio. They explicitly stated that moist heat should be used as an adjunct to other elements of treatment, but they emphasized its benefits in relieving

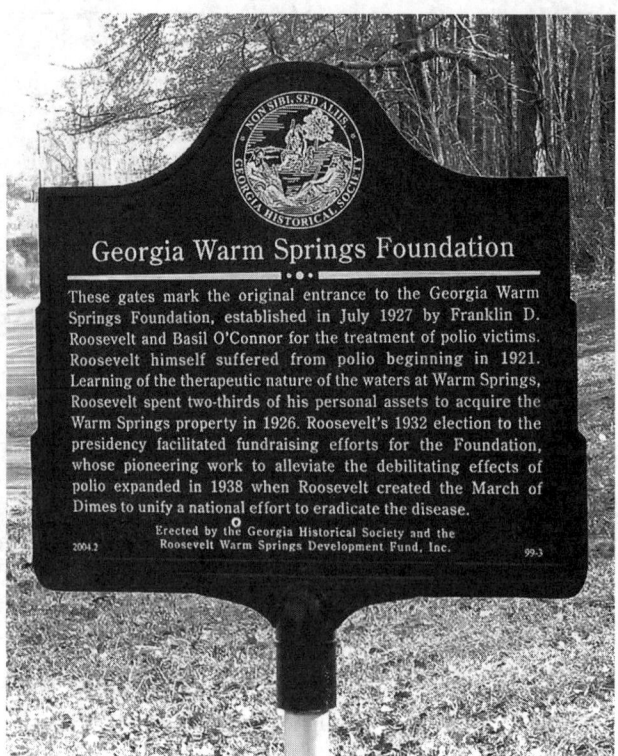

Sign at the entrance to Georgia Warm Springs Foundation.
David Seibert, courtesy of Debbie Bauch Seibert.

pain and relaxing tense muscles. Gucker had been studying the effects of various forms of heat on skin and muscle temperatures, and he and Green also showed that a hot pack applied for 20 minutes could increase a muscle's temperature for up to three hours.

Also in 1949, Gucker delivered a presentation with Green and Margaret Anderson (Green's research associate in the Growth Clinic) on the "Circulatory Changes in the Extremities, Associated with Infantile Paralysis and the Relation to the Occurrence of Shortening" at the Annual Meeting of the American Orthopaedic Association. (This was some seven years before Dr. Arthur Trott's studies of circulatory changes in poliomyelitis; see the section on Trott in this chapter.)

In 1950, Gucker left Boston for Georgia, where he spent six years as an associate surgeon at the Georgia Warm Springs Foundation. Two years later Gucker became a member of the American Academy of Orthopaedic Surgeons. Around this same time, he published research in which he found that light plaster shells prevented knee and heel cord contractures if used for prolonged periods. He also published his results with tendon transfers in the hand in quadriplegic patients and tendon transfers in the lower extremities in patients with polio:

> It is unwise to consider tendon transfers early in poliomyelitis; it is preferable to wait eighteen months or longer after the onset of paralysis and until the child is over five years of age… with the problem of progressive calcaneus and the very great difficulty of trying to control it by the usual conservative means of manipulation, retention splints, or braces. For that reason, therefore, it might be well to consider, as early as a year after onset, transference of the strongest of the deforming tendons posteriorly to the os calcis, even a number of years in advance of the age for stabilization. At the proper age, stabilization by triple arthrodesis will be necessary…[and] appropriate remaining tendon transfers can be done. The second consideration concerns the selection of the tendon for transference.
>
> May I present to you a problem that occasionally arises, which we find most difficult to analyze—specifically, the patient who has a partial foot-drop in combination with poor take-off, due to weakness of the gastrocnemius soleus group…we have found the analysis of this situation difficult when presented by a patient who has a tendo achilles contracture…an equinus which masks the truly deficient power of the gastrocnemius…In several instances we have observed patients who were treated for a fixed equinovalgus deformity…by heel-cord lengthening…triple arthrodesis, transference of both peroneals to the anteromedial tarsus, who then presented with a calcaneovarus deformity, which was more disabling than the equinovalgus. When the difficulties of evaluating the power of the gastrocnemius are so great…if adequate or even reasonable fair toe-extensor power remains to help dorsiflex the foot, and especially when heel-cord lengthening is necessary, it is wiser as a rule to transfer the peroneals to the os calcis…to avoid development of talipes calcaneus. This is particularly important when there is concomitant quadriceps weakness which is all the more exaggerated by a calcaneus gait. (T. Gucker 1952)

In 1956, Gucker left Georgia and:

> returned to Philadelphia as Associate Surgeon at the Hospital of the University of Pennsylvania and Associate Professor of Orthopaedic Surgery at the University of Pennsylvania School of Medicine. During 1956 and 1957, he was also a Fellow in Rehabilitation at the Hospital of the University of Pennsylvania. Gucker [then] moved to Los Angeles with his family to become the Medical Director of Rehabilitation and Assistant Medical Director of Orthopaedic Hospital in Los Angeles…He was also associated with the Muscular Dystrophy Association Clinic…[and] subsequently became Director of the one in Los Angeles…He served as Director for twenty-two years, until his retirement from the hospital. (J. D. H. 1987)

Gucker published ~20 papers, most on polio, neuromuscular disorders, and rehabilitation. Many were published in non-orthopaedic journals. In one such later publication, he reported the effects of spine fusion, the Milwaukee Brace, and the use of corrective casts on pulmonary function in 49 patients:

> Before treatment the mean sitting vital capacity was found to be 64 per cent of the predicted normal in patients with paralytic scoliosis and 80 per cent of normal in the patients with idiopathic scoliosis…Correction…by wedging or localizer casts produced a mean loss of vital

capacity of 21 per cent in patients with paralytic scoliosis and 29 per cent in patients with non-paralytic scoliosis...The use of a Milwaukee frame for correction was found to have less detrimental effect on vital capacity... of the twenty-one patients [treated by spine fusion], only three showed 10 per cent or more improvement in the predicted vital capacity.
(T. Gucker 1962a)

In 1976, about 15 years after settling in Los Angeles, Gucker, along with John Hsu, presented a one-day course on the diagnosis and care of patients with neuromuscular disease at the Los Angeles Orthopaedic Hospital. During that time, Gucker also held a faculty position at the University of Southern California. When he retired, he was named emeritus clinical professor of orthopaedic surgery.

Various groups acknowledged "his contributions in the field of orthopaedic rehabilitation" (J. D. H. 1987), including the National Rehabilitation Association, from which he received the W.F. Faulkes Award; and the Los Angeles Chamber of Commerce, which bestowed the Milestone Award; and the Muscular Dystrophy Association of America.

He is considered a pioneer in orthopaedic rehabilitation. He served on and represented both the orthopaedic surgeon and the handicapped person on numerous local and national committees, including the National Rehabilitation Association, the Arthritis Foundation, the Governors Committee for Employment of the Handicapped, the Medical Advisory Committee, the Muscular Dystrophy Association of America and the Committee on Orthopaedic Rehabilitation of the American Academy of Orthopaedic Surgeons. He was named Physician of the Year by the California Governor's Committee for Employment in 1980.
(J. D. H. 1987)

One of Gucker's patients in Los Angeles was inspired to become an orthopaedic surgeon. Robert D. Schlens, born in 1935, had gotten polio when he was 10 years old—just one year before Salk introduced his polio vaccine—and survived 9 months of his childhood in an iron lung. His paralysis was so extensive that his doctors told him he'd never walk again, but after Gucker performed several surgeries, Schlens was able to walk with crutches while wearing a brace. But Gucker's influence on Schlens' life didn't end there. Schlens went on to graduate with honors from Indiana University, and despite initial rejections from various medical schools because of his disability, he was eventually accepted into the medical school at Indiana University. He completed an internship and Gucker, then new to Los Angeles, actively swayed the leadership at Orthopedic Hospital to accept Schlens into the residency program there. Schlens finished his residency, became certified by the American Board of Orthopaedic Surgery, and went on to practice in Los Angeles for 50 years.

In 1979, Gucker was persuaded to write about "the historical aspects of poliomyelitis, which was a lifelong study and interest of his...This gave his colleagues, especially his students and others who may have some physical disability, a window into his life as well as some of his thoughts, words of wisdom and inspiration" (J. D. H. 1987).

Gucker retired from Orthopaedic Hospital a year later, in April 1980. "The day of his retirement from Orthopaedic Hospital...was unique in that it was attended not only by members of the staff...his colleagues, students and friends, but also by hundreds of his patients who presented him with good wishes and gifts" (J. D. H. 1987). After his retirement, he continued his work in the role of consultant in orthopaedic rehabilitation at the New Hope Pain Hospital in Alhambra. He died in August 1986 in Los Angeles, leaving behind his wife, Harriet, and their three sons. "Dr. Gucker will be remembered by all of those whose life he has touched" (J. D. H. 1987).

LLEWELLYN HALL

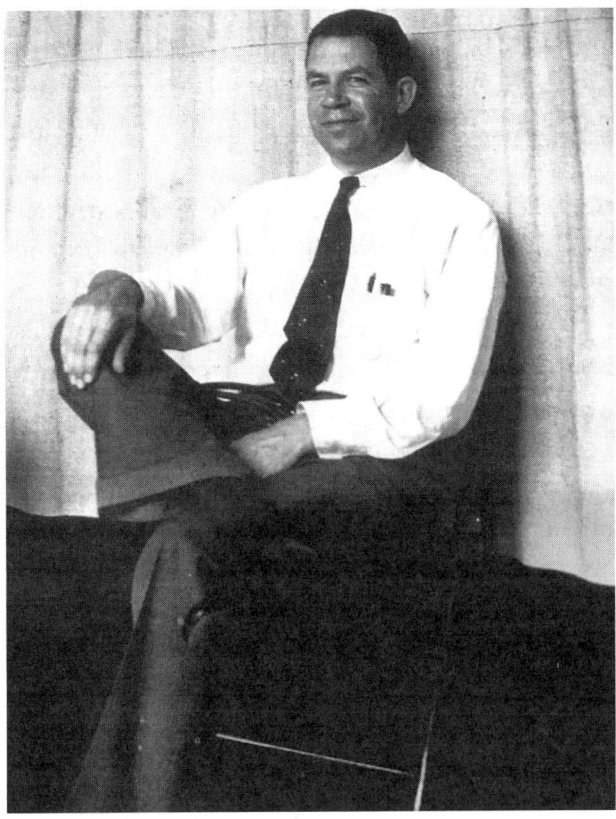

Llewellyn Hall. Courtesy of Dr. Robert S. Hall.

Physician Snapshot

Llewellyn Hall
BORN: ca. 1899
DIED: 1969
SIGNIFICANT CONTRIBUTIONS: On staff at Boston Children's Hospital when Dr. Robert Osgood was chief; changed career, becoming plant physician for Arlington Mills, followed by associate medical director of the Phoenix Mutual Insurance Company

Llewellyn Hall was born in Turners Falls, Massachusetts, and apparently grew up in Annapolis, Maryland. He graduated from Harvard College in 1920 and Harvard Medical School in 1924. In 1926, after successfully completing the national board examination, he registered with the Massachusetts Board of Medicine. At the time, he was a clinical assistant in the orthopaedic department at Boston Children's Hospital. He became a member of the Massachusetts Medical Society in 1930.

While on the staff at Boston Children's Hospital, he became the plant physician for Arlington Mills, a large textile manufacturer on the banks of the Spicket River in Northeast Massachusetts. Around 1930, "the only change in the staff [BCH] has been the acceptance of the resignation of Dr. Llewellyn Hall who has accepted a position on the staff of the Truesdale Hospital in Fall River." ("Annual Report of the Children's Hospital," Vol. 1926–1930, 250).

That same year Hall became the associate medical director of the Phoenix Mutual Insurance Company in Hartford, Connecticut. While he was an employee at Phoenix Mutual, the company pioneered many innovations, including advertising, for the first time, to potential customers. He retired in 1965 after 35 years at Phoenix Mutual.

Hall was a member of several professional organizations including the AMA, the Twentieth Century Club, the Harvard Club of Connecticut, the Hartford Medical Society, and the Society of Descendants of the Founders of Hartford. He served as president of both the Greater Hartford Tuberculosis Respiratory Disease Association and the Harvard Club of Connecticut. He died on June 6, 1969, at the age of 70 in Hartford Hospital. He was survived by his wife (Caroline Doane Hall), two sons, two daughters and his mother (Mrs. L. W. Hall) of Wellesley Hills, Massachusetts.

PAUL W. HUGENBERGER

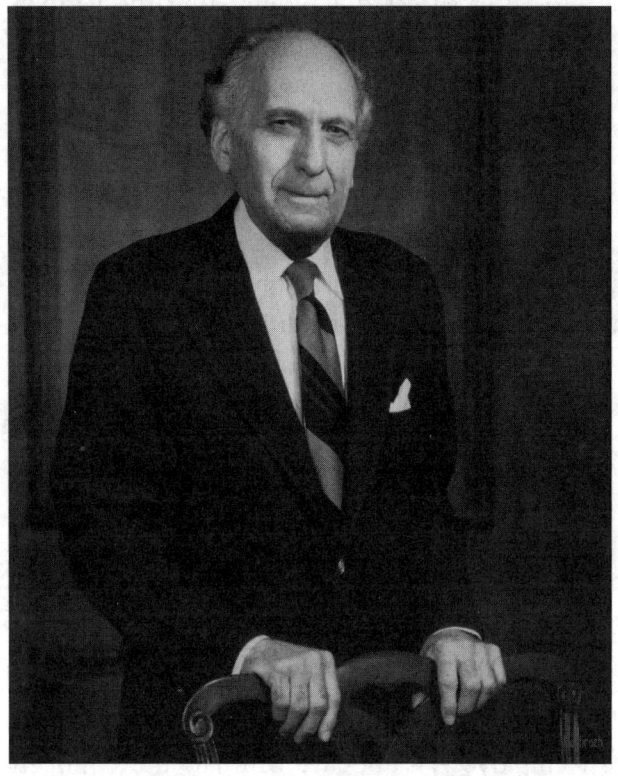

Paul W. Hugenberger.
Photo by James Koepfler/Boston Children's Hospital. Portrait by Bachrach Studios, reprinted by permission of Louis F. Bachrach.

Physician Snapshot

Paul W. Hugenberger
BORN: 1903
DIED: 1996
SIGNIFICANT CONTRIBUTIONS: Chief of orthopaedics at Salem Hospital; surgeon-in-chief at the New England Peabody Home for Crippled Children; president of the Boston Orthopaedic Club, 1965

Paul Willard Hugenberger was born in Portsmouth, Ohio, on June 12, 1903. His father, Herman, worked as a shoe laster (one who shaped and joined together the body of a shoe and the sole) and farmer. Paul sometimes worked in shoe stores but more often performed chores on the family's farm. As a farmer, Herman Hugenberger would frequently purchase an old, rundown farm, rehabilitate it, and then sell it. (He sold one such farm to John Dillinger's father. John was the same age as Paul, and they attended high school together.) Thus, Paul and his brothers, Franklin and Arthur, and their sister, Helen, moved about 13 times before their teens. Paul's children believe that such moves made it difficult for them to form close friendships. As a result, Paul and Franklin (only one-and-a-half years apart) formed an extremely close bond. Years later, Paul confided in his children that he and his brother noticed that in every town they moved to, the doctor had the nicest house, and that this influenced both brothers to become physicians.

Herman Hugenberger died at age 57, when Paul was 17. Paul and Franklin graduated from Stivers High School in Dayton, Ohio, and both attended Ohio State University. Elizabeth, their mother, bought and ran a boarding house near the university, renting rooms to students; in this way she supported the three boys and Helen throughout college. Paul graduated with a bachelor of arts degree in 1925, one year earlier than Franklin. Because both wanted to attend medical school together, Paul stayed at Ohio State University, getting a master of arts degree in psychology in 1926 and joining the US Army Reserves. With intentions to return to practice in Ohio, Paul and Franklin moved to Boston and attended Harvard Medical School, from which they graduated together in 1930—the first brothers to do so in the same class.

The brothers both trained in Boston—Franklin in obstetrics and Paul in orthopaedics. Franklin, however, decided to return to Ohio, whereas Paul remained in Boston. For seven months (September 30, 1930–April 31, 1931), Paul Hugenberger was an intern in bone and joint. He then spent five months (May 1–September 31, 1931) as an intern in pathology at Massachusetts General Hospital (MGH), immediately after which he became the first resident in pathology there (that residency lasted seven months). As a resident in pathology, he participated in two Cabot Case Records from the MGH: "Cholecystitis with Cholelithiasis" and "Abdominal Enlargement with Unusual Physical Findings," both published in the

New England Journal of Medicine. For the next 20 months, he was an intern in surgery at Boston City Hospital, during which time he also worked at Boston City Hospital Relief Station in Haymarket Square. During that surgical internship, Hugenberger appeared in an article in the *Daily Boston Globe* about a teenager who had struck his head while diving from the North End Park pier. After lifeguards pulled him from the water, they spent two hours trying to resuscitate him with a pulmotor. Hugenberger had arrived from the Haymarket Relief Station and examined the teenager throughout the efforts, though he eventually declared the boy dead. On December 15, 1933, Hugenberger began an eight-month internship in orthopaedic surgery at Children's Hospital and then moved directly into an eight-month internship in orthopaedic surgery at MGH; he completed the second on April 30, 1935. His training wasn't over: for one year beginning September 1, 1935, he was a resident in orthopaedic surgery at Children's Hospital. His teaching career began then, too, with an appointment as an assistant in orthopaedic surgery at Harvard Medical School.

Although Dr. Harvey Cushing at the Peter Bent Brigham Hospital pursued Hugenberger in attempts to get him to become a neurosurgeon, Hugenberger remained dedicated to practicing orthopaedics "because the outcomes were so much better and the mortality rates, so much lower in those days" (G. Hugenberger and J. Hugenberger, personal interview with the author, 2015). After completing his training, Hugenberger became an assistant to Dr. Frank Ober. He joined Ober's office at 234 Marlborough Street. Other orthopaedic surgeons who practiced out of that office included Drs. Joseph Barr (chapter 38), Albert Brewster, Charles Sturdevant (both discussed elsewhere in this chapter), Eugene Record, and Thomas DeLorme (both are discussed in chapter 40); the group was known as the Marlborough Medical Associates. In 1960, Drs. Barr, Record, and DeLorme resigned from the group, and eventually Hugenberger became the senior orthopaedic surgeon in the group. He moved his practice to 164 Beacon Street in 1974.

Beginning in 1960, Hugenberger opened an office in the Salem Hospital Medical Office Building. He "had an extensive private practice both in Boston and in Salem and was among the first orthopedic surgeons to practice in the North Shore Area" ("Other Orthopaedic Surgeons at Children's Hospital," n.d.). He practiced both adult and pediatric orthopaedics. At Salem Hospital his first appointment (as a member of the medical staff) was in 1940. He served as chief of orthopaedics there from 1955 to 1967, and, on January 1, 1969, he was named an emeritus staff member. On the North Shore, Hugenberger was a consultant orthopaedic surgeon at North Shore Children's Hospital in Salem, at the Anna Jacques Hospital in Newburyport, and at the Mary Alley Hospital in Marblehead.

In Boston, Hugenberger continued to practice at Children's Hospital, becoming an associate orthopedic surgeon in 1947, an orthopedic surgeon in 1959, senior associate in orthopedic surgery in 1962, and finally emeritus in 1991. He was appointed associate in orthopedic surgery to the Peter Bent Brigham Hospital in 1936, remaining on the active staff there until 1975, when Dr. Clement Sledge (then chief of the Orthopaedic Department) appointed him to emeritus status for another five years, during which time Hugenberger worked in the Industrial Accident Clinic.

According to his daughter Joan, one institution that Hugenberger greatly loved was the New England Peabody Home for Crippled Children in Newton. He joined the staff in 1937 and remained as a senior orthopaedic surgeon until it closed in 1961. Hugenberger also served as the hospital's surgeon-in-chief during its last few months of operation. In his 1961 annual report, he wrote that:

> with the resignation of our renowned Surgeon-in-Chief, Dr. Joseph S. Barr, on January 1, 1961, the New England Peabody Home lost a great leader and teacher, and it marks the beginning

of our end...Dr. Barr clearly summarized... that there was no longer a need for the Peabody Home...The Board of Trustees publicly announced that the present facilities on Oak Hill in Newton Center would be closed within a year and that the funds would be used to establish an Orthopedic Professorship at Harvard Medical School and a Peabody Clinic at the Children's Hospital Medical Center. This is, therefore, my first and presumably last Annual Report of the Chief of Staff...I consider it an honor to be the Chief of this famous institution even for a few months...our Monthly Staff Conference[s]...were originally started by Dr. Nathaniel Allison in 1925...Improved medical care over the years accounts for a major reduction in the length of stay in the home. For example, Streptomycin was first used in the treatment of bone and joint tuberculosis at the Peabody Home in February 1948 and since that time all cases of tuberculosis have been treated with chemotherapy with better results and much less time in the hospital... We have treated over the years a total of 86 cases of coxa plana or Legg Perthes Disease... and since non weight bearing over a long period of time is essential for a good result, the facilities of the Peabody Home have been ideal in the treatment of these cases...We are at the present time making a follow-up study on these cases and have examined and had x-rays on 55 cases...This has been a very interesting, and worth-while project. (P. W. Hugenberger 1961)

Hugenberger then called "attention to a few of those great men who have made New England Peabody Home for Crippled Children famous" and who would "never be forgotten," including Robert Lovett, Robert Soutter, Nathaniel Allison, Frank Ober, Joseph Barr, Albert Brewster, Edwin Cave, and Ralph Ghormley, "as well as scores of other devoted men and women who have contributed greatly in wealth and time to our beloved Peabody Home" (P. W. Hugenberger 1961).

The professorship mentioned in Hugenberger's report—endowed by the trustees of the Peabody Home—was first awarded to Dr. William T. Green. I was not able to find any published articles about the cases of Legg-Perthes disease that Hugenberger mentioned.

Hugenberger was involved with many other institutions. In 1949, he worked on at least two different occasions at the Georgia Warm Springs Foundation. For a brief time, he was on staff at Hahnemann Hospital in Brighton (1975–76); was an orthopaedic consultant to the Massachusetts Mental Health Center; was on the courtesy staff at Mount Auburn Hospital in Cambridge; was an orthopaedic consultant to St. Mark's School in Southborough; and was an orthopaedic consultant to the Dr. J. Robert Shaughnessy Rehabilitation Hospital, the West Roxbury Veteran's Administration Hospital (1975–80), and the Developmental School of the North Shore in Peabody (part of the United Cerebral Palsy Association).

At Harvard Medical School, Hugenberger was promoted from assistant to clinical instructor in orthopedic surgery in 1949, then to lecturer of orthopaedic surgery in 1960, a role he held for nine years. He was an associate at Brigham and Women's Hospital until 1975 and a senior associate at Children's Hospital until 1982. He held a position as a senior attending at North Shore Children's Hospital and as an orthopaedic surgeon at Anna Jacques Hospital until 1987. He served on the Harvard Medical School reunion committees in 1979 and 1984, and he was secretary to the Harvard Combined Orthopaedic Residency Program Alumni at the American Academy of Orthopaedic Surgeons annual meeting in 1983. He was a member of the board of trustees of the Peabody Foundation until 1988. He continued in private practice at his Beacon Street office until 1991, and at his medical office at Salem Hospital until 1993.

Hugenberger was frequently on service at Children's Hospital for more than 40 years. I can recall him leading evening rounds, which were long; he examined every patient, frequently watching a child walk, analyzing their gait, and often recommending conservative, nonoperative treatment. The physical therapists at Children's Hospital "loved him…he came in monthly…frequently attending grand rounds where he would sit in the second row [Dr. Green sat in the first row]. He was a mild-manner[ed] man…[. He] enjoyed discussing patients with a bad gait…after lots of discussion, Dr. Hugenberger would get up, look at the bottom of the patient's shoes and comment that 'he [the patient] needs a lateral or medial heel wedge and not surgery'" (C. McCarthy and M. Casella, personal interview with the author, 2012). Joan Hugenberger, Hugenberger's daughter, agreed with the physical therapists: "Dad was a man of few words—at least to us. He was also very kindly. He never lifted a hand to punish us" (G. Hugenberger and J. Hugenberger, personal interview with the author, 2015).

In 1950, Hugenberger presented a lecture, "The Problems of Infancy and Childhood," at the fifth Postgraduate Lecture Course of the Massachusetts Medical Society. I could not find any other lectures or papers presented by Hugenberger at professional meetings. He published one article in *Pediatric Clinics of North America* and three chapters in the series *Current Pediatric Therapy*, all between 1967 and 1973. Each chapter and the article were reviews of leg deformities, dislocations, torticollis, and congenital muscular defects. In 1983, at the annual Osgood Program, Dr. Thornton Brown presented the Osgood lecture, "Two-hundred Years of Harvard Orthopaedics." At that meeting, at the request of Dr. Henry Mankin, Hugenberger presented a brief talk on the early days at Children's Hospital in which he made special remarks about Dr. Frank Ober.

Hugenberger also "participated in the first clinical studies that established the relationship between pressure on the spinal cord and referred pain, and in the first clinical trials of spinal fusion surgery. He also perfected a surgical technique for lengthening legs" ("Dr. Paul W. Hugenberger 92" 1996).

Another of Hugenberger's lifelong contributions was as a consultant to the Division of Family Health Services for Handicapped Children with the Massachusetts Department of Public Health. For more than 30 years, he attended a monthly clinic in Salem; he only retired in August 1977 because he had reached the mandatory retirement age of 70.

Both Hugenberger and Albert Brewster acquired through their practice a collection of books and manuscripts from both Lovett and Ober, which they donated to the Boston Medical Library in 1976; at that time the library was part of the Francis A. Countway Library of Medicine at Harvard Medical School. The collection included "some of Dr. Lovett's diaries, dating from the mid-1880's, when he started practice, and a box of manuscript letters and materials documenting the treatment by him and other physicians of the illness from poliomyelitis of the late Franklin Delano Roosevelt" (R. J. Wolfe 1976). I believe that this was most likely the source of President Roosevelt's letters to Lovett, including his description of and drawings about his experiences getting about his boat. (See chapter 16).

According to Joan Hugenberger, her father treated many famous people, including the

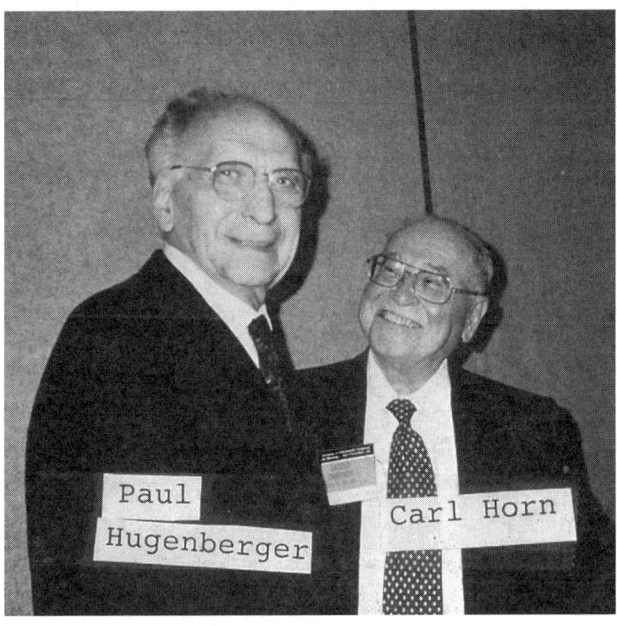

Dr. Hugenberger with Dr. Carl E. Horn (Sacramento) at an AAOS meeting. MGH HCORP Archives.

playwright, poet, Nobel Laureate in Literature, and Pulitzer Prize Winner Sylvia Plath; Academy Award–winning actress and direct descendant of Paul Revere, Anne Revere; Edward R. Morrow; and Howard Johnson. In February 1951, the playwright Eugene O'Neill left his home without his cane after quarreling with his wife and tripped over a rock covered by snow, breaking his leg. A physician making house calls saw O'Neill and brought him to Salem Hospital, where Hugenberger treated him and put him in a cast. Hugenberger said of O'Neill:

> He never complained of his disability or pain; he didn't try to make you feel sorry for him. After a couple of weeks, the cast was reduced, a painful procedure, but he took it gamely, even though he didn't have any anesthesia. I found him delightful, in spite of his low spirits at first. I used to spend some time with him in my visits. The circumstances of his accident were peculiar, and we considered the possibility that he intended suicide, but we couldn't come to any definite decision. It was only conjecture. (L. Sheaffer 1973)

I could not find any documented evidence of Hugenberger caring for the other notable individuals mentioned above, including Sylvia Plath. Plath did fracture her fibula in a fall while skiing at Saranac Lake, New York, on December 28, 1952, and she was treated in a cast for two months. She was a junior at Smith College at the time. She wrote in her journal: "I saw Dick, went to Saranac with him and broke my leg skiing. Now midyears approach. I have exams to work for, papers to write. There is snow and ice and I have a broken leg to drag around for two hellish months" (quoted in K. V. Kukil 2010). Later she described her leg after the cast was removed, saying that the doctor "lifted the white plaster lid like a gravedigger opening a sealed coffin. The corpse of my leg lay there, horrible, dark with clotted curls of black hair, discolored yellow, wasted shapeless by a two month internment…and the x-rays showed it wasn't completely mended" (quoted in K. V. Kukil 2010). Plath described her experience in her fictionalized autobiography *The Bell Jar* and nine years later wrote the poem "In Plaster" about it.

Hugenberger was a fellow of the American College of Surgeons, a diplomate of the American Board of Orthopaedic Surgery (1938), and a member of the American Academy of Orthopaedic Surgeons, the American Medical Association, the Massachusetts Medical Society, and the Boston Orthopaedic Cub; for the latter, he served as secretary/treasurer for seven years, and as president in 1965. He was a member of the Harvard Club of Boston and the Skating Club of Boston, where his children frequently skated. Married for 56 years to Janet (McMullin) Hugenberger, a talented landscape painter and musician, they had seven children, including Gordon Hugenberger, PhD, the senior pastor at the historic Park Street Church in Boston.

Children's Hospital Department of Orthopaedic Surgery honored Hugenberger in 1984 by dedicating the orthopaedic library in his name. A plaque honoring him in the Hugenberger Orthopaedic Library reads: "for years of loyal and dedicated service to the Orthopaedic Department of the Hospital." In 1987, he was named an honorary member of the medical staff at Anna Jacques Hospital, and the following year he was elected an honorary trustee of the Peabody Foundation. On September 23, 1989, Hugenberger received from the Brigham and Women's Hospital a certificate of appreciation for 50 years of devoted service signed by the president, H. Richard Nesson.

Hugenberger lived in Wellesley the last 52 years of his life. At age 89, he completed the 6.2-mile Salem Hospital Cancer Walk-a-Thon. He died at his home on January 31, 1996, at the age of 93. He will be remembered for his compassion for his patients. Joan, who had worked in her father's office, told me that he was very humble and always patient with them. As one patient said in a letter to Dr. Hugenberger, shared with me by his daughter Joan for this book: "I shall never forget the compassion and concern you showed for your patient and the confidence and trust you place in the other doctors. Your profound humility, patience and mature understanding and your enthusiasm for the work to which you are so dedicated made me realize that I was privileged to have known 'true greatness.' A man as tireless as yourself who gives so much of himself to his work is loved by all and should be told about it" (I. S. Walsh 1953).

MIRIAM G. KATZEFF

Physician Snapshot

Miriam G. Katzeff
BORN: 1899
DIED: 1989
SIGNIFICANT CONTRIBUTIONS: Possibly the first woman orthopaedic surgeon on staff at Children's Hospital, and one of the first in Massachusetts

Miriam Gertrude Katzeff was born in Boston on June 12, 1899. Both her parents (Mendel Katzeff and Frieda Felfnick) were from Lithuania. Little is recorded of her early history and education. She graduated from the Boston University School of Medicine in 1925. Boston University had established the Boston University School of Medicine in 1873 by assuming the debt of the New England Female Medical College, which itself had opened in 1848 and taught conventional medical treatment as well as a homeopathic approach. While a medical student, Katzeff participated in a series of weekly lectures given before the entire student body. Both faculty and medical students gave these lectures, covering medical history and biographies. Katzeff's lecture was entitled "Moses and the Early Jewish Medicine."

Details about Katzeff's internship and training as an orthopaedic surgeon are unknown, but she received appointments at Children's Hospital

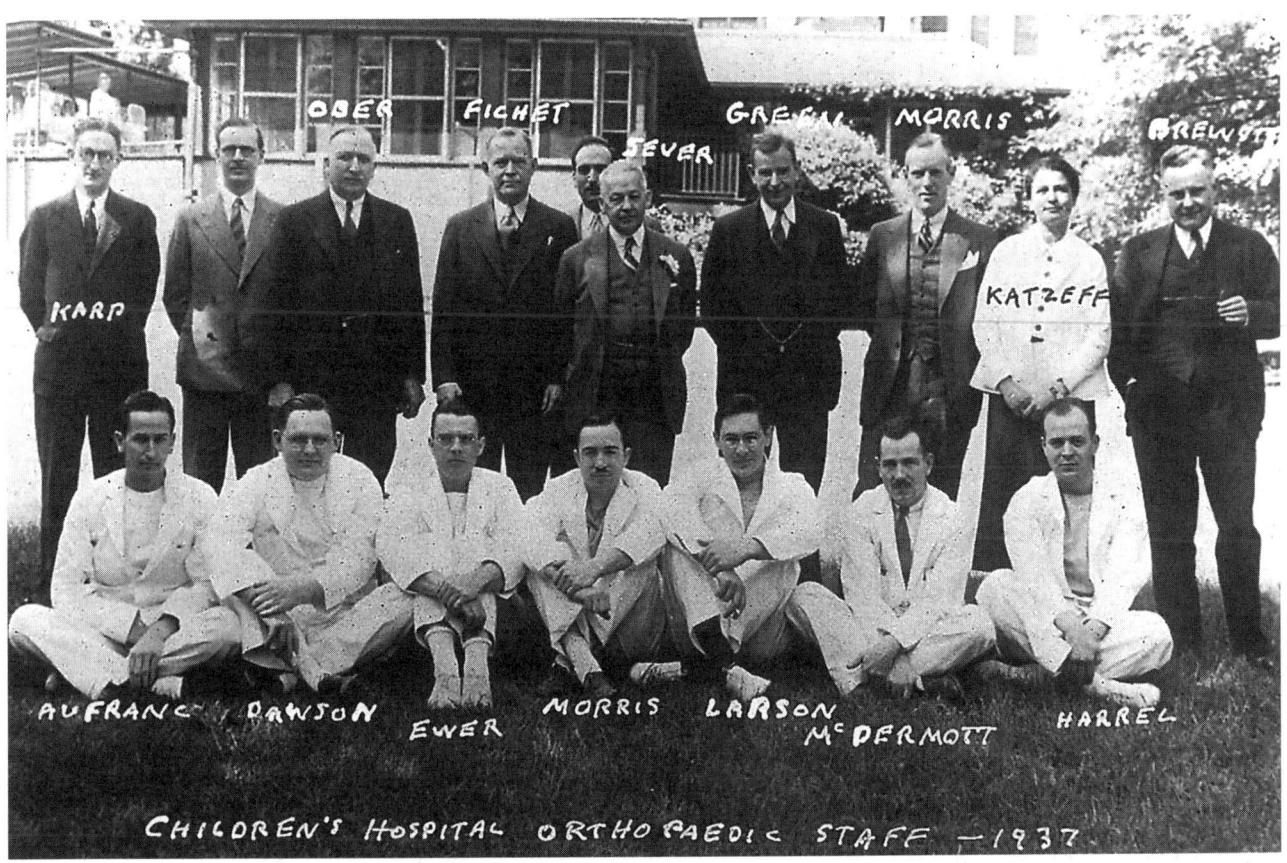

Orthopaedic Staff at BCH, 1937. Dr. Katzeff is standing in the back row, second from the right. MGH HCORP Archives.

early in her career, first as an assistant surgeon in the orthopaedic outpatient department in 1926 and then as junior assistant surgeon in the orthopaedic department in 1929. The duration of these appointments is also unknown. She worked with Drs. John Kuhns and Robert Joplin in the outpatient department; associate visiting surgeons were Drs. William Green and Robert Morris, and visiting surgeons were Drs. Albert Brewster, Seth Fitchet, Arthur Legg, and James Sever. Robert Osgood was the chief of the orthopaedic service. As a junior assistant surgeon, in addition to the aforementioned orthopaedic surgeons, she worked with Drs. Frank Ober, Henry FitzSimmons, Joseph Shortell, and Frederick C. Bost.

Katzeff also worked as an orthopaedist at the New England Hospital for Women and Children (later named the New England Hospital), as a clinical assistant in the orthopaedic outpatient department of Cambridge Hospital, and as a consultant at the Danvers State Hospital. She taught anatomy at the Boston University School of Medicine and occasionally attended the posture clinic for children at Wellesley College on Saturday mornings.

Case 23.5. Arthrogryposis Multiplex Congenita

"R.S., a boy aged 3 weeks, was admitted to the outpatient department of the Children's Hospital in Boston, Aug. 29, 1940, for the treatment of deformed upper and lower extremities, noted at birth. The father, aged 32 years, had diabetes. The mother, aged 22 years, was well except for occasional attacks of dermographia. The patient was the only child…The parents reported no deformities in their families.

"At the birth of the child…no instruments were used at delivery, although there was some type of manual manipulation to improve the position…Immediately after birth it was noted that the baby had deformities of the shoulders, elbows and hands, contracted knees and clubfeet.

"On examination both shoulders were adducted with passive abduction to 90 degrees. The deltoid muscles were small, with very little muscle that was palpable. The elbows were extended to the extreme degree and permitted passive flexion of 45 degrees on the right and 80 degrees on the left. Supination of the forearm was not possible on the left; 15 degrees was obtainable on the right. Pronation of the forearm on the left was 20 degrees, that on the right was 15 degrees. Extension of the wrist on the left was 20 degrees; that on the right, 20 degrees. Flexion of both wrists was possible to 50 degrees. Knees were permanently flexed to 25 degrees, with further flexion to 120 degrees. Both feet were in rigid equinovarus position.

"Roentgenograms of the upper and lower extremities showed deficiency of the muscle tissue shadows. The capsules and the ligaments appeared thickened. The bones were normal except for the deformities in the clubfeet.

"The child was given outpatient care, consisting of manipulation of the upper and lower extremities with weekly changes of casts to the feet, for a period of ten months…The infant at 10 months of age was admitted to the hospital for surgical correction of his feet and further manipulation of his upper extremities. Lengthening of both heel cords and posterior capsulotomy were done, and casts were applied with the feet in marked dorsiflexion, abduction and eversion. Following an uneventful convalescence of three weeks, the boy was again followed in the outpatient department…physical therapy was given to the upper extremities three times weekly. Bivalved casts were used between treatments. At 16 months of age he began to walk in corrective shoes. His feet were manipulated daily at home, and Dennis-Brown shoe splints were used during his day and night sleeping periods…

"[At aged] 2 years…[he] is attending a nursery school… His last examination, in November 1942, showed a good hand grasp, with some weakness…no contractures of fingers or wrists; the elbows had active flexion of 90 degrees and extension of 160 degrees, shoulder abduction was, active, 60 degrees; passive 90 degrees. Both feet were flexible and corrected 10 degrees beyond neutral in dorsiflexion, abduction and eversion. He walked and ran well and easily. His arms swung freely but not completely."

(M. G. Katzeff 1943)

Katzeff became a member of the Massachusetts Medical Society in 1927. She spoke infrequently at local and regional meetings, though throughout her career (mostly from 1932 through 1951) she gave lectures and presented case reports or discussions on a variety of orthopaedic topics—syphilis, pathological fractures in bone cysts, bone tumors of the knee, orthopaedic problems of the newborn, early treatment of club feet, postural problems in children, first aid, and eosinophilic granuloma. She published only two articles. The first, in 1933, was part of a tribute to Robert Osgood in the *New England Journal of Medicine*. Katzeff wrote an article entitled "Tuberculosis in Infancy and Childhood. A Statistical Study." She made the remarkable statement: "Gentlemen, I wish to call your attention to the fact that today this orthopaedic ward does not contain a single case of tuberculosis. This is a very different picture from that of not so many years ago when it was not a difficult task to select tuberculosis cases for student demonstration" (M. G. Katzeff 1933). She reviewed the statistics of patients with tuberculosis who had been admitted to Children's Hospital during the 47-year period from 1884 to 1931, compiling relevant graphs, concluding: "This study of tuberculosis cases at the Children's Hospital has confirmed the impression that tuberculosis of the osseous system is a disappearing disease and that this form of tuberculosis responds more favorably than the non-orthopaedic forms to the measures of preventive medicine" (M. G. Katzeff 1933). Her second publication was entitled "Arthrogryposis Multiplex Congenita," published in 1943. In it, she reviewed 18 patients treated at Children's Hospital from 1925 to 1942 (see **Case 23.5**). She made the following observations:

> Histologically there is atrophy and fat replacement of the involved muscles…In general, the younger patients were treated in this order: (1) manipulations without anesthesia, (2) supports, (3) anesthesia, manipulations and supports and (4) surgical corrections. The older patients were treated by operative procedures selected as most suitable for the correction of the individual deformity. These procedures were fasciotomy, capsulotomy, lengthening of tendons, open reduction of hips and arthrodesis for the correction of club feet. The end results varied…the best results were obtained with the early institution of corrective measures. These badly disabled children, presenting at birth a discouraging picture, were definitely improved by treatment. (M. G. Katzeff 1943)

I believe that Katzeff was the first woman on the orthopaedic department staff at Children's Hospital—and perhaps one of the first in Massachusetts. In 1962, she moved her office from 270 Commonwealth Avenue to 483 Beacon Street.

Katzeff never married. She spent much time advocating and encouraging medicine in Israel, and she volunteered there as a physician during Israel's wars. In 1942, she began spending summers at Wingaersheek Beach in West Gloucester. At that time, she most likely purchased her home in Gloucester, at 16 Grape Vine Road. She remained there until her death from intra-abdominal sepsis at Addison Gilbert Hospital on December 30, 1989. She was 90 years old.

JAMES G. MANSON

> **Physician Snapshot**
>
> James G. Manson
> BORN: 1931
> DIED: 2009
> SIGNIFICANT CONTRIBUTIONS: Ran the hemophilia clinic at Children's Hospital for ~20 years; chief of orthopaedics Mount Auburn Hospital; chief of orthopaedic services MIT Medical Clinics

James Gavin Manson was born to Scottish parents—his father was a physician—in Melton Mowbray, Leicestershire, England, on June 6, 1931. Melton Mowbray, 20 miles southeast of

Nottingham, is known as the "Rural Capital of Food" and is home to a famous pork pie; Stilton cheese originated nearby. After graduating from the Uppingham School, James completed his medical degree at Cambridge University in 1957, receiving bachelor's degrees in both medicine and surgery; he was 26 years old. During his postgraduate training at Guy's Hospital in London, he met Mary Lyon, who at the time was attending Harvard and in London writing a dissertation. They married in 1958 and then moved to the United States, settling in Cambridge, Massachusetts. She later became an English teacher at Windsor School, a private college preparatory school in Boston. Manson completed the orthopaedic residency program at Children's Hospital and MGH.

In 1963, Manson became a member of the part-time staff of MIT Medical, a clinic in Cambridge affiliated with MIT. By 1965, he was also an assistant in orthopedic surgery at Harvard Medical School and a junior associate in orthopedic surgery at Children's Hospital. Manson was actively involved in teaching the residents at Children's Hospital during rounds, but I don't recall him operating there (though he probably did so). He was in private practice and operated at Mount Auburn Hospital, where he was chief of orthopaedics from 1972 to 1984; he became president of the medical staff there in 1976. Beginning in the 1970s (after I had completed my own training at Children's Hospital), Manson ran a hemophilia clinic there; he operated it for ~20 years.

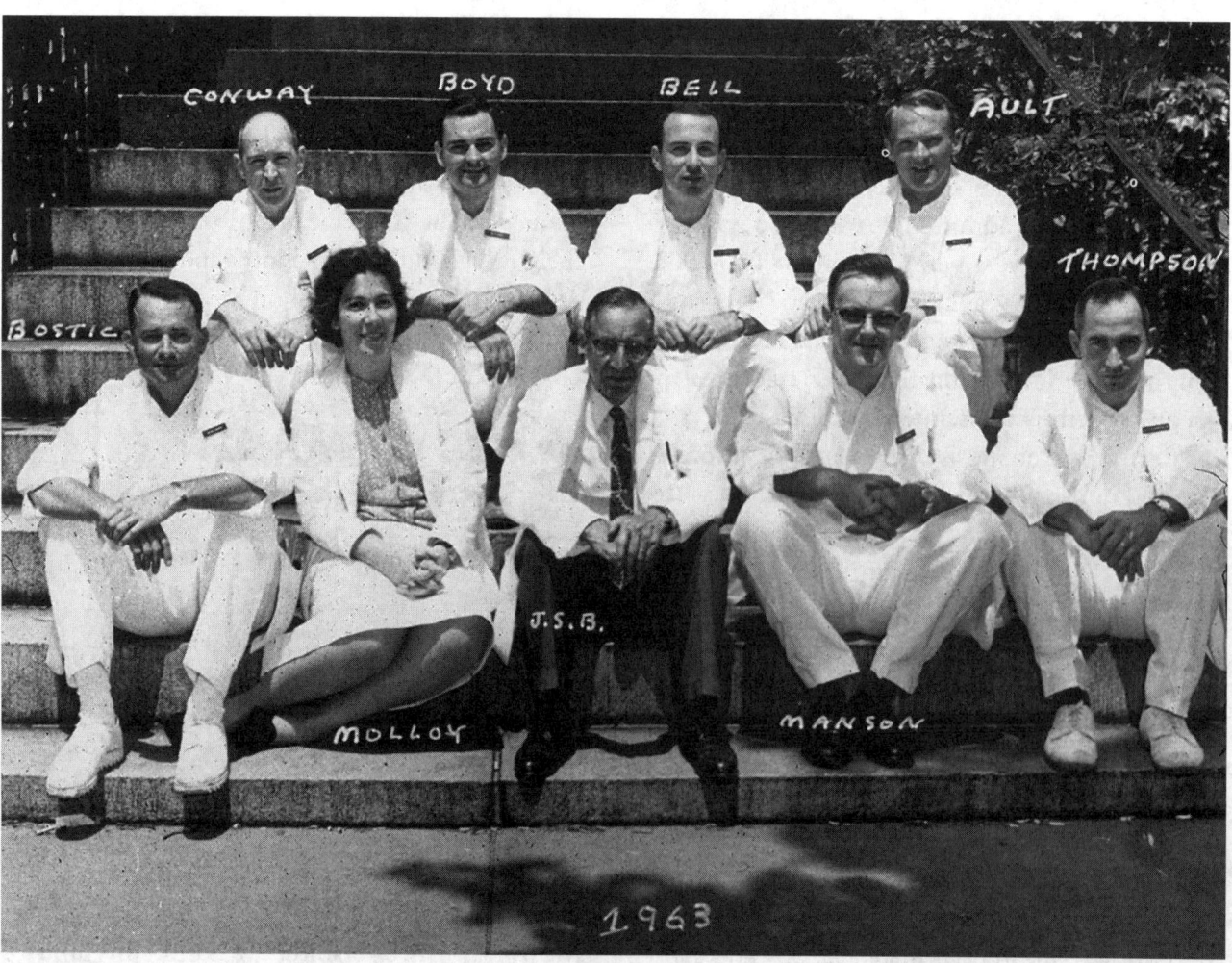

James G. Manson, resident at MGH, 1963. Dr. Molloy was the first known female resident in the HCORP. MGH HCORP Archives.

His work at MIT, which had begun in the MIT Medical clinic, spanned 22 years (he retired from the school in 1999). He was chief of the orthopedic services there, working with Drs. Robert Runyon, Elliott Thrasher, and Ronald Geiger. They worked in both the orthopaedic services and the sports medicine clinics. By 1969, he had become an associate in orthopedic surgery at Children's Hospital. Dr. Art Pappas was acting orthopaedic surgeon-in-chief at the time. His wife recalled that he continued to do "more and more work at MIT" and that "he became very fond of MIT and his experience there was very, very happy" (quoted in A. C. Waugh 2010).

I could not find any publications by Dr. Manson. In the sixth edition of her book *The Encyclopedia of Women's Health*, first published in 1983, Dr. Christine Ammer acknowledges Manson's orthopaedic contributions. In 1983, he cared for Elliot Forbes, the Fanny Peabody Professor of Music at Harvard, who at age 66 fell and fractured his hip while entering Memorial Church to attend a Sunday services.

Around 6:00 p.m. on March 5, 2008, Manson experienced some kind of medical emergency near the Fresh Pond reservoir in Cambridge. Later Chief Reardon wrote in the Cambridge Fire Company's Journal that Manson effusively thanked the emergency responders with the Fire Company and EMS team, who according to Manson provided him with "excellent care" (C. G. Reardon 2008).

Manson spent his leisure time in athletic pursuits. In 1992, at age 68, Manson rowed in the Head of the Charles Regatta in the veteran singles class. He was a member of the Riverside Boat Club in Cambridge. He also enjoyed music, particularly classical music, and this seems to have transferred to his daughter, Anne. She had initially been a premed student at Harvard but then switched to the music program. She trained as a conductor at the Royal College of Music in London and became an internationally recognized conductor, especially in opera. Manson traveled extensively worldwide to see her conduct various orchestras and operas. Manson lived in Deering, New Hampshire, and he spent much of his free time outdoors. He was, according to one source, "devoted" to his family (A. C. Waugh 2010): a son and three daughters, and seven grandchildren.

Manson died at age 78 on December 23, 2009. In the guest book at Manson's memorial service at Christ Church in Cambridge, fellow physician Lyn Dombromski noted that he had spent many years working with Manson in the operating rooms at Mount Auburn Hospital, and he said that Manson was among the "kindest surgeons" he knew ("Dr. James Gavin Manson," n.d.). Dr. William M. Kettyle, Medical Director at MIT Medical, referred to Manson as an "orthopaedic generalist" who sometimes operated but most often evaluated and provided ongoing care for patients with musculoskeletal problems. According to Kettyle, Manson "was an outstanding clinician, caregiver and colleague who served the MIT community for over 30 years" (quoted in A. C. Waugh 2010).

JOHN B. MCGINTY

Physician Snapshot

John B. McGinty
BORN: 1930
DIED: 2019
SIGNIFICANT CONTRIBUTIONS: The first to use a camera at the end of an arthroscope; one of the founders of the Arthroscopy Association of North America and its first president; president of AAOS 1990 and a main leader in the formation of the Academy's Learning Center

John (Jack) B. McGinty was born in the Jamaica Plain neighborhood of Boston November 19, 1930. He was raised by a single mother and attended Boston Latin School. He graduated from Harvard College in 1952 and Tufts University School of Medicine in 1956. While in medical school he was elected into Alpha Omega Alpha. He married Beth A. Dignan the year he graduated from Tufts; with one child already (he and

Beth would eventually have two more), he joined the National Guard to support his family while training to be a surgeon. He was paid $3,000 per year. By contrast, as an intern at Yale's Grace New Haven Hospital in New Haven, Connecticut, he was paid $25 per month. After two years in a general surgery residency at New Haven Hospital, he switched to orthopaedics: "The orthopaedic residents let me do everything" (J. B. McGinty, personal interview with the author, 2009). He applied to the Massachusetts General Hospital/Children's Hospital program; Dr. David Grice interviewed him in Dr. William Green's absence (at the time Green was probably traveling in his role as president of the AAOS). McGinty was accepted and began the three-year program in January 1959. He signed up for the army's deferred service program to obtain financial support and received a captain's salary during his orthopaedic residency; four years after completing his residency, however, he had to repay the army with a year's service for each year in training, plus an additional year.

At the time, the MGH/Children's Hospital residency was a three-year program. McGinty spent the first year at Children's Hospital and the second at MGH; the third year was divided: six months at Children's and six months at the Peter Bent Brigham Hospital (PBBH). When I interviewed him in 2009, McGinty said he received "zero pay" while he was at Children's Hospital. He spent the last six months of his orthopaedic residency at the PBBH and finished in 1961. He recalled that,

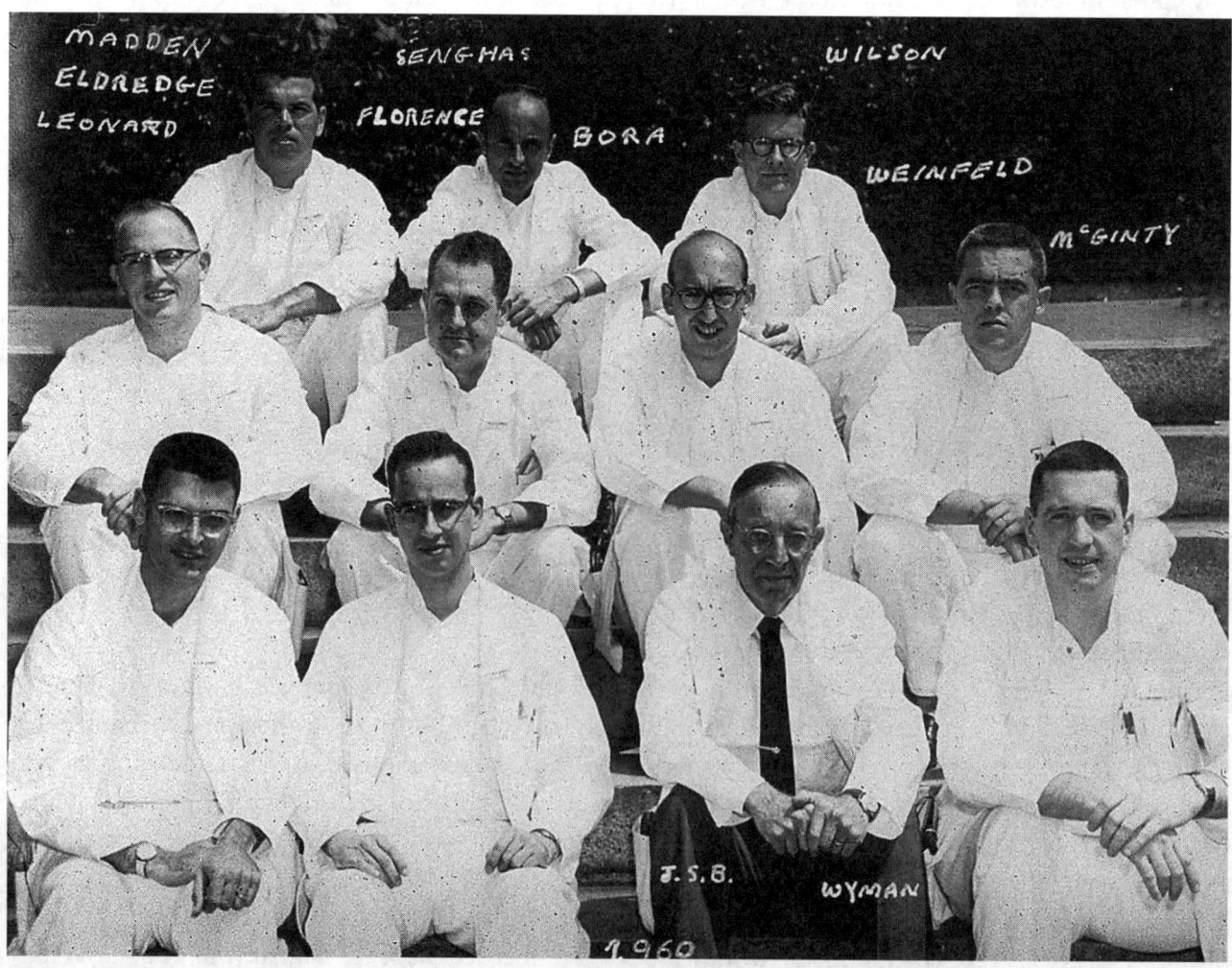

Residents at the MGH with Dr. Barr, 1960. Dr. McGinty is in the second row, on the far right. MGH HCORP Archives.

while at PBBH, "Henry Banks ran the Orthopaedic Service for Dr. Green" (J. B. McGinty, personal interview with the author, 2009), who was the chief of the service and made weekly rounds there. McGinty also worked with Dr. Thomas "Bart" Quigley, who McGinty recalled was a general surgeon who did orthopaedics in the Army and focused on orthopaedic trauma and sports injuries at the PBBH.

McGinty completed his military obligation, spending four years in Frankfurt, Germany, and the fifth and last year at Valley Forge Army Hospital in Phoenixville, Pennsylvania, where he was chief of the orthopaedic service from October 1964 to December 31, 1965. He was discharged with the rank of major in 1966. He was certified by the American Board of Orthopaedic Surgery in 1964.

McGinty returned to Boston after his discharge from the army, and Green asked him to join his practice. He also became the part-time chief at the Veterans Affairs Hospital, started a private practice at Newton-Wellesley Hospital, and joined the part-time staff at Children's Hospital. I was a junior and senior resident at Children's Hospital shortly after McGinty came on as a junior associate of orthopaedic surgery with Dr. Zeke Zimbler. He frequently participated in our daily evening walk rounds; he was an excellent teacher and always helpful to the residents.

McGinty, who was interested in the new technology of arthroscopy, visited his good friend Dr. Robert Jackson in Toronto in 1967. Jackson had learned the technique of arthroscopy when visiting Dr. Masaki Watanabi at Tokyo University. After his return to Toronto, Jackson hired a new associate, Dr. Isso Abe, and together they performed numerous arthroscopic procedures. McGinty did his first operation with an arthroscope at the VA Hospital, after which he began to use arthroscopy in his practice at Newton-Wellesley Hospital. He believes he was the first person to use a camera at the end of an arthroscope, and he reported his experiences in 1975 at the Annual Meeting of Society of the

> ### Arthroscopy of the Knee
> EVALUATION OF AN OUT-PATIENT PROCEDURE UNDER LOCAL ANESTHESIA*
> BY JOHN B. MCGINTY, M.D.†, AND RICHARD A. MATZA, M.D.‡,
> NEWTON LOWER FALLS, MASSACHUSETTS
> THE JOURNAL OF BONE AND JOINT SURGERY
> VOL. 60-A, NO. 6, SEPTEMBER 1978

Title of McGinty's article on knee arthroscopy under local anesthesia. *Journal of Bone and Joint Surgery* 1978; 60: 787.

International Congress of Orthopedics and Traumatology and published an article in the *French Journal of Rheumatology* (all the photographs were black and white.) In 1978, McGinty and R. A. Matza published an arthroscopy procedure done under local anesthesia in the *Journal of Bone and Joint Surgery* (**Box 23.7**).

McGinty continued on the part-time staff at Children's Hospital and the VA Hospital until Dr. John Hall became chief at Children's and Dr. Clement Sledge arrived as chief of orthopaedics at the two Brigham hospitals, in 1971. He remained at Newton-Wellesley Hospital as chief of orthopaedics from 1975 through 1984, and he joined Banks at Tufts University, where he was appointed as a clinical professor of orthopaedic surgery. (Banks had previously left the PBBH to become chief of orthopaedics at Tufts.)

McGinty published ~34 papers during his career; 8 of those were published while he was in Boston. Fourteen were about arthroscopy. He also published two textbooks: The first was the fifth volume of the *Techniques in Orthopaedics* series, entitled *Arthroscopic Surgery Update*, published in 1985. The second, published in 1991, was *Operative Arthroscopy*, which he cowrote with Richard B. Caspari, Robert W. Jackson, and Gary G. Poehling; with a second edition published in 1996 and a third edition in 2003, this was a "classic book, by an international faculty of experts,

Box 23.7. McGinty and Matza's Procedure for Arthroscopy of the Knee

"**Procedure**: With the patient supine, the operating surgeon stands on the same side as the involved knee, and places enough padding under the extended knee to flex it 30 degrees. Ten milliliters of 0.5 per cent Xylocaine without epinephrine is injected into the skin, subcutaneous tissue, joint capsule, and knee joint at a point one centimeter proximal to the joint line, lateral and adjacent to the patellar tendon. A transverse incision one centimeter long is made down to the capsule. The sheath of the arthroscope, with the sharp trocar in place, is introduced 45 degrees from the vertical, horizontal, and coronal planes. It is directed proximally, aimed at the intercondylar notch, and passed through the capsule but not through the synovial membrane. This is accomplished by grasping the sheath in one hand and rotating it with an oscillating motion. The index finger is braced firmly against the skin to prevent plunging the arthroscope too deeply. A definite, sudden release can be felt as the tip of the instrument penetrates the capsule. The sharp trocar then is removed and the sheath with the blunt obturator is pushed through the synovium into the intercondylar notch inferior to the patella. The sheath is passed under the patella into the suprapatellar pouch. The obturator is then removed, and the synovial fluid is allowed to drain off into a basin. The appropriate bridge is attached to the sheath and the arthroscope is inserted and locked into position. Failure to use a bridge is the most common cause of damage to the arthroscope because its end then protrudes beyond the sheath. Prior to attaching the inflow and outflow tubing, ten milliliters of 0.5 per cent Xylocaine is instilled, followed by ten milliliters of 0.5 per cent Marcaine injected directly into the sheath.

"The problems we have encountered during this procedure are as follows:

1. Pain on passage of the sharp trocar through the capsule. For this, more Xylocaine is injected along the outside of the sheath with a spinal needle.
2. Difficulty in entering the knee with the blunt trocar because the patient tightens the quadriceps muscle. This can be overcome by asking the patient to relax and by passively hyperextending the knee while the patella is manipulated.
3. Pain during the procedure. More Xylocaine is instilled in the inflow tubing after the fluid in the knee is evacuated and the outflow valve is closed. The outflow valve is connected to wall suction and is in the open position only when the knee is being evacuated. The inflow valve is open throughout the examination.

"A compression dressing is applied after the arthroscopy, and the patient is discharged from the hospital immediately on leaving the operating room. Crutches are rarely required, and significant postoperative effusion is seldom seen. The patient is advised to remove the compression dressing in forty-eight hours and then to cover the wound with a Band-Aid. The patient can usually return to work on the day following arthroscopy, and is instructed to return in one week for suture removal and for detailed planning of definitive treatment based on the lesion encountered at arthroscopy.

"We have had no difficulty in maneuvering the arthroscope in the knee of a conscious patient. All of our anxious patients were reassured by an explicit explanation and description of the procedure and a confident approach. We now perform arthroscopy routinely under local anesthesia unless an operative procedure is planned immediately thereafter. We avoid the use of a tourniquet because the fiberoptic arthroscopes afford adequate irrigation for good visualization, and the natural color and character of the synovium is more clearly delineated if it is not ischemic. Bleeding was never so excessive as to interfere with visualization. There were some limitations to the procedure as far as seeing the entire knee was concerned, but our view of the lesion was at least as good as with most arthrotomy approaches and equal to that obtained at arthroscopy with general or spinal anesthesia."

—McGinty and Matza 1978

Title of McGinty's AAOS presidential address.
Journal of Bone and Joint Surgery 1990; 72: 482.

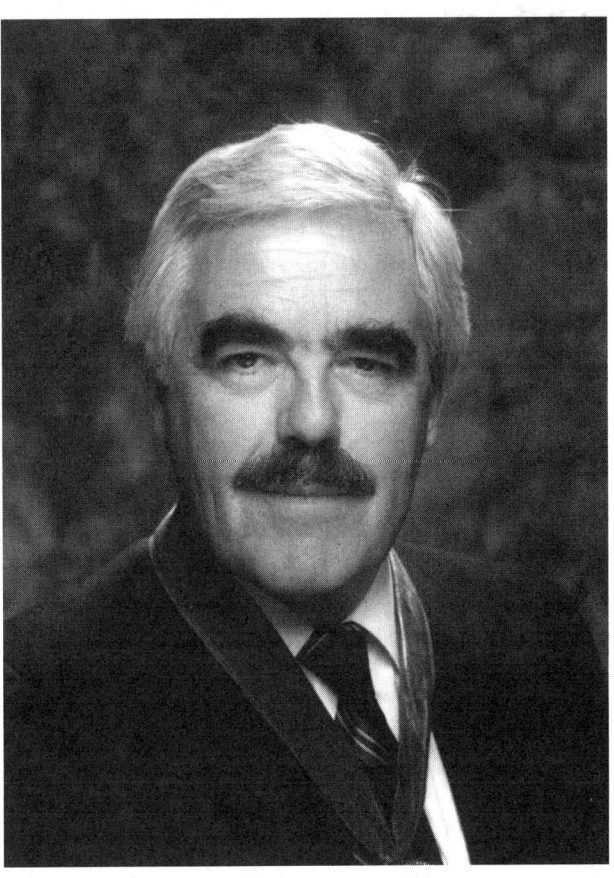

Jack McGinty, AAOS President, 1990. J.C.R., "John B. McGinty, MD 1930-2019," *Journal of Bone and Joint Surgery* 2020; 102: 731.

[which] will continue to serve as the gold standard in operative arthroscopy for quite some time" (W. D. Stanish 1997).

McGinty was for many years the chairman of the American Academy of Orthopaedic Surgeons course titled "Arthroscopy and Arthrography of the Knee." He served as president of three professional organizations: the Arthroscopy Association of North America (1982, one of its founders in 1981), the International Arthroscopy Association (1984–1987), and the American Academy of Orthopaedic Surgeons (1990). He gave the American Academy of Orthopaedic Surgeons First Vice-President's Address in 1990, which was titled "Winds of Change." He addressed major social and economic forces that were affecting orthopaedic practice, including quality assurance, proof of competence, orthopaedic unity and physician reimbursement. Eight years later, in his welcoming remarks to the AAOS class of 1998—"A Single Constant in a World of Change"—he stated: "I don't believe that any of us, at that time [1990], realized just how hard the winds were blowing and how profound the changes in the practice of medicine in this country, and therefore, the practice of orthopaedics, would be in the ensuing eight years" (J. B. McGinty 1998).

In 1984, McGinty left Boston for Charleston, South Carolina, where he became a professor of orthopaedic surgery and the chairman of the Department of Orthopaedic Surgery at the Medical University of South Carolina. Throughout his career, he had been active in numerous orthopaedic associations, including the American Orthopaedic Association, the Association of Bone and Joint Surgeons, the American Medical Association, the American Orthopaedic Society for Sports Medicine, the Eastern Orthopaedic Association, and the Southern Orthopaedic Association. He also served as chief editor of *Orthopaedics Today* (1993–2003).

McGinty remained at the Medical University of South Carolina until his retirement in 1994, when he moved to Mobile, Alabama. There he served as executive vice-president of the Arthroscopy Association of North America from 1995 to 2000. He died in Alabama on November 30, 2019.

ROBERT H. MORRIS

> **Physician Snapshot**
>
> Robert H. Morris
> BORN: 1892
> DIED: 1971
> SIGNIFICANT CONTRIBUTIONS: President of the St. Botolph Club in Boston; president of the medical staff at New England Baptist Hospital; chancellor of King's College Nova Scotia, 1964–69

Robert Hartshorne Morris was born in Shelbourne, Nova Scotia, Canada, on October 8, 1892. His father was a canon in the Church of England. At age 23, Robert enlisted in the Canadian Infantry (112th Battalion) on July 12, 1916, and served in Europe during World War I. After the war, he attended King's College in Halifax and graduated from the University of Toronto Medical School in 1922 at the age of 30.

Little is known about Morris's life. He had completed an internship in Buffalo, New York, and had worked at Doctor's Hospital in New York City before moving to Boston, where he joined a private practice at 319 Longwood Avenue. In 1929, he married Miriam Morss, and they lived on Beacon Hill at 58 Brimmer Street.

He was on the staff at Children's Hospital for many years. During my research, I found only that Morris had been named a junior assistant orthopaedic surgeon in 1926, after volunteering as an assistant in the outpatient department for a few years. In 1929, he worked under Dr. S. M. Fitchet. Associate surgeons at Children's Hospital at that time included Drs. Arthur Legg (chapter 18), James Sever (chapter 17), Henry FitzSimmons (described earlier in this chapter), and Frank Ober (chapter 20). Morris then became an associate visiting surgeon with Dr. William Green, during Dr. Robert Osgood's tenure as chief of the Orthopaedic Service.

By 1933, Morris had been promoted to assistant orthopaedic surgeon at Children's Hospital and instructor in orthopaedics at Harvard Medical School. In that year, he published his only article in the literature: "Foot Stabilization: A Review of Fifty-Two Operations." This article was part of the *New England Journal of Medicine*'s tribute to Dr. Osgood. Morris analyzed in detail the outcomes of 52 arthrodesis procedures: subastragalar arthrodesis, Hoke stabilization, and triple arthrodesis. Summarizing Dr. Hoke's four requirements for a foot to be considered stabilized, Morris (1933) suggested that they could be:

> summed up by good function and good appearance…In this series every good-looking foot is a good functioning foot. There are, however, thirty-one operated feet which have good function, but owing to some deformity were not so good-looking…the question to be answered is, would these thirty-one operated feet have functioned better without the deformity. The answer seems to be strongly in the affirmative. In other words, the better the appearance, the better the function.
>
> A perfect postoperative foot must of necessity vary from the normal in two ways. One, the foot will look short. Two, the relationship of the malleoli and astragalus to the calcis will be slightly anterior to the normal.

Morris (1933) explained a unique observation he had recognized while reviewing patients' records:

> the postoperative deformities have been considered with great care and perhaps too great severity, so that a casual glance at the chart gives the impression that the results are very unsatisfactory. However, a closer inspection shows the reverse to be true…Sixteen (30%) of all operated feet show no postoperative deformity and are considered perfect both as regards appearance and function. These perfect feet all have good backward displacement, solid bony fusion and perfect or almost perfect muscle balance, laterally and anteroposteriorly…Absence

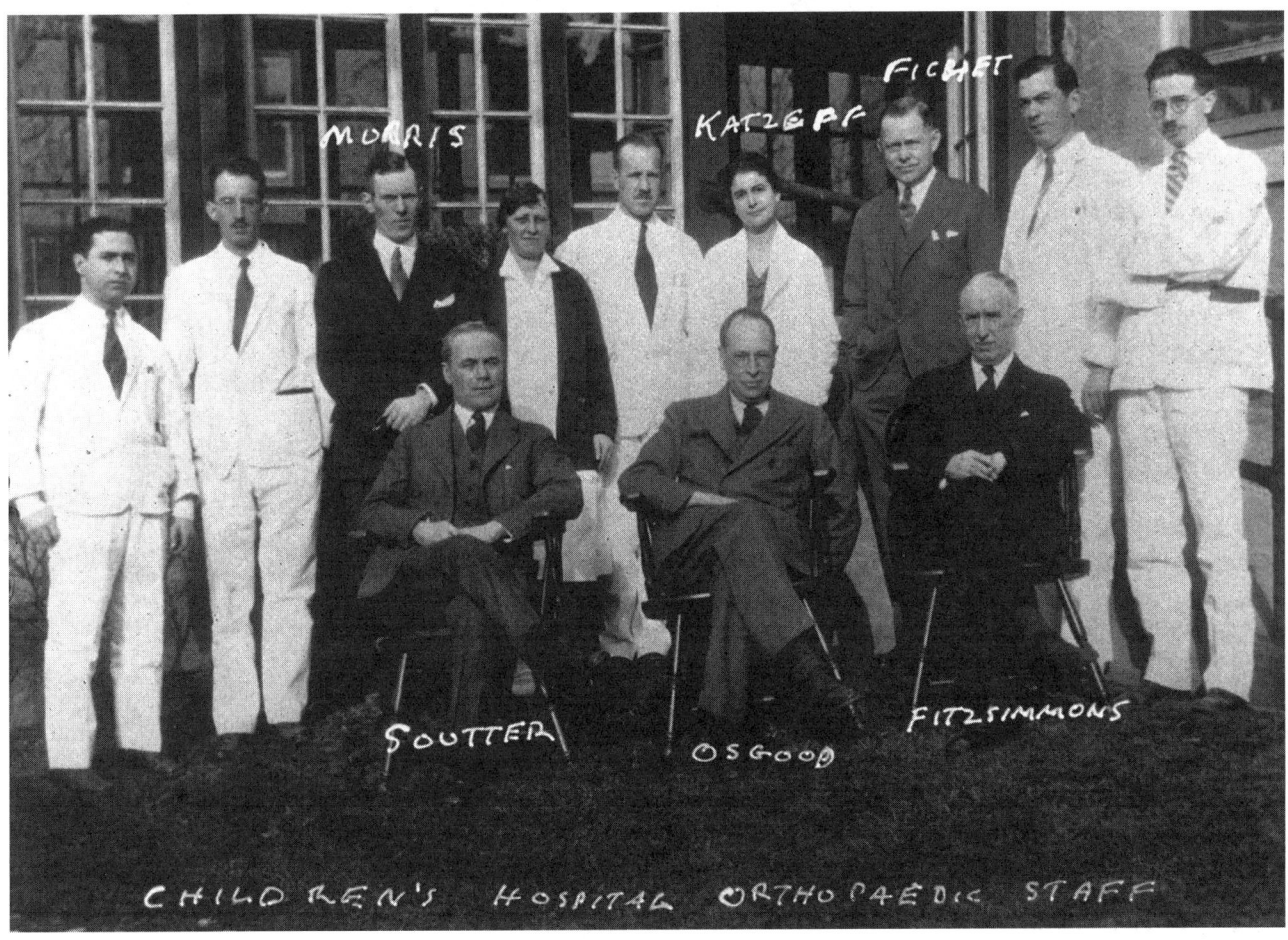

Orthopaedic staff at BCH. Robert H. Morris is standing in the back row, third from the left. MGH HCORP Archives.

of backward displacement, failure of complete fusion and imperfect muscle balance account for all the deformities.

In that publication, he also described two methods surgeons at Children's Hospital used to "assure maintenance of backward displacement – 1. Postoperative repositioning of the foot as advocated by Dr. Hoke when he devised his operation for foot stabilization. 2. Counter-sinking the astragalus into the os calcis as devised by Dr. A. H. Brewster in his modification of Dr. Hoke's procedure" (R. H. Morris 1933).

Morris (1933) documented that solid fusion was obtained in 90% of the cases clinically, but in only 80% when considering evidence on roentgenograms: "ten per cent have fibrous union so solid that manipulation cannot produce lateral mobility. Ten per cent…show complete failure to fuse both clinically and by x-ray." For Morris (1933), "This failure to obtain fusion is due to 1. Insufficient removal of cartilage at time of operation. 2. Inadequate immobilization following the operation." He also noted that some surgeons at the time doubted the value of balancing the foot with tendon transplantations, and he reported 32 successful transplantations with an arthrodesis: "It is shown that the anterior and posterior tibial muscles as well as the peroneals can be used as dorsi-flexors of the foot or placed in the os calcis to act as plantar-flexors. In only three cases is it impossible to demonstrate muscle action in the transplanted tendon…It is…nevertheless most gratifying to find that not a single patient complains of pain" (R. H. Morris 1933).

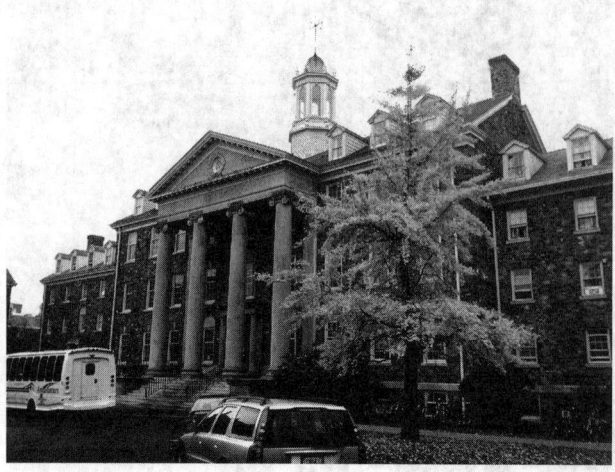

King's College, Nova Scotia. Mathew Ingram/Wikimedia Commons.

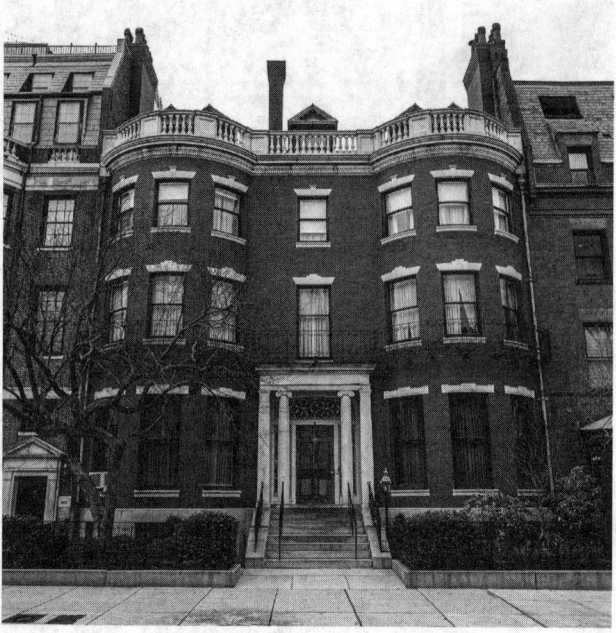

St. Botolph Club, Boston. Kael E. Randall/Kael Randall Images.

At the end of the article, Morris (1933) made the following conclusions:

1. A good-looking foot is a good functioning foot.
2. A perfect postoperative foot must have
   a. Good backward displacement
   b. Solid fusion
   c. Perfect or nearly perfect muscle balance
2. Failure to maintain backward displacement is the greatest single cause of postoperative deformity.
3. Slight muscle imbalance is of no consequence in a well-fused and backwardly displaced foot. Whereas with non fusion, slight muscle imbalance will cause marked deformity with sometimes great overgrowth of new bone.
4. That arthrodesis combined with tendon transplantation is an ideal method for procuring good function and good appearance in a stabilized foot.

Morris eventually moved to an office at 253 Newbury Street. In addition to being on the staff at Children's Hospital, he was an orthopaedic surgeon at the Long Island Hospital and a member of the Board of Medical Advisors for the Industrial School for Crippled Children. Early on, in 1937, he joined the corporation running the New England Baptist Hospital, and almost 30 years later (1964–65) he served as president of its medical staff.

Dr. William Green, in his annual department report in 1960, stated: "Dr. Albert H. Brewster and Dr. Robert Morris, long senior members of our staff, were each promoted to Orthopedic Surgeon, Emeritus, after many years of service to the Hospital. The Hospital is indebted to them. They gave much to it over the years and we will miss their active participation." From 1964 to 1969, Morris was chancellor of King's College in Nova Scotia. He had been an active member of the American Medical Association, the American Academy of Orthopaedic Surgeons, and the American College of Surgeons. He was also a trustee of the Berwick Academy in Berwick, Maine. He also had served as president of the St. Botolph Club in Boston.

Morris died at age 78 on August 2, 1971, at the New England Baptist Hospital. He left behind his second wife, Katherine, whom he married in 1957 (his first wife had predeceased him), a daughter, and six grandchildren.

ARTHUR M. PAPPAS

Physician Snapshot

Arthur M. Pappas
BORN: 1931
DIED: 2016
SIGNIFICANT CONTRIBUTIONS: Pioneered sports medicine in the US by beginning the first athletic injury clinic at Children's Hospital (with Quigley and Boland); founding chair of the Department of Orthopaedics and Physical Rehabilitation at University of Massachusetts

Arthur Michael Pappas was born July 3, 1931, in Auburn, Massachusetts. His parents had immigrated from Albania, and he was the youngest of three children (Alex was nine years older, and Athena was eight years older). Their "father farmed the land and ran a grocery store" (quoted in C. K. Harris 2010). Arthur attended public schools in Auburn, and in high school he played numerous sports, and he played them well. He graduated in 1949. He received a football scholarship to Harvard College, and he played on the team with Ted Kennedy. Arthur played on the freshman football team, the Yardlings, and in a 1949 game against Army, the team "scored their first touchdown in the second period on a short buck by Art Pappas." They went on to defeat Exeter, 27–7. In Harvard's last game against Army—an ongoing rivalry since 1895—Arthur scored in the second half when he recovered a teammate's fumble inside Army's end zone. Harvard won, 22–21—only its 17th victory in the 49-year series.

Arthur graduated from Harvard in 1953 with a bachelor of arts degree and went on to the University of Rochester Medical School. He received his MD degree in 1957 and promptly joined the US Navy; he was assigned to serve at the Naval Hospital in Bethesda, Maryland. In a 2010 article for the *Auburn Daily Voice*, reporter C. K. Harris interviewed Pappas, who remembered well his time there: "It was excellent. I was in charge of a program devoted to tissue grafting."

He reported the results of his research at Bethesda in a paper he presented at the Surgical Forum of the American College of Surgeons in 1959 and subsequently published in 1961 as "Acceleration of Skin Graft Closure." He had spread a regenerated collagen film on wounds in animals that had been treated with cortisone (to delay wound healing). This film essentially ignored the cortisone and the defects closed to an extent similar to that in animals that hadn't received cortisone. He also observed—by applying cultured cells onto the collagen film—substantial wound closure occurred even in the presence of cortisone, and to an extent that exceeded the amount of closure in non-cortisone-treated animals.

After two years at Bethesda Naval Hospital, Pappas moved to Boston to become a resident in the Boston Children's Hospital/Massachusetts General Hospital orthopaedic training program. In his first role as an assistant resident, he worked in the orthopaedic laboratories at Children's Hospital (July–December 1960), where his interest in research continued. Over the next 10 years, Pappas would publish 15 basic science papers on topics ranging from congenital malformations, toxicity of metal particles, and bone grafting and bone storage to the treatment of fat embolism and gas gangrene and the effect of delayed manipulation on fracture healing.

Pappas began his orthopaedic clinical training at Children's Hospital on April 1, 1961. After rotations at the MGH, Children's, and the Peter Bent Brigham Hospital, he completed his training and, in 1965, joined the staff at the Children's Hospital (as a junior associate in orthopedic surgery) and at the Peter Bent Brigham Hospital, where he stayed for 10 years. In addition to his research publications during this period, he also published a few articles on pediatric orthopaedics.

Upon the retirement of Dr. William Green in the late 1960s, Dr. Leonard Cronkhite, the president of Children's Hospital and a friend of Pappas's, named Pappas the interim orthopaedic surgeon-in-chief (about 1969). During his stint as

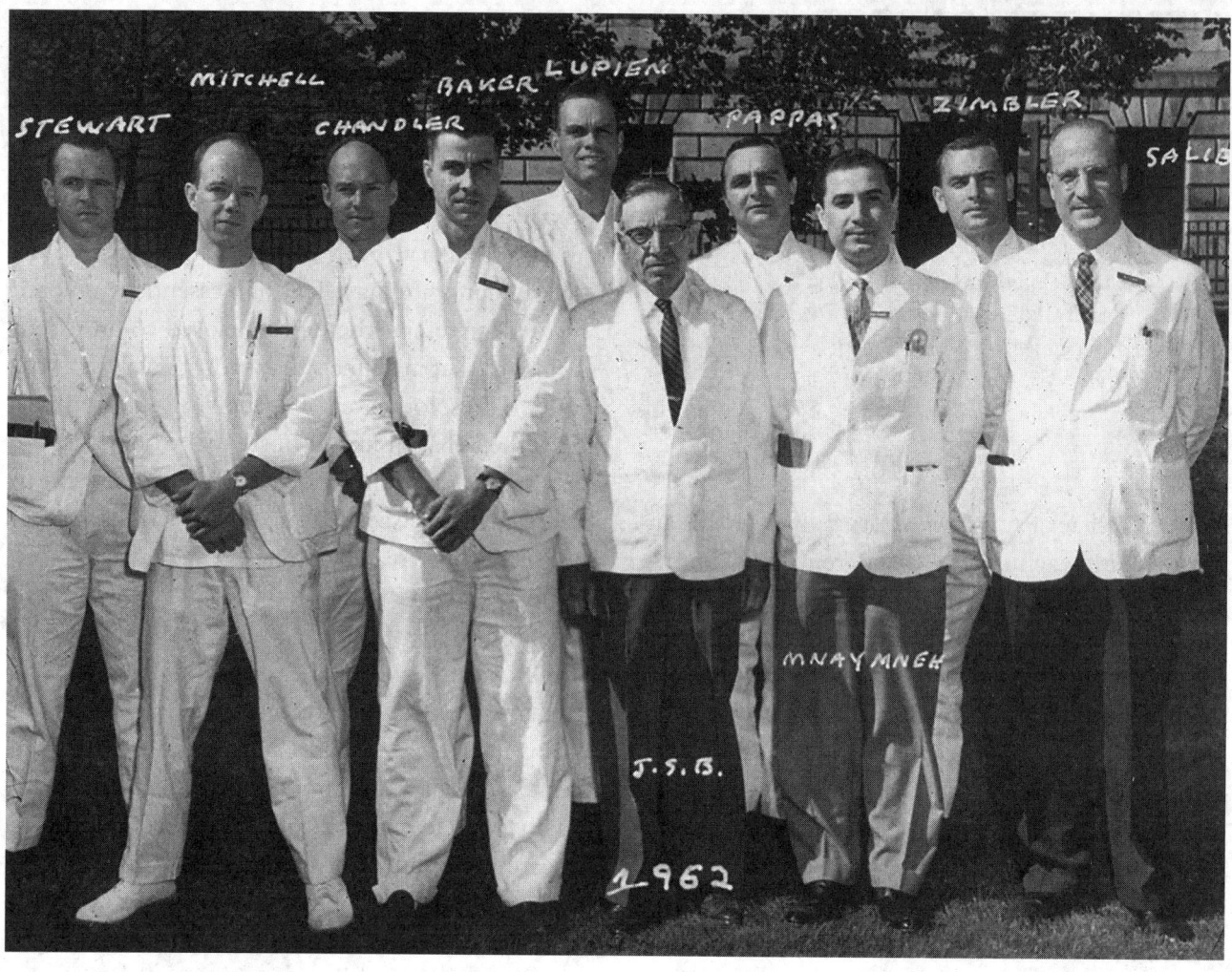

Orthopaedic residents with Dr. Barr, 1962. Dr. Pappas is in the back row, second from the right. MGH HCORP Archives.

interim chief, Pappas hired Drs. Robert Keller and Ben Bierbaum. Many years later, an interviewer asked Dr. Arthur Trott about Green's choice for his successor. (Trott was, at the time, on the full-time staff at Children's with Green, Pappas, and Griffin; his biography is included in this chapter.) Trott replied:

> Actually, he couldn't make up his mind… he recommended a successor, I guess. He picked Paul Griffin and Arthur Pappas as co-administrators. That didn't work out too well…There was always friction between the two…Eventually that broke up and Griffin left. Then finally Pappas left…They were both good surgeons. But Pappas saw the writing on the wall: This dual approach wasn't going to work out. So, he went to the University of Massachusetts and made a great name for himself there. (D. Dyer 1993)

In the end, Dr. Mel Glimcher became the new orthopaedic surgeon-in-chief and Dr. John Hall was recruited from Toronto as the clinical chief of the department; Edward Riseborough was recruited from MGH at that time as well. Pappas remained on the clinical staff at Children's for about six months, and although he had a huge practice and co-existed well with the new leadership, he left Children's to head the orthopaedic department at the University of Massachusetts.

THE EFFECT OF DELAYED MANIPULATION UPON THE RATE OF FRACTURE HEALING

ARTHUR M. PAPPAS, M.D., and ERIC RADIN, M.D., Boston, Massachusetts

Surgery, Gynecology & Obstetrics · June 1968

Title of Pappas' article on the positive effect on fracture healing by delayed manipulation. *Surgery, Gynecology and Obstetrics* 1968; 126: 1287.

Experimental Congenital Malformations of the Motorskeletal System*

ARTHUR M. PAPPAS, M.D.

Clinical Orthopaedics and Related Research
Number 59
July-August, 1968

Title of Pappas' research article on congenital malformations. *Clinical Orthopaedics and Related Research* 1968; 59: 249.

I worked with Pappas in the late 1960s. He was a favorite of the residents. When they were responsible for evaluating complex patients or planning a presentation of those patients at grand rounds or to Dr. Green's chief's clinic, they would often ask Pappas for assistance. He had great recall of many of these complex cases, including the patients' history and previous treatments. For example, Pappas cared for a patient who was born in April 1968 with severe arthrogryposis multiplex congenita and rushed to Children's Hospital not a day after he had been born and was admitted for the entirety of the next three months. With pins in his legs and placed in traction, daily physical therapy, casts on his extremities until age eight months, the child's family relied on Pappas during his treatment, which continued at the University of Massachusetts after Pappas moved there. The patient's parents said that often "only Dr. Pappas seemed to know what to do" (Reese and Reese 1995). The patient continued to received care from Pappas, along with prolonged physical therapy and a rare surgery, until he was 26, had graduated from Western New England College, and was married and working.

While at Children's Hospital, Pappas was a consultant for the Massachusetts Department of Public Health's crippled children's clinics in Haverhill with Dr. Green and in Lowell with Dr. Albert Brewster. In 1970, Pappas, Dr. T. B. Quigley, and Dr. Art Boland started an athletic injury clinic at Children's Hospital, "the only clinic of its kind in New England" ("Notices" 1970). These three surgeons also cared for the Harvard athletic teams at Dillon Field House. Interestingly, Pappas initially was of the opinion "that a sports clinic wouldn't work" (Lyle Micheli, personal interview with the author, 2011), mainly because he believed that every orthopaedist thought they could do everything.

Although this clinic was the first pediatric sports medicine clinic in the nation, it wasn't until the mid-1980s that sports medicine, with the support of Dr. John Hall, developed at Children's Hospital with the formation of a sports foundation by Dr. Lyle Micheli. Pappas's interest in sports increased rapidly. Clare McCarthy, head of physical therapy and an ice skater, recalled a patient she helped to see Pappas. That patient, also an ice skater, was having "difficulty landing jumps and had seen everyone in Boston" (McCarthy and Cassella, personal interview with the author, 2012). Pappas was just out of his residency. "He operated on her for a Morton's neuroma and she got back to skating" (McCarthy and Cassella, personal interview with the author, 2012). Pappas soon began seeing national and international skaters, and he often went to their rinks to watch them skate. By the time Pappas left Children's Hospital, he had published just one paper in sports medicine.

Career after Children's Hospital

Pappas left Children's for the University of Massachusetts around 1973; there he was appointed as a professor of orthopaedic surgery—the first at the university's medical school. In 1976, he was named the first chairman of the Department of Orthopaedics and Physical Rehabilitation. Once there, he continued to make a name for himself in sports medicine. He also became a limited partner in the Boston Red Sox. Beginning in 1977—and for the next 25 years—Pappas was the team's medical director, caring for the players and running the health-care-related resources at Fenway Park. Claire McCarthy recalled that Pappas approached her in the late 1970s about possibly giving a talk on normal shoulder anatomy and function before he presented a lecture on shoulder and elbow injuries to the Physical Therapy Association. That reconnection, years after Pappas had left Children's Hospital, provided a chance for McCarthy to evaluate shoulder injuries among the Boston Red Sox pitchers. Somewhat controversial in his role as medical director and his limited partnership with the Red Sox, Pappas treated many famous players—Roger Clemens, "Oil Can" Boyd, Nomar Garciaparra, Marty Barrett, Andre Dawson, Dennis Eckersley, Jim Rice, and many others—and he often made headlines.

He stepped down as chairman of the UMass Department of Orthopaedics and Physical Rehabilitation in 2001. During his tenure in that role and as a medical director of the Red Sox, he published an additional 11 papers on pediatric orthopaedic topics and 17 articles on sports medicine that concentrated mainly on pitching and the associated mechanics, and problems related to the shoulder, elbow, and wrist. In 1996, he coedited a book with Janet Walzer, *Upper Extremity Injuries in the Athlete*. Dr. Michael Wirth, in his 1996 review of the book, stated: "An exceptionally well written chapter is devoted to the physically challenged athlete...This book...provides the necessary guidelines for proper diagnosis, preventive measures, and rehabilitation, but it falls short in its coverage of operative treatment and could be enhanced by including the author's preferred operative technique for some of the more common injuries.

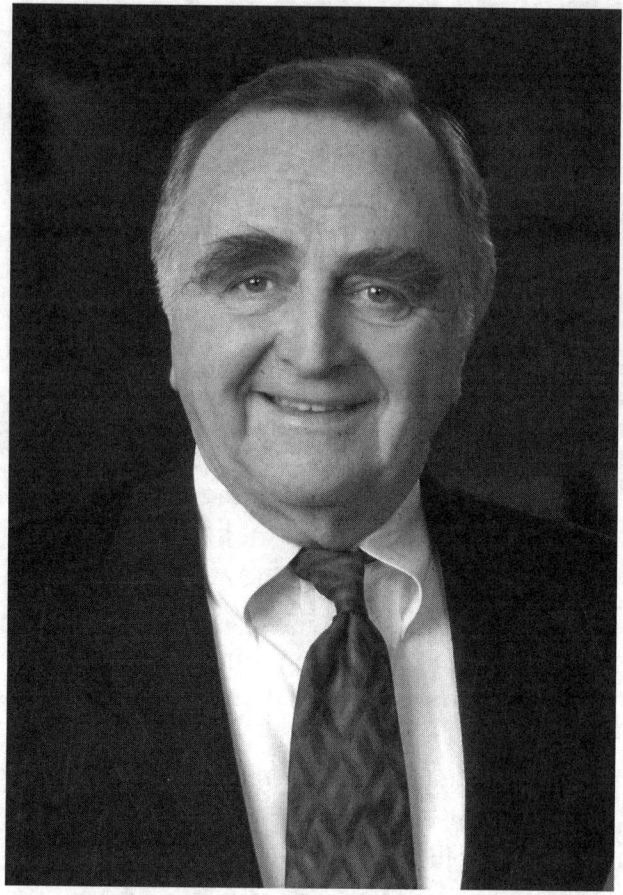

Arthur M. Pappas. Courtesy of University of Massachusetts Medical School.

Title of Pappas' article on the mechanics of pitching. *American Journal of Sports Medicine* 1985; 13: 216.

Box 23.8. Some of Arthur Pappas's Professional Leadership Positions

- President, Board of Directors of the Amateur Sports Foundation
- President, Association of Professional Baseball Physicians
- Chairman, Board of Trustees of the Massachusetts Hospital School for Handicapped Children
- Acting Director of Family Services, Massachusetts State Health Department
- President, Orthopedic Section of the American Academy of Pediatrics
- Member, Board of Overseers of the Jimmy Fund, Dana Farber Cancer Institute

Pappas served in numerous leadership positions (**Box 23.8**). He and his wife, Martha, received numerous individual and combined awards in their community and the region. Martha Pappas had a PhD in education and taught high-school English. She became department chair of the Career Exploration Program and wrote a book, *Heroes of the American West*. Living in Auburn, where they had met while in high school, they contributed enormous amounts of money and time to the area. For example, Pappas was awarded a Lifetime Achievement Award from the Massachusetts Medical Society in 2011, and the Worcester State College 2008 Community Service Award was given to Dr. Arthur and Dr. Martha Pappas because they "exemplify extraordinary leadership in community involvement in education, medicine, athletics, recreation and culture" (Ashley 2011).

Pappas died on March 22, 2016, at the University of Massachusetts Medical Center. He was 84 years old. Millis remembered Pappas as a "good clinician [who was] very thoughtful and knew his patients well" and noted that Pappas had been "very supportive of education and patient care" (Millis, personal interview with the author, 2012).

ROBERT C. RUNYON

Physician Snapshot

Robert C. Runyon
BORN: 1928
DIED: 2012
SIGNIFICANT CONTRIBUTIONS: Strong interest in the field of sports medicine; team physician for the Boston University football team; on the medical staff of the MIT orthopaedic and sports clinics

Little information is recorded about Dr. Robert Chase Runyon. He was born on September 13, 1928. He graduated from Columbia College in 1950 with a bachelor of arts degree, and from Cornell Medical College in 1954. After a year-long surgical internship at Bellevue Hospital, his residency training was complex and varied because he was unable to decide on a specialty: general surgery, neurosurgery, or orthopaedic surgery. He completed a second year of surgical training at Bellevue and then switched to the neurosurgery program (Cornell Service) at Bellevue for yet another year. From 1959 to 1960, he was a fellow in neurology at New York Hospital; following that, he spent two years (through 1962) as a resident in surgery there.

It was during that time that he applied for a residency in orthopaedic surgery through the Massachusetts General Hospital/Children's Hospital Program. He was accepted, and his subsequent orthopaedic training included 18 months (July 1962 to July 1963 and July to December 1964) at Children's Hospital and 24 months (July 1963 to July 1964 and January through December 1965) at Massachusetts General Hospital.

Runyon was 37 years old when he started his private practice in Boston, at 319 Longwood Avenue; he lived in Concord, about 25 miles northwest of Boston. In 1966, he was admitted into the Massachusetts Medical Society. Runyon was Board Certified by the American Board of Orthopaedic Surgery and a fellow of the American College of Surgeons. He held staff positions at Children's

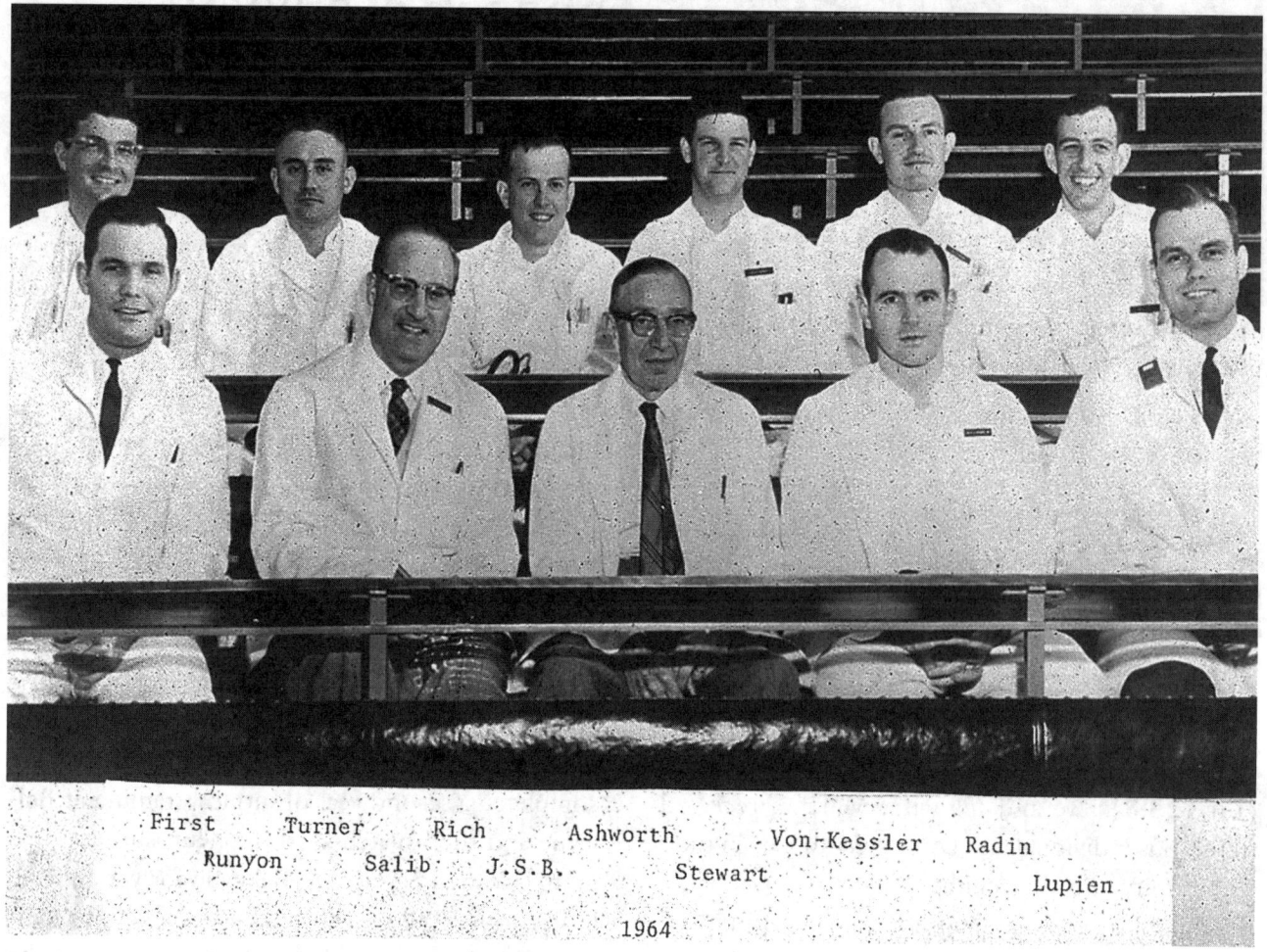

Orthopaedic residents at MGH with Dr. Barr, 1964. Robert C. Runyon is in the front row, far left. MGH HCORP Archives.

Hospital, Brigham and Women's Hospital, and the New England Baptist Hospital. He occasionally admitted patients to Children's Hospital while I was a resident there. He was a slow, meticulous, and often indecisive surgeon.

Runyon had been interested in sports medicine since he began his training, and he eventually became the team physician for the Boston University football team. In 1976, he admitted a 20-year-old sophomore linebacker to Children's Hospital; the player had broken his left leg in a game, which Runyon had treated in a temporary cast. The next day, the patient unexpectedly experienced a high fever upon receiving anesthesia; he died from acute hyperthermia, caused by an uncommon genetic condition that causes such an adverse reaction to anesthesia.

Runyon began on the medical staff at MIT in 1968 and remained there for more than 25 years. His appointment was half-time, and he provided clinical care in the Orthopedic Services and Sports Medicine clinics; during that time, he practiced with Drs. James Manson (described earlier in this chapter), Elliott Thrasher, and Ronald Geiger. "In 1982, when MIT realized the clinic was overstaffed" (*Runyon v. Massachusetts Institute of Technology* 1994), it reduced the orthopaedic staff in its clinics, retaining Runyon, Thrasher, and Geiger in the Sports Medicine Clinic but only Manson continued in the Orthopedic Services Clinic. Six years later, in 1988, MIT again had to reduce staff in the Sports Clinic; just two orthopaedic surgeons—Thasher and Geiger—were retained:

in view of their record of timeliness, cross-coverage, and continuity of treatment...[and because they also] worked out of the same office at Mount Auburn Hospital...Although Runyon provided evidence that his performance was timely and effective, MIT contends that he would often run late and that some athletes, refusing to wait for Runyon, would leave the clinic without seeing an orthopaedist...In 1988 Runyon underwent coronary bypass surgery and...went on leave for two months. When [he]...returned to work, he was told of the decision to consolidate the clinic...in September 1988...and Runyon was removed from his duties related to the Sports Medicine Clinic, but continued to work in MIT's Medical Department on a half-time basis...In the late 1980s the Medical Department Planning Committee...concluded that the Medical Department was overstaffed [and] reduce[d] each specialty area by one half-time appointment...[T]he Planning Committee then decided to eliminate Runyon's half-time position. (*Runyon v. Massachusetts Institute of Technology* 1994)

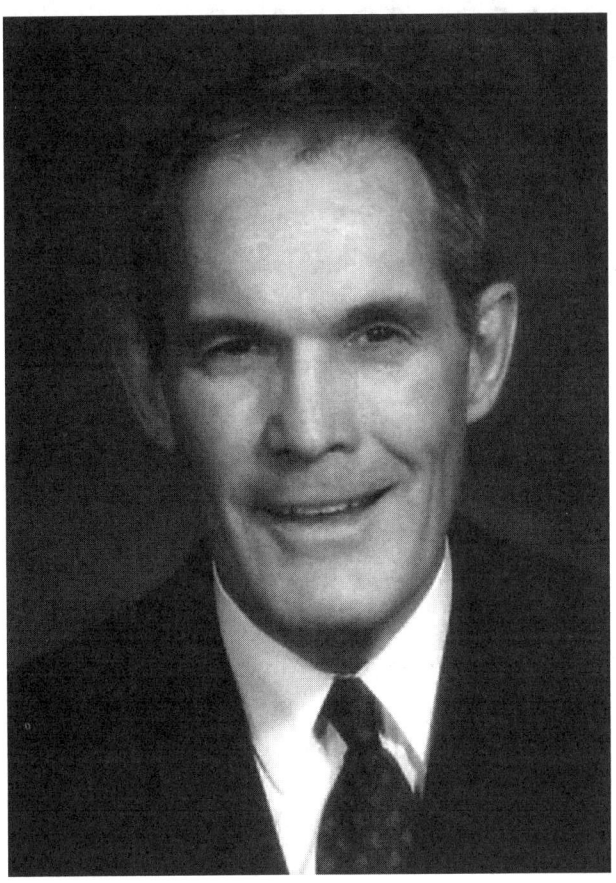

Robert C. Runyon. Courtesy of Dr. Scott Runyon.

Concerned about his retirement benefits, Runyon began negotiations with MIT. MIT stated that in September 1991, he "would be placed on a leave of absence...[but hold] a half-time appointment for purposes of benefits...He works on an emergency on-call basis only...On September 10, 1990, Runyon filed an administrative complaint against MIT with the Massachusetts Commission Against Discrimination...alleging age and handicap discrimination...He commenced this civil action in March 1992 (*Runyon v. Massachusetts Institute of Technology* 1994). On December 27, 1994, the US District Court ruled that the defendant's (MIT's) "summary judgment must be granted" (*Runyon v. Massachusetts Institute of Technology* 1994).

During his career, Runyon published only one paper (while he had been interested in general surgery), and practiced only orthopaedics for more than 50 years. Runyon's son Scott followed in his father's footsteps and attended Weill Cornell Medical College. He recalled that his father "instilled in him a commitment to compassionate medical care...[and that if Cornell Medical School] gave him [Robert] the sense of altruism and integrity that he had his whole life, that's where I wanted to be" ("Scott Runyon" 2013). Scott also remembered his father's slow decline from dementia in his later years, when he experienced memory loss and paranoia and "was in need of the same compassionate care he had provided to decades of patients" ("Scott Runyon" 2013).

Runyon died on January 16, 2012, at the age of 84, survived by his wife, Lucia; four children; and three grandchildren. He is remembered as "a man of impeccable character, integrity and kindness...[and] helped to usher in sports medicine to numerous Boston institutions" ("Obituaries: Robert Chase Runyon" 2012).

ROBERT SOUTTER

Physician Snapshot

Robert Soutter
BORN: 1870
DIED: 1933
SIGNIFICANT CONTRIBUTIONS: Developed procedures for treating hip contractures in poliomyelitis and a dislocated patella; designed a portable traction device for treating fractures and for use in operations on the lower extremity; designed an apparatus for correcting scoliosis; published his only book, *Technique of Operations on the Bones, Joints, Muscles and Tendons*, in 1917

Robert Soutter was born October 4, 1870, and raised in Kingston, New York, the son of Robert and Charlotte (Lamar) Soutter. Educated at Harvard, he graduated from Harvard Medical School in 1898. After graduation, he described his surgical training for the school report of the medical school class of 1898: "I have been house officer at the Children's Hospital. I am now House Surgeon at the Boston City Hospital, [and] my service of two years will end in July" (Caustic and Claflin 1902). Soutter returned to Children's Hospital after his training, where he practiced for his entire career, which spanned more than 30 years. He partnered in private practice with Dr. Edward Bradford, who was also on staff at Children's. Soutter's office was at 133 Newbury Street; he lived at 53 Hereford Street in Boston and had a summer home at Four Winds Farm, Walpole.

He held other appointments at Boston-area institutions, including as surgeon-in-chief at the House of the Good Samaritan and the Massachusetts Hospital for Cripples, orthopaedic surgeon at both the Long Island Hospital and the New England Peabody Home for Crippled Children, and district physician at the Boston Dispensary. He was also a member of various professional organizations (**Box 23.9**). He served as vice president of the American Orthopaedic Association in 1933. He was also a member of the Harvard Tennis and Racquet Club and the Union Club.

Box 23.9. Robert Soutter's Professional Memberships

- Massachusetts Medical Society
- American College of Surgeons
- American Orthopaedic Association
- American Medical Association
- Société des Chirurgie
- Société Internationale de Chirurgie Orthopedique
- Boston Surgical Society
- Boston Orthopedic Society
- Eastern Interurban Orthopedic Society
- Boston City Hospital Alumni Association
- Boston Children's Hospital Alumni Association

Soutter was married to Helen E. Whiteside of Cedar Island, Lake Champlain, New York, and they had four children: Robert Jr., Lamar, James, and Anne. Lamar became a successful surgeon and educator (**Box 23.10**).

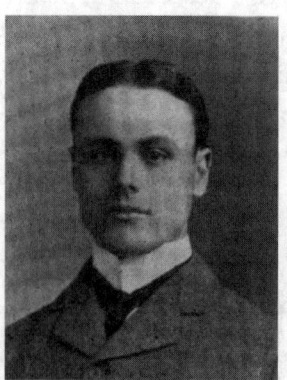 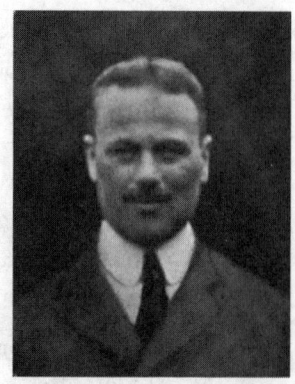

Robert Soutter as a young man and later in life.
Robert Soutter Photographs. Class of 1894—25th Anniversary Report. HUD 294.25. Harvard University Archives.

Box 23.10. Lamar Soutter

Lamar Soutter, Robert Soutter's second son, was born in 1909. Like his father, he graduated from both Harvard College (1931) and Harvard Medical School (1935). He received training in thoracic surgery in New York. He returned to Boston on the surgical staff at MGH where he founded the blood bank and became its first director.

Lamar served active duty during World War II, and "he was awarded the Silver Star for actions at the Battle of Bastogne" in Belgium ("Lamar Soutter" [Wikipedia], n.d.). After the war, he was an associate professor of surgery at Boston University School of Medicine, where he became associate dean in 1955 and then dean in 1960. In 1963, he was recruited to become the founding dean of the University of Massachusetts Medical School. In 1968, he presented the Annual Discourse to the Massachusetts Medical Society; it was entitled "Medical Education and the University (1901–1968)." In 1981, the UMass Medical School Library was named in his honor.

Innovation and Research

Soutter actively presented and published new contributions in various areas of orthopaedic surgery. His first publications were in 1906, a few years after he started practicing. He wrote a detailed critical analysis of shoes and their effects on feet and gait, stating: "A very large proportion of trouble with feet is caused by shoes…Notice on the street how few people walk unconscious of their feet and how awkwardly because of shoes…The shoe should be flexible. Heavy and stiff soles should be avoided" (R. Soutter 1906a).

That year he also reported 25 consecutive cases of subtrochanteric osteotomy in adults to correct severe deformity, especially flexion/adduction contractures secondary to hip disease:

> The operation consisted of linear osteotomy… abduction to nearly 45° without flexion and without outward rotation was the position for

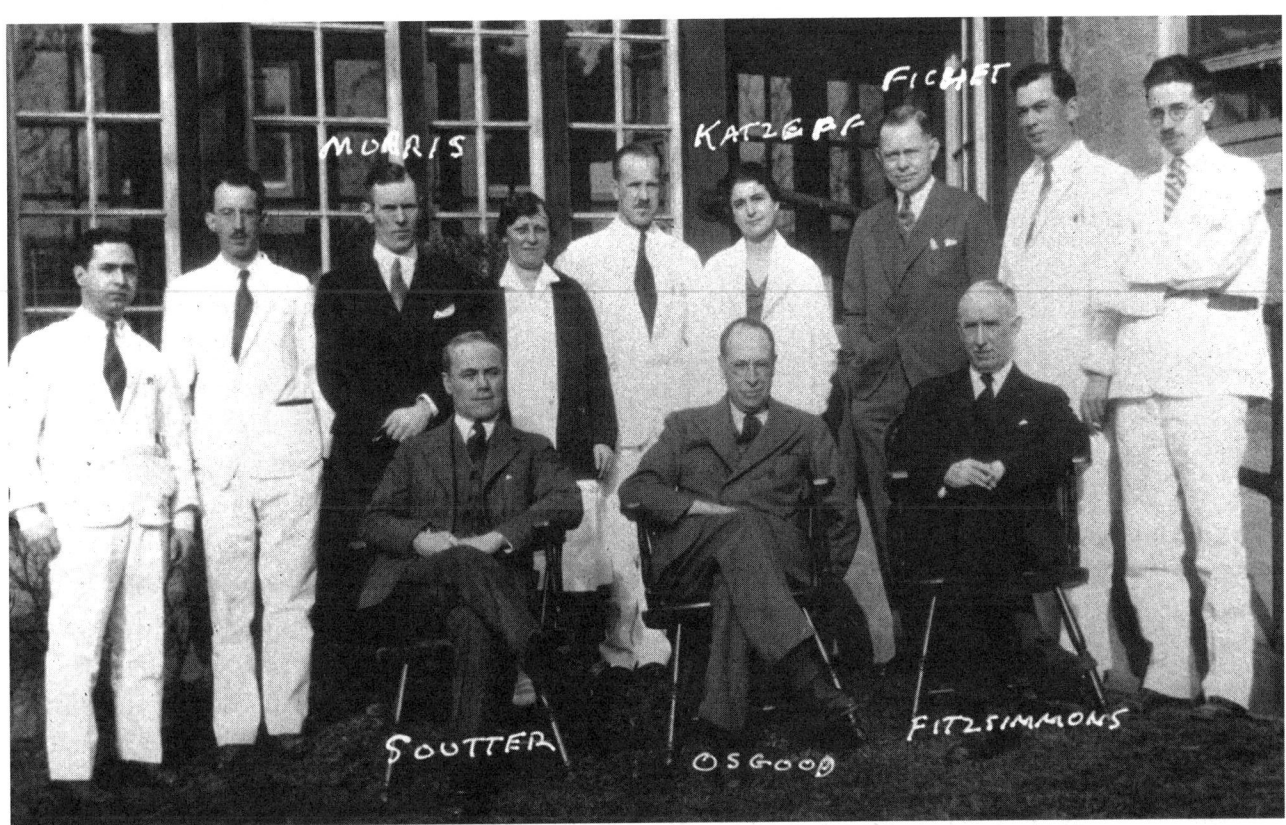

Orthopaedic staff at BCH. Dr. Soutter is seated in the first row, on the far left. MGH HCORP Archives.

the first plaster which extends from the nipples to the toes…The after-treatment consisted of recumbent position for six weeks, then a short pelvic plaster allowing the knee to bend. After the second six weeks…leg exercises…continued for six months…There was no pain or discomfort in any case eighteen months after operation…On the average in six months the patient was free from all discomfort. Patients could bear weight on the leg without cane or crutches from one and one-half to twelve months after operation, the average being 4 months. Walking was possible in 5 weeks to 10 months…Standing was easy three to nine months after operation. (R. Soutter 1906b)

On average, the patients had been disabled for 14 years. All healed after the procedure and eventually returned to work.

In 1912, he read a paper at the Boston Orthopedic Club describing his initial research efforts. He reported early results of 24 cartilage transplantations that he had performed in the surgical laboratories of Harvard Medical School. In one instance, he had also completely transplanted a joint. His results were inconclusive. I was unable to find any publication describing the final results of Soutter's research on cartilage transplantation.

New Surgical Procedures

Innovative in his surgical approaches, Soutter described two original operations. In 1914, he reported on a new operation to treat hip contractures in poliomyelitis (see **Box 23.11**). He emphasized the importance of postoperative care:

It is very important in the after treatment that the head, shoulders and buttocks should rest on a level, being held in this way on a Bradford frame. The legs are hyperextended backward below the frame. This position is more comfortably maintained by a plaster of Paris… from the nipple line to the toes…This position is maintained for eight weeks. The patient is then gotten up gradually and encouraged to walk with a short light plaster and crutches. Later braces if necessary are applied and the hyperextended position used for two or three hours a day only. A plaster shell and a Bradford frame is [sic] used during the hours of hyperextension; this makes it possible to obtain the correct position each time…This operation has been found of great value and the deformity is not apt to recur, for the lengthening of the muscles is definite and permanent. (R. Soutter 1917)

Many subsequent authors noted the beneficial effects of Soutter's operation, and it became "used more extensively than any other procedure" (J. E. Thomson 1924). But Winthrop Phelps reported in 1957 that "the Soutter operation gave poor results unless strong hip extensors were present." Carl Yount (1926) noted that with Soutter's operation, "hip flexion only is influenced directly, the knock-knee being unaffected because the zone of correction is so removed from the seat of the deformity and also because the intermuscular septa arising from the fascia lata…intimately connected with the ilio-tibial band, prevent[s] any appreciable amount of correction of the knee deformity." Nine years later Dr. Willis Campbell would modify Soutter's early pioneering procedure.

In 1933, Soutter described another new procedure, this one for treating a dislocated patella. In his book *Technique of Operations on the Bones, Joints, Muscles and Tendons*, published in 1917, he had written that he preferred Goldthwait's method of splitting the patellar tendon and transferring the lateral half to the medial side of the tibia. With his own technique, however, Soutter (1933) stated: "It is so much simpler than changing the angle of the condyle…cutting half of the patella ligament and transplanting half [as in Goldthwait's procedure], reefing the capsule which is useless, and many elaborate methods which involve alteration in the existing tissues or opening the joint." In his procedure, after an interior incision:

Box 23.11. Soutter's Procedure to Treat Hip Contractures in Poliomyelitis

"In poliomyelitis the usual contractures of the soft tissues at the hip hold the thigh flexed and abducted and involve a shortening of more or less all the soft tissues on the outer and anterior aspect of the region of the hip. The deformity may be slight, considerable or extreme. It is usually accompanied by a compensatory lumbar lordosis which on account of the flexibility of the spine here makes complete correction more difficult.

"Contractures of the soft tissues at the hip…are sometimes easily overcome by manipulation and stretching. When they are of long standing they may not yield to tenotomies of the tendons and of the tensor fascia femoris, and myotomies are necessary. The severe contractures that need myotomies require some surgical experience on account of the vascularity and the amount of muscle tissues that must be cut before the hip will come down…

"For these difficult cases and also some of the milder ones the following operation has been devised: First a longitudinal incision is made three inches long, parallel with the long axis of the body, with its middle two inches posterior to the anterior superior spine. It is carried down to the fascia. By retracting the subcutaneous tissue the fascia is exposed from the anterior superior spine back to the trochanter. Second, the fascia is incised at right angles to the skin incision, cutting all its fibres transversely from the anterior superior spine back to the great trochanter. Third, the skin incision is next retracted in such a way as to expose the anterior superior spine. By means of an osteotome, the attached muscles and fascia are removed from the anterior superior spine subperiosteally on the inside, on the outside and below; they are all pushed downward. The hip is hyperextended backwards, pulling the tissues down with it. If the tension is great the soft tissues are pushed down by means of gauze or blunt dissector, clearing off the periosteum and soft tissues from that part of the pelvis below the anterior superior spine.

"Following the operation a plaster of Paris bandage is applied to the whole leg. The hip is hyperextended in order to correct the lumbar lordosis usually present in these cases. It is also adducted slightly to stretch the lateral contractures. The plaster of Paris extends from the nipple line in front and from the lower waist behind to the toes of the foot operated upon. A window may be cut in the plaster over the abdomen. The patient is put on a Bradford Frame elevated to allow the legs to drop to a lower level than the hips and shoulders. The advantages of this method of procedure are as follows: There is practically no bleeding, the operation does not require much surgical skill and the contracture is definitely relieved. The muscles are not cut across; their periosteal attachment is simply moved one and one-half or two inches downward. The anterior superior spine will be found to be practically moved downward."

—R. Soutter, "A New Operation for Hip Contractures in Poliomyelitis." *Boston Medical and Surgical Journal*, 1914

the patella is tunneled obliquely from above downward and from without mesially. At about the middle of this tunnel a window is opened in the top. A similar tunnel is made in the tibia in approximately the same line and well to the mesial side of the tibia…a window is cut down to…[the tibial tunnel] through the overlying fascia as described above for the patella. The ligament in the patella is passed from the mesial side of the tunnel upward and the loose end, as it emerges from the outer side of the patella, is folded over the top of the patella and tucked in through the window, emerging below at the entrance to the tunnel on the mesial side of the patella…In a similar way the fascial ligament is tucked in on the outer side of the tibial tunnel. It emerges at the mesial side of the knee. The loose end is then brought out at the mesial side of the tibia…folded over and tucked in through the window and merges at the outer side of the tunnel. The two loose ends being then approximated, are passed through each other and sutured twice with catgut…An incision is made over the outer side of the thigh of the good leg, or, of the affected leg, down to the fascia lata. A strip is removed 1¼" or 1½" broad. The necessary length is carefully measured so that it will reach twice the distance between the farther side of the tunnel in the tibia to the farther side of the tunnel in the patella. (R. Soutter 1933)

He reported satisfactory results in both children and adults after immobilization in a cast for three weeks.

Scoliosis

With a long interest in scoliosis since beginning his practice, Soutter published scoliosis-related articles with Bradford and others. In 1906, with the assistance of Professor Thomas Dwight, Dr. John Warren, and others in the Department of Anatomy at Harvard Medical School, he studied the effects of pressure on the curve and rotation of the spine in the cadavers of two children, one who had been 5 and the other 12 years old. From his studies he concluded that:

> the spinal column can be rotated by pressure on the ribs. Slight pressure causes flattening with lateral bulging of the ribs. More pressure causes flattening and lateral bulging of the ribs, and a rotation of the spine...Pressure on ribs rotates the spine, but not the spinous tips to the same extent. In other words, the inter-vertebral disks play an important part in allowing curvature and rotation...It was impossible to get a twist without some slight lateral deviation...Lateral deviation was greatest in the lower dorsal and lumbar spine...For obtaining rotation, the recumbent position yielded more for a given pressure... Head pull is especially helpful for high rotation... suspension with toes touching is especially good for equal correction of both high and low rotation at the same time. A lying position is the most advantageous for getting the maximum correction with a minimum force. (R. Soutter 1906)

In patients with long-standing scoliosis and severe structural changes, Soutter recommended, in addition to exercise, the use of both a corrective jacket and an apparatus to obtain maximum correction of the curve and the rotational deformity:

> In the forcible correction of curvature, head pull and shoulder pull, varying with the patient, from 100 lb. to nearly 150 or more, facilitates the correction of the curve and the rotation by means of pressure...A cast is made from the jacket applied [while in the apparatus]; it is modeled to obtain the points of correction that were necessarily omitted at the time of applying the plaster to the patient. The patient is kept recumbent and successive corrective jackets applied either from remodeling the cast or from newly applied jackets. (R. Soutter 1911)

A patient would initially wear the jackets day and night for two to four months. Then, after maximal correction, the patient wore a retentive jacket for another two to six months. During this treatment period, patients were instructed in exercises to enhance strength and flexibility. Of the 182 patients treated, "Sixty-five, or one third, were greatly corrected, 97 were improved; 20 while benefited [sic] in strength, endurance and health, their curves were not improved" (R. Soutter 1911).

In 1913, in a scoliosis symposium at the 27th Annual Meeting of the American Orthopaedic Association, Soutter, recognized Dr. James Sever's work at Children's Hospital, stating, "with these difficult structural cases [Sever] has been so wonderfully successful that I think we should record it at this time. He [Sever] used a method of traction on the head and corrective gymnastics" ("Reports of Societies" 1913).

Soutter also designed some new devices to aid treatment of patients with orthopaedic problems. One was a unique apparatus for correcting scoliosis using a pendulum seat, traction and rotation straps, a brace for postural scoliosis, a plaster swathe, and

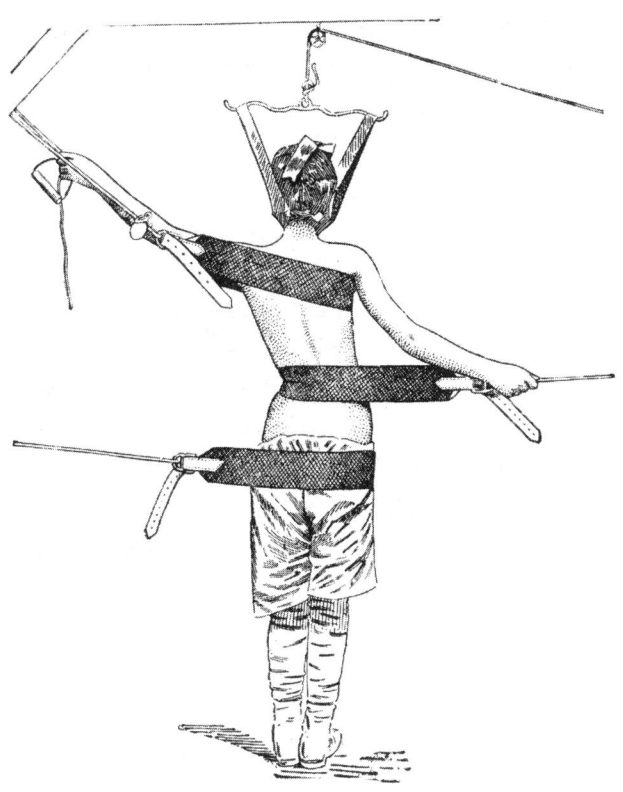

Apparatus used for self-correction of a scoliosis at BCH.
Treatise on Orthopedic Surgery, 2nd edition, by Bradford and Lovett. New York: William Wood and Company, 1899. Columbia University Libraries/Internet Archive.

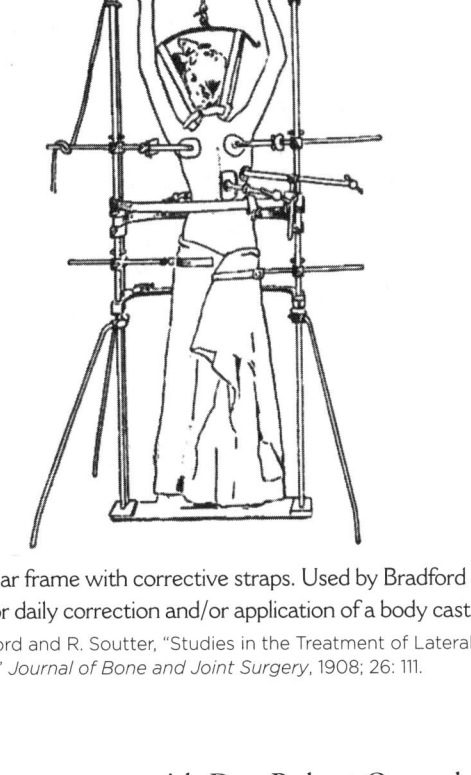

Rectangular frame with corrective straps. Used by Bradford and Soutter for daily correction and/or application of a body cast.
E.H. Bradford and R. Soutter, "Studies in the Treatment of Lateral Curvature," *Journal of Bone and Joint Surgery*, 1908; 26: 111.

a plaster-of-Paris bar or rope that orthopaedists still use today to strengthen cast windows and reinforce a limb mobilized in plaster attached to a body cast, i.e., a spica cast. He also designed a portable traction device for use in treating fractures or in operations on the lower extremity, as well as a minimally invasive technique of stabilizing fractures in infants and young children.

The *Boston Medical and Surgical Journal* frequently published articles in a series called "Recent Progress in Orthopedic Surgery," which provided periodic updates on new developments in orthopaedic surgery. The series began in 1879 and continued for 52 years. Bradford, either alone or with coauthors, published most of these reports. In 1919, Soutter cowrote one with C. Hermann Bucholz and others, and, in 1903, he published one he wrote alone. Soutter's involvement in the series continued, and, from 1912 through 1919, he cowrote reports with Drs. Robert Osgood, C. Herman Bucholz, Murray Danforth, and Harry Low. Soutter's final report, published in 1924, was cowritten with Osgood, Nathaniel Allison, Low, Danforth, Bucholz, Lloyd Brown, Philip Wilson, Marius Smith-Petersen, and Loring Swaim. The last article in the series was written in 1931 by William Rogers and Edwin Cave.

Technique of Operations on the Bones, Joints, Muscles and Tendons

Dr. Soutter published his only book in 1917. He dedicated it to Bradford, who at the time was a professor of orthopaedic surgery at and the dean of Harvard Medical School. It spoke to the high regard in which Soutter held Bradford, and their close relationship: "This volume is dedicated as a token of appreciation of his [Bradford's] clear-minded judgment, his high surgical skill and professional ideals, all of which have been a constant source of inspiration during the intimate association of fifteen years partnership" (R. Soutter 1917).

The book was uniquely organized into seven parts, each for a specific area of the anatomy: hip, knee, foot and ankle, shoulder, elbow, wrist, and "miscellaneous operations." The chapters in each part described the procedures or techniques in the particular area sequentially, starting with number 1 in chapter 1 and ending with number 347 in chapter 3 of part 7. Each chapter briefly described the technique for the specific procedure.

Cover of Soutter's book, Technique of Operations on the Bones, Joints, Muscles and Tendons. Internet Archive/Columbia University Libraries.

The American Journal of Orthopedic Surgery published a review of the book:

Dr. Soutter reviews his own book when he says in the preface: "I have not planned to compile an encyclopedia but to present a ready reference for the technic of the more practical operations on the upper and lower extremities. The operative procedures useful in infantile paralysis are dealt with at length, and the tried-out methods are here recommended, rather than every possible operation." It is a book some three hundred pages, written by an orthopedic surgeon of wide operative experience. It is typical of the present stage of development of orthopedic surgery as a specialty. By this statement I mean that the book takes up in detail orthopedic operative procedures and postoperative treatment, while fractures and operations, which heretofore have been considered part of the work of the general surgeon, are not gone into to the same extent.

In reading the book one misses, decidedly, the absence of references to original articles. A book that is supposed to be used for ready references surely ought to contain references to original articles, for anyone who may want to go into the operative procedure in greater detail than given in Dr. Soutter's book.

It is a book of distinct value, and is full of suggestions as to operative and non-operative treatment. Post-operative treatment is taken up in considerable detail, and although very few orthopedic surgeons agree as to this phase of the treatment, it gives a good sound working basis, especially for those who have not had sufficient experience to have an opinion of their own. It is a valuable book both to the orthopedic surgeon and to the general surgeon. ("Technic [sic] of Operations" 1918)

A Tragic End

In 1933, Soutter was an instructor in orthopaedic surgery at Harvard Medical School. On Wednesday,

February 15, 1933, Soutter scratched his thumb while operating on a child. He gave it no thought, but that evening "the toxic effects of the poison became apparent" ("Dr. Robert Soutter Dies" 1933). He was rushed to MGH (Baker Memorial), where he received two blood transfusions and the next day underwent an operation (likely incision and drainage of the thumb)—all without success. He died from blood poisoning on February 21, 1933. The *New York Times*, in an article about his death, called Soutter "one of the country's foremost orthopedic surgeons" ("Dr. Soutter Dead" 1933). He was survived by his wife and children.

NOTED SURGEON DIES OF BLOOD POISONING

Dr Robert Soutter Infected During an Operation

Infected while operating on a child last Wednesday, Dr Robert Soutter, noted orthopedic surgeon, died from blood poisoning at the Baker Memorial of the Massachusetts General Hospital yesterday.

Twice since he scratched his thumb during the operation. Wednesday he was given blood transfusions, and on Thursday an operation was performed.

Dr Soutter was one of the best known orthopedic surgeons in the United States. For several years he had been the partner of Dr E. H. Bradford, who established the department of orthopedic surgery at the

Continued on the Seventeenth Page

Article in the Daily Boston Globe announcing Dr. Soutter's premature death. From *The Boston Globe*. © 1933 Boston Globe Media Partners. All rights reserved. Used under license.

CHARLES L. STURDEVANT

Physician Snapshot

Charles L. Sturdevant
BORN: ca. 1913
DIED: Unknown
SIGNIFICANT CONTRIBUTION: Consultant at the Clinics for Crippled Children with the Massachusetts Department of Public Health in Greenfield

Little is known about Dr. Charles L. Sturdevant. He graduated from the University of Nebraska College of Medicine in 1936. By 1940, he was an assistant in orthopaedic surgery at Harvard Medical School. In Dr. Frank Ober's annual departmental report at Children's Hospital in 1941, he wrote that Sturdevant served as both a resident orthopaedic surgeon and a junior assistant surgeon (along with Dr. John F. Bell [who is described earlier in this chapter] and Drs. Leo J. McDermott and Eugene E. Record). The orthopaedic house officers at the time included David S. Grice (chapter 22), John F. Bell (in this chapter), and Vincent Zechino. In 1946, Sturdevant was among those from Middlesex South District who applied for a fellowship with the Massachusetts Medical Society.

Sturdevant remained an assistant in orthopaedic surgery at Harvard Medical School from 1940 to at least 1955, if not longer. He served as a consultant with the Clinics for Crippled Children run by the Massachusetts Department of Public Health in Greenfield. His office was located at 234 Marlborough Street in Boston; there he practiced at Marlborough Medical Associates with Drs. Frank Ober (chapter 20), Albert Brewster and Paul Hugenberger (both described earlier in this chapter), Joseph Barr (chapter 38), and Eugene Record and Tom DeLorme (both described in chapter 40). He remained in the practice after Barr, Record, and DeLorme resigned from the group.

I was unable to find any publications by Sturdevant, but in the presentation "Osteochondritis Dissecans in Children" by Drs. William Green and Henry Banks at the 1952 Annual Meeting of the American Academy of Orthopaedic Surgeons, Green mentioned Sturdevant in his concluding remarks: "I merely want to thank the discussors [*sic*] for being kind, and to mention that Dr. Charles Sturdevant and Dr. George Beattie assisted in the follow-up of these cases" (Green and Banks 1953).

MIHRAN O. TACHDJIAN

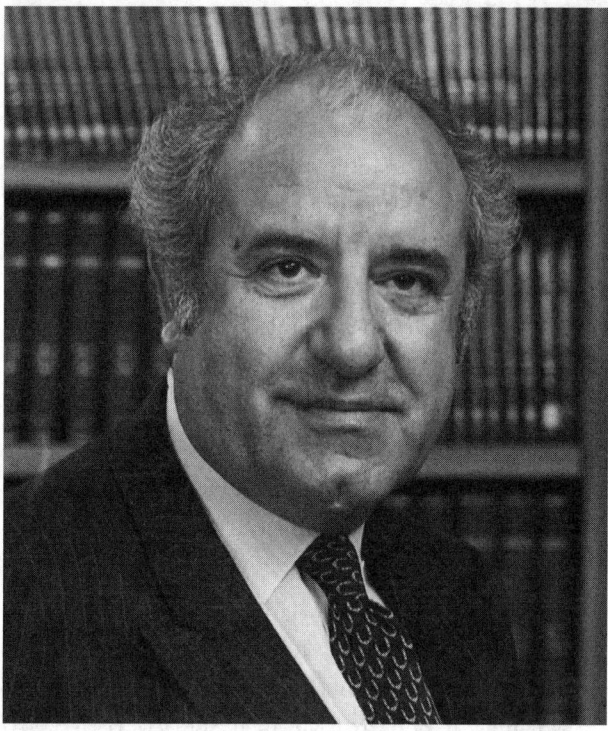

Mihran O. Tachdjian. POSNA Archive c/o Texas Scottish Rite Hospital for Children. POSNA.Archivist@tsrh.org. 214-559-8545.

Physician Snapshot

Mihran O. Tachdjian
BORN: 1927
DIED: 1996

SIGNIFICANT CONTRIBUTIONS: Developed the pediatric orthopaedic fellowship program at Chicago's Children's Memorial Hospital; wrote the classic two-volume text *Pediatric Orthopaedics*; founded in 1975 and subsequently directed the Pediatric Orthopaedic International Seminars; helped to internationalize the field of pediatric orthopaedics through the Pediatric Orthopaedic International Seminars and the International Pediatric Orthopaedic Think Tank; one of 12 members who chartered the Pediatric Orthopaedic Society

Mihran "Myke" Tachdjian, originally from Beirut, Lebanon, was born June 12, 1927. After studying piano and music in Paris as a teenager, he returned to Beirut and attended the American University of Beirut. After graduating in 1948, he went to the medical school there, earning his MD in 1952.

At that point, Tachdjian came to the US to continue his training. After an internship at Wesley Memorial Hospital in Chicago, he completed a residency in orthopaedic surgery at Northwestern University Medical School, rotating at Wesley Memorial Hospital; at St. Francis Hospital in Evanston, Illinois; and at Carrie Tingley Hospital in Truth or Consequences, New Mexico—at the time the children's hospital affiliated with Northwestern's orthopaedic residency program. It was during his pediatric orthopaedic rotation at Carrie Tingley Hospital that he recognized his passion for pediatric orthopaedics. In 1957, Tachdjian received a master of science degree from Northwestern. "He then became associated with Dr. Edward Compere, Professor of Orthopedic Surgery at Northwestern" (Children's Hospital Archives), whom he joined in practice on the faculty at Northwestern.

He published his first two papers on children with cerebral palsy, whom he encountered during his experience at Carrie Tingley Hospital: the first, "Hip Dislocation in Cerebral Palsy," published in 1956, and the second, "Sensory Disturbances in the Hands of Children with Cerebral Palsy," published in 1958. In the first one, he reviewed 590 patients, of whom 25 (4%) showed evidence of subluxation or dislocation of the hip. He concluded that "dislocation of the hip in cerebral palsy is preventable" and "stress[ed] the importance of prophylactic tenotomy of the spastic hip adductors and strengthening the motor power of the cerebral-zero hip abductors by automatic reflex" (Tachdjian and Minear 1956) to avoid the development of coxa valga. In the second paper on cerebral palsy, he reviewed the records of 800 children with cerebral palsy and reported on 96 patients in whom he had performed a sensory examination of their hands:

The end-result determination was made from one to nine years after surgery [muscle releases, tendon transfers, wrist fusion and first to second metacarpal bone graft block], with an average of three and one-half years...The extremely impaired sensation in these hands [n=15] no doubt adversely affected the outcome of the surgery. Before undertaking surgery on the hand affected by cerebral palsy, the motor and sensory status of the involved upper extremity and of the patient as a whole should be carefully evaluated. (Tachdjian and Minear 1958)

Soon after receiving his master of science degree he enlisted in the US Army (probably around 1958). After his discharge in 1960, Tachdjian became an assistant in orthopaedic surgery at Children's Hospital, where he worked closely with Dr. William Green for four years. He was promoted to associate in orthopaedic surgery in 1962, along with Frank Bates and Paul Griffin. Senior associates at the time included Henry Banks, Jonathan Cohen, Arthur Trott, and Paul Hugenberger.

Tachdjian was very productive during his four years on the staff at Children's Hospital. In 1962, Green wrote about Tachdjian's contributions:

Dr. Mihran O. Tachdjian discussed "Fractures of the Neck of the Femur in Children" at the April 1962 meeting of the State Trauma Committee of the American College of Surgeons here in Boston...Dr. Griffin along with Dr. Tachdjian presented a scientific exhibit at the American Academy of Orthopaedic Surgeons meeting in January 1962 on "Pauci-articular Arthritis in Children" and read a paper on the same subject at the meeting of the America Medical Association in June 1962. Dr. Tachdjian was the co-author of a motion picture presentation... on cerebral palsy at the meeting of the American Academy for Cerebral Palsy in St. Louis in October, 1961, and read a paper on "Intermetacarpal Bone Block for Thenar Paralysis" at the Meeting of the American Orthopaedic Association in May 1962...Dr. Tachdjian, along with Dr. Banks and their associates, has been concerned with developing an objective method of recording motor performance in cerebral palsy. His other activities include a study of fractures of the neck of the femur in the child, and the orthopedic manifestations of spinal cord tumors. Dr. Tachdjian assisted me in writing the orthopedic section of a textbook of surgery soon to be published. (W. T. Green 1962)

In addition to these presentations and research activities, Tachdjian published five papers, including a large consecutive series of intraspinal tumors in children, cowritten with Dr. Donald Matson (**Case 23.6**). They reviewed 115 patients treated at Children's Hospital over a 30-year period. In their article they emphasized "the importance of early diagnosis and treatment before the development of extensive neuromuscular damage...[and that] 83 percent of all patients required orthopaedic care because of musculoskeletal abnormality...[They hoped] that their presentation will alert all physicians to the possibility of spinal-cord tumor whenever a child is found to have torticollis, scoliosis, unexplained limp, weakness of an extremity, sphincter disturbance, or an obscure pain in the trunk or an extremity" (Tachdjian and Matson 1965).

Sensory Disturbances in the Hands of Children with Cerebral Palsy

BY MIHRAN O. TACHDJIAN, M.D., CHICAGO, ILLINOIS
AND WILLIAM L. MINEAR, M.D., PH.D., ALBUQUERQUE, NEW MEXICO

THE JOURNAL OF BONE AND JOINT SURGERY
VOL. 40-A, NO. 1, JANUARY 1958

Title of Tachdjian's article on the importance of sensory deficits in the hands of children with cerebral palsy.

M. O. Tachdjian and W. L. Minear. "Sensory disturbances in the hands of children with cerebral palsy," *Journal of Bone and Joint Surgery*, 1958; 40:85.

Case 23.6. Orthopaedic Aspects of Intraspinal Tumors in Children

> "M.D., a white girl, three and one-half years old, was admitted to the Children's Hospital with the diagnosis of traumatic subluxation of the second on the third cervical vertebra and paralysis of the right upper extremity caused by a fall from a kitchen stool six months previously. Treatment with head-halter traction by an orthopaedic surgeon in another state was complicated by a pressure sore on the chin; traction with Crutchfield tongs was then substituted, but a decubitus ulcer developed over the occiput which eventually required débridement and skin-grafting to heal.
>
> "On admission, she had obvious atrophy of the right upper extremity with weakness of all muscles and torticollis on the right. Any passive motion of the cervical spine was painful and restricted. There was hypesthesia to light touch and pinprick over the fourth through the seventh cervical dermatome. Deep tendon reflexes in both lower extremities were hyperactive but equal; her gait was broad-based and ataxic.
>
> "Roentgenograms of the cervical spine showed marked widening of the spinal canal from the first cervical to the first thoracic level, with no evidence of erosion, bone destruction, subluxation or dislocation. The roentgenographic diagnosis was that of a widened spinal canal, apparently of long standing, caused by an intraspinal expansile lesion.
>
> "Myelograms showed marked widening of the cervical spinal canal extending from the first cervical to the first thoracic vertebra with almost complete block between the second and fifth cervical vertebrae. Total proteins of the cerebrospinal fluid were elevated (109 milligrams per 100 milliliters). At laminectomy, a cystic astrocytoma (Grade I-II) of the spinal cord was found. The cyst was aspirated, and a large amount of solid tumor was removed. Postoperatively, there was some return of motor function in the right upper extremity. A Thomas cervical collar was applied for support. Roentgenograms, made about one year after surgery, showed no evidence of instability of the cervical spine. Clinically the patient was asymptomatic and there was further return of muscle strength in the right upper extremity."
>
> (Tachdjian and Matson 1965)

In his annual chairman's report, Green mentioned Tachdjian's resignation from Children's: "Losses from our active staff were Dr. Mihran Tachdjian...[who] resigned August 1, 1964, to become Orthopedic Surgeon-in-Chief of the Children's Memorial Hospital in Chicago and Associate Professor of Orthopaedic Surgery at Northwestern University." Green was reportedly very upset at the loss of Tachdjian, who had been recruited to Northwestern by Dr. Orvar Sevenson, professor of surgery and surgeon-in-chief at Children's Memorial Hospital in Chicago. Sevenson had been a house officer at Children's Hospital and the Peter Bent Brigham Hospital, and had remained on the staff at Harvard Medical School for 12 years (1938–50), so Green would have known and worked with him. In an interview sponsored by the Pediatric History Center of the American Academy of Pediatrics, Sevenson stated that orthopaedics was fairly underdeveloped at Northwestern and Children's Memorial Hospital, and so, at the urging of the pediatricians there, he used a gift bequeathed to the Department of Surgery to start a full-time orthopaedic program. He used a stipend from the bequest to recruit Tachdjian, and he said that Green called and "excoriated" him for stealing Tachdjian from Children's.

Tachdjian's exemplary career in pediatric orthopaedics continued at Children's Memorial Hospital. He focused fully on improving the hospital's teaching program and developed a fellowship program. He was well respected by residents and fellows, who recognized Tachdjian's dedication to their training in all aspects of orthopaedic surgery.

He also published an additional 30 articles and, with pediatric orthopaedic leaders at the time—Lynn Staheli, Sherman Coleman, Robert Hensinger, John Ogden, and Robert Salter—developed an instructional course on congenital hip dysplasia for the American Academy of Orthopaedic

Surgeons (1984). His contributions, however, were most significant in two areas. First, he published seven books and two symposia on topics in pediatric orthopaedics (**Box 23.12**), and second, he gave his popular and well-attended annual international seminars in pediatric orthopaedics.

Box 23.12. Tachdjian's Books and Symposia Publications

- *Congenital Dislocation of the Hip* (1982)
- *The Child's Foot* (1985)
- *Clinical Pediatric Orthopedics: The Art of Diagnosis and Principles of Management* (1997)
- *Atlas of Pediatric Orthopedic Surgery* (1994)
- *Pediatric Orthopedics* (1972)
- Two separate symposia on pediatric orthopaedics in *Orthopedic Clinics of North America* (1978 and 1980)

His *Pediatric Orthopedics* is a popular classic and is still in print today (as *Tachdjian's Pediatric Orthopaedics*, in its fifth edition as of 2013). One 1996 article in the *Chicago Tribune* called it the "international standard" of pediatric orthopaedics (K. Heise 1996). Another writer said that the book "consolidated our specialty" (A. H. Crawford 1991). Initially published in two volumes in 1972, Tachdjian wrote the entirety of the text. The first edition was "beautifully organized...[with] at least one important operative procedure for every surgical condition...presented in detail...The two volumes are a must for any orthopedist who does a good deal of children's orthopedics" (R. K. Ashley 1973). The second edition, published 18 years later in 1990, was updated to include four volumes. "Although the book has been written by a single author [Tachdjian], he acknowledges assistance from many experts and credits the participation of the faculty of his annual international seminars in pediatric orthopedics...[The] book...is best used as a reference" (S. A. Wasilewski 1991). Hugh G. Watts, writing about the history of pediatric

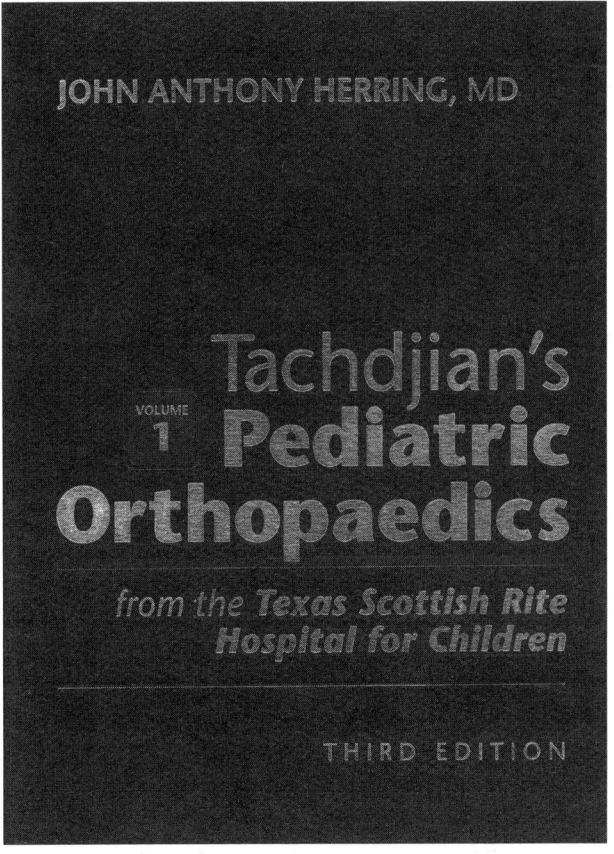

Cover of Tachdjian's classic book, Pediatric Orthopaedics.
Reprinted from *Tachdjian's Pediatric Orthopaedics*, 3rd edition, Vol. 1, John Anthony Herring, MD, 2001.

orthopaedics as a specialty in the US, commented that Green, Tachdjian's mentor during his time at Children's Hospital in Boston, may have had hard feelings about Tachdjian's publication of *Pediatric Orthopaedics*, just as he had when Albert Ferguson had published his *Orthopaedic Surgery in Infancy and Childhood* in 1957. Green had felt that many of the patients Ferguson had described were cases from Children's Hospital and had expected Ferguson (and possibly Tachdjian) to either ask permission or list Green as a coauthor (see chapter 21). Green never published his own textbook.

Tachdjian did recognize Green—he dedicated the first edition of *Pediatric Orthopaedics* to him. He also frequently mentioned Green in the text, through references to Green's articles and through beautifully detailed drawings that demonstrate many of the procedures Green had developed or modified. It also included copies of Green's and Anderson's growth charts and orthoroentgenographic techniques from their previous publications; Tachdjian gave appropriate credit and suggested that readers read the relevant papers by Green and Anderson. In the preface Tachdjian (1972) explained his "ambitious" and "complex" book, noting that his experience and education drove the inclusion of the various preferred treatments. A review of the more recent fourth edition, published in 2008, noted that because of the quality, comprehensiveness, and wide acceptance of this classic text:

> the compilation of the Tachdjian textbook devolved to Herring and colleagues as an ongoing project, the initial product was an in-house work written entirely by contributors at the Texas Scottish Rite Hospital in Dallas. The new, fourth edition (the second by the group at Texas Scottish Rite Hospital) includes contributions from Boston to supplement those by the local authors…[the] new features…[include] a set of two DVDs that portray several surgical procedures…[and] access to the publisher's only web site, which enables the purchaser to view the entire text and figures online…[T]his volume continues to honor Dr. Mihran Tachdjian as a high quality, well-written, well referenced, and excellently illustrated work on pediatric orthopaedics. (R. D. Blasier 2008)

The obituary for Tachdjian published in the *Journal of Pediatric Orthopaedics* notes that throughout his three-decade-long career, Tachdjian aimed to teach and to care for children with orthopaedic conditions worldwide.

In 1975, Tachdjian founded, with his colleagues Paul Griffin, Dean MacEwen, and Douglas McKay, the Pediatric Orthopaedic International Seminars program. Two years earlier they had begun discussing—over good meals—the need for better teaching in pediatric orthopaedics. They came up with the idea for a course as a way to

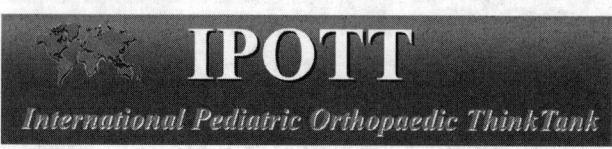

Logo of the International Pediatric Orthopedic Think Tank (IPOTT). Courtesy of IPOTT.

both further education in the specialty and generate income. It became an annual occasion, which Tachdjian directed (attendees called it "the Tachdjian course"). Originally held in Chicago and then moved to San Francisco, Tachdjian used his connections to include orthopaedic surgeons from around the world in the Seminars, thereby helping to expand and develop the specialty worldwide. These seminars are still held today.

Tachdjian also helped to develop and enhance orthopaedic education through the International Pediatric Orthopedic Think Tank (IPOTT). First held in 1996 in Paris, France, 50 leaders in the field, from both the US and Europe, came together to discuss the pediatric orthopaedic specialty.

Tachdjian was one of the 12 charter members of the Pediatric Orthopedic Society, founded in 1971. He served as its president in 1977. In his manuscript about pediatric orthopaedics in the US and Canada, Hugh Watts interviewed various players in the field. Dr. Anthony Bianco Jr. told Watts in 1995 that Tachdjian had been "the real spark plug in putting the organization together…He did the early hard work and kept us all interested" (quoted in H. G. Watts, n.d.). Dr. John Hall shared with Watts an anecdote about Tachdjian and a Society dinner: "Mike Tachdjian was the chairman. He arranged a dinner at a very fine restaurant and I remember everyone remarked what a fine wine he had chosen. It wasn't until later that we would find out why it was so good, when we discovered that the dinner had bankrupted the society" (quoted in H. G. Watts, n.d.).

In addition to the Pediatric Orthopedic Society, Tachdjian was a member of various other organizations, and he received numerous awards for his contributions to the field (**Box 23.13**).

Box 23.13. *Mihran Tachdjian's Professional Memberships, Honors, and Awards*

Memberships

- Pediatric Orthopaedic Society
- American Academy of Pediatrics
- American Academy of Orthopaedic Surgeons
- Pediatric Orthopedic Society of North America (POSNA)
- Society of the International Congress of Orthopedics and Traumatology (SICOT)
- Societé Française de Chirugie Orthopédique et Traumatologique (SOFCOT)

Honors and Awards

- Gold Medal from the British Orthopaedic Association (1982)
- The Stinchfield Award from the Hip Society (1983)
- "Member of Honor" award from the French Orthopedic and Traumatology Society
- The Berg Medal from the University of Göteberg in Sweden

On December 2, 1996, Tachdjian died unexpectedly at Northwestern Memorial Hospital after a major heart attack. He was 69 years old. Dr. Norris Carroll, then the chief of orthopaedics at Children's Memorial Hospital, said, "It's a terrible shock to us all…We've lost a dear friend and an esteemed colleague. He was going full bore. Next to his family Myke's love was pediatric orthopaedics" (quoted in N. Steinberg 1996). Another physician at Children's Memorial, James Conway, said of Tachdjian: "He loved children — just loved them" (quoted in K. Heise 1996). "Myke had a wonderful charm in dealing with people and was an excellent clinician, one who gave you the time and who made the effort" (K. Heise 1996). He was survived by his wife, Vivian; his son, Jason; and his four siblings.

AUGUSTUS THORNDIKE

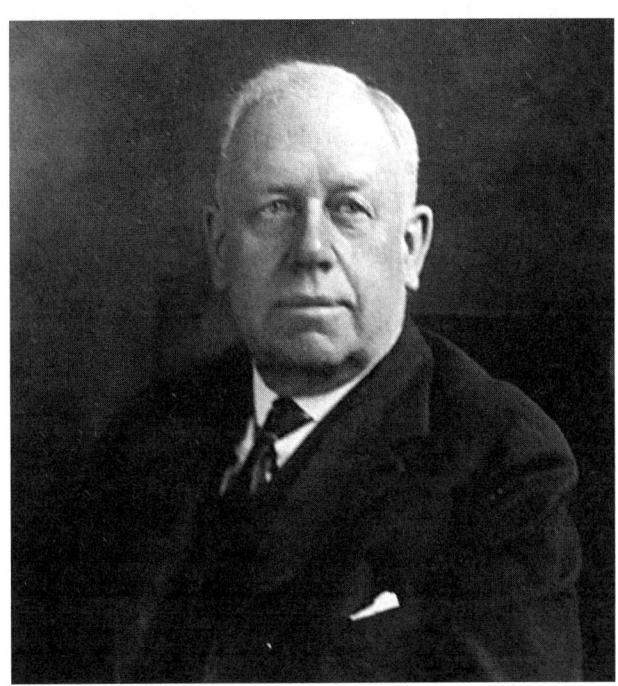

Augustus Thorndike (senior). Courtesy of Joan I. Thorndike.

Physician Snapshot

Augustus Thorndike
BORN: 1863
DIED: 1940
SIGNIFICANT CONTRIBUTIONS: Founded, with Dr. Edward Bradford, the Industrial School for Crippled and Deformed Children (1893); helped to establish the State Hospital School for Children in Canton, Massachusetts (1907); president of the American Orthopaedic Association (1910)

Although Augustus Thorndike was born in Paris in 1863, his family came to Boston during his early years, and Augustus went to Nobles School in the city. Commonly known as "Nobles," Nobles Classical School was a relatively new institution, founded in 1866, when Augustus Thorndike was three. Initially, when Thorndike attended, it was a boy's preparatory day school for Harvard; it later became the Noble and Greenough Country Day and Board School, located in Dedham, Massachusetts, since 1922. A. Lawrence Lowell, who was president of Harvard from 1909 to 1933, graduated from Nobles in 1873, seven years before Thorndike did.

Augustus went on to Harvard College after Nobles, graduating in 1884, and then continued further, graduating from Harvard Medical School in 1888. At Harvard he was a member of the Hasty Pudding Club.

He then completed three internships: one at the Massachusetts General Hospital on the West Surgical Service (1888–89), another at Boston Lying-In Hospital, and a third at the House of the Good Samaritan. We know that Thorndike was a house pupil at MGH in 1888, because he arranged the hospital records for a case report, published in the *Boston Medical and Surgical Journal* by Dr. J. W. Elliot, who was temporarily in charge of the wards of Dr. John Homans. The patient had aspirated a peanut, was admitted to MGH on June 2, 1888, and died of gangrenous pneumonia 17 days later in spite of a tracheotomy and failed efforts to retrieve the peanut (including holding the patient upside down while trying to capture it with long A forceps).

During his internship at the House of the Good Samaritan, Thorndike:

> became interested in the special care necessary in the treatment of the crippled child. At that time a large proportion of the cases were tuberculous, and, because of the fact that hospital equipment was then meager, these children required a great deal of careful attention and personal supervision from those who were in surgical charge. From the beginning of his work [there]…Dr. Thorndike showed his capacity of conscientious care and his sympathy for these children, which were demonstrated by the success which he had with these difficult and protracted cases. ("Augustus Thorndike 1863–1914" 1940)

After his internship, he remained at the House of the Good Samaritan, as a member of the active staff, for ~28 years until his retirement. During his time there, the institution often did not have adequate equipment, but Thorndike patiently cared for the very sick children with tuberculosis there, and his abilities were "evidenced by the success which he had with these difficult cases" (*New England Journal of Medicine* 1940).

Early in his career, after completing his internships, Thorndike worked at the Boston Dispensary. Founded in 1796:

> the Boston Medical Dispensary…has afforded the means of relief to many necessitous persons, among others, whose feelings would have been hurt by an application for assistance from the alms house; as they are by this charity attended free of any expense by an able physician, either at their own houses, or at the Dispensary, as they may require and furnish with whatever medicine they may need, and with wine, if necessary. This institution is supported by subscriptions; the payment of 5 dollars annually entitling the subscriber to recommend two patients constantly to the care of the Dispensary. The town is divided into three districts; the Southern…the Middle…[and] the Northern. (*The Boston Directory* 1807)

Many physicians trained at the Boston Dispensary during its time in operation: Oliver Wendell Holmes, Henry Bowditch, Buckminster Brown, and others. After ~170 years, the Dispensary became part of the Floating Hospital for Children and the Tufts Medical Center Hospital.

In 1890, Thorndike was 1 of 11 district physicians at the Dispensary. Dr. Charles L. Scudder headed its Orthopedic Department, which treated a total of 91 patients that year, including 43 children. Thorndike continued to volunteer at the Boston Dispensary as a surgeon at least until 1895. Orthopaedic surgery remained an interest for his entire career.

Following Robert Lovett in 1893, Thorndike became secretary of the Harvard Medical Alumni Association. He was also active in the Massachusetts Medical Association, becoming chairman of

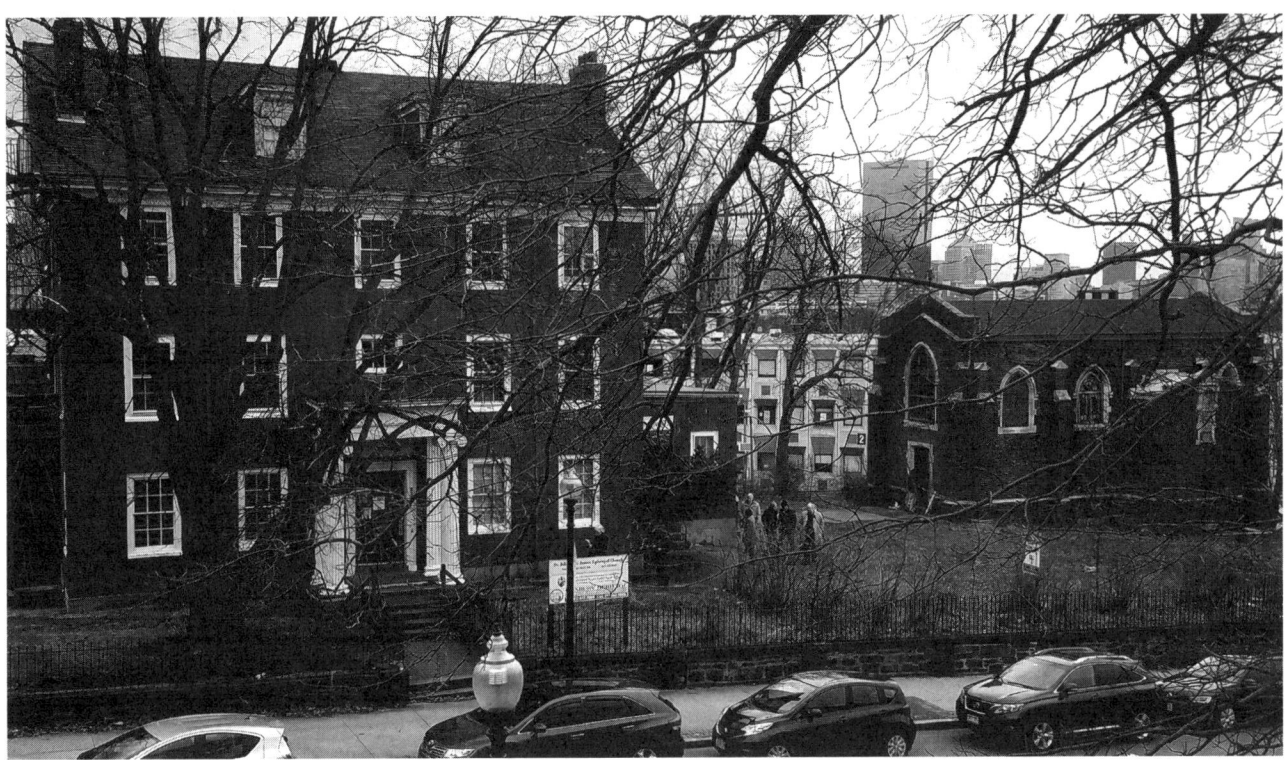

St. Luke's Home for Convalescents (Ionic Hall) and St. Luke's Chapel. Courtesy of Historic Boston Incorporated.

its Committee on Arrangements in 1896. It was at that meeting in Mechanics Hall in Boston that "an exhibition of orthopedic apparatus…such as any blacksmith could make" ("Massachusetts Medical Society" 1896) was held. and Dr. Ernest Codman gave the membership "a chance to examine patients with the fluoroscope, to see shadowgraphs and to study the methods employed in their production" ("Massachusetts Medical Society" 1896)—this was probably the first time this equipment was shown publicly.

Thorndike was also a visiting surgeon at St. Luke's Home for Convalescents to which he also "gave freely of his time and effort" ("Augustus Thorndike 1863–1914" 1940). But it was Boston Children's Hospital "to which he devoted the greatest amount of his time and energy. Such a service, at that time, to be performed faithfully, required devotion and sacrifice of personal interests, and his contribution to this Hospital was a very prominent feature. It was characterized by his unusual dependability and by his careful and painstaking attention, not only to the surgical care of the children but also to their general interest, and he was untiring in his efforts to bring the best to this group of children" ("Augustus Thorndike 1863–1914" 1940). He joined the active staff of Children's Hospital after completing his internships, in 1889. That same year he, along with Edward H. Nichols, John Dane, and James S. Stone, was elected as a junior assistant surgeon at Children's. He was affiliated with the orthopaedic department at Children's since the beginning of his time there, and he was promoted to associate surgeon in 1914.

He also began as an assistant in orthopaedics at Harvard Medical School in 1897. From 1909, he was an instructor in orthopaedics, and, in 1913, he was promoted to associate in orthopaedic surgery.

He focused much of his attention on caring for children with physical disabilities:

> Dr. Thorndike was always especially interested in the problem of the crippled child, and

occupied himself very largely with its solution, – not only as to medical and surgical care, but toward providing opportunities to offset the loss of those advantages of which they were so often deprived because of their infirmities. He was particularly interested also in the provision for their education and for manual training [occupational], to be given with the object of fitting them for some gainful occupation. He was one of the incorporators of the Boston Industrial School for Crippled Children and served as a member of its Board of Directors as well as of the medical staff during the early period of its establishment, and he was influential in the conduct of its affairs in its later growth. ("Augustus Thorndike 1863–1940" 1940)

Educating Physically Disabled Children

One major effort developed from Thorndike's interest in these children, particularly in answer to the need to provide them with an education when their physical problems precluded them from going to school. In 1893, Thorndike and Dr. Edward Bradford, the chief orthopaedic surgeon from Children's Hospital, established the Industrial School for Crippled and Deformed Children—the first school for physically disabled children in the US. A new building was opened at 241 St. Botolph Street in Boston in 1904, at which time eight teachers taught up to 150 students. An outdoor classroom was built in 1912. The school continued to expand over the subsequent decades, during which time it was renamed Cotting School. Both Thorndike and Bradford were members of the school's board of directors—Bradford until 1924 and Thorndike until 1940. In 1946, Augustus Thorndike Jr. began serving on the board as well; he remained a member until 1972, and then was an emeritus member from 1973 to 1985. After 80 years in Boston, because of expensive repairs needed to the Botolph Street building, the school moved to Lexington, Massachusetts, in 1988.

Thorndike "also took part in the establishment of the State Hospital School for Children at Canton which was organized [in 1907] some years after the incorporation of the School for Crippled Children" ("Augustus Thorndike 1863–1940" 1940). It was originally founded to provide medical care and schooling to children with polio — and was distinct from other state institutions for the mentally ill. Eventually the Massachusetts Hospital School expanded its population to include young adults—its patients ranged in age from 6 to 22 years—and to care for patients with conditions other than polio, including cerebral palsy, muscular dystrophy, myelodysplasia, spina bifida, brain injury, and other physically disabling and neuromuscular disorders. Located at 3 Randolph Street in Canton, Massachusetts (~20 miles south of Boston), it had an inpatient capacity of 93 beds. Arthur M. Pappas was chairman of the school's board of trustees for more than 40 years; in fact, the school is now named for him: the Pappas Rehabilitation Hospital for Children.

Clinical Research

Before 1897, Thorndike had published three articles in *Transactions of the American Orthopedic Association*, the first in 1893, and two papers in the *Boston Medical and Surgical Journal*, one of which he had presented to the Boston Society for Medical Improvement, and the other to the Massachusetts Medical Society. All dealt with pediatric-orthopaedics-related topics, ranging from tubercular arthritis, treatment of club foot, and tenotomy of the hand in cerebral palsy to modification of a long traction splint for use in young infants.

In his largest paper, "Joint-Disease in Infancy," he reviewed 11,291 records of children under the age of two years treated at Children's Hospital over a 13-year period (1883–96). He identified 210 cases of tuberculosis: 120 with spinal tuberculosis (spinal caries), 61 with tuberculosis of the hip, and 29 with tuberculosis of the knee ("white swelling of the knee" or "tumor albus" [A. Thorndike 1898a]). These cases together comprised "1.8 per cent of all the surgical out-patients" (A. Thorndike 1898a). In summarizing his findings, he stated:

> spinal caries was twice as common as hip-disease and four times as common as tumor albus. It occurred at any age from birth up; the dorsal region was affected in almost three-quarters of the cases. There was frequently much pain. Abscesses were common...Paralysis occurred in one-seventh and was sometimes a grave symptom. The death rate was high...In hip-disease the onset was usually gradual and painless but was acutely painful in one-quarter of the cases. Night-crisis occurred in one-half; abscess in almost one-third. Atrophy and shortening were usually considerable, and fatal results were not uncommon. The death rate is high...general tuberculosis and tubercular meningitis are to be dreaded in infantile hip-disease. Tumor albus in infancy was far less common than the other two affections, of a milder type, and more amenable to treatment. Tubercular joint disease in infancy, therefore, seems to present the following distinctions: It is frequently attended by great pain and acute symptoms, and is more apt to result in general dissemination or infection with tubercle bacilli than in older children. (A. Thorndike 1898a)

More than 25 years later, Felipe Muro reviewed cases of spinal tuberculosis at Children's Hospital in the 10-year period from 1913 to 1922. In that review, he commented on Thorndike's earlier findings: "Thorndike found 87 in the dorsal region, or 75.6 percent...17 cases with paralysis stating that four of these had complete paralysis...Thorndike found two deaths from tuberculous meningitis, three from general tuberculosis, and one from bronchitis...[With regard to treatment...it] is well known that the system most in practice at the Children's Hospital makes use of the recumbent position with hyperextension on a posterior plaster-shell" (F. Muro 1924).

In 1897, Thorndike presented a paper entitled "Spina Bifida Rupture during Birth, Recovery" at a meeting of the Boston Society for Medical Improvement held in the Boston Medical Library. The following year, he published a paper on four cases of rupture of a spina bifida sac (see **Case 23.7**), asking:

> What conclusions are we to draw? Should we temporize? Should we operate?...[T]he testimony so far is certainly in favor of early operation...In meningoceles the operation of excision can be performed with comparative safety... In meningo-myelocoles [sic], the sac should be opened and the nerves separated from it and replaced before closing off the spinal canal; the neck of the sac should either be sutured or ligated and the skin closed over the stump...The prognosis in cases which rupture is bad; death is the rule, usually in three or four days. Still a few cases survive. (A. Thorndike 1898a)

Thorndike frequently presented papers on clinical pediatric conditions at annual meetings of the American Orthopaedic Association—13 over a 10-year period. "[T]he welcome accorded him at [those] meetings was evidence of the high esteem in which he was held" ("Obituary Augustus Thorndike" 1940). In 1910, Thorndike was president of that association. His presidential address was entitled, "Our Relations with the Community and Especially with Medical Men." He began his address by stating the lofty goals of both physicians and orthopaedic surgeons:

> The duty of the physician is plain. First, foremost, and all the time, his duty is to care for his patient—to cure him...This duty is paramount; it is above all other duties and above all other calls on his time and attention...his duty to his patient is an inheritance down through the generations...It is the same with the orthopedic

Case 23.7. Rupture of the Spina Bifida Sac

> "Case III was seen with Drs. J.E. Cleaves and N.F. Chandler in Medford on April 9, 1897. Dr. Cleaves has given me the following notes of the confinement: The labor was a rapid one, and the child was born a few minutes before Dr. Cleaves arrived. As soon as the placenta and perineum were attended to the baby was seen and the sac discovered ruptured and collapsed. After washing with bichloride it was dressed with corrosive gauze. As the sac was quite long (six inches) it was folded over in the dressing and a snug bandage applied. I operated five hours later. The child, a large, healthy-looking baby, was slightly etherized lying with its stomach on a hot-water bottle (the water at 110° F.) and well covered to keep it warm. The dressing, which was perfectly dry, was removed, uncovering a pedunculated sac completely collapsed, covered with healthy skin except at a spot at the apex where there was a small tear. It was translucent, and no bands were seen or felt; I therefore assumed that no nerves were involved, that is, that it was a simple meningocele, and, surrounding the base by an elliptical incision, the sac wall was tied with a silk ligature, cut off, and the skin wound closed with four silk sutures. This took but a few minutes and, after applying a large sterilized dressing, the baby was put in a warmed bed with heaters, and given with the medicine-dropper ten drops of brandy well diluted. Brandy was given every half-hour for four hours, then three times a day for three days. The wound united by first intention; there was no shock, and the baby nursed well.
>
> "I again saw the baby November 14th, aged seven months. Save for one attack of diarrhea in the summer, it has been well and is fat. The parents told me that, after healing, two little pimples had appeared near the wound, and discharged until July, when the silk ligature was removed and it healed."
>
> —A. Thorndike
> "Four Cases of Rupture of Spina Bifida Sac, Three During Childbirth." *Boston Medical and Surgical Journal*, 1898

surgeon, for is he not a physician? His paramount duty is to his patient, first, foremost, and all the time, his duty is to cure deformity safely, quickly and pleasantly if he can, to make the crooked straight, the lame walk, run and leap like his brothers, and when perfect restoration is not to be, to minimize the disability and ameliorate the condition…there has arisen a strong popular sentiment which insists on the supervision and in future the treatment…so that deformities may be discovered early, and made to grow straight before they become severe and incurable. (A. Thorndike 1910a)

He then argued for orthopaedic supervision in public and private schools, but he recognized that, because of their small numbers, orthopaedic surgeons must delegate these responsibilities to other physicians and nurses. He also recognized the need for orthopaedic supervision in sports, stating that "there seems to be a growing demand for trained medical supervision, and, if possible, orthopedic supervision of all gymnasium work and training for athletic sports. Here again, the opportunity is far too large for the thin ranks of orthopedists to cover the ground unaided and means must be devised to instruct others how to do much of this work" (A. Thorndike 1910a). Interestingly, this early observation by Thorndike would later be realized in his son's (Augustus Thorndike Jr.) surgical practice: he specialized in sports medicine and acted as chief surgeon for both the Department of Hygiene and the Harvard Athletic Association (see chapter 12).

In his speech, Thorndike commented briefly on three other issues he felt strongly about. The first was the importance of schools for disabled children, with the goal of "securing such a healthy development of the cripple as will strengthen him, straighten his deformity, and minimize his physical disability…[T]he primary aim should be to teach the cripple some useful trade or occupation, in order to make him…self-supporting and self-reliant…[so he is able] to compete with his

Title of Thorndike's AOA presidential address. *American Journal of Orthopedic Surgery* 1910; 8: 1.

fellow men in the struggle for a living afterward" (A. Thorndike 1910a). Second, he emphasized what orthopaedists should give to and what they need from "other medical men":

> [He needs] their friendship and co-operation to accomplish the orthopedic good of the community, and to gain it he must first give them his...He should...read and defend in the meeting of [a] society a paper on some orthopedic subject of general interest...In doing this quasi-missionary work, the orthopedist is not advertising himself, he is educating his medical brethren and if he does it in the best and surest way he does it without their knowing it... [including] another class of our medical brethren whom we are bound to help in every possible way—the medical students, both graduate and undergraduate...[their] teaching of our specialty falls rightly to us. (A. Thorndike 1910a)

Third, Thorndike concluded that "the community demands and ever will demand of us, first and foremost, our full duty to the patient. Orthopedic surgery stands for conservatism, for the cure of deformity and the restoration of function in disabled limbs. Much of our work is mechanical and the orthopedic surgeon must ever remain a master of the art of designing, making, and fitting splints and braces for the correction or amelioration of deformities. The community looks to us for this, and ever will" (A. Thorndike 1910a).

In 1907, Thorndike published his book, *A Manual of Orthopedic Surgery*. It was 401 pages and included 191 illustrations with radiographs, drawings, and photos of patients. He dedicated the book to: "My colleagues past and present at the Children's Hospital and especially to my teachers and friends, E.H. Bradford, M.D. and R.W. Lovett, M.D. in grateful acknowledgement of their kindness and patience" (A. Thorndike 1907). The book consisted of five parts: "I: Deformities originating before or during birth. Malformations, Fetal Diseases; II: Deformities caused by the influence of external forces acting upon the growth of the skeleton; III: Affections of bones and joints; IV: Acquired diseases of the nervous and muscular systems with deformities; V: Plaster bandages and orthopedic apparatus" (A. Thorndike 1907).

A Manual of Orthopedic Surgery was a required text at numerous medical schools. The *Boston Medical and Surgical Journal* published a review of it in 1908:

> There has been for some time a demand for a reliable small "handy volume" on orthopedic surgery, presenting to beginners and to busy practitioners the essential facts of this branch. This need has been met in a most admirable manner by Dr. Thorndike's publication...written by a surgeon of experience and excellent mature judgment, who writes after a careful study of all that has been written and taught, revised by a just critical spirit developed from personal experience and investigation, the result cannot fail to be of great value. The work is one which can be recommended without hesitation to all students, practitioners and specialists. ("Review. A Manual of Orthopaedic Surgery" 1908)

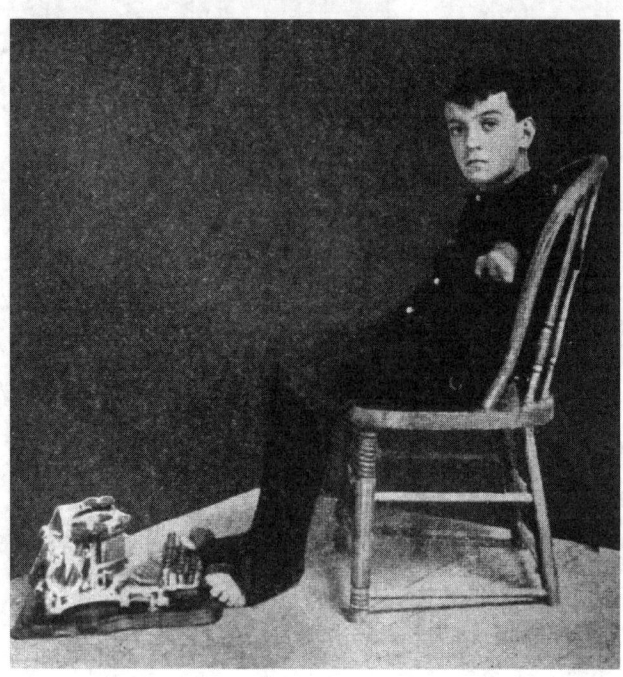

A boy without arms using a typewriter at Cotting School (formerly Industrial School for Crippled and Deformed Children).
A Manual of Orthopedic Surgery by A. Thorndike. Philadelphia: P. Blakiston's Son & Co., 1907. Library of Congress/Internet Archive.

Cover of Thorndike's book, A Manual of Orthopedic Surgery. Library of Congress/Internet Archive.

Later Career and Retirement

Throughout his career Thorndike "was an active member of many societies in and about his home, — the Massachusetts Medical Society, the Boston Medical Benevolent Society and the Society of Medical Sciences, [the American Medical Association, and the American College of Surgeons,] and he was also interested in the Boston Medical Library" ("Obituary Augustus Thorndike" 1940). He retired from active practice in 1918, at age 55 years: "The Hospital has lost the services of Dr. Augustus Thorndike, who retired from work after having given many years of devoted service to the Hospital" (Children's Hospital Archives, Annual Report 1917).

The Thorndike family had a summer house in Bar Harbor, Maine, and Thorndike had been president of the Bar Harbor Medical and Surgical Hospital. His wife, Alice, died in 1938, two years before him; they had been married more than 35 years and had five children. [Thorndike] died suddenly on August 23, 1940, at his summer home… at the age of seventy-seven years." ("Obituary Augustus Thorndike" 1940).

An obituary published in the *Journal of Bone and Joint Surgery* praised Thorndike's care for others—not only his patients but also his colleagues:

Dr. Thorndike's helpful attitude toward his associates, and particularly with his coworkers, was an outstanding feature of his character, and he gave freely of himself. He was just in his estimate of people, free from criticism, and tolerant toward the opinions of others…He had the faculty of bringing out the best in those with whom he worked. He had definite and strong convictions but was always kindly and tolerant toward the opinions of others even when differing from them…He was a good friend and had a philosophy of life that drew all to him. ("Augustus Thorndike 1863–1940" 1940)

ARTHUR W. TROTT

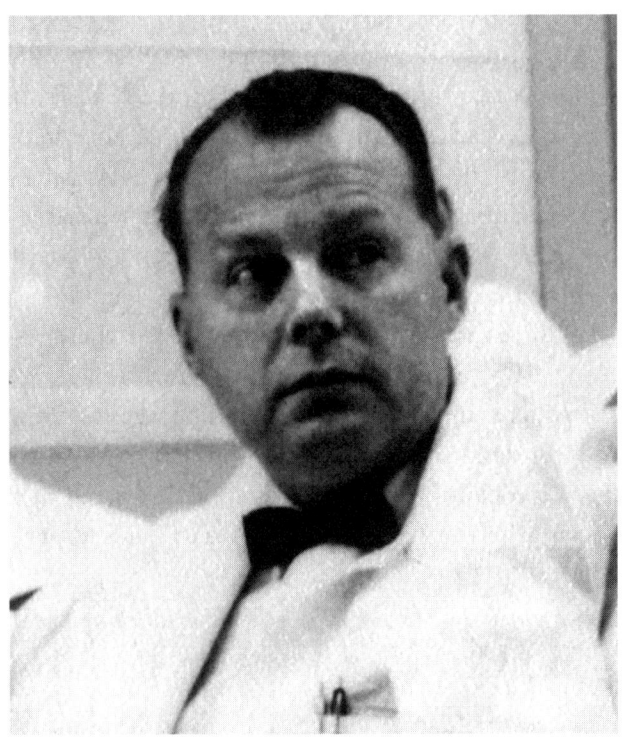

Arthur W. Trott. Boston Children's Hospital Archives, Boston, Massachusetts.

Physician Snapshot

Arthur W. Trott
BORN: 1920
DIED: 2002
SIGNIFICANT CONTRIBUTIONS: Worked tirelessly during the 1949 and 1955 polio epidemics in Boston; March of Dimes campaign director; president of the American Orthopaedic Foot and Ankle Society in 1997

Arthur Warren Trott, born in 1920, grew up in Wollaston, Massachusetts. He graduated from Harvard College in 1941 and from Harvard Medical School in 1944. In 1942, he received one of the scholarships offered by Harvard Medical School. In a 1993 interview with the Winthrop Group, Trott recalled that he graduated during World War II, and thus, after completing a surgical internship at the Boston City Hospital, which lasted nine months, he immediately joined the US Navy; he served in the Pacific theater. He returned to active duty a few years later, when he served at the Naval Hospital in Chelsea, Massachusetts, near the Boston Navy Yard, during the Korean War. After being discharged from the navy, he returned to Harvard Medical School to take refresher courses before completing two residencies in orthopaedics, one at Boston City Hospital and then a second at the West Roxbury Veterans Administration Hospital. He then had a year-long chief residency at the Cushing VA Hospital. He continued with an assistant residency and then another chief residency, both at Children's Hospital. He completed this last residency in 1950, and then joined the staff at Children's, where he advanced to a senior associate in orthopaedic surgery and spent the rest of his 35-year career (until 1984). At Harvard Medical School he advanced to clinical professor of orthopaedic surgery. During this time, Trott married Dorothy Crawford of Milton, Massachusetts. They had two children and three grandchildren. They lived in Wollaston their entire married life together.

Trott joined the full-time practice of Drs. William Green and David Grice, who were based at Children's Hospital. Arthur Pappas and Paul Griffin, as well as Drs. William Elliston, Frank Ober, and Meier Karp, were also members of that practice, but they had offices elsewhere and came to the hospital as consulting staff, going on rounds with residents and helping them during surgeries. All of them simultaneously cared for patients on the wards in the hospital and for their own private patients.

Trott, like most of the other orthopaedists at Children's, was also on the staff at the Peter Bent Brigham Hospital. As at Children's, he had to spend a particular amount of time there each year. His practice comprised mostly children, though ~30 percent of his patients were adults. Apparently, Green insisted that all his surgeons be a "well-rounded orthopedic surgeon and not pigeonholed in any one area," requiring that they be "well-trained in all aspects of orthopedics" (quoted in D. Dyer 1993).

Trott was a surgical consultant for almost 20 years at the naval hospitals in Chelsea and in

Newport, Rhode Island. He covered a consultation clinic for crippled children in Fall River, Massachusetts, where he sometimes worked with Drs. Paul Griffin and Benjamin Bierbaum.

At the 1957 annual meeting of the American Academy of Orthopaedic Surgeons, during which Green was president, Trott, Dr. Henry Banks, Dr. John Leidholt, and Dr. Richard Kilfole were elected as new members. Trott was then 37. In 1964, a new curriculum for the third- and fourth-year students at Harvard Medical School included a required clerkship in orthopaedic surgery, which Trott developed. At that time, Trott was the administrative officer for the orthopaedic teaching program at Children's Hospital.

Expertise in Polio

During Boston's polio epidemics of 1949 (1,728 people contracted polio that year) and 1955, Trott worked ceaselessly to treat patients. At the time, Grice was the assistant director of the Massachusetts Infantile Paralysis Clinic and Trott was director of the Respiratory Unit of Children's Medical Center in Wellesley. During the 1955 epidemic ~4,000 patients with polio were treated there; of those, 125 required treatment in an iron lung. As the patients improved, they would be weaned from the iron lung (or "tank respirator," as Trott called it) to a rocking bed. In patients being treated in a rocking bed, "the abdominal organs slide down,

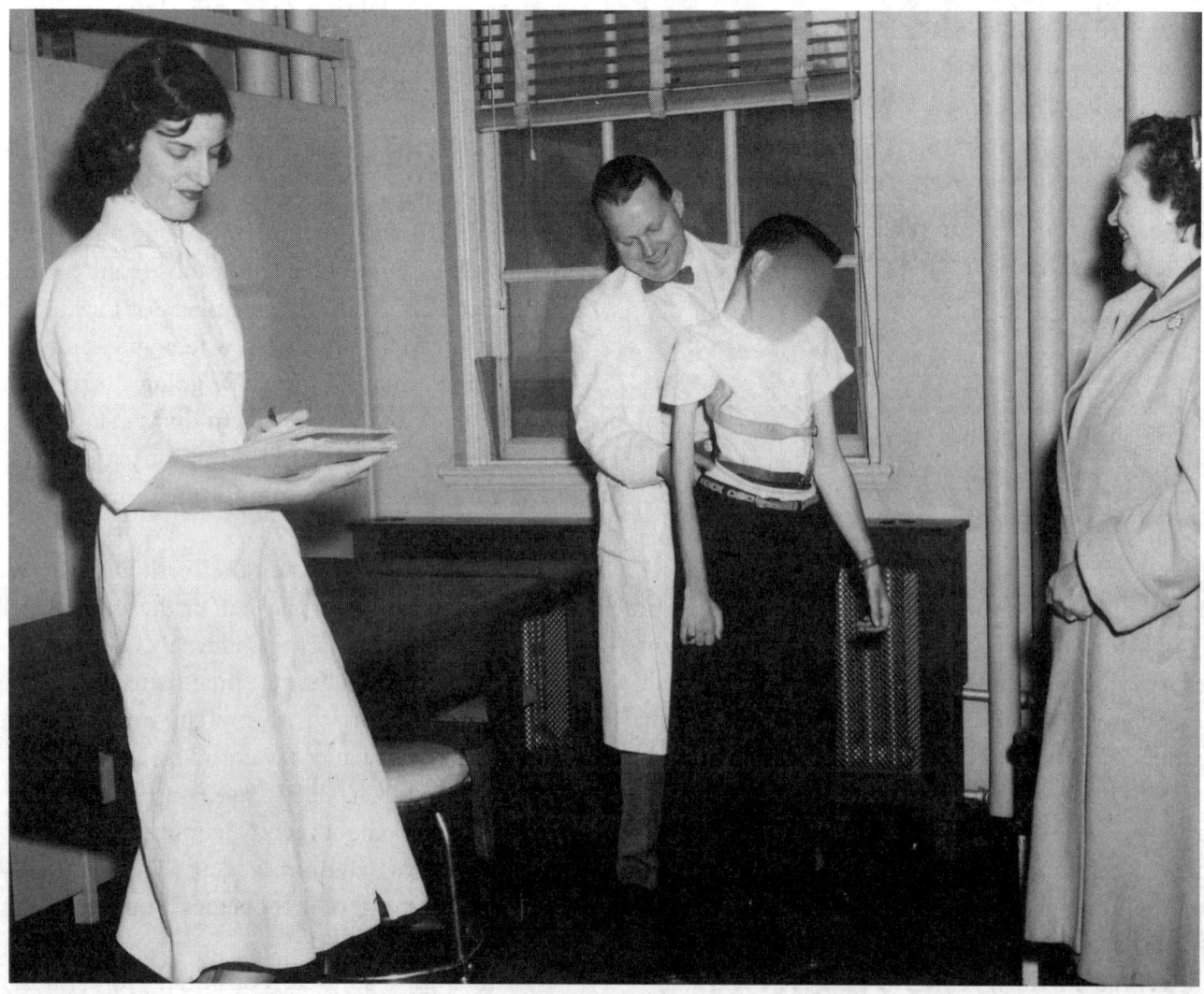

Dr. Trott examining the spine of a patient in the polio clinic. Boston Children's Hospital Archives, Boston, Massachusetts.

and in doing so they pull the diaphragm down, so that air sucks in" (quoted in D. Dyer 1993). These patients then would be treated with "things like the chest respirator...a plastic body that could ventilate...eventually you could get a good proportion of the patients free of the respirator" (quoted in D. Dyer 1993).

At Children's Hospital, Trott was required to evaluate every patient with polio who was admitted. Because of the risk:

> When you were examining an acute polio patient, you would wear a mask...Three times during the polio season we each had to give a blood sample to see if there was a change in the antibody titer. It turned out that none of the personnel got polio, just through using simple hand-washing techniques and a mask in case the patient coughed. We had one nurse who got polio, but she wasn't involved in the admitting. (quoted in D. Dyer 1993)

Trott didn't only treat patients with polio at Children's:

> I had a bunch of polio cases at the Peter Bent Brigham, about six respiratory cases. I was handling the service at the Peter Bent Brigham during the 1949 epidemic. Later on, when they had a big epidemic in Brazil around 1958 or 1959, Ben Ferris was there. He was a respiratory physiologist from the Harvard School of Public Health and worked with me at the Mary MacArthur. Ben went to Brazil because all their medical personnel were coming down with polio, too. They just never washed their hands. All he had to do was introduce the simple technique of washing your hands. It cut down the number of personnel getting polio. (quoted in D. Dyer 1993)

During the peak of these polio epidemics, Trott and Grice oversaw a large polio clinic three mornings a week (Tuesday, Thursday, and Friday)

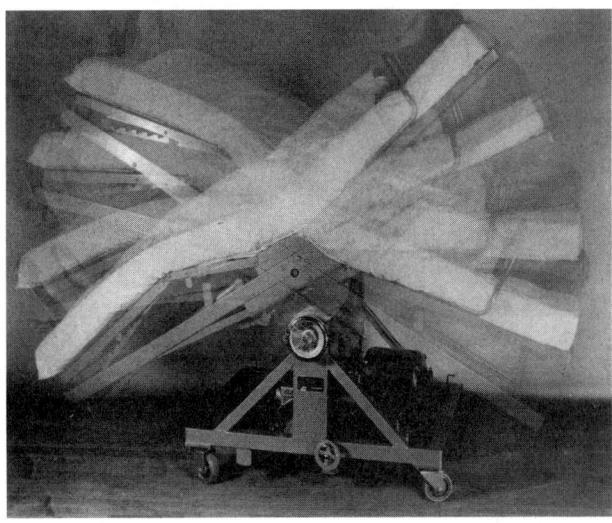

Rocking bed—time-elapsed image. Division of Medicine and Science, National Museum of American History, Smithsonian Institution.

at Children's; Trott took charge when Grice moved to Philadelphia in 1958 but before that Trott also managed the Mary MacArthur Memorial Respiratory Unit in Wellesley. This unit was named in memory of the daughter of theater actress Helen Hayes, who in 1949 died of polio: "We developed a good relationship with Helen Hayes. Every time she came to town, my wife and I got front row tickets. I got to know Helen Hayes very well" (quoted in D. Dyer 1993).

Albert Sabin visited Boston as a guest of the Boston chapter of the March of Dimes in 1962—just one year after he had developed the oral polio vaccine. Massachusetts was the first state to conduct an extensive immunization program. Trott represented the Massachusetts Medical Association at a luncheon held in Sabin's honor. Speaking at a press conference after the luncheon, Trott praised Sabin for his major discovery and the March of Dimes for its continual support in fighting polio and supporting victims of the disease. Trott would later become the campaign director for the March of Dimes.

In 1954, Trott attended, with Dr. Vern Nickel, a meeting of the Mary MacArthur Memorial Respiratory Centers in Houston, Texas. Most of the attendees at the meeting were respiratory therapists, so Trott and Nickel gravitated toward the local orthopaedists who were present. Trott described a novel treatment they learned of from Paul Harrington at one of the sessions:

> Harrington...had developed this technique of putting in a rod with a hook at one end to hook into the bone, and at the other end there was a ratchet. You could ratchet this thing up, jump from one step upwards and straighten out the spine, right on the spot. He was doing that in polio patients at the time...His idea at the time...was new. It wasn't even in the literature at the time. Vern Nichol [sic] and I were fascinated...So when I came back from Houston I told Dr. Green about it. He said, "Well, keep your eye on it."
>
> About two years or so after that, it really became feasible. It was on the market. We did a lot of those at the time...about 1954 or 1955. (quoted in D. Dyer 1993)

Trott described the method orthopaedists at Children's Hospital used to correct severe curves in patients with scoliosis before they began using Harrington rods:

> In the early days we had to put these patients in a big plaster cast involving one leg down to just above the knee, and one arm to the elbow. This covered the entire body. Then we would put in what we called a turnbuckle type of thing, and make a cut in the cast so it would allow the spine to be brought back into a straight alignment...a several-week problem before you could get the spine straight and then operate on the patient to fuse the spine in the corrective position, which was amazing because we did the operation through the cast; we didn't take the cast off, just cut holes in it...a patient with scoliosis, say in 1949 or 1950, was spending up to six months in a cast including one arm to the elbow and one leg to above the knee... [N]ow they come in, get operated on, put in a nice plastic jacket, and home they go. The time of treatment and hospitalization has markedly decreased. (quoted in D. Dyer 1993)

This quick treatment was definitely in use when Trott was interviewed in 1993, but when I was a resident at Children's Hospital in 1967 and 1969, most patients with scoliosis were still receiving tibial osteoperiosteal grafts while wearing turnbuckle casts with maximally corrected spine alignment. I still remember attending grand rounds as a senior resident and hearing Dr. Robert Keller, a young attending physician at the time, present the first case in which he used a Harrington rod in a patient with scoliosis.

Trott published five papers, coedited one book, and wrote seven book reviews. Two of his articles focused on circulatory changes in the lower extremities of patients with poliomyelitis, which he first reported to the Orthopaedic Research Society in 1956. At the time, some reports named peripheral vasospasm as being responsible for the cold and clammy skin and the peripheral cyanosis that often occurred in patients with polio. Trott and his colleagues, measuring both skin and muscle temperatures in 40 patients during the first 40 days of their illness, found no significant changes in the involved extremities from the temperatures in the limbs of normal patients during bed rest.

In a 1958 study involving 153 patients, Trott and his coauthors concluded that such vasoconstriction did not occur until well into the disease—five or six months after onset—and then only intermittently and to a nominal extent. As the disease progressed, however, the affected extremities became colder in patients with extensive paralysis. Their findings showed a correlation between skin and muscle temperature and extent of paralysis.

Clinical Interest in the Foot and Ankle

Trott was program chairman for the 1976 meeting of the American Orthopaedic Foot Society (AOFS), now named the American Orthopaedic Foot and Ankle Society (AOFAS). He was elected

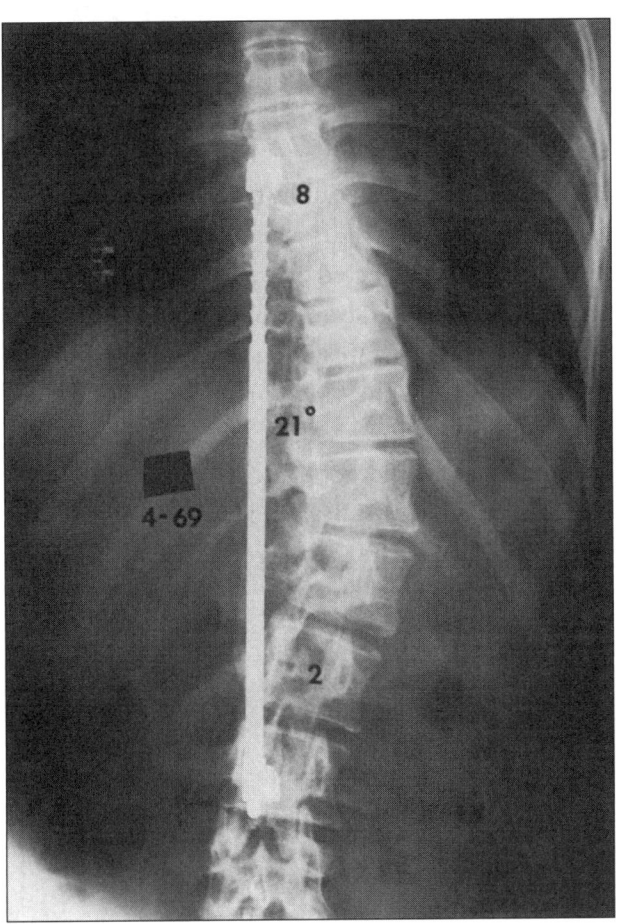

Example of the original Harrington rods.
Scoliosis and Other Deformities of the Axial Skeleton by E. Riseborough and J. Herndon. Boston: Little, Brown & Co., 1975. Courtesy of the author and publisher.

as the ninth president of the society in 1977. At that time, its membership totaled 212. Dr. N. Giannestras served as his program chair during that year's meeting. The year 1977 was a big one for the AOFS: its annual meeting that year was approved for the first time as a category 1 continuing medical education (CME) credit by the Liaison Committee for Continuing Medical Education, and the American Board of Orthopaedic Surgery agreed to include at least one question about the foot during the oral examinations for certification.

Trott made several statements about feet and shoes during his presidency. One was about the arch. He stated that normally low arches cannot be raised by strengthening or stretching muscles, as bones and ligaments—not muscles—determine one's arch. Another statement concerned improper fit: not only incorrect sizing but tight toes in shoes and backless shoes can lead to injury.

He made two public statements about high-heeled shoes. In the first, he described how they destabilize the foot and can result in sprains or fractures. They cause pain (because just the metatarsals have to support the weight of the body) as well as bunions and corns (because they squeeze the foot). For Trott, a "proper" shoe has a "light and flexible" sole and adjusts to the shape of the foot. In the second, Trott again emphasized how they destabilize the whole foot, sometimes resulting in muscle sprains and fractures, and negatively affect the normal posture that is necessary for balance.

After his year as president of AOFS, Trott, along with Dr. James E. Bateman (president of the AOFS two years before Trott), published a selection of papers from the 1977 and 1978 meetings in a book, *The Foot and Ankle*. Dr. Andrea Cracchiolo reviewed the book for the *Journal of Bone and Joint Surgery* in 1981, stating, "Over-all the papers present a compendium of information that generally is not commonly available in the orthopaedic literature. Thus, although the book resembles a hard-cover 'journal,' it is a worthwhile collection of important knowledge on the foot."

Professional Relationship with Dr. William Green

In his 1993 interview with the Winthrop Group, Trott was asked about Dr. William T. Green. Obviously a fan and friend of Green, Trott described him as a warm and friendly person who did not have a temper, although "the residents all feared him, because if they didn't do things correctly, he might make a rather caustic comment" (quoted in D. Dyer 1993). I recall one event that occurred while I was in an operating room with Trott. The procedure was a distal femoral stapling to treat a leg length discrepancy. Trott, as he often did, was allowing me to insert the staples. At the time, I was a first-year orthopaedic resident (a "pup"), though I had already completed two years of surgical training. Green entered the room and immediately demanded that I stop stapling and angrily criticized Trott for allowing a "pup" to operate. Green told me to leave the room (though I was able to return later and assist Trott).

Trott believed Green had a sense of humor and was "a great host. He had a big place in Duxbury…Every Fourth of July he'd have the staff members, the residents and their families there for the day" (quoted in D. Dyer 1993). Trott didn't recall that Green had any interests outside of work, except for occasionally going sailing. Green "ran a fairly tight ship. He was on top of things. I ended up as the hatchet man, unfortunately, because if something came up, he'd send me off to find out what was happening, and I'd have to come back and report to him so he could make his decision" (quoted in D. Dyer 1993). According to Trott, Green was a hard worker: "He spent long hours at the hospital. He wouldn't go home until 8:00 at night sometimes. He had to be in early in the morning, so he expected everybody else to do it…I used to spend long days there" (quoted in D. Dyer 1993). I remember residents and staff staying in the hospital until they saw Green's car gone from its reserved parking space. Once Green had left, everyone else would go home.

Trott died at the Brigham and Women's Hospital on May 18, 2002, at age 82. His wife, Dorothy, died 10 years later, on August 1, 2012; she was 92 years old.

CHAPTER 24

Melvin J. Glimcher

Father of the Bone Field

Melvin Jacob Glimcher was born to Aaron Glimcher and Clara Finkelstein on June 2, 1925, in Brookline, Massachusetts. His family owned a garment factory in Chelsea where he grew up. He attended Chelsea High School there, working as a night sports reporter for the local newspaper, the *Chelsea Record*. Later in life, he felt that experience, along with playing in a violin duo in high school, to be one of his prized memories. After graduating at age 17, he enlisted in the Marine Corps in 1942. He never saw active duty during WWII, but he was instead sent to study science and engineering at Duke University, later attending Purdue University. He graduated with highest honors from Purdue in 1946 in two different fields, mechanical engineering and physics. In 1950, he received his medical degree from Harvard Medical School (HMS), graduating magna cum laude. He completed his honors thesis on lower limb orthopaedic brace research in cooperation with the Department of Civil Engineering at the Massachusetts Institute of Technology (MIT). He won both the Soma Weiss Prize and the Borden Research Award for his research.

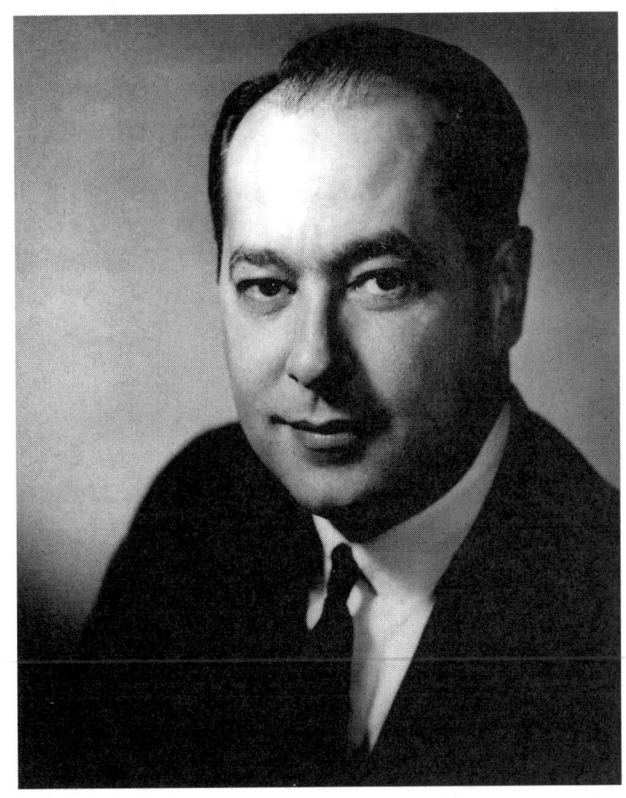

Melvin J. Glimcher. Massachusetts General Hospital, Archives and Special Collections.

Physician Snapshot

Melvin J. Glimcher
BORN: 1925
DIED: 2014
SIGNIFICANT CONTRIBUTIONS: Discovered the physiology of mineralization; clarified the pathophysiology of avascular necrosis of the femoral head; developed the "Boston Arm," a myoelectric prosthesis

EARLY ORTHOPAEDIC TRAINING AND CAREER

Glimcher was a surgical intern at Strong Memorial Hospital 1950–1951 at the University of Rochester in New York. He then returned to Harvard,

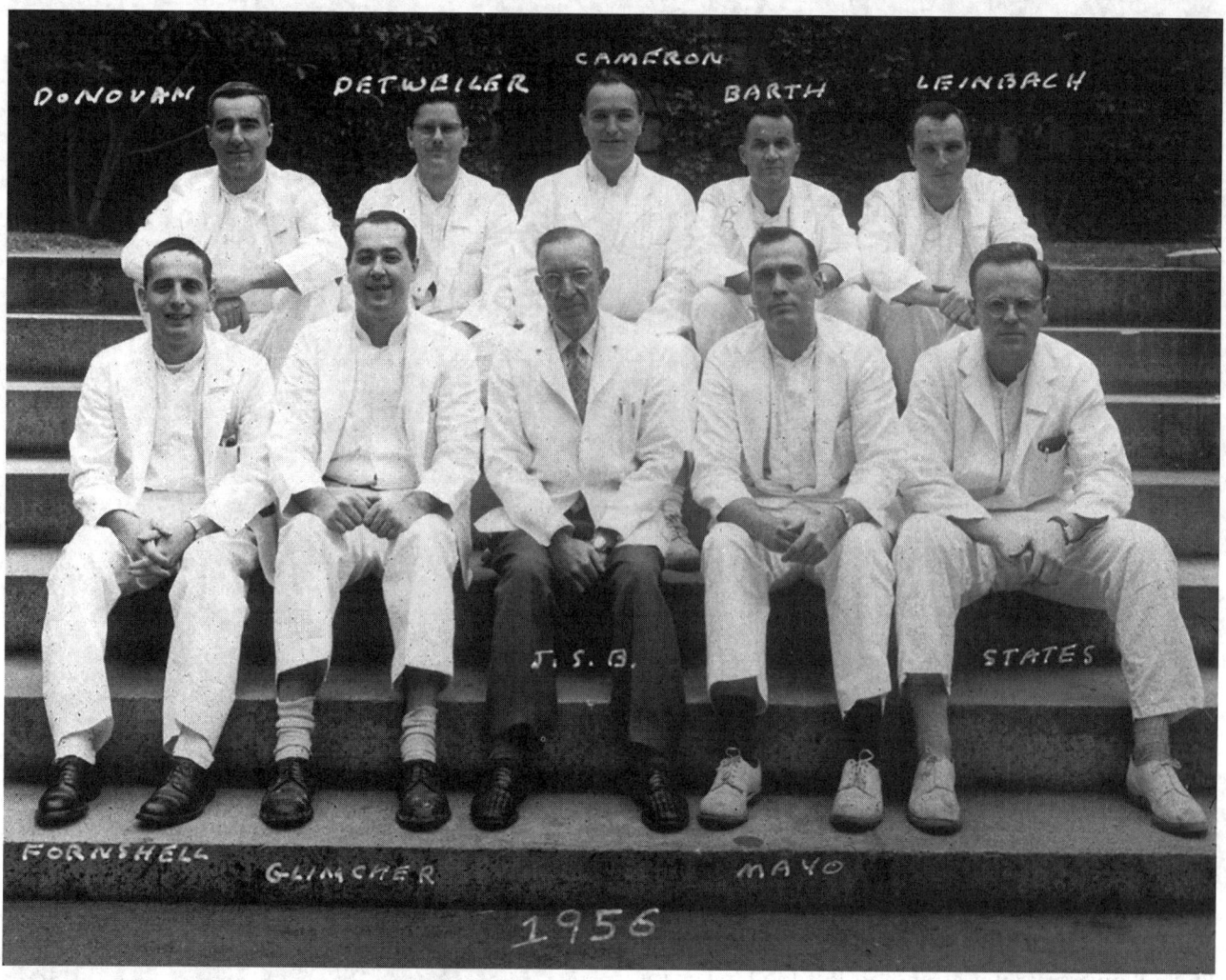

Residents at MGH with Dr. Barr, 1956. Dr. Glimcher is in the front row, second from the left. MGH HCORP Archives.

first as an assistant resident in surgery at Massachusetts General Hospital (MGH) for one year, and then again as an orthopaedic resident in the MGH/Boston Children's Hospital Orthopaedic Residency Program for three years. From 1955 to 1956, he was a chief resident at both MGH and Boston Children's Hospital. As a junior resident in surgery at MGH, he participated in two weekly clinicopathologic exercises founded by Dr. Richard C. Cabot and led at the time by Dr. Benjamin Castleman. In the first, he discussed his findings on physical examination of a patient with abdominal pain and a mass in the right upper quadrant in the emergency department. He described the mass as ill-defined during the case presentation, but, in his characteristic sharp and critical response, he stated:

"I suppose the reason the mass was termed ill-defined in the protocol is that only half the physicians who examined the patient could palpate it. To those of us who did feel it, it was anything but ill defined" ("Case 38842. Presentation of a Case" 1952). At surgery, the patient was found to have a large adenocarcinoma at the head of the pancreas. In the second case, a 33-year-old patient had undergone an uneventful left hip cup arthroplasty but had then developed acute abdominal pain and vomiting on the sixth postoperative day. Glimcher clarified three points about the patient's course that were not raised in the discussion. During a second operation, the same patient was found to have acute cholecystitis with impaction of the gall-bladder ampulla in the foramen of Winslow, not a small bowel obstruction or acute pancreatitis as had been suspected by the surgeons.

During his orthopaedic surgery training, Glimcher became increasingly fascinated with the structure of bone, and he changed the direction of his career. He began to focus on understanding the basic structure, function, and properties of bone. He published his first case report in the *New England Journal of Medicine* in 1955 on epiphyseal injuries on a child's hand after frostbite (see **Case 24.1**). By 1957, he published his second paper as lead author after only one year into an NIH-sponsored research fellowship at the Massachusetts Institute of Technology (MIT). His paper, titled "Macromolecular Aggregation States in Relation to Mineralization: The Collagen-Hydroxyapatite System as Studied in Vitro," published in the "Proceedings of the National Academy of Sciences of the USA," became a seminal work on the calcification of bones (it specifically analyzed long chain protein collagen), and it is still cited today. During the course of his four-year fellowship, Glimcher researched connective tissues in a lab and was mentored by Professor Francis O. Schmidt; he pursued studies in advanced biochemistry, biophysics, and engineering during this time. That same year, Glimcher became a fellow of the Massachusetts Medical Society, and by 1958, he presented his first paper to the Orthopaedic Research Society, titled "The Specificity of the Macromolecular Aggregation State of Collagen in Calcification." He was one of 12 other individuals elected into membership at that meeting. Glimcher did "more than enough" to have earned his PhD, but he elected to leave MIT before receiving the degree (Martin 2014). He may have felt fully confident in his research skills and prepared to move into the new position awaiting him at MGH.

DIRECTOR OF THE MGH ORTHOPAEDIC RESEARCH LABORATORIES

In 1959, he returned to Harvard as an assistant professor of orthopaedic surgery and to MGH as an assistant orthopaedic surgeon and director of the soon-to-be-built Orthopaedic Research Laboratories. He was director during the planning, fundraising, and construction of the labs. Upon his return, he established a strong research collaboration with Dr. Stephen Krane, chief of the arthritis unit at MGH and well-known for his contributions to the bone and mineral field and to rheumatology. They wrote articles together on apatite crystals and the incorporation of organic phosphate by collagen fibrils. Their research suggested "that the phosphorus ion of the mineral is the linking atom which binds together the crystals with the protein organic matrix. It had been commonly thought previously that calcium atoms did this" (Black 1965). Glimcher continued his basic research on bone, teeth, and enamel, doing:

> intricate studies that took many years, Dr. Glimcher and his colleagues showed that an entirely different process is at the root of bone mineralization. It is actually a process akin to cloud-seeding, in which crystals form in the clouds because of the presence of molecules of silver iodide that serve as nuclei to promote the crystal formation. In the case of the body's mineralized tissues, the nuclei for crystal formation are in the collagen, the most common protein in bone. (Schmeck 1988)

Dr. Joseph Barr, Chief of the Orthopaedic Department at the time, valued Glimcher's

---

MACROMOLECULAR AGGREGATION STATES IN RELATION TO
MINERALIZATION: THE COLLAGEN-HYDROXYAPATITE
SYSTEM AS STUDIED IN VITRO*

BY MELVIN J. GLIMCHER,† ALAN J. HODGE, AND FRANCIS O. SCHMITT

DEPARTMENT OF BIOLOGY, MASSACHUSETTS INSTITUTE OF TECHNOLOGY, CAMBRIDGE, MASSACHUSETTS

Communicated August 28, 1957

Title of Glimcher's article in which he described the process of mineralization. *Proceedings of the National Academy of Sciences USA*, 1957; 43:860.

Case 24.1. Epiphyseal Injures Following Frostbite on a 7-year-old Patient's Hand

> "E.N. (M.G.H.), a 7-year old girl was first seen in the Orthopedic Outpatient Department in January, 1955, because of finger deformities. In March, 1950, at the age of 2 ½ years she wandered out of the house with her dog and onto a snow-covered road in Saskatchewan at 5 p.m. when the temperature was below 0. When found about 2 hours later, she was wearing woolen leggings and a sweater but was without hat or gloves; her left hand was in a pocket. Her father immediately noticed that fingers of both hands, particularly the right, were white and the tissues stony hard. Ice could be scraped from the skin surface. There was no apparent pain. The hands were thawed in cold water for 60 to 90 minutes, after which there was considerable pain, worse in the right hand than the left, and the tissues gradually became swollen and developed a mottled pink to blue discoloration. The attending physician applied a bland salve and wrapped each finger and hand separately.
>
> "On the following day, vesiculation extending from their tips to the proximal interphalangeal joints appeared in the skin of the 2d, 3d, 4th and 5th fingers of the right hand. During the next several weeks, the swelling, blistering and pain subsided, but the skin over these fingers became dry and hard and turned a dark brownish black. The only treatment was a daily application of ointment and change of dressing.
>
> "At about the 3d week, the fingernails of the involved 4 fingers became detached, and the skin down to the proximal interphalangeal joints 'peeled off, like a glove,' revealing a delicate covering of pink skin. At no time was there any evidence of infection. The left hand showed none of these changes.
>
> "Five or 6 months after the frostbite, the mother noticed flexion deformities of the distal interphalangeal joints of the 2d through 5th fingers of the right hand; these have progressed very gradually. About a year later, it was first noted that the fingers of the right hand, especially the distal phalanges, were shorter than those of the left. No difference in function between the 2 hands and no change in color after exposure to cold had been observed. The patient never complained of cold sensitivity of the fingers, and, in fact, the mother believed that the right hand usually felt warmer than the left.
>
> "Physical examination showed a co-operative, healthy-appearing girl. The color, temperature and pulses of both hands were equal and normal, and there was no evidence of increased or decreased sweating of either hand. The left hand appeared normal. With the right hand at rest, there was slight flexion of the distal interphalangeal joints of the 2d through 5th fingers, most marked in the 3d and 5th fingers. There was also some radial deviation of the distal phalanges of the 4th and 5th fingers. The distal phalanges of the 3d, 4th and 5th fingers appeared clinically shorter and broader than those on the left, as did the middle phalanges of the 4th and 5th fingers. The distal interphalangeal joints

research brilliance and had arranged for the first orthopaedic research laboratories at MGH to be built on the third and fourth floors of the White Building. Financial support for construction of the laboratories came from funds left over from Dr. Joel Goldthwait's effort to build the hospital's first orthopaedic ward in 1903 and from the hospital's 1961 development fund on its 150th anniversary with the blessing of the hospital's trustees. Dr. Edward D. Churchill, the chief of surgery, strongly supported the orthopaedic laboratory. Goldthwait was still alive and approved the use of the funds raised by him for Ward 1. David Crockett of the development office raised matching funds from the foundation, grants and individuals.

Initially, four laboratories were opened under the direction of Dr. Glimcher. They included Dr. Joel E. Goldthwait, the biochemistry laboratory; Dr. Robert B. Osgood, the crystal laboratory; Dr. Armin Klein, the histology laboratory; and Dr. Marius N. Smith-Petersen, the physical chemistry laboratory. After the unveiling, there was a luncheon and tour of the new laboratories,

> of these fingers were thickened, and there was dorsal prominence of the 3d distal phalanx at the proximal end.
>
> "Actively, the distal interphalangeal joints of the 2d through 5th fingers on the right lacked 5, 30, 20 and 60° of full extension respectively. All these joints, however, could be passively extended to neutral and the radial deviations could be passively corrected. There was full flexion of all the joints, and function was excellent with smooth motion and no grating or crepitus. Although the patient could distinguish sharp from dull pain, there was moderate hypesthesia over the volar aspect and minimal hypesthesia over the dorsal surface of the distal phalanges of the 2d through 5th fingers, more marked in the 4th and 5th fingers.
>
> "X-rays examination was reported as follows:
>
> "The bone age is approximately 6 years and 10 months, according to Todd's standards, which corresponds to the stated chronologic age of 7 years. Bone density and architecture of the left hand appear to be entirely normal. There are, however, striking abnormal changes in the right hand. The distal phalanges of the 3d, 4th and 5th fingers are shorter than those of the left hand; the middle phalanges of the 4th and 5th fingers are also shorter and broader than their opposite members. The trabecular pattern is accentuated. The most significant change is the complete absence of the epiphyses normally accompanying the distal phalanges of the 3d, 4th and 5th fingers, as well as that of the middle phalanx of the 5th finger. A tiny fragment of the secondary ossification center of the epiphysis of the distal phalanx of the 2nd finger is present and also a portion of secondary ossification center of the epiphysis of the middle phalanx of the 4th finger, which is partially fused with the shaft. In addition, at the articular surfaces there are numerous small, rounded areas of demineralization of a 'punched-out' nature. There is flexion deformity of the distal interphalangeal joints of the 2d through 5th fingers on the right, more marked in the 3d and 5th fingers. The remaining bones of the right hand are normal.
>
> "X-ray measurements of phalangeal length were made by means of posteroanterior and lateral films, the latter to obviate the error due to flexion contractures of the distal phalanges. These measurements showed that the distal phalanges of the index fingers were of equal length, the distal phalanges of the right 3d and 4th fingers and the middle phalanx of the right 4th finger were 0.3 cm. shorter than the left, the distal phalanx of the right 5th finger was 0.25 cm. shorter than the left, and the middle phalanx of the right 5th finger was 0.4 cm. shorter than the left. Measurements were made to include the entire ossified portion of the phalanx, which included secondary ossification centers where present."
>
> (Dreyfuss and Glimcher 1955)

attended by 200 members of the orthopaedic department, HMS faculty, faculty of other medical schools, MGH staff and staff at other hospitals, government officials, and representatives of philanthropy organizations. A program of speeches was presided over by MGH trustee and MIT professor, Dr. Francis O. Schmidt, who stated: "With some basic biophysical and biochemical research going on in a hospital, you have at one end the molecules, at the other end, Man" (Burns 1960). Dr. Barr added, "In Dr. Glimcher the hospital has [a] laboratory as this [which] has no place in a hospital...If we fail, this laboratory will be placed in the medical school or MIT, but we already had some breakthroughs and some unexpected breakthroughs. We may find the need for bone surgery diminishing [and] rediscover the kinship between all living things" (Burns 1960). Dr. Glimcher concluded, "We are examining the tissue of the bone with special x-rays, the electron microscope and other scientific techniques that give detailed information about the way the atoms of the molecules in the bones are arranged and how these molecules are placed in the positions that give bone its structure and strength" (Burns 1960). The research team, under the direction of Dr. Glimcher, included:

- Dr. Lawrence C. Bonar, crystallographer
- Dr. Eton P. Katz, physical chemist
- Dr. Gerald L. Mechanic, biochemist
- Dr. Dorothy F. Travis, biophysicist
- Dr. Philip T. Levine, dentist and oral biologist

Dr. George Packer Berry, Dean of HMS, made the following comments:

> Orthopedics is on the threshold of developments of unpredictably great value to the disabled and injured [and] if the resources can be found to build for orthopedics the academic triad of teaching, research and patient care. In these research facilities…physical scientists and orthopaedic surgeons will work together and the resources of Harvard Medical School, the MGH and the MIT will come to focus on orthopedic problems. (Burns 1960)

At the time, Dr. Thornton Brown (a professor at HMS and interim chief of orthopaedics at MGH following Barr's retirement) also stated:

> Boston has been referred to as the cradle of orthopedics in surgery [and] [f]or many years many of the nation's professors of orthopedics had been trained here. Orthopedics reached its peak of development in technical progress under Smith-Petersen in this hospital. (Burns 1960)

Glimcher was also appointed an Albert List Scholar in Medical Sciences at HMS from 1961 until 1964 and then chief of the Department of Orthopaedic Surgery at MGH in 1965. At the time of his appointment, he had published over

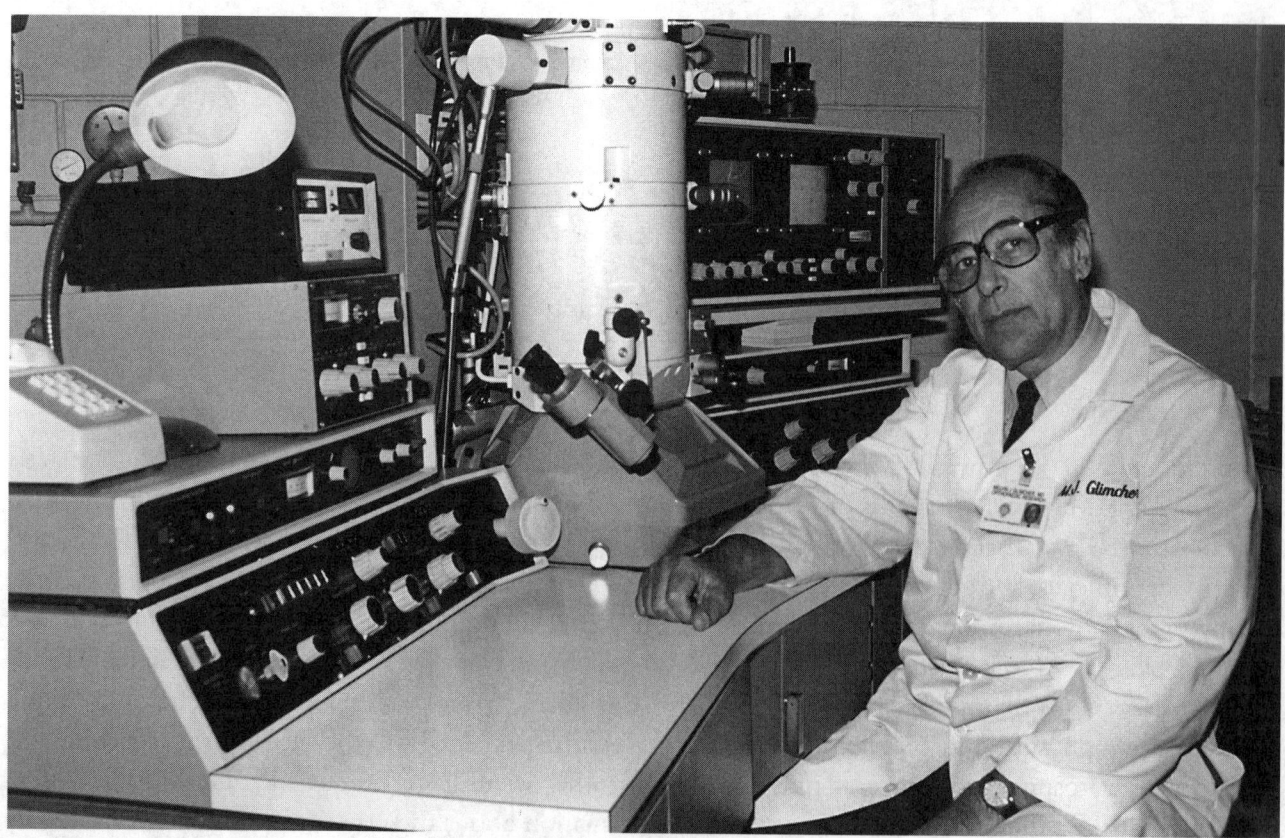

Dr. Glimcher in his laboratory, seated at an electron microscope. *Images of America. Children's Hospital Boston.* Charleston, SC: Arcadia Publishing, 2005. Boston Children's Hospital Archives, Boston, Massachusetts.

Author Recollections

I was an intern at the University of Pennsylvania from 1965 to 1966 when I interviewed at Boston Children's Hospital and MGH for a position in the orthopaedic residency program. I still recall my tour at MGH provided by Dr. Kirby Von Kessler, the chief resident at the time. On a roof balcony overlooking the Charles River, I asked Von Kessler about who was being considered for the new chief position at MGH. Dr. Joseph Barr had retired for health reasons. Von Kessler mentioned that two were in competition for the top job: one a clinician (Dr. Otto Aufranc) and the other a research orthopaedic surgeon scientist in the lab (whose name he could not recall). He did not know who would be selected, but he commented that the faculty were divided with many of the clinicians, especially the hip surgeons, favoring Aufranc. Only some months later did I learn that Dr. Glimcher was appointed the chief of the Department of Orthopaedic Surgery at MGH—demonstrating support for continued research in orthopaedics—and later the Edith M. Ashley Professor of Orthopaedic Surgery at HMS, positions he held until 1970.

During my residency at MGH, I found Glimcher to have a ubiquitous sense of directness and fervent support for his convictions. On one occasion during the chief's weekly meetings with the residents, I recall Glimcher's defense of a salary increase for the residents to the hospital's board of trustees. We were paid a minimal stipend in those days, and Glimcher angrily addressed the trustees, stating that residents were professionals and not shoe salesmen. We deserved a better salary. He was very angry, almost shouting, when recalling his meeting with the trustees to us. On another occasion, before advancing to a chief resident's position, he instituted a series of six, one-half-hour examinations for the residents before individual faculty. I can't remember all six of my examiners but do recall two, Dr. Harris and Dr. Glimcher. Both were demanding and difficult. I only remember Dr. Glimcher's questions to me. They dealt with the biomechanics of Harrington Rod fixation in the scoliotic spine, for an entire one-half hour.

---

56 articles in leading research journals, including a paper in *Science*, and he had received several major awards, including:

- the Kappa Delta Award for outstanding research
- the International Association for Dental Research Award (first recipient) for his research on biological mineralization
- the Claude Bernard Medal in Physiology from the University of Montreal for his research on the structure and function of bone
- the Ralph Pemberton Award from the American Rheumatism Society (Philadelphia Branch)

Not long after, Glimcher was elected a Fellow of the American Academy of Arts and Sciences in 1966, and in an interview with the *Boston Globe* he stated, "Orthopedics in the future will not be simply surgery, or medicine…but a contribution of both plus knowledge of the whole area of skeletal structure, its biology, chemistry, and biomechanics" (Stickgold 2014).

Glimcher published his first article for orthopaedic surgeons on the organization of mineralized tissues in 1968. Using x-ray diffraction and electron microscopy and MRI, which he had learned to apply during his MIT research fellowship, Glimcher wrote:

One of the striking features of most of the biologically mineralized tissues is the highly ordered and organized arrangement of the mineral phase [which] vary from tissue to tissue [,and] it is... likely that the formation of the first solid phase is dependent on a co-operative event involving the interactions between a number of ions, ion clusters, matrix-bound mineral components, and the surfaces within the holes of the collagen...the induction of the mineral phase by collagen fibrils is highly dependent on the presence of hydrated spaces within the collagen fibrils. (Glimcher 1968)

Eric Radin, one of Glimcher's former research colleagues, "called [him] 'an intellectual giant' who intuitively saw a need to bring engineering principles to medicine. 'He understood that from very early on when none of the rest of us did'" (Martin 2014).

Not only did he study the development of bone, but that same year he was "a leading developer of... the 'Boston Arm': an artificial limb that responds to commands from the brain" (Stickgold 2014). Dr. Glimcher was a consultant to Liberty Mutual Insurance Company, a large workman's compensation insurer at the time. He, along with Professor Robert W. Mann at MIT (Mechanical Engineering) and Dr. Alden L. Cudworth, director of the Liberty Mutual Research Center, and with other engineers began to develop an upper extremity prosthesis that would respond to electromyographic (EMG) signals; not relying on active motions of the shoulder or elbow to drive the prosthesis and originally conceived in the United Kingdom and Russia. The concept of this type of prosthesis:

> grew out of talks in 1960 between Dr. Glimcher and the late Dr. Norbert Weiner of MIT, originator of the theory of cybergenetics, or the study of control and communication in the animal and the machine (1948). An important factor in cybergenetics is the feedback principle, in which an operating organism or machine senses the effects of its actions automatically and adjusts accordingly. The Boston Arm makes use of this principle with its weight-sensing mechanism...a force-sensing element detects fluctuations in weight...[and] automatically adjusts the voltage level of the electrical energy being supplied to the arm, thus controlling the force the arm exerts in lifting. (Stevens 1968)

They developed a prototype and fitted two amputees successfully. "This is where the Boston Arm is truly ingenious. Its secret lies in the principle of feedback—the technique of feeding back a part of a resulting reaction to control the initial reaction" (Freese 1968). This initial project, originally supported by Liberty Mutual, eventually was turned over to Liberating Technologies, Inc., an independent company located in Holliston, Massachusetts. Liberating Technologies, Inc., has further developed the myoelectric prosthesis, first the Boston Digital Arm and now the LTI Digital™ Arm Systems for Adults which includes a variety of hands, elbows, wrist, and shoulder components.

ORTHOPAEDIC SURGEON-IN-CHIEF AT BOSTON CHILDREN'S HOSPITAL

Glimcher resigned as chief of orthopaedics at MGH in 1970 in order to become orthopaedic surgeon-in-chief at Boston Children's Hospital

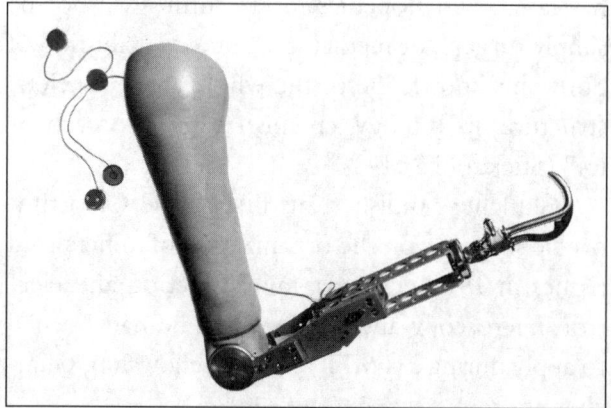

The "Boston Arm." Courtesy of Bruce Petersen.

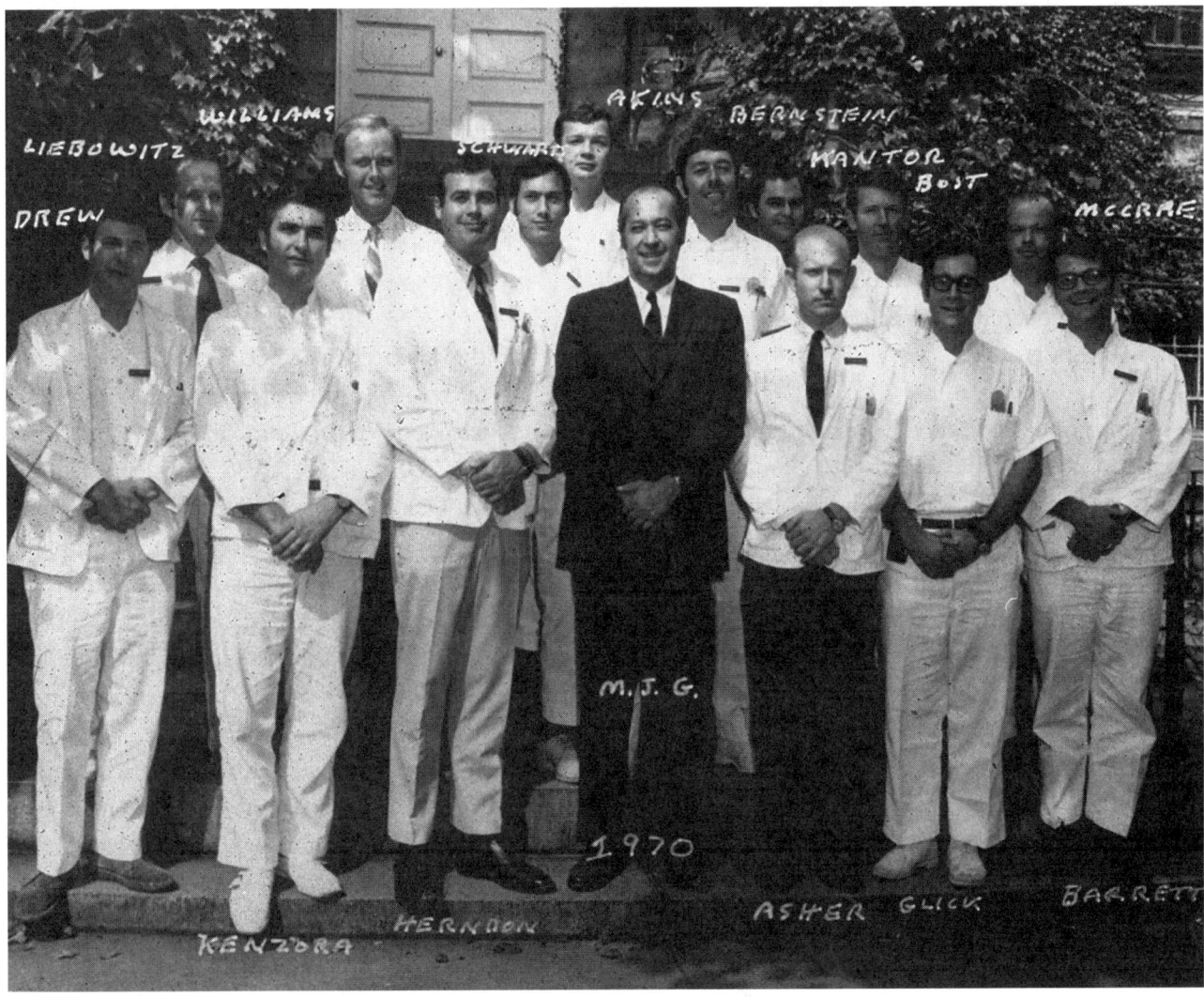

Residents at MGH with Dr. Glimcher, 1970. MGH HCORP Archives.

Medical Center, replicating a similar move made by Dr. Robert Osgood 42 years earlier. He also was named the Harriet M. Peabody Professor of Orthopaedic Surgery at HMS. He had chaired the Department of Orthopaedic Surgery at HMS 1968–1971, but he then moved his laboratories to Boston Children's Hospital. In 1971, he was also elected president of the Orthopaedic Research Society. In 1972, he published two papers, one in the "Proceedings of the National Academy of Sciences" and the other in the *New England Journal of Medicine*, both concerning a heritable disease of connective tissue. Analyzing tissue samples of bone, cartilage, and skin, Glimcher and his coauthors:

speculated that Type II collagen, the major collagen component in cartilage, contains a normal amount of hydroxylysine, while Type I collagen [found in skin and bone], which is the major source of the crosslinks, is hydroxylysine-deficient [and] the deficiency of hydroxylysine in the collagen of these patients…suggest that at least some skeletal and connective tissue abnormalities are directly related to underlying molecular pathology. (Eyre and Glimcher 1972)

He then reported cases of two sisters with severe scoliosis, recurrent joint dislocation, and hyperextensible skin and joints. He stated:

Amino acid analysis of dermal collagen revealed marked decreased in hydroxylysine content; skin from a clinically normal older sister and from the parents were normal in amino acid content. Collagen fibrils were normal morphologically... the defect is probably inherited as an autosomal recessive and due to a deficiency of enzymatic hydroxylation of lysine in collagen, which in turn results in decreased structural integrity of this important protein. (Pinnell et al. 1972)

Combining his interests in biomechanics and biochemistry of connective tissue, Glimcher along with Dr. Brickley-Parsons studied collagen in the intervertebral discs of normal adolescents and adults, and in scoliotic patients who underwent a Dwyer procedure for scoliosis by Dr. John Hall. Orientation of the discs was carefully marked as to the position of the annulus fibrosis on either the convex or concave aspects of the curve. They remarked:

From adolescence to mature adulthood, the most significant change is an increase in the content of Type I collagen at the expense of genetically distinct Type II collagen in the outer lamella of the posterior quadrant, while just the reverse is true of the anterior quadrant. These changes are accompanied by similar but smaller alterations in the total collagen content and in the crosslink hydroxylysinohydroxynorleucine. The same differences in the distribution of Types I and II collagens occur in the annuli on the concave and convex sides of the scoliotic curves. Together, these data establish that active cellular activity and tissue remodeling occur in the annuli fibrosi and suggest that the specific changes are initiated in response to overall increase in compressive loading on the concave side and tensile loading on the convex side of the spine and...changes they induce in the magnitude and distribution of internal stresses within the annuli the biologic behavior of annuli fibrosi to mechanical forces appears to follow Wolff's law...While Wolff's law was formulated originally to describe the adaptive response of bone to externally applied mechanical forces, there is no a priori reason why the same biological principles do not apply to other skeletal structures like the annulus fibrosus whose major functions are also mechanical in nature. (Brickley-Parsons and Glimcher 1984)

For this research, they received the 1983 Volvo Award in Basic Science from the International Society for Study of the Lumbar Spine.

In 1974, Glimcher received the Silver Anniversary Kappa Delta Prize from the AAOS for the best research on bone for the previous 25 years, and, by 1978, he received the Nicholas Andry Award for Most Outstanding Basic Research Related to Clinical Orthopaedics by the Association of Bone and Joint Surgeons. Another major interest of Glimcher's was the biology of osteonecrosis of the femoral head. He received the award for three papers he published with Dr. John Kenzora (initially a research fellow in Glimcher's lab and later chief of orthopaedics at the University of Maryland) in *Clinical Orthopaedics and Related Research*, including "Tissue Biology," "The Pathologic Changes in the Femoral Head as an Organ and in the Hip Joint," and "Discussion of the Etiology and Genesis of the Pathological Sequelae; Comments on Treatment." They studied approximately 150 femoral heads, noting in summary that:

NICOLAS ANDRY AWARD

The Biology of Osteonecrosis of the Human Femoral Head and its Clinical Implications:

I. Tissue Biology

MELVIN J. GLIMCHER, M.D. AND JOHN E. KENZORA, M.D.

Title of Glimcher's article describing the pathophysiology of osteonecrosis of the femoral head. *Clinical Orthopaedics and Related Research*, 1979; 138: 284.

The hallmark of the repair of the coarse cancellous bone is the formation of new, living bone on the surfaces of the dead trabeculae. The extent of this reaction varies depending on the underlying basis of the osteonecrosis...the repair of dead coarse cancellous bone consists of 2 distinct and apparently independent phenomena: (1) cell proliferation and spreading of the repair tissue throughout the femoral head; (2) differentiation of undifferentiated mesenchymal cells, initially to osteoblasts...which form new bone on the surfaces of the dead trabeculae, and considerably later to osteoclasts...The repair tissue of coarse cancellous bone following Av.O. [avascular necrosis] usually spreads and forms new bone more rapidly and extensively than in I.O. [idiopathic osteonecrosis]...once the repair tissue has crossed the subcapital fracture line... The extension of this fibrous tissue and fibrocartilage between the dead trabeculae of the necrotic segment of the adjacent bone, and especially the continued motion of the fracture fragments and the further propagation of the intracapital fractures in Av.O., results in extensive resorption of dead trabeculae and their replacement with fibrous tissue and fibrocartilage, rather than new bone formation...In contrast to the repair of coarse cancellous bone, the repair of the compact bone of the subchondral plate is highlighted by bone resorption which far outdistances the relatively small amount of new living bone formed to replace the resorbed dead bone. This results in a marked local loss of bone substance subchondrally...Cell death (necrosis) per se does not lead directly to physical disruption or disintegration of bone... 'Dead' bone may function mechanically for many years without gross structural failure. The pathological sequelae which occur in the femoral head... intracapital fractures, collapse and deformation...are produced by changes in the structural properties of the bone...as a result of the action of living cells during the repair process...the fracture is propagated...at the junction between the dead bone and the living, repaired, compacted bone where the stress is concentrated due to differences in the elastic moduli and the compliance of the dead coarse cancellous bone and the living, compacted, repaired bone tissue...During the early stages, the articular cartilage cells remain viable and function normally despite the osteonecrosis and its repair...Later with the development of osteoarthritis, there is an absolute and relative loss of the proteoglycans. Massive cartilage cell necrosis does not occur as a primary event in osteonecrosis. (Glimcher and Kenzora 1979)

He received the Faculty Scholar Award from the Joseph F. Macy Jr. Foundation in 1979, the same year he was the first CNRS-Harvard visiting professor at the University of Paris VII, Laboratoire d'Anatomi Comparee and l'Hospital de Enfants Malades. In 1980, he was named director of the Laboratory for the Study of Skeletal Disorders and Rehabilitation, with a staff of about 100 researchers. The next two years (1980–1982), he was also president of the Boston Orthopaedic Club.

Glimcher remained very productive in his laboratory at Boston Children's Hospital. He coauthored papers on cartilage repair; the use of solid-state MRI, which "provides direct images of the calcium phosphate constituents of bone substance and is a quantitative measurement of the true volumetric bone mineral density of bone" (Wu et al. 1979); basic studies on the role of the osteoporotic cytokine (Eta-1); the first study to establish that bone collagen in chickens contains γ-glutamyl phosphate, writing that "possible functions of the γ-glutamyl phosphate can only be speculative at this time: direct involvement in the process whereby a solid phase of calcium phosphate is deposited in bone (heterogenous nucleation, oriented overgrowth, crystal size and shape, and so forth), or indirectly in mineralization or other tissue functions by conferring an enzymatic activity to the collagen molecules or fibrils, such as the ATPase activity noted previously in decalcified bone and reconstituted collagens" (L. Cohen-Solal et al. 1979).

Later in his career, he collaborated in research with his daughter, Laurie Glimcher, a Harvard-trained immunologist. In 1996, they discovered that activating transcription factor-2 (ATF-2) is vital to the development of the skeletal and nervous systems. They reported in *Nature* that certain mice with a mutation in this transcription factor had a defect in bone growth—similar to human hypochondroplasia—occurring at the epiphyseal plates. Father and daughter published many articles together, and in 2006, they published in *Science* an article on a mechanism regulating bone growth. He was 81 at the time. They showed "that Schnurri-3 (Shn3), a mammalian homolog of the Drosophila zinc finger adapter protein, is an essential regulator of adult bone formation... We propose the Shn3 belongs to the small group of factors that regulate postnatal osteoblastic activity. Compounds designed to block Shn3/WWP 1 function may serve as therapeutic agents for the treatment of osteoporosis" (Jones et al. 2006).

LEGACY

Dr. Melvin Glimcher trained many scientists in his laboratory throughout his illustrious career. I remember, when returning to Boston in 1998, as chairman of the Partner's Department of Orthopaedic Surgery, that he still had his NIH training grant, the longest-renewed training grant in the history of the National Institutes of Health. Dr. Henry Kronenberg—who worked with Glimcher at MGH and who had called him the "father of the bone field"—recalled that Glimcher had "cared a lot about bringing people into the bone field...That was his *modus operandi*: He was very supportive of young people in the sciences... That's part of him not everyone knows about... [and] brought very rigorous chemistry and vigorous thinking [to his work and research]...He was a very rigorous man...a great leader that people

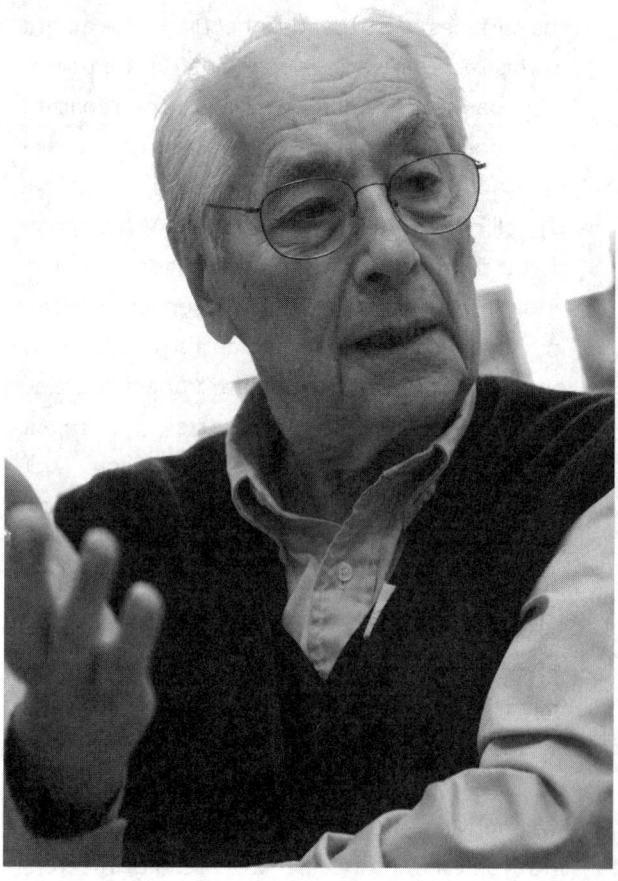

Melvin J. Glimcher. Photo by Stephanie Mitchell/Harvard University.

admired. He was always honest in telling people what he thought. That's very useful in a scientist" (Stickgold 2014).

Glimcher was a prolific writer and published about 400 papers and edited several books/proceedings. He received numerous additional awards, including the first Bristol-Myers Squibb/Zimmer Award for distinguished achievement in orthopaedic research (1988), a MERIT Award from the National Institutes of Health: Arthritis and Musculoskeletal and Skin Diseases (1991), the William F. Neuman Award for distinguished achievement in the field of bone and mineral research (1996) of the American Society for Bone and Mineral Research, the Dr. Marian Ropes Physician Achievement Award for excellence in arthritis research (1996) by the Arthritis Foundation, and in 1997 the Alfred Rives Shands Jr. Award for Outstanding Research by the Orthopaedic Research Society. In 2004, he was recognized by his alma mater, Purdue University, with an honorary doctorate in engineering: "Melvin J. Glimcher has distinguished himself as one of the most productive and creative scientists concerned with the general field of biologically mineralized tissues, such as bone and tooth…[using new advanced tools and high technology] to contribute a significant number of original seminal concepts" (*Purdue University News* 2004).

In addition to the Orthopaedic Research Society, the American Academy of Orthopaedic Surgeons and the Boston Orthopaedic Club, Dr. Glimcher was also a member of the Electron Microscopic Society of America, the Biophysical Society, Sigma Xi, the International Society of Cell Biology, the American Orthopaedic Association, SICOT, the Ohio Academy of Science, the American Society for Bone and Mineral Research, the North American Subcommittee of the International Committee on Prosthetics and Orthotics. He was a member of the advisory board of the Massachusetts Association of Paraplegics, chairman of the Research Committee of the Medical Foundation, a member of the Medical Foundation's board of directors and the board of trustees of the Hospital for Special Surgery. He served also as a trustee of the New England Peabody Home for Crippled Children, the Forsyth Dental Center and New England Sinai Hospital. He was an honorary member of Omega Kappa Upsilon (Dental Honor Society).

At age 88, he died in his home in Manhattan on May 12, 2014. He was survived by three daughters, six grandchildren, and one great-grandchild. Two daughters are tax attorneys; the third, Laurie, the former Irene Heinz Given Professor of Immunology at HMS and current dean of Cornell's Weill College of Medicine, was selected to replace Dr. Edward Benz as CEO of the Dana-Farber Center. She was the one to confirm his death. She stated that her father:

> had a restless curiosity and energy well into his later years, and would sleep only four hours a night… "Dr. Glimcher drove himself," she said. She recalled once stalking out of her Harvard lab because her experiments were not working and running into her father. He scoffed, saying that 98 percent of experiments fail, and urged her to return. "It's when the experiments are not going well that you dig in and you don't give in and you work, and you work," he told her.
> (Martin 2014)

She further recalled, "He was a very inventive scientist and a brilliant man," (Stickgold 2014), and she went on to say that he was tireless in his pursuit of new knowledge and understanding, not satisfied to repeat earlier experiments. He never gave up in the face of failure but was only spurred onward by his passion to innovate. That innate curiosity and drive continues to pave the way for further innovation today.

CHAPTER 25

John E. Hall
Mentor to Many and Master Surgeon

John Emmett Hall was born April 23, 1925, to Emmett Matthew Hall and Isabelle Mary (Parker) Hall and raised in Saskatoon, Saskatchewan, Canada. Saskatoon's downtown area, located along the South Saskatchewan River, is similar in appearance to Pittsburgh's central business district at the confluence of the Allegheny and Monongahela Rivers, with numerous bridges allowing access to both cities. Hall's early education at the University of Saskatchewan was interrupted by World War II, during which he served as a bomber pilot in the Royal Canadian Air Force (RCAF). After the war, Hall returned to the University of Saskatchewan, receiving his BA degree in 1948.

EARLY CAREER AND CLINICAL CONTRIBUTIONS

Hall had decided on a career in medicine; his "A" average and his bachelor's degree assured him of acceptance to McGill University, his medical school of choice. He received his MD, CM degree in 1952. Newly married to Francis "Frankie" Norma Walsh, Hall began his surgical training immediately after graduation. He completed a one-year rotating internship in 1953 and spent 1954 as a senior surgical intern at St. Joseph's Hospital in Toronto.

From 1954 to 1956, Hall was an orthopaedic registrar at the Royal National Orthopaedic Hospital in London. It was there that he first met J. I. P.

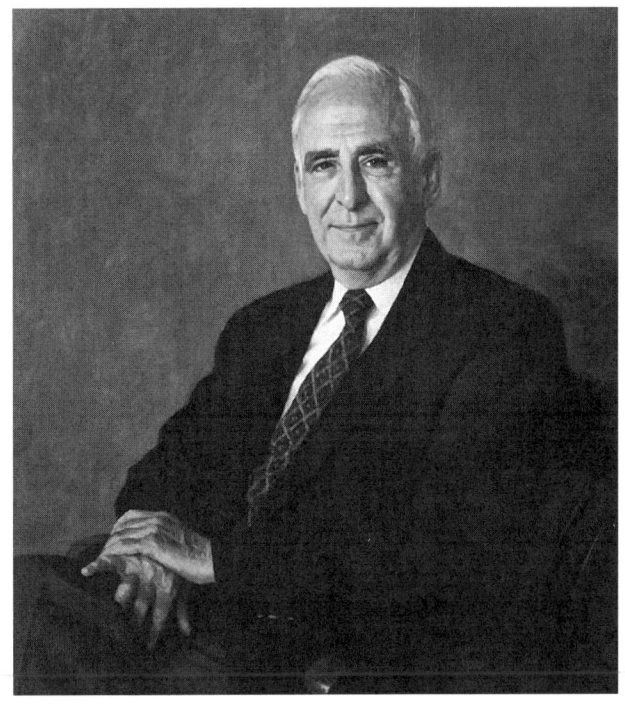

John E. Hall. J.B.E., M.B.M., and R.M.S. "John E. Hall 1925–2018." *Journal of Bone and Joint Surgery* 2018; 100: 2092.

Physician Snapshot

John E. Hall
BORN: 1925
DIED: 2018

SIGNIFICANT CONTRIBUTIONS: Advanced the operative and nonoperative treatment of scoliosis; created a surgical frame to minimize blood loss during spinal fusion; collaborated with Bill Miller to develop the Boston bracing system; organized orthopaedic staff and developed salary structure for orthopaedic surgeons at Children's Hospital.

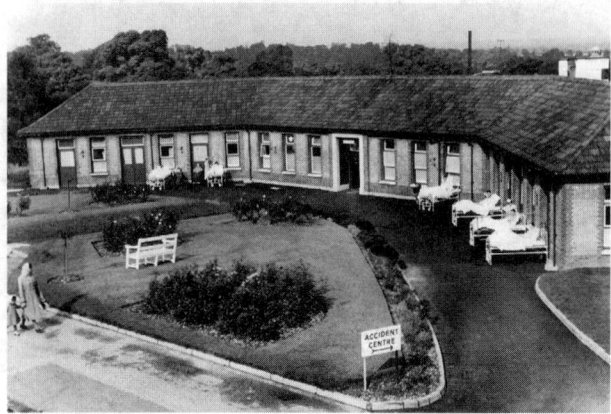

Royal National Orthopaedic Hospital, 1950s. Courtesy of the Royal National Orthopaedic Hospital NHS Trust.

James, who treated patients with severe scoliosis (curves >100°). Hall referred to James as the "guru of scoliosis" (Hall 1998). The Royal National Orthopaedic Hospital had two divisions. The town division could treat up to 100 patients with acute conditions; it had one operating room. The county arm was larger, with two operating rooms and almost 500 beds, some of which were reserved for patients with orthopaedic conditions such as polio (200 beds), tuberculosis (100 beds), scoliosis (50 beds), and osteomyelitis (20 beds). In the mid-1950s, such patients with scoliosis might remain in a cast as inpatients for up to one year. Poor outcomes included pseudarthrosis (50%) and deep infection (35%), and no patients maintained correction. After his experience at the Royal National Orthopaedic Hospital, Hall was emphatic that he would not have a future in treating scoliosis.

Upon returning to Canada, Hall entered the orthopaedic program at the University of Toronto, first as a Duncan Fellow in orthopaedics at Toronto General Hospital (1956–1957), then as an orthopaedic resident at Sunnybrook Hospital (1957), and finally as chief resident at the Hospital for Sick Children (1958). Dr. Robert Salter, who had been recently named chief of the division of orthopaedic surgery at the Hospital for Sick Children, hired Hall as his first staff member. Despite Hall's earlier emphasis that he would never treat patients with scoliosis, once he had accepted the position with Salter, Salter assigned him that very challenge. In addition, he was named chief of the amputee clinic at Ontario Crippled Children's Center. He also received an academic appointment at the University of Toronto, first as a clinical teacher (1958–1963) and then as an associate in surgery.

Hall remained at the Hospital for Sick Children for 14 years (1958–1971). While there, "in the early 1960s when the brief but disastrous use of thalidomide led to several hundred cases of phocomelia, Dr. Hall used his mechanical aptitude to [become] a respected authority in the prosthetic and surgical treatment of the child with a limb deficiency" (Millis and Emans 1999). Early in his career, also while at the Hospital for Sick Children, he, along with anesthesiologist J. E. S. Relton, developed an operational frame designed to reduce blood loss during spinal fusion. The frame became the standard apparatus for scoliosis surgeries and other time-consuming procedures on the spine. In 1967, Hall and Relton reported on the use of their frame in 38 cases of posterior spine fusion with internal metallic fixation for scoliosis. They compared their blood lost during those procedures in patients with congenital and idiopathic scoliosis (566 mL) with that reported by Relton and Conn for a similar series in 1963 (1800 mL).

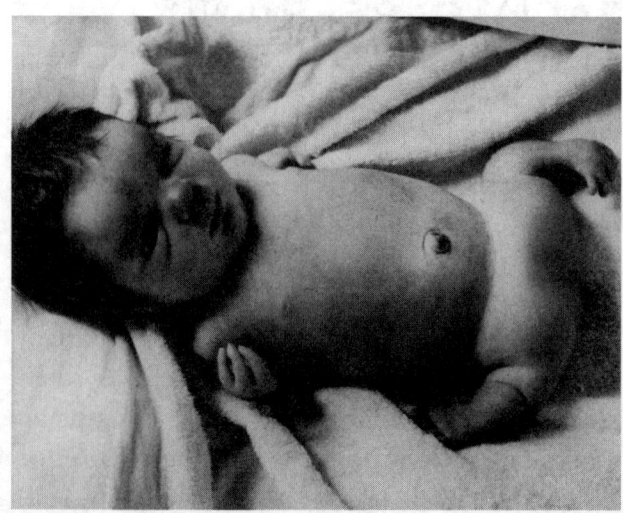

Birth abnormalities after exposure to thalidomide. Science History Images/Alamy Stock Photo.

Title of Relton & Hall's article describing their newly designed frame to support the patient during a posterior spine fusion.
Journal of Bone and Joint Surgery [Br] 1967; 49B: 327.

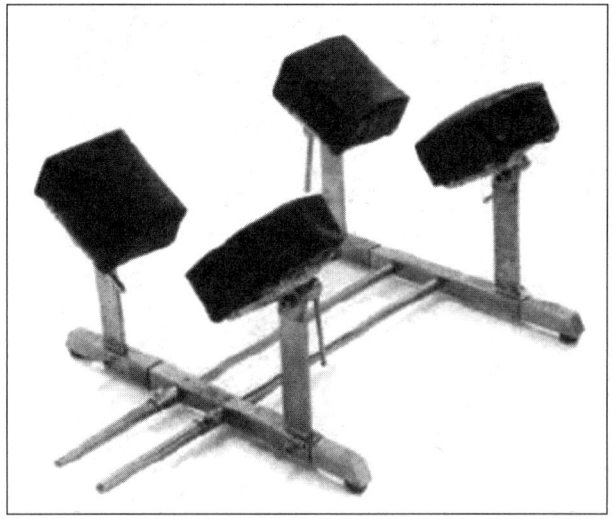

Relton Hall Frame.
J. E. Relton and J. E. Hall, "An operation frame for spinal fusion. A new apparatus designed to reduce haemorrhage during operation," *Journal of Bone and Joint Surgery [Br]* 1967; 49B: 327.

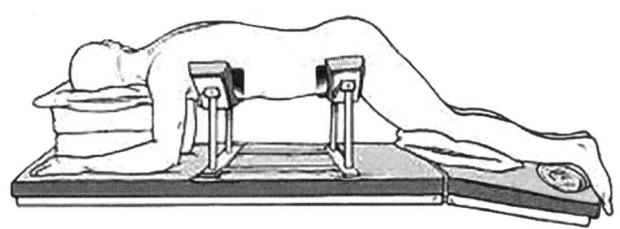

Drawing of a patient in the prone position on the Relton Hall Frame. A. Schubert, "Positioning Injuries in Anesthesia: An Update," *Advances in Anesthesia* 2008; 26: 46.

In patients with scoliosis and neuromuscular disease, Relton and Hall reported a mean blood loss of 942 mL, whereas Relton and Conn reported a mean loss of 1995 mL. Advantages of Relton and Hall's approach included allowing the abdominal contents to hang free with no pressure applied to the abdomen by the frame because the patient was prone and the chest and abdomen were supported on the sides. This avoided any pressure on the great vessels, especially the vena cava and the aorta. The frame also provided firm and stable support for the patient and permitted correction of the spinal deformity. They note that their frame is safe as well; though because it causes lordosis, they discouraged its use in patients with disc protrusion who are undergoing laminectomy. The frame is still manufactured today by the Imperial Surgical Company in Toronto, Canada.

During 1966–1968, he also served as both president of the medical staff and chair of the medical advisory board of the Prosthetic Research and Development Unit at the Ontario Crippled Children's Center. The staff "visited Germany and other countries to learn more about how they were coping with their large numbers of deformed children" (Hall 2000). Meanwhile, the same year that Hall and Relton reported on use of their frame, Salter was made surgeon-in-chief of the Hospital for Sick Children. Salter appointed Hall chief of the division of orthopaedic surgery, a role in which he remained until 1971 when he moved to Boston.

Having seen only J. I. P. James care for patients with severe scoliotic deformities using "very antiquated techniques" in the mid-1950s, and now faced with the responsibility of leading the scoliosis program at the Hospital for Sick Children, Hall visited several leaders in the development of scoliosis treatments in the US. He visited Paul Harrington, who was beginning to treat scoliosis with internal fixation of the spine; John Moe, then the leader in scoliosis treatment in North America; and, in Los Angeles, Joseph Risser, who bucked the conventional measures of confining patients to bed in a body cast for a year and instead made them ambulate in a plaster turnbuckle jacket (developed by John R. Cobb) soon after surgery. He also visited Dr. Wally Blount in Milwaukee, Wisconsin,

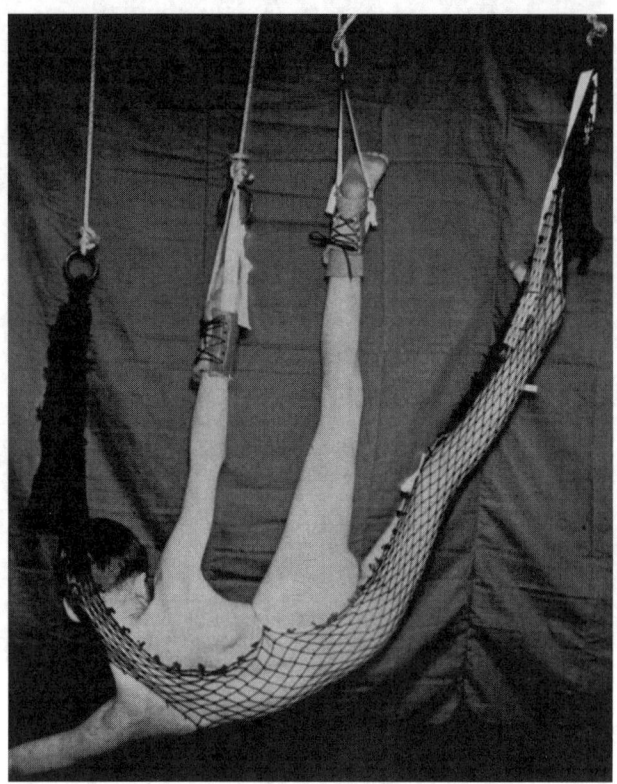

Patient suspended in fish net to correct spinal deformity before application of a body cast.

A. B. LeMesurier, "A method of correcting the deformity in scoliosis before performing the fusion operation," *Journal of Bone and Joint Surgery* 1941; 23: 521.

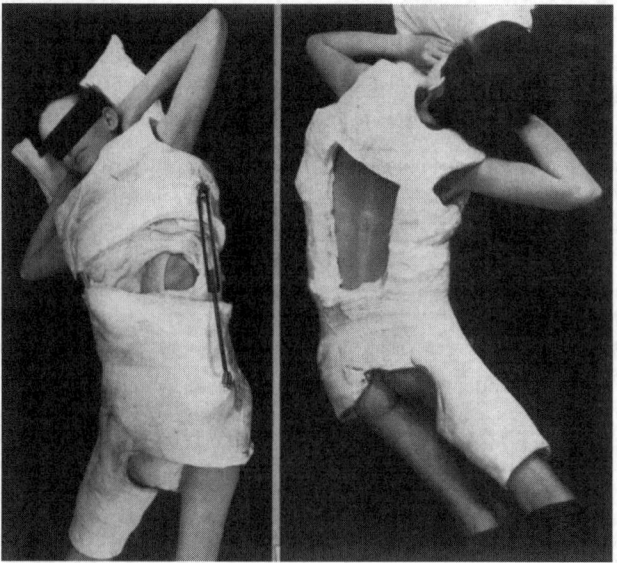

Example of a turnbuckle cast to treat a scoliosis.

J. I. P. James, "The Management of Scoliosis," *Postgraduate Medical Journal* 1952; 28: 386.

Title of Hall's article on the use of Dwyer instrumentation.
Journal of Bone and Joint Surgery 1981; 63: 1188.

to learn about the nonoperative management of scoliosis with the Milwaukee brace. Throughout his career, Hall also visited other scoliosis experts around the world to learn new surgical techniques, including Allen Dwyer, who "first performed his anterior instrumentation of scoliosis [in 1964], and by 1969 he [had] published his preliminary results" (Millis and Emans 1999). In 1968, Hall invited Dwyer to the Hospital for the Sick Children "to demonstrate his technique, which Dr. Hall quickly mastered and improved upon, with certain important changes in screws and inserting equipment. As with the Harrington instrumentation, Dr. Hall's mastery of anterior techniques of instrumenting the spine became renowned" (Millis and Emans 1999). Hall also invited other experts to Toronto, using funds from a rehab symposium in Toronto, including "Arthur Hodgson from Hong Kong, who pioneered the anterior approach to the spine for tuberculosis" (Hall 2000). Through his consultations with experts worldwide and his own extensive practice, "Dr. Hall quickly became a master in the techniques of posterior spinal instrumentation[,] doing five to six instrumentations a week through the 1960s" (Millis and Emans 1999).

MAKING WAVES IN BOSTON

Dr. Mel Glimcher, then chief at Boston Children's Hospital, invited Hall to Boston in 1971. "The years Dr. Hall spent in Toronto had seen the rapid evolution, not only of his medical career, but also the rapid growth of his family, from two children that John and Frankie had when they returned from England to seven children by the time Dr. Hall received [the] intriguing job offer" (Millis and Emans 1999). Hall was undecided, first planning to go learn about the program, then changing his mind—then changing it yet again and actually visiting. He began work at Children's Hospital later that year.

ROCKY TENURE AS CHIEF AT CHILDREN'S HOSPITAL

Hall was appointed chief of clinical services of the Department of Orthopaedic Surgery (a new leadership position in the department) and professor of orthopaedic surgery at Harvard Medical School. He was also made an associate in orthopaedics at the Brigham and Women's Hospital. Glimcher retained the title of orthopaedic surgeon-in-chief at Children's Hospital and the Harriet M. Peabody professorship at Harvard, both of which had also been held by his predecessor, Dr. William Green. The first eight years at Children's Hospital were difficult for Hall. He was responsible for leading the clinical service but lacked the authority to do so. He decried the culture that supported only "one way to do things" with regard to clinical problems (Emans, pers. comm., 2011), and he set out to change it. He emphasized principles in orthopaedics and favored the use of the Socratic method in teaching. Although the transition was difficult, "the department evolved over the years to Hall's way" (Emans, pers. comm., 2011).

The hospital administration fought Hall on many things: bringing in new staff, determining the staff's clinical privileges, and changing clinicians' salary structure and source. Hall later recalled (at his retirement exit interview in 2006) that when he began his tenure, a large staff of clinicians ran the private clinic, caring for inpatients and performing surgeries, whereas residents provided care in the public clinic. This disconnect carried over into the treatment the patients received. (At that time, the same private/public system functioned throughout the rest of the hospital as well.) Hall began overhauling the system: staff either could take on a full-time clinician position, being required to be present in the clinic and see every patient or at least approve all patient treatment decisions, or they could leave; and the private/public wards transitioned to a system based on patient age (1–5 years and ≥6 years old).

In addition to the difficult staff issues, which were sometimes disruptive, Hall was not given oversight and control of the department's finances. All faculty, including Hall, were full-time salaried employees. The department lacked coding experts; the hospital did the billing, though it was inexperienced and inefficient in billing and collecting for physicians. The hospital did not make its finances, including endowments, transparent to faculty. Faculty did not even have pension plans. Dr. Emans later noted that "the surgeons were busy, but not paid well" (Emans, pers. comm., 2011). The administration and Hall had major disagreements in this regard.

Despite his complex relationship with the administration, he was responsible for the sudden and extensive advancements in spinal surgery that developed at Children's Hospital in the 1970s; a significant change from the previous centennium. In 1870, when the orthopaedic service at Children's Hospital began operating year-round, among 83 total admissions, only 8 were for an orthopaedic condition (morbus coxae); upon discharge patients were graded as "well relieved," "not relieved," or "dead," indicating that outcome-based care was in effect by that time. Ten years later, in 1880, total admissions had increased to almost 200; 69 were related to musculoskeletal diseases, 16 of which affected the spine. **Table 25.1** presents such changes in orthopaedic treatment at Children's Hospital since the turn of the twentieth century, highlighting the increase in spinal surgery under Hall's leadership in the 1970s

Table 25.1. Orthopaedic Surgery at Children's Hospital Over the Twentieth Century

Year	Commonly treated conditions	No. of orthopaedic procedures
1902	Orthopaedic conditions (792 admissions)	459 total 1 (1 Albee spinal fusion)
1941	Orthopaedic conditions (admissions unknown)	478 total (4 spinal fusions)
1965	Primary idiopathic scoliosis, including 1 case of postirradiation scoliosis and 1 case of myelomeningocele scoliosis (Orthopaedic conditions not included)	1209 total, including 55 in situ spinal fusions for scoliosis and 2 spinal fusions with Harrington instrumentation
1975	Scoliosis (idiopathic or congenital, or related to cerebral palsy, myelomeningocele, sacral agenesis, or myopathy) (Orthopaedic conditions not included)	1617 total, including 226 surgeries for scoliosis 1 fusion with anterior-posterior instrumentation and fusion in one stage 9 posterior osteotomies 10 in situ spinal fusions 19 fusions with anterior release 20 fusions with Dwyer instrumentation 22 halo-femoral traction 145 fusions with Harrington instrumentation
2010	Scoliosis, fractures, congenital deformities, birth palsies, sports injuries and others. (Orthopaedic conditions not included)	4309 (339 surgeries for scoliosis; 3970 unspecified inpatient orthopaedic procedures)

(Karlin 2012).

and the later drastic upsurge in orthopaedic care provided by the early 2000s. From the table, we can intuit that spinal surgery began to transform after 1965, with these cases increasing from about 57 in 1965 to about 226 in 1975. These changes stem in part from advances in surgical instrumentation, e.g., the Harrington rod, and wider sharing of knowledge, e.g., through the Scoliosis Research Society, initiated in 1966. At Children's Hospital, Hall embraced new procedures and techniques, and encouraged his staff to implement and even upgrade them. His leadership gave Children's Hospital its reputation as a leading spinal care facility.

Nevertheless, by 1979 the administration had reached irreconcilable differences with Hall and fired him from his position as chief of the orthopaedic clinical service. His successor at Children's Hospital, Paul Griffin, had the same ideas as Hall and thus the same issues with the administration, and he left soon after taking over. That year, Hall became an associate in orthopaedics at the New England Baptist Hospital, and he later entered private practice as well. The Harvard plan—which limited income for full-time employees of the university and its teaching hospitals—no longer applied and his income tripled. He served as acting chief at Children's until Griffin was hired in 1981, continuing with all his previous responsibilities at Children's until that time. Drs. Lyle Micheli, Michael Millis, and John Emans joined Hall in private practice in 1981, each under their own professional corporation. The other surgeons remained as full-time staff at the hospital. The interruption in Hall's tenure lasted approximately seven years; he was acting chief for approximately two of those years. Some on the staff called this period "the private practice era" (Emans, pers. comm., 2011). As of 1986, the hospital administration remained unchanged. After Griffin resigned, Hall was acting chief again for a brief period before the same president who had fired him years earlier asked him to take on the title of chief again. He said, "I had to tell them that they were crazy, that I was still the same person. I wanted the same things, but this time I got them" (Heskel 2006).

Authority to Change the Orthopaedic Department at Children's Hospital

During his second term as chief, Hall enjoyed more harmony in the department. The new members committee and the financial committee began to operate more fully. When asked later whether it was difficult to implement changes during this period, Hall responded that he initially received pushback, but he believed that everyone recognized that patient separation—for example, based on town of residence (affluence) or ability to pay—was no longer necessary. Public and private patients might be in beds next to each other. Large rooms with 12 beds ended with a new building (it's unclear from the records whether Hall was referring to the expansion of the Farley surgery and radiology pavilion in 1970 or if he was referring to the 1987 expansion of a new inpatient building but the latter is most likely). And someone was always on call. When asked about the extent of the staff changes, Hall recollected that at the time, about 15 staff spent limited time at the hospital. Hall encouraged to stay those he wanted to stay, and he made leaving attractive for those he wanted to leave. Only a few staff remained after that, and those newly hired were brought on because they were the best for the position. Hall explained that clear communication and the inclusion of all staff in committee decisions (a new member committee and a financial committee) allowed the team to work well for 35 years—most had been there since the beginning of the new system.

When the same exit interviewer asked Hall if it had been easier to accomplish his goals after returning as chief, Hall responded with an emphatic yes. He had required the changes he wanted be included in his contract, and the administration adhered to it. Although the resolution was not the norm, things were changing, particularly with regard to surgeon salaries: they were now paid through a hospital-affiliated foundation, disconnecting their tight ties to the hospital administration (this is now widespread practice). Hall stated that "times change. If you're a little bit ahead, you get thumped for it" (Heskel 2006). Hall was unflagging in his leadership and championship of new ideas and advancements until he voluntarily stepped down as chief in 1994.

CLINICAL CONTRIBUTIONS

Hall had continued to make numerous contributions to the management of scoliosis and the study of spinal deformity and kyphosis throughout his tenure as chief at Boston Children's Hospital.

Scoliosis and Spinal Deformity

Shortly after his arrival at Boston Children's Hospital, he "brought the gifted orthotist, Bill Miller, from the Midwest. Their collaboration resulted in the Boston bracing system, perhaps the most widely used scoliosis orthosis in the Western world" (Millis and Emans 1999). Hall and Miller first reported their concept of brace management of scoliosis (the Boston bracing system) in 1975. The main design elements of the system—"1) a prefabricated, symmetric thoracolumbar–pelvic module with 2) built-in lumbar flexion or antilordosis, 3) areas of 'relief' or 'voids' opposite areas of pressure" (Emans et al. 1986)—haven't changed since it was introduced, and an exercise program is still required with use. Later in his career, Hall and Miller, now with Emans and others, reported results in 1986 from 295 patients whom they followed for a minimum of one year after treatment. They concluded that:

- the bracing system significantly improved curves measuring between 30 and 45 degrees in children who had not yet reached skeletal maturity
- the bracing system corrected or controlled idiopathic scoliosis in ~80% of patients
- bracing outcomes were affected by patient age and curve severity, as well as initial correction while wearing the brace
- poor control was achieved in those with curves greater than 45°, multiple curves (>2) and when the height of the curve is above T7
- control achieved with brace superstructure was similar to that obtained without it in patients with curves at a level below T7

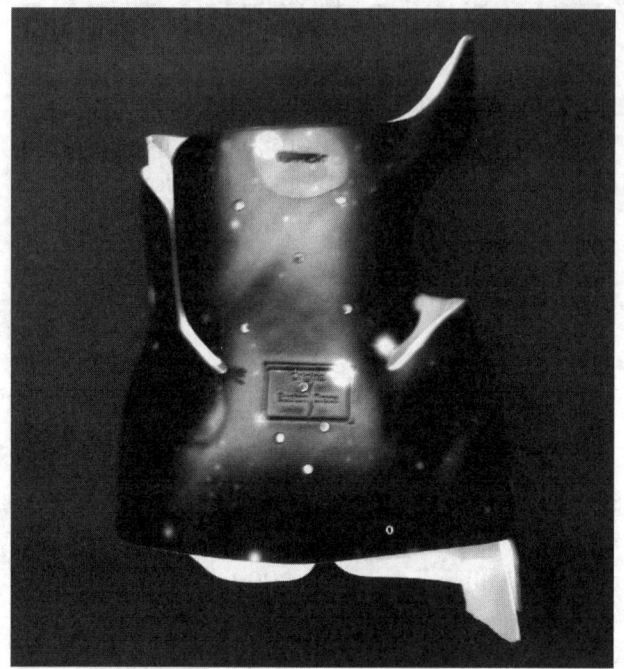

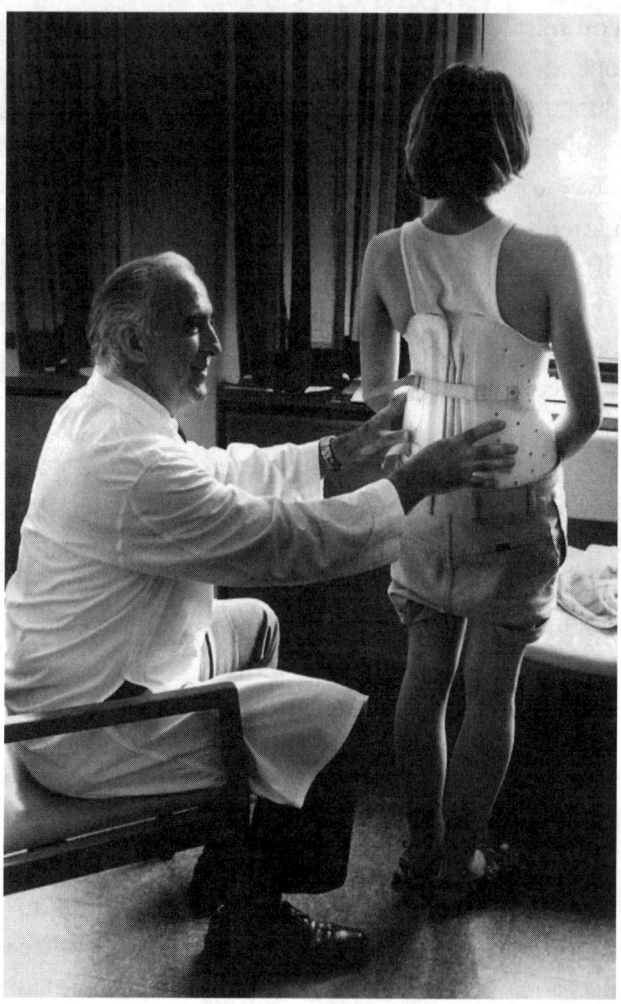

Dr. Hall checking a patient in a Boston brace. Boston Children's Hospital Archives, Boston, Massachusetts.

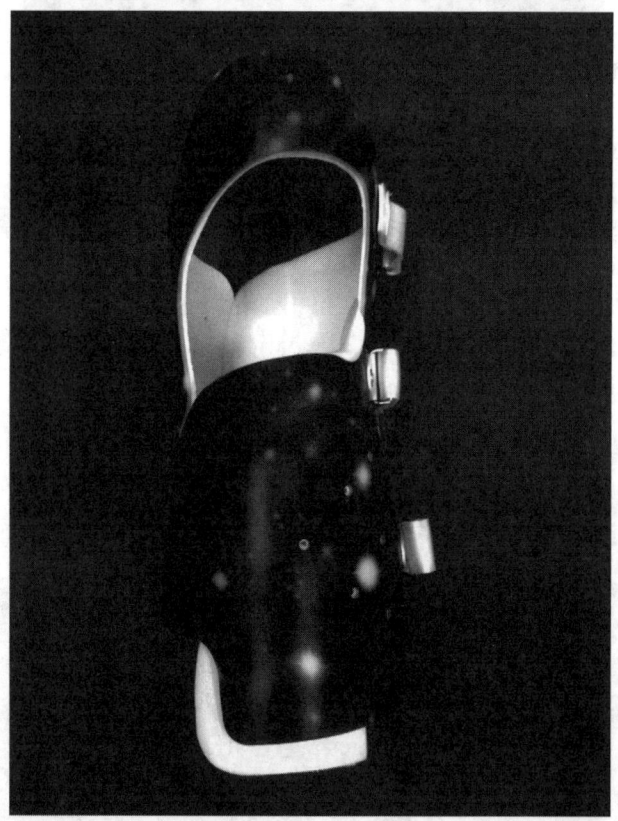

Boston Brace. Courtesy of Boston Orthotics & Prosthetics.

Hall was also a strong proponent of implementing the wake-up test during spinal fusion with Harrington instrumentation in patients with scoliosis. Drs. C. Vauzelle, P. Stagnara, and P. Jorevinroux first proposed the use of this test in 1973, and Hall began using it at Children's Hospital in January 1975 when a 15-year-old girl experienced partial short-term paraplegia immediately upon awakening in the operating room (see **Case 25.1**). Hall et al. reported their overall experience with the test in 1976. It proved safe: they found no neurologic abnormalities in 42 patients; and patients' movements did not dislodge the Harrington rod. Two years later, they reported additional experiences with the test, describing 166 consecutive patients. Among those, three patients (1.2%) had neurologic deficits upon awakening. They noted that this rate was:

a much higher rate than would be expected from the reports to the Scoliosis Research Society Morbidity Committee (0.56 per cent)...The high incidence in our series might be explained by the fact that our series was not composed predominantly of patients with the usual idiopathic scoliosis. Of our three patients with a neural deficit at wake-up, one had idiopathic thoracic scoliosis, one had congenital scoliosis, and the third had a previously damaged spinal cord. The correlation of low potential in the evoked cortical response and loss of voluntary muscle power in this patient is of special interest, since it suggests that the two monitoring methods give comparable results. The important finding in this study was the fact that the

Case 25.1. Posterior Spinal Fusion in Idiopathic Scoliosis

"A 15-year old girl was admitted with a diagnosis of idiopathic scoliosis which had been detected during a routine physical examination. She had no cardiorespiratory symptoms attributable to scoliosis. Neurologic findings were benign. Standing roentgenograms showed a right thoracic curve of 57° from 6th dorsal to 1st lumbar vertebras and a left lumbar curve of 43° from 1st lumbar to 5th lumbar vertebras. Hematocrit was 43.3% and urinalysis, electrolytes, prothrombin time, and partial thromboplastin time were normal. Chest x-ray and pulmonary-function tests showed moderate restrictive lung disease.

"The patient was scheduled for posterior spinal fusion from 5th dorsal to 3rd lumbar vertebras with iliac bone graft and Harrington-rod instrumentation. Premedication consisted of pentobarbital, 2 mg/kg orally at 0500 hr, and atropine (0.015 mg/kg), and morphine (0.15 mg/kg) IM, 90 minutes before operation, which was at 0800 hr. Anesthesia was induced with thiopental (5 mg/kg) and succinylcholine (1.5 mg/kg) IV, followed by endotracheal intubation with a 7-mm cuffed tube. Anesthesia was maintained with N2O-O2-curare and morphine. Anesthetic course throughout the operation was uneventful.

"At the end of the procedure, the patient was turned supine on a Striker frame, with the endotracheal tube in place. Muscle relaxants were reversed with atropine and neostigmine. The N2O was discontinued and 100% O2 was administered. The patient opened her eyes and was awake within a few minutes.

"As the anesthesiologist was preparing to extubate the patient, one of the surgeons asked the patient to move her feet. She was able to move her right foot but not her left. A sensory deficit was noted on the right side up to the midthoracic level. The patient also had urinary incontinence. At this time, she was conscious enough to raise her head, both arms and right foot, but still could not move her left foot.

"With the patient reanesthetized and placed prone on the operating table, the surgical incision was reopened and the Harrington rod removed. Fifth dorsal to 3rd lumbar interspaces were explored, but no abnormality could be detected. The incision was closed and the patient was again awakened in the supine position, but was still unable to move her left foot. Immediate postoperative neurologic examination demonstrated a ban of sensory loss below the left nipple, loss of motor function in the left lower limb and sensory loss in the right lower limb.

"Progressive neurologic improvement was noted over the next 12 hours. A myelogram on the 1st postoperative day was negative. The patient remained incontinent of urine for the next 8 days and required intermittent catheterization (12 hourly). On the 9th postoperative day, urinary residual increased, and a cystometrogram showed a hypotonic autonomous bladder with denervation hypersensitivity to bethanechol chloride (Urecholine). Intermittent catheterization was continued.

"Treatment by localizer cast reduced her dorsal curve to 37° and lumbar curve to 23°. She was discharged to recumbency at home on the 23 postoperative day. At followup 3 months later, a repeat cystometrogram was normal and the patient was found to have complete motor and sensory recovery except for a patch of sensory loss on the left side of the chest."

(Sudhar, Smith, Hall, and Hansen 1976)

neural impairment due to distraction is immediately reversible in its early phase. (Hall et al 1978)

The authors identified that there was an increased rate of an abnormal wake-up test in patients with congenital scoliosis and in patients with a previously damaged spinal cord than had been reported by the Scoliosis Research Society.

Over the next decade, spine surgeons began to increasingly monitor somatosensory evoked potentials (SSEPs) in adults. Dr. Sandra Helmers and Hall reported their experience with SSEPs in children: they found the technique to be useful intraoperatively, especially in children with mental disabilities or who were unable to cooperate during a wake-up test. The cortices were the main point of monitoring, but the results from that location could be inaccurate, so they also recorded through the cervical spine, popliteal fossa, and scalp. Helmers and Hall drew attention to some technical difficulties among 343 patients who underwent surgery for a wide variety of spinal deformities and diseases. In particular, they noted waveform changes while inserting instrumentation or excising a tumor (in nine of their patients); to avoid this they changed the instrumentation or procedure. They also highlighted issues that conferred high risk to these patients, including preexisting neurological disabilities or previous extensive operations. Too, the fact that these patients were children, not adults, brought its own challenges, including short stature and underlying conditions that precluded their ability to respond while under anesthesia. To counter the latter, they used an inhaled anesthetic.

Never content, he continued to travel and study new advancements and techniques. Hall noted, "A session in Paris with my friends Yves Cotrel and Jean Dubousset in the early 1980s opened new vistas with their double rod rotating system. They laid the groundwork for the amazing proliferation of the currently used spinal instrumentation systems" (Hall 2000). Hall had a "reputation as a master clinician with world renowned surgical skills" (Millis and Emans 1999). Hall was an early advocate for the use of Dwyer instrumentation with anterior fusion. He wrote a review article in 1981 summarizing his thoughts and those of other surgeons who reported their experiences at meetings of the Scoliosis Research Society and other organizations:

> The general consensus of opinion is that Dwyer instrumentation and anterior spine fusion are not recommended for routine use in simple spinal deformities. The procedure is most valuable as a supplement to posterior correction and stabilization in the severe paralytic curve, in the absence of posterior elements, and in cerebral palsy. It still is my personal preference to manage idiopathic thoracolumbar and lumbar curves in patients with trunk imbalance by Dwyer instrumentation in order to obtain complete correction with a shorter fusion area. (Hall 1981)

Hall et al. (1981) reported general truths related to their experience in surgically treating congenital scoliosis:

> Proper treatment of congenital scoliosis requires early recognition of curves that have already progressed or will certainly do so. Fusion without instrumentation then is sufficient. If correction is necessary, staged procedures (halo-femoral traction, anterior release, and posterior fusion) may be required for severe curves. For the less severe curves, instrumentation as the primary means of obtaining correction proved to be safe and effective in this small series, but should only be attempted by experienced surgeons at institutions with all of the necessary facilities.

Hall published his experience with scoliosis in patients with neurofibromatosis; spinal deformities in patients with myelomeningocele; spinal fusion in children with spondylolysis and spondylolisthesis, and in those with spinal muscular atrophy; and osteotomy and refusion in patients with a previously fused spine but with a progressive painful deformity and trunk imbalance. He also reported the outcomes of adult patients who underwent procedures to treat idiopathic scoliosis. Of 45 such adults, Hall and his colleagues wrote:

> One striking feature of all published studies on adults in whom scoliosis is surgically treated is the substantial rate of complications (33 to 57 percent), however experienced the surgeon or surgeons may be. The high incidence was confirmed in our series. More than half of the patients had one or more complications, and a patient…died [from pulmonary embolism]. The rate of pseudoarthrosis in our patients (approximately 10 percent)…When averaged for all the patients who were operated on, the major and minor complications necessitated three days of additional hospitalization…In addition…our patients showed a significant decrease in the lordosis and the mobility of the lumbar spine postoperatively. Although some measures of pain and function showed improvement, we noted their lack of correlation with the radiographic and the clinical factors we studied… thus adult patients who are considering surgery…should be counseled that regardless of the radiographic appearance of the spine, the likely result is a decrease in the peak and constant levels of pain with no change in frequency, no changes in occupation or recreation activities, improvement in appearance and no change in pulmonary function. (Sponseller et al. 1987)

The authors reported that adults who have a spine fusion for scoliosis have a higher rate of complications—almost double that in children. Adults should expect a decrease in the intensity of their pain, but not full relief, and improvement in appearance and function, but not any change in their capacity for work and recreational activities. These outcomes were the same in experienced and less experienced surgeons.

Hall made numerous other contributions in the field of spinal deformity, maintaining an unquenchable thirst for knowledge and understanding throughout his career. In the early 1990s, Hall even went to Korea to visit Se Il Suk, who was achieving excellent outcomes with the use of pedicle screws in both the thoracic and lumbar spine; this use became ubiquitous at the turn of the century.

Kyphosis

In 1978, Dr. R. B. Winter and Hall had published a review of kyphosis in childhood and adolescence. They noted that kyphosis has emerged as a challenging problem; left untreated it can cause paraplegia. They mentioned that bracing does not always resolve kyphosis, and anterior fusion is often necessary; not infrequently with anterior cord decompression. Winter and Hall pointed out that although kyphosis and other conditions that were historically considered difficult can now be treated, physicians require more education about such management options.

By the early 1980s, Hall and colleagues reported the use of staged anterior and posterior procedures to treat Scheuermann kyphosis and other major spinal deformities such as "severe rigid kyphosis…a major thoracolumbar or lumbar scoliotic curve with trunk imbalance to marked pelvic obliquity, congenital scoliotic curves associated with a hemivertebra or anterior unsegmented bar, absent posterior elements associated with severe scoliosis or kyphosis… [and] failed anterior fusion" (Floman et al. 1982). Anterior release was done through a:

> transthoracic [approach], retroperitoneal [approach,] or a combination of both [that] involves transverse sectioning of the anterior longitudinal ligament, excision of the intervertebral discs as well as the vertebral end plates, and the placement of interbody bone graft…In cases with a severe kyphotic deformity…the vertebral body resection is completed and the posterior longitudinal ligament is visualized…a strut graft is placed at this stage…Following the anterior

procedure, the patient is kept in halo-femoral or halo-pelvic traction and after about two weeks, a posterior spine fusion and instrumentation are performed. Shortly after the posterior fusion, a body cast is applied, and the patient starts ambulating...The overall complication rate was high (32/73 patients). (Floman et al. 1982)

The authors described an extensive anterior release of the spine in severe kyphosis—including the anterior longitudinal ligament, vertebral discs and endplates and if necessary, a vertebral body—followed by a period in halo-femoral traction and finally a posterior spine fusion with instrumentation.

In view of this high completion rate, throughout the rest of the 1980s and 1990s—as he had throughout his surgical career—Hall improved his surgical technique by combining staged anterior release and fusion followed by posterior fusion into a one-stage operation, performing both at the same time. Initially, his approach was the same one that he used for hemivertebra excision with spinal stabilization and fusion. With the patient in the lateral decubitus position, he used an anterior approach through a transthoracic or thoracoabdominal incision, and a posterior approach through a standard midline posterior incision. One publication reported that "with the technique discussed in this study [including surgical procedures performed over 1993–1996], the authors were able to obtain a 77% improvement in curve magnitude and preserve as many motion and growth segments as possible...the average number of motion segments fused was two...The amount of correction obtained...and the lack of complications suggests that early operative intervention (average age, 18 months) may provide better correction with less neurologic risk than suggested in the literature" (Lazar and Hall 1999).

Six years later, Daniel Hedequest, Hall, and Emans reported the results of this procedure in another series of patients treated between 1996 and 2000. They described benefits achieved with the combined approach (anterior and posterior) during hemivertebra excision. The surgeon is able to:

- retain control of the spine
- easily identify various anatomical landmarks in the spine, cord and nerves
- with total visualization the surgeon can provide a corrective force anteriorly while using a compression apparatus posteriorly

They believed that the use of state-of-the-art instruments can help retain the correction achieved during the procedure. They reported a "minimal" complication rate, a 71% curve correction rate, and a 100% fusion rate.

In his Harrington Lecture to the Scoliosis Research Society in 1998, Hall described instances when operations may need to be performed through an anterior approach, such as to relieve frontal spinal

Title of Lazar and Hall's article describing their technique of combining the anterior and posterior procedures into one single operation. *Clinical Orthopaedics and Related Research* 1999; 364: 76.

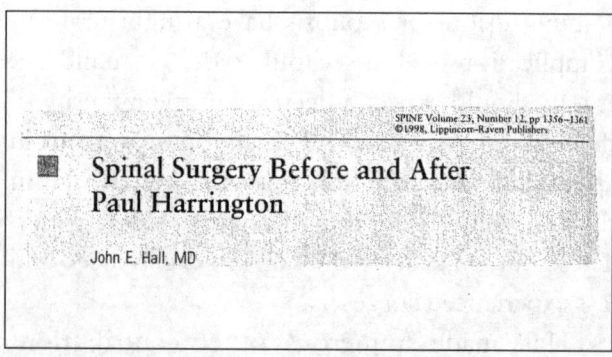

Title of Hall's Harrington Lecture in 1998. *Spine*, 1998; 23: 1356.

cord compression, to achieve stability through spinal fusion or anterior release in patients with kyphosis or severe scoliosis, to avoid "crankshafting" with growth in children who require posterior fusion, and to correct moderate thoracolumbar curvature. Advantages of anterior procedures include the ability to save portions of the lumbar spine that aid in movement, and that they can be performed at the same time as posterior procedures.

Hall and his colleagues made 5 key points in their 2001 report of congenital kyphosis:

- congenital kyphosis responds best to early surgical intervention
- posterior fusion can be performed in patients with no neurological deficiency and less than 60° of kyphosis
- in situ posterior fusion in young children can correct kyphosis over time as the child grows
- hemivertebra excision can safely and immediately correct kyphosis in children
- neurological damage is more likely in children with kyphosis who undergo anterior and posterior fusion, particularly older children, those with more severe kyphosis, and those with other preexisting spinal cord conditions

In another report of children with kyphosis secondary to irradiation or after laminectomy, Hall and his coauthors found "no role for bracing in preventing progression of kyphosis. Although flexible deformities can be treated by posterior instrumentation alone, severe rigid kyphoses require combined anterior release combined with spinal fusion and posterior instrumentation combined with spinal fusion to achieve the best correction and maintain it" (Otsuka et al. 1998).

RECOGNITION OF HALL AS DOCTOR AND MENTOR

Hall extensively improved his patients' lives over his more than 40 years in practice: "[He treated]

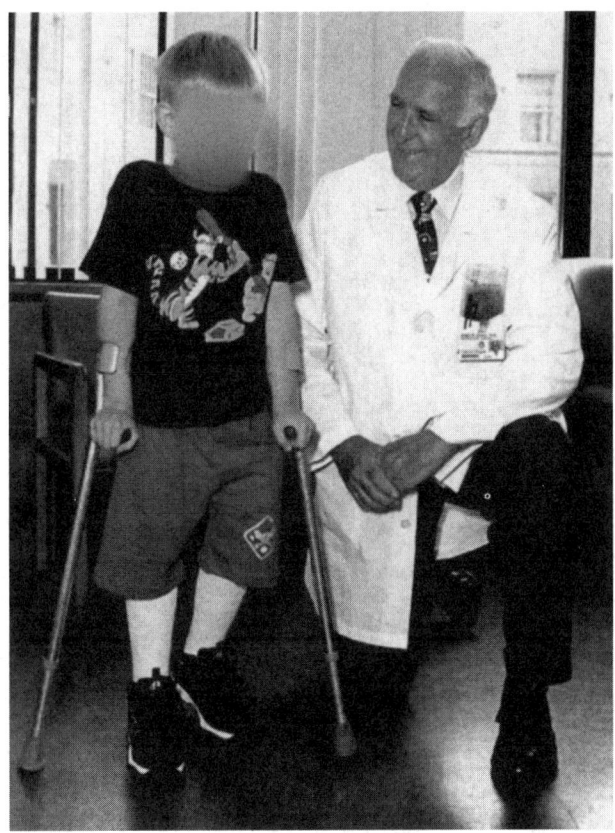

Dr. Hall enjoying a moment with one of his patients.
Images of America. Children's Hospital Boston. Charleston, SC: Arcadia Publishing, 2005. Boston Children's Hospital Archives, Boston, Massachusetts.

thousands of patients with various severe orthopaedic problems…many coming from great distances. These patients knew his reputation as a master clinician with world renowned surgical skills" (Millis and Emans 1999). Approximately one-third of his publications dealt not with spinal deformity, but with various pediatric problems and diseases, trauma, and amputations. Examples of such conditions include congenital pseudoarthrosis of the tibia, congenital absence of the tibia (treated with the Brown procedure), proximal femoral focal deficiency (treated with the Van Nes rotational osteotomy), slipped femoral epiphysis, and hereditary multiple exostoses. He also studied the role of innominate and Chiari osteotomies, treatment of fractures of the femoral neck and supracondylar fractures of the humerus, and management of chronic Monteggia lesions.

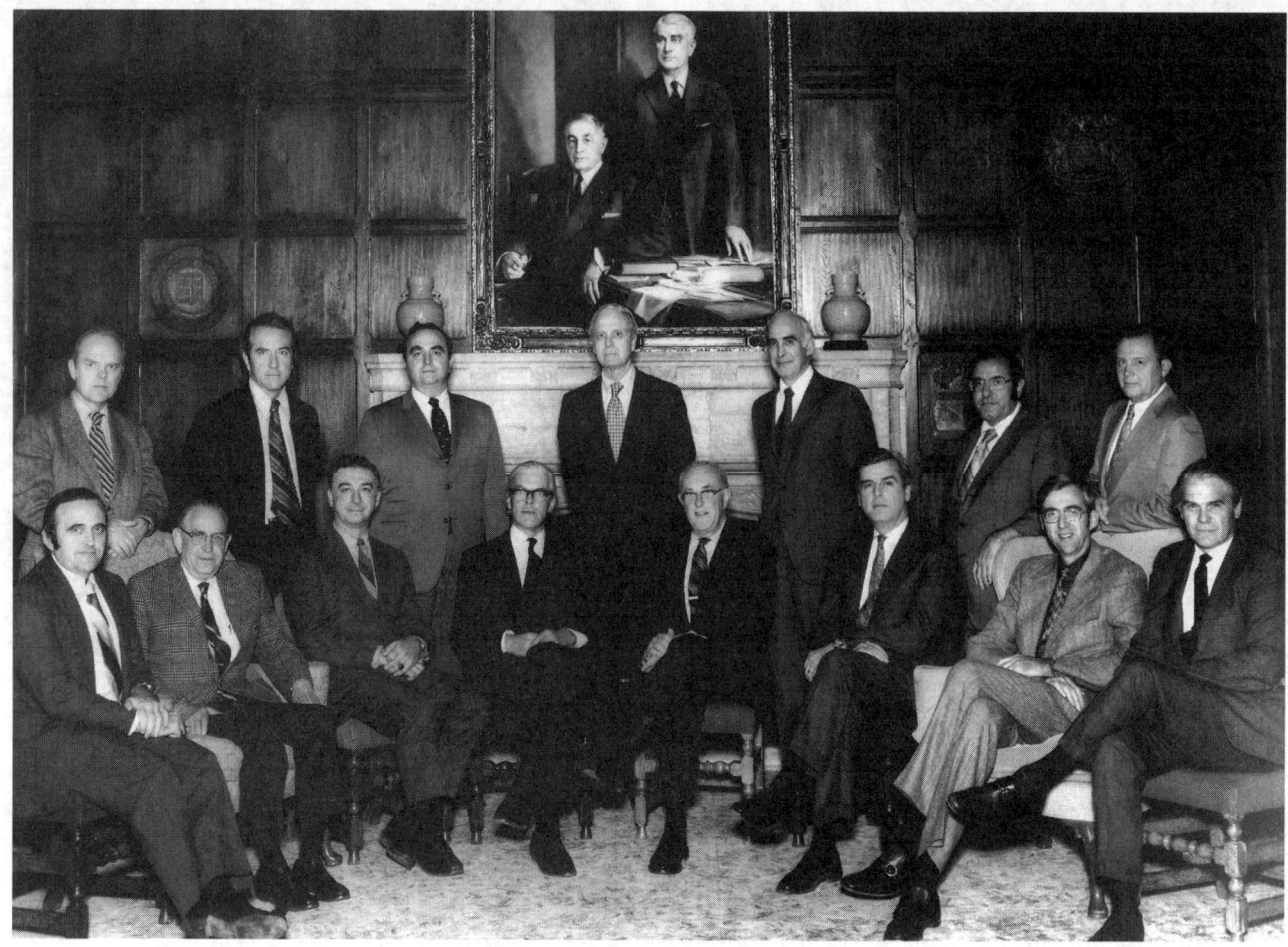

Founding members of the Pediatric Orthopaedic Society of North America. Dr. Hall is standing, third from the right.
POSNA Archive c/o Texas Scottish Rite Hospital for Children. POSNA.Archivist@tsrh.org. 214-559-8545.

In volume 2 of the *Orthopaedic Journal at Harvard Medical School*, Dr. Tony Herring (2000) wrote a dedication to Hall:

Dr. Hall is a special individual who has been an exemplary role model for us all. When I think of the word "surgeon," I think of Dr. John Hall. He is strong, yet compassionate. He is a skilled technician...His innovative techniques in pediatric spinal surgery have revolutionized the way we...care for children with spinal deformities. However, it is his gift for teaching and caring for children that are his most admired traits. As young physicians in an ever-changing world, we have learned a great deal about the honor and the responsibility of being a surgeon from Dr. Hall. When asked why we chose pediatric orthopedic surgery for a career, my peers and I usually answer with two words—John Hall...It was his intangible qualities that led us into the field...First, he insisted on striving to achieve perfection during surgery. He was absolutely intolerant of half-hearted or unskilled efforts... He taught us surgery based on fact and careful study of results rather than by personal dogma or tradition. His view of surgery as constantly changing and improving inspired us to change and improve rather than to rely on old habits. His message was clear: Each time as we enter the operating room, we seek to improve our understanding of technique and anatomy, learn from our mistakes and shortcomings, and thus, continue to advance our art...Dr. Hall taught us that the patient always comes first, and that all

Author Recollections

I recall two personal experiences with Hall that testify to his generosity and support; having only met him on a few occasions. When I became chair of orthopaedics at Brown and Rhode Island Hospital, I engaged in creating a new academic department—a difficult cultural change for any institution. Hall called me one day and offered his support; he said he was willing to come to our hospital and speak to the board of trustees, to help them understand what I was attempting to do and why the change was necessary. In my experience, his offer was not a common one.

On another occasion I was asked to see an 18-year-old man with neurofibromatosis who, after his third posterior cervical decompression, awoke with quadriplegia and no bony elements remaining in his posterior cervical spine. I immediately placed him in a halo to straighten his severely flexed neck, and within hours he had regained motor and sensory function. I recalled a case that Hall had reported a few years earlier in which he used a Kocher approach (mandible and tongue splitting) to the spine in a patient with progressive kyphosis and quadriparesis following a wide posterior laminectomy. I called him the next day, hoping I could transfer the patient to him. In a confident and supportive manner, he suggested that I do the procedure myself. I did, with his consultation. The patient underwent an extensive anterior cervical fusion and remained in a halo cast until the fusion healed. The man walked out of the hospital after a full neurologic recovery. He graduated from college the following year.

Hall was a special person. He left a lasting impression on me, and he was a mentor to many.

---

of our decisions must be aimed to achieve the best outcome for each child. He believed that a patient's family must be heard and that their concerns must be addressed openly and honestly. He respected, and taught us to respect the dignity of children.

Hall held leadership positions in several professional organizations. He was founder and the first chair of the Canadian Board of Certification for Prosthetics and Orthotics, on which he served from 1966 to 1971. He was a founding member of the Scoliosis Research Society and served as its president from 1968 to 1970. In 1980, he was elected president of the Pediatric Orthopaedic Society. A fellow of the Royal College of Surgeons in Canada, he was also certified by the American Board of Orthopaedic Surgery and was an examiner with that board for many years.

Approximately 10 of his former fellows became chiefs of pediatric orthopaedics or departments of orthopaedic surgery. Millis and Emans (1999) described Hall's impact on his colleagues and students, and an especial honor he received from them:

> In 1996, 80 of Dr. Hall's past and present colleagues, chief residents and fellows organized and attended a symposium in his honor at the Children's Hospital in Boston...and announced the funding of the John E. Hall Professorship in Orthopaedic Surgery at Harvard Medical School, a position now funded in perpetuity to partially support the present and future orthopaedic surgeon-in-chief at the Children's Hospital...Those of us who have been fortunate enough to learn from Dr. Hall and work with him continue to marvel at his unique combination of support, generosity, and kindness to patients and colleagues alike, and his delightful open mindedness to new ideas and techniques at a stage in his career when most would retreat into the comforts of the familiar.

They went on to say:

Recognizing another of John Hall's many skills, as a Chevalier du Tastevin [an exclusive fraternity of Burgundy wine enthusiasts; originally founded in 1703 and revived in 1934, it has chapters worldwide; its members meet to eat elaborate meals and sample Burgundy wines], we figuratively raise our glasses in a toast [to] celebrate Dr. Hall's gifts to generations of grateful patients…and to colleagues…[T]he orthopaedic nurses have placed [a small gold plaque] on the wall in Room Nine, Dr. Hall's room, in the surgical suite at the Children's Hospital. It reads as follows: "The Dr. John Hall Room. Dedicated to excellence, compassion, and respect." (Millis and Emans 1999)

Hall voluntarily stepped down as chief in 1994, at age 69 years. He remained active in clinical care for another 12 years. He fully retired in 2006 when he and Frankie returned to Toronto, the city where his academic orthopaedic career had begun some 36 years before. Dr. Hall died on March 22, 2018, at the age of 92; he was predeceased by Frankie by only a few weeks.

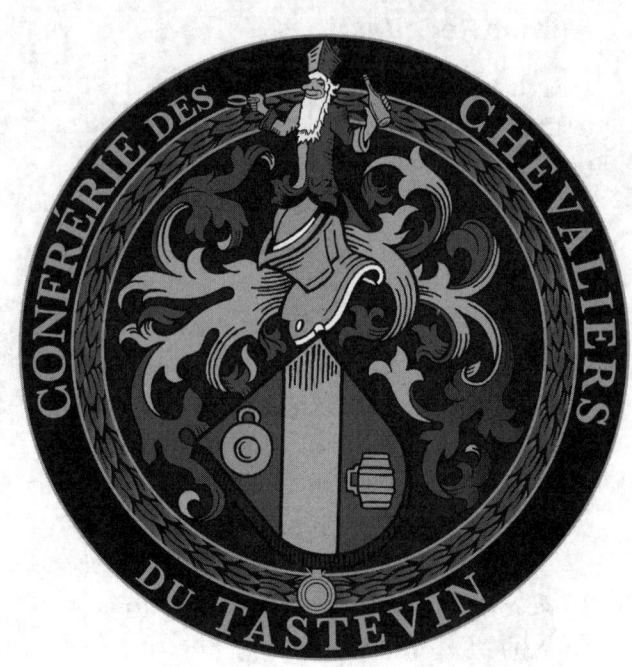

Seal of the Chevaliers du Tastevin. Courtesy of the Confrérie des Chevaliers du Tastevin.

CHAPTER 26

Paul P. Griffin
Southern Gentleman and Disciple of Dr. William T. Green

Paul Putnam Griffin was born on February 4, 1927, to Jesse Christopher (a minister) and Bertha Mae Dail Griffin in the small town of Goldsboro, North Carolina. He met his wife, Margaret Braswell, while he studied medicine at Bowman Gray School of Medicine and she worked as a laboratory technician. He had previously graduated magna cum laude with his bachelor of science in 1949 from Wake Forest University, and after medical school, Dr. Griffin interned between 1953 and 1954 at the University of Michigan. He later completed his residency at both North Carolina Baptist Hospital and Boston Children's Hospital, and, "after an outstanding performance as Chief Resident, joined the staff as Assistant Orthopedic Surgeon" in 1959 (Children's Hospital Archives, Annual Report 1960).

Griffin spent the next 10 years at Boston Children's Hospital and Harvard Medical School (HMS). In 1962, he was promoted to instructor of orthopaedic surgery at HMS and then to associate in orthopaedic surgery in 1963 at Boston Children's Hospital. In 1963, he also assumed a role as an examiner on the American Board of Orthopaedic Surgery, just four years after completing his chief residency. Griffin was especially intrigued by "the study of pauci-articular arthritis in children, septic joints in the child and bone tumors" (Children's Hospital Archives, Annual Report 1962), and that same year he coauthored a publication with Drs. Green and Tachdjian

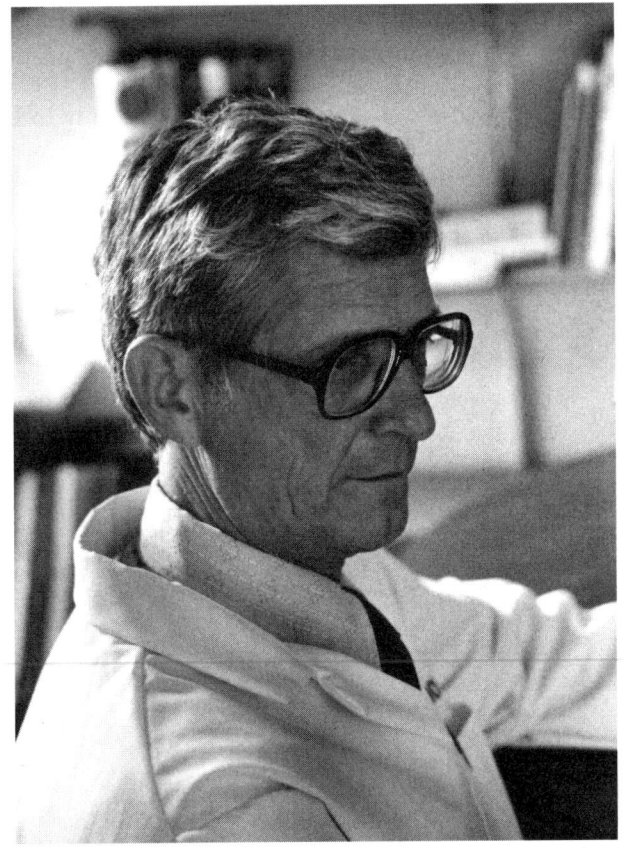

Paul P. Griffin seated at his desk. Boston Children's Hospital Archives, Boston, Massachusetts.

Physician Snapshot

Paul P. Griffin
BORN: 1927
DIED: 2018
SIGNIFICANT CONTRIBUTIONS: Dedicated educator; co-founder of the Pediatric Orthopaedic Society

titled "Pauciarticular Arthritis in Children." They reviewed 78 cases treated at Boston Children's Hospital, and used the term "pauciarticular" (a descriptor previously coined by Green in the late 1930s) to designate the distinctive form of pediatric arthritis studied (involving four or fewer joints) from more severe pediatric rheumatoid arthritis, now called juvenile idiopathic arthritis. They concluded that "the disorder may very well be a mild form of rheumatoid arthritis, since the reactions in the synovium, articular cartilage, and joint fluid are similar to those seen in rheumatoid arthritis, but the extent and severity of these changes are much less in pauciarticular arthritis [and] adequate local treatment is the most important, as this is the only one which we physicians can control" (Griffin and Green 1963).

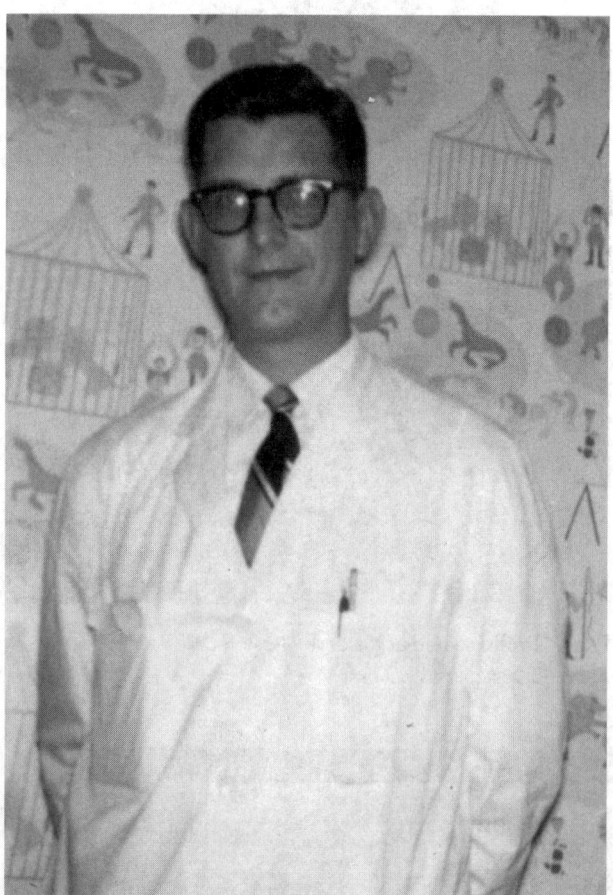

Paul Griffin during his early years as an attending orthopaedic surgeon at BCH. Boston Children's Hospital Archives, Boston, Massachusetts.

Quickly thereafter, he was promoted to clinical associate in orthopaedic surgery at HMS in 1966 and to senior associate in 1968 at Boston Children's Hospital. I was a junior and a senior resident during this period, and Griffin was an excellent teacher in the clinic, on walk rounds, and in the operating room. He obviously enjoyed teaching and was always the "southern gentleman." During this period, he also published two other papers in addition to his discussion of the treatment of a child with a dislocated hip at Massachusetts General Hospital in a *JAMA* "Fractures of the Month" series (**Case 24.2**). He published an American Academy of Orthopaedic Surgeons (AAOS) instructional course on "Treatment of Fractures in Children," and he coauthored a second paper, "Fractures of the Shaft of the Femur in Children," with Drs. Green and Margaret Anderson. It became a "classic paper on managing the child's fracture femur, elucidating prudent original observations that have become standard knowledge" (Gross and Tate 1997). Leg length discrepancies were frequent at the time in 1972, with overgrowth following a fractured femur. Allowing the fracture fragments to override was popular, but the amount recommended varied from a low of one centimeter to a high of three centimeters. In their review of 95 cases treated at Boston Children's Hospital between 1955 and 1963, Griffin, Anderson, and Green concluded that:

- If the original deformity of the "fracture fragments is less than 20 degrees" and the femur is stable: there should be no abnormalities
- If pediatric patients are younger than two years of age or are prepubescent: bony fragments should not be allowed to overlap and shorten the total length of the bone
- If pediatric patients are "between two years and ten years of age": the fracture may be allowed to overlap no more than 1.0 to 1.5 cm to allow for future overgrowth. (Griffin, Anderson, and Green 1972).

In 1969, Griffin left Boston and went on to accept the position of professor of orthopaedic surgery at George Washington University and chief of the Department of Orthopaedics at the Children's Hospital of the District of Columbia. After three years, he became chairman of the Department of Orthopaedics and Rehabilitation of Vanderbilt University School of Medicine and chief of the Department of Orthopaedics at Vanderbilt University Hospital, positions he held for 10 years. During this period, he published an additional 23 papers—all covering different aspects of pediatric orthopaedics, and he went on to establish the Pediatric Orthopaedic Society (POS) with Drs. Douglas McKay and Mihran Tachdjian in 1971. They elected Green as the society's first president, and they appointed Griffin treasurer and later president in 1978. The purpose of the society was to bring pediatric orthopaedists together to discuss issues of special relevance to their specialty. Their first meeting included Griffin, McKay, Tachdjian, and Green as well as Drs. Burr Curtis and Frank Stelling. Because POS limited their membership to by invitation only, younger pediatric orthopaedists formed their own separate organization in 1974, which they called the Pediatric Orthopedic Study Group (POSG). Eventually a movement for unification developed and in 1981, when Dr. Hall was president of the POS, he "made a very eloquent but simple talk encouraging amalgamation [and] he said we [the members] could either look towards the progress of our specialty and approve amalgamation or we could say 'pull up the gang plank, Jack, I'm aboard'" (Watts 1996). The result was the formation of the Pediatric Orthopedic Society of North America (POSNA) in 1984.

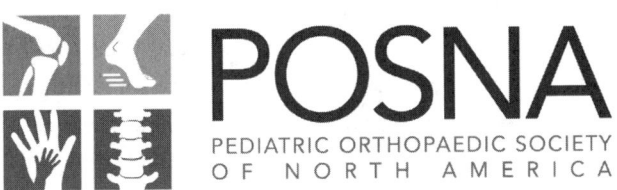

Logo of POSNA (Pediatric Orthopaedic Society of North America). Courtesy of POSNA.

Title of Green, Beauchamp, and Griffin's article supporting the importance of femoral head extrusion in Legg-Calvé-Perthes Disease. *Journal of Bone and Joint Surgery* 1981; 63: 900.

In the meantime, while still in Tennessee, Griffin—along with Neil Green and Richard Bauchamp—had published an article in July of 1981 that described a prognostic index for Legg-Perthes Disease. In a review of 221 patients with Legg-Calvé-Perthes disease in the hip, the authors concluded:

> Catterall's classification of the extent of involvement for the femoral head...has prognostic value, as does age at onset. However, there are exceptions, since some children who are less than four years old at onset have a poor result and some other children have a good result. Containment treatment also definitely influences the prognosis. Epiphyseal extrusion is a simple assessment of the amount of subluxation of the femoral head; and when this factor is considered along with the patient's age and the amount of involvement of the femur head, the outcome of the disease can be predicted accurately. (Green et al. 1981)

For example, if greater than 20% of the femoral head was extruded, i.e., not covered by the acetabulum, the results were recorded as poor in their series.

By September of that same year, Griffin returned to Boston Children's Hospital as orthopaedic surgeon-in-chief and to HMS as professor

Case 24.2. Recurrent Traumatic Dislocation of the Hip in a Child

"Dr. William Harris: A 6 ½-year old boy was brought to the emergency ward of the Massachusetts General Hospital because of pain in his right hip. He had been sitting on his bed, leaning forward to tie his shoe, when he slipped off the edge of the bed. He landed on his right knee with his right thigh in a position of adduction and flexion and was unable to rise from the floor.

"Examination of his hip showed that the right thigh was adducted, internally rotated, and flexed, and the femoral head could be felt in the right buttock. There was full motion and motor power throughout the right lower extremity below the hip. Sensation and circulation were intact. X-ray examination of the hip showed complete dislocation of the right hip.

"This was not the first episode of dislocation of the right hip that this young boy had experienced. At the age of 3 he had fallen from a fence and sustained a dislocation of the right hip. X-ray films taken at the time revealed no evidence of abnormality of the femur or acetabulum. After closed reduction had been carried out at another hospital, he was treated in traction for five days and then a spica cast for six weeks. Following removal of his cast, he was kept at bed rest for an additional month. After resuming full activity the patient had done well and walked without a limp, but had complained periodically of pain in the right hip after mild trauma.

"Two years prior to his current dislocation at the age of 4 years, he had been pushed off his feet in a playground and again noted the sudden onset of acute pain in his right hip. He had been able to walk after this episode, but because of his limp and the persistent pain in his right hip he had been brought to the hospital. X-ray films confirmed the clinical diagnosis of dislocation of the right hip. These films revealed no evidence of abnormality of the acetabulum or femoral head.

"On that admission he was given morphine and pentobarbital (Nembutal) in the emergency ward and placed in the prone position for a Stimson maneuver. This maneuver was not successful, and a general anesthesia was required to obtain a closed reduction. He was then placed in a 1½ spica in the frog position.

"His spica was removed at six weeks and again x-rays, including acetabular views and views of the posterior acetabulum, showed no evidence of osseous abnormality…

"It was the recommendation of the majority of the staff at that time that an arthrogram should be done, but this was deferred by those treating the patient.

"He had been completely well from that episode until his current admission. Following his recovery from his dislocation at age of 4, he was noted to have normal muscle power in his right hip and was fully active. He had a full range of motion but no evidence of ligamentous laxity."

"Dr. Aufranc: We have Dr. Paul Griffin from the Children's Medical Center here to discuss this case with us today."

"Dr. Griffin: This is a very interesting case, and I am privileged to discuss it. Three problems are presented by this case: First, why does he have recurrent dislocation of the hip? Second, how can further dislocations be prevented? And third, what is the prognosis for the hip?

"It is often said that traumatic dislocation of the hip in children is so rare that no one surgeon has enough personal experience to be dogmatic in his principles of treatment. This is even more true in recurrent traumatic dislocation of the hip, as it is indeed rare.

"This child demonstrates the ease with which the hip in a young child can be dislocated for certainly none of his injuries were severe. In the very young child a moderate force directed through the long axis of the femoral shaft with the hip flexed and adducted will dislocate the hip posteriorly. More severe trauma is usually necessary for dislocating the hip anteriorly, or into the obturator foramen, or into the sciatic notch. In older children, a greater force is necessary to dislocate the hip, and the incidence of associated fractures of the acetabulum becomes greater.

"Recurrent dislocation of the hip should more likely occur in the very young child, in patients with structural abnormalities of the hip, in children with ligamentous laxity, or in the presence of a local defect in the joint capsule. The patient presented here has no x-ray evidence of a structural abnormality of the hip, and does not have ligamentous laxity. Unless he had a local defect in the capsule of the hip, one would have to assume that the recurrent dislocations were due to the degree and direction of the forces on the hip in a young child. I would recommend an arthrogram to rule out the presence of a local defect in the capsule. If the arthrogram failed to demonstrate an abnormality of the capsule, I would treat this patient conservatively.

Although I would not be critical of the previous treatment of this patient, I would, on this occasion, recommend more prolonged protection, and maintain immobilization of the hip in a spica cast in abduction for three or four months. After removing the spica, I would continue to protect the hip by a partial weightbearing crutch gait for an additional six to eight weeks.

"If the arthrogram showed an abnormality in the capsule, I would recommend that the capsule be repaired and reefed. Before doing this, however, I would give the hip two- or three-weeks rest in a bi-valved spica cast in abduction to allow the synovium to recover from the trauma of dislocation. During the last week of this period of time, I would exercise the hip gently in abduction. Post-operatively the hip should be held in a bi-valved spica, and after three weeks gentle exercises in abduction should be started. Eight weeks after the reduction he could be started on a partial weight-bearing crutch gait.

"The most common complication of dislocation of the hip is avascular necrosis. In the very young child it occurs rarely, but in older children the incidence of avascular necrosis ranges from 10% to 30%. The frequency of this complication is greater in those patients in whom treatment is delayed for more than 24 hours, and in those patients who require open reduction. Open reduction should seldom be needed in children, but is occasionally necessary when treatment has been delayed or when the head of the femur is trapped in a button-hole defect in the capsule.

"I think the prognosis in this child should be good, because treatment was not delayed, and I assume that the hip was reduced by closed manipulation. If a capsulorrhaphy was performed, it adds some risk, but if it were done several weeks after closed reduction, the risk should be slight."

"Dr. Aufranc: If it were necessary to repair a capsular tear, would you deliberately dislocate the hip to see the ligamentum teres?"

"Dr. Griffin: I would think that the ligamentum teres must have been ruptured. I would want to inspect the acetabulum and femoral head carefully and this would require dislocation."

"Dr. Jones: What approach would you use?"

"Dr. Griffin: A defect in the capsule would most likely be posterior, but could be superior. A Gibson skin incision would provide excellent exposure for the repair."

"Dr. Harris: With the patient under general anesthesia, the hip reduced with ease, with one click, and once the hip had been extended there was a second click. After the reduction, there was a full range of passive motion while the patient was under anesthesia, and gentle pressure on the knee in the direction of the hip, with the hip in a position of moderate flexion and moderate abduction, did not redislocate the hip. The patient was placed in a 1½ spica cast.

"A week after the manipulative reduction, exploration of the hip was carried out through a posterior approach, splitting the fibers of the gluteus maximus. In the aureolar tissue covering the short external rotators, a large pouch of synovium was identified. This pouch arose from the posterior aspect of the capsule of the hip joint, and extruded in the space between the quadratus and the inferior gemellus. The defect in the posterior capsule of the hip joint extended about one third of the circumference of the head and was about 1 cm from the acetabular attachment of the capsule. It was oriented generally in a saggital direction. The synovial pouch was closed with silk sutures in a "vest-over-pants" manner. The hip was not dislocated. The sciatic nerve lay in its normal bed, and had normal appearance. The patient was then kept for six weeks in a spica cast, and then started on partial weightbearing, using crutches. Arthrograms had been attempted prior to the surgery, but the arthrogram on his right hip was not successful.

"One year following his surgery he had a full range of motion on the right hip except that his external rotation in flexion was 80°, compared to 90° on the left, and internal rotation in flexion was 60°, compared to 80° on the left. Films showed normal development of the capital femoral epiphysis and the acetabulum."

"Dr. Robert Brendze: We need to watch for three additional complications in this patient other [than] avascular necrosis. They are coxa magna, degenerative arthritis, and premature epiphyseal fusion."

"Dr. Griffin: While he has shown no avascular necrosis during the first year, this possibility remains. Cases have been reported in which avascular necrosis first appeared four and five years after the injury."

(Aufranc et al. 1964)

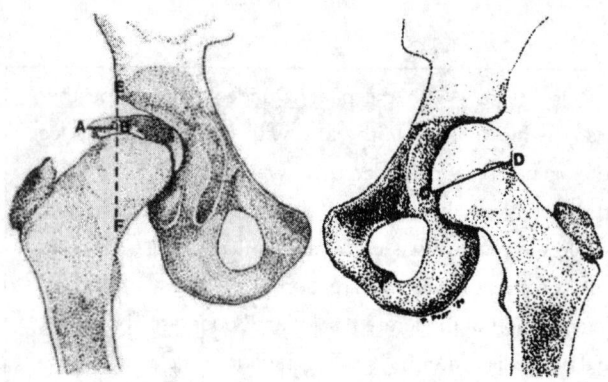

Method of measuring the epiphyseal extrusion: Extrusion=% of head (lateral to Perkin's Line E-F) uncovered (A-B) by the width of the opposite femoral head (C-D).

N. E. Green, R. D. Beauchamp, and P. P. Griffin, "Epiphyseal extrusion as a prognostic index in Legg-Calvé-Perthes disease," *Journal of Bone and Joint Surgery* 1981; 63: 902.

of orthopaedic surgery. According to an interview with Dr. James Kasser, Griffin had always hoped to return there because he considered it "the greatest place in the world," and he wished to return to the culture that Green had previously established within the orthopaedics department (Kasser, pers. comm., Nov. 7, 2014). In another interview, Griffin stated, "Children's Hospital has a long and very distinguished history in the field of orthopedics. Many of the hospital's first patients had orthopedic problems, especially scoliosis and tuberculosis of the spine" (Griffin 1981). Griffin had been heavily influenced in his decision to return by Dr. Sledge, as well as Dr. Robert Maslin and Dr. William Berenberg—two of the more senior pediatricians. Griffin described his goals in a statement:

> ...to reinstitute the growth study originated at Children's Hospital by Dr. Green...We want to build on Dr. Green's work...to look at growth abnormalities in children of short stature; and gather data about normal growth in children of the 1980s, as compared with children of the 1930s and 1940s. We know children are larger.
> (*Focus*, Children's Hospital Bulletin)

He planned for Dr. Frederic Shapiro to lead these new growth studies.

In his new appointment, Griffin was responsible for overseeing the outpatients and inpatients in all subspecialties of pediatric orthopaedics, including: scoliosis, cerebral palsy, arthritis, clubfoot, growth problems, injuries, limb deformities and myelodysplasia, the gait lab, the brace shop, and the division of sports medicine. However, at the time of his return, the orthopaedic service was in disarray, and it did not have an active chief. Dr. Glimcher was devoted fulltime to his laboratory research and did not attend clinical conferences, and Dr. Hall, who had been hired as chief of clinical orthopaedics in 1971, entered private practice. Hall's three associates—Drs. Millis, Emans, and Micheli, who were all independent private corporations—and other recent hires remained on staff, including Drs. Shapiro, Rosenthal, Simon, and Thompson. Griffin quickly hired Dr. Richard Gross in early 1982 and Dr. James Kasser by midsummer.

Although the hospital had promised Griffin his authority, they did not provide any financial support except for some salaries and the charge that he should establish a foundation model for the orthopaedic clinicians. This became the first of a new model for departmental clinical practices desired by the hospital's administrative leadership. Although Griffin was an outstanding educator, he was not so successful with his foundation model. There were numerous reasons for this, but they included lack of knowledge of orthopaedic funds at Boston Children's Hospital, inability to control any of the indirect support from external grants (controlled by the hospital), internal staff disruptions, and legal suits among other issues. Essentially, Griffin had the responsibilities of a chief of service at Children's Hospital and professor of orthopaedic surgery at Harvard Medical School, but without true authority. His full-time staff was on hospital salaries and clinical income was insufficient, so the department continued to increase its indebtedness to the hospital.

In a letter to Dr. Griffin in 1983, Dr. Sledge described his meeting with some of the faculty at Children's to determine if he could help improve the contentious situation in the orthopaedic department. Sledge made the following suggestions to Griffin:

1. [regarding] the inter-relationship between the Foundation and the hospital. They [faculty] are loathe to enter into a practice mode that depends upon the good will of the hospital since the past has not demonstrated that good will is invariably present nor with any guarantees about the future. It would be an enormous step forward if it were possible for you to restructure your Foundation along the lines of the… Foundations here [BWH] and probably the Anesthesia's Foundation at Children's, that is, free-standing with an external Board composed of Layman but not chosen by the hospital…

2. …I had urged Mr. Weiner and Luskia to erase the debt so that the Foundation could start off debt-free. It is my impression that that is possible…

3. [The faculty's] perception that your multiple duties, both locally and nationally, preclude the attention to detail…desirable in terms of business management. Their suggestion was that the Foundation hire a business manager…a forceful spokesperson for you and your department in the relationships with a sometimes hostile world, including your own hospital…[and] conserve your energies for more important matters and also coopt the reluctant staff into joining with you in the battle. (Sledge 1983)

In an earlier letter to the president of the hospital, Sledge also stated:

I am convinced that we have the best possible person in the job…because of everything I learn from the residents…[what is] happening educationally in the institution…[and] there is a superb group of orthopedic surgeons currently at Children's Hospital…I humbly suggest that you consider writing off the department's debt so that the new Departmental Group Practice can start out on even ground, rather than "in the hole." (Sledge 1983)

By 1986, Dr. Griffin found himself unsuccessful and depressed in these endeavors, and he resigned from his most prized position at Children's and moved to Chicago Shriner's Hospital as chief of staff. A subsequent move to the Medical University of South Carolina allowed him to rejoin his clinical partnership with Dr. Gross. Eventually, Dr. Griffin retired from academics and settled in the Greensboro area as a pediatric consultant. Throughout the duration of his career, he had also served on the board of visitors at his alma mater, Wake Forest University; the university honored him with the Distinguished Alumni Award (an award for outstanding commitment to service). Dr. Richard Gross, a long-time colleague of Griffin's at Boston Children's Hospital, summed up Griffin's illustrious career with the following words:

I have had the privilege of being a partner of Paul Griffin for most of the past 15 years… Those years of daily exposure to an inquisitive mind, to a master diagnostician and clinician, to a knowledgeable but self-critical student of the field, to a committed teacher, and to a scrupulously ethical human being have made me a better physician than I might have been… it is a pleasure to acknowledge Paul Griffin as a true academician; one who probes, practices, and most important teaches…The late Mihran Tachdjian…and Paul Griffin served together as residents at the Children's Hospital in Boston… Dr. Tachdjian recalled Paul Griffin as "methodical, thorough, and dedicated, with sympathy and concern for the child." These qualities were balanced with insistence that "the resident must know the patient and the literature." Edwin

Wyman…served as a junior resident under Paul Griffin at The Children's Hospital. Dr. Wyman recalled that at the time of his residency in the late 1950s learning was largely through intimidation. Some teachers used grinding techniques to educate house staff, "like the way a tin plate assumes the shape of a hubcap when placed in a hubcap press." Paul Griffin encouraged "younger residents with a dry sense of humor and complete approach to medicine." Although Paul Griffin does not use grinding techniques, there is no doubt when he is not pleased. There is no worse feeling than to give a presentation, then hear Paul Griffin intone "I guess you could do it that way. I've heard of it being done that way; I wouldn't do it that way" …His bedside teaching and physical examination techniques are excellent. His approach of taking a history and performing a physical examination harkens back to an earlier, less hurried era, when direct patient contact, not high technology tests, made the diagnosis. In the operating room, he is all business. Surgery proceeds efficiently and he is constantly teaching and pointing out important aspects of the particular cases. His skills are superb. [His]…dedication to teaching and to patients is unchanged from the earliest portion of his career…His example of lifelong learning, unending curiosity, and overall excellence serves as an inspiration for all who have worked with him. (Gross and Tate 1997)

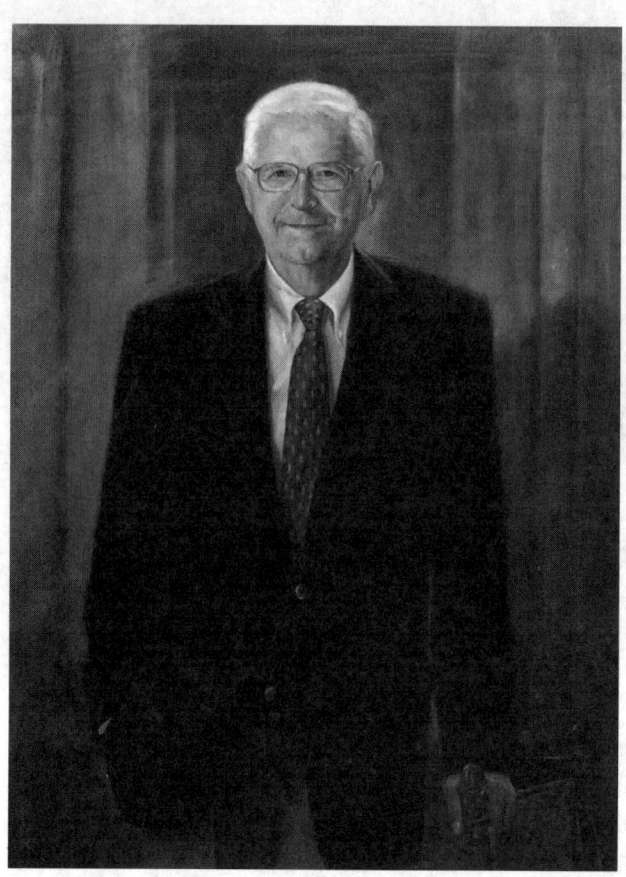

Portrait of Dr. Griffin. James Koepfler/Boston Children's Hospital.

After over 50 years of dedicated service to the field, Griffin died on June 4, 2018.

CHAPTER 27

BCH Other Surgeon Scholars

(1970–2000)

Orthopaedic surgeons at Boston Children's Hospital continued to influence the fields of surgery and medicine throughout the 1900s. As the twentieth century came to a close, new generations of these clinicians—whom Harvard referred to as "surgeon-scholars"—had proven themselves to be worthy additions to the ranks of the surgeons and physicians who had preceded them in practice and laid the foundations for their work. The 15 surgeon-scholars described here are some of those who had a lasting influence at Boston Children's Hospital. They include:

John B. Emans	357
M. Timothy Hresko	364
Lawrence I. Karlin	369
Robert B. Keller	371
Mininder S. Kocher	376
Lyle J. Micheli	383
Michael B. Millis	388
Edward J. Riseborough	395
Robert K. Rosenthal	401
Frederic Shapiro	402
Sheldon R. Simon	405
Brian D. Snyder	409
Sandra J. Thompson	412
Peter Waters	414
Hugh G. Watts	420

JOHN B. EMANS

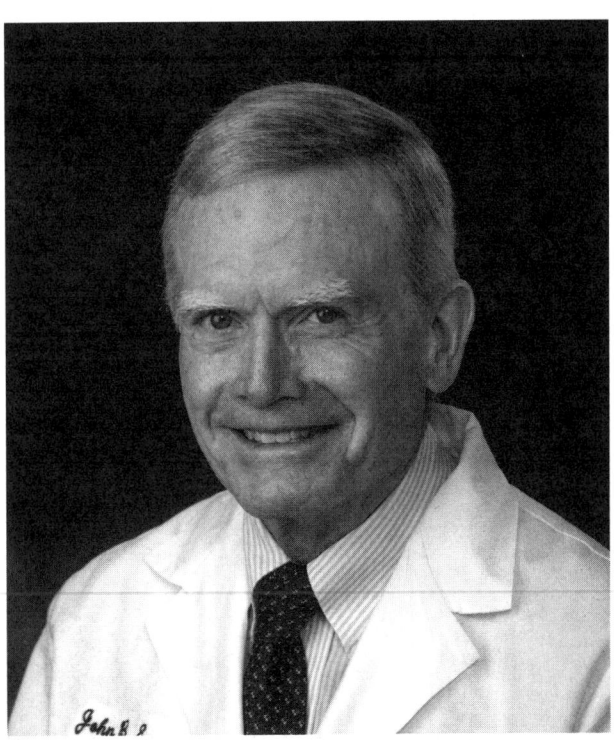

John B. Emans. James Koepfler/Boston Children's Hospital.

Physician Snapshot

John B. Emans
BORN: 1944
DIED: —

SIGNIFICANT CONTRIBUTIONS: Made many modifications to the Boston bracing system; director spine surgery service and myelodysplasia program; helped develop and disseminate the HCORP core curriculum

John B. Emans was born in Washington, DC, and grew up in Schenectady, New York. He received his bachelor of arts degree in biochemistry from Harvard in 1966 (he was a classmate of Mike Millis, whose career is described later in this chapter). While an undergraduate, Emans was a member of the ski team and Kirkland House. Upon graduation, he entered Harvard Medical School; he received an MD degree in 1970.

He remained in Boston for his residency (a surgical internship and a one-year general surgical residency at the Peter Bent Brigham Hospital), followed by an orthopaedic surgical residency in the Harvard Combined Orthopaedic Residency Program, which he completed in 1976. He was chief resident and a fellow in pediatric orthopaedics at Children's Hospital from January to July 1976, at which time he entered the army because of his commitment to the Berry Plan. For two years, he served as chief of the orthopaedic service at Cutler Army Hospital at Fort Devens, Massachusetts.

Returning to civilian life in 1978, Emans joined the faculty at Children's Hospital under Dr. John Hall's leadership, and he has remained on staff there since. In that same year he also began a five-year tenure (1978–83) at Parker Hill Hospital, which closed in the early 1980s, at which time he became a staff member at Kennedy Memorial Hospital (1983–87). He is currently on the courtesy staff at the Brigham and Women's Hospital, the New England Baptist Hospital, and the Newton Wellesley Hospital.

He has held various faculty appointments at Harvard, moving from instructor (1978–87) to assistant clinical professor of orthopaedic surgery (1987–95), then associate professor of clinical orthopaedic surgery (1995–98), associate professor of orthopaedic surgery (1998–2000), and then full professor in 2001. Initially on the full-time faculty, Emans went into private practice but remained on the clinical staff at Children's Hospital when Hall stepped down; when Hall was reinstated as chief of the orthopaedic department, Emans also returned to the staff full-time.

Since 1979, Emans has been director of the Boston Brace Instructional Courses. Hall had established the Boston bracing system for scoliosis early during his time at Children's Hospital, and, in his 2014 curriculum vitae, Emans described his own engagement in modifying elements of that system over the subsequent three decades. In 1986, Emans, M. E. "Bill" Miller, Hall, and others described the use of the Boston bracing system in 295 patients with idiopathic scoliosis. They concluded that among the children in their study, the

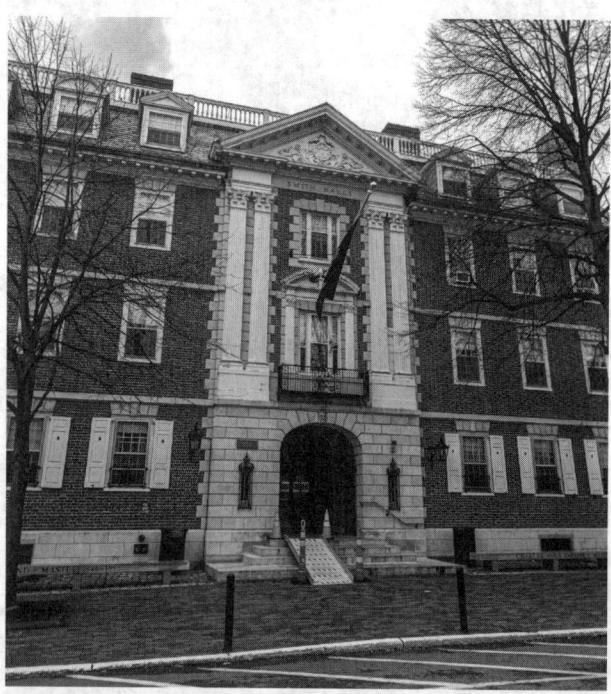

Kirkland House, Harvard. Kael E. Randall/Kael Randall Images.

Title of Emans et al. article on their results with the Boston brace. *Spine*, 1986; 11: 792.

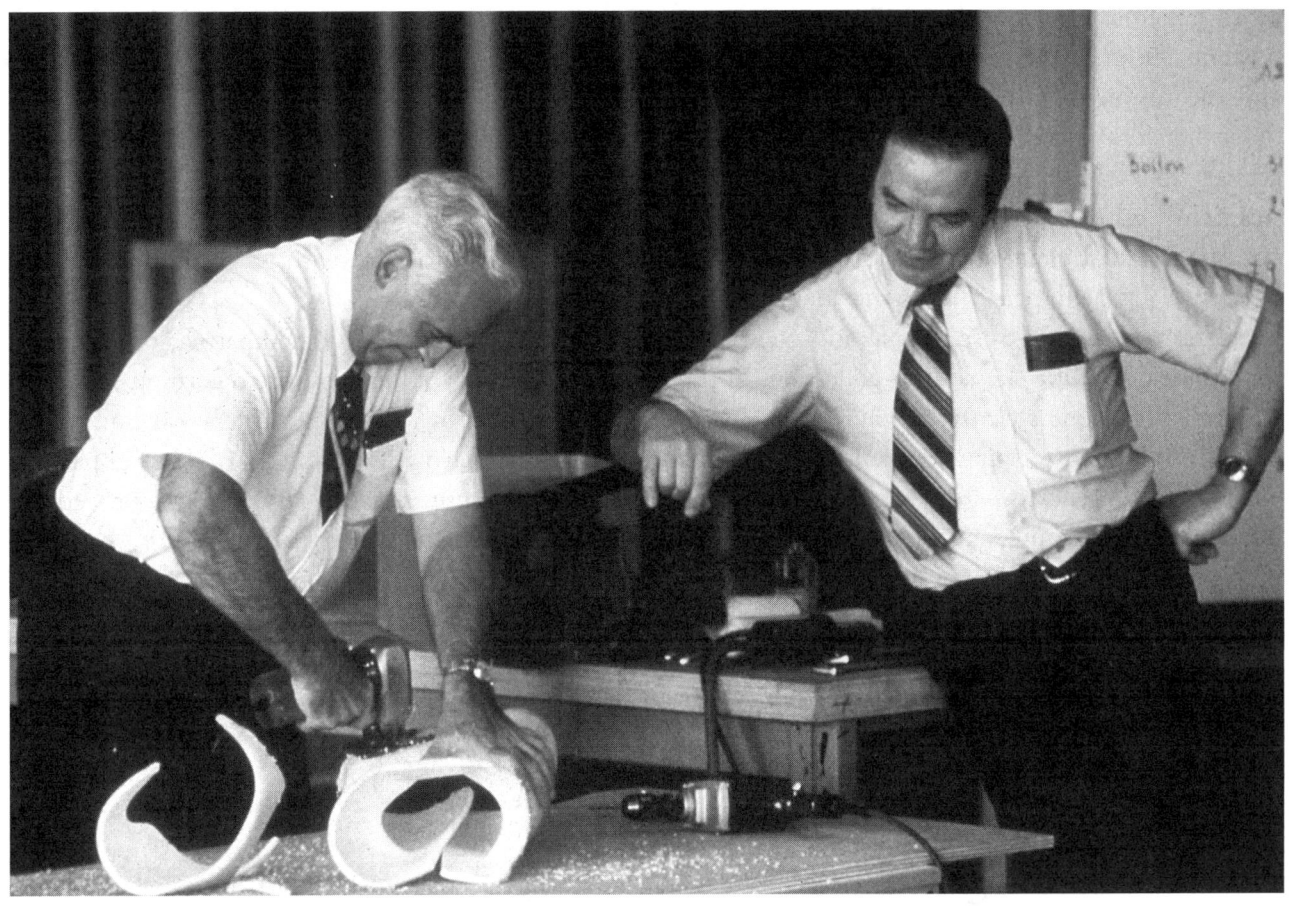

John Hall and Bill Miller during a presentation about the Boston brace. James Koepfler/Boston Children's Hospital Archives, Boston, Massachusetts.

system improved 30- to 45-degree curves, and the scoliosis was controlled or corrected in ~80% of their patients. For patients with curves below the level of T7, addition of the superstructure to the brace did not seem to make a difference in the result. The results presented in that report have come to represent achievable standards after using braces to treat idiopathic scoliosis. Emans noted that his study caused orthopaedists at Children's Hospital to begin to avoid treating some conditions, such as high thoracic curves, and to consider acute in-brace curve correction when determining prognosis.

Since 1984, Emans has been director of the Myelodysplasia Program at Children's Hospital, which is the largest such program in the region. His goal has been for the multidisciplinary clinic to provide compassionate, skillful, and integrated care. In his 2014 curriculum vitae, Emans described both his use of pedicle screws and his improvements to "eggshell" partial vertebrectomy for correction in patients with myelodysplasia spine deformity. In 2001, Emans became director of the Spinal Surgery Service at Children's Hospital.

Emans has published more than 106 articles, 77 of which are on the spine and scoliosis, seven on myelodysplasia, and three on the Boston bracing system. His other articles discuss various additional pediatric orthopaedic topics, including six on trauma. He's also published 10 book chapters and a manual on the Boston brace, which includes a syllabus and instructional guide.

Emans' first paper on the spine was written with Dr. William Herndon, Dr. Lyle Micheli, and Hall in 1981. It dealt with surgical treatment of the spine in Scheuermann kyphosis in a small series of 13 patients. They concluded that anterior and posterior fusion is a requisite for acceptable results, and the fusion must comprise the whole of the deformity. They noted that although reduced pulmonary function could result, function would be sufficiently normal.

Another of Emans' main areas of interest has been special growth preservation in patients requiring surgery for early-onset spinal and chest-wall deformities. In 2005, he and his colleagues in the Clinical Effectiveness Center at Children's Hospital published their experience treating 31 patients with fused ribs, chest wall deformity with thoracic inefficiency syndrome, and spine deformity. In such patients, the thorax can become constricted on one or both sides, and thoracic insufficiency syndrome can occur. The authors recommended expansion thoracostomy and use of VEPTR (Vertical Expandable Prosthetic Titanium Rib), which together have three main benefits: reduces chest-wall constriction, increases lung volume, and corrects spinal deformity, without restricting thoracic spine growth.

Emans, with Behrooz Akbarnia, published in 2012 a review of the literature regarding complications with growth-sparing surgery—including the insertion of growth rods and VEPTR—in patients with early onset scoliosis (EOS). Such procedures aim to affect deformities of the chest and spine and reduce the extent of thoracic insufficiency

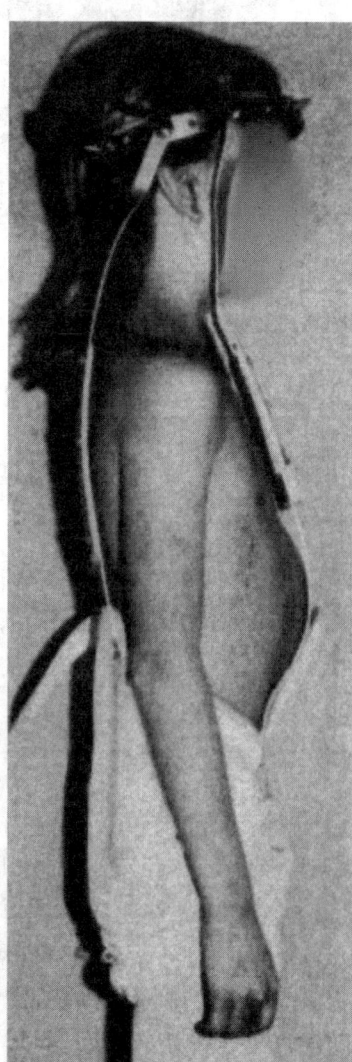

Original Boston brace with attached halo to stabilize the head and neck.
H. G. Watts, J. E. Hall, and W. M. Stanish, "The Boston Brace System for the Treatment of Low Thoracic and Lumbar Scoliosis by the Use of a Girdle Without Superstructure," *Journal of Bone and Joint Surgery* 1977; 126: 89.

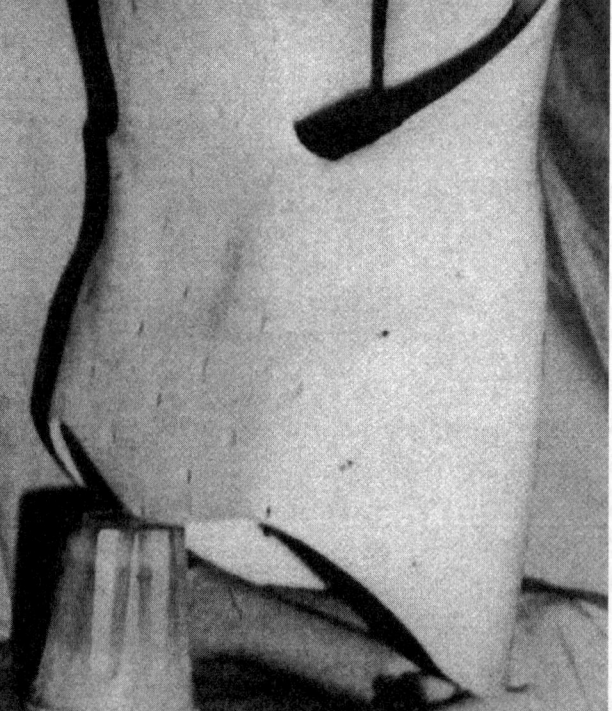

Original Boston brace; shaped from a prefabricated module.
H. G. Watts, J. E. Hall, and W. M. Stanish, "The Boston Brace System for the Treatment of Low Thoracic and Lumbar Scoliosis by the Use of a Girdle Without Superstructure," *Journal of Bone and Joint Surgery* 1977; 126: 88.

syndrome in these patients. Akbarnia and Emans noted that surgeons must know when to perform these procedures and which is best for each particular patient. In determining this, surgeons must consider potential complications, which occur often, aiming for optimal patient health and the most appropriate technique in order to reduce the incidence of any complications.

Nutrition is an important factor affecting success in these complex cases. Emans, as part of the Chest Wall and Spinal Deformity Study Group, evaluated patients' nutritional status and

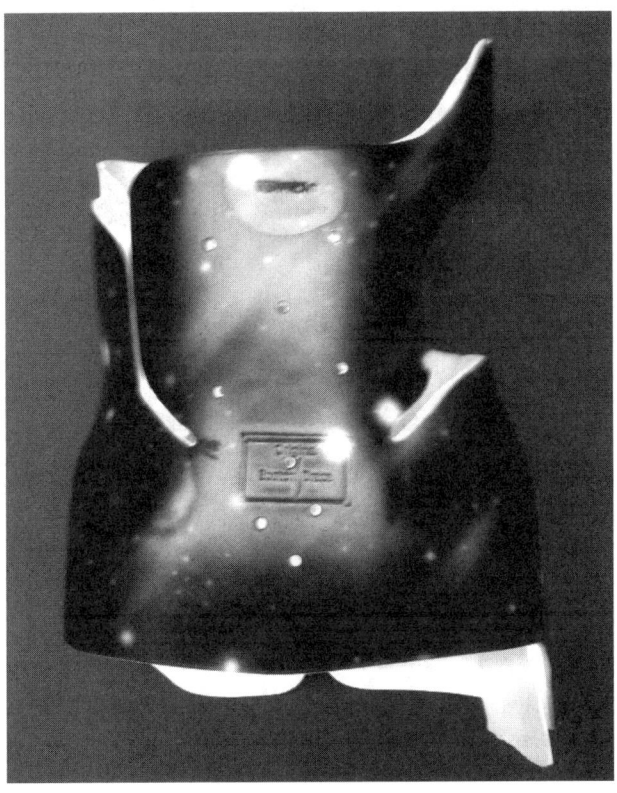

Modern Boston brace. Courtesy of Boston Orthotics & Prosthetics.

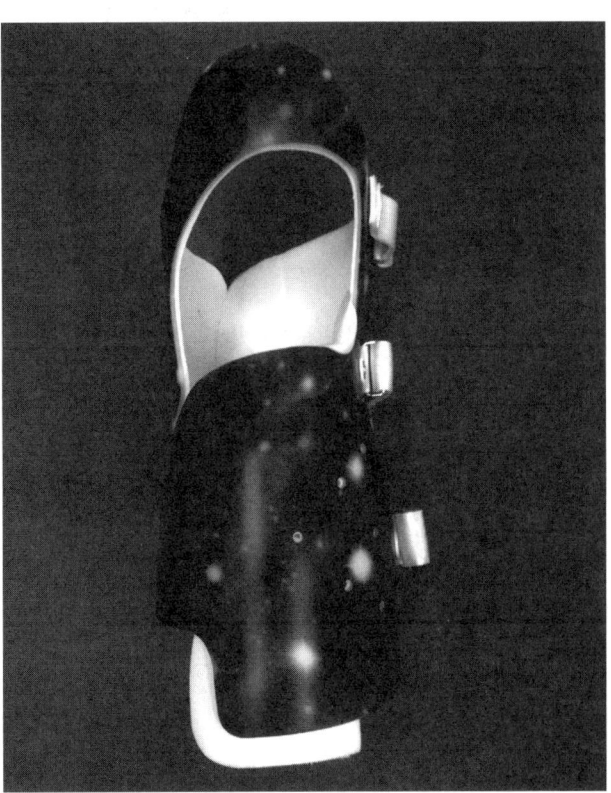

Modern Boston brace; lateral view. Courtesy of Boston Orthotics & Prosthetics.

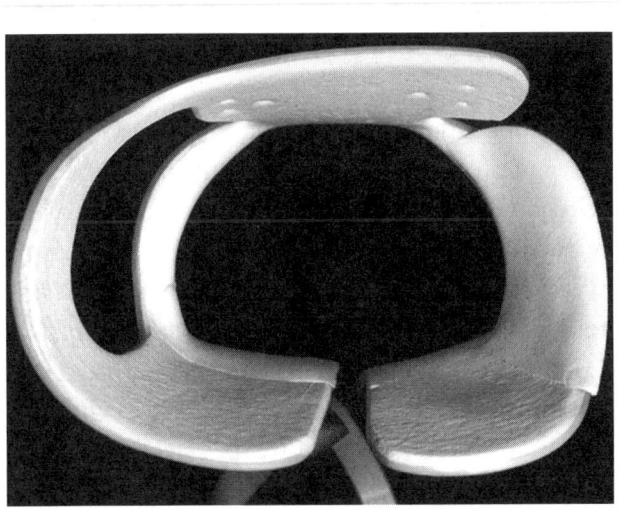

Original Boston brace with additive asymmetry to the brace. Courtesy of Boston Orthotics & Prosthetics.

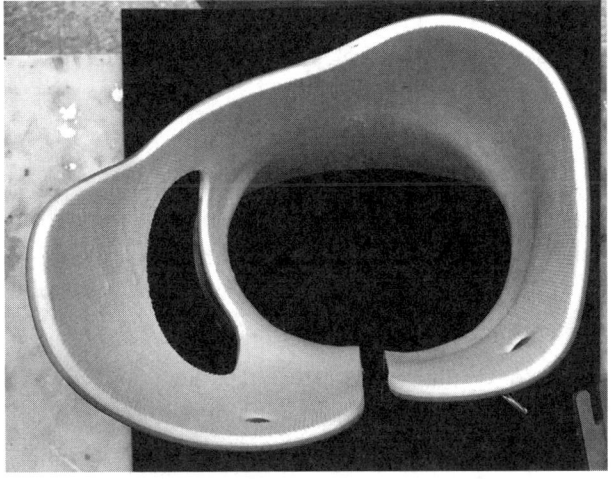

Modern Boston brace with asymmetry built in the brace. Courtesy of Boston Orthotics & Prosthetics.

Title of Emans et al. article reporting their results with use of the prosthetic titanium rib for spine and chest wall deformities. *Spine* 2005; 30: S58.

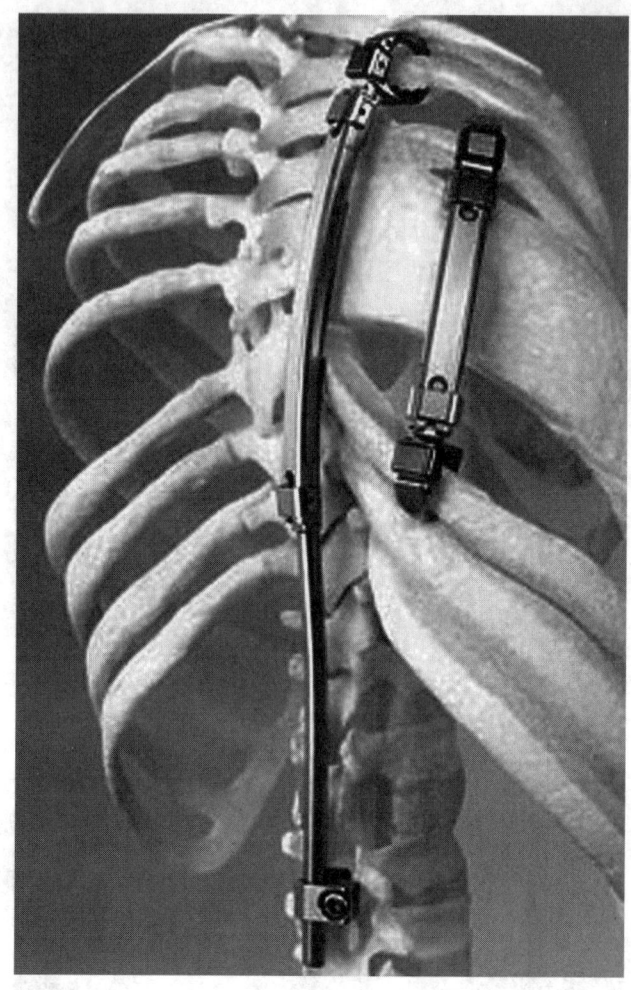

Vertical expandable prosthetic titanium rib (VEPTR).
Courtesy of Children's Hospital of Philadelphia.

improvement following growing rod surgery. The study group concluded that nutrition improved in half of patients, lending credence to the idea that this treatment helps improve the health of patients with EOS.

As a member of the Chest Wall and Spinal Deformity Study Group, he participated in a 2011 study in which Vitale et al. evaluated expert surgeons' choice of treatment in 12 patients with early-onset scoliosis (EOS). The authors described their results:

> [We] found poor intraobserver and fair interobserver agreement...[because] we lack precise indicators for surgical constructs available to treat EOS, including spinal fusion, hemiepiphysiodesis with staples or tethers, growing rods, and the VEPTR™ [a vertical expandable prosthetic titanium rib used to treat both spine and chest wall deformity during growth]... [For spine implants,] intraobserver agreement was only fair and interobserver agreement substantial when surgeons decided to use the VEPTR™ bilaterally...Treatment options... reflect individual preferences and opinions... [and] Our study highlights the difficulty in choosing among treatments optimal in children with EOS...Better evidence needs to be developed to help surgeons formulate optional strategies...and develop and validate classification systems that can guide operative indications. (Vitale et al. 2011)

In one large multicenter study, Emans and his colleagues evaluated complications in 147 consecutive patients with severe spine deformity who had vertebral column resections (VCRs) performed by seven senior-level pediatric orthopaedic surgeons over seven years. The VCR procedure was described as "3-column circumferential vertebral osteotomy creating a segmental defect with sufficient instability to require provisional instrumentation" (quoted in Lenke et al. 2013). The surgeons corrected the deformity with VCR in all planes under direct observation, which subsequent

Box 27.1. John Emans's Professional Memberships

- American Academy of Orthopaedic Surgeons
- Pediatric Orthopaedic Study Group (1979–83)
- Pediatric Orthopaedic Society of North America
- American College of Sports Medicine (1978–90)
- American Academy for Cerebral Palsy and Developmental Medicine (1986–2000)
- SICOT (International Society of Orthopaedic Surgery and Traumatology)
- Group Internationale de Cotrel Dubousset (1989–99)
- American Medical Association
- International Society for the Study of Spina Bifida
- American Orthopaedic Association
- Massachusetts Medical Society
- New England Orthopedic Society
- Massachusetts Orthopedic Society
- Boston Orthopaedic Club
- Scoliosis Research Society

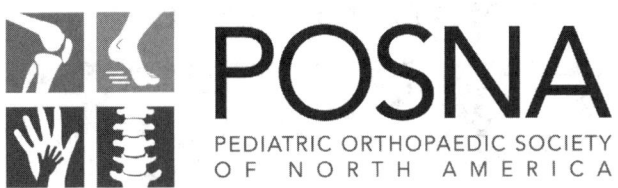

Logo of POSNA (Pediatric Orthopaedic Society of North America). Courtesy of POSNA.

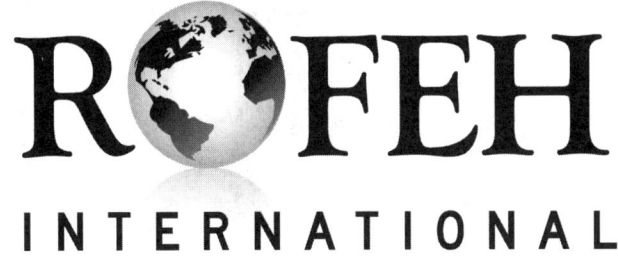

Logo of ROFEH International. Courtesy of ROFEH International.

radiographs proved to provide excellent results: Within the study sample, 86 patients (59%) experienced complication and 39 patients (27%) experienced a neurological event during the procedure. None of the VCRs resulted in complete permanent paraplegia, and no patients died.

Emans has been a member of many professional organizations throughout his career; these are listed in **Box 27.1**. He was an allied fellow of the American Academy of Pediatrics from 1995 to 2002, and he served on the board of directors of the Scoliosis Research Society from 1997 to 1999 and as secretary from 1999 to 2003.

Emans has received several awards, including the 1992 Huene Award for best clinical paper presentation, from the Pediatric Orthopaedic Society of North America. In 1999, he was nominated for the Harvard Medical School Excellence in Teaching Award. In 2013, he received the ROFEH International Award. ROFEH International is a nonprofit Jewish humanitarian organization whose mission is to help the sick in all walks of life. It supports patients and families.

In the narrative on his 2014 curriculum vitae, Emans recognized the "tradition of clinical excellence" in the orthopaedic department at Children's Hospital, and its clinicians' "passion for teaching," and he noted his own extensive role in developing and disseminating the core curriculum for residents in the HCORP. "I have had the privilege to associate with a series of department chiefs who have each epitomized this tradition, and who have been generous in granting me unique opportunities and responsibilities to carry on this tradition" (Emans 2014).

M. TIMOTHY HRESKO

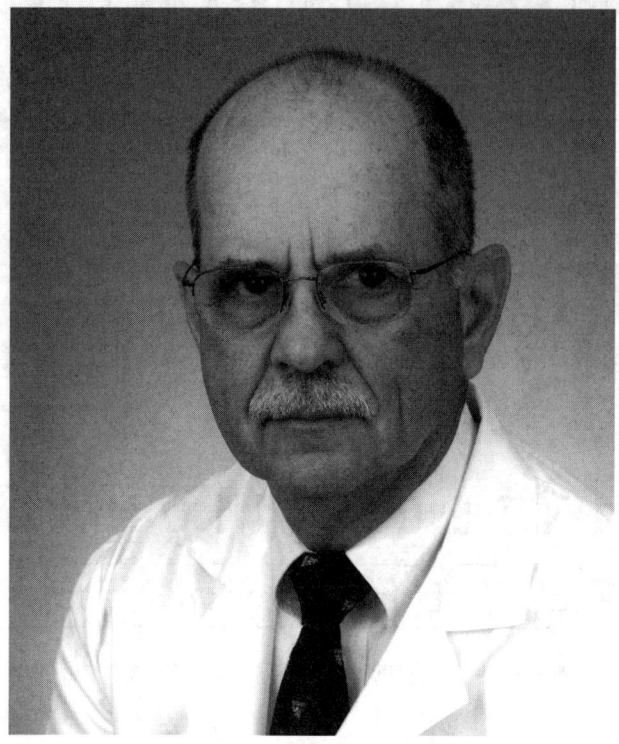

M. Timothy Hresko. James Koepfler/Boston Children's Hospital.

Physician Snapshot

M. Timothy Hresko
BORN: 1954
DIED: —
SIGNIFICANT CONTRIBUTIONS: Performed extensive clinical research regarding scoliosis and spine deformity in pediatric patients

Michael Timothy "Tim" Hresko was born and raised in Flint, Michigan. He spent his undergraduate years at Harvard College, and, in 1976, he received a bachelor of arts degree cum laude in biology. With the support of a Rotary Foundation fellowship, Hresko spent one year doing research in the Department of Social Administration at the London School of Economics, after which he entered the Columbia University College of Physicians and Surgeons, from which he received an MD degree in 1981. After a surgical internship and a year-long general surgical residency on the Harvard Surgical Service at the New England Deaconess Hospital, he spent six months (July through December 1983) as a research associate in orthopaedics at Tufts University, and he completed an orthopaedic surgery residency there in June 1987. During the last six months of his residency he was a chief resident at the New England Baptist Hospital. From July 1, 1987, through June 30, 1988, he was a fellow in pediatric orthopaedic surgery at Boston Children's Hospital.

Hresko stayed in Massachusetts after completing his fellowship. He joined the faculty at the University of Massachusetts, where he was appointed assistant professor of orthopaedic surgery in 1988; four years later he received a secondary appointment as assistant professor of pediatrics. He was on the active staff of the University of Massachusetts Medical Center, a consultant in orthopaedics at Memorial Hospital, and a consultant in pediatric orthopaedics at the Massachusetts Hospital School. While at the University of Massachusetts, he was director of the spina bifida clinic, course director of pediatric orthopaedics for the orthopaedic residency program, and course director of diagnostic therapeutic advances in pediatric orthopaedics.

In 1992, Dr. James Kasser recruited Hresko to join the faculty at Boston Children's Hospital, where he remains today. After 17 years as an assistant professor at Harvard Medical School, he was promoted to associate professor in 2009. In addition to being on the active staff at Children's Hospital, Hresko is a consultant at the New England Baptist Hospital, Newton Wellesley Hospital, and Beth Israel Deaconess Medical Center. Since 2002, he has been an affiliate pediatrician in newborn medicine at the Brigham and Women's Hospital.

Active in the Pediatric Orthopaedic Society of North America, Hresko was chairman of the program committee in 2002 and served on the historical archivists committee from 2006 to 2007.

Clinical and Research Interests

Hresko's main clinical interests are scoliosis and spinal deformity. He has been a member of the

Spinal Deformity Study Group since 1999 and was elected a fellow of the Scoliosis Research Society in 2000. He has also studied trauma in pediatric patients. He has published more than 55 articles and ~7 book chapters—most about scoliosis (see **Case 27.1**) and spine deformity, and approximately one-third on trauma.

Case 27.1. Latent Psoas Abscess After Anterior Spinal Fusion

"A 14-year, 7-month-old female patient presented with a left lumbar scoliosis of 55° from T11 to L4 and trunk imbalance of 3 cm to the left of the midline. An anterior spinal fusion from T12 to L2 with Dwyer instrumentation was recommended. A left thoracoabdominal incision through the 10th rib allowed exposure for the three-level fusion and placement of the Dwyer instrumentation on the convexity of the curve. Over the fused segment, 8° of overcorrection was obtained by the procedure, to reduce the total lumbar curve from 55° to 31°. The surgery was uncomplicated, with an estimated blood loss of 1,100 ml. Persistent drainage from the chest tube insertion site responded to local wound care after a retained subcutaneous suture was removed. Her subsequent recovery was otherwise unremarkable. Four years after surgery, during a routine yearly examination, she described occasional stiffness and nonlocalized low-back pain with damp weather as the only difficulties associated with her spinal surgery. She was able to carry out all activities without fear of back pain. In addition, she noted cold intolerance in her left leg since her spinal surgery. No focal findings were discovered on her examination. Roentgenograms of the spine at that time showed no changes from the postoperative period.

"Over the next 4 weeks she developed severe, progressive low-back pain that did not improve with bed rest, the use of spinal orthosis, and nonsteroidal anti-inflammatory medication. Her pain and dysesthesia along the left anterior thigh became aggravated by stance. She was afebrile. Repeat physical examination was now remarkable for the tenderness along the left lumbar sacral junction, pain on lumbar extension, and hyperesthesia along the anterior medial thigh. The Laseque maneuver and the remainder of the neurologic examination were normal. Further diagnostic studies were performed in light of the patient's severe, incapacitating pain. A bone scan revealed diffuse increased uptake over the area of old fusion, with no focal increase in uptake. A computed tomography (CT) scan of the fusion area and the lumbar spine was initially misinterpreted as negative. Several days passed without significant improvement in her condition. The physical examination became remarkable for a hip flexion deformity, intolerable pain on passive extension of the hips, and left flank tenderness on percussion. Although she remained afebrile, her white blood cell count was 17,600, with a shift to the left, whereas the sedimentation rate was 54. A secondary review of the CT scan suggested the presence of a fluid-filled collection in the left psoas muscle. Ultrasonic examination of the retroperitoneum confirmed that a sausage-shaped collection within the psoas muscle extended from the upper lumbar spine to the junction with the iliacus. Percutaneous drainage under ultrasonic guidance evacuated 450 ml of purulent material, which cultures showed to be a methicillin-resistant *Staphylococcus aureus* infection. On exploration of the left retroperitoneum, the genitofemoral nerve was found to be adherent to the anterior aspect of the abscess cavity. The spine was solidly fused from T12 to L2, and the Dwyer instrumentation was removed. Deep suction catheters were left in place, then advanced out of the abscess after drainage ceased 1 week after the operation. Parenteral vancomycin was administered for 6 weeks. Recurrence of left leg dysesthesia required an additional percutaneous drainage of a sterile collection of 80 ml. Prompt relief of her pain was obtained from the procedure. After 6 weeks on the vancomycin, a CT scan of the retroperitoneum showed no recurrence of the fluid collection, and no destructive lesions in the vertebrae. She has had no further back or leg pain. The cold intolerance in her leg, which had appeared after her original surgery, was no longer present."

(Hresko and Hall 1992)

Scoliosis and Spinal Deformities

In 1997, at Children's Hospital, Hresko and his collaborators treated seven children with segmental spinal dysgenesis, a rare and complex congenital condition, three of whom lost motor control before they had undergone surgery. They recognized that in these unusual cases treatment is controversial and the role of surgery unclear, and they recommended that surgeons do not wait for evidence (clinical or radiographic) that the dysgenesis has progressed to perform surgery, as this could allow the patient's neurological status to decline. Surgeons should provide prompt treatment once the dysgenesis has been diagnosed, including anterior and posterior fusion, and anterior decompression. They did, however, recognize the difficulty of the procedure and the risks that come with using instrumentation in such cases.

In an important 2001 paper on the surgical treatment of congenital kyphosis, Hresko and his colleagues made various key points:

1. Intervention achieves the best results when performed early.
2. Posterior fusion can be done when the patient has a kyphosis <60° and no neurological issues, and when instrumentation was used, pseudoarthrosis did not often occur when the fusion mass was augmented.
3. In children three years old or younger who undergo posterior in situ fusion, kyphosis may resolve gradually, as the child grows.
4. In young children, hemivertebral excision can be used to immediately correct kyphosis, but neurological injury could occur in those who undergo anterior and posterior fusion, particularly those who are older, have a more extensive deformity, and in whom the spinal cord is involved.

In an attempt to measure motion of the spine in adolescent girls with scoliosis, in 2006 Hresko and his colleagues reported the evaluation of three noninvasive measurement methods: a tape measure (the modified Schober method), dual inclinometers, and a three-dimensional electrogoniometer. They concluded that such methods are not adequate for fully measuring the amount of motion in scoliosis, and that surgeons should use "preoperative side-bending radiograph[s]" to aid in determining the appropriate surgical plan.

In a clinical practice review article for the *New England Journal of Medicine*, Hresko (2013) summarized key clinical points about idiopathic scoliosis in adolescents:

- The diagnosis of scoliosis is suspected on the basis of physical examination and is confirmed by radiography while the patient is in a standing position...[revealing] a spinal curvature of 10 degrees or greater.
- Idiopathic scoliosis is present in 2% of adolescents... [and they] should have a thorough

Title of Hresko et al. article on the surgical treatment of congenital kyphosis. *Spine* 2001; 26: 2251.

Title of Hresko's idiopathic scoliosis review article. *New England Journal of Medicine* 2013; 368: 834.

physical examination to rule out hereditary connective-tissue disorders, e.g., Marfan's syndrome, neurofibromatosis, or neurologic conditions.
- Most adolescents with nonprogressive idiopathic scoliosis can be seen by a primary care physician and do not require active treatment…data are lacking from randomized trials to show that screening results in improved outcomes.
- Bracing is commonly recommended in patients with an immature skeleton with curve progression of 25 to 45 degrees… It requires adherence to the recommended number of hours of treatment (usually ≥ 12 hours daily) until the skeleton is mature.
- Surgical treatment is recommended in patients with an immature skeleton who have progressive scoliosis greater than 45 degrees.

In a large, multicenter, prospective registry study centered at Children's Hospital in Boston in 2013, Hresko participated with the division of pain medicine in evaluating the prevalence of pain in patients after spine fusion surgery. Their results showed that approximately one-third had preoperative pain that was either moderate or severe. Those with functional limitations preoperatively, causing them to frequently miss work or school, had persistent pain. Although 15% continued to experience moderate to severe pain 2–5 years after undergoing surgery, most patients had less pain postoperatively. Whether a patient experienced pain did not seem to affect the patient's mental health or body image, but the authors noted that such factors, as well as parental factors; e.g., distress, responses to behavior; required further study.

In 2014, with Dr. Hillard Spencer and others, Hresko reported increases in spinal height among patients who underwent surgical procedures to correct idiopathic scoliosis. Spencer et al. (2014) noted that the "mean spinal height gain due to surgery [spinal instrumentation and fusion] was 2.7 centimeters," which is a "substantial gain [in] spinal height in relation to the magnitude of surgical correction, the numbers of spinal levels involved, and preoperative stature. Moderate continued spinal growth can be observed in many cases by two years after surgery and is related to shorter fusions, early Risser stages, male sex, and younger age."

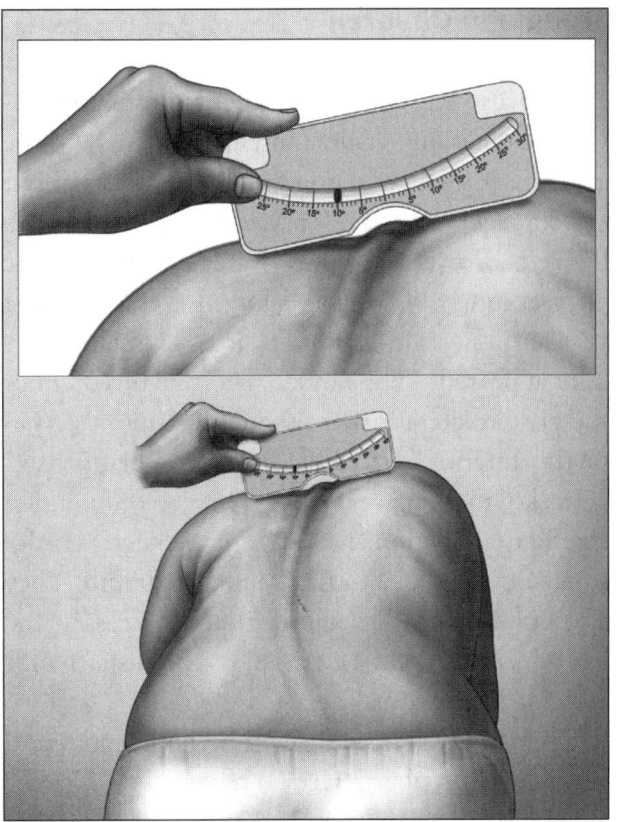

Drawing of the forward flexion test of Adam. With the use of an inclinometer, Hresko reported that rotation of <5 degrees is associated with a 95% probability that the curve is < 30 degrees. Hresko, "Idiopathic Scoliosis in Adolescents," *New England Journal of Medicine* 2013; 368: 836.

Pain Prevalence and Trajectories Following Pediatric Spinal Fusion Surgery

Christine B. Sieberg,*,[†] Laura E. Simons,*,[†] Mark R. Edelstein,*,[§] Maria R. DeAngelis,* Melissa Pielech,* Navil Sethna,* and M. Timothy Hresko[‡]
*Division of Pain Medicine, Department of Anesthesiology, Perioperative and Pain Medicine, Boston Children's Hospital, Boston, Massachusetts.
[†]Department of Psychiatry, Harvard Medical School, Boston, Massachusetts.
[‡]Department of Orthopaedic Surgery, Boston Children's Hospital/Harvard Medical School, Boston, Massachusetts.
[§]Boston University School of Medicine, Boston, Massachusetts.

Hresko et al. article that reported a significant number of patients had continued pain after spine fusion.
Journal of Pain 2013; 14: 1694.

Trauma in Children

Hresko also has cowritten some interesting observations regarding trauma in children. In 1989 he and Kasser drew attention to physeal arrests about the knee in 10- to 12.5-year-old patients who injured a lower extremity: "Recognition of the physeal injury was delayed for an average of one year and ten months until a gross angular deformity appeared...The physeal arrest involved either the posterolateral part of the distal femoral physis or the anterior part of the proximal tibial physis" (Hresko and Kasser 1989). They recommended careful examination and x-rays of the knee in order to recognize injury to the traumatized limb. They also noted that if skeletal traction is necessary, the traction pin should be placed in the distal femur and not the proximal tibia.

Ten years later, with Drs. Arthur Pappas and Benjamin Rosenberg, Hresko reported on 25 adolescent patients with stiff painful radiocapitellar joints secondary to developmental deformities or trauma. They suggested excising the radial head in patients <18 years old, which can provide benefits in up to 70%. Patients must, however, be informed that they may require subsequent revision surgery to remove bone deposited on the radial neck, which does not resolve as the patient achieves skeletal maturity.

In the 2000s, with Dr. Mininder Kocher and others at Children's Hospital, Hresko participated in a prospective randomized trial comparing medial and lateral versus lateral pin placement in treating completely displaced Gartland type 3 supracondylar humeral fractures. They concluded that "both pin-fixation techniques appear[ed] to be effective" (Kocher et al. 2007). Five years later they reevaluated their results and found that after the trial, most surgeons placed bicolumnar lateral pins. Of the eight surgeons, five changed the way they placed pins, showing that level 1 evidence can help drive changes in practice patterns.

Hresko also cowrote other interesting papers about orthopaedics. In one, he and Drs. Joseph McCarthy and Michael Goldberg reviewed ambulation ability among 65 adult patients with Down syndrome. They noted that at the time the literature did not delineate the functional disabilities of adult patients with Down syndrome, though such patients were living longer. Their 65 patients had a mean age of 40 years (range 14–70 years) and either lived in community housing or required institutional care. Hresko et al. reported on hip disease in such patients: 18% of the patients in their sample had hip dysplasia, and 66% of those experienced gross subluxation or dislocation. This progression to more severe disease negatively affected the patients' ability to walk, which in turn affected their ability to remain in their community living facilities. As the patients aged, they became less able to walk as well. Among 13 of their patients who had normal radiographs of the hip, 12 could walk at age 40, but this declined greatly to just six walking at age 60–70, and most of their patients couldn't walk after age 30.

Current Role

Hresko is currently a busy clinician who performs more than 250 major surgical procedures each year. He lives in Chestnut Hill, Massachusetts. For many years he has volunteered as both a baseball coach and a basketball coach in the Brookline Youth Leagues.

LAWRENCE I. KARLIN

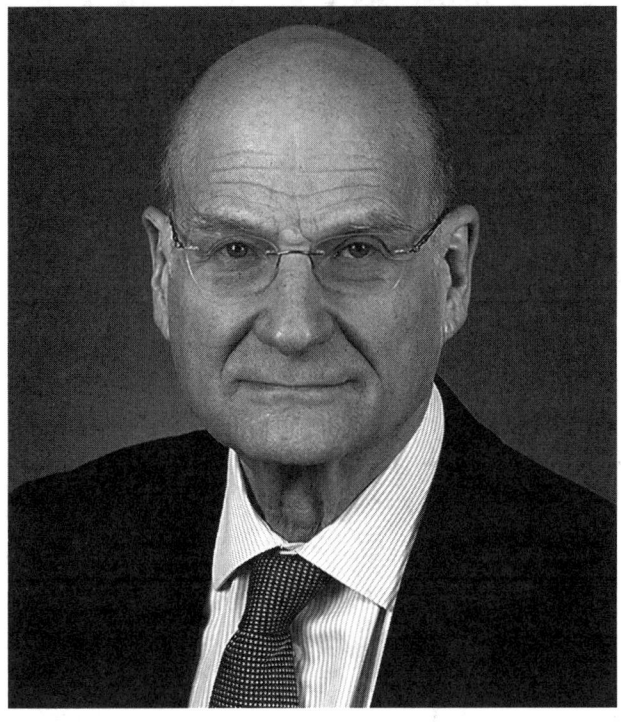

Lawrence I. Karlin. James Koepfler/Boston Children's Hospital.

Physician Snapshot

Lawrence I. Karlin
BORN: 1945
DIED: —
SIGNIFICANT CONTRIBUTIONS: Introduced the Isola spinal instrumentation technique to Children's Hospital

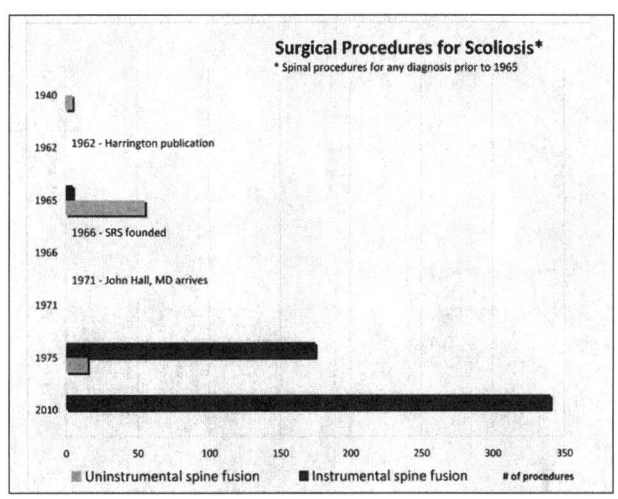

Surgical procedures for scoliosis at BCH, 1940–2010.
Courtesy of Dr. Lawrence Karlin.

Originally from Washington, DC, Lawrence Ira Karlin graduated in 1967 with a bachelor of arts degree from Hamilton College in upstate New York. He received an MD degree from Tufts University School of Medicine in 1971, winning the medical school's Anatomy Award. After two years of surgical training at Case Western Reserve University Hospital followed by two years as a general medical officer in the US Air Force, he completed a three-year orthopaedic residency program in the Tufts University Combined Program in 1979. In 1981, he finished a fellowship in pediatric orthopaedic surgery at Boston Children's Hospital.

After his fellowship, Karlin joined the faculty of Tufts University School of Medicine as an instructor of orthopaedic surgery and became a member of the orthopaedic staff at Kennedy Memorial Hospital/Franciscan Children's Hospital. He was also on staff at the Lemuel Shattuck Hospital and the Newton-Wellesley Hospital. In 1982, he was promoted to assistant professor of orthopaedic surgery at Tufts, and, in 1989, he was named chief of the pediatric orthopaedic division of the orthopaedic department there, a position he held for eight years.

In 1993, during Karlin's time at Tufts, a reporter from the Boston Globe interviewed Karlin after Dr. Arnold Schiller, a surgeon at the New England Baptist Hospital, performed a two-level spinal fusion—a five-hour procedure—on the professional basketball player Larry Bird. Karlin described the procedure, including its differences from Bird's previous surgery. The fusion required a larger incision and caused more bleeding and edema, and some of the effects Bird would experience after the procedure, including up to 20% less flexibility. Karlin noted that had Bird planned to continue playing basketball after the procedure, his abilities may have been substantially affected by this loss.

In 1997, Dr. James Kasser recruited Karlin to Boston Children's Hospital. Karlin went to Children's, along with seven other physicians (five cardiologists and two geneticists) that same year,

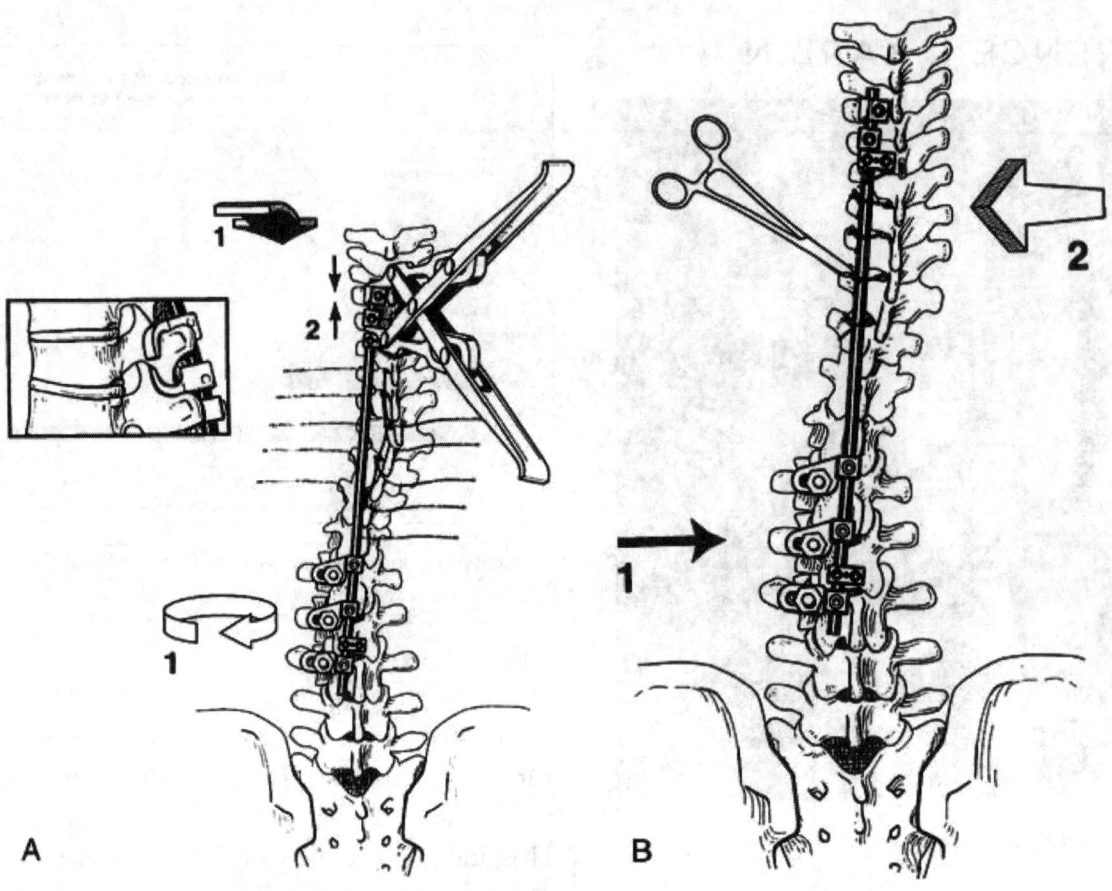

ISOLA Implants. M. A. Asher and D. C. Burton, "A Concept of Idiopathic Scoliosis Deformities as Imperfect Torsion(s)," *Clinical Orthopaedics and Related Research* 1999; 364: 17.

from Floating Hospital, during the turmoil of the nationwide shift to managed care. According to a 1998 *Boston Globe* article, this "exodus" was devastating for Floating Hospital.

Karlin has remained at Children's since his move there from Tufts. He was initially a lecturer in orthopaedic surgery at Harvard Medical School; since 2002 he's been an assistant professor. His clinical activities in pediatric orthopaedics—he mainly focuses on spinal deformities in cerebral palsy and Down syndrome, spina bifida, and congenital abnormalities—engage him full-time. He also attends related clinics at Children's and the National Birth Defects Center.

Karlin is board certified (1973) and an active member of numerous professional organizations:

- American Academy of Orthopaedic Surgeons
- American Academy of Pediatrics (Orthopaedic Section)
- Scoliosis Research Society
- American Orthopaedic Association
- Pediatric Orthopaedic Society of North America
- American Academy for Cerebral Palsy and Development Medicine Massachusetts Orthopaedic Society
- Massachusetts Medical Society

In the Scoliosis Research Society, Karlin has been a member of the Poster Exhibit Committee and the Neuromuscular Scoliosis Outcome Committee, and chairman of both the Patient Based Outcomes Committee (2007–8), and the Growing Spine Committee (2010–11).

He has given numerous lectures and presentations. In 2006, Karlin was named the Arthur A. Thibodeau Lecturer at Tufts University School of Medicine. He has lectured for the Maine Orthopaedic Review Course for more than a decade.

Karlin has published 29 articles and 9 book chapters, the majority of which focus on the spine, scoliosis, and congenital deformities of the spine. He was the lead investigator on a multicenter study of the surgical treatment of Scheuermann kyphosis, and he is active in the Isola Study Group. In fact, he introduced the Isola spinal instrumentation technique to Children's Hospital.

ROBERT B. KELLER

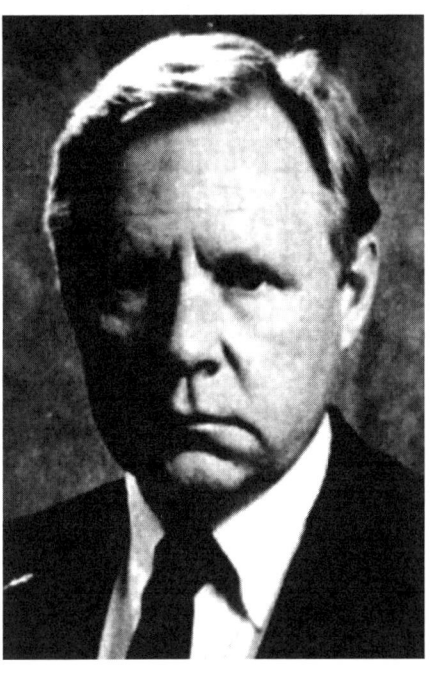

Robert B. Keller. "Belfast orthopedic surgeon named to national physician payment panel," *Bangor Daily News*, March 13, 1990.

Physician Snapshot

Robert B. Keller
BORN: ca. 1937
DIED: —
SIGNIFICANT CONTRIBUTIONS: Led the Maine Medical Assessment Foundation; used variation analysis and long-term outcomes of operative and nonoperative treatments for musculoskeletal disorders in order to establish clinical practice guidelines

Robert B. Keller graduated from Cornell University Medical School in 1961. After two years of training in general surgery at the Dartmouth-Hitchcock Medical Center (1961–63), he entered the Massachusetts General Hospital/Boston Children's Hospital Orthopaedic Residency Program, graduating in 1969. That same year, he was appointed instructor of orthopaedic surgery at Harvard Medical School (a position he held until 1973), and he joined the staff at Children's Hospital (at that time Dr. Arthur Pappas was the interim chief). Residents considered Keller to be a specialist in scoliosis and spine surgery. I remember Keller presenting, during grand rounds, one of the first cases in which Harrington rod fixation was used in a patient with scoliosis. The discussion was lively and almost confrontational.

When Pappas moved to the University of Massachusetts to become chairman of the orthopaedic department, Keller accompanied him. In 1972, Keller was appointed assistant professor at the University of Massachusetts Medical School. In 1975, he was promoted to associate professor (an appointment he held until 1998). Keller entered private practice in 1979 in Belfast, Maine, and was concurrently on the active staff of the Waldo County General Hospital there.

Keller was a principal investigator on a study of low-back pain for the Agency for Healthcare Research and Quality and for the large national Spine Patient Outcomes Research Trial (SPORT), led by Dr. James N. Weinstein at Dartmouth Medical School. From 1991 until 2001 he was an adjunct professor of family and community medicine and surgery at the Dartmouth-Hitchcock Medical Center.

Keller's clinical interest in spine surgery continued, but his career took a different direction, moving toward health care policy, particularly small-area regional variations in care, practice guidelines, outcomes, and costs. Active in the American Academy of Orthopaedic Surgeons as a member of the Council on Health Policy and Practice, Keller was also a member of the Back Problems Guideline Panel, along with Drs. Stanley Bigos, Richard Deyo, Matthew Laing, Malcolm Pope, James Weinstein, and others. In 1994, the group wrote the clinical practice guidelines on acute low-back problems in adults.

Work with the Maine Medical Assessment Foundation

The Maine Medical Assessment Foundation, an organization within the Maine Medical Association, was formed around 1975 under the leadership of Dr. Daniel F. Hanley (executive director of the Maine Medical Association) and his longtime friend, Dr. Jack Wennberg (a health care researcher at Dartmouth), with the goal of encouraging physician interest in and examination of patient outcomes and care differences. Keller became executive director of the foundation in the 1980s and led it for many years.

Under Keller's leadership, the Maine Medical Assessment Foundation formed eight study groups to investigate variations in medical practice. Each group comprised practicing physicians and surgeons who were able to disseminate to practitioners information on area variations of care, specifically epidemiologic data. Practitioners' buy-in has, as a result, changed practice patterns, thereby greatly improving quality of care and reducing health care resource utilization.

In 1990, Keller and his coauthors, Drs. D. Soule, J. Wennberg, and D. Hanley, published the experience of the Maine Medical Assessment Foundation's Orthopaedic Study Group in evaluating variations in rates of hospitalization for five orthopaedic conditions (hip fractures, ankle fractures, forearm fractures, knee derangement, and lumbosacral sprain) and five orthopaedic procedures (total hip replacement, total knee replacement, disc excision, reduction of forearm fracture, and bunion excision). They concluded that:

> the variation in decision-making by orthopaedists was least for fractures of the ankle and fractures of the hip and was greatest for fractures of the forearm, derangement of the knee, and lumbosacral sprain. The rates in an area tended to be consistently high or low for these same treatments. The major reasons for the variations appeared to be related to lack of agreement about optimal treatment. Feedback of data to physicians on variations in patterns of practice reduced the variation. (Keller et al. 1990)

Keller et al. (1990) were optimistic that research on outcomes among both physicians and patients "will help to resolve many of the uncertainties that are part of current orthopaedic practice."

Throughout the 1990s, Keller published numerous articles on the accomplishments of the Maine Medical Assessment Foundation. He documented practitioners' participation in advancing their own knowledge of quality improvement, mainly through self-assessment and education, thereby resulting in altered practice patterns. He organized specialty groups to study health care utilization data and evaluation guidelines and findings in the literature; these groups performed outcomes studies, educated patients, and presented their findings. These study groups expanded into New Hampshire and Vermont and were aimed at creating a practice guideline to standardize care for patients with chest pain and for treating low-back pain, and reducing caesarian section rates.

Keller et al. article on geographic variations in orthopaedic hospital admissions. *Journal of Bone and Joint Surgery* 1990; 72: 1286.

The Maine Lumbar Spine Study

One such study group—the Maine Lumbar Spine Study Group, which comprised both orthopaedic surgeons and neurosurgeons—was of special interest to Keller as a specialist in spine surgery. In 1996—six years before the Spine Patient Outcomes Research Trial was published—the study group published, in three parts, the Maine Lumbar Spine Study in the journal *Spine*. Part 1 described the prospective cohort study design and their innovative method of including enrolled and non-enrolled patients. That article stressed the importance of participation by community-based physicians and patients. Part 2 analyzed the outcomes among 507 patients with sciatica who had been treated nonoperatively (n = 232) or with open discectomy (a few percutaneously [n = 275]). No spine fusions were performed. All patients received follow-up at one year. The group concluded that back and leg pain improved more in patients who underwent a surgical procedure; 71% noted a "definite improvement." The benefits of surgical treatment were similar to those of nontreatment among patients who had only minor symptoms. Whether patients received state workers' compensation had little effect: only 5% of those treated surgically and 7% of those treated nonsurgically were unemployed one year later. Part 3 analyzed the outcomes of 148 patients with lumbar spinal stenosis who had been treated either nonoperatively (n = 67) or with a laminectomy, with occasional fusion without instrumentation (n = 81); those in the latter group showed more severe stenosis on radiographs and had more severe symptoms and a worse functional status. At the one-year follow-up, almost twice as many patients who underwent surgery noted a "definite improvement."

Dr. Alf Nachemson wrote a "Point of View" for *Spine* about these three articles, in which he enumerated three main concerns: (1) the use of a prospective cohort design, rather than a randomized controlled trial; (2) the relatively small study populations; and (3) the fairly short follow-up duration (only one year). Keller and his coauthors responded, addressing all three issues. First, they disagreed that a randomized controlled trial was necessary because their focus was the effectiveness of the surgical procedures within community settings, which cannot be controlled like the settings in randomized controlled trials. They agreed with his second concern regarding the low enrollment, and described how they randomly asked patients who were not enrolled in the study but who were undergoing a surgical procedure during the study's enrollment period to take the survey in order to obtain additional data. Regarding the third concern about the short follow-up (one year), the study group mentioned that they were continuing to follow their patients but believed other physicians would be intrigued by the one-year results, which would, they hoped, point those physicians toward an appreciation for and perhaps participation in effectiveness research at the community level.

Overall, Keller aimed to educate clinicians about future trends in health care, particular those that would allow the public to recognize the quality of care a physician provides. This was tied into what became known as "physician profiling" by health insurance companies. Keller wanted

---

The Maine Lumbar Spine Study, Part I. Background and concepts
R B Keller [1], S J Atlas, D E Singer, A M Chapin, N A Mooney, D L Patrick, R A Deyo

The Maine Lumbar Spine Study, Part II. 1-year outcomes of surgical and nonsurgical management of sciatica
S J Atlas [1], R A Deyo, R B Keller, A M Chapin, D L Patrick, J M Long, D E Singer

The Maine Lumbar Spine Study, Part III. 1-year outcomes of surgical and nonsurgical management of lumbar spinal stenosis
S J Atlas [1], R A Deyo, R B Keller, A M Chapin, D L Patrick, J M Long, D E Singer

Keller et al. articles (n=3) reporting outcomes of surgical and nonsurgical treatment of patients with sciatica and spinal stenosis at one year after treatment. *Spine* 1996; 21: 1769-1787.

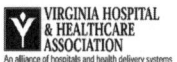

Title page of *The Dartmouth Atlas of Health Care in Virginia*.
AHA Press/The Trustees of Dartmouth College, 2000.

physicians to identify and report their own outcomes in order to help them succeed in what he called the "age of accountability."

The lead authors, who were at the General Medicine and Clinical Epidemiology units at the Massachusetts General Hospital, the Center for the Evaluative Clinical Sciences at Dartmouth, and the Center for Cost and Outcomes Research at the University of Washington, followed the patients in the sciatica and lumbar spinal stenosis studies (described in parts 2 and 3) for another 8–10 years. They published those long-term outcomes in 2005, three years after the Maine Medical Assessment Foundation closed.

On the basis of their 10-year follow-up on the treatment of sciatica, in which they evaluated 84% of the original cohort, they concluded that surgery relieved leg pain more extensively and better improved patients' function, and it increased the patients' satisfaction with the general outcome. They did note, however, outcomes regarding symptoms, physical disability, and ability to work were similar between those who underwent surgery and those who did not. During that 10-year period, 25% of surgically treated patients had at least one additional spine operation, and 25% of the patients who were initially treated nonoperatively had a spine operation. Nevertheless, the authors recognized the difficulties inherent in evaluating end results among patients with a lumbar disc herniation who receive different treatments.

The group advocated for shared decision making between patients and their surgeons when determining which treatment is most appropriate. Among patients who had been treated for lumbar spinal stenosis, 23% of the surgically treated group had another spine operation and 39% in the nonsurgical group had undergone surgery during that same 10-year period. The long-term follow-up of these patients (79% of the original study population) indicated both similarities and differences between those who were initially treated surgically or nonsurgically: low-back pain was alleviated and symptoms improved to a similar extent in both groups, and the patients' satisfaction with their current function was comparable. Those patients who had undergone surgery at the start of the study, however, reported less leg pain and better back function.

Participation in Other Study Groups/Research

With early successful research in small-area regional variations of care, Jack Wennberg produced the famous "Dartmouth Atlas of Health Care" in 1996. The science of small-area variations of care was also part of the 1993 Health Security Act ("Hillarycare"). In 1994, Wennberg and Keller wrote a commentary on regional professional foundations, as laid out in section 5008 of then-president Bill Clinton's Health Security Act. They noted that these regional professional foundations, comprising groups of physicians, medical educational institutions, and professional associations, were meant to create projects with four main goals: "to improve the quality and appropriateness of medical care; to participate in outcomes research; and to develop innovative ways to increase patients' participation in their choices of medical care...[and] to ensure the timely dissemination of information about quality improvement programs, practice guidelines, research findings, and ways of using health professionals most effectively." Despite the positive aims of this act, it was controversial from the beginning, and the nation was in turmoil over the president's planned reforms. By 1994 the Health Security Act was dead.

In 2000, Keller assisted in the publication of the Dartmouth Atlas of Health Care in Virginia Working Group, a cooperative effort of the Center for the Evaluative Clinical Sciences at Dartmouth and the Maine Medical Assessment Foundation.

Other Orthopaedic Interests

Carpal Tunnel Syndrome

Through outcome studies and small-area variation analyses, Keller has also focused on carpal tunnel syndrome. He was the lead author on a study of small-area variations that found that rates of carpal tunnel release were divergent (up to 3.5-fold) among various service areas. The mean release rate in Maine was 1.44 per 1,000; rates were higher than this mean in four areas and lower in two areas. The study concluded that variations in practice patterns among physicians—particularly decision-making methods and "beliefs and practice styles" (Keller 1998)—are the main reason for these differences.

In 1998, Keller, Drs. Jeffrey Katz and Barry Simmons from Brigham and Women's Hospital, and other coauthors described a prospective, observational, community-based study of 2.5-year outcomes of carpal tunnel syndrome treated surgically or nonsurgically. Among 429 patients, 270 received surgical treatment, 125 received medical treatment, and 34 who were initially in the nonsurgical group crossed into the surgical group. Patients who were treated surgically showed improved outcomes, whereas those who did not showed no or minimal improvements. Among those who did undergo surgery, the outcomes of open and endoscopic procedures did not differ. Patients receiving Workers' Compensation had worse outcomes than those who did not receive such financial benefits. These findings led them to determine that carpal tunnel release is effective when performed in community settings.

> **Maine Carpal Tunnel Study: Small Area Variations**
>
> Robert B. Keller, MD,
> Anne Marie Largay, MPH, David N. Soule, BA,† Manchester, ME,
> Jeffrey N. Katz, MD, Boston, MA
>
> The Journal of Hand Surgery / Vol. 23A No. 4 July 1998

Keller et al. article on communities' outcomes after surgical and nonsurgical treatment of carpal tunnel syndrome.
Journal of Hand Surgery 1998; 23: P692.

Health Care Issues in the US

In 1996, Keller gave the Kennedy Lecture at the interim meeting of the American Orthopaedic Society of Sports Medicine. His lecture was titled "Unstable Knees in Unstable Times." He focused on four main issues confronting health care in the United States at the time: (1) the changing face of medical practice, (2) physician profiling, (3) outcomes research, and (4) the physician workforce. He concluded that these four issues can have extensive negative effects on medical practice and orthopaedics, mainly because of health systems' focus on profit rather than quality and on pushing patients toward "in-network" physicians, as well as faulty and flawed research and too many physicians.

Title of Keller's 1996 Kennedy Lecture at the meeting of the American Orthopaedic Society of Sports Medicine. *American Journal of Sports Medicine* 1996; 24: 570.

To counter these issues, he recommended deliberate evaluation of *how* physicians practice, initiate collaborative outcomes research, and acknowledge the various dilemmas and concerns confronting physicians in various (sub)specialties.

Keller has been a member of the orthopaedic group of the medical review board of Healthwise. Healthwise is a nonprofit organization that provides "evidence-based, easy-to-understand health information[;] innovative technology solutions...[;] and expert guidance on...behavior change and shared decision making" to "the top health plans, health systems and hospitals, care management companies, and consumer health portals" in order to "help people make better health decisions and manage their health" (Healthwise 2020).

He has also been a member of the Performance Advisory Committee of the American Medical Association, and of the Maine Health Policy Advisory Council. In 1989, he served as president of the Maine Medical Association. In 1990, he was appointed to the 12-member National Physician Payment Review Commission (replacing Gail R. Wilensky, who became administrator of the Health Care Financing Administration in the US Department of Health and Human Services). In 1990, he also was on the board of directors of the Maine Medical Mutual Insurance Company. He has participated in workshops of the Office of Technology Assessment of the Congress of the United States and has been an active participant in the federally funded Patient Outcome Research Team program, which is funded by the Agency for Healthcare Research and Quality.

Around 2003, Keller left his private practice in Belfast and joined the Maine Medical Practice of Neurosurgery and Spine in Scarborough, Maine. In 2013, he chaired the Advisory Council of the Dirigo Health Agency's Maine Quality Forum, and he remains active in health care improvement changes in Maine.

MININDER S. KOCHER

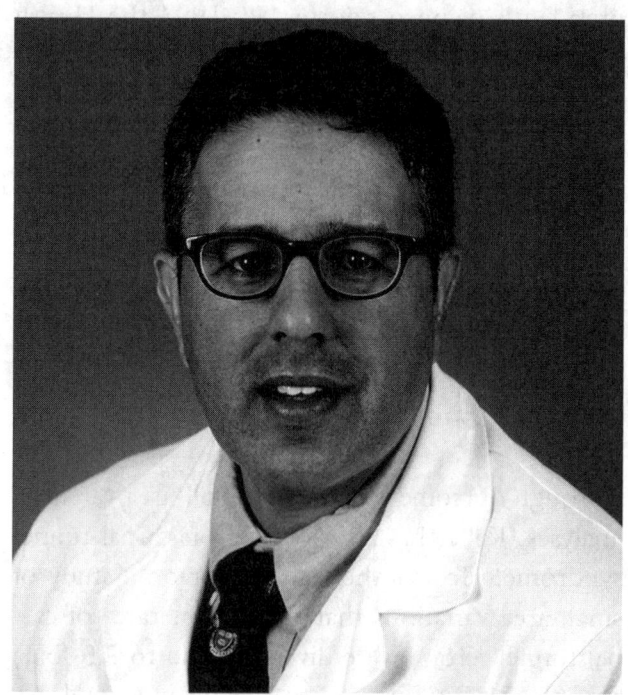

Mininder (Min) S. Kocher. James Koepfler/Boston Children's Hospital.

Physician Snapshot

Mininder S. Kocher
BORN: 1966
DIED: —

SIGNIFICANT CONTRIBUTIONS: Leader in outcomes research in pediatric orthopaedic conditions, especially sports injuries, using epidemiological tools

Mininder "Min" Singh Kocher grew up in Rochester, New York. In 1989, he graduated from

Dartmouth College with a bachelor of arts degree in biology and psychology. As an undergraduate, he was very bright and successful, receiving, among other major four-year scholarships, the National Merit Scholarship. He was a Rufus Choate Scholar, graduated magna cum laude, and was elected into Phi Beta Kappa. At Dartmouth, he was a member of the Nathan Smith Society.

Kocher then entered Duke University School of Medicine. While at Duke, he demonstrated an early interest in orthopaedics and sports medicine, receiving the Glaxo Medical Student Research Award for his research entitled "Proprioception Following Anterior Cruciate Ligament Reconstruction." He also received the Wilburt C. Davison Award for Clinical Excellence.

From 1993 to 1994, Kocher was a surgical intern at the Beth Israel Hospital in Boston. In 1994 he received the 25th annual Harris S. Yett Award for clinical excellence in orthopaedics. For the next four years, he was a resident in the Harvard Combined Orthopaedic Residency Program, graduating in 1998. His continued drive to contribute to and excel in his chosen profession is evidenced in the host of additional awards he received while a resident and fellow (**Box 27.2**).

Kocher was a chief resident at Boston Children's Hospital; followed by a one-year fellowship in pediatric orthopaedics there. In 2000, he completed another one-year fellowship in sports medicine and arthroscopy at the Steadman Hawkins Clinic in Vail, Colorado. Six months preceding his sports medicine fellowship, Kocher began a master's program in public health, majoring in clinical epidemiology at the Harvard School of Public Health. He achieved his master's degree in 2001. At that time, he received a Health Services Research Fellowship from the American Academy of Orthopaedic Surgeons.

Ready to begin his practice, Kocher joined the faculty at Children's Hospital and the Brigham and Women's Hospital in 2000, where he remains today. He is also on staff at the New England Baptist Hospital (since 2002) and the Beth Israel Deaconess Medical Center (since 2004). At Harvard Medical School, he has held appointments as an instructor (2000–2003), assistant professor (2003–2006), and associate professor of orthopaedic surgery (2006–2012). He has been a professor of orthopaedic surgery since 2012.

Kocher is a thesis advisor for graduate students in the Harvard School of Public Health and is an active participant in medical student and orthopaedic resident education.

Box 27.2. Awards Granted to Kocher During His Residency/Fellowship

- Smith and Nephew Resident Research Award (1997)
- Arthroscopy Association of North America Resident Award (1997)
- Von L. Meyer Award for house staff at Children's Hospital (1998)
- Best Paper Award of the American Orthopaedic Association's 32nd annual Residents' Conference (1999)
- Richard Kilfoyle Award for Research of the New England Orthopaedic Society (1999)
- Resident/Fellow Clinical Research Essay Award of the Arthroscopy Association of North America (2000)
- Vernon Thompson Research Award of the Western Orthopaedic Association (2000)
- Resident/Fellow Clinical Research Award of the Eastern Orthopaedic Association (2000)
- Resident/Fellow Clinical Research Award of the Arthroscopy Association of North America (2001)

Focus on Research

Kocher has received grants for his clinical research from the Orthopaedic Research and Education Foundation, American Orthopaedic Society for Sports Medicine, Boston Children's Hospital, and others. He has published

> **Evidence-based Pediatric Orthopaedics: An Introduction, Part 1**
> *James G. Wright, MD, MPH, FRCSC,* Mininder S. Kocher, MD, MPH,† and James O. Sanders, MD‡*
>
> **Evidence-based Pediatric Orthopaedics: An Introduction, Part 2**
> *James G. Wright, MD, MPH, FRCSC,* Mininder S. Kocher, MD, MPH,† and James O. Sanders, MD‡*
>
> *J Pediatr Orthop* • Volume 32, Number 2 Supplement, September 2012

Title of articles on evidence-based pediatric orthopaedics by Wright, Kocher, and Sanders. *Journal of Pediatric Orthopedics* 2012; 32: S83-S91.

165 peer-reviewed scientific articles, four books, and 70 book chapters. The main themes of his research focus on sports medicine in children, e.g., anterior cruciate ligament (ACL) injuries and knee and shoulder problems; trauma in children; pediatric orthopaedics; and various other issues such as ethics, statistics, publication bias, evidence-based guidelines, conflicts of interest, and ghost surgery.

In 2012, he cowrote two papers with Drs. James Wright and James Sanders on "Evidence-based Pediatric Orthopaedics." They acknowledged that evidence-based medicine (EBM) was at the time a recent notion and a matter of contention, and so they provided advice on how clinicians could apply an evidence-based approach to their practice. In their second paper, they highlighted the importance of physicians being educated about factors that can affect study results, including study design, confounding, and bias, and they reiterated that EBM focuses not just on results but also on the quality of a study.

As a fellow in sports medicine at the Steadman Hawkins Clinic, Kocher began a prospective study of 201 patients undergoing ACL reconstruction. He followed the cohort for a minimum of two years, with the goal of determining patients' satisfaction with their outcomes. He and his coauthors concluded that:

> The most robust relationships of patient satisfaction with the outcomes...were subjective measures of symptoms and function. Pain, swelling, giving-way, locking noise, stiffness [especially lack of extension], and limp had highly significant associations with dissatisfaction. Similarly, walking, squatting, ascending or descending stairs, running, cutting, jumping, twisting, activities of daily living, sports activity, work activity and activity without symptoms had highly significant associations with satisfaction...Although patient satisfaction is an important outcome measure in its own right...a comprehensive assessment of outcomes after a treatment intervention would include a generic measure of health-related quality of life, a condition-specific measure of knee function and a measure of patient satisfaction. (Kocher et al. 2002)

Kocher, with Drs. Sumeet Garg and Lyle Micheli, wrote several papers on ACL reconstruction and preservation of bone growth in patients with immature skeletons. In 2005, they reported on 44 skeletally immature patients who underwent intra-articular and extra-articular reconstruction of the ACL with an autogenous iliotibial band graft between 1980 and 2002; the mean follow-up was 5.3 years. They concluded that "this technique provided excellent functional outcome with a low revision rate and no growth disturbance...Although nonanatomic, it provided for a stable knee with excellent function in children who returned to sports that involved cutting and pivoting...[and] this technique has functioned as the definitive reconstruction for most of our patients" (Kocher, Garg, and Micheli 2005). Two years later, Kocher, Micheli, and others reported on another series of 59 patients (61 knees)—these were older (mean chronological age 14.7 years) than the cohort described in their

2005 publication (10.3 years)—in whom they reconstructed the ACL with a transphyseal graft of autogenous quadrupled hamstring tendons with metaphyseal fixation. They reported "a low revision rate (3%), with excellent functional outcomes, few complications, and no cases of growth disturbance" (Kocher et al. 2007). Using the Tanner system for determining biologic age, they "advocate[d] a treatment algorithm for skeletally immature patients with ACL insufficiency based on the amount of growth remaining…according to three categories: prepubescent children with substantial growth remaining, prepubescent adolescents with a variable amount of growth remaining[, and] older adolescents approaching skeletal maturity with minimal growth remaining" (Kocher et al. 2007). It is important to note that in the children with extensive growth remaining, they used physeal-sparing intra-articular and extra-articular reconstruction with an autogenous iliotibial band graft, whereas in the adolescents with variable growth remaining they used transphyseal reconstruction with an autogenous quadrupled hamstring tendon graft with metaphyseal fixation.

In 2011, Kocher, Dr. Won Joon Yoo, and Micheli, reported their long-term follow-up (up to three years) of growth plate disturbances after transphyseal reconstruction. They evaluated the disturbances in 43 adolescents using magnetic resonance imaging, which showed a focal physeal disruption in 5 patients (11.6%), but no associated altered growth. In light of this, they concluded that transphyseal ACL reconstruction might not be appropriate for use in young children that have years of growing ahead of them.

In 2007, closed reduction and percutaneous pin fixation composed the accepted method for treating displaced supracondylar humerus fractures, although no consensus existed regarding the most appropriate pin placement. Kocher, with other faculty at Children's Hospital, led a prospective randomized clinical trial of pin placement in displaced supracondylar humerus fractures. Fifty-two patients completed the study. Kocher et al. (2007) concluded that two pin-fixation methods—lateral entry and medial and lateral entry—"appear to be effective…For medial and lateral entry pin fixations, the lateral pin was placed first, the elbow was extended to a position of < 90°, and a small incision was made over the medial epicondyle to protect the ulnar nerve…For effective lateral entry pin fixation, the pins must be placed in both the lateral and the central column of the distal part of the humerus."

Five years later, the group assessed their practice patterns to determine whether they had changed from using medial and lateral entry pins to only lateral entry pins. They reviewed the cases of 141 patients treated before the trial and 126 patients treated after the trial, and indeed noted a statistical difference in the type of pins used. Eight surgeons used more lateral entry pins for patients treated after the trial; for five of those surgeons, this pointed to a statistically significant change. Importantly, these changes did not affect patient outcomes.

Kocher, with Drs. James Pace and David Skaggs, published a review of evidence-based practices applied in managing open pediatric fractures. They touched on antibiotic use (choice and duration of treatment), nonoperative treatments, operative treatments (timing of surgery, wound irrigation, and wound management), and wound cultures. The evidence they evaluated indicated for them that no standardized treatment process—nor much level 1 evidence—exists for treating such fractures. They concluded that all the topics they described in their article could benefit from additional research, including on patient outcomes, although much of this work would have to be done through prospective cohort studies.

Outcomes Research

Outcomes research has been an important topic of interest of Kocher. He has published papers on the outcomes of patients with juvenile osteochondritis dissecans treated with transarticular arthroscopic drilling and patient satisfaction after rotator cuff surgery, and he has critically evaluated the reliability, validity, and responsiveness of the Subjective Shoulder Scale, from the American Shoulder and Elbow Surgeons (ASES). He and his coauthors "found that the ASES subjective shoulder scale demonstrated acceptable psychometric performance for patients with shoulder instability, rotator cuff disease, and glenohumeral arthritis...but may not be the optimal outcome measure. Reliability was acceptable, but may not be precise enough... on an individual basis" (Kocher et al. 2005).

He also published outcomes after the treatment of slipped capital femoral epiphysis and addressed the controversial decision of prophylactically pinning the opposite hip, in light of potential adverse events such as chondrolysis and osteonecrosis. He and his coauthors at Children's Hospital recommended "pinning of the contralateral hip...when the probability of contralateral slip exceeds 27% or when reliable follow-up is not feasible" (Kocher et al. 2004). They noted, "For a given patient, the optimal strategy depends not only on the probabilities of the various outcomes, but also on personal preference" and thus they "advocate[d] a model of shared decision-making...considering both outcome probabilities and patient preferences" (Kocher et al. 2004).

Other Research Interests

Another main pediatric interest of Kocher's has been the long-standing clinical problems related to diagnosis and early management of transient synovitis of the hip versus the more emergent issue, septic arthritis of the hip. Since 1999, he has published at least four articles on the topic. One such study, published in 2015, noted that, in their research published in 1999, Drs. Kocher, Zurakowski, and Kasser had:

> demonstrated that the greater the number of four different risk factors present—specifically fever, refusal or inability to bear weight, elevated ESR [40 mm/hr], and elevated serum WBC count [>12,000 cells/mm^3]—the more likely the patient was to be ultimately diagnosed with SAH [septic arthritis of the hip] instead of TSH [transient synovitis of the hip]. Therefore they proposed an algorithmic approach to the workup of such patients, recommending that those with no or one risk factor be observed without aspiration, those with two risk factors undergo hip aspiration with ultrasound guidance, and those with three or four risk factors undergo hip aspiration in the operating room...the algorithm remains a valuable and widely utilized tool. (Heyworth et al. 2015)

Kocher has participated in the Multicenter Arthroscopy of the Hip Outcomes Research Network (MAHORN), which developed a self-administered quality-of-life outcome measurement tool, including a shorter version (the 12-item International Hip Outcome Tool) validated for routine use in clinical practice. He has helped evaluate the reliability and validity of the Lysholm Knee Scoring Scale and the Tegner Activity Scale in patients with meniscal injuries and in patients with ACL injuries. He and his colleagues modified

ETHICS IN PRACTICE

GHOST SURGERY: THE ETHICAL AND LEGAL IMPLICATIONS OF WHO DOES THE OPERATION

BY MININDER S. KOCHER, MD, MPH
THE JOURNAL OF BONE & JOINT SURGERY · JBJS.ORG
VOLUME 84-A · NUMBER 1 · JANUARY 2002

Title of Kocher's article about the ethical and legal issues associated with ghost surgery. *Journal of Bone and Joint Surgery* 2002; 84: 148.

the International Knee Documentation Committee (IKDC) Subjective Knee Form for children, which research has proven to be a reliable and valid instrument for accessing the outcomes of knee disorders in children between the ages of 10 and 18 years. He published a similar study evaluating the Simple Shoulder Test.

Regarding ethical issues, Kocher published a timely paper on ghost surgery, discussing the legal issues and ethical implications of three cases when a surgeon's partner performed a reoperation on the surgeon's patient, and he described two cases involving residents performing an operation while supervised by an attending surgeon; in these instances the patient was either not informed of the switch or was told only immediately before the procedure. Kocher (2002) wrote:

> The substitution of an authorized surgeon by an unauthorized surgeon or the allowance of unauthorized surgical trainees to operate without adequate supervision constitutes "ghost surgery." These practices are legally and ethically iniquitous. Ghost surgery flies in the face of case law and violates an individual's right to control his or her own body and violates that person's right to information needed to make an informed decision. Such practices breach the fiduciary doctor-patient relationship and may, therefore, be a cause of action against the unauthorized surgeon for battery and against the authorized surgeon for malpractice or fraud. Assistance by a surgical trainee with adequate supervision does not constitute "ghost surgery" when there has been adequate disclosure and truly informed consent. Adequate supervision entails active participation by the attending surgeon during the essential parts of an operation.

He has also written about publication bias in orthopaedic research and the association of higher publication rates with financial conflict of interest and level of evidence.

Honors and Awards

Kocher is a member of many professional organizations and has given many lectures, some of which are listed in **Box 27.3**.

Kocher has continued to win awards as his career has progressed. In 2004, he received the second annual Angela M. Kuo Award of the Pediatric Orthopaedic Society of North America, given for excellence and promise in research. In 2005, he and his colleagues David Zurakowski and James Kasser received the OREF Clinical Research Award of the American Academy of Orthopaedic Surgeons for their research project titled "Septic Arthritis of the Hip in Children: An Evidenced-based Approach to Improving Clinical Effectiveness." In 2011, he received the Oded Bar-Or Award, from the Council on Sports Medicine and Fitness, for his paper "Treatment of Posterior Cruciate Ligament Injuries in Pediatric and Adolescent Patients." That award is named for Dr. Oded Bar-Or, a pioneer in the field of exercise physiology in children and a member of the faculty of McMaster University in Hamilton, Ontario, Canada.

ETHICS IN PRACTICE

The Legal and Ethical Issues Surrounding Financial Conflict of Interest in Orthopaedic Research

By Kanu Okike, BA, and Mininder S. Kocher, MD, MPH
THE JOURNAL OF BONE & JOINT SURGERY · JBJS.ORG
VOLUME 89-A · NUMBER 4 · APRIL 2007

Title of Okike and Kocher's article about the ethical and legal issues surrounding conflicts of interest in orthopaedic research. *Journal of Bone and Joint Surgery* 2007; 89: 910.

Box 27.3. Kocher's Professional Memberships, Team Physician Positions, and Invited Lectures

Organizational Memberships
- American Academy of Orthopaedic Surgeons (has been a member of the board of directors)
- ACL Study Group
- Academic Children's Orthopaedic Resource Network
- American Association of the History of Medicine
- American College of Sports Medicine
- American Orthopaedic Association
- American Orthopaedic Society for Sports Medicine (has been a member of the board of directors)
- American Medical Association
- Hawkins Shoulder Society
- Herodicus Society
- International Orthopaedic Think Tank
- International Society for Hip Arthroscopy
- Massachusetts Orthopaedic Association
- Pediatric Orthopaedic Society of North America (has been a member of the board of directors)
- Steadman Hawkins Sports Medicine Foundation

Team Physician Positions
- Head team physician for Babson College, Boston Public Schools, Dover-Sherborn Regional High School, Lasell College, and Noble and Greenough School
- Assistant physician to the Boston Ballet
- Finish-line physician for the Boston Marathon
- Orthopaedic consultant for Northeastern University
- Team physician for Roxbury Latin School
- Physician for USA Track and Field and the US Figure Skating Association
- Assistant team physician for the US Men's and the US Women's Alpine Ski Team and the US Disabled Ski Team

Lectures
- Thomas B. Dameron Lecture at Wake Forest School of Medicine
- Michael Demerich Memorial Lecture at Albany Medical College
- Joseph C. Wilson Visiting Professor at Los Angeles Children's Hospital
- Robert Johnson Visiting Lecture at the University of Vermont
- David Trevor Visiting Professor at Children's Hospital of Philadelphia
- Kern Visiting Professor at the University of Washington
- 25th Eugene Regola Visiting Professor at Montreal Children's Hospital

LYLE J. MICHELI

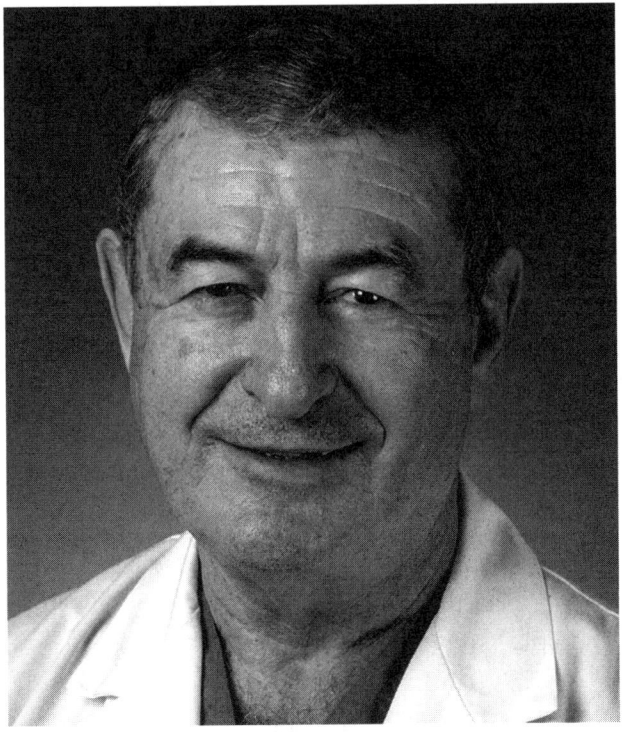

Lyle J. Micheli. James Koepfler/Boston Children's Hospital.

Physician Snapshot

Lyle J. Micheli
BORN: 1940
DIED: —
SIGNIFICANT CONTRIBUTIONS: Established the sports medicine division and sports medicine fellowship at Children's Hospital; instrumental in bringing to the attention of the public the importance of preventing and appropriately treating sports injuries in young athletes

Lyle Joseph Micheli was born in LaSalle, Illinois, on August 19, 1940, to Prodie and Margaret Garcia Micheli. In high school and as an undergraduate at Harvard College, Lyle participated in various sports, including rugby, football, and boxing. He was a Harvard National Scholar during 1959–61, and he received his bachelor of arts degree cum laude in general studies from Harvard College in 1962. Remaining at Harvard, he went on to earn an MD degree from the medical school in 1966. He completed his surgical internship in 1967 and then a year of surgical residency in 1968 at the University Hospital of Cleveland. Returning to Boston in 1968, he entered the Massachusetts General Hospital/Boston Children's Hospital Orthopaedic Surgery Residency Program, which he finished in 1972.

From 1972 through 1974, Micheli served the obligatory two years as a major in the US Air Force (USAF). He was stationed at the Malcolm Grow USAF Medical Center (named after the first surgeon general of the USAF) on Joint Base Andrews near Washington, DC. In 1973, while still in the Air Force, Micheli received a Berg-Sloat Traveling Fellowship in pediatric orthopaedic surgery from the Orthopaedic Research Society. That same year he received his certification from the American Board of Orthopaedic Surgery and held the position of assistant clinical professor of orthopaedic surgery at George Washington University School of Medicine.

When Micheli's military obligation was complete, he returned to Boston as a junior associate in orthopaedic surgery at Children's Hospital and an assistant clinical professor of orthopaedic surgery at Harvard Medical School. Throughout his training and military service, and even while practicing at Children's Hospital, Micheli continued to play rugby for various clubs, including the Boston Rugby Football Club, the Cleveland Blues, and the Washington Rugby Club. He even coached members of the Mystic Rugby Club. In 1984,

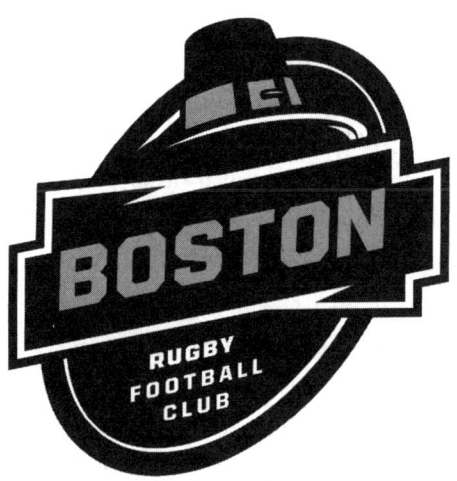

Logo of the Boston Rugby Football Club. Courtesy of Boston Rugby Football Club.

he became a member of the US Rugby Football Foundation's board of directors and chaired the USA Rugby Football Union's Medical and Risk Management Committee.

Focus on Sports Medicine

In 1974, his first year on the staff at Children's Hospital, Micheli, with the help of Dr. Art Boland and the support of Dr. John Hall, then chief of orthopaedics, established a division of sports medicine, which included a clinic treating sports injuries in young people—the first of its kind. In 1975, the hospital began offering a fellowship in sports medicine. Micheli acted as the director of both the division and the fellowship. "[He] was also one of the first, if not the first, doctor to sound the alarm bells about overuse injuries in youth sports. He has seen first hand how year-round sports and early specialization have taken their toll on the bodies of our kids, and has worked tirelessly over the years to make youth sports safer" (MomsTeam Institute of Youth Sports Safety 2018).

I interviewed Micheli in 2011. He observed that in the mid-1970s, "every orthopaedic surgeon thought they could do everything"—an admittedly controversial opinion. With regard to the sports medicine program, Micheli recalled that "Dr. [Arthur] Pappas said, 'a sports clinic won't work'; Dr. J. Drennan Lowell spoke against it at grand rounds and Dr. [Henry] Mankin [apparently] said, 'the *American Journal of Sports Medicine* is an orthopaedic comic book'" (Micheli, interview with the author 2011). Despite this, Micheli was not deterred from his vision of sports medicine as a discipline, particularly with regard to preventing injuries. "In the first year, only 80 patients were seen; but now [2011] over 700 patients are seen each week" (Micheli, interview with the author 2011). Micheli initially treated both adults and children, but later he focused mainly on pediatric patients.

As the 1970s continued, Micheli became an associate orthopaedic surgeon at the Massachusetts Hospital School in Canton, an associate orthopaedic surgeon at Beth Israel Hospital (now Beth Israel Deaconess Medical Center) and the Brigham and Women's Hospital, an orthopaedic staff surgeon at the New England Baptist and Brookline Hospitals, a member of the courtesy staff at Milton Hospital, a consultant at Braintree Hospital, and an active staff member at the New England Deaconess Hospital (now Beth Israel Deaconess Medical Center). Micheli was promoted to associate in orthopaedic surgery at Children's Hospital in 1976.

In 1977, Micheli became the attending physician for the Boston Ballet—a position he still holds today, more than 40 years later—and a medical consultant to the Boston Ballet School. He became a member of the Boston Ballet's board of trustees in 1985, and, in 1994, he received the Medal of Honor from the Boston Ballet. He is also a member of the Rudolph Nureyev Foundation Medical Board.

In 1990, Micheli was promoted to associate clinical professor of orthopaedic surgery at Harvard Medical School. In 2005, he received the title of Joseph O'Donnell Family Professor of Orthopaedic Sports Medicine at Children's Hospital.

In addition to carrying a large clinical load, participating in many organizations, and giving frequent lectures, Micheli has made numerous guest appearances in national and local media, including a *Good Morning America* episode and an NBC television special about sports medicine, as well as in articles in both *People* magazine and *USA Today*. The 1980 *People* magazine article quoted Micheli regarding the potential dangers of extensive focus on youth training and sports: "I don't know of a culture…that systemically organizes children's sports

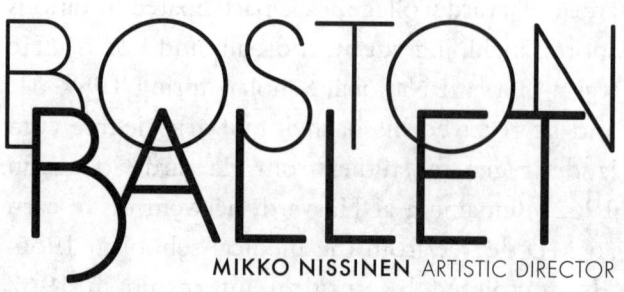

Logo of the Boston Ballet. Courtesy of Boston Ballet.

to the degree we do…An increasing portion of this trauma is caused by organized competitive sports for children…[and] organized team sports[,] in the past dominated by young adult males, are being played increasingly by boys and girls under 12."

Extensive Publications

Micheli has to his name more than 200 peer-reviewed publications and numerous book chapters and commentaries. He has cowritten four books, including *The Sports Medicine Bible* in 1995 (a Book-of-the-Month-Club selection) and *The Sports Medicine Bible for Young Athletes* in 2001, and has co-edited 11. About half of his books are aimed at physicians and sports specialists; the other half are written for the general public, parents, coaches, trainers, and athletes. Dr. T. Berry Brazelton, a noted pediatrician, author, and founder of the Child Development Unit at Children's Hospital, wrote the foreword for Micheli's *The Sports Medicine Bible for Young Athletes*. In it, he noted that the book was for all those who have any "interest in children's sports."

In 1974, the year he started his practice at Children's Hospital, Micheli published two papers that focused on his early interests: "The Management of Spine Deformities in the Myelomeningocele Patient," written with John Hall, and "The Incidence of Injuries in Rugby Football," written with Dr. Edward Riseborough (also an active rugby player; his career is described later in this chapter). Into the mid-1980s, he continued to publish articles about spine problems in children—~35 of them—related to conditions, e.g.; Down syndrome, Larsen syndrome, diastematomyelia, cerebral palsy, and torsional dystoni; equipment (the Boston brace); and procedures (anterior and posterior fusion in Scheuermann kyphosis), in addition to trauma and, occasionally, sports issues (see **Case 27.2**).

As the 1980s continued, he began writing about spine problems in athletes. His first such paper, titled "Back Injuries in Dancers," was published in 1983. Throughout the next 30 years, Micheli's publications focused primarily on sports issues and injuries in children and adolescents. They covered the full gamut of topics related to sports medicine in young athletes; a few examples are overuse injuries, acute knee injuries in immature athletes, injuries to the spine and feet in dancers, use of anabolic steroids, compartment syndrome, anterior cruciate ligament reconstruction, strength training, autologous chondrocyte implantation, concussion injuries, and strengthening and injury prevention programs.

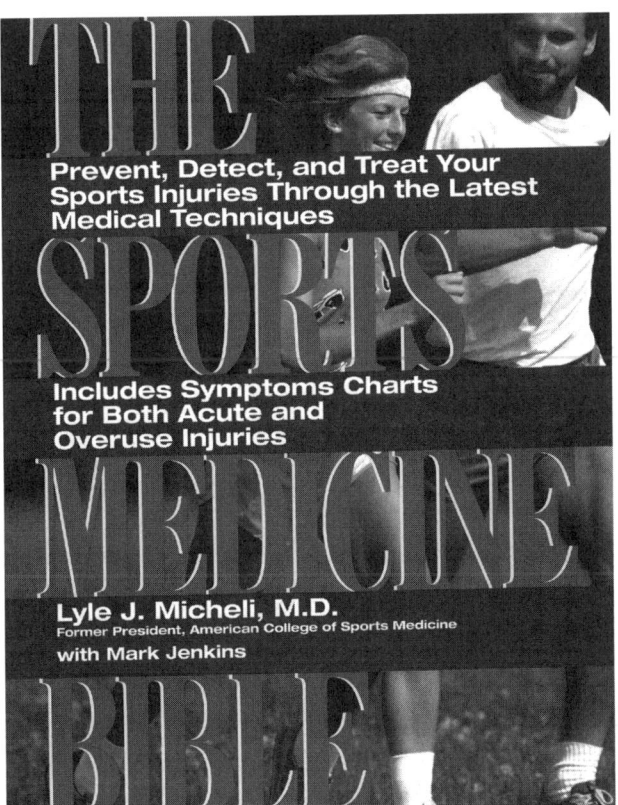

Cover of Micheli's book, *The Sports Medicine Bible*.
The Sports Medicine Bible by Lyle J. Micheli. Copyright © 1995 by Lyle J. Micheli and John Boswell Management, Inc. Used by permission of HarperCollins Publishers.

Micheli et al. article describing his technique for ACL reconstruction in the immature athlete. *Clinical Orthopaedics and Related Research* 1999; 364:40

Case 27.2. Avulsion of the Posterior Cruciate Ligament in an Eleven-Year-Old Boy

"K.S., an eleven-year-old black boy, sustained a hyperextension injury to the right knee while jumping on a trampoline. He was immediately brought to the Emergency Department complaining of pain. Physical examination showed a moderate amount of effusion and there was posterior swelling extending over the gastrocnemius muscle. There was tenderness over the medial collateral ligament at the joint line, a mildly positive anterior drawer sign, and a more extensive posterior drawer sign. No circulatory or neural deficits were noted. The routine anteroposterior and lateral roentgenograms showed an effusion, with no fracture visible.

"The following day, examination under anesthesia showed marked anterior and posterior drawer signs. The medial and lateral collateral ligaments were intact but the tibia could be subluxated posteriorly on the femur with the knee flexed 90 degrees and the tibia internally rotated.

"Arthrotomy through a medial incision revealed that the posterior cruciate ligament had been avulsed from its femoral insertion with a circumferential rim of bone and cartilage. The ligament was reattached by sutures passed through drill holes across the medial condyle. A rent in the posteromedial capsule was repaired by advancement and the medial meniscus, which had been detached posteriorly, was reattached. The insertion of the tendon of the semimembranosus was advanced.

"The patient was discharged wearing a long cast with the knee in 20 degrees of flexion and neutral rotation, non-weight-bearing. He failed to keep his appointments and returned for the first time four months later, at which time the sutures were removed. The patient had removed the cast himself after an indeterminate period. The knee lacked 15 degrees of extension but was stable. He was then lost to follow-up until a year after the injury, at which time he gave no history of instability and was able to participate in athletics without apparent disability. Examination revealed a posterior sag of the tibia on the femur and there was posterolateral rotator instability. Additionally, there was straight anterior instability and minimum anterolateral rotator instability as shown by positive anterior drawer tests in both neutral and internal rotation. There was no significant medial or lateral instability. The pivot-shift test was negative."

(Mayer and Micheli 1979)

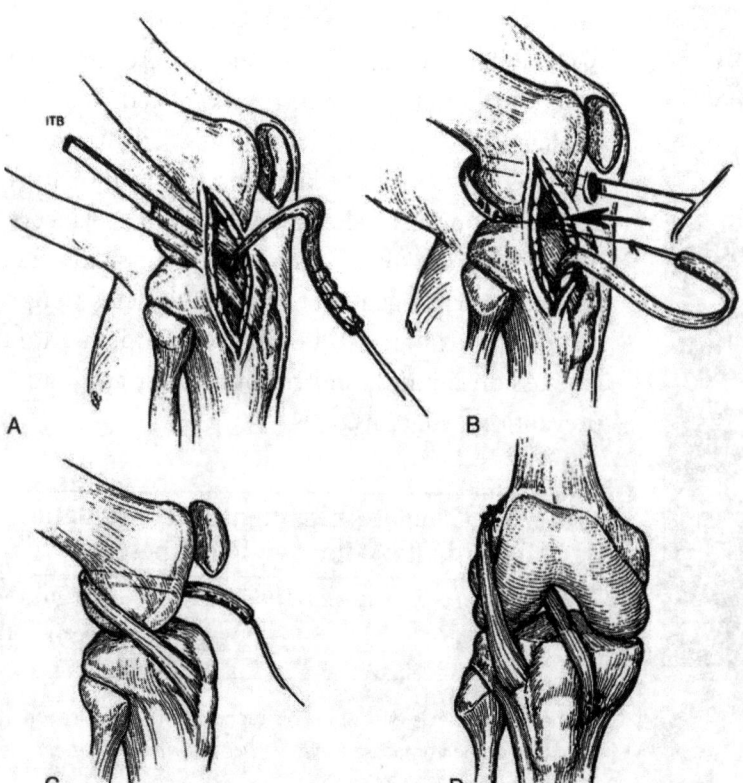

Drawings of Micheli's technique of ACL reconstruction using the iliotibial band. The band is passed around and over the top of the lateral femoral condyle and through a notch in the distal femur, distal to the epiphysis. The graft is then sutured proximally at the superior aspect of the lateral femoral condyle and distally to the periosteum on the medial side of the tibial tubercle. The epiphyseal plates in the distal femur and the proximal tibia are not penetrated.

L. J. Micheli, B. Rask, and L. Gerberg, "Anterior Cruciate Ligament Reconstruction in Patients Who Are Prepubescent," *Clinical Orthopaedics and Related Research* 1999; 364: 42.

Box 27.4. Lyle Micheli's Leadership Roles and Honors and Awards

- Past president (1989–90), American College of Sports Medicine
- President, New England Chapter, American College of Sports Medicine (1980)
- American College of Sports Medicine representative in the selection process for the Sports Science Award, International Olympic Committee (since 1988)
- Chairperson, Massachusetts Governor's Committee on Physical Fitness and Sports (1991–2004)
- Member (1990) and chair (1995–98) of the Education Commission, member of the executive board (1998), and secretary general (2010), International Federation of Sports Medicine
- Co-chair of an International Olympic Committee subcommittee that wrote the "IOC Consensus Statement on the Health and Fitness of Young People through Physical Activity and Sport"
- President, Herodicus Society (1990)
- Member, board of directors, National Youth Sports Safety Foundation (since 1988)
- Member, board of directors, American College of Sports Medicine Foundation (since 1993)
- Member, board of advisors, Jimmie Heuga Foundation (since 1983)
- Dudley Allen Sargent Centennial Lecture, Boston University (1980)
- Medicine Honor Award from the New England Chapter of the American College of Sports Medicine (1988)
- David G. Moyer Award, Eastern Athletic Trainers Association (1988)
- Moore Lecture, Philadelphia Orthopaedic Society (1989)
- Citation Award, American College of Sports Medicine (1993)

Micheli has served in various leadership roles in numerous professional organizations (**Box 27.4**). He also has received much recognition for his contributions to adolescent and child athletes; some of these are also listed in **Box 27.4**.

Currently, Micheli continues to focus his work on the prevention of pediatric sports-related injuries, specifically risk factors for and the occurrence of injury. He is mainly interested in rowing, ballet, long-distance running, and rugby.

In an interview in 2009, Micheli was asked how sports medicine training helps physicians treat knee injuries. His reply emphasized the importance of a safe return to play and complete rehabilitation:

Our training in Sports Medicine helps us treat injuries in so far as the whole goal of sports medicine is early but safe return to sports participation with complete rehabilitation. We have taught our colleagues and ourselves that it's not enough to simply diagnose and treat the injury be [sic] also the very careful and focused rehabilitation in order to return to a level of fitness and training that will allow safe participation is an equally important part of the whole training of the athlete. ("Kneel Hero" 2009)

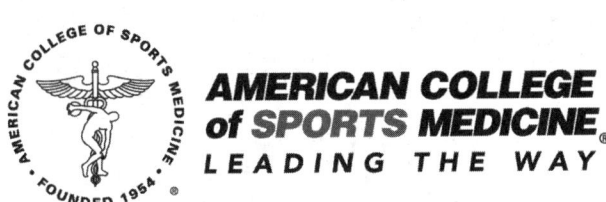

Logo of the American College of Sports Medicine. Courtesy of the ACSM.

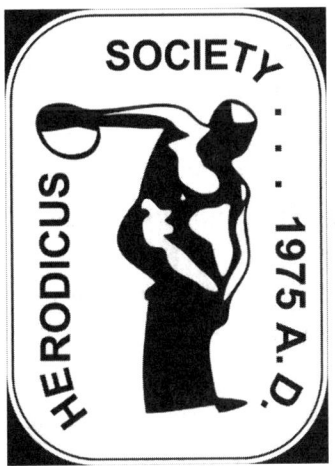

Logo of the Herodicus Society. Courtesy of the Herodicus Society.

MICHAEL B. MILLIS

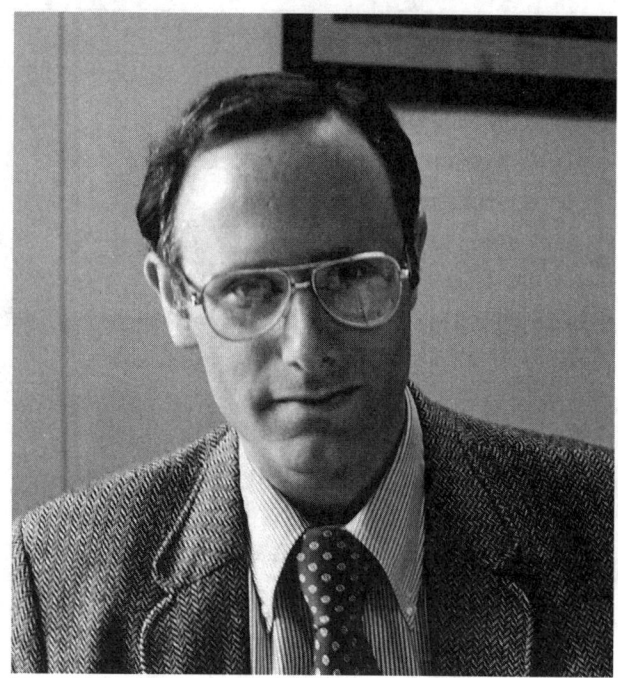

Michael B. Millis. Boston Children's Hospital Archives, Boston, Massachusetts.

Physician Snapshot

Michael B. Millis
BORN: 1944
DIED: —

SIGNIFICANT CONTRIBUTIONS: Co-developed a method to measure acetabular dysplasia; codeveloped, with a team at Children's Hospital, the "Boston concept," a modification of the Bernese periacetabular osteotomy; trained >25 orthopaedic fellows, who now have successful careers in pediatric orthopaedics

Michael Brian Millis was born and raised in Victoria, Texas. He received a bachelor of arts degree cum laude from Harvard College in 1966 (he attended with John Emans, the first physician described in this chapter). As an undergraduate, he was a member of Dunster House, a biology major, and captain of the golf team. He stayed on in Boston and received an MD degree from Harvard Medical School in 1970.

After completing a surgical internship and a year (1972) as a junior resident in surgery at Case Western University Hospital in Cleveland, he went back to Boston and entered the Harvard Combined Orthopaedic Residency Program (1972–75). From 1975 to 1976 he was chief resident and a clinical fellow in pediatric orthopaedics at Children's Hospital. After finishing his residency Millis needed to complete his military obligation, and he served as a lieutenant commander in the US Naval Medical Corps at the Naval Regional Medical Center in Charlestown, South Carolina (1976–78). He received an appointment as an instructor in orthopaedic surgery at the Medical University of South Carolina during his time in the navy.

In 1978, after being discharged from the navy, Millis was hired by Hall as an instructor in orthopaedic surgery at Children's Hospital and as a tutor in medical sciences at Harvard Medical School. In 1979, he received an AO International Fellowship in Hip and Joint-Preserving Surgery with Professor Heinz Wagner at the Wickernhaus Hospital and Clinic in Altdorf/Nuremburg, Germany. For

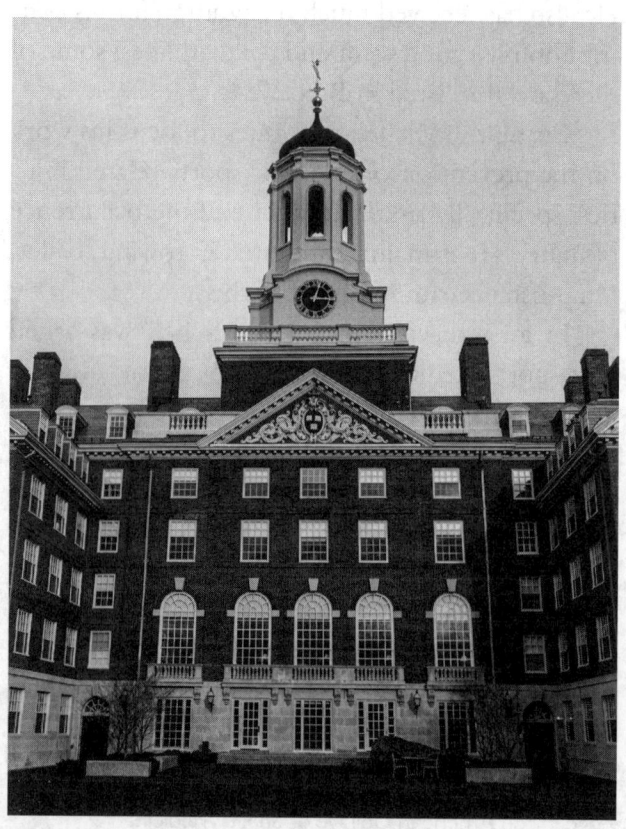

Dunster House, Harvard. Kael E. Randall/Kael Randall Images.

12 years (1982–94), he was a visiting fellow in hip surgery with Wagner at the Krankenhaus Rummelsberg in Germany.

Millis has remained at Children's and Harvard throughout his career. Because of political turmoil in the department at Children's, however, he had left the full-time staff in 1980, becoming a clinical instructor in orthopaedic surgery at Harvard and remaining in private practice at Children's. In 1989, he was promoted to assistant clinical professor, and, in the 1990s, he returned to full-time staff. From 1995 until 1998, he was an associate professor of clinical orthopaedic surgery. In 1998, he was promoted to associate professor, and he became a full professor in 2010.

In addition to his staff position as an associate in orthopaedics at Children's Hospital, he has been an associate in orthopaedics at the Brigham and Women's Hospital, the New England Baptist Hospital, and the Beth Israel Deaconess Medical Center. Since 2001, he has served as director of the adolescent and young adult hip unit at Children's.

Research Focus on the Hip and Pelvis

Millis has published more than 110 articles, has cowritten two books, and has written ~eight book chapters and several American Academy of Orthopaedic Surgeons Instructional Courses. His expertise, clinical research, and practice have focused on the hip and pelvis, especially periacetabular osteotomy; 32 of his papers have dealt with this topic, for example, its use in preserving the hip joint and preventing the development of osteoarthritis. Although he has published articles in other areas of pediatric orthopaedics, including slipped capital femoral epiphysis, Legg-Perthes disease, scoliosis, fractures, Down syndrome, and developmental hip dysplasia, Millis has focused his academic contributions to the hip: more than 90 of his published articles have concentrated on the hip and pelvis—topics such as acetabular dysplasia, the role and safety of the surgical dislocation of the femoral head, femoral acetabular impingement, imaging techniques to determine articular cartilage status, acetabular morphology.

His first paper involving the hip, which he co-wrote with Hall, was published in 1979. He and Hall described the use of a modified innominate osteotomy to lengthen one of the lower extremities and restore postural balance. In 20 patients, they achieved a mean increase in length of 2.3 cm, allowing 14 of the patients to cease use of their shoe lift.

In the mid-1980s, Millis collaborated with Drs. Steven Murphy, Sheldon Simon, and others to study computer-simulated planning of reconstructive orthopaedic surgery. Further collaborations with the Joint Center for Radiation Therapy and the Department of Radiation Therapy at Harvard Medical School led to a publication in 1990 describing a method to measure acetabular dysplastic deformity and an attempt to predict the anatomic result of various osteotomies of the hip joint. Their study described:

> methods of quantifying hip-joint geometry in three dimensions based on computed tomography and magnetic resonance studies, and of simulating pelvic osteotomy to correct the deformity. The study analyzes 49 normal hip joints and 20 dysplastic hip joints. The results show that the normal acetabulum is nearly a full hemisphere, which is anteverted 20° and abducted 53°. The normal lateral center-edge angle is 37°. The dysplastic acetabulum is not anterolaterally maldirected, as has been assumed, but is globally dysplastic…[with] a wide variability. Some patients were deficient

---

Acetabular Dysplasia in the Adolescent and Young Adult

STEPHEN B. MURPHY, M.D., PETER K. KIJEWSKI, PH.D.,* MICHAEL B. MILLIS, M.D., AND ANDREW HARLESS, A.B.*

Title of Murphy, Kijewski, Millis, and Harless article for which they received the Hip Society's Frank Stinchfield Award.
Clinical Orthopaedics and Related Research 1980: 261; 214.

globally, some anterolaterally, and some posterolaterally. (Murphy et al. 1999)

Case 27.3 describes one of the patients they included in that study. Millis and his coauthors received the Frank Stinchfield Award from the Hip Society for their contribution.

Millis and Murphy continued to collaborate over the next approximately nine years. Together with Dr. Robert Poss, they gave two Academy Instructional Course Lectures (in 1992 and 1996) on osteotomies of the hip to prevent osteoarthritis; they delivered a third lecture with Ganz and Dr. Young-Jo Kim in 2006. They published eight papers together, including what they called the "Boston Concept," a periacetabular osteotomy through a direct anterior approach, allowing an arthrotomy of the hip joint to be performed during the procedure.

The Boston Concept

Methods such as Salter's innominate osteotomy, La Coeur's triple osteotomy, and Wagner's dial or spherical osteotomy presented many difficulties for surgeons. To help avoid these difficulties, Professor Reinhold Ganz at the University of Berne, Switzerland, "developed a new periacetabular osteotomy in 1983 based on a series of osteotomies on bone models in addition to operations on cadaveric specimens" (Ganz et al. 1988). It had five main advantages:

(1) one approach [Smith-Petersen] is used; (2) a large correction can be obtained in all directions including the medial and lateral planes; (3) blood supply to the acetabulum is preserved; (4) the posterior column of the hemipelvis remains mechanically intact, allowing

---

Case 27.3. Acetabular Dysplasia in the Young Adult

"A 29-year old woman who had been treated nonoperatively for congenital dysplasia of the right hip was referred for evaluation. She had noted increasing right groin pain over the previous ten years…Her hip roentgenogram shows a CT image through the roof of the acetabulum.

"A preoperative geometric analysis was performed… [It] demonstrated that the acetabulum was excessively abducted (10° above normal) and that containment was severely and globally deficient. The deficiency was greater anteriorly than posteriorly. Specifically the lateral CE angle was +5.2° (normal 37.5°), the anterior CE angle was -75.5° (normal -27.5°), and the posterior CE angle was – 6.9° (normal, 14.5°), The containment angles were 14°-45° below normal. The patient's acetabulum formed only one-third of a hemisphere rather than a nearly complete hemisphere as in the normal acetabulum.

"The Salter innominate and Dial osteotomies were simulated preoperatively to predict the normalizing effects of these proposed procedures. The innominate osteotomy was simulated by dividing the pelvis from the right sciatic notch to the right anterior inferior iliac spine. The distal pelvic fragment, which includes the acetabulum, was rotated 30° around an axis defined by the pelvic symphysis and the right sciatic notch…

"The Dial osteotomy was simulated by dividing the acetabulum from the surrounding pelvis using a spherical cut with a 4-cm radius centered at the center of the joint surface of the femoral head. The free acetabular fragment was abducted 29° and retroverted 20°…

"Results of the 30° innominate osteotomy simulation demonstrated that although the acetabular abduction would be improved by 13°, the global acetabular deficiency was so severe that the lateral CE angle would still only be 18.4°. Results of the simulated Dial osteotomy demonstrated dramatic improvement in the lateral CE angle from 5.2° to 37.5°, and anterior and posterior deficiencies were more balanced. For these reasons the Dial osteotomy was elected and performed in this particular case."

—Murphy, Kijewski, Millis, and Harless
"Acetabular dysplasia in the adolescent and young adult"
Clinical Orthopaedics and Related Research, 1990

immediate crutch walking with minimal internal fixation and without the use of external fixation; and (5) the shape of the true pelvis is unaltered, permitting normal child delivery, a factor of importance in that many patients with these dysplasias are young women…Indications for this periacetabular osteotomy are in adolescent or adult dysplastic hips that require correction of congruency and containment…[and] it provides a more anatomic reconstruction. (Ganz et al. 1988)

Ganz et al. reported excellent results in 75 patients, noting that since 1984 they had performed this osteotomy—which they now called the Bernese periacetabular osteotomy—on more than 700 patients in their hospital. In 1999, they published the long-term follow-up of those original 75 patients and reported the results from 71 of them:

> In 58 patients (82%) the hip joint was preserved…with a good to excellent result in 72%. Unfavorable outcome was significantly associated with higher age of the patient, moderate to severe osteoarthritis at surgery, a labral lesion, less anterior connection, and a suboptimal acetabular index. Major complications were encountered in the first 18 patients including an intraarticular cut in two, excessive lateralization in one, secondary loss of correction in two and femoral head subluxation in three patients. (Siebenrock et al. 1999)

> Orthopade. 1998 Nov;27(11):751-8.
>
> **[The Boston concept. peri-acetabular osteotomy with simultaneous arthrotomy via direct anterior approach]**
>
> [Article in German]
> M B Millis [1], S B Murphy

The "Boston Concept": a periacetabular osteotomy and hip arthrotomy performed together through a direct anterior approach. *Orthopade* 1998; 11: 751.

In 1999, Millis worked again with Murphy and Hall to review three acetabular redirection operations: the Salter innominate osteotomy, the Wagner spherical osteotomy, and the Bernese periacetabular osteotomy. For them, "the modified Bernese periacetabular osteotomy is the authors' current preferred method of treating acetabular dysplasia, even in the presence of mild to moderate secondary osteoarthrosis" (Murphy, Millis, and Hall 1999). They defended this preference by describing issues encountered with the other methods. For the Salter innominate osteotomy:

> the limited correction achieved…suggests this procedure should be reserved for younger patients with mild dysplasia…Based on the preliminary experience with the Salter innominate osteotomy at the author's institution [Children's Hospital], by the middle to late 1970's, the need for a pelvic osteotomy that allowed for more freedom of correction became clear. The faculty of the orthopaedic department thought that the triple osteotomy of Steele was not an adequate alternative for several reasons. (Murphy, Millis, and Hall 1999)

With regard to the Wagner spherical acetabular osteotomy, they:

> considered [it] to be a potentially attractive alternative because the osteotomies were close to the acetabulum, that permitted large, individualized corrections while leaving the posterior columns intact. After one of the authors (MBM) learned the technique from Wagner [Millis completed his fellowship under Wagner in 1979–80], the osteotomy became the primary method of correcting high grade hip dysplasia at Children's Hospital in 1980… The osteotomy was performed through the Smith-Petersen (iliofemoral) exposure by dissecting the abductors from the lateral iliac wing…[but the authors found] several limitations to the procedure. First, because of

concern about blood supply to the acetabular fragment, the hip joint was not explored... Second, the periacetabular bone in adults with dysplasia can be hard and brittle...[and] therefore it can be difficult to perform a spherical cut with a curved osteotomy...Third, since the osteotomies are introduced from a lateral position, the pelvic origin of the tensor and abductors have to be dissected...which makes the postoperative rehabilitation slower and more difficult. (Murphy, Millis, and Hall 1999)

As Millis and his surgical colleagues at Children's began to identify the limitations of Wagner's method, Ganz was perfecting the Bernese periacetabular osteotomy. Murphy, Millis, and Hall (1999) did note that Wagner's "spherical acetabular osteotomy and the Bernese periacetabular osteotomy essentially are variations of the same operation in principle. In practice, however, the Bernese periacetabular osteotomy has numerous advantages...The need to open the joint at the time of acetabular redirection...was apparent [leaving large labral lesions unaddressed]...Arthrotomy at the time of...osteotomy did not lead to acetabular osteonecrosis." Thus, in order to avoid "dissection of the origins of the tensor and abductors...[and] cracking of the posterior column into the lesser sciatic notch" (Murphy, Millis, and Hall 1999), the team at Children's Hospital developed a modification—direct anterior exposure (referred to as the Boston approach by Millis, Murphy, and Hall) that allowed:

a combined exposure...This technique combines the medial portion of the iliofemoral exposure with the lateral portion of the ilioinguinal exposure. The two can be combined by osteotomizing the anterosuperior iliac spine and reflecting the sartorius and inguinal ligament inferiorly...performing the entire osteotomy without abductor dissection...[and use] of the second window of the ilioinguinal exposure...had several advantages. First access to the superior pubic ramus is far superior...[and] makes the superior pubic ramus osteotomy easier to perform, gives better control to mobilize the acetabular fragment and facilitates bone grafting in this area...Second, better access to the deep true pelvis medially facilitates performance of the last and deepest osteotomy across the ischium...without cracking the posterior column, leaving a stronger pelvis. (Murphy, Millis, and Hall 1999)

The modified Bernese periacetabular osteotomy (the Boston concept) became the authors' choice of a redirection periacetabular osteotomy with a simultaneous arthrotomy if required.

Soon after reporting their "Boston experience" with the history and development of acetabular redirection osteotomies, Millis and Murphy continued to publish and make contributions regarding this specific surgical technique, albeit separately.

Other Contributions in Hip Disease

Millis's contributions to the understanding of hip disease have continued throughout his career. A few examples include his work in acetabular morphology in slipped capital femoral epiphysis; hip instability and use of the periacetabular osteotomy in patients with Down syndrome; blood supply to the femoral head in Legg-Perthes disease; hip dysplasia in Charcot-Marie-Tooth disease; and, more recently, the mechanical loading and matrix composition of articular cartilage after periacetabular osteotomy. He has enormous experience with periacetabular osteotomy, allowing him to report on its successful use in patients older than 40 years of age with hip dysplasia and only mild or no arthrosis. He reported a high rate of femoroacetabular impingement in males after a Bernese periacetabular osteotomy.

Millis is a member of the Academic Network for Conservational Hip Outcomes Research (ANCHOR) Group, which includes both European and United States surgeons and operates

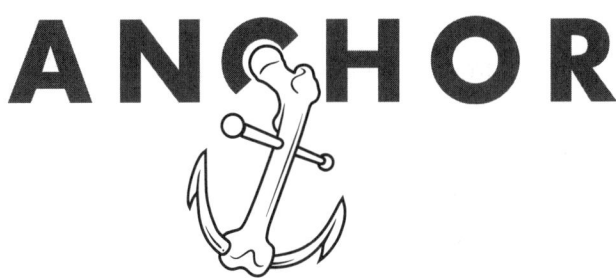

Logo of the Academic Network for Conservational Hip Outcomes Research (ANCHOR) Group. Courtesy of the ANCHOR Group.

under an agreed-upon set of ethical guidelines for research. The ANCHOR Group uses the Clavien-Dindo classification in general surgery, "a standardized, objective complication grading scheme…for reporting complications associated with hip preservation surgery [because it] has interobserver and intraobserver reliabilities" (Sink et al. 2012). This classification method "endeavors to facilitate standardization of complication reporting and may be useful for all orthopaedic procedures…it is applicable to future outcomes analysis of hip preservation surgery because of (1) any long-term morbidity from the complication…is critical to the risk/benefit analysis of the procedure; and (2) the magnitude of treatment… required to manage the complication…is important to the overall cost to the patient, third party insurer and hospital" (Sink et al. 2012).

In 2012, in describing "Prevention of Nerve Injury after Periacetabular Osteotomy," the ANCHOR group, including Millis, reported: "Thirty-six of the 1760 patients (2.1%) had a major nerve deficit of the sciatic or femoral nerve…Seventeen of the 36 patients had complete recovery. The median time to recovery or plateau was 5.5 months…Full recovery can be expected in only ½ of the patients and more commonly with injuries of the femoral nerve. If direct nerve injury is suspected, we believe exploration may be warranted." The authors of that study were unable to identify any risk factors.

In 2014, members of the ANCHOR group (Millis was an author) again reported on periacetabular osteotomy—this time related to complications of the procedure:

> Major complications (grade III or IV) occurred in twelve patients (5.9%)…Nine…required a second surgical intervention, including repair for acetabular migration or implant adjustment… incision and drainage for a deep infection… and heterotopic bone resection, contralateral peroneal nerve decompression, and posterior column fixation…There were no vascular injuries, permanent nerve palsies, intra-articular osteotomies and/or fractures, or acetabular osteonecrosis. The most common grade-I or II complication was asymptomatic heterotopic ossification.

All of the 205 consecutive procedures were performed by experienced surgeons.

In 2004, the journal *Orthopedics* published an interview with Millis. In it he updated the journal's readers on the current state of periacetabular osteotomy:

> This kind of surgery is highly effective if patients are diagnosed in time and referred to appropriate specialists. Our experience in Boston with the Bernese acetabular osteotomy is approximately 700 hips, and only 22 of those hips so far have gone on to total hip replacement (THR) during our 15 years of experience…we use the Bernese osteotomy because it allows extensive corrections to be done without disturbing the abductor muscles. It also allows medialization as well as rotation in three planes, so it is a versatile operation that can be done through several different surgical approaches… [it] also allows one to simultaneously do an arthrotomy and deal with intra-articular problems such as labral tears…it is a good operation for young active people. It allows them to get back to doing all of their activities almost without restriction, which does not occur with a routine THR. The inclusion criteria are a

mature patient with congruous acetabular dysplasia severe enough to cause symptoms of, or the future risk of, osteoarthritis. The exclusion criteria include patients with dysplasia so mild that they do not need the procedure or someone in whom the osteoarthritis is so far along that the procedure will not help them. Immature patients who have open growth centers… should be excluded as well…absolute absence of symptoms is a contraindication for the procedure…The potential complications include all of those associated with any major hip surgery…[including] damage to adjacent nerves… femoral or sciatic nerve, as well as the obturator nerve and lateral femoral cutaneous nerve; damage to major blood vessels, osteonecrosis of the acetabular fragment or femoral head; intra-articular fracture; and thromboembolic phenomena, mainly blood clots in the legs… The progression of osteoarthritis may also occur if the procedure is done…with osteoarthritis that is too advanced…[if done improperly] the potential exists for either lengthening the ipsilateral limb or shortening it, or for translocating the fragment anteriorly, which would make patients seem as if they had a long leg when they sit…[Postoperatively] patients are on two crutches for 6-12 weeks…The physical therapy program is not aggressive. Mostly it is a gentle range of motion with strengthening exercises…It is rare for patients to develop more pathologic pain or any significant problems with nerve-based weakness…[which] can occur in approximately 1% of patients. [Regarding a role for computer navigation] as approaches become much more minimally invasive, we probably will be using more computer navigation. ("Michael B. Millis on periacetabular osteotomy" 2004)

Well Loved by Patients and Students

One of Millis's patients created "What's the Hip Fix?", an active blog about hip dysplasia and its treatment. In their posts they praise Millis, calling him "affable" and "enthusiastic." One of their "favorite qualities" about Millis is his willingness to spend time with his patients, explaining imaging studies, results, procedures—what the blogger called "geek[ing] out…about the science of surgery." In one comment, another of his patients said he was a "straight shooter." Since 2008 many patients have shared their stories of Millis on this blog.

Millis has trained more than 25 fellows, five of whom are now chiefs of pediatric orthopaedics. In his curriculum vitae, Millis (n.d.) described himself and his practice:

> I am a pediatric orthopaedist by classical training, with a particular interest as a clinician and a clinical researcher in developmental hip problems that play out over a lifetime. The focus of my orthopaedic practice has been on the large adolescent and young adult patient population with structural hip abnormalities predisposing to painful osteoarthritis. These patients lie in the watershed zone between the specialty care offered by the pediatric orthopaedist and the total hip replacement care for destroyed hip joints provided by the adult orthopaedist. Their clinical problems have been relatively understudied and undertreated, despite the great therapeutic potential for preventing future morbidity in this population…I am and have been privileged to learn from and to collaborate with world-class authorities here and abroad, developing and employing powerful therapeutic and diagnostic techniques relevant to developmental hip disease. I see my primary role as a very active academic clinician with unusual extensive hip joint-preserving experience…to improve the treatment methods of both pediatric orthopaedists and adult orthopaedists in caring for patients with various developmental hip deformities.

EDWARD J. RISEBOROUGH

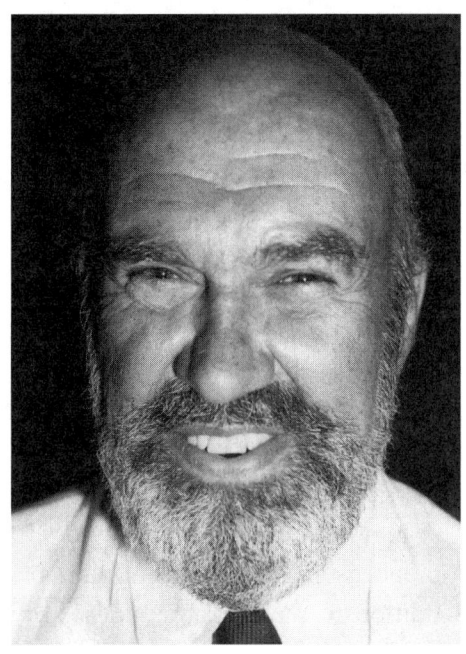

Edward J. Riseborough. Boston Children's Hospital Archives, Boston, Massachusetts.

Physician Snapshot:

Edward J. Riseborough
BORN: 1925
DIED: 1985
SIGNIFICANT CONTRIBUTIONS: Humanitarian and committed teacher; mentor to residents and an expert in scoliosis

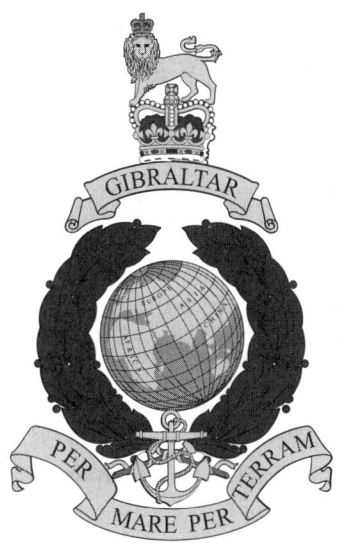

Logo of the British Royal Marines. Wikimedia Commons.

Edward "Ted" J. Riseborough was originally from South Africa, born in Cape Town on April 15, 1925. After graduating from the Rondebosch Boys High School in 1942:

> He entered the British Royal Marines in 1943 [at age 18] and served with them [during World War II] in southeast Asia and the Pacific through 1947. On returning to Cape Town, he received his B.S.C. degree from the University of Cape Town in 1949 and his M.B.Ch.B. degree from the same university in 1952. Dr. Riseborough then served as a medical and surgical house officer in the Pietermaritzburg Hospital in Natal, South Africa, and as senior officer at the Stals Memorial Sanatorium in Cape Town. He continued his training in London in 1954, serving as a registrar from 1955 to 1957 and as a senior orthopaedic registrar at the Heatherwood Hospital, Ascot, England from 1958 to 1960. Dr. Riseborough came to this country [the United States] in 1960 and served as a Fellow in the Department of Orthopaedic Surgery at the Massachusetts General Hospital from 1960 to 1961. He was also a fellow in the Department of Orthopaedic Surgery at the University of Minnesota during 1967.
> ("Edward J. Riseborough, MD" 1986)

After completing his fellowship in Minneapolis, Riseborough returned to MGH in 1967 as an assistant in orthopaedic surgery at MGH; he was also named an instructor in orthopaedic surgery at Harvard Medical School. In all, he "served on the staff of the Massachusetts General Hospital from 1960 to 1971," where he built a scoliosis practice "and was associated with Dr. Joseph Barr" ("Edward J. Riseborough, MD" 1986).

Interests in Scoliosis and Trauma

While at MGH, Riseborough published ~15 papers. His first, "Treatment of Low Back and Sciatic Pain in Patients over 60 Years of Age. A Study of 100 Patients," was cowritten with Barr in 1963. (All 100 patients were treated in Barr's private practice.) They enumerated four conclusions:

1. Patients over the age of 60 who have prolonged low back and sciatic pain need to have a careful history, physical examination and roentgenograms taken before a diagnosis is made and treatment is undertaken. Other tests such as myelography are occasionally indicated.

2. The causes of low back pain with sciatica in patients over 60 fell into 4 main groups...local lesions of the intervertebral disk, spondylolisthesis, muscular/ligamentous low back strain and generalized disease of the lumbar spine.

3. The majority of patients recovered on a conservative program aimed at relieving pain and muscle spasm, followed by a rehabilitation regimen.

4. Only 9 per cent came to surgery. After adequate conservative treatment, a laminectomy was performed in all cases, and the nerve roots explored. Only those patients required spinal fusions who were likely to lead active postoperative lives or in whom such a large part of the dural arch had been removed at the surgery that it appeared that the lumbar spine would be unstable. (Barr and Riseborough 1963)

Riseborough was one of several coauthors with Barr on two other papers, including an end-result study of the treatment of patients with herniated discs.

In 1967, Riseborough wrote a review of the treatment of scoliosis at the time in a Current Concepts article for the *New England Journal of Medicine*, in which he stated: "With the development of the Milwaukee brace, Harrington instruments and the more effective cast techniques described by Risser ['eliminating the difficult application and constant supervision necessary with the use of the turnbuckle cast'], an aggressive approach to the treatment of scoliosis has replaced the time-honored 'watchful-waiting' method. Watching scoliosis gradually progress in children is no longer tenable" (Riseborough 1967 [explanatory quotes in brackets from later in the same article]). He also published three papers on abnormal lung function and ventilation perfusion deficits in patients with kyphoscoliosis.

In addition to scoliosis, trauma was of interest to Riseborough. He cowrote, with Dr. Eric Radin, two classic papers that are frequently quoted today. The first paper was a 1966 review of cases of fracture of the radial head. Using the Mason classification, they examined 100 patients at least two years after they had been treated. At the time: "Opinions... [varied] as to whether the radial head should be excised in treatment of fractures of the radial head. The issue is further complicated by fear of causing inferior radio-ulnar subluxation by radial-head excision" (Radin and Riseborough 1966). They believed that: "The controversy surrounding the treatment of radial-head fractures is based...on the failure to separate undisplaced, displaced, comminuted, complicated and pediatric fractures" (Radin

Title of Barr and Riseborough's article on the management of back pain in patients >60 years of age. *Clinical Orthopaedics and Related Research* 1963; 26: 12.

Title of Radin and Riseborough's article on management of radial head fractures. *Journal of Bone and Joint Surgery* 1966; 48: 1055.

and Riseborough 1966). On the basis of their classifications determined two years after treatment, they described four main findings: "(1) Early motion may displace otherwise undisplaced fractures; (2) if more than one-third of the radial head is displaced, limitation of motion will probably result; (3) the range of motion depends on the anatomical result; (4) inferior radio-ulnar subluxation does occur, but it is of so little significance that it can be ignored as an argument against excision of the radial head" (Radin and Riseborough 1966). They also made recommendations for treating undisplaced and displaced fractures: "We would treat undisplaced fractures involving less than one-third of the radial head with active motion as soon as the patient is comfortable...Displaced fractures involving less than two-thirds of the radial head should...be treated by early active motion...Displaced fractures involving more than two-thirds...should be treated by early total excision, as should all comminuted fractures" (Radin and Riseborough 1966).

In the second article, published in 1969, they classified intercondylar T fractures of the humerus into four categories. After reviewing the outcomes of 27 patients (among a series of 52) who had been treated operatively and nonoperatively, they concluded that:

> The treatment of intercondylar fractures in adults should be determined on the basis of the amount of rotator deformity and comminution. Severely comminuted factors do not lend themselves to open reduction and are best treated with skeletal traction and gentle closed manipulation...In the minimally displaced fractures, good results can be obtained by immobilization in a plaster cast... findings in this small series suggest that fractures with significant rotatory deformity...are more likely to have a good result when skeletal traction is used rather than open reduction and internal fixation. Open reduction and adequate internal fixation are not easy...[and] open reduction is very rarely indicated. (Riseborough and Radin 1969)

Another focus in trauma for Riseborough was the fat embolism syndrome. He, along with Drs. Josef Fisher, Roderick Turner, and myself, reported in 1971 on the use of massive steroid therapy in severe cases of fat embolism syndrome: among 17 patients treated at MGH, none died. With increased interest in this complex pathophysiologic event, Riseborough and I completed a prospective study including 164 unselected patients with lower-limb fractures who had been admitted to MGH. More than half of the 118 patients who completed the study:

> exhibited hypoxemia as well as a decrease in the hematocrit and platelet counts with a concomitant increase in platelet adhesiveness... [T]hose patients with hypoxemia showed increased fibrinogen degenerative product

---

Intercondylar T Fractures of the Humerus in the Adult

A COMPARISON OF OPERATIVE AND NON-OPERATIVE TREATMENT IN TWENTY-NINE CASES*

BY EDWARD J. RISEBOROUGH, M.D.†, AND ERIC L. RADIN, M.D.†, BOSTON, MASSACHUSETTS

From the Orthopedic Service, Massachusetts General Hospital, and Harvard Medical School, Boston

JBJS, 1969, Volume 51, Issue 1

Title of Riseborough and Radin's article on management of Intercondylar fractures of the humerus in adults. *Journal of Bone and Joint Surgery* 1969; 51: 130.

Alterations in Pulmonary Function, Coagulation and Fat Metabolism in Patients with Fractures of the Lower Limbs

EDWARD J. RISEBOROUGH, M.B., CH.B.* AND JAMES H. HERNDON, M.D.**

Clinical Orthopaedics and Related Research
Number 115
March-April, 1976

Title of Riseborough and Herndon's article describing physiologic changes in the fat embolism syndrome. *Clinical Orthopaedics and Related Research* 1976; 115: 248.

levels indicating increased fibrinolysis...[N]onesterified fatty acid levels rose sharply over the first three days following trauma associated with an increase in serum lipase...[F]at emboli with adherent platelets and other vascular elements are formed...[that] would lodge in the capillaries and small vessels of the lung, thereby producing a physiological shunt. An increase in the A-aDo2 confirmed this hypothesis and was associated with a decrease in the arterial oxygen level in over half the patients studied. Although 58 of our patients showed evidence of hypoxemia...not one of them showed clinical signs and symptoms of the fat embolus syndrome. This study suggests that a subclinical form of fat embolism does exist... The majority of our patients spontaneously returned to normal within 5 days. (Riseborough and Herndon 1976)

Riseborough "had a great warmth as a teacher and loved to steer the student along the path of learning" ("Edward J. Riseborough, MD" 1986). After working closely with Ted in his office (brief locum tenens) at MGH, I couldn't agree more with this statement. As described above, we wrote several papers together about our clinical research on fat embolism. Riseborough also had a "keen interest in scoliosis" ("Edward J. Riseborough, MD" 1986), and I was enormously surprised and moved when he requested that I help him write a book on the topic; each of us would write a chapter and then edit the other's chapter. I will be forever grateful for his generous sharing. Our collaboration, *Scoliosis and Other Deformities of the Axial Skeleton*, was published in 1975. In the foreword to the book, Arthur R. Hodgson, a professor in and the chairman of the Department of Orthopaedics and Traumatology at the University of Hong Kong, wrote:

> Scoliosis and Other Deformities of the Axial Skeleton is the first book in which all types of spinal deformity are considered, and this is a very important step forward. The days when orthopedic surgeons should specialize in scoliosis alone are gone. The specialization should be in spinal deformities. The authors present a book that is a product of accurate and intelligent clinical observation...It is an unusual book also in that it has a chapter on anesthesia in patients with spinal deformities. This demonstrates the authors' breath of vision. (Riseborough and Herndon 1975)

I still remember a very difficult case I handled as a senior resident with Riseborough while we were both at MGH: A teenage girl had an advanced osteosarcoma of the proximal humerus. To complicate matters, as Jehovah's Witnesses, she and her family refused any blood transfusions. Riseborough assisted me with the case as he always did—staying hands off, but providing moral support (a gift that few attending surgeons possess). The patient chose to undergo forequarter amputation. Riseborough also almost always allowed residents to operate with

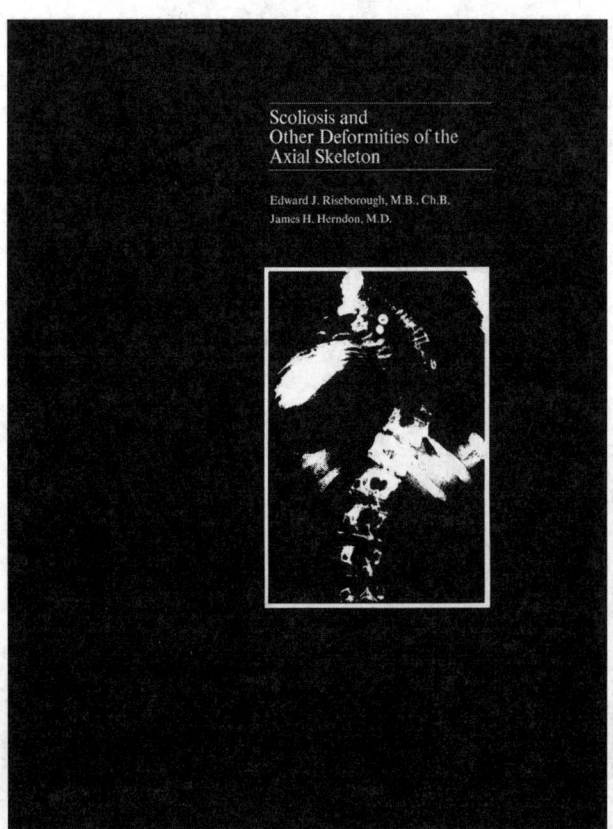

Cover of Riseborough and Herndon's book, *Scoliosis and Other Deformities of the Axial Skeleton*. Little, Brown & Co., 1975.

him assisting, and so I performed this complex procedure. To add to my tension, Dr. Hardy Hendren entered the operating room during the amputation and began to quiz me about the anatomy. It is, therefore, no surprise that I can recall this case after 45 years. The patient lost a minimal amount of blood; she didn't need a transfusion and left the hospital after recovery, with no complications.

Soon after I completed my chief residency at MGH in 1970 and entered the US Army (I had been drafted but deferred service under the Berry Plan), Riseborough moved from MGH to Children's Hospital in order to join Dr. John Hall, who had just arrived in Boston from Toronto. Riseborough became a senior associate in orthopaedic surgery at Children's Hospital and an assistant clinical professor in orthopaedic surgery at Harvard Medical School. He was also on the medical staff of the Peter Bent Brigham Hospital and the Newton-Wellesley Hospital.

During his time at Children's he continued to publish on trauma and on scoliosis (another ~12 papers); the scoliosis-related topics he discussed were significant and varied: the development of scoliosis, kyphoscoliosis and kyphosis after irradiation for Wilms tumors, scoliosis in patients with neurofibromatosis (occurring in 26% of such patients), thoracolumbar kyphosis and growth disturbances in patients with dwarfism and achondroplasia, and the anterior approach to the spine. (**Case 27.4** provides an excerpt from one of his publications on kyphosis.) He also wrote two papers with Hall and others about combined anterior and posterior fusions, and osteotomy of the fusion mass in patients with an unbalanced spine after fusion.

In 1973, Riseborough published an article with Dr. Ruth Wynne-Davies, an orthopaedic geneticist in J. I. P. James's orthopaedic department at the University of Edinburgh. They based their study on a genetic survey of children in Boston with idiopathic scoliosis, and: "the data suggested a multifactorial mode of inheritance" (Riseborough and Wynne-Davies 1973). They demonstrated a differing prevalence of early-onset scoliosis in

Case 27.4. Transthoracic Vertebral Excision and Halo-Femoral Traction in Congenital Kyphosis

> "A 13-year-old girl with congenital kyphosis secondary to a wedged fifth dorsal vertebral body (D-5) underwent right transthoracic excision of the vertebral body. The defect was strutted with rib grafts. Absorbable gelatin sponge was used to control epidural bleeding on the right side of the vertebral canal behind the posterior longitudinal ligament, the pleura closed over the area, and the lung field fully re-expanded. No antibiotics were used. Postoperatively the patient did well and was placed in halo-femoral traction with increasing weights. On the seventh postoperative day she developed a Brown-Séquard syndrome with a sensory level on the left at D-5 and urinary incontinence. Her anal sphincter was relaxed. Reduction of weight led to no relief and she was promptly reexplored. Upon opening the pleura a yellow-white fluid gushed out under pressure from the area of the sponge packing. Gram stain showed a few polymorphonuclear leukocytes, but no bacteria. All cultures were negative.
>
> "The patient recovered fully neurologically in six days. She was returned to halo-femoral traction and later underwent posterior spine fusion without difficulty."
>
> —Herndon, Grillo, Riseborough, and Rich
> *Archives of Surgery*, 1972

two regions—the United Kingdom and New England—where the populace of both locations has a "similar genetic background." In addition to genetics, they also evaluated various "environmental factors" that could have an effect, e.g., prone or supine positioning.

In 1980, he and his colleagues reported that diastematomyelia was present in 60% of patients with congenital scoliosis. They recommended using "myelography…in [determining] the diagnosis, particularly prior to any procedure that might cause traction on the spinal cord. Laminectomy for removal of the spur was indicated when neural deficits were progressive or before corrective surgery on the spine…Observation of patients with diastematomyelia who have no neural deficit or a

> A Genetic Survey of Idiopathic Scoliosis in
> Boston, Massachusetts
> BY EDWARD J. RISEBOROUGH, M.D.*, BOSTON, MASSACHUSETTS, AND
> RUTH WYNNE-DAVIES, F.R.C.S.†, EDINBURGH, SCOTLAND
> THE JOURNAL OF BONE AND JOINT SURGERY
> VOL. 55-A, NO. 5, JULY 1973

Title of Riseborough and Wynne-Davies article in which they reported a possible multifactorial inheritance in idiopathic scoliosis. *Journal of Bone and Joint Surgery* 1973; 55: 974.

stable, non-progressing deficit is recommended" (Hood et al. 1980).

With Drs. Ian Barrett and Frederic Shapiro, he published in 1983 a review of growth disturbances in the femur after distal femoral physeal fractures. Among 66 patients, 37 had "lower-extremity leg length discrepancies in excess of 2.4 centimeters...angular deformity of more than 5 degrees or requiring osteotomy...[and] central arrest...in thirteen patients...[The radiographic sign of central arrest] had excellent predictive value for the development of limb-length discrepancy...We believe that the final results would be improved by anatomical reduction and greater use of internal fixation in type-II, III, and IV injuries" (Riseborough, Barrett, and Shapiro 1983).

Professional Memberships and Other Interests

Riseborough was a founding member of the Scoliosis Research Society. He was also "a member of the British Orthopaedic Association, the American Orthopaedic Association, the Pediatric Orthopaedic Study Group, the Pediatric Orthopaedic Society and the American Academy of Orthopaedic Surgeons" ("Edward J. Riseborough, MD" 1986). He had held leadership positions in the Boston Rugby Football Club and the British Officers Club of Boston, and he was in the Harvard Club.

According to an April 2, 1985, *Boston Globe* article, Riseborough was "a man of varied interests." He loved jazz music and opera; cultivated an interest in ships (particularly shipbuilding and sailing); collected stamps and orchids; and appreciated ancient Mayan art. The article also referred to him as a "humanitarian" who focused on others' needs before his own, describing as a case in point Riseborough's work in Guatemala City in 1976, after an earthquake caused extensive damage. Riseborough went with six other physicians from New Orleans; he spoke Spanish, which helped him communicate there. Riseborough described it as "a ghastly sight...there were bodies all around the hospital and all over the place...[It was] just like a nightmare" (quoted in Dwyer 1976). The article also mentioned a 14-day mission trip to Ethiopia he took in 1985 with Jennifer, his wife and a nurse.

Riseborough experienced a heart attack on March 31, 1985, and died suddenly and unexpectedly. At the time, he had been in New York visiting some of his children. He was survived by his wife and eight children, as well as a brother and sister, who still lived in Cape Town.

The obituary published in the *Journal of Bone and Joint Surgery* ("Edward J. Riseborough, MD" 1986) noted Riseborough as having "a great desire to help other people succeed." That article quoted a poem Riseborough's son Bruce had written about his father:

My father loved the sun
He would wake up early to watch it rise
He loved what it would do to his orchids,
Reaching up like him to its warmth.

Most of all, like the warmth of the sun.
The security in knowledge. His dexterity with tools.
His music, his patients – he loved life.

—B. Riseborough

ROBERT K. ROSENTHAL

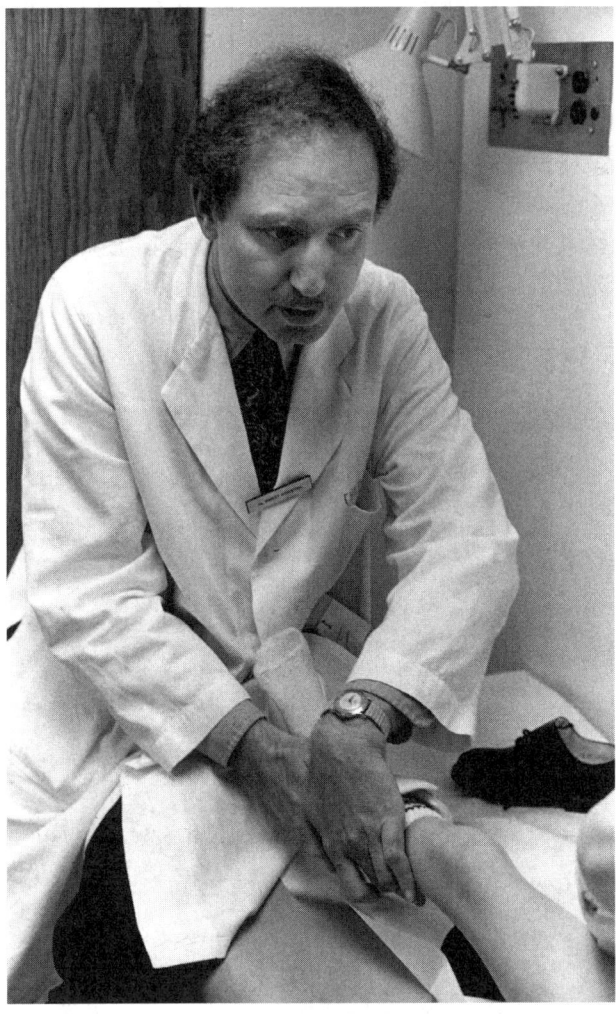

Robert K. Rosenthal examining a patient's foot in the cerebral palsy clinic. Boston Children's Hospital Archives, Boston, Massachusetts.

Physician Snapshot

Robert K. Rosenthal
BORN: 1936
DIED: 2021
SIGNIFICANT CONTRIBUTIONS: Studied cerebral palsy throughout career; chief of the Cerebral Palsy Clinic at Children's Hospital from 1971 to 1983

Robert Kenneth Rosenthal, a Boston native, graduated from Boston University with a BA in 1958 and then with an MD degree from Tufts University School of Medicine in 1962. After a surgical internship at the New England Medical Center, he was on active duty in the United States Air Force (1963–65). Following his discharge from the Air Force, Rosenthal was an assistant resident in surgery at the New England Medical Center for one year. He then completed an orthopaedic residency comprising one year (1966) at Metropolitan Hospital in New York and two years (1967–69) at St. Joseph's Hospital in Patterson, New Jersey. After his residency he held two fellowships, one as a fellow in orthopaedics at the Hospital for Special Surgery (1969–71), and then a clinical fellow at Boston Children's Hospital (1972–73) through the United Cerebral Palsy Association.

After completing his cerebral palsy fellowship, he remained on staff at Children's Hospital, as an attending surgeon. Appointed as an instructor in orthopaedic surgery at Harvard Medical School in 1972, he was promoted to assistant professor in 1978. A year later his appointment was changed to assistant clinical professor—a role he would continue in for the next 35 years. In 2014, he was again named an assistant professor of orthopaedic surgery, though then he taught only part-time.

Rosenthal was interested in cerebral palsy early in his career, and he published four papers on the topic, specifically about the etiology of the disorder, femoral head changes in patients with dislocated hips, the use of levodopa to treat cerebral palsy, and scoliosis—all based on his experiences as a fellow at the Hospital for Special Surgery. His

Levodopa therapy in athetoid cerebral palsy

A preliminary report

Robert K. Rosenthal, M.D., Fletcher H. McDowell, M.D., and William Cooper,* M.D.

Title of Rosenthal et al. article on the use of Levodopa in cerebral palsy. *Neurology* 1957; 22: 1.

Title of Rosenthal et al. article on the use of a fixed ankle short leg brace to treat spastic genu recurvatum.
Journal of Bone and Joint Surgery 1975; 57: 545.

interest in the disorder continued at Children's Hospital, where he was chief of the Cerebral Palsy Clinic from 1971 to 1983; during that time, he also staffed the hospital's Myelodysplasia Clinic. During his first 20 years in the Children's Hospital Cerebral Palsy Clinic, he published various papers: five on the knee, two on the hip, and one each on the spine, foot and ankle, and leg-length discrepancy. He also published one book chapter. In addition to publishing on cerebral palsy, he also published one paper on adductor transfers in myelodysplasia and one book chapter on myelodysplasia.

As chief of the Cerebral Palsy Clinic, he and Dr. John Hall offered a one-year pediatric orthopaedic fellowship (1972–80). It focused on "the area of neuromuscular disorders, including cerebral palsy and myelodysplasia. It will give the Fellow an opportunity to study in depth one or two specific orthopaedic problems, as well as to participate with other members of the staff of the Children's Hospital in the areas of scoliosis, hip disorders and general pediatric conditions" ("A Clinical Fellowship" 1973).

Rosenthal has been an active member of the American Academy for Cerebral Palsy and Developmental Medicine, serving on many committees and, in 1995–96, as president. He served on its Endowment Committee. Certified by the American Board of Orthopaedic Surgery, he was a member of the American Academy of Orthopaedic Surgeons, the Pediatric Orthopaedic Society of North America (a past member of its Pediatric Orthopaedic Study Group), the Societé Internationale de Chirurgie Orthopédique et de Traumatologie, and the Boston Orthopaedic Club. In 1979, he received the United Cerebral Palsy Research and Education Foundation Research Award. Rosenthal was a board member of the Barrington Stage Company in Pittsfield, Massachusetts, and was on the honorary board of the Longwood Symphony Orchestra in Boston.

FREDERIC SHAPIRO

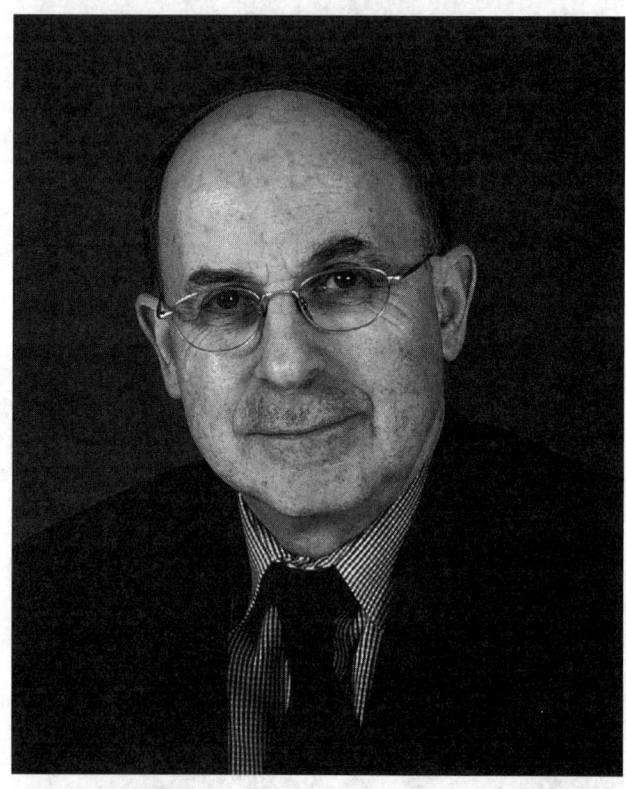

Frederic Shapiro. James Koepfler/Boston Children's Hospital.

Physician Snapshot

Frederic Shapiro
BORN: 1942
DIED: —

SIGNIFICANT CONTRIBUTIONS: Published extensively on the basic science of orthopaedics, particularly the three-volume compendium *Pediatric Orthopaedic Deformities*

Frederic Shapiro was born and raised in Toronto, Canada. He completed his premedical undergraduate courses at the University of Toronto in 1962, then went on to receive a medical degree from the Faculty of Medicine there in 1967. After an internship at Toronto General Hospital, he completed a year of training in general surgery on the Harvard Surgical Service at the Boston City Hospital. From 1969 to 1972, he was an orthopaedic resident in the McGill University–Montreal General Hospital program in Montreal, Quebec, Canada. After graduating in 1972, Shapiro held a two-year research fellowship in the Department of Orthopaedic Surgery at Boston Children's Hospital Medical Center and Harvard Medical School.

After completing his research fellowship at Children's Hospital (1973–75), Shapiro joined the staff there as an attending orthopaedic surgeon (an assistant in orthopaedic surgery), and as an instructor at Harvard Medical School. His appointments at Children's Hospital and Harvard Medical School are listed in **Box 27.5**.

Shapiro has written more than 125 original publications, mainly in broad categories of basic science, including bone development, bone repair, cartilage repair, osteopetrosis, osteogenesis imperfecta, osteosarcoma and hereditary multiple exostoses, epiphyseal growth, leg length discrepancies in juvenile rheumatoid arthritis, inherited muscular diseases, and other unusual bone diseases such as Ollier disease. He published the textbook *Pediatric Orthopedic Deformities: Basic Science Diagnosis, and Treatment* in 2002 (953 pages), which was republished later as *Pediatric Orthopedic Deformities*—the first volume in 2016 and the second in 2019 (volume 3 has not yet been published), which together come in at more than 1600 pages. Dennis Wenger, in his review of Shapiro's book in 2003, noted that despite "its special focus," students of pediatric orthopaedics would do well to begin their studies with a text like Shapiro's, with its wide coverage of the basic science of orthopaedic conditions in children.

With more than 40 years of clinical experience, Shapiro has been head of the New England

Box 27.5. Frederic Shapiro's Research and Teaching Appointments

Children's Hospital

- Research assistant, Orthopaedic Research Laboratory (1976–1981)
- Research associate in the Laboratory for the Study of Skeletal Disorders/Orthopaedic Research Laboratory (1982–1997)
- Research associate in the Orthopaedic Research Laboratory (since 1988)

Harvard Medical School

- Instructor in orthopaedic surgery, 1976
- Assistant professor of orthopaedic surgery, 1981
- Associate professor of orthopaedic surgery, 1988

Muscular Dystrophy Association Clinic Directors; a member of the Duchenne Muscular Dystrophy Care Considerations Working Group and the head of their Orthopaedic Management Group; and a member of the International Standard of Care Committee for Congenital Myopathies, heading up that committee's Orthopaedic/Rehabilitation Management Group. In 2007, he participated with other orthopaedic surgeons at the Osteogenesis Imperfecta Foundation's sixth annual meeting on "Clinical Care Strategies in Osteogenesis Imperfecta."

His overall average patient rating has been excellent: he continually receives five-star reviews. He has received three patient care awards from the health care database company Vitals: the Patient Choice Award (in 2008, 2009, 2011, 2012, and 2014), the Compassionate Doctor Recognition award (in 2012 and 2014), and the On-Time Doctor Award (in 2014). In 1993, Shapiro won the Arthur H. Huene Award from the Pediatric Orthopaedic Society of North America, which is given to "an outstanding researcher for excellence and promise in pediatric orthopedics" (POSNA website), and, in 1995, along with his coauthors, he received the John

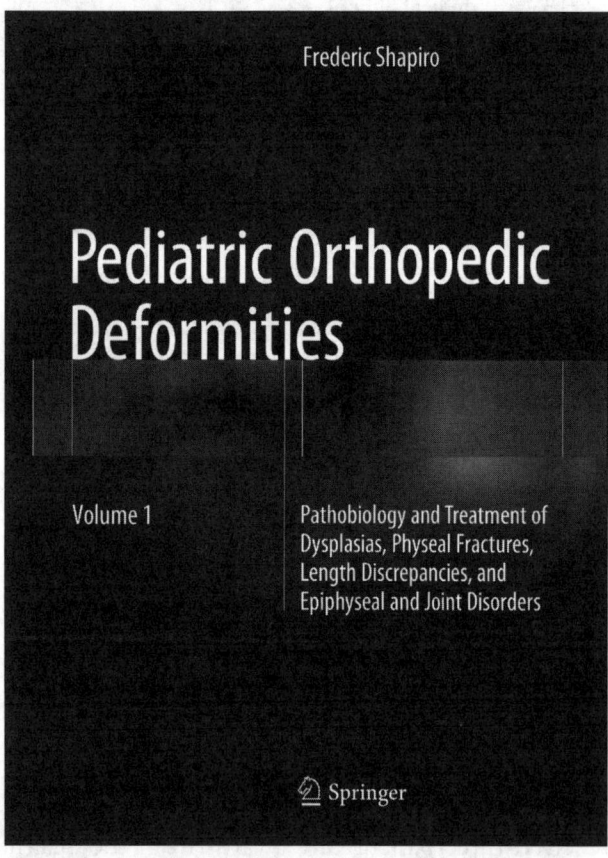

Title of Shapiro, Simon, and Glimcher's article, "Hereditary Multiple Exostoses." *Journal of Bone and Joint Surgery* 1979; 61: 815.

Cover, *Pediatric Orthopedic Deformities*, Volume 1. Courtesy of Springer Nature.

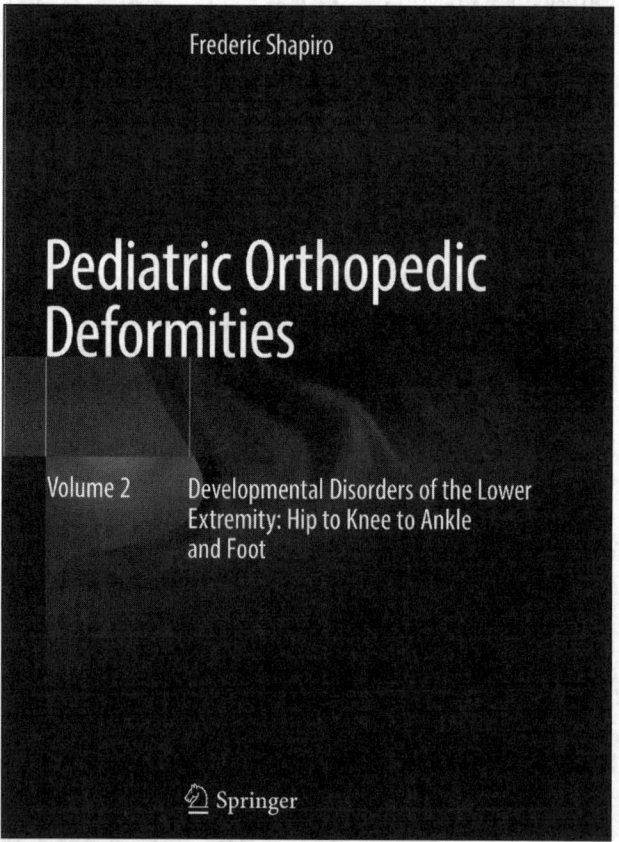

Title of Shapiro and Specht's article on diagnosing and treating inherited muscle diseases. *Journal of Bone and Joint Surgery* 1993; 75: 439.

Cover, *Pediatric Orthopedic Deformities*, Volume 2. Courtesy of Springer Nature.

Caffey Award from the Society for Pediatric Radiology for the paper titled "Evaluation of Perfusion of the Normal and Ischemic Cartilaginous Epiphysis by Using Gadolinium-enhanced MR Imaging."

Shapiro is certified by the American Board of Orthopaedic Surgery and is a fellow of the American Academy of Orthopaedic Surgeons and the Royal College of Surgeons of Canada, and a member of the Pediatric Orthopaedic Society of North America and the American Society for Bone and Mineral Research. He served as a consulting editor for research for the *Journal of Bone and Joint Surgery* (1986–2001) and was on the editorial board of the *Journal of Calcified Tissue International* (2000–2004). From 1997 to 2002, he served on the medical advisory board of the Ollier/Maffucci Self-Help Group.

Sandy Ho, a patient with osteogenesis imperfecta who received care at Children's Hospital, wrote in her blog about being treated by Shapiro:

> Having a care team that knows what has worked for me in the past (and what hasn't) matters a lot...Dr. Frederic Shapiro has been my orthopedic doctor and go-to-guy ever since birth. My family and I have tried many times to play the "guess how old Dr. Shapiro is?" game, but no one really knows. The point being, I dread that day when he tells me he is going to retire...Will Dr. Shapiro's replacement be as flexible about how and when we communicate[?]...But as much as I love Dr. Shapiro and Boston Children's, I can't deny that there are parts of me that required adult health care at this point...I appreciate the friendly nudging [by my health care team] into the boring world of adult hospitals...I will miss the sounds, noise, colors and clowns of Boston Children's...[but] part of being an adult means doing what's right for you, even it's not the easiest option...I'll get there eventually...I just wish I could take Dr. Shapiro with me.
>
> —Sandy Ho
> "What Will Happen When My Doctor Retires?" 2012

SHELDON R. SIMON

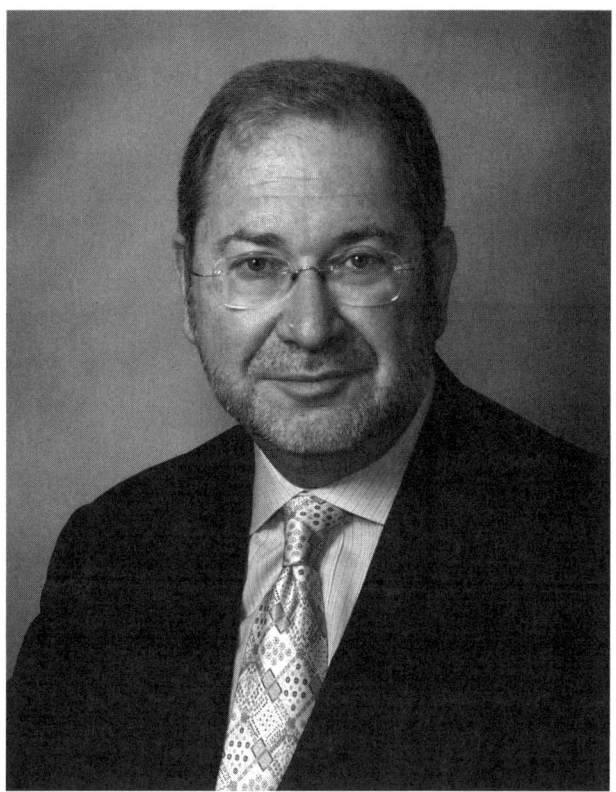

Sheldon R. Simon. Courtesy of Dr. Sheldon Simon/Mount Sinai Health System.

Physician Snapshot

Sheldon R. Simon
BORN: 1941
DIED: —
SIGNIFICANT CONTRIBUTIONS: Led the first modern gait laboratory at Boston Children's Hospital

Sheldon R. Simon was born August 19, 1941, and raised in Brooklyn, New York. He recalled that after graduating in 1962 with an engineering degree from the New York College of Engineering, he decided to apply to medical school because he had friends who did so. He attended New York University School of Medicine, graduating in 1966. During his time there, he recognized how the fields of engineering and medicine overlapped. Though his initial work in medicine dealt with heart valves, he eventually became interested in orthopaedics. Following an internship at the New

Simon et al. article titled, "Genu Recurvatum in Spastic Cerebral Palsy." *Journal of Bone and Joint Surgery* 1978; 60: 882.

The Frank Stinchfield Award paper: "Internal Rotation Gait in Spastic Cerebral Palsy." *Hip* 1982; 89.

York Bellevue Hospital Medical Center, he spent an additional year there as a resident in general surgery, finishing in 1968.

In an interview he gave when he was inducted into the Hall of Fellows of the Rehabilitation Engineering and Assistive Technology Society of North America, Simon recalled, "Melvin Glimcher, MD, recruited me into the orthopaedic program at Harvard. He believed my engineering skills could be effectively applied to orthopaedics." Simon began his orthopaedic residency at the Massachusetts General Hospital in September 1968. After his first year as an assistant resident, he became a research fellow, spending another year at MGH under the supervision of Glimcher. He spent nine months (October 1970 through June 1971) as an assistant resident in orthopaedics at Children's Hospital, after which he returned to MGH. He spent the next two years as assistant resident and resident there, finishing on June 30, 1973. He then spent six months as chief resident at the West Roxbury Veterans Administration Hospital, completing his training there on December 31, 1973.

In April 1972, through a traveling fellowship with the AO Foundation Simon visited Professor Martin Allgöwer, in Basel, Switzerland, for a six-week elective rotation to study the Swiss method of surgically treating fractures. Simon also received a Cave Traveling Fellowship, which he spent analyzing gait at Rancho Los Amigos Hospital and Shriners Hospital for Crippled Children in San Francisco.

After Simon completed his training and traveling fellowships, Glimcher hired him as an assistant in orthopaedic surgery at Children's Hospital and Harvard Medical School. He also received a faculty appointment as visiting associate in the Department of Mechanical Engineering at MIT. Glimcher funded a gait laboratory ($100,000) for Simon at Children's Hospital; today that lab works directly with the hospital's Cerebral Palsy and Spasticity Center, "using multiple cameras to measure gait-pattern abnormalities and determine the most appropriate treatments" for the center's patients ("Cerebral Palsy and Spasticity Center" 2020). In 1978, Simon published his first paper on cerebral palsy based on data from his gait laboratory, a study of spastic patients with genu recurvatum. In 1979, he published two papers on gait analysis in patients who had ankle surgery (either arthrodesis or total ankle replacement). Simon recalled that William Berenberg, chief of the Cerebral Palsy Clinic at Children's in the 1970s, helped Simon deepen his knowledge of neuromuscular disorders and had an important role in establishing the Rehabilitation Engineering Research Center, a collaboration between Harvard and MIT.

During the next 13 years, which Simon spent as a full-time faculty member at Children's Hospital and Harvard Medical School, he published ~35 papers on orthopaedics and biomechanics. His first articles, published in 1973 and cowritten with Drs. Eric Radin (Simon's colleague at Children's and

Harvard), Igor Paul, and Robert Rose (the latter two, both professors of mechanical engineering at MIT), focused on impact loading and friction and wear of total hip prostheses. Using a simulator, they demonstrated that metal/polyethylene prostheses had a lower coefficient of friction and, therefore, a lessened tendency for loosening with 1,000 hours of walking, than did metal-on-metal prostheses. Overall, he published nine publications about various biomechanical aspects of the hip and hip replacement prostheses.

In all, he has published 21 articles on normal and abnormal gait. One of these, titled "Internal Rotation Gait in Spastic Cerebral Palsy," which Simon cowrote with C. Tylkowski and J. Mansour, was awarded the Frank Stinchfield Award in 1982 by the Hip Society.

Simon has been active clinically throughout his career, and in addition to cerebral palsy he has focused his attention on foot and ankle problems in both children (at Boston Children's Hospital) and adults (at Brigham and Women's Hospital). In one 1987 study of abnormal gait in children who were learning to walk, funded by the shoemaking company Stride Rite, he found that those children who wore flexible shoes with a leather sole were more stable and experienced fewer falls than did the children who wore sneakers.

Simon's research has been funded by grants from the National Institutes of Health and other government agencies, as well as various industry players including the United Cerebral Palsy Research and Education Foundation, the Orthopaedic Research & Education Foundation, the Hearst Foundation, and the Orthopaedic Research & Education Foundation. He is certified by the American Board of Orthopaedic Surgery and is a fellow of the American Academy of Orthopaedic Surgeons. Various of his other memberships and awards are listed in **Box 27.6**.

Simon left Boston Children's Hospital and Harvard Medical School in 1986, when he accepted the position of chief of the Division of Orthopaedics in the Department of Surgery at the Ohio State University School of Medicine. He also was appointed as an adjunct professor with the Graduate Faculty of Industrial and Systems Engineering at Ohio State, and he served on the board of directors of the Ohio State University for Ergonomics. He remained chief for 12 years, leaving in 1998. (The following year the Division of Orthopaedics became an independent

Box 27.6. Sheldon Simon's Various Memberships and Honors and Awards

Professional Roles

- Member, Pediatric Orthopaedic Society of North America
- Member, American Foot and Ankle Society.
- Member, National Institutes of Health Orthopedic Study Section
- Member, American Orthopaedic Association
- Chairman, Easter Seals Research Board
- Chairman, AAOS Basic Science Committee

Honors and Awards

- Isabelle and Leonard H. Goldenson Award for Research in Medicine and Technology Relating to Cerebral Palsy, from the United Cerebral Palsy Research and Education Foundation
- Visiting professor and guest speaker, European Symposium on Clinical Gait Analysis
- Founding member in 1979 of the Rehabilitation Engineering Society of North America (RESNA), and past treasurer and president
- Member of the American Institute for Medical and Biological Engineering (1992) Named in 2004 as one of America's Top Physicians by the Consumer Research Council of America
- Received in 2008 the Lifetime Member Award from the Cambridge Who's Who Registry of Executives, Professionals and Entrepreneurs

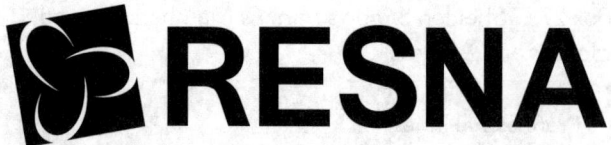

Logo of the Rehabilitation Engineering and Assistive Technology Society of North America (RESNA). Courtesy of RESNA.

department.) While at Ohio State, Simon published ~14 papers, seven of which discussed gait, for example, after total knee replacement, in obese men, in patients with low back disorders, and in those who had experienced stroke. At this time, he was publishing more on adult clinical problems than children's issues.

In 1999, Simon moved to New York, where he took up the positions of professor of clinical orthopaedic surgery at Albert Einstein College of Medicine and division chief of pediatric orthopaedics in the Department of Orthopaedics and Sports Medicine at Beth Israel Medical Center, where he continues to practice today. He is also an adjunct professor of orthopaedic surgery at the New York Downstate Medical Center, division chief of pediatric orthopedics at Long Island College Hospital in Brooklyn, and director of the Gait Analysis Laboratory at the Stanley S. Lamm Institute for Developmental Disabilities at Long Island College Hospital. He is on the staff of many hospitals in the New York area and has served as president of the medical board of the Beth Israel Medical Center.

He continues to publish on gait, though less so since his move to New York. His work since 2000 includes an article on the biomechanical and metabolic effects of backpack loads while marching. In 2004, Simon published a paper about the benefits and limitations of gait analysis in clinical problems. In it, he acknowledged technological developments that have allowed kinesiology to advance, but he lamented the lack of gait analysis within clinical settings, noting that this lack likely is a result of the expense of equipment and the time required to evaluate such analyses. For Simon, in order to resolve such issues and increase the clinical use of gait analysis, technology must continue to evolve and engineers and clinicians must better connect.

The Rehabilitation Engineering and Assistive Technology Society of North America (RESNA) (founded in 1979) provides on its website a biography of each of its fellows, who are selected on the basis of their work in advancing assistive technology and in furthering the efforts of RESNA. Simon (along with Dr. William Berenberg, of Boston Children's Hospital, and Dr. Robert E. Toom, a Tennessee orthopaedist) was elected into the RESNA Hall of Fellows in 1989. He eventually served as president of RESNA in 1986. In the online RESNA Hall of Fellows, Simon described the importance of his work:

> My work in human motion and gait analysis has been important in order to make sense of the treatments we were using. There was no biomechanical basis for many of the treatments we were using and no objective ways of measuring results. I have focused my work primarily in gait analysis and the clinical problems of gait of neuromuscular and orthopaedic disorders...
>
> I believe the greatest successes have been the number of engineers who received PhDs through our programs...The application of computer science, statistics, and artificial intelligence to the problems of gait analysis have been major contributions. We developed sophisticated computer programs...[putting] the science of gait analysis on a solid foundation, bringing it into the electronic and computing age. I contributed to the commercialization of motion analysis systems with the Vicon system. We also contributed to the ability to merge additional data with the gait data such as the EMG. I also contributed to the development of the AMT force plate.
>
> I was the only medical doctor among the original founders of RESNA.

BRIAN D. SNYDER

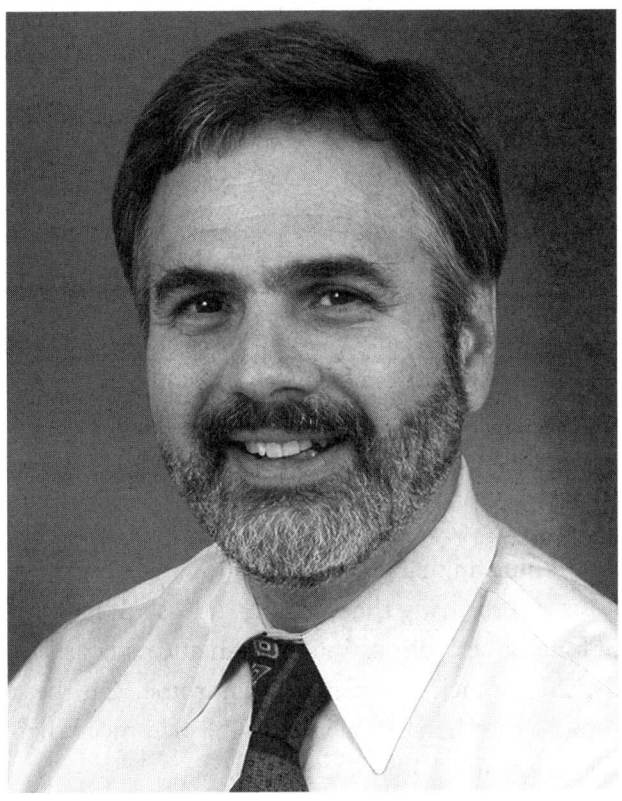

Brian D. Snyder. James Koepfler/Boston Children's Hospital.

Physician Snapshot

Brian D. Snyder
BORN: 1957
DIED: —
SIGNIFICANT CONTRIBUTIONS: Clinician-scientist investigating biomechanics of bone; established criteria for predicting fracture risk in benign neoplasms of bone and bone metastases using quantitative CT-based rigidity analysis (CTRA)

Brian Dale Snyder was born in 1957 in Philadelphia, Pennsylvania, where he received most of his education. He completed a BS degree in bioengineering at the University of Pennsylvania in 1980, followed by a MS degree in 1982. After graduating with an MD degree from Penn in 1986, he completed his PhD degree in biomechanics (1991) there and in the National Institutes of Health Medical Scientist Training Program during his orthopaedic residency.

In 1986, Snyder moved from Philadelphia to Boston, where he has remained since. After a surgical internship on the Harvard 5th Surgical Service at the New England Deaconess Hospital, he completed the Harvard Combined Orthopaedic Residency Program (1988–92). In 1992, he was chief resident in orthopaedic surgery at the Brigham and Women's Hospital, then was a fellow in pediatric orthopaedics at Children's Hospital (1993–94). As a National Institutes of Health research fellow in 1985 and 1987 at the Orthopaedic Biomechanics Laboratory (headed by Toby Hayes, PhD), Snyder completed his research for his PhD thesis, "Multiaxial Structure-Property Relationships in Trabecular Bone." He presented his thesis to Penn's Department of Biomedical Engineering on April 24, 1991.

Upon completing his clinical training, Snyder remained on staff at Children's Hospital, as an attending physician, and was appointed instructor in orthopaedic surgery at Harvard Medical School. He also currently holds hospital appointments at the Franciscan Children's Hospital (since 1993), Brigham and Women's Hospital (an associate position since 1994), Beth Israel Deaconess Medical Center (a member of the courtesy staff since 1995), the Massachusetts Hospital School (on the consulting staff since 2003), and St. Elizabeth's Hospital (on the affiliate staff since 2005). At Harvard Medical School, he was promoted to assistant professor in 1999, associate professor in 2007, and full professor in 2015.

In his curriculum vitae, updated in 2015, Snyder stated:

> I am...director of the Cerebral Palsy Clinic at Children's Hospital where my practice focuses on musculoskeletal deformity related to neuromuscular diseases affecting the spine, hip and appendicular skeleton...[My] laboratory is a multi-disciplinary core research facility associated with the Harvard Medical School, the Harvard Combined Orthopaedic Residency Program, and the Departments of

Bioengineering at Harvard University, Massachusetts Institute of Technology and Boston University Graduate School of Engineering... My work has focused on improving the practice of orthopaedic surgery by applying quantitative engineering analysis to clinical problems. I have been the principal investigator of NIH/NCI/NIAMS ROI, NIH/NIAMS R21, NASA, DOD, and numerous private foundations (Whitaker, OREF, Susan B. Komen, AO/ASIF, Coulter, POSNA, SRS) as well as industry sponsored grants.

He also describes in his curriculum vitae the focus of his research to date:

My applied research that has led to several clinical innovations has focused on the biomechanics of the musculoskeletal system including: 1) characterizing bone structure property relationships; 2) predicting and preventing pathologic fractures as a consequence of metabolic bone diseases, benign or metastatic neoplasms; 3) development contract-enhanced, quantitative CT arthrography to non-invasively evaluate the biochemical and biomechanical properties of hyaline cartilage using anionic and cationic iodinated contrast agents that function as mobile ionic probes; 4) creating an animal model of early onset scoliosis to parametrically evaluate the effect of expansion thoracoplasty on the growth and development of the spine, thorax and lungs for treating thoracic insufficiency syndrome...5) developing a portable, dual probe, ultrasound system to measure the static and dynamic mechanical properties of cervical spine functional spine units...to identify occupational related causes of degenerative spine disease in subjects performing work place activities.

Snyder is productive in clinical research and in performing clinical trials and numerous basic research activities in the laboratory, including

> **PREDICTING FRACTURE THROUGH BENIGN SKELETAL LESIONS WITH QUANTITATIVE COMPUTED TOMOGRAPHY**
> By Brian D. Snyder, MD, PhD, Diana A. Hauser-Kara, PhD, John A. Hipp, PhD, David Zurakowski, PhD, Andrew C. Hecht, MD, and Mark C. Gebhardt, MD
> *Investigation performed at Children's Hospital and the Orthopaedic Biomechanics Laboratory, Beth Israel Deaconess Medical Center, Boston, Massachusetts*
> The Journal of Bone & Joint Surgery · JBJS.ORG
> Volume 88-A · Number 1 · January 2006

Snyder et al. article describing a method of using quantitative CT to predict fracture risk in benign bone lesions.
Journal of Bone and Joint Surgery 2006; 88: 55.

developing animal models to study early-onset scoliosis and studying the strength and risk of fracture of long bones, lubrication in traumatic osteoarthritis, the thoracic insufficiency syndrome. On these topics and others, Snyder has published more than 75 papers and 10 book chapters.

In 2006, he was the lead author on a paper titled "Predicting Fracture through Benign Skeletal Lesions with Quantitative Computed Tomography." At the time several different risk factors for fracture had been reported, including lesions with a diameter larger than 2.5 cm and destruction of more than 50% of the bone's cortex. Snyder and his coauthors (2006) found that the literature that reported those risk factors contained "large errors in estimating the load-bearing capacity of the affected bone." They concluded that "the combination of the ratios of bending and torsional rigidities as determined with computed tomography-based structural analysis of... affected and normal bones provides a sensitive [100%] and specific [94%] method for accurately predicting fracture risk in children with a variety of benign neoplasms of the skeleton" (Snyder et al. 2006). They also demonstrated that quantitative computed tomography "was more accurate (97%) for predicting pathologic fracture through benign bone lesions in children than were standard radiographic criteria (42% to 61% accuracy)" (Snyder et al. 2006). As a result of that study, quantitative "CT based rigidity analysis (CTRA)...is now used routinely at Boston Children's Hospital to assess children with benign neoplasms...[that] require surgical stabilization" (Snyder 2015).

With these biomechanical guidelines in place, Snyder and his colleagues completed a prospective clinical trial, published as "Computed Tomography-Based Structural Analysis for Predicting Fracture Risk in Children with Benign Skeletal Neoplasms" in 2010. They studied 41 patients and concluded that "quantitative computed tomography-based rigidity analysis is more specific (97% specificity) than criteria based on plain radiographs [in lesions involving more than 50% of the cortex] (12% specificity) for predicting the risk of a pathologic fracture...[and that] indices based on lesion size alone fail to account for the compensatory remodeling of the host bone that occurs in response to the presence of the lesion in a growing child" (Leong et al. 2010).

A year earlier, Snyder et al. had published a paper on fracture risk in patients with metastatic breast disease, "Noninvasive Prediction of Fracture Risk in Patients with Metastatic Cancer to the Spine." They evaluated 94 patients in a prospective observational study to determine the effectiveness of CTRA in predicting vertebral fractures. They concluded that, when compared with standard x-ray criteria, CTRA had similar sensitivity but was significantly more specific for predicting vertebral fractures. Using specified thresholds, the authors continued to investigate predictive factors in a larger multicenter study. Published in 2015, the study included 124 patients. At follow-up they found that seven fractures occurred among patients who did not receive fixation, CTRA was sensitive (100%) and specific (90%) in predicting these fractures—much more so than the Mirels' method, which was [based on location, pain, and lesion type and size]. On the basis of these results, they suggested that CTRA might be beneficial in screening for pathologic fractures. Snyder and his colleagues received the 2004 Ann Doner Vaughn Kappa Delta Award for their work on predicting the risk of fracture in patients with metastatic disease to the skeleton.

Snyder's other significant contributions include work on contrast-enhanced computed tomography of cartilage, joint lubrication, neuromuscular scoliosis, classification of early-onset scoliosis, use of growing rods, and other clinical problems such as progeria, cerebral palsy, fractures, and slipped femoral capital epiphysis. His recent interests include the use of platelet-rich plasma in an animal model of ACL injury and the use of stem cells to produce bonelike tissue.

Snyder has also received other awards, including the Russell Hibbs Award for outstanding basic science research, from the Scoliosis Research Society, and the A. Clifford Bayer Excellence in Mentoring Award from Harvard Medical School, which he received for overseeing 35 predoctoral and 13 postdoctoral trainees in his biomechanics

---

Computed Tomography-Based Structural Analysis for Predicting Fracture Risk in Children with Benign Skeletal Neoplasms

Comparison of Specificity with That of Plain Radiographs

By Natalie L. Leong, BS, Megan E. Anderson, MD, Mark C. Gebhardt, MD, and Brian D. Snyder, MD, PhD

Investigation performed at the Department of Orthopedic Surgery, Children's Hospital Boston, Boston, Massachusetts

Leong et al. article reporting the results of a prospective clinical trial, comparing quantitative CT to plain radiographs, in predicting fracture risk in children with benign bone lesions. *Journal of Bone and Joint Surgery* 2010; 92: 1827.

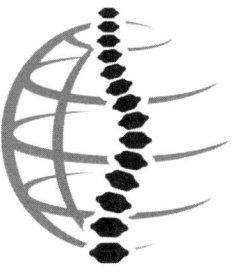

Logo Scoliosis Research Society (SRS). Courtesy of SRS.

laboratory at Beth Israel Deaconess Medical Center.

Active in numerous National Institutes of Health/National Institute of Arthritis and Musculoskeletal and Skin Diseases study sections, he is also a member of the Small Business Orthopaedic and Skeletal Biology panel and a current member of the Tissue Engineering Study panel. He is active in many professional societies, including the Orthopaedic Research Society, acting as program chairman in 2015; and the American Academy of Orthopaedic Surgeons, where he serves on the Research Committee of the Board of Specialty Societies and is their designee to the Orthopaedic Device Forum. He has served on the US Food and Drug Administration's pediatric clinical trials panel, on the medical advisory committee for the Families of Spinal Muscular Atrophy, and as a member of the advisory board of the University of Pennsylvania's Department of Bioengineering. He holds two patents on modular spinal instrumentation devices.

SANDRA J. THOMPSON

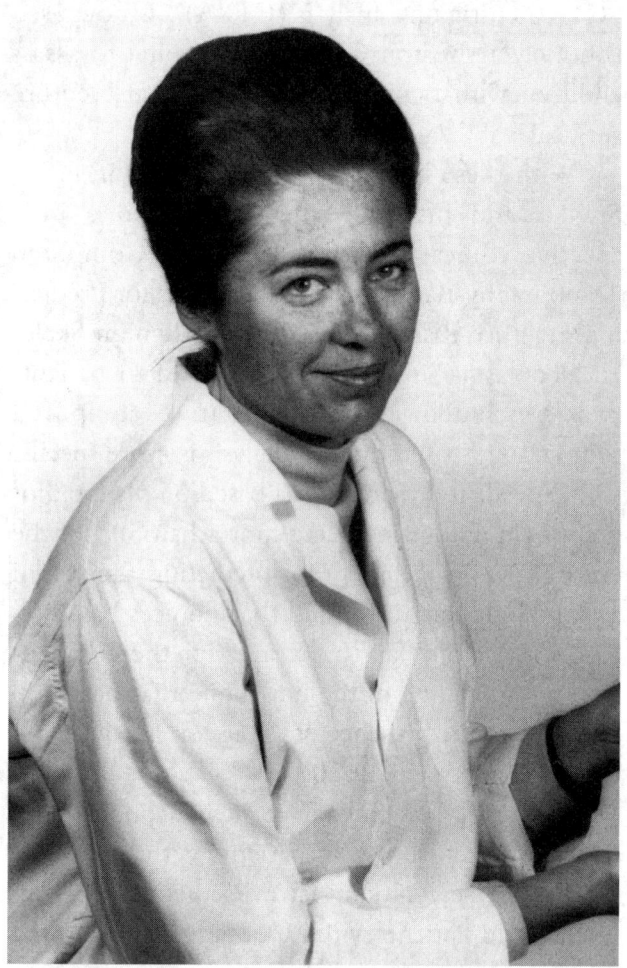

Sandra J. Thompson. Boston Children's Hospital Archives, Boston, Massachusetts.

Physician Snapshot

Sandra J. Thompson
BORN: ca. 1937
DIED: 2003
SIGNIFICANT CONTRIBUTIONS: Founding member of the Ruth Jackson Orthopaedic Society

Born in Boston, Sandra J. Thompson was raised in Osterville, in the town of Barnstable along the Nantucket Sound. She attended Newton College of the Sacred Heart, graduating in 1958, and then the Women's Medical College of Pennsylvania, graduating in 1962.

After an internship at the Boston City Hospital, she trained in orthopaedic surgery at the

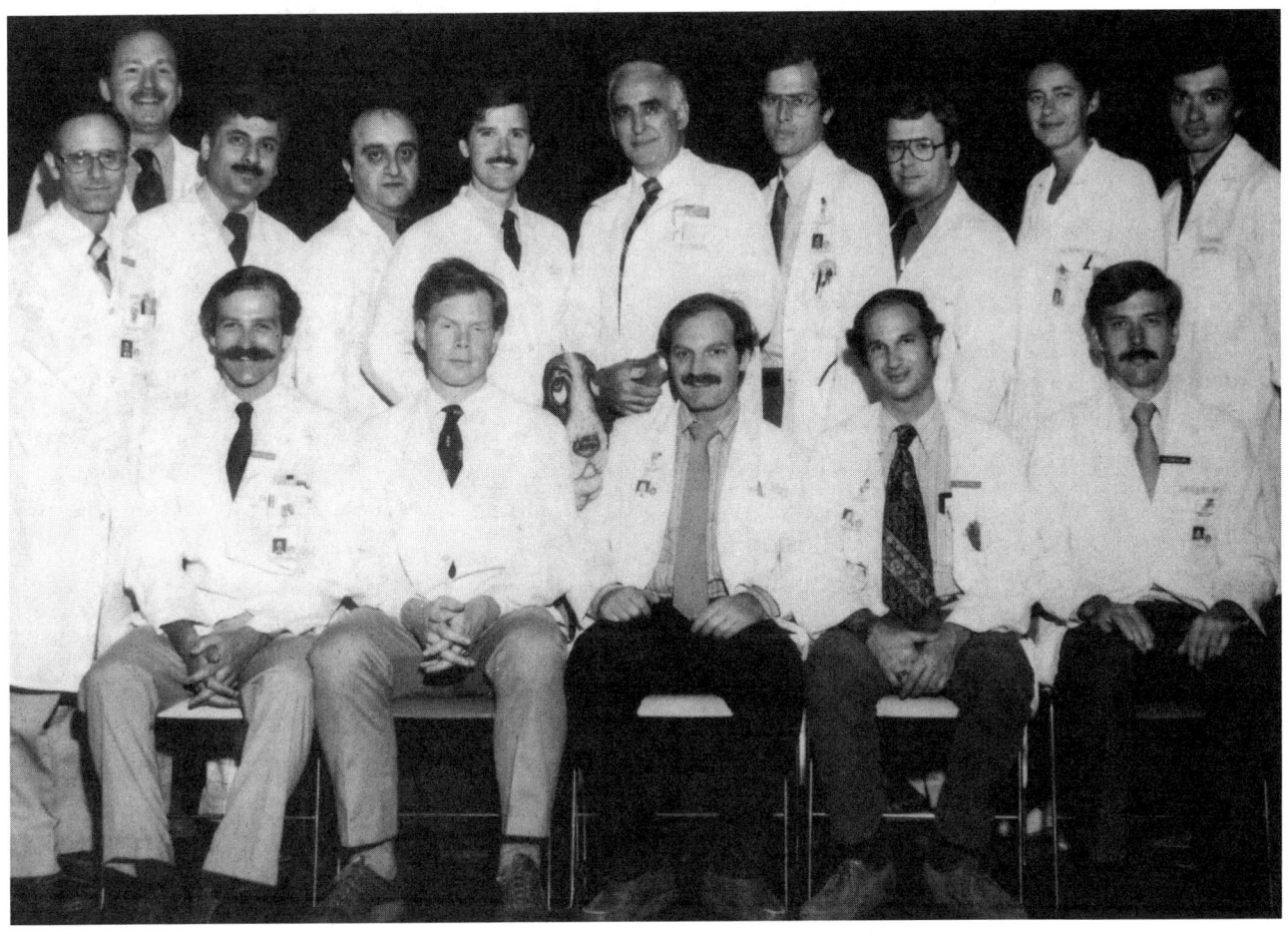

Residents at Boston Children's Hospital with Dr. Hall. Sandra Thompson is standing in the back row, second from the right.
MGH HCORP Archives.

Lahey Clinic. She received further training in pediatric orthopaedics, and in 1969 she became an assistant in orthopaedic surgery at the Children's Hospital Medical Center in Boston. She took a fellowship at the Institute for Children with Thalidomide Induced Limb Deformation in Germany in 1971.

Thompson remained on the orthopaedic staff at the Children's Hospital Medical Center, eventually becoming an associate in orthopaedic surgery. She also took a position as assistant clinical professor at the Harvard Medical School's Laboratory for Skeletal Disorders and Rehabilitation. She staffed both the arthritis clinic and the prosthetic clinic with Dr. Paul Griffin (chapter 26).

Thompson gave anatomy lectures at Simmons College and lectures on special education at Boston College during the 1970s. She took numerous groups of students to Haiti on "humanitarian missions." A friend noted that "'it wasn't in Dr. Thompson's nature…to call attention to work there. She would be very understated about it… She would consider it inappropriate to say, look at what I've done'" (quoted in Krauss 2003).

In 1983, Thompson became a founding member of the Ruth Jackson Orthopaedic Society, whose purpose is to "promote professional development of and for women in orthopaedics throughout all stages of their careers" (Ruth Jackson Orthopaedic Society 2019), with a focus on four strategic domains: professional development, membership, research, and organizational excellence. She was certified by the American Board of Orthopaedic Surgery, was a fellow of the American

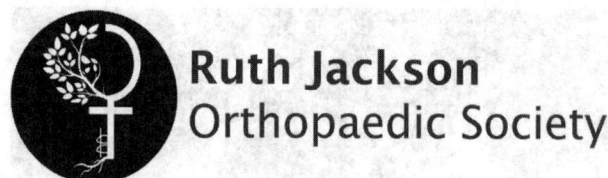

Logo Ruth Jackson Orthopaedic Society. Courtesy of Ruth Jackson Orthopaedic Society.

Academy of Orthopaedic Surgeons and the American Academy of Pediatrics and was active through the member relations committee of Bay State Health Care.

Thompson served as a trustee at Boston College from 1977 to 1985. She was reappointed to that role in 1988, along with such notable figures as Peter Lynch, a senior vice president at Fidelity Investments, and Warren Rudman, a Republican junior senator from New Hampshire.

One of Thompson's longtime friends, Maureen Riley, recalled that Thompson "was always going to be a surgeon" and that she "devoted her life to children" (quoted in Krauss 2003). She was a specialist in pediatric rehabilitation, working closely with disabled children until she retired in the 1990s. She was greatly attached to Cape Cod, and she spent much time at her residence in her hometown of Osterville.

In 2003, Thompson was at home in Brookline when she died of heart failure. She was 66 years old. Although her obituary notes that she published widely on subjects such as amputation and pediatric surgery, I was unable to find any such publications.

PETER WATERS

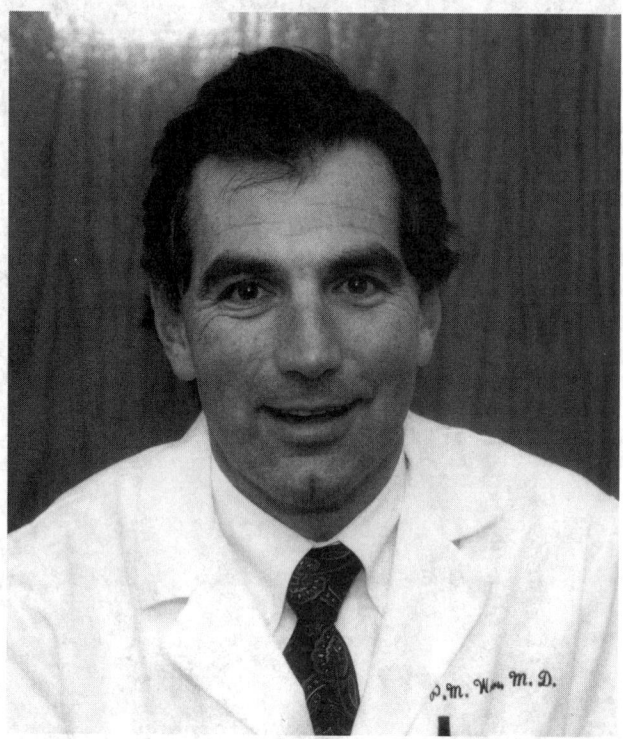

Peter Waters. Boston Children's Hospital Archives, Boston, Massachusetts.

Physician Snapshot

Peter Waters
BORN: 1955
DIED: —

SIGNIFICANT CONTRIBUTIONS: Defined anatomical changes in the humeral head and glenoid from birth palsies using new imaging technologies; described a method for classifying these deformities

Peter M. Waters was born in Syracuse, New York, in 1955. His father was a pediatric hematologist and oncologist, and Peter planned early to follow his father with a career in pediatrics. He graduated summa cum laude from Tufts University in 1977, and he received an MD degree from Tufts University Medical School in 1981. True to his original career plans, he entered the pediatric residency program at Massachusetts General Hospital. He completed two years of the program, but he found instead that his "life path" lay in pediatric hand surgery. After a year of surgical training at the Santa Barbara Cottage Hospital, he entered the Harvard Combined Orthopaedic Residency Program in 1984. In 1988, he was chief resident at Boston Children's Hospital, and then he completed a year-long (1988–89) fellowship in hand and upper extremity surgery at the Brigham and Women's Hospital and Children's Hospital.

Waters began his academic career at Children's Hospital and Harvard after his training and has since remained affiliated with both institutions; **Box 27.7** outlines his career track at each institution.

Waters has been very active at Children's Hospital—serving on numerous committees, on the board of directors of the Pediatric Physicians' Organization, and as chair of the Standardized Clinical Assessment and Management Plan executive committee—and in many professional organizations (**Box 27.8**). He's given numerous lectures, held a number of visiting professorships, and has taken an active role as an educator (**Box 27.8**). He has also received several awards: the Richard Kilfoyle Award in 1994, given by the New England Orthopaedic Society for the best paper on clinical practice written by a resident; the Robert Salter Award (1995), given by the Pediatric Orthopaedic Society for excellence in orthopaedic education; and the Sumner Koch Award (2014), given by the American Society for Surgery of the Hand for outstanding research.

Clinical Research in Birth Palsies

Waters has published more than 150 articles—mainly in clinical research related to trauma in the hand and upper extremity in children (>100 articles) and to the brachial plexus (22 articles). He's also published four books and written more than 55 book chapters.

Following in the footsteps of Drs. James Sever, Robert Lovett, and William Green at Children's Hospital, and Dr. J. H. Stevens at Tufts and Harvard, Waters has made major contributions to the understanding of the pathophysiology, treatment, outcomes, function, and classification of brachial plexus birth palsies.

Research on birth palsies began in the late nineteenth century. In 1918, Sever reported the results of a procedure for soft-tissue release (named after him) in patients with brachial plexus birth palsies. In contrast to Dr. Fairbank, who in 1913 reported his method of releasing the subscapularis and the anterior capsule together, Sever released the pectoralis major and subscapularis, but left the shoulder capsule intact. He reported observing more severe contractures after the shoulder capsule was released anteriorly. He also wrote that he had not observed any posterior dislocations, but he noted later, in 1925, that some older babies had a

Box 27.7. Waters' Career Path

At Children's Hospital

- Associate in orthopaedic surgery (1989–2007)
- Associate chief of orthopaedics (2007–2008)
- Clinical chief of orthopaedics (2008–2013)
- Orthopaedic Surgeon-in-Chief (replacing Dr. James Kasser in 2013)

At Harvard Medical School

- Instructor in orthopaedic surgery (1989–93)
- Assistant professor (1993–99)
- Associate professor (1999–2005)
- Co-director (with Dr. Barry Simmons) of the Harvard Hand Surgery Fellowship (1999–2004)
- Professor (2005–2009)
- Named the John E. Hall Professor of Orthopaedic Surgery in 2009

At Other Institutions

- Assistant in orthopaedic surgery at Brigham and Women's Hospital, Faulkner Hospital, New England Baptist Hospital, and Beth Israel Deaconess Medical Center

Box 27.8. Waters's Lectures and His Roles in Professional Organizations

Visiting Professorships and Named Lectures

- Bertrich Memorial Lecture (Albany Medical College)
- John Banta Lecture (Connecticut's Children's Medical Center)
- Lee Ramsay Straub Lecture (Hospital for Special Surgery)
- Wavering Lecture (Northwestern University)
- Ochsner Memorial Lecture (Robert Wood Johnson Medical School)
- Crawford Campbell Annual Lecture (Albany Medical Center, Albany, NY)
- Robert Salter Visiting Professor (The Hospital for Sick Children, Toronto)
- 33rd John C. Wilson Sr. Visiting Professor (Children's Hospital, Los Angeles, CA),
- Smith Day Orator (Massachusetts General Hospital)
- Brandon Carrell Visiting Professor (Texas Scottish Rite Hospital)
- Jesse T. Nicholson Visiting Professor (Children's Hospital of Philadelphia)
- Neil Green Lecture (Vanderbilt University)
- Carroll B. Larson Lecture (University of Iowa)
- Annual Burton Professor (University of Rochester)
- Henry B. Lacey Visiting Professor (Nationwide Children's Hospital, Columbus, Ohio)
- Stromberg Memorial Lecture (Chicago Society for Surgery of Hand)
- Integra Visiting Professor (University of Michigan)

Professional Organizations / Leadership Positions

- Chair of the Program Committee (1999) and the Basic Science Research Committee, American Society for Surgery of the Hand
- President, Pediatric Orthopaedic Society of North America Board of Directors (2011–12)

Roles as an Active Educator

- Contributor to Instructional Course Lectures, the Summer Institute, the Comprehensive Review Course, and annual meeting symposia for the American Academy of Orthopaedic Surgeons
- Lectured in the regional review courses and instructions courses for the American Society for Surgery of the Hand
- Lectured at international pediatric orthopaedic symposia
- Member of the International Pediatric Orthopaedic Think Tank

Memberships

- 20th Century Orthopaedic Association
- American Bone and Joint Surgeons
- American Orthopaedic Association
- Boston Hand Club
- Boston Orthopaedic Club
- Certificate of Added Qualifications (CAQ) in Surgery of the Hand (2005–2006)
- Interurban Orthopaedic Society
- Irish American Orthopaedic Society
- Kiros Hand Research Society (a nonprofit organization that awards research grants)
- Massachusetts Medical Society
- Massachusetts Orthopaedic Association
- New England Hand Society
- New England Hand Surgery Study Group (1994–98)
- Pediatric Orthopaedic Society of North America
- Pediatric Orthopedic Society

flattened glenoid fossa associated with a posterior subluxation.

In 1934—16 years after Sever's paper had been published—Dr. Joseph L'Episcopo reported a modification of Sever's procedure, the goal of which was to restore muscle balance in the shoulder. In addition to anteriorly releasing the pectoralis major and subscapularis tendon, he also released the anterior capsule of the glenohumeral joint. Posteriorly, he released the latissimus dorsi and teres major tendons, and then transferred them to the posterolateral aspect of the proximal humerus, making them external rotators rather than internal rotators of the shoulder.

After another 30 years, in 1963, Drs. William Green and Mihran Tachdjian reported another modification of the Sever procedure/L'Episcopo's operation: Z-lengthening of the pectoralis major and latissimus dorsi, release of the subscapularis, and transfer of the latissimus dorsi and teres major to a cleft in the proximal lateral humerus. I remember this as the procedure of choice at Children's Hospital, where it was called the Sever-L'Episcopo procedure. Although the date of the first use of this name is unknown, a colleague of Sever's recalls its use as early as the 1940s. In their 1963 publication, Green and Tachdjian did not give it a particular name, but simply stated that their modification was "based upon the Sever and L'Episcopo procedures" (Green and Tachdjian 1963).

Waters' first publication, written with S. Troum and W. Floyd III in 1993, described two posterior shoulder dislocations associated with a birth palsy (see **Case 27.5**). In the subsequent years, aided by new imaging techniques—computerized tomography and magnetic resonance imaging—Waters and his colleagues defined in great detail the changes that occur in the humeral head and glenoid fossa. In 1998, they reported such changes in 42 children, concluding that these imaging modalities, "as well as analysis of functional parameters, demonstrated an association between persistent palsy and glenohumeral deformity in patients who had residual functional deficits secondary to persistent brachial plexus birth palsy" (Waters, Smith, and Jaramillo 1998). They "made the point that glenohumeral deformity occurs along a spectrum of severity, with less severe changes being potentially reversible with soft-tissue joint relocation procedures" (Bennett and Allen 1999). This work by Waters et al. led to a method of classifying glenohumeral deformity by Bae and Waters based on imaging findings and the Severin classification of developmental hip dysplasia (**Table 27.1**).

Not surprisingly, since their original publications, numerous modifications of Sever's procedure, and of L'Episcopo's and Green's modifications of that procedure, have been described—as have other soft-tissue releases, transfers, and bony procedures. Treatment of brachial plexus birth palsies has evolved greatly since Sever's report

---

Brachial Plexus Birth Palsy: The Boston Children's Hospital Experience

Donald S. Bae, M.D.[1] and Peter M. Waters, M.D.[1]

Bae and Waters article describing their x-ray classification of glenohumeral deformities in brachial plexus birth palsies.
Seminars in Plastic Surgery 2004; 18:275.

Glenohumeral Deformity Secondary to Brachial Plexus Birth Palsy

BY PETER M. WATERS, M.D.†, GARTH R. SMITH, M.D.†, AND DIEGO JARAMILLO, M.D.†, BOSTON, MASSACHUSETTS

Investigation performed at Children's Hospital, Harvard Medical School, Boston

THE JOURNAL OF BONE AND JOINT SURGERY
VOL. 80-A, NO. 5, MAY 1998

Waters et al. article describing abnormalities in the humeral head and glenoid in patients with a brachial plexus palsy.
Journal of Bone and Joint Surgery 1998; 80: 668.

Case 27.5. Posterior Dislocation of the Femoral Head in an Infant with Obstetrical Paralysis

> "A female infant who had a history of a left Erb paralysis, a high birth weight, and a difficult delivery was first seen by us at the age of six months. Although the child was otherwise healthy, physical examination revealed that abduction and external rotation of the left shoulder were limited, there was a 20-degree flexion contracture of the elbow and the palm could not be brought to face upward (in a plane parallel to a transverse plane of the body) when the forearm was passively supinated maximally while the shoulder was passively flexed. The strength of the biceps brachii was normal, and the strength of the deltoid and external rotators of the shoulder was good (grade 4 of 5). Extrinsic and intrinsic muscles distal to the left forearm appeared intact. Both lower limbs and the right upper limb were normal.
>
> "Anteroposterior radiographs demonstrated hypoplasia of the left glenoid and delayed ossification of the humeral head. True lateral and axillary radiographs of the left shoulder demonstrated a posterior dislocation of the humeral head; its presence was confirmed by computerized tomographic scanning and magnetic resonance imaging. Electromyographic findings were consistent with a left Erb palsy with partial reinnervation of the fifth and sixth cervical levels.
>
> "Open reduction was performed when the patient was nine months old. Through a deltopectoral approach to the shoulder, the conjoined tendon was incised at its origin from the coracoid process and the contracted subscapularis muscle was released just medial to its humeral insertion. The joint could not be reduced before the subscapularis was released. Through a posterior incision, the infraspinatus was divided just medial to its humeral insertion. The posterior part of the shoulder capsule was identified and noted to be loose and redundant. The humeral head, which was palpable and dislocated posteriorly, could be easily reduced. A longitudinal incision was made in the posterior aspect of the capsule approximately one centimeter parallel to its scapular original. The glenoid was hypoplastic; the capsule was not thickened or tight anteriorly. The glenohumeral joint was reduced and the posterior aspect of the capsule was imbricated: after plication of the capsule, the shoulder could no longer be easily dislocated. The infraspinatus was reattached to its insertion and the conjoined tendon was reattached to the coracoid process. The subscapularis was not repaired. The shoulder was immobilized in abduction and external rotation in a spica cast.
>
> "One month after the operation, the immobilization was discontinued and range-of-motion exercises were begun. The shoulder remained reduced and stable. Twenty-six months after the operation, the patient could actively abduct the shoulder to 100 degrees. Active forward flexion was possible to 120 degrees, active external rotation to 50 degrees; and internal rotation, to the point where the hand could touch the sacrum. The patient could pronate and supinate the forearm fully, although a 10-degree flexion contracture of the elbow persisted. Radiographs revealed an ossified humeral head and a concentric glenohumeral joint."
>
> (Troum, Floyd, and Waters 1993)

in 1925, when the brachial plexus was explored without providing much benefit to the patient. Today, even though most patients recover spontaneously, many experience functional limitations and neurological deficits. Microsurgical repair/reconstruction is often performed.

To document the short- and long-term outcomes among patients undergoing such repairs and compare those with the natural history of such palsies, and with the results of soft-tissue and bony procedures about the shoulder (and the timing of such interventions), Waters and Dr. Donald Bae led a prospective multicenter trial in 2005, supported by grants from the Pediatric Society of North America and the American Society for Surgery of the Hand. They reported their results with soft-tissue balancing procedures, including lengthening of the pectoralis major and the subscapularis, open reduction of the glenohumeral joint, and transfers of the latissimus dorsi and teres major to

Table 27.1. Radiographic Classification of Glenohumeral Deformity Based on the Work of Bae & Waters

Type	Radiographic Features
I	Normal glenoid (a <5° difference in retroversion between the involved side and the contralateral side)
II	Minimal deformity (a <5° difference in retroversion between the involved side and the contralateral side)
III	Moderate deformity (posterior subluxation of the humeral head)
IV	Severe deformity (posterior subluxation of the humeral head and a false glenoid)
V	Infantile glenohumeral dislocation
VI	Arrest of growth in the proximal humerus

(Adapted from Bae and Waters 2004).

the rotator cuff. In 25 patients, they found that such transfers:

> combined with appropriate extra-articular musculotendinous lengthening, significantly improved global shoulder function, but led to only modest improvements in glenoid retroversion and humeral head subluxation. No profound glenohumeral remodeling occurs after these extra-articular rebalancing procedures, even when they are performed in patients of a young age…[They] halted the progression of, but not to have markedly decreased, glenohumeral dysplasia. (Waters and Bae 2005)

Waters and Bae described the indications for the aforementioned procedures, which:

> include brachial plexus birth palsy with persistent external rotation and abduction weakness, internal rotation contractures, and mild-to-moderate glenohumeral joint deformity (types III and IV according to the classification of Waters et al). In addition younger patients with progressive loss of passive external rotation despite physical therapy and evidence of joint subluxation and dysplasia on magnetic resonance imaging scans are candidates for this surgery. (Waters and Bae 2009)

They suggested a derotational humeral osteotomy for "patients more than five to seven years of age with external rotation weakness, internal rotation contractures, and advanced dysplasia (humeral head flattening, complete posterior dislocation, a convex or absent glenoid)" and noted that "a small subset of patients who are less than five years of age, but have marked glenohumeral deformity. If they were older, a humeral osteotomy would be indicated" (Waters and Bae 2009).

They also contradicted the trend toward reconstruction in young children:

> With the positive results of glenoid remodeling after arthroscopic and open reduction in younger children, there is a growing preference to perform a reconstructive rather than salvage operation. However, the degree of subscapularis and capsular release necessary to reduce the joint with either method can lead to loss of internal rotation power or even an external rotation contracture. In this small subset of patients, a combination of an external rotation humeral osteotomy in the range of 30°, along with joint reduction and tendon transfers, has been performed successfully. (Waters and Bae 2009)

EFFECT OF TENDON TRANSFERS AND EXTRA-ARTICULAR SOFT-TISSUE BALANCING ON GLENOHUMERAL DEVELOPMENT IN BRACHIAL PLEXUS BIRTH PALSY

By Peter M. Waters, MD, and Donald S. Bae, MD

Investigation performed at the Children's Hospital, Boston, Massachusetts

The Journal of Bone & Joint Surgery · JBJS.ORG
Volume 87-A · Number 2 · February 2005

Waters and Bae, "Effect of Tendon Transfers and Extra-Articular Soft-Tissue Balancing on Glenohumeral Development in Brachial Plexus Birth Palsy." *Journal of Bone and Joint Surgery* 2005; 87: 320.

In another 2009 study, Waters, again with Bae as well as other colleagues, quantified the cross-sectional areas of internal and external rotators in the shoulder in patients with a chronic brachial plexus birth palsy who had not had any surgery. They concluded that:

> The results do not suggest a linear relationship between an increasing magnitude of muscle imbalance and greater glenohumeral deformity. It is possible that there is a threshold that is reached at type III, as there appears to be a linear increase in muscle imbalance among types IV and V. There is, however, a clear increase in deformity from type II through type V...Magnetic resonance imaging assessment early in life may be more crucial in the determination of the need for and timing of surgical treatment. (Waters et al. 2009)

Dr. Waters continues his clinical research interests at Boston Children's Hospital. He succeeded Kasser as orthopaedic surgeon-in-chief in 2013.

HUGH G. WATTS

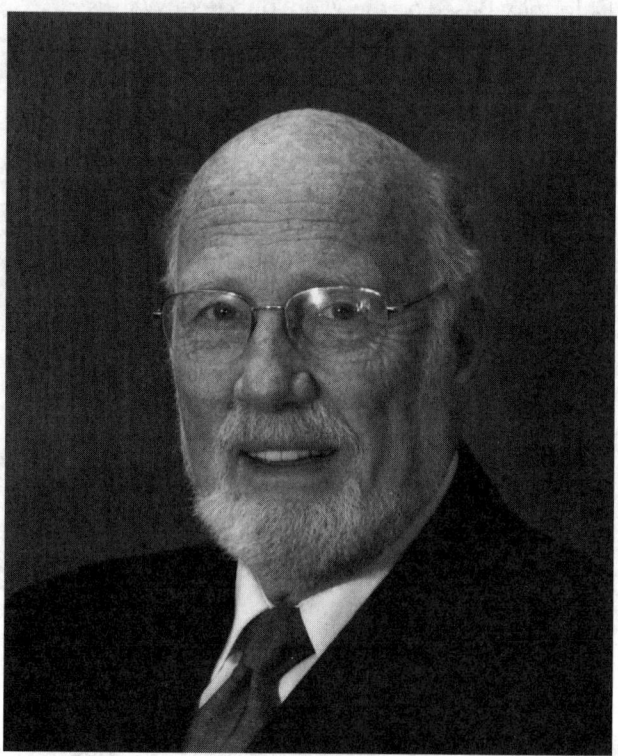

Hugh G. Watts. Courtesy of Dr. Hugh G. Watts.

Physician Snapshot

Hugh G. Watts
BORN: 1934
DIED: —

SIGNIFICANT CONTRIBUTIONS: Performed first limb-salvage procedure for osteosarcoma at Boston Children's Hospital; active teacher and clinician in global humanitarian initiatives

Born in Japan to missionary parents—his father was an Anglican bishop—Hugh Godfrey Watts and his family returned to Canada, their native country, when Hugh was seven years old. After his primary and secondary education, he came to the United States to attend Princeton University, graduating with a BA with honors in economics and sociology in 1956. In 1960, at age 26, he received an MD degree from Harvard Medical School. Returning to Canada, Watts served a rotating internship at the Royal Victoria Hospital in Montreal (1960–61).

What would become a life-long interest in health care in other countries was evident early in Watts's career. After his internship he volunteered for the nonprofit MEDICO, a humanitarian service organization, and spent almost two years (July 1961 through May 1963) at the Avicenna Hospital (Ibn Sina General Hospital) in Kabal, Afghanistan, named after the philosopher-physician Ali al-Hussain Abd-Ulla Ibn Sina (known in the West as Avicenna [980–1037]), Afghanistan's "prince of physicians."

In the summer of 1963, Watts began a surgical residency at the Peter Bent Brigham Hospital (PBBH). After six months there, he spent a year receiving surgical training at Boston Children's Hospital, finishing in November 1965. Apparently, while at the PBBH, he chose to change his training to focus on orthopaedic surgery. In a letter dated September 8, 1964, Dr. Frances Moore (Moseley Professor of Surgery at the Peter Bent Brigham Hospital) wrote to Dr. William T. Green, strongly supporting Watts: "We have found Hugh to be a devoted, willing, and able worker. He is a quiet, soft spoken and effective individual...I believe that he would do an excellent piece of work." Watts spent the next year (November 1965 to June 30, 1966) as a surgical research fellow at the PBBH.

He produced three publications during that research year: one on thyrocalcitonin, one on the use of scintiscanning of the thyroid and parathyroid glands with 75-selenomethionine, and one on the localizing parathyroid adenomas by using that scintiscanning technique.

After completing his surgical research fellowship, Watts began his orthopaedic training in the MGH/Children's Hospital residency program. His rotations included one year at Children's Hospital (July 1, 1966, through June 30, 1967), one year at MGH (July 1, 1967, through June 30, 1968), and 18 months at Children's Hospital and its affiliates (July 1, 1968, through December 30, 1969).

During his residency, in 1968, Watts published another paper, "Radiocalcium-47 Kinetic Studies in the Dog," cowritten with Dr. William Green Jr., Dr. Henry Banks, and others. This was his first from the Orthopaedic Department, and the research had been carried out in the surgical laboratories of the PBBH with Moore's approval and support.

During the last six months of Watts's chief residency at Children's Hospital, I was a senior resident there. Watts was a terrific chief and an excellent teacher and surgeon. He was also very thoughtful and generous. Toward the end of my

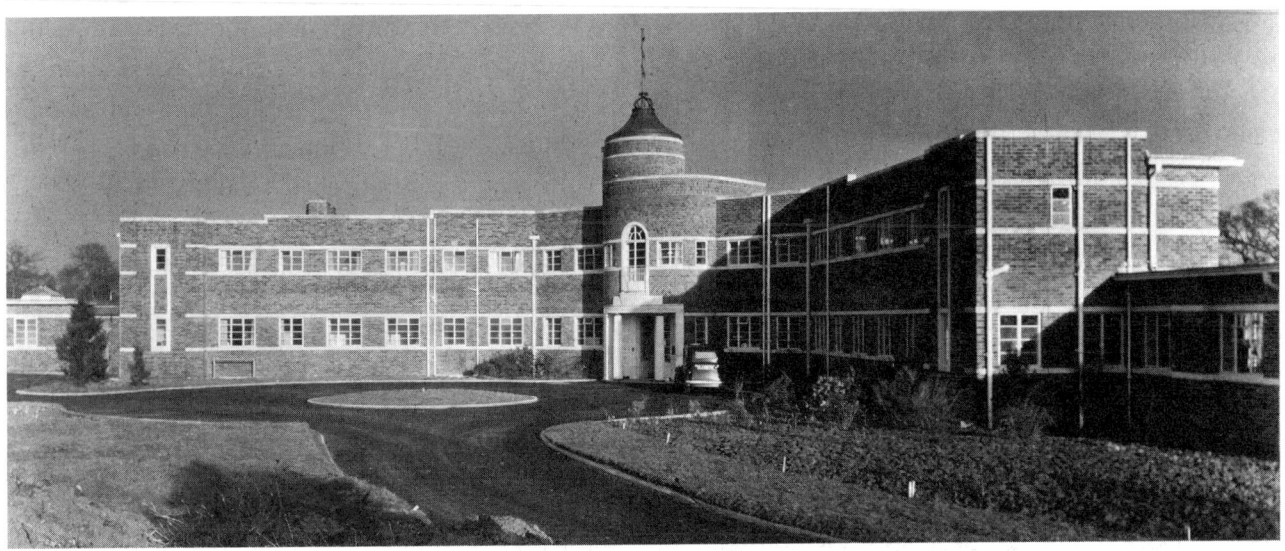

Queen Victoria Hospital. Copyright: Queen Victoria Hospital NHS Foundation Trust/East Grinstead Museum

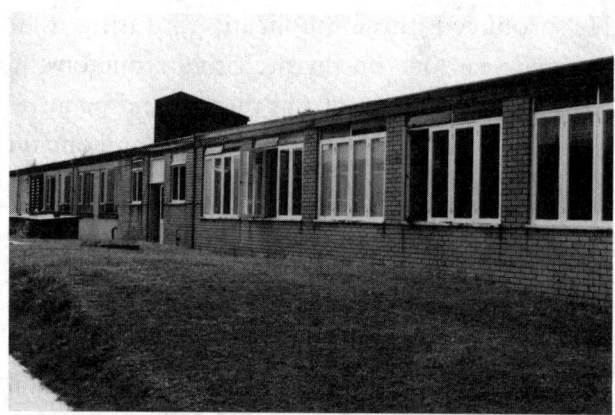

McIndoe Research Centre. Copyright: Queen Victoria Hospital NHS Foundation Trust/East Grinstead Museum

residency I had scheduled a week-long vacation; my wife and I had planned to drive to Nova Scotia, but our car had been seriously damaged in a hit-and-run accident just before our trip—another driver ran a red light at the intersection of Brookline Avenue and Riverway, hitting us broadside. Without a car, our trip to Nova Scotia would be impossible. Watts came to the rescue, generously offering us the use of his station wagon, which had a mattress in the back his children used. We had a wonderful time in Nova Scotia and even slept in the car for a few nights when lodging was unavailable—all thanks to Hugh Watts.

After completing his residency, Watts traveled overseas again—this time to England. He spent two years researching transplant immunology at the McIndoe Memorial Research Unit in Queen Victoria Hospital in East Grinstead, about 27 miles south of London. He published approximately six papers on transplantation, antibodies, graft-versus-host disease, and the role of cyclic AMP in immunocompetent cells. He then returned to Children's Hospital as a staff orthopaedic surgeon; he remained there for about seven years. He also joined the faculty at Harvard Medical School. At that time Dr. Melvin Glimcher was chairman of the Orthopaedic Department and Dr. John Hall was the chief of the Clinical Service in Orthopaedics. In the 1977 annual report of Boston Children's Hospital, Watts was listed as an associate in orthopaedic surgery at Children's Hospital and an assistant professor of orthopaedic surgery at Harvard Medical School. He also started a one-year fellowship in pediatric orthopaedics while at Children's.

Watts had a very busy clinical practice at Children's Hospital, focusing mainly on treating children with sarcomas, but he also treated children with scoliosis and other problems. In 1976, he presented to the American Academy of Orthopaedic Surgeons his early results with the use of high-dose methotrexate with citrovorum rescue in children two weeks after surgical removal of an osteosarcoma. At that time, other reports had:

Jaffe, Watts, et al. "Local En Bloc Resection for Limb Preservation." *Cancer Treatment Reports* 1978; 62: 217.

> confirmed that chemotherapy has substantially improved the prognosis in patients with osteosarcoma...high-dose methotrexate with citrovorum-factor 'rescue' and Adriamycin... [were] the major drugs [used, along with amputation, but] the advantage is the use of chemotherapy preoperatively to reduce the bulk of the tumor as well as to control the disease...so that resection of the tumor rather than amputation is feasible. (Jaffe and Watts 1976)

Dr. Emil Frei III and Dr. Norman Jaffe pioneered chemotherapy before limb-salvage surgery in children with osteosarcoma. This allowed surgeons to avoid amputation, gave the children a higher quality of life, and resulted in a higher overall rate of cure (see **Box 27.9**).

While at Children's Hospital, Watts published several papers on scoliosis, including the initial report introducing the Boston bracing system, cowritten in 1977 with Hall and Dr. William Stanish. They noted that since 1973, physicians at Children's Hospital had been developing:

a system of bracing [for] special deformities… which has become known as the "Boston Brace system"…[T]he orthotist's goal is to convert a partially prefabricated module, capable of fitting a number of patients into an individual brace designed to fit a specific patient and to correct

Box 27.9. Limb-Salvage Procedure Described by Watts et al. (1978)

"The limb preservation program comprised four basic components:

- Weekly courses of vincristine, high-dose MTX, and citrovorum factor (V-MTX-CF);
- intra-arterial ADR;
- local en bloc resection; and
- insertion of an internal prosthesis.

"Weekly V-MTX-CF…In the initial study, four weekly doses of V-MTX-CF were administered. Subsequently, after the safety of the procedure was determined and since, in several instances, a suitable endoprosthesis had not been manufactured after four weeks, the number of courses was extended to eight. Following the last V-MTX-CF course, a repeat angiographic study was performed.

"Intra-arterial ADR. In five patients, intra-arterial ADR was administered by a Harvard pump 24 hours preceding the first or final V-MTX-CF infusion. The doses varied from 45 to 75 mg/m2 and were administered over 6 hours in four patients and over 72 hours in the fifth patient.

"Local en bloc resection. This operation was performed 10–14 days after the completion of chemotherapy, provided the hemogram was normal and no complications had developed. Each tumor was resected with wide margins. Seven centimeters of bone proximal to femoral lesions or distal to tibial or humeral lesions were removed – the limit of the tumor was estimated by bone scan. The entire knee joint including the patella, all ligaments, and suprapatellar arch was removed in each lower-extremity tumor. Femoral lesions included the proximal tibia just proximal to the infrapatellar ligament. Tibial lesions included sufficient distal femur to be just proximal to the suprapatellar pouch. Active extension of the knee was made possible by transferring the hamstring muscles anteriorly. The humeral lesion was resected together with the scapula and shoulder joint and the proximal one half of the humerus.

"Internal prostheses. A variety of prostheses was used. Knee joints were modified Guepar knees with solid segments designed to replace the resected bone. Individual prostheses were made because of the varying sizes required for children. These prostheses took approximately 8 weeks for individual manufacture. The Guepar knee was chosen because it is intrinsically stable in extension. One tibial tumor in an obese boy (125 kg) was replaced with intramedullary Kuntscher rods plus steel mesh and methyl methacrylate cement. Following resection of the humeral lesion, the humerus was stabilized with a Buchholz shoulder prosthesis modified with a segment of Kuntscher rod to give adequate length for the resected bone and the glenoid component was cemented into the residual clavicle. Allografts were not used because our experience shows that bone grafts are extremely slow to heal when chemotherapy is used.

"Patients were treated with iv antibiotics during the operation and more recently postoperatively for 1 week. Oral antibiotics were then prescribed for varying periods of time until complete healing and the absence of infection were demonstrated, and chemotherapy was concluded. The limbs were immobilized for 2–3 weeks and gradually allowed motion. Full weight bearing was permitted as soon as the patients could stand comfortably, usually at 5–7 days. Adjuvant chemotherapy with V-MTX-CF-ADR was initiated 3 weeks after the operation. More recently, postoperative chemotherapy has been modified to include an intensive course of four weekly V-MTX-CF treatments before commencing V-MTX-CF-ADR."

—Watts, Jaffe, Fellows, and Vawter 1978

that specific patient's curves...[A] brace for the non-operative treatment of scoliosis constructed without a metal superstructure [Milwaukee brace] is preferred by teenage patients. Preliminary results show that a 50–60% correction can be achieved as measured on standing x-rays in the brace. Three quarters of these patients have no skin problems. (Watts, Hall, and Stanish 1977)

Long-term results allowed the eventual discontinuance of the Milwaukee brace in most cases.

In 1979, Watts moved to Philadelphia, where he became the chief of the Orthopaedic Department at the Children's Hospital of Philadelphia (CHOP) and a professor of orthopaedic surgery at the University of Pennsylvania School of Medicine. Watts had long been an active member of the team of cancer therapists at the Dana Farber Cancer Institute, who had published more than 20 papers on musculoskeletal sarcomas—work that continued for 10 years after Watts moved to Philadelphia.

Watts spent five years at CHOP and Penn, but his urge to travel resurfaced, and in 1984 he went to Saudi Arabia, where he spent five years helping to create the first Department of Orthopaedic Surgery at the King Faisal Specialist Hospital in Riyadh. With colleagues there he cowrote ~14 articles on various pediatric orthopaedic problems; three of those papers were published in the *Annals of Saudi Medicine*.

He returned to the US in 1989—now in Los Angeles, at the Shriners Hospital for Children. Watts continued to publish in his new roles there.

The Boston Brace System for the Treatment of Low Thoracic and Lumbar Scoliosis by the Use of a Girdle Without Superstructure

H. G. WATTS, M.D., J. E. HALL, M.D. AND WM. STANISH, M.D.

Watts et al. initial article introducing the Boston Brace System. *Clinical Orthopaedics and Related Research* 1977; 126: 87.

In 1994, Watts published an editorial on the use of gait laboratories to aid in preoperative decision making. He stated that such laboratories were, at that time, still only "research tool[s]," and that preoperative decisions for children with cerebral palsy should be made elsewhere. He backed up his criticism of gait labs by citing the large expense and the "unproven benefits."

He cowrote two Current Concepts Reviews for publication in the *Journal of Bone and Joint Surgery*. The first was titled "Tuberculosis of Bones and Joints." In their response to a letter to the editor about that review, Watts and Lifeso (1997) agreed with the correspondent regarding loss of disc space height, replying that "septic discitis in an adult begins as an inflammatory process in paravertebral soft tissues and probably in the adjacent vertebral body. The end plates... are then most likely penetrated by either inflammatory granulation tissue or actual septic foci...[leading to] loss of definition of the end plate...[and] as the disease progresses there is increasing loss of the disc space." The correspondent noted that such disc space loss is an early finding, but Watts and Lifeso (1997) disagreed: "It is more of a late finding...[The] use of magnetic resonance imaging...[has demonstrated that] the earliest finding... is rarefaction of the end plate." In response to the second letter that indicated a concern about sinus formation if wounds were not closed, Watts and Lifeso (1998) responded, "In our experience in Saudi Arabia, sinus formation was not a substantial problem...we do not recall ever seeing a persistent sinus after adequate débridement and prolonged antituberculosis chemotherapy."

Related to their second Current Concepts Review titled "Methods for Locating Missing Patients for the Purpose of Long-Term Clinical Studies," Dr. Marc Swiontkowski expressed concern about retrospective studies and patient confidentiality. Watts and Lifeso (1999) noted that "in our ongoing multi-institutional prospective trial on the treatment of Legg-Perthes disease, such information [new sources] was not part of the initial

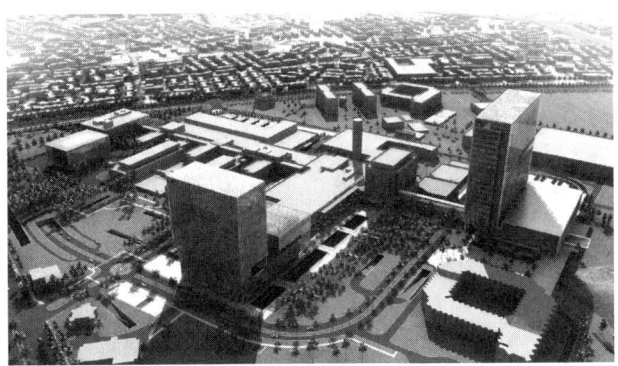

King Faisal Specialist Hospital. Courtesy of CannonDesign.

demographic data. When the patients had to be located fifteen years later, use of the internet greatly facilitated our search...[W]e are in complete agreement with Dr. Swiontkowski that an individual patient's privacy cannot be de-emphasized."

Watts was one of eight members of the Pediatric Orthopaedic Study Group (POSG), which was organized in 1982 with the goal of developing a long-term study of patients with Legg-Calvé-Perthes disease. The POSG eventually became the Legg-Perthes Study Group, comprising 39 members, including Dr. Seymour Zimbler of Boston Children's Hospital. The Legg-Perthes Study Group undertook a "large, controlled, prospective multicenter study...designed to determine the effect of treatment and other risk factors on the outcome in patients with this disorder" (Herring, Kim, and Browne 2004).

More recently, in 2013, Watts, along with Drs. John Lawrence and Katherine Au, wrote a letter to the editor regarding a paper on the Krukenberg procedure. They agreed with the authors of the article that the procedure helps patients to function independently, even those who experience blindness or may have had one or both hands amputated. They disagreed, however, that the procedure is most appropriate for patients who are blind and have had both arms amputated, calling those restrictions "outmoded" and "unnecessarily restrictive." Watts, Lawrence, and Au had performed the Krukenberg procedure in eight patients with unilateral amputations and noted that all of them had shown a benefit. The children whose arms had developed normally before their injury used their forearm muscles.

Watts is a clinical professor of orthopaedic surgery at the University of California, Los Angeles and an adjunct associate professor in the Division of Biokinesiology and Physical Therapy at the University of Southern California. His interest in global public health has continued: He led the formation of the Pediatric Orthopaedic Society of North America's Committee for International Activities. He has given lectures throughout the US and worldwide, including in Sweden, Germany, France, Italy, the Middle East, Argentina, and Australia. His work has taken him to Colombia, Ecuador, Guatemala, Liberia, Lithuania, Palestine, Sierra Leone. He has taught often in Gaza and the West Bank, and he is a member of the advisory board for the Palestine Children's Relief Fund. Watts works also with the Silver Service Children's Foundation in Buga, Colombia, and in Saudi Arabia.

CHAPTER 28

Boston Children's Hospital

Modernization and Preparation for the Twenty-First Century

The twentieth century witnessed a plethora of innovation and change at Boston Children's Hospital. At the time that orthopaedics separated from surgery in 1903, three equal departments were organized there: the Department of Orthopedic Surgery, the Department of Surgery, and the Department of Medicine. Even the hospital's name changed many times over subsequent years, from Children's Hospital, Boston; to Children's Medical Center; to the Children's Hospital Medical Center; to its present name, Boston Children's Hospital. For consistency, I have referred to it as Boston Children's Hospital (BCH) throughout this chapter and this book. There were numerous affiliations, mergers, and separations; among them the House of the Good Samaritan, Infants' Hospital, the appliance shop, New England Peabody Home, and Wellesley Convalescent Home. Annual service reports for the medical and surgical services began in 1894 (the first report included 1869–1894), followed by yearly annual reports of the hospital and individual departments as they developed. However, there is a paucity of information available within these reports and "only occasional reference to those whose faithfulness and sympathy continually contributed to the reputation for high standards of care" (Snedeker 1969).

HISTORICAL OVERVIEW OF THE TWENTIETH CENTURY

During the hospital's 32-year tenure at the Huntington Avenue location, the hospital had grown from an original 20-bed facility to 30 beds and then to 96 beds, with a new east wing addition in 1889. By the early twentieth century, hospital admissions had increased almost six-fold, from 862 (1883–1885) to 5,062 (1911–1913). Medical, surgical and orthopaedic conditions were the primary reasons for admission at the Huntington location, and tuberculosis was often the underlying cause of orthopaedic admissions. Other significant early changes included:

- 1900: opening of the first pediatric radiology department in the United States
- 1903: establishment of the hospital as a HMS teaching hospital
- 1914: organization of the first physical therapy department in the United States

The physical location on Huntington Avenue was made of brick and included a center building, two wings, and an outpatient building:

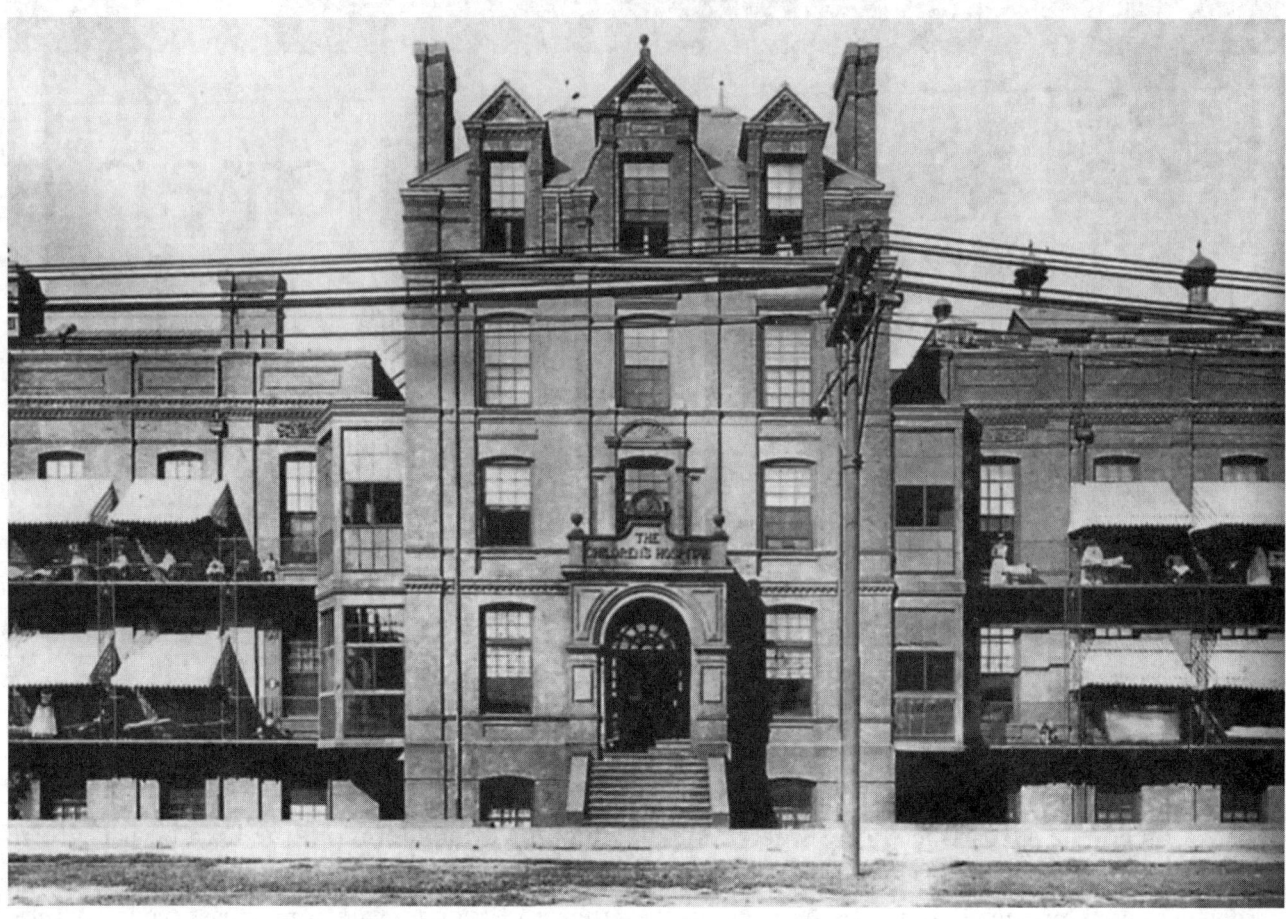

Children's Hospital on Huntington Avenue, 1913. *Images of America. Children's Hospital Boston.* Charleston, SC: Arcadia Publishing, 2005. Boston Children's Hospital Archives, Boston, Massachusetts.

The centre or administrative building contains, on the first floor, the managers' and staff room, reception rooms, sitting-rooms and dining-rooms for the house officers and Sisters, an operating room, an etherizing room, a dispensary, and a small ward, etc. The second floor of this building is devoted to the Sisters who have charge of the work. The third floor has five rooms for private patients, and the fourth floor accommodates the nurses…The west wing is devoted to the surgical patients, who are disposed of in two wards, of twenty beds each…The east wing is mostly set apart for medical cases…over these wards the space has been so utilized that a playroom is secured…The building for the outpatient department was especially erected for the purpose. The first floor has a large waiting-room for surgical out-patients…from this waiting-room extend a series of small rooms where children are prepared for observation, and apparatus is fitted. There is an operating-room, and a room for the application of massage and gymnastic exercise…A room for photography and a lecture-room complete the rooms on… [the second] floor. The upper floor, which is reached by a separate entrance, is devoted to…contagious cases…the basement is divided into rooms used for a large museum, a plaster-of-Paris workroom, a workshop for house officers, and a surgical appliance shop. (F. H. Brown, n.d.)

On March 3, 1914, BCH moved to 300 Longwood Avenue, to an expansive open field next to HMS's new buildings. Dr. Bradford was dean of HMS at the time. The new hospital had a capacity of 145 beds, including orthopaedics (48 were split

Boston Children's Hospital

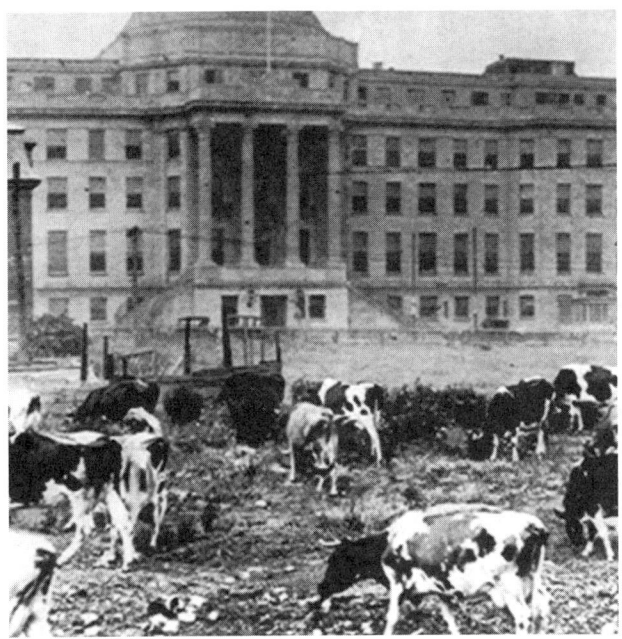

Children's Hospital, 1919. Cows grazing in the front of the hospital provided milk for the hospital's patients.
Images of America. Children's Hospital Boston. Charleston, SC: Arcadia Publishing, 2005. Boston Children's Hospital Archives, Boston, Massachusetts.

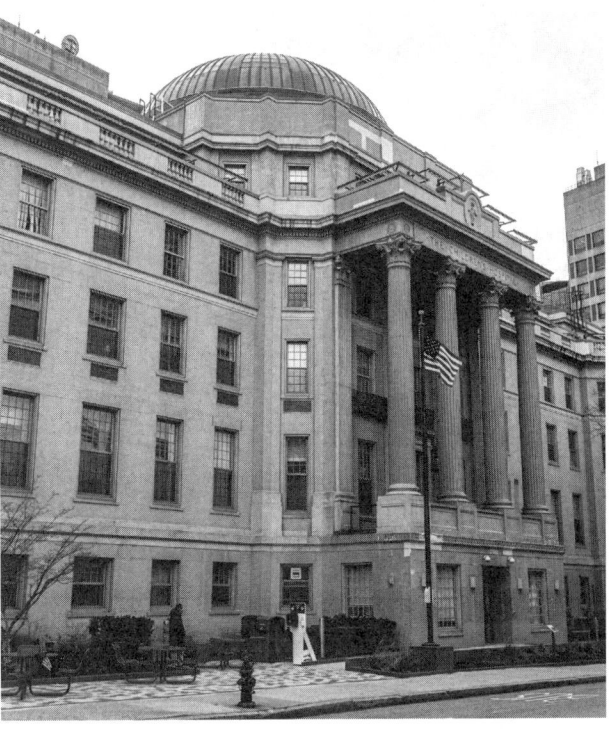

Entrance to the hospital (Hunnewell Building). Kael E. Randall/Kael Randall Images.

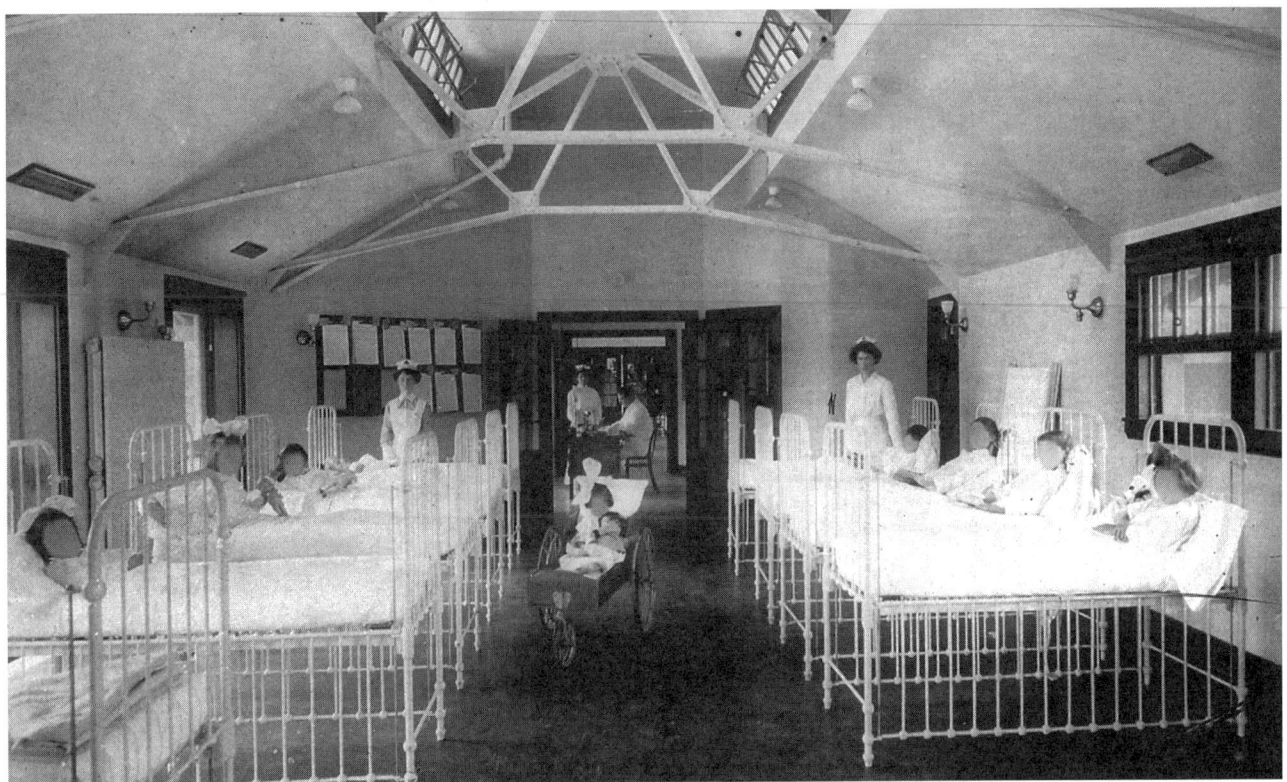

Interior of a standard ward with 10 patient beds, ca. 1914. Small wards were built to maximize air and light and minimize the spread of infectious diseases. *The Children's Hospital of Boston: Built Better Than They Knew* by Clement A. Smith. Boston: Little, Brown and Co., 1983. Boston Children's Hospital Archives, Boston, Massachusetts.

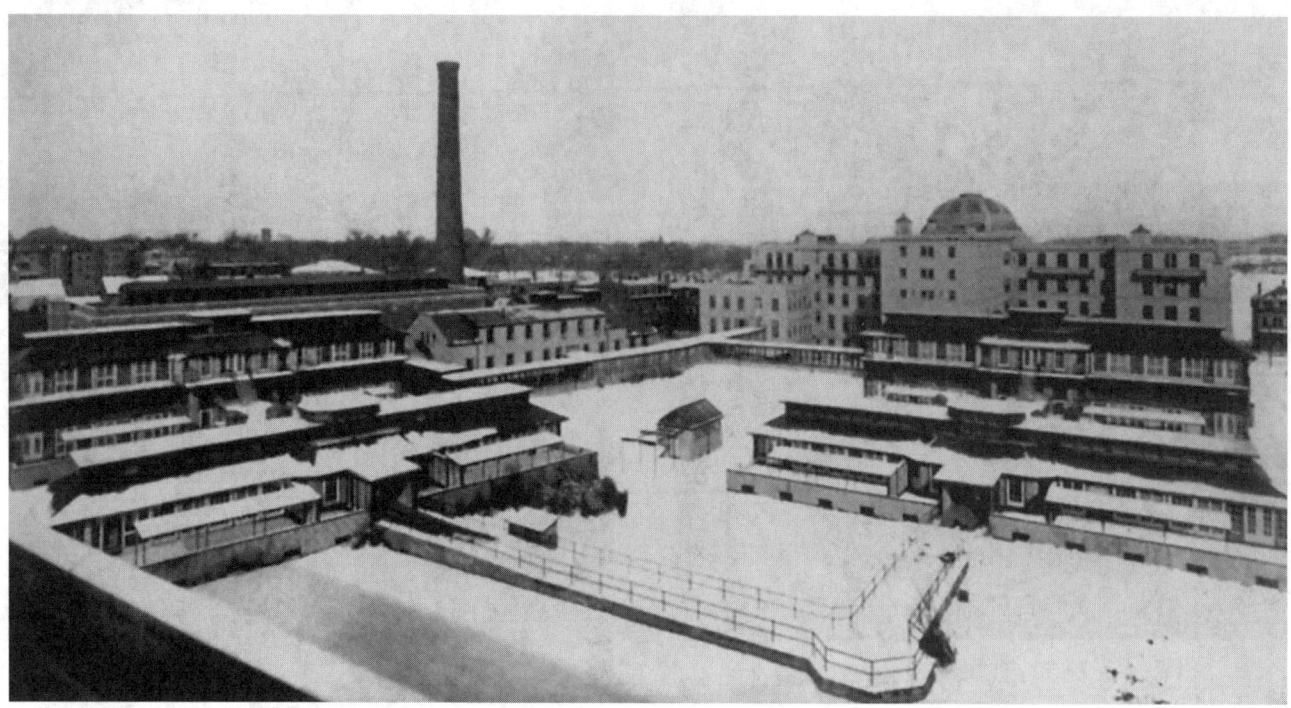

Children's Hospital in the winter, ca. 1920. *Images of America. Children's Hospital Boston*. Charleston, SC: Arcadia Publishing, 2005. Boston Children's Hospital Archives, Boston, Massachusetts.

between two floors), medicine (47), and surgery (50). Covered walkways with abundant light and ventilation connected the administration building and other buildings, called pavilions. Liberal facilities included numerous offices and examination rooms, an x-ray department, a dispensary, plaster rooms, a location for private patients, and even an isolation room and a gymnasium. The interior of the wards was similar. There was no elevator, only stairs existed between the upper and lower floors of orthopedics. Hospital staff had to hand carry patients to the appropriate ward, even patients in full body casts. The Annual Report by the Children's Hospital's Orthopaedic Department (1914) describes the move to the new location as:

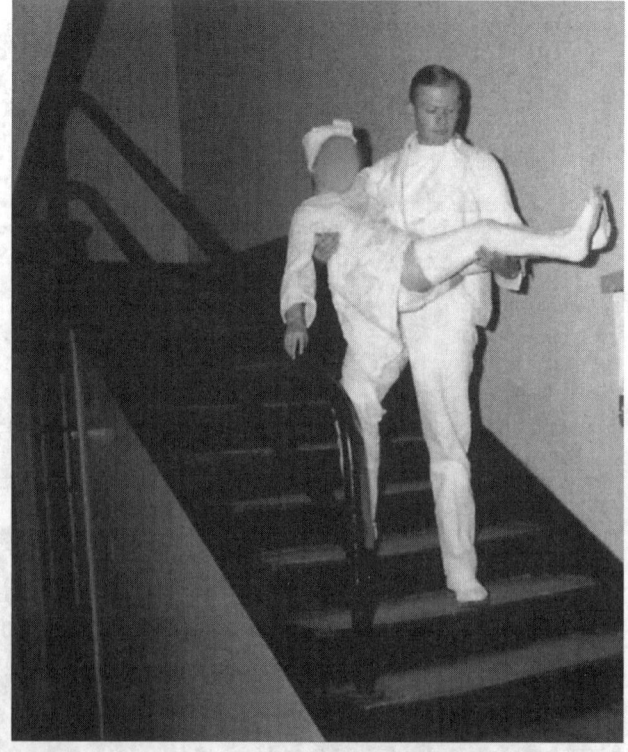

Without the presence of elevators residents had to carry patients in casts up and down stairs, ca. late 1920s.
Images of America. Children's Hospital Boston. Charleston, SC: Arcadia Publishing, 2005. Boston Children's Hospital Archives, Boston, Massachusetts.

> the greatest possible benefit to the orthopedic as to the other departments, and the work is now done under satisfactory conditions…the construction of the wards is particularly favorable for the treatment of orthopedic cases, because with the large number of cases of tuberculous joint disease that we necessarily have, the

present conditions make it possible for us to treat the children by out-of-door treatment… then danger of hospitalism seems much less, and we find that the children bear bed confinement much better than under the old conditions. The segregation of the children in ward units of ten has also affected favorably the occurrence of infectious disease whereas in the old hospital the orthopedic department was seriously handicapped—as a rule several times a year—by the presence of infection spreading among the children…no child in any unit is allowed to see a child in any other, and if a contagious disease breaks out, we are in a position to isolate the ward and continue the rest of the service. Formerly, with the children in the large wards, the service was greatly crippled, as happened for several weeks during the latter part of our stay in the old hospital. (Children's Hospital Archives)

At the time, the hospital admitted children two years and over, and Infant's Hospital admitted those children younger than two years of age. By 1923, Infant's Hospital had relocated on the campus of BCH and eventually it merged with them. The Ida C. Smith ward for infants with surgical problems was added later to the surgical ward. Ida Smith, RN, served as the Hospital's superintendent between 1917 and 1933, following the departure of the Sisters of St. Margaret. The year of the merger, individual cubicles of metal and glass had been installed on the upper floor of Ward V (orthopaedics). The process established for these cubicles greatly improved morale among the nurses and physicians. According to the 1923 Annual Report by the Children's Hospital's Orthopaedic Department:

All cases are admitted to these cubicles and no transfers are made to the lower ward until the children have been in the hospital two weeks [avoiding exposure to any contagious disease]… Wash basins have been placed in all the open wards in convenient and conspicuous places and the rule of washing the hands after touching any of the cases is rigidly observed. (Children's Hospital Archives)

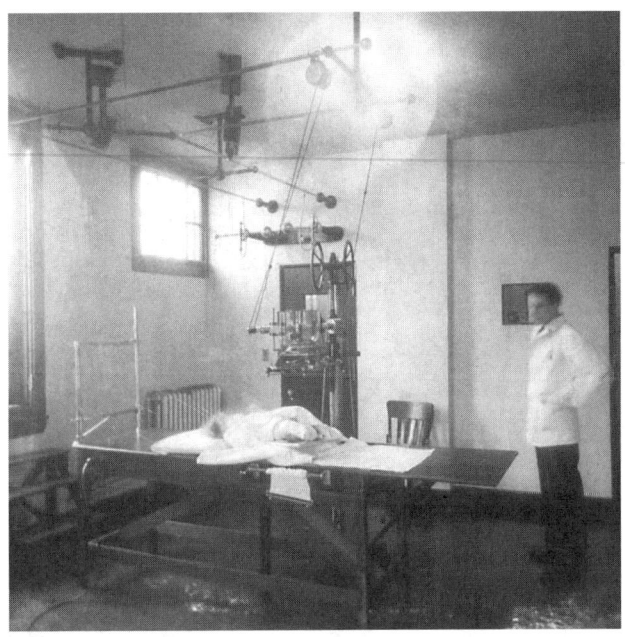

Radiology department, ca. late 1920s.
Images of America. Children's Hospital Boston. Charleston, SC: Arcadia Publishing, 2005. Boston Children's Hospital Archives, Boston, Massachusetts.

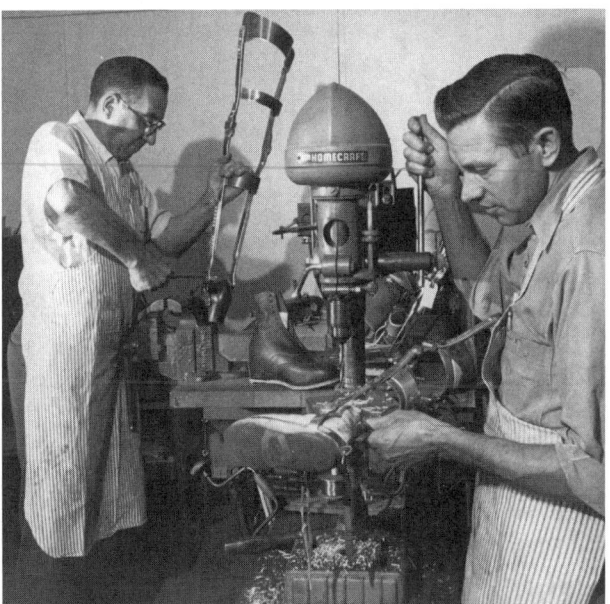

Appliance shop. Boston Children's Hospital Archives, Boston, Massachusetts.

By 1928, the new Bader building was completed for the care of children with neuromuscular diseases. The clinics of the Harvard Infantile Paralysis Commission were held in this building. Dr. William T. Green's growth study offices were also located in the Bader building. The top floor was a memorial to Dr. Legg, called the Functional Therapy Room. The Bader pool, however, closed in 1932 during the Great Depression. George von L. Meyer succeeded Ida Smith as the hospital director and administrator during the World War II years, and by 1944, the hospital established "a general plan for the development of the hospital [including] a Children's Medical Center covering all phases of pediatrics" (Children's Hospital Archives, Annual Report 1944). Dr. Robert M. Smith, who joined the staff at BCH in 1945 and served as the first chief of anesthesia from 1946 to 1980, recalled there were four operating rooms when he arrived. There were also individual pavilions designated for orthopaedics, infants, older children, and operations.

Throughout the twentieth century and into the first quarter of the twenty-first century, BCH

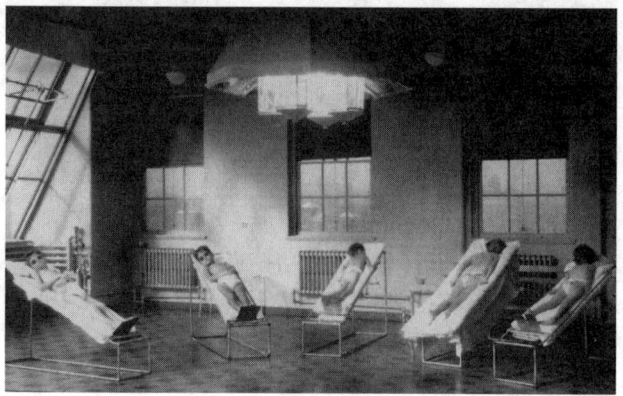

The Bader Solarium, 1930s.
Images of America. Children's Hospital Boston. Charleston, SC: Arcadia Publishing, 2005. Boston Children's Hospital Archives, Boston, Massachusetts.

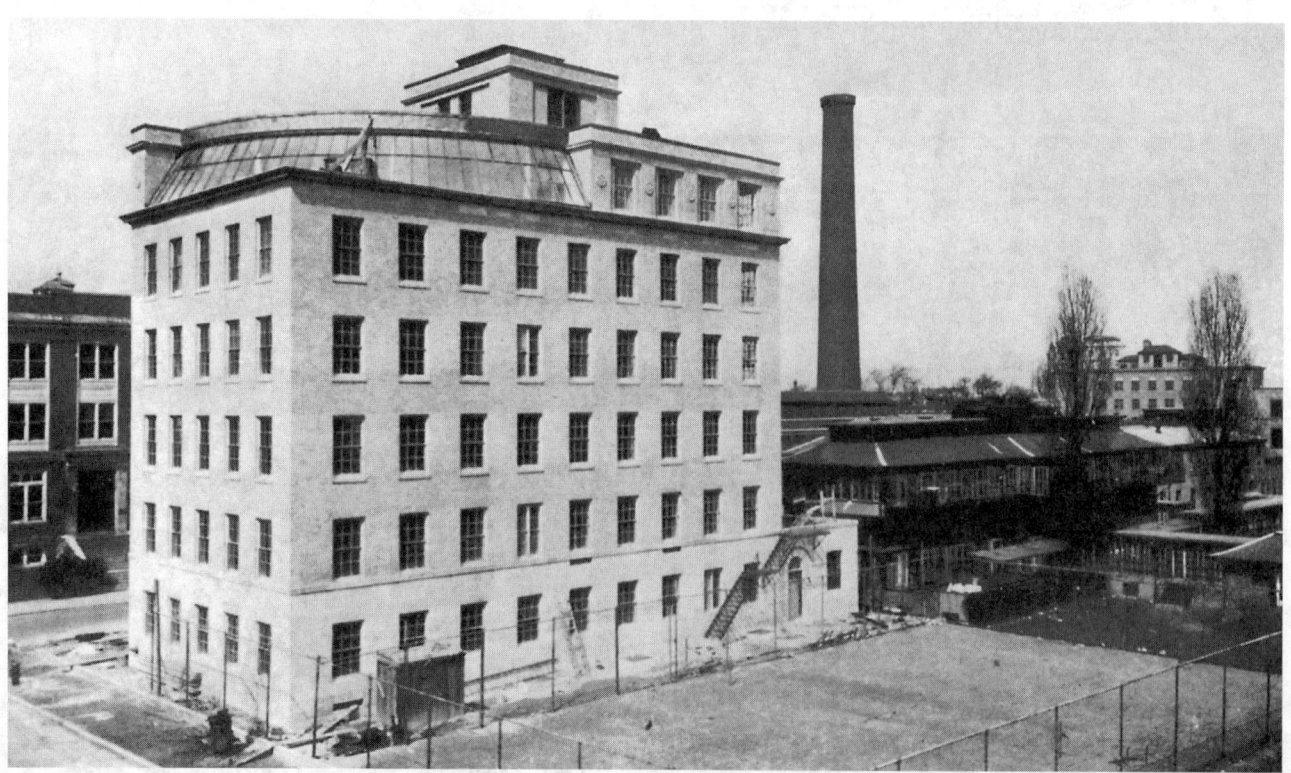

Bader Building, 1930. Built next to Orthopedic Ward 5. It contained a special unit for children with neuromuscular diseases, physical therapy, a solarium, and an exercise pool. *Images of America. Children's Hospital Boston.* Charleston, SC: Arcadia Publishing, 2005. Boston Children's Hospital Archives, Boston, Massachusetts.

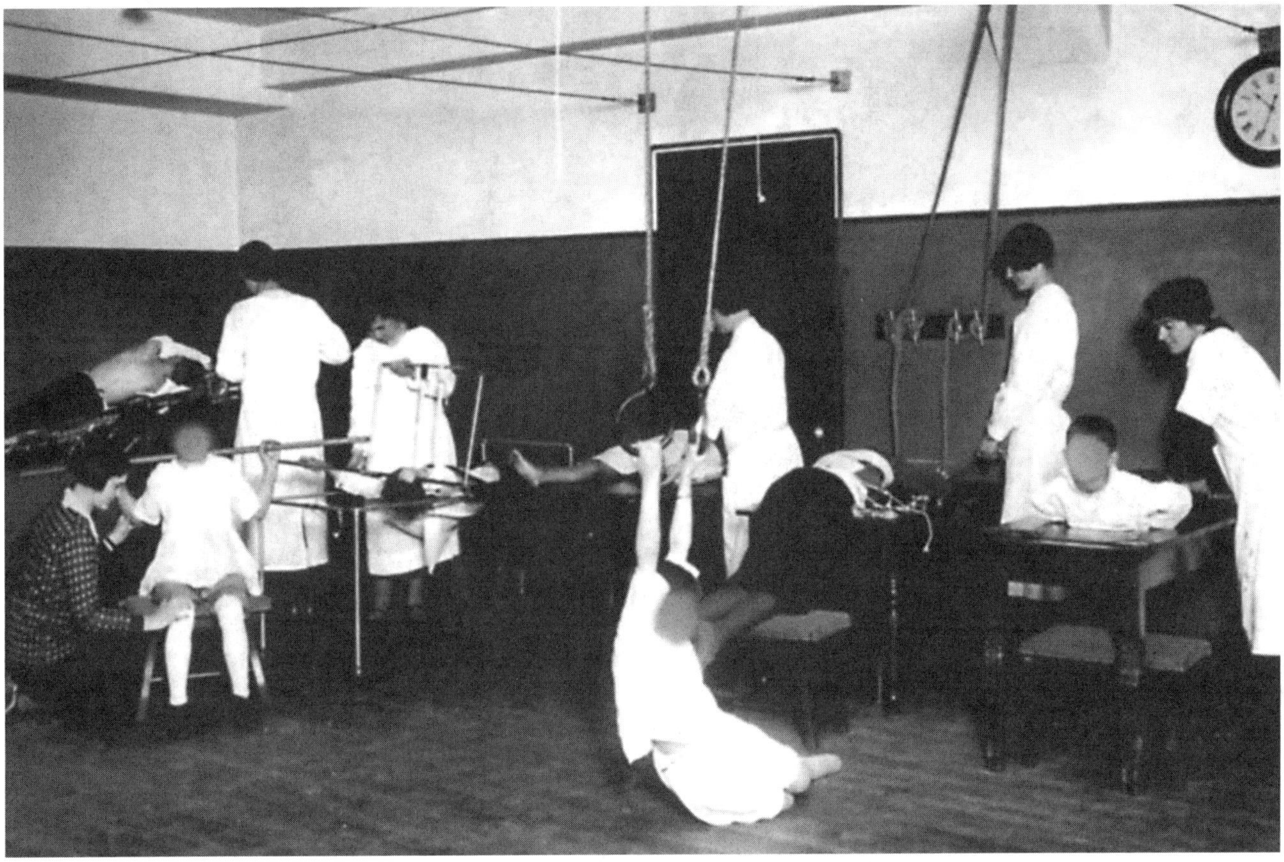

The Gymnasium, Orthopedic Ward 5, ca. 1925. *Images of America. Children's Hospital Boston.* Charleston, SC: Arcadia Publishing, 2005. Boston Children's Hospital Archives, Boston, Massachusetts.

continued to expand its facilities with new buildings in the Longwood area and satellites in the Boston area. By 1958, the Hospital and Convalescent Home for Children (Wellesley) had closed, but that same year they developed a new division of laboratories consisting of 12 units, including orthopaedics and the orthopaedic research laboratories. By 1967, the new Fegan building was completed (at the time, I was a junior resident at Boston Children's). It was a high-rise, ambulatory-care facility that centralized the hospital's specialty clinics. Before its completion, orthopaedics and other specialty clinics were scattered along Brookline and Longwood Avenues. That year the House of the Good Samaritan was also legally incorporated into the BCH. **Table 28.1** demonstrates the enormous growth at BCH over a 50-year period.

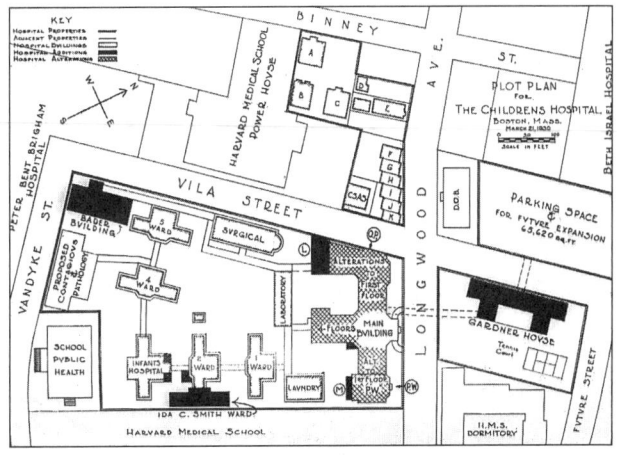

The Expansion Plan, 1930. Modernization of the hospital's physical plant included the Bader Building, the Gardner House (School of Nursing), and the Ida C. Smith Ward for additional surgical beds.

Images of America. Children's Hospital Boston. Charleston, SC: Arcadia Publishing, 2005. Boston Children's Hospital Archives, Boston, Massachusetts.

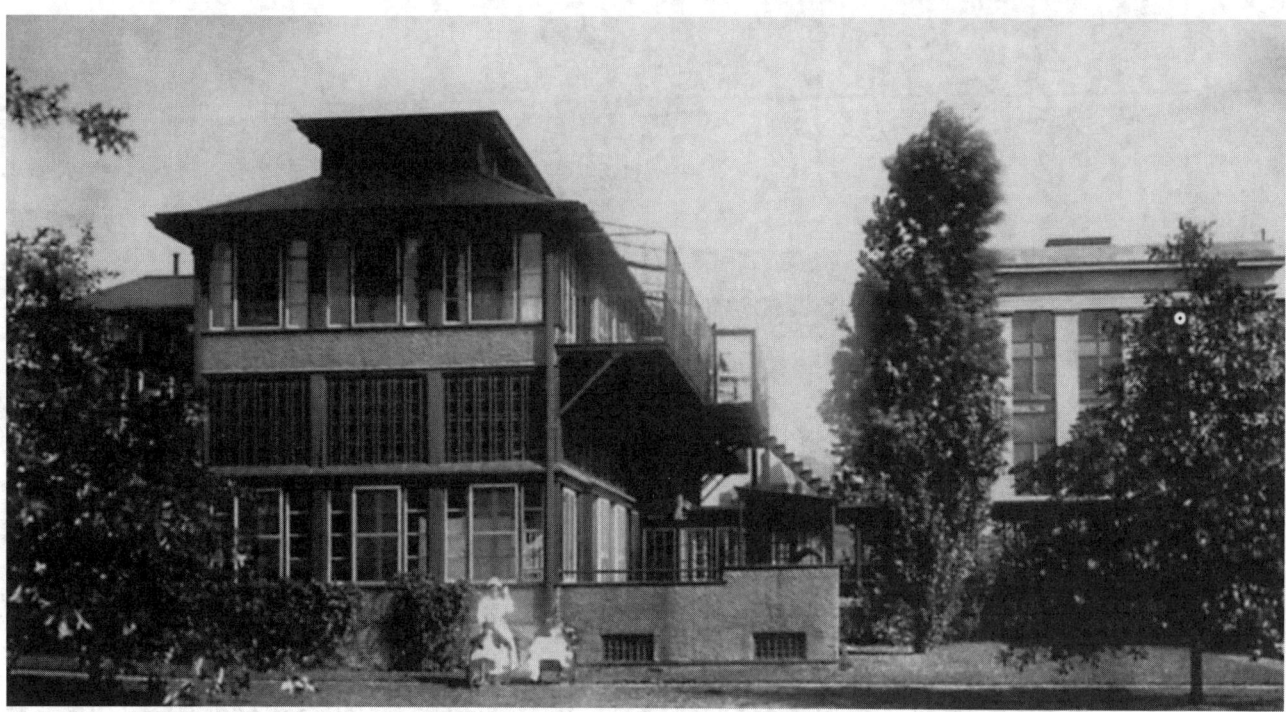

Ward I, ca. 1930. Medical Ward I and Orthopedic Ward 5 were two stories each, while Surgical Wards 2 and 4 were one story each.
Images of America. Children's Hospital Boston. Charleston, SC: Arcadia Publishing, 2005. Boston Children's Hospital Archives, Boston, Massachusetts.

Table 28.1. Fifty Years of Exponential Growth at Boston Children's Hospital: 1932–1982

	1932	1982
Admissions	6,681	12,659
Physicians	68	340
Nurses	63	711
X-ray technicians	5	38

(C. A. Smith 1983).

DEPARTMENT OF ORTHOPAEDIC SURGERY: CONTINUED GROWTH AND PROFITABILITY

Dr. Melvin J. Glimcher's laboratories received federal grant support, but before he took over as orthopaedic surgeon-in-chief (OSIC) in 1971, the new research building was half empty. During Dr. John E. Hall's initial tenure and before Dr. Paul P. Griffin's arrival, Glimcher's laboratories had expanded to occupy three floors of the building, and during his peak activity, there were approximately 50 scientists, staff, and postdoctoral students. However, both before Griffin's arrival as OSIC in 1981 and after his departure in 1986, the clinical cost center of the orthopaedic department was in debt to the hospital. During Hall's tenure as OSIC (Griffin's successor), the department followed Harvard's academic salary guidelines, and the full-time staff in the new foundation were all clinically busy and performed well financially.

Griffin had originally hired Dr. James R. Kasser in 1982 as a staff orthopaedic surgeon and instructor at HMS, and Hall later named Kasser—who was very interested in administrative work—associate chief of the orthopaedics department. Kasser had graduated from Tufts Medical School and completed his orthopaedic residency there, followed by a pediatric orthopaedic fellowship at the Alfred I. DuPont Institute in Wilmington, Delaware. Kasser represented Hall at numerous committee meetings, but at the time, the department's endowment fund lacked transparency,

Boston Children's Hospital

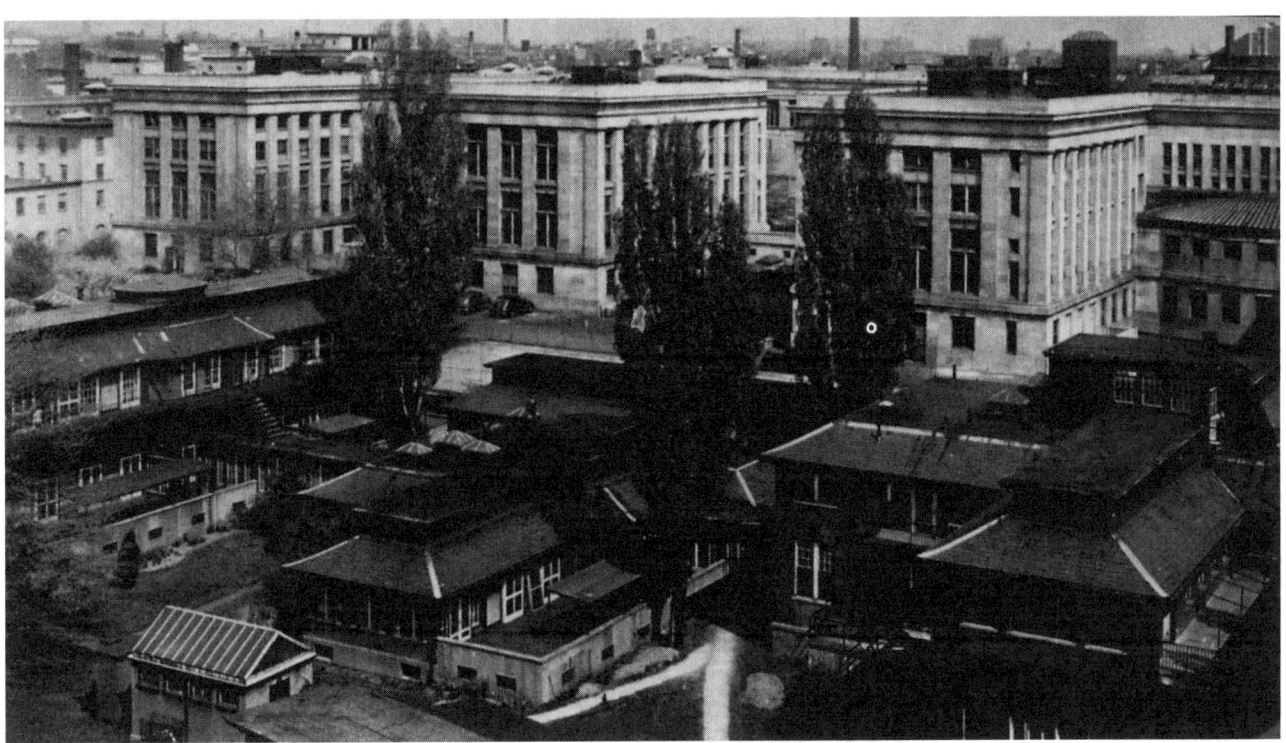

Children's Hospital Pavilion Wards, 1953. These old cottage wards eventually became antiquated. *Images of America. Children's Hospital Boston*. Charleston, SC: Arcadia Publishing, 2005. Boston Children's Hospital Archives, Boston, Massachusetts.

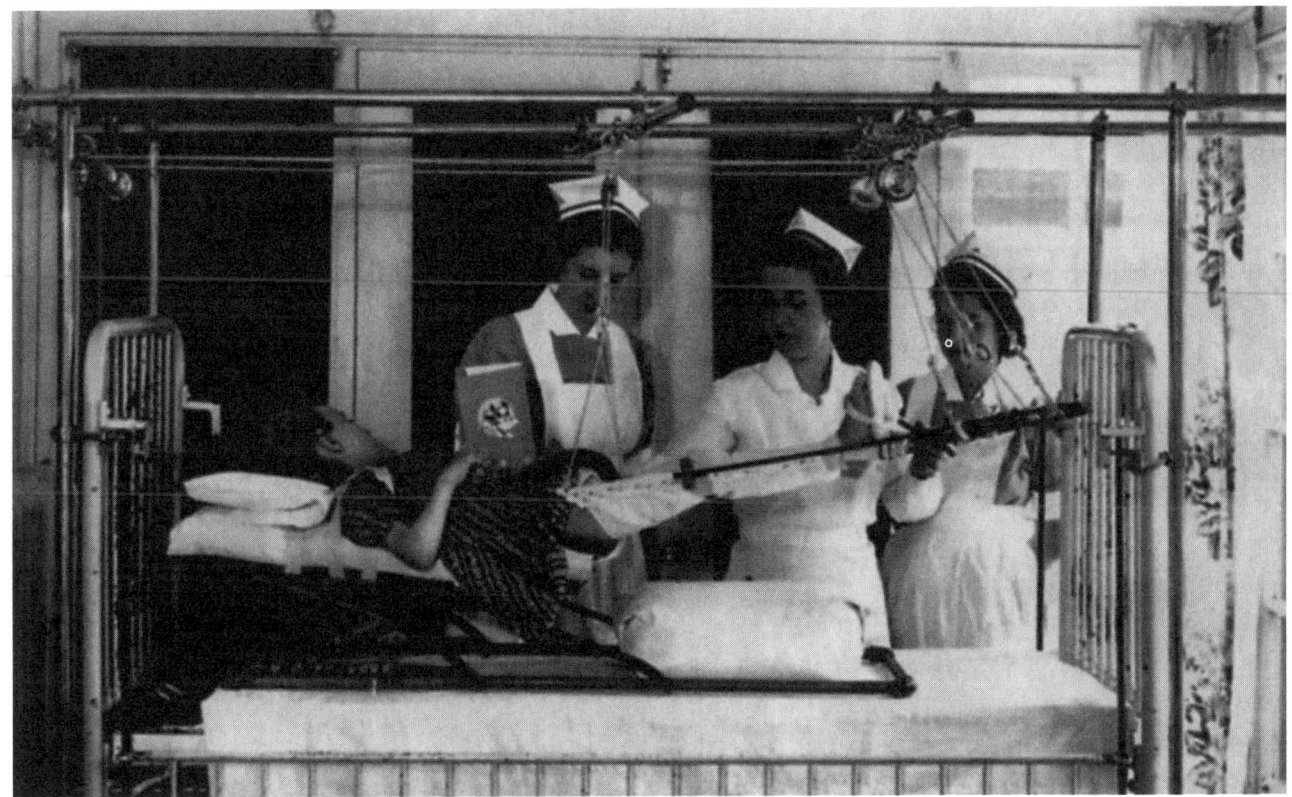

Bedside teaching was the hallmark of physician and nursing education at Children's Hospital. *Images of America. Children's Hospital Boston*. Charleston, SC: Arcadia Publishing, 2005. Boston Children's Hospital Archives, Boston, Massachusetts.

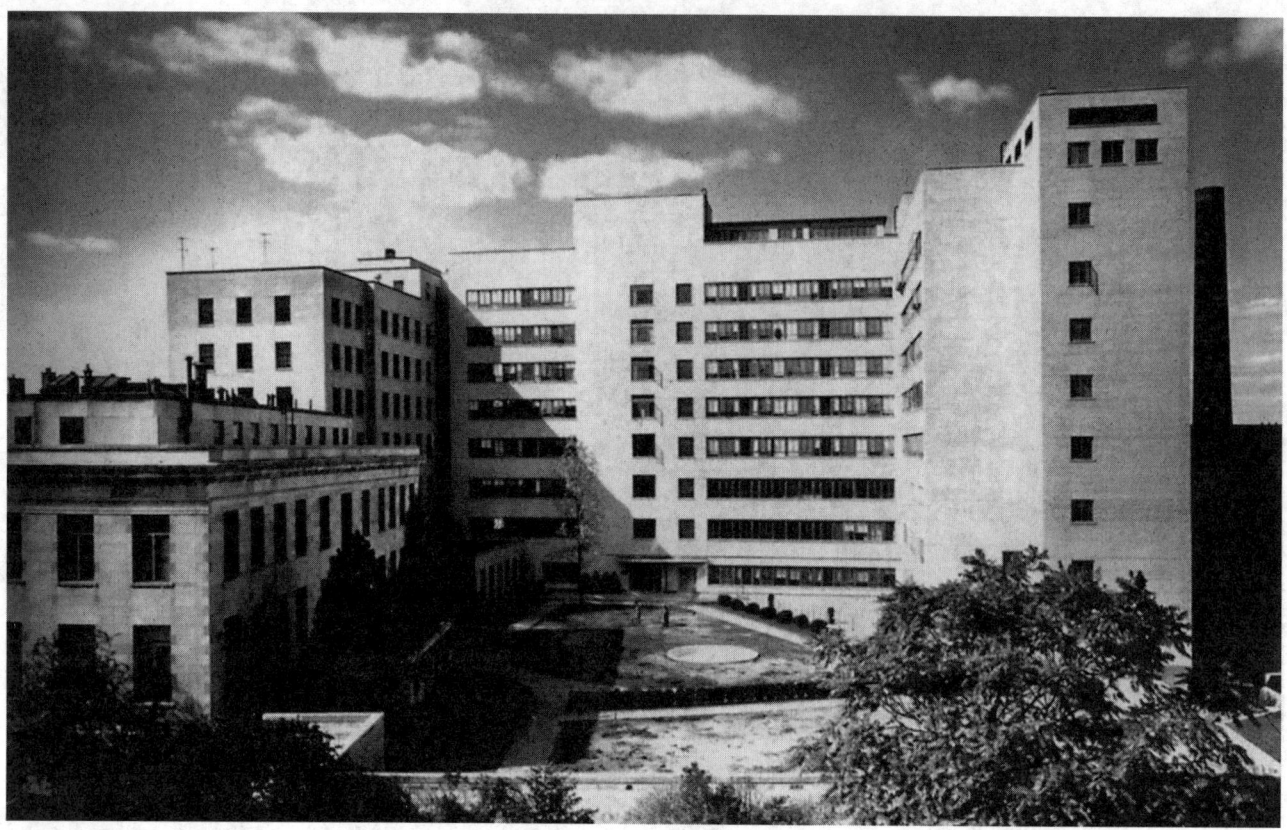

Children's Hospital Medical Center, 1955. New buildings replaced the old pavilion wards and surrounded an open space that became the Prouty Garden. *Images of America. Children's Hospital Boston.* Charleston, SC: Arcadia Publishing, 2005. Boston Children's Hospital Archives, Boston, Massachusetts.

and the staff were unaware of its existence. When Hall had been named OSIC, the department's foundation—originally formed by Griffin—was closed. Although Dr. Lyle Micheli's sports' foundation (an independent professional corporation) remained, Drs. Hall, Kasser, Millis and Emans opened a new foundation. Hall headed the organization, and under his leadership, its membership continued to grow. Even after Hall's retirement in 1994, and Kasser's promotion to OSIC and associate professor at HMS, the foundation remained. The hospital turned over control of the department's endowment funds to Kasser in 1994. The new foundation's practice plan included a tax system, most of the faculty were directors of the foundation, and transparency existed regarding revenue, expenses, and funding flow. Existing funds included the Peabody Fund supporting Glimcher's chair and his research program, the Ober Research Fund, the William T. Green Fund, and an Infantile Paralysis Fund. Kasser eventually combined the funds into two major funds, a clinical teaching fund and a basic research fund.

BCH also developed guidelines for medical practices in the institution. They determined that optimal operation included designating all physicians across departments as full-time and centrally located with all staff working toward a shared mission. During an interview with the Winthrop Group in 1993, President and CEO David Weiner explained:

> We ultimately came up with three different models of organization that each clinical department could consider and adopt. That was a major breakthrough [about 1980]…it took the better part of five years cajoling, demonstrating how key factors had been successfully

implemented in other institutions, etc....after the first couple of years of experience with it, it was becoming clearer and clearer to the chiefs of the clinical departments as well as to the administration that we really had found our way into the new era, and we were working together... for the first time. This kind of organizational charge took not only a joint planning effort between the management group and a group of chiefs who had the respect of their colleagues, but ultimately required strong background on the part of the board of trustees to mandate the change and ascribe a timetable for implementation...the board went through several iterations of change when they recognized that the original board structure was not working well... that a board membership over 100 was no longer capable of effective governance...the resulting board comprised fifteen members including the physician-in-chief, the surgeon-in-chief, the president, and twelve lay trustees. That has turned out to be an optimum-sized leadership group for policy and strategy development here at Children's. (D. Dyer 1993)

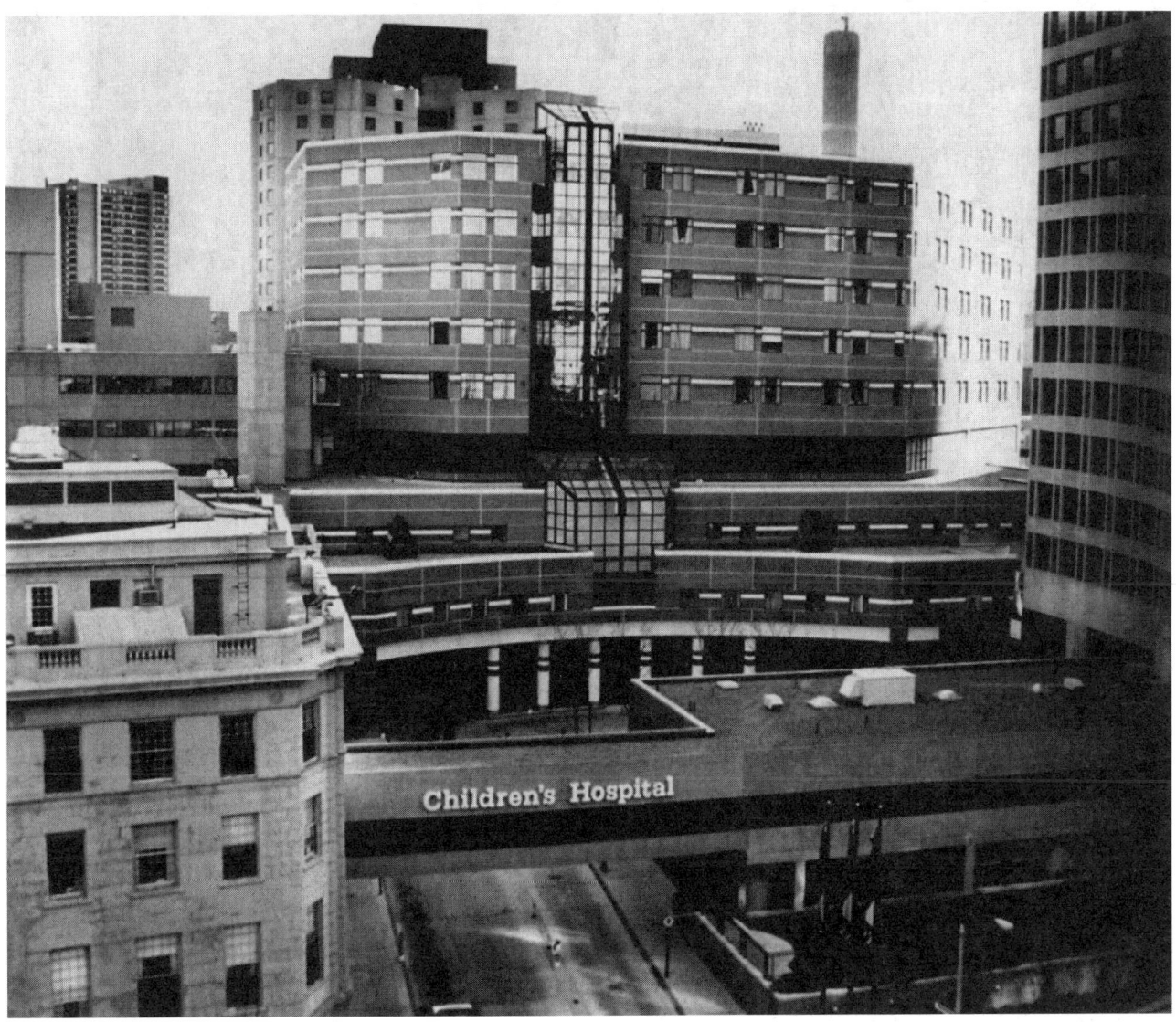

Children's Hospital, 1987. The center 10-story building had 325 inpatient beds. It began the major expansion of BCH into the twenty-first century. *Images of America. Children's Hospital Boston.* Charleston, SC: Arcadia Publishing, 2005. Boston Children's Hospital Archives, Boston, Massachusetts.

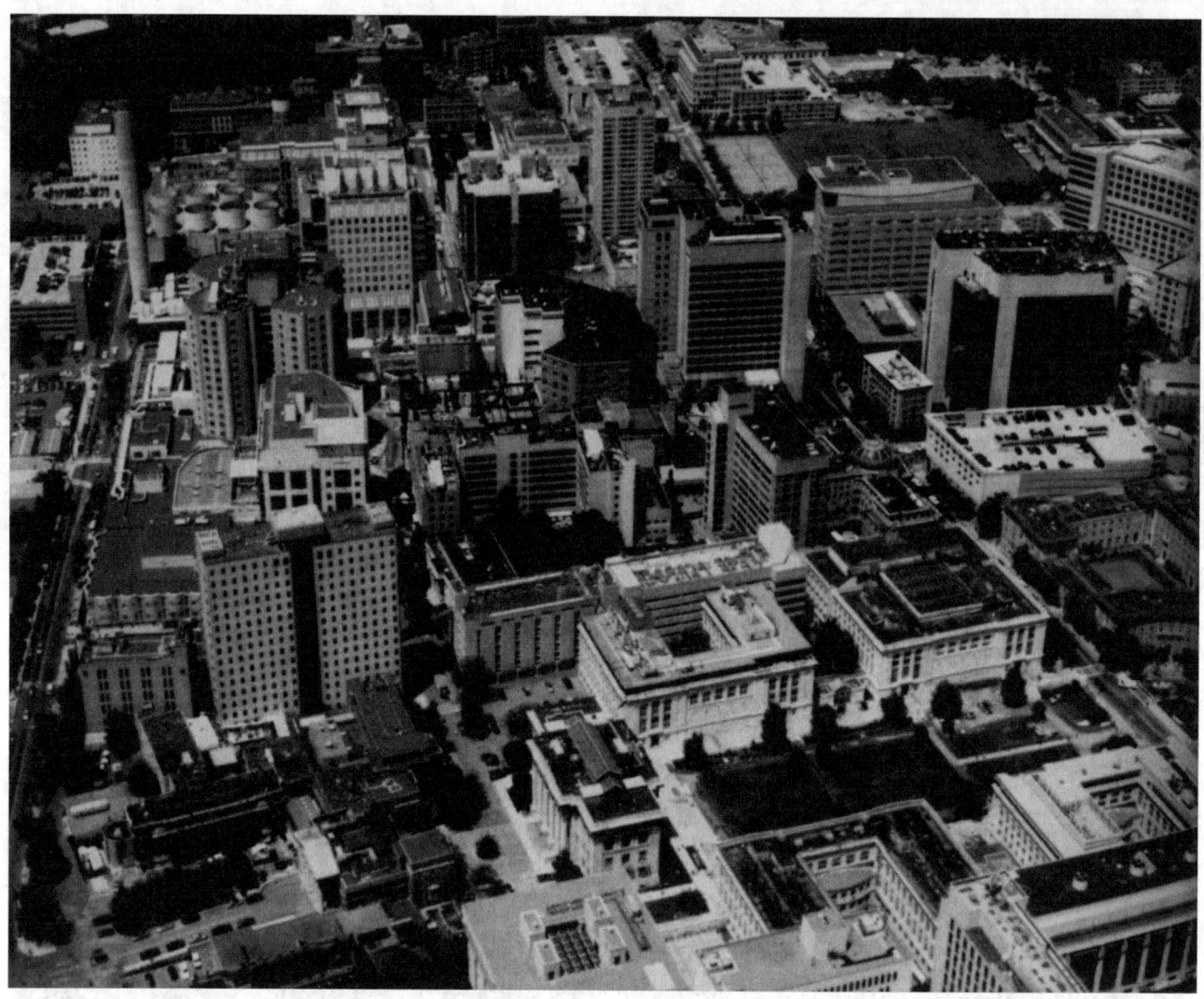

Aerial view of BCH (center), 2003. HMS is in the right foreground; BWH is in the left side of the photograph; and BIDMC is in the upper right of the photograph. *Images of America. Children's Hospital Boston.* Charleston, SC: Arcadia Publishing, 2005. Boston Children's Hospital Archives, Boston, Massachusetts.

During the latter part of the twentieth century, new faculty were hired; some left for other positions (**Box 28.1**). Some of those who practiced at Children's for a short time before leaving are not discussed or mentioned only briefly in this book; an incomplete list includes Benjamin Bierbaum, R. Plato Swartz, W. P. Cotting, G. K. Carpenter, Robert J. Cook, J. S. Stone, Leo J. McDermott, Nathan Rudo, Ascar S. Staples, Richard Gross, Raymond Morrissey, Tony Herring, Fred Ralph Zeiss, Charles L. Scudder, John Michael Allen, G. Wilbur Weston, and Peter Garbino. As the orthopaedic department transitioned to the twenty-first century, the faculty has grown to become what was likely the largest pediatric orthopaedic department in the United States. It included four endowed Harvard professorships: Harriet M. Peabody (the oldest), Frederick W. and Jane M. Ilfeld, Catharina Ormandy, and John E. Hall; it was also home to the Joseph O'Donnell Family in Orthopedic Sports Medicine professorship. The department has numerous individual funds, including the orthopedic fellow education fund and the Children's sports injury prevention fund to name only two.

So, too, has the research laboratory transitioned from Dr. Cohen's initial lab evaluating the biologic response to metal implants, to Dr. Simon's gait laboratory, to Dr. Glimcher's laboratory for the study of skeletal disorders and rehabilitation concentration on the study of tissue mineralization, to the current orthopaedic laboratories. The transition to the twenty-first century has ushered in a focus on molecular biology and the genetics of musculoskeletal diseases, led by Dr. Matthew Warman, the director of the lab. Dr. Mathew Harris studies animal mutation models to identify mechanisms of skeletogenesis. Dr. Martha Murray conducts translational research, which focuses on intra-articular healing of the anterior cruciate ligament. A breakthrough in the understanding, healing, and biologic treatment of the injured anterior cruciate ligament has enormous potential for the treatment of all athletes. The Department of Orthopaedic Surgery at BCH is well-prepared to continue its clinical and research and modern educational programs throughout the twenty-first century.

Box 28.1. Boston Children's Hospital's Endowments and Professorships

Professorships

- John E. Hall Professorship in Pediatric Orthopaedic Surgery
  - James Kasser, 1998–2009
  - Peter Waters, 2009
- Frederick W. and Jane M. Ilfeld Professorship in Orthopedics
  - Mark Gebhardt, 1998
- Catharina Ormandy Professorship
  - Matt Warman, 2006–2009
  - James Kasser, 2009
- Harriet M. Peabody Fund
  - William T. Green, 1962–1968
  - Melvin J. Glimcher, 1971–2009
  - Matt Warman, 2009

Chair

- Joseph O'Donnell Family Chair in Orthopedic Sports Medicine
  - Lyle Micheli, 2005

Named Funds

- Lloyd Alpern–Dr. Rosenthal Physical Therapy Fund
- Children's Sports Injury Prevention Fund
- Musculoskeletal Imaging Fund
- Orthopaedic Fellow Education Fund
- Orthopaedic Surgical Advancement Fund
- Dr. Robert K. Rosenthal Cerebral Palsy Fund in Orthopaedics
- Sports Medicine Fund
- Harold and Anna Snider Ullian Orthopaedic Fund

Active Staff

- Mark C. Gebhardt, MD
- Peter Gerbino, MD
- John E. Hall, MD
- M. Timothy Hresko
- Lawrence I. Karlin, MD
- James R. Kasser, MD
- Young–Jo Kim, MD
- Mininder S. Kocher
- Lyle J. Micheli, MD
- Michael B. Millis, MD
- Leela Ragaswamy, MD
- Frederick Shapiro, MD
- Bryan, Schneider, MD, PhD
- Peter M. Waters, MD
- Seymour Zimbler, MD

Index

Illustrations are indicated by page numbers in *italics*. Page numbers followed by t and b indicate tables and boxes.

Page numbers are formatted as: Volume: page

A

AAOS. *See* American Academy of Orthopaedic Surgeons (AAOS)
AAOS Council on Education, 4: 173
AAOS Diversity Committee, 1: 239
AAST. *See* American Association for the Surgery of Trauma (AAST)
Abbott, Edward Gilbert, 1: 59; 2: 87–88
Abbott, Josephine Dormitzer, 2: 97
Abbott, LeRoy C., 1: 189, 197; 2: 77, 110, 160, 183; 3: 180, 229; 4: 473
Abbott Frame, 4: 232, *232*
"Abscesses of Hip Disease, The" (Lovett and Goldthwait), 2: 52
abdominal surgery, 1: 81; 3: 18, 108
Abe, Isso, 2: 279
Abraham, John, 4: 190b
absorbable animal membrane research, 3: 166, *166*, 167, *171*
Academy of Medicine, 4: 324
Accreditation Council for Graduate Medical Education (ACGME), 1: 200, 213, 217, 237–239
acetabular dysplasia, 2: 389, *389*, 390
"Acetone" (Sever), 2: 84
ACGME. *See* Accreditation Council for Graduate Medical Education (ACGME)
Achilles tendon
    club foot and, 2: 25, 29, 145
    gastrocnemius paralysis and, 2: 150
    injury in, 3: 272
    sliding procedure and, 2: *198*
    subcutaneous release of, 2: 29, 36
    tenotomy, 1: 100–101, 106; 2: 25
achillobursitis, 2: 89
Ackerman, Gary, 1: 217b
acromioclavicular joint dislocation, 1: 268, 277
acromioplasty, 3: 191, 239
ACS Committee on Fractures, 3: 64; 4: 324
activating transcription factor-2 (ATF-2), 2: 330
acute ligament injuries, 1: 277
acute thigh compartment syndrome, 3: 417, *417*, 418
Adams, Frances Kidder, 3: 228
Adams, Helen Foster, 3: 228, 236
Adams, Herbert D., 3: 275
Adams, John, 1: 8–10, 14, 18
Adams, John D.
    back pain treatment, 4: 358
    Boston Dispensary and, 4: 358–359
    education and training, 4: 357–358
    HMS appointment, 4: 360
    Massachusetts Regional Fracture Committee, 3: 64
    Mt. Sinai Hospital and, 4: 204
    New England Medical Center and, 4: 360
    occupational therapy and, 4: 358–359
    patellar turndown procedure, 4: 373–374
    private medical practice, 4: 358
    professional memberships, 4: 360
    publications and research, 4: 359, *359*
    scaphoid fracture treatment, 4: 359–360
    Tufts Medical School appointment, 4: 360
Adams, John Quincy, 1: 10
Adams, M., 3: 133
Adams, Nancy, 3: 236
Adams, Samuel, 3: 236
Adams, Samuel (1722–1803), 1: 13, 15–17
Adams, Zabdiel B. (1875–1940), 3: *228*
    AOA Commission on Congenital Dislocation of the Hip and, 3: 232, *232*, 233–234
    Base Hospital No. 6 and, 4: 433–434
    Boston Children's Hospital and, 2: 247; 3: 228
    Boston City Hospital and, 4: 305b
    CDH treatment, 3: 233–235
    death of, 3: 236
    early life, 3: 228
    education and training, 3: 228
    fracture management and, 3: 61
    HMS appointment, 3: 232
    Lakeville State Sanatorium and, 3: 235
    marriage and family, 3: 228, 236
    Medical Reserve Corps and, 3: 232
    memberships and, 3: 235–236
    as MGH house officer, 1: 189
    as MGH orthopaedic surgeon, 3: 228, 235, 266, 268
    military surgeon training and, 2: 42
    New England Deaconess Hospital and, 4: 225

441

publications and research,
  3: 228–232
 scoliosis treatment and, 2: 84,
  86; 3: 229–232
 World War I and, 3: 232; 4: 412
Adams, Zabdiel B. (father), 3: 228
Adam's machine, 2: 86
Affiliated Hospitals Center, Inc.,
  4: 42, 113–114, 118, 120, 127,
  132
Agel, Julie, 1: 287
Agency for Healthcare Research and
  Quality, 2: 371
Aitken, Alexander P. (1904–1993),
  4: *350*
 BCH Bone and Joint Service,
  4: 353, 356, 380*b*
 Boston City Hospital and, 4: 350
 Boston University Medical School
  appointment, 4: 350
 Chelsea Memorial Hospital and,
  4: 350
 classification of epiphyseal fractures, 4: 355–356
 death of, 4: 356
 education and training, 4: 350
 epiphyseal injury treatment,
  4: 350–352, 355–356
 fracture of the proximal tibial epiphyseal cartilage case,
  4: 355
 fracture research and, 4: 354
 hospital appointments, 4: 356
 legacy of, 4: 356
 Liberty Mutual Insurance Rehabilitation Clinic and, 4: 352–
  353, 356
 Massachusetts Regional Fracture
  Committee, 3: 64
 Monson State Hospital and,
  4: 350
 private medical practice, 4: 356
 professional memberships,
  4: 352, 356
 publications and research,
  4: 350–355
 rehabilitation of injured workers
  and, 4: 350, 352–354
 ruptured intervertebral disc treatment, 4: 350, 352–353
 Tufts Medical School appointment, 4: 353
 workers' compensation issues,
  4: 353–354
Aitken, H. F., 1: *89*
Akbarnia, Behrooz, 2: 359, 361
Akeson, Wayne, 3: 382
Akins, Carlton M., 1: 217*b*
Alais, J., 1: *34*

Alan Gerry Clinical Professor of
  Orthopaedic Surgery, 3: 224, 464*b*
Albee, F. H., 3: 157; 4: 406
Albert, E., 3: 95
Albert, Todd J., 4: 266*b*
Albert Einstein College of Medicine,
  2: 408
Alden, Eliza, 2: 231
Alden, Louise, 2: 241
Alder Hey Hospital (Liverpool),
  4: 401
Aldrich, Marion, 3: 164
Allen, Arthur W., 3: 60*b*, 315;
  4: 208
Allen, John Michael, 2: 438
Allen, L., 3: 133
Allen Street House (MGH),
  3: 17–18
Allgemeines Krankenhaus, 1: 81
Allgöwer, Martin, 2: 406
Allied Relief Fund, 4: 363
Allison, Addie Shultz, 3: 163
Allison, James, 3: 163
Allison, Marion Aldrich, 3: 164
Allison, Nathaniel (1876–1932),
  3: *163, 174*; 4: *417*
 absorbable animal membrane
  research, 3: 166, *166*, 167, *171*
 adult orthopaedics and, 2: 157
 AEF splint board, 4: 416–417
 American Ambulance Hospital
  and, 2: 119
 animal research and, 3: 165–167,
  170, *171*
 AOA Committee on war preparation, 2: 124
 AOA preparedness committee,
  4: 394
 as AOA president, 3: 172
 army manual of splints and appliances, 2: 126
 arthroplasty research,
  3: 165–166
 as BCH house officer, 3: 163
 on bone atrophy, 3: 170
 Chicago University orthopaedics
  department, 3: 175
 death of, 3: 176
 Department for Military Orthopedics and, 4: 405–406
 Diagnosis in Joint Disease,
  3: 175, 289, *290*
 early life, 3: 163
 education and training, 3: 163
 *Fundamentals of Orthopaedic Sur-
  gery in General Medicine and
  Surgery*, 2: 135–136
 on hip dislocations, 3: 164, 175
 HMS appointment, 3: 173

 knee derangement treatment,
  3: 165
 legacy of, 3: 176–177
 on Legg-Calvé-Perthes disease,
  3: 165–166
 low-back pain research, 3: 175
 marriage and, 3: 164
 memberships and, 3: 176, 176*b*
 MGH Fracture Clinic and,
  3: 60*b*, 314, 371
 MGH house officers and, 1: 189
 as MGH orthopaedics chief,
  1: 152; 2: 133–134; 3: 11*b*,
  173–174, 227
 military orthopaedics and, 2: 128
 New England Peabody Home for
  Crippled Children and, 2: 270;
  3: 174
 orthopaedic research and,
  3: 164–167, 170, 174–175
 on orthopaedics education,
  2: 134; 3: 170–173
 private medical practice, 2: 146
 "Progress in Orthopaedic Surgery" series, 2: 297
 publications and research,
  4: 102, 225–226, 372
 on sacroiliac joint fusion, 3: 185
 on splints for Army, 3: 167–168,
  168, 169, 169*b*
 synovial fluid research, 3: 174,
  174, 175
 Walter Reed General Hospital
  and, 4: 452
 Washington University orthopaedic department and, 3: 163–
  165, 170; 4: 419
 World War I and, 3: 157,
  166–169; 4: 417
Allison, Nathaniel (grandfather),
  3: 163
allografts
 bone banks for, 3: 386, 396,
  433, 440–441
 distal femoral osteonecrosis and,
  3: 433
 femoral heads and, 3: 442
 infection and freeze-dried,
  3: 440
 irradiation and, 3: 435
 knee fusion with, 3: 435
 long-term study of, 3: 433, 435
 malignant bone tumors and,
  3: 389
 osteoarticular, 3: 442
 osteosarcomas and, 3: 433
 transmission of disease through,
  3: 442–443, *443*
Alman, B. A., 2: 212
Alqueza, Arnold, 4: 190*b*

Index

Alqueza, Arnold B., 3: 463*b*
Altman, Greg, 4: 285–286
Altschule, Mark D., 1: 171, 239
AMA Committee on the Medical Aspects of Sports, 1: 274, 280
AMA Council on Medical Education and Hospitals, 1: 146, 196–197, 199, 211
Amadio, Peter C., 3: 431
Ambulatory Care Center (ACC) (MGH), 3: 396
Ambulatory Care Unit (ACU) (MGH), 3: 399
American Academy for Cerebral Palsy, 2: 176, 196–198
American Academy of Arts and Sciences, 1: 29, 61
American Academy of Orthopaedic Surgeons (AAOS), 1: xxv, 213; 2: 176, 201–203; 3: 90; 4: 337
American Ambulance Field Service, 2: 118
American Ambulance Hospital (Neuilly, France), 2: 119; 4: 386
    Harvard Unit and, 2: 118–120; 3: 166, 180, *180*; 4: 386, *387*, 389*b*, 391
    Osgood and, 2: 117–120; 4: 386, 391–393
    Smith-Petersen and, 3: 180
American Appreciation, An (Wilson), 3: 369
American Association for Labor Legislation, 4: 325–326
American Association for the Surgery of Trauma (AAST), 3: 65, 315, *315*; 4: *319*, 349
American Association of Medical Colleges (AAMC), 1: 168–169
American Association of Tissue Banks, 3: 386, 442–443, *443*
American Board of Orthopaedic Surgery (ABOS), 1: xxv, 197–200, 211, 213, 215–216, 231; 2: 317; 4: 173, 377–379
American British Canadian (ABC) Traveling Fellow, 3: 218
American College of Rheumatology, 4: 57–58
American College of Sports Medicine, 2: *387*
American College of Surgeons (ACS), 2: 158; 3: 112, *112*, 113*b*, 131, 310, 367; 4: 102, 324, 354
American College of Surgeons Board of Regents, 3: 62–63
American Expeditionary Forces (AEF)
    base hospitals for BEF, 4: 420, 426
    Division of Orthopedic Surgery, 4: 410*b*, 417, 439, 453–454
    Goldthwait and, 4: 416
    Johns Hopkins Hospital Unit and, 2: 221
    medical care in, 4: 417
    orthopaedic treatment and, 4: 409, 410*b*
    Osgood and, 2: 124, 126, 128; 4: 417, 421*b*
    physician deaths in, 4: 425
    Shortell and, 4: 338
    splint board and, 4: 416
    standardization of splints and dressings for, 2: 124; 3: 168
    Wilson and, 3: 370
American Field Service Ambulance, 4: 386, *386*, 387, *387*, 388
American Hospital Association, 1: 211
American Jewish Committee, 4: 203
American Journal of Orthopedic Surgery, 4: 226
American Medical Association (AMA), 1: xxv, 69, 189–191, 211, 213; 2: 42, 124; 3: 35, 131
American Mutual Liability Insurance Company, 3: 314, 316
American Orthopaedic Association (AOA), 4: 463
    Barr and, 1: 158
    Bradford and, 2: 24–26, 34, 43
    Buckminster Brown and, 1: 111
    Committee of Undergraduate Training, 2: 183
    founding of, 1: 114; 2: 48, *48*, 49
    graduate education study committee, 1: 196–197
    investigation of fusion on tubercular spines, 3: 157–158
    Lovett and, 2: 51
    military surgeon training and, 2: 65
    orthopaedic surgery terminology, 1: xxiv, xxv
    orthopaedics residencies survey, 2: 160–161
    Osgood and, 1: xxii; 2: 137
    Phelps and, 1: 193
    preparedness committee, 4: 394
    scoliosis treatment committee, 2: 87–88
    World War I and, 2: 64, 124
American Orthopaedic Foot and Ankle Society (AOFAS), 2: 316
American Orthopaedic Foot Society (AOFS), 2: 316–317; 3: 295, 298
American Orthopaedic Society of Sports Medicine (AOSSM), 1: 286, 289; 2: 163, 375; 3: 360
"American Orthopedic Surgery" (Bick), 1: 114
American Pediatric Society, 2: 15
American Public Health Association, 4: 439
American Radium Society, 1: 275–276
American Rheumatism Association, 2: 137; 4: 41*b*, 57–58, 63, 169
American Shoulder and Elbow Surgeons (ASES), 2: 380; 3: 415, *415*
American Society for Surgery of the Hand (ASSH), 2: 251; 3: 316, 428, *428*, 429, *430*; 4: 168, 186
American Society for Testing and Materials (ATSM), 3: 210
American Society of Hand Therapists, 4: 168
American Surgical Association, 1: 87; 2: 43; 3: 58
American Surgical Materials Association, 3: 210
American Whigs, 1: 11
AmeriCares, 3: 416
Ames Test, 4: 171
Ammer, Christine, 2: 277
amputations
    blood perfusion in, 3: 287
    economic importance and, 4: 419
    ether and, 1: 61
    fractures and, 1: 50, 54
    geriatric patients and, 3: 330
    Gritti-Stokes, 3: 374
    guillotine, 4: *469*
    John Collins Warren and, 1: 52–53, 61
    kineplastic forearm, 4: 360
    kit for, 1: *60*
    length and, 3: 374
    malpractice suits and, 1: 50
    military wounds and, 1: 23; 4: 418–419
    mortality rates, 1: 65, 74, 84
    osteosarcoma and, 3: 391
    research in, 3: 373, *373*
    results of, 3: 374*t*
    sepsis and, 3: 373
    shoulder, 1: 23
    skin traction and, 4: *419*
    suction socket prosthesis and, 1: 273
    temporary prostheses and, 3: 374
    transmetatarsal, 4: 276
    trauma and, 3: 373
    tuberculosis and, 3: 374

without anesthesia, 1: 10, 36, 65
wounded soldiers and,
  4: 446–447
Amputees and Their Prostheses (Pierce and Mital), 3: 320
AMTI, 3.224
Amuralt, Tom, 3: 463
Anatomical and Surgical Treatment of Hernia (Cooper), 1: 36
Anatomy Act, 1: 52
Anatomy of the Breast (Cooper), 1: 36
Anatomy of the Thymus Gland (Cooper), 1: 36
Anderson, Gunnar B. J., 4: 266*b*
Anderson, Margaret, 2: 170, 191–194, 264, 304, 350
Anderson, Megan E., 4: 287
Andrews, H. V., 3: 133
Andry, Nicolas, 1: xxi, xxii, xxiii, xxiv; 3: 90; 4: 233
anesthesia
  acetonuria associated with death after, 3: 305
  bubble bottle method, 4: 323
  charting in, 3: *95*, 96
  chloroform as, 1: 62–63, 82
  Cotton-Boothby apparatus, 4: *320*, 323
  ether as, 1: 55–58, 60–62, *63*, 64–65, 82
  hypnosis and, 1: 56, 65
  nitrous oxide as, 1: 56–59, 63
  orthopaedic surgery and, 2: 15
  surgery before, 1: 6, 10, 23, 36, 74
  use at Boston Orthopedic Institution, 1: 107, 118
  use at Massachusetts General Hospital (MGH), 1: 57–62, 118
anesthesiology, 1: 61
ankle valgus, 2: 212
ankles
  arthrodesis and, 3: 330
  astragalectomy and, 2: 93–94
  athletes and, 3: 348
  central-graft operation, 3: 368
  fractures, 4: 313–315, *315*, 316
  gait analysis and, 2: 406–407
  instability and Pott's fracture, 4: *317*, 318
  lubrication and, 3: 324
  sports injuries and, 1: 281
  stabilization of, 2: 148
  tendon transfers and, 2: 148
  tuberculosis and, 1: 73
  weakness and, 2: 150
ankylosis, 4: 64
Anna Jacques Hospital, 2: 269, 272

Annual Bibliography of Orthopaedic Surgery, 3: 261
anterior cruciate ligament (ACL)
  direct repair of, 2: 91
  growth plate disturbances, 2: 379
  intra-articular healing of, 2: 439
  intra-/extra-articular reconstruction, 3: 448
  outpatient arthroscopic reconstructions, 4: 255
  reconstruction of, 2: 91, 378–379, *386*
  skeletally immature patients and, 2: 378–379
  Tegner Activity Scale and, 2: 380
  young athletes and, 2: 385, *385*, 386
Anthology Club, 1: 29
antisepsis
  acceptance in the U.S., 1: 118
  carbolic acid treatment, 1: 82–83
  Coll Warren promotion of, 1: 85
  discovery of, 1: 55
  Lister and, 1: 55, 81, 84; 3: 45
  orthopaedic surgery and, 2: 15
  prevention of infection and, 1: 84–85
  surgeon resistance to, 1: 85
  trench warfare and, 4: 385
Antiseptic surgery (Cheyne), 1: *83*
AO Foundation, 3: 409, *409*
AOA. *See* American Orthopaedic Association (AOA)
apothecary, 1: 184
Appleton, Paul, 3: 410; 4: 288
Arbuckle, Robert H., 4: 163, 193
Archibald, Edward W., 3: 26, 50
Archives of Surgery (Jackson), 3: 35
Arlington Mills, 2: 267
Armed Forces Institute of Pathology, 4: 126
arms
  Bankart procedure and, 3: 359–360
  Boston Arm, 2: 326
  carpal tunnel syndrome, 2: 375
  compartment syndrome, 2: 249–250
  cubitus varus deformity, 2: 229
  dead arm syndrome, 3: 359–360
  distal humerus prosthesis, 2: 250
  kineplastic forearm amputation, 4: 360
  Krukenberg procedure, 2: 425
  tendon transfers and, 3: 428
  Volkmann ischemic contracture, 2: 200–201, 249–250
  x-ray of fetal, 3: 97, *97*
Armstrong, Stewart, 4: 41*b*

Arnold, Benedict, 1: 19, 33
Arnold, Horace D., 1: 250; 3: 122
arthritis. *See also* osteoarthritis; rheumatoid arthritis
  allied health professionals and, 4: 28
  experimental septic, 2: 79
  femoroacetabular impingement, 3: 189
  forms of chronic, 4: 55
  Green and, 2: 171
  growth disturbances in children, 4: 56
  hand and, 4: 96
  hip fusion for, 3: 156*b*
  hips and, 2: 380
  juvenile idiopathic, 2: 171, 350
  Lovett Fund and, 2: 82
  MGH and, 2: 82
  nylon arthroplasty and, 4: 65–66, 66*b*, 69
  orthopaedic treatment for, 2: 171; 4: 32–33
  pauciarticular, 2: 171, 350
  pediatric, 2: 349–350
  prevention and, 4: 60–61
  psoriatic, 4: 99
  rheumatoid, 2: 82, 171, 350; 3: 239
  roentgenotherapy for, 4: 64, *64*
  sacroiliac joint fusion for, 3: 184–185
  synovectomy in chronic, 4: 102, 371–372
  treatment of, 4: 32–33, 43, 54–55
  Vitallium mold arthroplasty and, 3: 239
Arthritis, Medicine and the Spiritual Law (Swaim), 4: 58, *58*
Arthritis and Rheumatism Foundation, 4: 39
Arthritis Foundation, 3: 279
arthrodesis procedures
  ankles and, 3: 330
  central-graft operation, 3: 368, *368*
  joints and, 3: 165
  MCP joint, 4: 97
  Morris on, 2: 282
  rheumatoid arthritis and, 4: 166
  rheumatoid arthritis of the hand research, 4: 167
  sacroiliac joint and, 3: 183–185
  wrists and, 3: 191, 239; 4: 166–167
arthrogram, 3: *99*
arthrogryposis multiplex congenita, 2: 274–275, 287

Index

arthroplasty. *See also* mold arthroplasty
  absorbable animal membrane research, 3: 165–167
  advances in, 4: 43
  of the elbow, 3: 64, 341; 4: 63
  hip and, 3: 181, 242, 242*t*, *242*, 243
  implant, 4: 99–100
  of the knee, 4: 64, 70*b*–71*b*, 93–94, 103, 179*t*
  metacarpophalangeal, 4: 97
  nylon, 4: 64, *65*, 66, 66*b*, 93
  release of contractures, 4: 166
  silicone flexible implants, 4: 166, *167*, *168*
  total knee, 4: 129–130, 131*t*
  using interpositional tissues, 4: 64
  volar plate, 2: 248
  wrist and, 3: 191

Arthroscopic Surgery Update (McGinty), 2: 279

arthroscopy
  cameras and, 2: 279
  knee injuries and, 1: 279; 4: 129
  knee simulator, 4: 173
  McGinty and Matza's procedure, 2: 279, 280*b*, 281
  operative, 3: 422–423
  orthopaedics education and, 1: 220, 230

Arthroscopy Association of North America, 2: 281; 3: 422, *422*

arthrotomy, 3: 165, 165*b*, 166, 351

Arthur H. Huene Award, 2: 403

Arthur T. Legg Memorial Room, 2: *106*, 107

articular cartilage
  allografts and, 3: 389–390
  chondrocytes and, 3: 444
  compression forces and, 3: 326
  cup arthroplasty of the hip and, 3: 244
  degradative enzymes in, 3: *401*
  dimethyl sulfoxide (DMSO) and glycerol, 3: 442
  gene transfer treatment, 3: 445
  histologic-histochemical grading system for, 3: 384, 385*t*, *385*
  lubrication and, 3: 326–327
  osteoarthritis and, 3: 387–388
  preservation of, 3: 442, *442*
  repair using tritiated thymidine, 3: 383
  sling procedure and, 3: 296

Aseptic Treatment of Wounds, The (Walter), 4: 106, *106*, 107*b*

Ashworth, Michael A., 4: 22

assistive technology, 2: 408

Association of American Medical Colleges (AAMC), 1: 211; 2: 158

Association of Bone and Joint Surgeons, 3: 436, *436*

Association of Franklin Medal Scholars, 1: 31

Association of Residency Coordinators in Orthopaedic Surgery, 1: 238

astragalectomy (Whitman's operation), 2: 92–94

Asylum for the Insane, The, 1: 294

athletic injuries. *See* sports medicine

Athletic Injuries. Prevention, Diagnosis and Treatment (Thorndike), 1: 265, *266*

athletic training. *See also* sports medicine
  dieticians and, 1: 258
  football team and, 1: 248, 250–253, 255–256, 258
  over-training and, 1: 251, 265
  scientific study of, 1: 250–251, 265–266

athletics. *See* Harvard athletics

Atsatt, Rodney F., 1: 193; 2: 140

ATSM Committee F-4 on Medical and Surgical Materials and Devices, 3: 210

Attucks, Crispus, 1: 14

Au, Katherine, 2: 425

Aufranc, Otto E. (1909–1990), 3: *236*, *245*, *273*, *300*
  AAOS and, 2: 215
  accomplishments of, 3: 241–242
  Boston Children's Hospital and, 3: 237
  Boston City Hospital internship, 3: 237
  Bronze Star and, 3: 240, 240*b*, *240*
  Chandler and, 3: 277
  Children's Hospital/MGH combined program and, 3: 237
  Constructive Surgery of the Hip, 3: 244, *246*
  on Coonse, 4: 372–373
  death of, 3: 247
  early life, 3: 236–237
  education and training, 3: 237
  Fracture Clinic and, 3: 60*b*, 241–242, 245
  "Fracture of the Month" column, 3: 243, *243*
  hip nailing and, 3: 237
  hip surgery and, 3: 238–243; 4: 187
  HMS appointment, 3: 241–242
  as honorary orthopaedic surgeon, 3: 398*b*
  honors and awards, 3: 245*b*
  Knight's Cross, Royal Norwegian Order of St. Olav, 3: *245*
  kyphosis treatment, 3: 239–240
  legacy of, 3: 247
  MGH Staff Associates and, 3: 241
  as MGH surgeon, 1: 203–204; 2: 325; 3: 74, 192, 217, 238–239, 241, 246
  mold arthroplasty and, 3: 192, 218, 238–239, 241–243, 243*b*, 244, 292*b*, 456*b*
  New England Baptist Hospital and, 3: 246–247
  Newton-Wellesley Hospital, 3: 240
  patient care and, 3: 244
  PBBH and, 4: 373
  private medical practice, 3: 238–240; 4: 158
  publications and research, 1: 286; 3: 191–192, 218, 239–244, 246, 302; 4: 161, 373
  rheumatoid arthritis research, 2: 137; 3: 239
  6th General Hospital and, 4: *476*, 482, 483*b*
  Smith-Petersen and, 3: 237–240
  Tufts appointment, 3: 247
  World War II service, 3: 239–241

Aufranc, Randolph Arnold, 3: 247

Aufranc, St. George Tucker, 3: 247; 4: 163, 193

Augustus Thorndike Professor of Orthopaedic Surgery, 3: 450, 464*b*

Augustus White III Symposium, 4: 265, 266*b*

Austen, Frank F., 4: 42, 114, 119, 128, 132

Austen, R. Frank, 4: 68–69

Austen, W. Gerald, 3: 256, 287, 397

Austin Moore prosthesis, 3: 213, 241, 354*b*

Australian Civil Constitution Corps (CCC), 4: 489

Australian Orthopaedic Association, 3: 360

Avallone, Nicholas, 4: 190*b*

Avicenna Hospital, 2: 421

Awbrey, Brian J., 3: 460*b*, 464*b*

Axelrod, Terry S., 3: 431

Aycock, W. Lloyd, 2: 82

Ayres, Douglas K., 4: 287

B

Babcock, Warren L., 4: 429, 433, 437
Bach, Bernard R., Jr., 1: 284, 288–289; 3: 379
back disabilities. *See also* sciatica
   industrial accidents and, 2: 92; 4: 358
   laminectomy and, 3: 204, 206–208
   low-back pain, 2: 371–372, 396; 3: 175, 204–206, 250b–252b
   lumbago and, 3: 203
   lumbar spinal stenosis, 2: 373–374
   MRI and, 3: 255
   Norton-Brown spinal brace and, 3: 318, 318tg, 319
   Ober Test and, 2: 151–152
   psychiatric investigation and, 3: 258
   ruptured intervertebral disc, 3: 204, *204*, 205–207, *207*, 208; 4: 352–353
   sacroiliac joint and, 3: 184
   Sever on, 2: 92
   spine fusion and, 3: 207–208
   treatment of, 3: 203
Back Problems Guideline Panel, 2: 371
"Back Strains and Sciatica" (Ober), 2: 151–152
Bader Functional Room, 2: *106*
Bae, Donald S., 2: *417*, 418–419, 419t, *419*; 4: 190b
Baer, William S., 2: 126; 3: 158, 166–167; 4: 416
Baetzer, Fred H., 3: 87
Bailey, Fred Warren, 2: 78
Bailey, George G., Jr. (unk.–1998)
   Boston City Hospital and, 4: 360
   death of, 4: 360
   education and training, 4: 360
   kineplastic forearm amputation case, 4: 360
   Mt. Auburn Hospital and, 4: 360
   professional memberships, 4: 360
   publications and research, 4: 360
Baker, Charles, 2: 39
Baker, Frances Prescott, 3: 308
Balach, Franklin, 4: 41b
Balch, Emily, 3: 142
Balch, Franklin G., Jr., 4: 193
Balkan Frame, 3: 317, 357b
Ball, Anna, 1: 95
Ballentine, H. Thomas, 3: 314
Bancroft, Frederic, 3: 316
Bankart, A. S. Blundell, 3: 449

Bankart procedure, 3: 351–354, 357–358, 358t, *359*, 360, 450
Banks, Henry H. (1921–), 1: *202*, 205, 207; 4: 72, 342
   AAOS and, 2: 314
   Aufranc and, 3: 247
   on BCH residencies, 4: 377
   BIH Board of Consultants, 4: 262–263
   Boston Children's Hospital and, 1: 204–206; 2: 233, 301; 4: 72
   Boston City Hospital and, 4: 297
   on Carl Walter, 4: 108
   cerebral palsy research and treatment, 2: 196–200; 4: 74, 76–77
   education and training, 4: 72
   flexor carpi ulnaris transfer procedure, 2: 188
   on Green, 2: 168, 204–205
   Grice and, 1: 206
   hip fracture research, 4: 74–78
   Little Orthopaedic Club and, 4: 74
   on Mark Rogers, 4: 229–230
   metastatic malignant melanoma fracture case, 4: 77–78
   MGH and, 1: 203–204
   on Ober, 2: 149
   Orthopaedic Surgery at Tufts University, 4: 77
   on osteochondritis dissecans, 2: 195
   PBBH and, 1: 204–205; 4: 19–20, 22, 72, 73b–74b, 128
   as PBBH chief of orthopaedics, 4: 22, 43, 76, 116b, 196b
   on PBBH research program, 4: 75b
   professional memberships, 4: 76–77
   publications and research, 4: 72, 75–77
   on Quigley, 1: 276–277, 282
   RBBH and, 4: 36, 40
   residency training under Green, 1: 202–203
   as Tufts University chair of orthopaedics, 4: 22, 76–77, 116
   US Army Medical Corps and, 4: 72
   on Zimbler, 4: 250
Bar Harbor Medical and Surgical Hospital, 2: 312
Barber, D. B., 2: 172
Barlow, Joel, 1: 292–293
Barnes Hospital, 3: 165; 4: 125
Barr, Dorrice Nash, 3: 247

Barr, Joseph S. (1901–1964), 1: *205*; 2: 249, 278, 286, 290, 320; 3: 142, *201*, 213
   as AAOS president, 3: 210
   appointments and positions, 3: 202b
   on audio-visual aids in teaching, 1: 161
   back pain and sciatica research, 3: 203–208
   Brigham and Women's Hospital and, 4: 195b
   as chair of AOA research committee, 3: 209, *209*
   as clinical professor, 1: 158
   Committee of Undergraduate Training, 2: 183
   death of, 3: 214
   development of research at MGH, 1: 180
   early life, 3: 201
   education and training, 3: 201
   Ferguson and, 2: 188
   Glimcher and, 2: 321–322
   on herniated disc and sciatica, 3: 184
   HMS appointment, 2: 223; 3: 202; 4: 61
   John Ball and Buckminster Brown Professorship, 3: 202, 453b, 464b; 4: 195b
   Joint Committee for the Study of Surgical Materials and, 3: 210
   leadership of, 3: 453, 453b–456b
   legacy of, 3: 212–214
   Marlborough Medical Associates and, 2: 146, 269, 299
   marriage and family, 3: 214
   memberships and, 3: 212–213
   as MGH orthopaedics chief, 3: 11b, 202, 227, 241, 277
   MGH residents and, 3: *212*, 217, 238, 254, 278, 285, 323, 377, 456; 4: *161*, 245
   MGH Staff Associates and, 3: 241
   as MGH surgeon, 3: 187, 201
   New England Peabody Home for Crippled Children and, 3: 209
   New England Society of Bone and Joint Surgery, 4: 347
   orthopaedic research and, 3: 210–212
   on orthopaedics curriculum, 1: 207
   PBBH 50th anniversary, 4: 21
   polio research, 3: 209, 331–333
   private medical practice, 3: 454b
   as professor of orthopaedic surgery, 1: 158, 179–180

Index

publications and research, 2: 152, 250; 3: 202–211, 302, 331
rehabilitation planning and, 1: 272
resident training by, 1: 199, 203, 206–207
retirement of, 2: 325
ruptured intervertebral disc research, 3: 204; 4: 352
scoliosis treatment, 2: 396; 3: 208–209
on shoulder arthrodesis, 2: 154
slipped capital femoral epiphysis research, 4: 237
on the surgical experiment, 3: 210
US Navy and, 3: 201
Barr, Joseph S., Jr. (1934–), 3: *247, 461*
  ankle arthrodesis case, 3: 330
  Boston Interhospital Augmentation Study (BIAS) and, 3: 248–249
  Boston Prosthetics Course and, 1: 217
  Children's Hospital/MGH combined program and, 3: 248
  early life, 3: 247
  education and training, 3: 248
  Faulkner Hospital and, 3: 248
  Glimcher and, 3: 248
  Halo Vest, 3: 321
  HMS appointment, 3: 248
  on Leffert, 3: 413
  on low-back pain, 3: 250*b*–252*b*
  as MGH clinical faculty, 3: 464*b*
  as MGH surgeon, 3: 214, 248, 398*b*
  professional memberships and, 3: 249
  publications and research, 3: 249
  sailing and, 3: 249, 252
  Schmidt and, 3: 248
  spine treatment and, 3: 460*b*
  US Naval Medical Corps and, 3: 248
Barr, Mary, 3: 214
Barrell, Joseph, 3: 9
Barrett, Ian, 2: 400
Barron, M. E., 4: 199
Bartlett, John, 1: 41; 3: 3, 5
Bartlett, Josiah, 1: 293
Bartlett, Marshall K., 3: 241; 4: 475, 482*b*
Bartlett, Ralph W., 2: 34
Barton, Lyman G., Jr., 2: 119; 4: 389*b*
Baruch, Bernard M., 1: 272
Baruch Committee, 1: 272–273

base hospitals. *See also* military reconstruction hospitals; US Army Base Hospitals
  AEF and, 4: 417, 419–420
  amputations and, 4: 418
  Boston-derived, 4: 420*t*
  Camp Devens, 4: 452
  Camp Taylor, 4: 452
  field splinting and, 4: 408
  Harvard Units and, 4: 419–420, 437–438
  injuries and mortality rates in, 4: 424
  organization of American, 4: 419–420
  orthopaedics surgery and, 4: 406, 412, 417–419, 440, 443, 445, 451–453
  training in, 4: 420–421
  US and British medical staff in, 4: 422
  wounded soldiers and, 4: 385, 414, 416–417
basic fibroblast growth factor (bFGF), 3: 445
Bateman, James E., 2: 317; 3: 295
Bates, Frank D. (1925–2011)
  Boston Children's Hospital and, 2: 301
  Brigham and Women's Hospital and, 4: 193
  Korean War and, 2: 218
  PBBH and, 4: 20, 22, 116, 128
  Winchester Hospital and, 3: 299
Battle of Bunker Hill, 1: *17, 18, 18*, 19, 22
Battle of Lexington and Concord, 1: 17–18, 22
"Battle of the Delta, The," 1: 245–247
Baue, Arthur, 1: 90
Bauer, Thomas, 4: 174
Bauer, Walter, 2: 82, 171; 3: 335
Bayne-Jones, Stanhope, 4: 405*b*
Beach, Henry H. A., 2: 24; 3: 40
Bean, Harold C., 2: 230
Bearse, Carl, 4: 208
Beattie, George, 2: 300
Beauchamp, Richard, 2: 351, *351*
Bedford Veterans Administration Hospital, 3: 314
Beecher, Henry K., 1: 171, 239; 3: 96
Begg, Alexander S., 1: 88
Bell, Anna Elizabeth Bowman, 2: 219
Bell, Emily J. Buck, 2: 220
Bell, Enoch, 2: 219
Bell, J. L., 1: 24
Bell, John, 1: 37

Bell, John F. (1909–1989)
  Boston Children's Hospital and, 2: 299
  club foot treatment, 2: 208
  Crippled Children's Clinic and, 2: 221
  Crotched Mountain Foundation, 2: 221
  death of, 2: 221
  disabled children and, 2: 221
  education and training, 2: 219, 220*b*
  Journal of Bone and Joint Surgery editor, 2: 221
  marriage and family, 2: 220
  Ober and, 2: 220
  Palmer Memorial Hospital and, 2: 219–220
  PBBH and, 2: 220
  pediatric orthopaedics and, 2: 221
  publications of, 2: 208, 220–221
  University of Vermont and, 2: 220–221
  Vermont Department of Health and, 2: 221
Bell, Joseph, 1: 84
Bell, Sir Charles, 1: 37, 73, 76
Bellare, Anuj, 4: 194
Bellevue Medical College, 2: 63
Bemis, George, 1: 307, 317
Bender, Anita, 4: 81
Bender, Ralph H. (1930–1999), 4: *80*
  on back pain, 4: 80
  Beth Israel Hospital and, 4: 247
  death of, 4: 81
  education and training, 4: 80
  hospital appointments, 4: 80
  marriage and family, 4: 81
  private medical practice, 4: 80
  professional memberships, 4: 81
  RBBH and, 4: 41*b*, 68, 80, 102
  US Air Force and, 4: 80
Benet, George, 4: 389*b*
Bennet, Eban E., 2: 72, 74–75
Bennett, G. A., 3: 335
Bennett, George E., 2: 77–78, 119; 4: 473
Benz, Edward, 2: 331
Berenberg, William, 2: 196, 213, 354, 406, 408
Bergenfeldt, E., 4: 356
Berlin, David D.
  Beth Israel Hospital and, 4: 361
  Boston City Hospital and, 4: 361
  education and training, 4: 361
  publications and research, 4: 361
  scaphoid fracture treatment, 4: 361

Tufts Medical School appointment, 4: 361
Bernard, Claude, 1: 82; 3: 142
Bernard, Francis, 1: 8, 13
Bernese periacetabular osteotomy, 2: 391–392
Bernhardt, Mark, 4: 263
Bernstein, Fredrika Ehrenfried, 4: 220
Bernstein, Irving, 4: 220
Bernstein, J., 1: 168
Berry, George P., 1: 180; 2: 183, 324; 3: 202, 334; 4: 113, 303
Bertody, Charles, 1: 60
Berven, Sigurd, 3: *278*
Beth Israel Deaconess Medical Center (BIDMC)
   Augustus White III Symposium, 4: 265, 266*b*
   Bierbaum and, 1: 233–234
   CareGroup and, 4: 281
   Carl J. Shapiro Department of Orthopaedics, 4: 288
   East Campus, 4: *213, 287*
   Emergency Department, 4: 286
   financial difficulties, 4: 283–284
   formation of, 4: 214, 223, 270, 281, 283
   HCORP and, 4: 284, 288
   as HMS teaching hospital, 4: 214
   Kocher and, 2: 377
   orthopaedics department, 1: 171; 4: 284–288
   orthopaedics department chiefs, 4: 289*b*
   orthopaedics residencies, 1: 223–224, 234, 236, 242; 4: 285–288
   West Campus, 4: *213, 280*
Beth Israel Hospital Association, 4: 204–205
Beth Israel Hospital (BIH)
   affiliation with Harvard Medical School, 4: 213–214, 251
   affiliation with Tufts Medical School, 4: 213–214, 214*b*, 228
   Brookline Avenue location, 4: 211, *211*, 228
   continuing medical education and, 4: 208
   establishment of new location, 4: 210, 210*b*, 211
   facilities for, 4: 207–208, 210
   financial difficulties, 4: 210–211, 281
   founding of, 4: 199
   growth of, 4: 209–210
   HCORP and, 1: 218; 4: 247–248
   HMS courses at, 1: 158
   house officers at, 4: 209*b*
   immigrant care in, 4: 283
   infectious disease fellowship, 1: 91
   internships at, 1: 196
   Jewish patients at, 4: 199, 205–206, 223
   Jewish physician training at, 1: 158; 4: 199, 283
   leadership of, 4: 206–211
   medical education and, 4: 213
   merger with New England Deaconess Hospital, 4: 214, 223, 270, 281, 283
   Mueller Professorship, 4: 263
   non-discrimination and, 4: 199
   opening of, 4: 205, 223
   operating room at, 4: *212, 228*
   Orthopaedic Biomechanics Laboratory, 4: 262
   orthopaedic division chiefs, 4: 223, 289*b*
   orthopaedic residencies at, 4: 247–248, 251
   orthopaedics department at, 4: 213, 247, 262–263
   orthopaedics department chiefs, 4: 289*b*
   orthopaedics surgery at, 2: 377; 3: 325; 4: 208, 208*b*
   sports medicine and, 4: 255
   surgeon-in-chiefs at, 4: 283, 283*t*
   surgical departments at, 4: 208
   Townsend Street location, 4: 205, *205, 206, 207*
Beth Israel Medical Center (NY), 2: 408; 4: 206
Bettman, Henry Wald, 3: 86
Bhashyam, Abhiram R., 3: 463*b*
Bianco, Anthony, Jr., 2: 304
Bick, Edgar M., 1: 101, 114; 4: 88
Bicknell, Macalister, 3: 192
BIDMC. *See* Beth Israel Deaconess Medical Center (BIDMC)
Bierbaum, Benjamin
   as BIDMC chief of orthopaedics, 1: 233–234, 236; 4: 284–286, 289*b*
   Boston Children's Hospital and, 2: 286, 438
   Brigham and Women's Hospital and, 4: 193
   Crippled Children's Clinic and, 2: 314
   hip surgery and, 4: 284
   HMS appointment, 4: 284–285
   New England Baptist Hospital and, 1: 233; 4: 284
   PBBH and, 4: 22, 116, 128, 163
   Tufts Medical School appointment, 4: 284
Biesiadecki, Alfred, 1: 82
Bigelow, Henry Jacob (1818–1890), 1: *137*; 3: *23, 30, 32, 46*
   as accomplished surgeon, 3: 39–41
   bladder stones treatment, 3: 41–42
   cellular pathology and, 3: 34
   Charitable Surgical Institution, 3: 30
   Chickahominy fever and, 3: 44
   Civil War medicine and, 3: 43–44
   code of conduct, 3: 47*b*, 48
   controversy over, 3: 44–45
   disbelief in antisepsis, 3: 45
   discounting of Warren, 3: 32–34, 36
   "Discourse on Self-Limited Diseases, A," 3: 12–13
   drawings of femur malunions, 3: *42*
   early life, 3: 23
   education and training, 3: 23–25
   ether and anesthetics, 3: 27–29, 31–34
   European medical studies, 3: 25
   excision of the elbow, 3: 34
   femoral neck fractures, 3: 38–39, *39*
   hip dislocations and, 3: 34–36, 38
   hip joint excision, 3: 34
   as HMS professor of surgery, 1: 137; 3: 34, 42–43, *43*, 44
   home in Newton, 3: *48*
   house on Tuckernuck Island, 3: *49*
   on the importance of flexion, 3: 38
   injury and death of, 3: 49–50
   "Insensibility During Surgical Operations Produced by Inhalation," 3: 27, *27*
   legacy of, 3: 45–48
   Manual of Orthopedic Surgery, 3: 25–26, *26*
   marriage and family, 3: 30, 34
   Mechanism of Dislocation and Fracture of the Hip, 3: 35, *35*, 38
   memberships and, 3: 48
   as MGH surgeon, 1: 84; 3: 15, 25–27, 30–31, *31*
   as MGH surgeon emeritus, 3: 45–46
   New England Peabody Home for Crippled Children and, 2: 230

nitrous oxide and, 1: 56
orthopaedic contributions, 3: 34–36, 37*b*, 38–39
orthopaedics curriculum and, 1: 140
posthumous commemorations of, 3: 50, 50*b*, 51, 51*b*
reform of HMS and, 1: 139; 3: 44–45
resistance to antisepsis techniques, 1: 85
as senior surgeon at MGH, 1: 86; 2: 20
on spinal disease, 2: 57
support for House of the Good Samaritan, 1: 124
surgical illustrations and, 3: 25
surgical instruments and, 3: 40–41
Tremont Street Medical School and, 3: 26, 42
ununited fractures research, 3: 34–35
on use of ether, 1: 57, 59, 61–62
Bigelow, Jacob, 1: 60, 296, 299–300, 302; 3: 12, 23, 42
Bigelow, Mary Scollay, 3: 23
Bigelow, Sturgis, 1: *61*
Bigelow, Susan Sturgis, 3: 30, 34
Bigelow, W. S. (William Sturgis), 3: 23, 34, 40–41, 47*b*, 48, 50
Bigelow Building (MGH), 3: 15–17
Bigelow Medal, 3: *49*, 50
Bigelow's septum, 3: 39
Bigos, Stanley, 2: 371
BIH/Camp International Visiting Lecture, 4: 263
Billroth, Theodor, 1: 81–82
Binney, Horace, 3: 237; 4: 420
Biochemistry and Physiology of Bone (Bourne), 3: 337
bioethics, 4: 324
Biography of Otto E. Aufranc, A, 3: *246*
Biomaterials and Innovative Technologies Laboratory, 3: 463, 464*b*
biomechanics
  backpack loads and, 2: 408
  bone structure property relations, 2: 410
  collagen in the intervertebral discs and, 2: 328
  CT arthrography and, 2: 410
  early study of, 1: xxii
  Harrington rods and, 2: 325
  hips and, 2: 407
  laboratory for, 3: 220
  orthopaedics education and, 1: 220, 230, 241

  osteoarthritis and, 3: 322, 326–328, 383–384
  posterior cruciate ligament injury and, 3: 448
  subchondral bone with impact loading, 3: 326–327
"Biomechanics of Baseball Pitching" (Pappas), 2: *288*
Biomotion Laboratory, 3: 463, 464*b*
biopsy, 3: 390–391
Bird, Larry, 2: 369
birth abnormalities, 2: 275, 334, *334*
birth fractures, 2: 172. *See also* congenital pseudarthrosis of the tibia
birth palsies research, 2: 415, 417, *417*, 418–420
Black, Eric, 4: 190*b*
Blackman, Kenneth D., 1: 178
bladder stones, 3: 41–42
Blake, John Bapst, 4: 291
Blake, Joseph A., 2: 118; 4: 416
Bland, Edward, 4: 482*b*
Bland, Edward F., 3: 241; 4: 22
Blazar, Philip, 3: 410; 4: 194
Blazina, M. E., 1: 279
blood poisoning, 2: 299
blood transfusions, 1: 23; 3: 313
Bloodgood, Joseph C., 3: 137
bloodletting, 1: 9, 23, 74
Bloomberg, Maxwell H., 4: 208*b*
Blount, Walter, 2: 176, 335
Blumer, George, 2: 158
Boachie-Adjei, Oheneba, 4: 266*b*
Bock, Arlie V., 1: 265; 2: 253
Bock, Bernard, 1: 217*b*
body mechanics, 3: 81, 91; 4: 82–83, 233, 236
Body Mechanics in Health and Disease (Goldthwait et al.), 3: 91; 4: 53, 62
Body Snatchers, 1: *32*
Bohlman, Henry H., 4: 266*b*
Böhm, Max, 3: 67, 71, 265–266
Boland, Arthur L. (1935–), 1: *283*, 285
  awards and honors, 1: 288–289
  Brigham and Women's Hospital and, 1: 284; 4: 163, 193
  Children's Hospital/MGH combined program and, 1: 283
  on concussions, 1: 286–287
  education and training, 1: 283–284
  Harvard University Health Service and, 1: 284
  as head surgeon for Harvard athletics, 1: 284–288; 3: 399
  as HMS clinical instructor, 1: 166, 284
  knee injuries and, 1: 287

  as MGH clinical faculty, 3: 464*b*
  as MGH surgeon, 3: 399
  PBBH and, 4: 116, 128, 163
  publications of, 1: 286, 288
  sports medicine and, 1: 284–289; 2: 384; 3: 448, 460*b*
  women basketball players and, 1: 285–286
Boland, Jane Macknight, 1: 289
Bonar, Lawrence C., 2: 324
bone and joint disorders
  arthrodesis and, 3: 165
  atypical multiple case tuberculosis, 2: 257
  bone atrophy and, 3: 170
  chondrosarcoma, 3: 406
  conditions of interest in, 3: 82*b*
  fusion and, 3: 368
  Legg and, 2: 110
  lubrication and, 3: 324–327
  mobilization of, 4: 27*b*
  PBBH annual report, 4: 13, 13*t*, 16
  sacroiliac joint treatment, 3: 183–184
  schools for disabled children, 2: 37
  subchondral bone research, 3: 326–327, *327*
  total disability following fractures, 3: *373*
  tubercular cows and, 2: 16
  tuberculosis in pediatric patients, 2: 308–309
  tuberculosis of the hip, 3: 148
  tuberculosis treatment, 2: 11, 25; 3: 166, 289
  use of x-rays, 3: 101–103
bone banks, 3: 386, 388, 396, 433
bone cement, 4: 129, 133, 171
bone grafts
  arthrodesis procedures, 3: 368
  Boston approach and, 2: 392
  chemotherapy and, 2: 423
  chronic nonunions of the humerus and, 2: *96*
  early study of, 1: xxiii
  flexion injuries and, 3: 348
  Grice procedure and, 2: 209–210
  injured soldiers and, 3: 336, *337*
  kyphosis and, 2: 343
  modified Colonna reconstructive method, 3: 194
  non-union fractures and, 2: 238; 3: 59
  posterior spinal fusion and, 2: 341
  radioactive calcium tracers in, 2: 237, 240
  spinal fusion and, 3: 208, 425

tibial pseudarthrosis in neurofibromatosis case, 2: 175–176
total hip replacement and, 3: 279
bone granuloma, 2: 171
bone growth
activating transcription factor-2
(ATF-2) and, 2: 330
Digby's method for measuring,
2: 170, 170t
distal femur and proximal tibia,
2: 191–192, *192*, 193
effects of irradiation on epiphyseal growth, 3: 331
epiphyseal arrest and, 2: 192,
192t, 193
Green and, 2: 170, 191–194
Green-Andersen growth charts,
2: 193, *193*, 194
Moseley's growth charts, 2: 194
orthoroentgenograms and,
2: 192–193
Paley multiplier method, 2: 194
research in, 2: 191–194
skeletal age in predictions, 2: 192
bone irradiation, 2: 237
Bone Sarcoma Registry of the American College of Surgeons, 4: 102
bone sarcomas, 3: 136–137, 137t,
138–140, 140b, 141–142
bones and teeth
apatite crystals and, 2: 321
collagen in, 2: 327–328
electron microscopes and,
2: 323, *324*
Haversian systems in, 2: 241
hydroxylysine and, 2: 327–328
mineralized crystals, 2: 325–326
research in, 2: 322–324
research in lesions, 2: 236
Bonfiglio, Michael, 3: 303
Boothby, Walter M., 4: 216, 323,
389b, 422b
Boott, Francis, 1: 59
Borden Research Award, 2: 319
Borges, Larry, 3: 420
Boron Neutron Capture Synovectomy, 4: 136
Bosch, Joanne P., 4: 183
Bost, Frederick C., 2: 274; 4: 60
Boston, Mass.
annual Christmas tree from Halifax, 3: 135, *135*
cholera epidemic, 1: 295; 4: 293
colonial economy in, 1: 10
Committee of Correspondence
in, 1: 16
Fort Warren, 1: 20
Halifax Harbor explosion aid,
3: 134–135
infectious disease in, 1: 7–9; 2: 4

inoculation hospitals, 1: 8–9
Irish Catholics in, 4: 200
Irish immigration to, 4: 293
Jewish immigration to, 4: 199–
200, 220
Jewish physicians in, 4: 199–200
Jewish Quarter, 4: 200, *200*
malnutrition in, 2: 4
maps, 1: *7, 114, 296*
military reconstruction hospital
and, 4: 444
need for hospital in, 1: 41; 3: 3;
4: 293–294, 294b
orthopaedics institutions in,
1: 189–190
Stamp Act protests in, 1: 11–13
tea party protest and, 1: 15–16
Townshend Act protests, 1: 13–14
Warren family and, 1: 4b
Boston Almshouse, 1: 29; 3: 3
HMS clinical teaching at, 1: 28,
40; 3: 4–5
house pupils at, 1: 80
inadequacy of, 1: 41; 3: 3–4
John Ball Brown and, 1: 96
medical care at, 2: 20; 3: 3–4
Boston Arm, 2: 326, *326*; 3: 287
Boston Association of Cardiac Clinics, 1: 129
Boston Ballet, 2: 384, *384*
Boston brace, 2: 339–340, *340*,
358–359, *359*–*360*, *361*, 423, *424*
Boston Brace Instructional Courses,
2: 358
Boston Bruins, 3: 348, 356–357,
357b, 397, 399, 448; 4: 342
Boston Children's Hospital (BCH),
1: *194*; 2: *177*, *437*, *438*
Act of Incorporation, 2: 7, *7*
astragalectomy at, 2: 93–94
bedside teaching at, 2: *435*
Berlin polio epidemic team,
2: 260, 264
Boston brace and, 2: 339–340,
423
Boston Concept and, 2: 392
cerebral palsy cases, 2: 171–172
Cerebral Palsy Clinic, 2: 402,
406, 409
charitable surgical appliances,
2: *14*
children with poliomyelitis and,
1: 191; 2: 163
children's convalescence and,
2: 9
clinical service rotations, 1: 198
clinical surgery curricula
at, 1: 141, 143, 147, 151,
155–157, 162
cows and, 2: *429*

decline in skeletal tuberculosis
admissions, 2: 16, 16t
Department of Medicine, 2: 427
Department of Orthopaedic Surgery, 1: 171–172, 189–190;
2: 10–13, 15–16, 40, *98*, *133*,
156, *177*, *200*, *222*, *252*, *255*,
283, *293*, 354–355, 427, 434,
438–439, 439b; 3: 67
Department of Surgery, 2: 427
endowed professorships, 2: 438,
439b
founding of, 1: 123; 2: 3–9
Growth Study (Green and Anderson), 2: 193
HCORP and, 1: 213, 215
hip disease and, 2: 52
House of the Good Samaritan
merger, 1: 130; 2: 433
house officers at, 1: 184, 189
house officer's certificate, 2: *41*
impact of World War II on,
4: 468
Infantile Paralysis Clinic, 2: 79
innovation and change at,
2: 427–428, 430–434,
436–439
internships at, 1: 196
Massachusetts Infantile Paralysis
Clinics, 2: 188–189
military surgeon training at,
1: 151, 191; 4: 396
Myelodysplasia Clinic, 2: 359,
402
named funds, 2: 436, 439b
nursing program at, 2: 13–14
objections to, 2: 8–9
organizational models,
2: 436–437
orthopaedic admissions at,
2: 15t, 40, 40t
orthopaedic chairpersons, 2: 15b
orthopaedic surgeries, 2: 9–12,
12t, 13, *13*, 14–15, 39–40,
337–338, 338t
orthopaedics residencies, 1: 186–
187, 199, 202–207, 211,
217–218, 224–225; 2: *413*
outpatient services at, 1: 190;
2: 11–12
patient registry, 2: *10*
PBBH and, 4: 10, 14
pediatrics at, 2: 3
polio clinics at, 2: 78–79, 188
private/public system in, 2: 313,
337, 339
psoas abscesses and, 2: 54
radiology at, 2: 16, *16*, 17, 17t,
431
Report of the Medical Staff, 2: 9

Index

resident salaries, 1: 206, *206*
scoliosis clinic at, 2: 35–36, 84–86
Sever-L'Episcopo procedure, 2: 417
Spanish American War patients, 4: *311*
specialization in, 2: 11
Spinal Surgery Service, 2: 359
spinal tuberculosis and, 2: 11, 308–309
sports medicine and, 2: 287, 384
Statement by Four Physicians, 2: 6–7
surgeon-scholars at, 2: 217, 357
surgical procedures for scoliosis, 2: *369*
surgical training at, 1: 188–189
teaching clinics at, 1: 194; 2: *62*
teaching fellows, 1: 192–193
tuberculosis patients, 2: 275
20th century overview of, 2: 427–428, 430–434, 436–439
use of radiographs, 2: 54
Boston Children's Hospital (BCH). Facilities
   appliance shop at, 2: 22, *22*, 431
   Bader building, 2: 432, *432–433*
   Bader Solarium, 2: *432*
   Boy's Ward, 2: *14*
   expansion of, 2: 9–11, 13, *433*, *434t*
   Fegan building, 2: *433*
   Functional Therapy Room, 2: *432*
   gait laboratory, 2: 107, 406
   Girl's Surgical Ward, 2: *15*
   gymnasium, 2: *433*
   Hunnewell Building entrance, 2: *429*
   on Huntington Ave., 2: 11, *11*, 12, *12*, 427–428, *428*
   Ida C. Smith ward, 2: *431*
   Infant's Hospital, 2: *431*
   lack of elevators in, 2: 430, *430*
   on Longwood Avenue, 2: 64, 428, 430–431
   Medical Center and Prouty Garden, 2: *436*
   orthopaedic research laboratory, 2: 234
   Pavilion Wards, 2: *435*
   research laboratories, 2: 234–236, 285, 434, 438–439
   standard ward in, 2: *144*, *429*
   Ward I, 2: *434*
   at Washington and Rutland Streets, 2: *11*
   in the winter, 2: *430*

Boston Children's Hospital/Massachusetts General residency program, 1: 210; 2: 144
Boston City Base Hospital No. 7 (France), 4: 301–302
Boston City Hospital (BCH), 4: *306*, *379*
   affiliation with Boston University Medical School, 4: 296–297, 303, 380
   affiliation with Harvard Medical School, 4: 296, 298, 302–303, 379–380
   affiliation with Tufts Medical School, 4: 228, 296–297, 303
   Base Hospital No. 7 and, 1: 256; 4: 301–302, 420t, 438–439
   Bone and Joint Service, 4: 306–307, 328, 333–334, 357, 377, 377t, 380b
   Bradford and, 2: 21; 4: 298, 303, 307
   Burrell and, 4: 298–299, *299*, 300–301, 307
   Centre building, 4: *295*
   clinical courses for Harvard students at, 4: 380t–381t
   compound fracture therapy at, 4: *335*, 337
   construction of, 4: 295
   end of Harvard Medical School relationship, 4: 380
   ether tray at, 4: *298*
   examining room, 4: *300*
   fracture treatment and, 4: 362
   Harvard Fifth Surgical Service at, 4: 275, 277, 297, 302–303, 305–306
   Harvard Medical Unit at, 4: 296–297, 303
   house officers at, 4: 305, 305b
   intern and residency training programs, 4: 303–306
   internships at, 1: 189, 196
   Joseph H. Shortell Fracture Unit, 4: 342, *342*, 357
   medical school affiliations, 4: 370–371
   merger with Boston University Medical Center Hospital, 4: 297
   Nichols and, 1: 174, 252; 4: 301–302
   opening of, 4: 295–296
   operating room at, 4: *298*, *301*
   orthopaedic residencies at, 1: 186, 199; 3: 237; 4: 377–380
   orthopaedic surgery at, 4: 307
   Outpatient Department, 4: *300*, 357
   Pavilion I, 4: *295*
   physical therapy room, 4: *308*
   planning for, 4: 293–295
   plot plan for, 4: *293*, *307*
   Relief Station, 4: *305*
   specialty services at, 4: 306–307
   staffing of, 4: 296
   surgeon-scholars at, 1: 174; 4: 333, 357
   Surgical Outpatient Department Building, 4: *295*
   surgical services at, 4: 297–303, 307, 370–371
   Surgical Ward, 4: *295*
   teaching clinics at, 1: 141, 143
   Thorndike Building, 4: *296*
   Thorndike Memorial Laboratory, 4: 297
   treatment of children in, 2: 4
   Tufts University Medical Service and, 4: 297
   undergraduate surgical education, 4: 303
   Ward O, 4: *296*
   wards in, 4: *301*
   West Roxbury Department, 4: 447–448
   women in orthopaedics at, 1: 200
Boston City Hospital Relief Station, 2: 269
Boston Concept, 2: 391, *391*, 392
Boston Dispensary, 1: 40, 96; 2: 20, 306; 3: 3; 4: 48, 311, *311*, 358
Boston Dynamics, 4: 173
Boston Hospital for Women, 4: 42–43, 69, 113–114, 119
Boston Infant's Hospital, 2: 242
Boston Interhospital Augmentation Study (BIAS), 3: 248–249
Boston Lying-in-Hospital, 1: 123; 4: 113–114
Boston Massacre, 1: 14–16
Boston Medical and Surgical Journal, 4: 293, 294b
Boston Medical Association, 1: 25, 38; 3: 25
Boston Medical Center (BMC), 4: 89, 297
Boston Medical Library, 1: 39, 59; 2: 271
Boston Medical Society, 4: 200, 202
Boston Organ Bank Group, 3: 386
Boston Orthopaedic Group, 4: 251, 285–286, 288
"Boston Orthopaedic Institution, The" (Cohen), 1: 114

Boston Orthopedic Club, 2: 171, 230, 294, 329; 3: 289; 4: 66
Boston Orthopedic Institution
  attraction of patients from the U.S. and abroad, 1: 99
  Buckminster Brown and, 1: 107, 118, 120–122
  closing of, 1: 121–122; 3: 30
  founding of, 1: xxiv, 99
  John Ball Brown and, 1: 99–100, 107, 113–114, 118–122
  long term treatment in, 2: 25
  origins and growth of, 1: 114–118
  scholarship on, 1: 114
  treatment advances in, 1: 118–120
  use of ether, 1: 107, 118
Boston Orthopedique Infirmary, 1: 99–100, 113. *See also* Boston Orthopedic Institution
Boston Pathology Course, 1: 216, 218
Boston Prosthetics Course, 1: 220
Boston Red Sox, 1: 258; 2: 288; 3: 348; 4: 345
Boston Rugby Football Club, 2: 383, *383*, 400
Boston School of Occupational Therapy, 4: 30, 32
Boston School of Physical Education, 3: 84
Boston School of Physical Therapy, 4: 30, 32
Boston Shriner's Hospital, 1: 123
Boston Society for Medical Improvement, 1: 61; 3: 44, 48, 150
Boston Surgical Society, 2: 69; 3: 50, 65
Boston University School of Medicine, 1: 239; 2: 273–274; 4: 67–68, 296
Boston Veterans Administration Hospital, 1: 71, 90; 3: 298
Bottomly, John T., 3: 116
Bouillaud, J. B., 4: 93
Bourne, Geoffrey, 3: 337
Bouvé, Marjorie, 4: 444
Bouvier, Sauveur-Henri Victor, 1: 106
Bowditch, Charles Pickering, 1: 82; 3: 142
Bowditch, Henry I., 1: 53, 73, 82, *82*; 2: 306; 3: 9, 97–98; 4: 3
Bowditch, Henry P., 2: 48; 3: 94
Bowditch, Katherine Putman, 3: 142
Bowditch, Nathaniel, 3: 15, 142, 146
Bowen, Abel, 1: *29*
Bowker, John H., 3: 299

Boyd, A. D., Jr., 4: 136
Boyd, Robert J. (1930–), 3: *254, 256*
  Barr and, 3: 255
  Children's Hospital/MGH combined program and, 3: 253
  education and training, 3: 253
  hip surgery and, 3: 253
  HMS appointment, 3: 254
  Lemuel Shattuck Hospital and, 3: 253
  Lynn General Hospital and, 3: 253
  MGH Staff Associates and, 3: 256
  as MGH surgeon, 3: 253, 256, 398*b*
  private medical practice, 3: 256
  Problem Back Clinic at MGH and, 3: 254
  problem back service and, 3: 388*t*
  publications and research, 3: 253–255, *255*
  Scarlet Key Society and, 3: 253
  Sledge and, 4: 127
  spine and trauma work, 3: 254–255, 420, 460*b*
  Trauma Management, 3: 62, 253
Boyes, Joseph, 3: 427
Boylston, Thomas, 3: 5
Boylston Medical School, 1: 138
Boylston Medical Society, 3: 25–26, 48
Bozic, Kevin J., 1: 225; 4: 266*b*
brachial plexus injuries, 2: 90–91, 96; 3: 412–414
Brachial Plexus Injuries (Leffert), 3: 414
brachioradialis transfer, 2: 153–154, *154*
Brackett, Elliott G. (1860–1942), 3: *147, 157*; 4: *394*
  Advisory Orthopedic Board and, 3: 157
  AOA meeting and, 2: 137
  Beth Israel Hospital and, 4: 208*b*
  Boston Children's Hospital and, 2: 13, 34, 40, 247, 264; 3: 147–148, 153
  Boston City Hospital and, 4: 305*b*, 308*b*, 406
  Bradford and, 3: 147, 150–151
  on Buckminster Brown, 3: 150
  chronic hip disease and, 3: 147, 151
  Clinical Congress of Surgeons in North America and, 3: 116

  Department for Military Orthopedics and, 4: 405–406
  early life, 3: 147
  education and training, 3: 147
  on functional inactivity, 2: 110
  on fusion in tubercular spines, 3: 148–149, 157–158, 158*b*
  on gunshot injuries, 3: 156, 156*b*
  HMS appointment, 3: 154
  HMS Orthopaedic surgery and, 1: 171
  hot pack treatment and, 2: 264
  House of the Good Samaritan and, 2: 114; 3: 148
  interest in the hip, 3: 148
  Journal of Bone and Joint Surgery editor, 3: 157–159, 160*b*, 161, 344
  legacy of, 3: 161–162
  marriage and, 3: 154
  memberships and, 3: 161
  as MGH orthopaedics chief, 2: 129–130; 3: 11*b*, 155, 227
  as MGH surgeon, 2: 99; 3: 153
  military surgeon training and, 2: 42; 4: 393, 395–396
  pathological findings in tubercular spine specimens, 3: 154–155
  Pott's Disease treatment, 3: 148–150
  private medical practice, 3: 154
  publications and research, 2: 56, 61; 3: 148, 151, 153–155
  RBBH and, 4: 406
  rehabilitation of soldiers and, 4: 396, 439, 444
  on sacroiliac joint fusion, 3: 185
  schools for disabled children, 2: 36; 3: 151, 161
  scoliosis treatment and, 2: 35, 56; 3: 151–152
  Section of Orthopaedic Surgery and, 4: 412
  treatment by Bradford, 3: 147
  US Army Medical Corps and, 4: 405
  use of orthopaedics apparatus, 3: 150–151
  Volunteer Aid Association and, 3: 152–153
  World War I and, 3: 156–157; 4: 404–405, 411
Brackett, Katherine F. Pedrick, 3: 154
Bradford, Charles F., 2: 19
Bradford, Charles Henry (1904–2000)
  Battle of Corregidor, 4: 363–364

Index

BCH Bone and Joint Service, 4: 367
Boston City Hospital and, 4: 362
Boston University Medical School appointment, 4: 366
Britten hip fusion technique and, 4: 363
civil defense and, 4: 364–366
Combat Over Corregidor, 4: *364*
Cotting School and, 4: 367
death of, 4: 368
education and training, 4: 361–362
Faulkner Hospital and, 4: 362
fracture treatment and, 4: 362
hospital appointments, 4: 364
legacy of, 4: 366–368
marriage and family, 4: 361
Massachusetts Medical Society lecture, 4: *365*, 366*b*, 367, 367*b*
Mt. Auburn Hospital and, 4: 362
poetry writing and, 4: 364
professional memberships, 4: 368
publications and research, 4: 352, 363, 365, *365*, 368
tibial spine fracture case, 4: 365
Tufts Medical School appointment, 4: 366
US Army Medical Corps and, 4: 363–364
World War II medical volunteers and, 4: 362–363
Bradford, Charles Hickling, 2: 42–43
Bradford, Edith Fiske, 2: 42; 4: 361
Bradford, Edward H. (1848–1926), 2: *19, 39, 44*
  AOA address, 2: 24–26
  as AOA president, 2: 43
  as BCH surgeon-in-chief, 2: 39–40, *41*
  Boston Children's Hospital and, 2: 10–11, 13, 15–16, 21, 29, 39–40
  Boston City Hospital and, 4: 298, 303, 307
  Boston City Hospital appointments, 2: 21, 24
  Bradford Frame and, 2: 27, *27*, 30–31, *31*, 32
  Buckminster Brown and, 2: 20; 3: 150
  on Burrell, 4: 298–299
  CDH treatment, 2: 32–33, *33*, 34
  club foot apparatus, 2: 22–23, *23*
  club foot treatment, 2: 22–24, 28, *28*, 29
  curative workshops and, 4: 403
  as dean of HMS, 1: 172–174; 2: 15, 41–42; 4: 324
  death of, 2: 43–44
  early life, 2: 19
  education and training, 2: 19–20
  European medical studies, 1: 186; 2: 20
  first craniotomy performed, 2: 24–25
  FitzSimmons and, 2: 255
  general surgery and, 2: 24
  hip disease treatment, 2: 21–22, 32
  HMS appointment, 2: 21, 40–41, 428; 4: 213
  House of the Good Samaritan and, 1: 128–130; 2: 21
  influences on, 2: 20, 22
  knee flexion contracture appliance, 2: *20, 21*
  knee valgus deformity, 2: *21*
  legacy of, 2: 42–44
  loss of eyesight, 2: 43
  Lovett and, 2: 49
  marriage and family, 2: 42
  on medical education, 4: 299–301
  memberships and, 2: 43
  method of reducing the gibbus, 3: *149*
  as MGH surgeon, 3: 266
  nose and throat clinic creation, 2: 40–41
  orthopaedic brace shop, 2: 22, *22*
  as orthopaedic chair, 2: 15*b*
  Orthopaedic Journal Club, 3: 369
  orthopaedic surgery advances, 2: 27, 36, 39–40
  Orthopedic Surgery, 4: 318
  osteotomies and, 2: 29, 34
  poliomyelitis treatment, 2: 264
  on Pott's Disease, 3: 148
  on preventative measures, 2: 36
  private medical practice and, 1: 176
  as professor of orthopaedic surgery, 1: 69, 111, 141, 143, 171
  "Progress in Orthopaedic Surgery" series, 2: 43, 297
  schools for disabled children, 2: 36–39, 67, 97, 308; 3: 151
  scientific study and, 1: 256
  scoliosis treatment, 2: 35, *35*, *36*, 58
  Sever and, 2: 92
  Soutter and, 2: 292, 297
  as surgical house officer at MGH, 2: 20
  teaching hospitals and, 1: 174, 187–188
  Treatise on Orthopaedic Surgery, A, 1: 108, 143; 2: 29–30, 43, 50, *50*, 51
  treatment of Brackett, 3: 147
  tuberculosis treatment, 2: 32
Bradford, Edward H., Jr., 2: 42
Bradford, Edward, Jr., 4: 361
Bradford, Eliza Edes Hickling, 2: 19
Bradford, Elizabeth, 2: 42; 4: 361, 368
Bradford, Gamaliel, 1: 96
Bradford, Mary Lythgoe, 4: 361
Bradford, Robert Fiske, 2: 42
Bradford, William, 2: 19
Bradford Frame, 2: 27, *27*, 30–31, *31*, 32
Bradlee, Helen C., 3: 18
Bradlee, J. Putnam, 3: 18
Bradley, Alfred E., 4: 416
Bradley, John, 3: 289
Braintree HealthSouth Hospital, 4: 194
Brase, D. W., 4: 167
Braswell, Margaret, 2: 349
Braunwald, Eugene, 4: 119
Brazelton, T. Berry, 2: 385
Breed's Hill (Bunker Hill), 1: 18, *18*
Breene, R. G., 4: 93
Bremer, John L., 4: 6
Brendze, R., 3: *461*
Brengle, Fred E., 3: 463
Brengle, Joan, 3: 463
Brewster, Albert H. (1892–1988), 2: *222*
  AAOS and, 4: 337
  Boston Children's Hospital and, 2: 222–223, 231, 252, 274; 4: 60, 338
  countersinking the talus, 2: 228, 283
  Crippled Children's Clinic and, 2: 230, 287
  death of, 2: 231
  donations to Boston Medical Library, 2: 271
  education and training, 2: 221
  foot deformity treatment, 2: 228–229
  grand rounds and, 2: 230
  HMS appointment, 2: 222–223; 4: 60
  Marlborough Medical Associates and, 2: 269, 299
  marriage and family, 2: 231
  New England Peabody Home for Crippled Children and, 2: 230–231
  Osgood tribute, 2: 136

PBBH and, 2: 222; 4: 16–18, 20, 110
private medical practice, 2: 146, 230, *230*
professional memberships and, 2: 230
publications of, 2: 79, 223, 225, 227–229; 4: 240
scoliosis treatment, 2: 223–228
on supracondylar fractures of the humerus, 2: 229
turnbuckle jacket and, 2: 223–224, *224*, 225, 227
World War I service and, 2: 221–222
Brewster, Albert H., Jr., 2: 231
Brewster, Elsie Estelle Carter, 2: 231
Brewster, Nancy, 2: 231
Brezinski, Mark, 4: 194
Brick, Gregory W., 4: 193, 195*b*
Brickley-Parsons, D., 2: 328
Bridges, Miss, 3: 133
Brigham, Elizabeth Fay, 4: vii, 1*b*, 23*b*, 24, 39*b*
Brigham, John Bent, 4: 1*b*
Brigham, Peter Bent, 4: 1, 1*b*, 2, 2*b*, 4–5, 22
Brigham, Robert Breck, 4: vii, 22, 23*b*, 24, 39*b*
Brigham, Uriah, 4: 1*b*
Brigham and Women's Hospital (BWH), 4: vii, *120*, *122*, *192*, *196*
  acute rehabilitation service, 4: 191
  Administrative Building, 4: *191*
  Ambulatory building, 4: *193*
  Ambulatory Care Center, 4: *193*, 194
  Bornstein Family Amphitheater, 4: *191*
  capitellocondylar total elbow replacements, 4: 146–147
  Carl J. and Ruth Shapiro Cardiovascular Center, 4: *195*
  carpal tunnel syndrome study, 2: 375
  Cartilage Repair Center, 4: 195*b*
  Center for Molecular Orthopaedics, 4: 194, 195*b*
  clinical and research faculty, 4: 195*b*
  Faulkner Hospital, 4: 194, *194*
  Foot and Ankle Center, 4: 194
  formation of, 4: 43, 113–114, 119–120, 127
  fundraising for, 4: 118
  HCORP and, 1: 213, 215
  Mary Horrigan Conner's Center for Women's Health, 4: *194*
  modernization of, 4: 191–196

  Musculoskeletal (MSK) Research Center, 4: 195*b*
  naming of, 4: 119, 123
  new facility construction, 4: 118–119, 122, 132
  opening of, 4: 121, *123*
  Orthopaedic and Arthritis Center, 4: 121, 123, 195*b*
  orthopaedic biomechanics laboratory, 4: 137–138
  orthopaedic chairmen at, 4: 196*b*
  orthopaedic grand rounds in, 4: 191
  orthopaedic research laboratory and, 4: 194
  orthopaedic surgery department, 1: 171; 4: 43, 113–115, 121
  orthopaedics fellowships, 1: 241
  orthopaedics residencies, 1: 217–218, 223–224, 241–242
  professional staff committee, 4: 132
  professorships at, 4: 195*b*
  RBBH as specialty arthritis hospital in, 4: 122–123
  research at, 4: 121
  Skeletal Biology Laboratory, 4: 195*b*
  staffing of, 4: 193–196
  surgeon-scholars at, 4: 143, 163, 193–194, 195*b*
  surgical caseloads at, 4: 194–195
  Tissue Engineering Laboratory, 4: 195*b*
  Total Joint Replacement Registry, 4: 141, *172*, 173
  transition period at, 4: 113–118, 132
  work with prosthetic devices at, 4: 122
Brigham and Women's Physician Organization (BWPO), 4: 192
Brigham and Women's/Mass General Health Care Center (Foxboro), 4: 194
Brigham Anesthesia Associates, 4: 22
Brigham Family, 4: 1*b*
Brigham Orthopaedic Foundation (BOF), 4: 123, 172, 191–192
Brigham Orthopedic Associates (BOA), 4: 123, 172, 191–192
British 31st General Hospital, 4: 485
British Base Hospital No. 12 (Rouen, France), 3: 166
British Expeditionary Forces (BEF)
  American Medical Corps and, 4: 420
  American medical volunteers and, 4: 405*b*, 425
  Base Hospital No. 5 and, 4: 420

  Harvard Unit and, 1: 256; 4: 10, 391, 438
  physician deaths in, 4: 425
  use of AEF base hospitals, 4: 420
British hospitals
  American surgeon-volunteers in, 4: 409
  documentation and, 4: 407
  general scheme of, 4: *414*
  increase in military, 4: 454
  orthopaedic surgery and, 4: 409
  registrars in, 4: 12
  World War I and, 4: 407, 409, 454
British Orthopaedic Association, 1: xxiv; 2: 137; 3: 345, 360; 4: 363, *404*
British Red Cross, 4: 399, 401
British Royal Army Medical Corps, 4: 393
British Society for Surgery of the Hand, 4: 95
Broderick, Thomas F., 3: 209, 332–333
Brodhurst, Bernard Edward, 1: 83, 106
Brodie, Sir Benjamin Collins, 1: 106
bronchitis, 2: 4
Bronfin, Isidore D., 4: 206, 209
Brooks, Barney, 3: 165–167, 170, *171*; 4: 178
Brooks, Charles, 1: 239
Brostrom, Frank, 2: 78, 110
Browder, N. C., 1: 259
Brower, Thomas D., 1: 162; 3: 382
Brown, Anna Ball, 1: 95
Brown, Arnold Welles, 1: 98
Brown, Buckminster (1819–1891), 1: *105*
  advancement of Harvard Medical School and, 1: 111
  advocacy for disabled children, 1: 107, 109, 126
  Boston Dispensary and, 2: 306
  Boston Orthopedic Institution and, 1: 107, 118, 120–122
  congenital hip dislocation treatment, 1: 108
  death of, 1: 111
  Edward H. Bradford and, 2: 20, 22
  European medical studies, 1: 105–106, 186
  forward-thinking treatment of, 1: 107–108
  House of the Good Samaritan and, 1: 107, 121–122, 125–128; 2: 49
  long-term treatment and, 2: 25
  marriage and, 1: 107

Index

orthopaedic specialization of,
  1: 99, 107–108
orthopaedic treatment advances,
  1: 118; 2: 26–27, 32
Pott's Disease and, 1: 97, 105,
  109
publications of, 1: 110b, 120,
  120, 121
scoliosis brace and, 1: 109
Brown, Charles H., Jr., 4: 193, 195b
Brown, Douglas, 2: 163
Brown, Francis Henry
  Boston Children's Hospital and,
    2: 5, *5*, 6, 9–10, 21
  on hospital construction, 2: 5
  orthopaedics expertise, 2: 9
Brown, George, 1: 98
Brown, Jabez, 1: 95
Brown, John Ball (1784–1862),
  1: *95*, *102*
  apparatus used for knee contracture, 1: *98*
  Boston dispensary and, 1: 293
  Boston Orthopedic Institution
    and, 1: 99–100, 107, 113–
    122; 3: 30
  club foot treatment, 2: 36
  correction of spine deformities,
    1: 97–98, 100
  death of, 1: 103, 122
  early telemedicine by, 1: 100
  education and training, 1: 95–96
  establishment of orthopaedics as
    specialty, 1: 95–96, 98–99,
    119
  founding of Boston Orthopedic
    Institution, 1: xxiv
  George Parkman and, 1: 296
  legacy of, 1: 102–103
  marriage and family, 1: 96–98
  opening of orthopaedic specialty
    hospital, 1: 99
  orthopaedic surgery and,
    1: 99–102, 113; 2: 25–26
  publications of, 1: 102b, 120,
    120, 121
  *Remarks on the Operation for the
    Cure of Club Feet with Cases*,
    1: 100
  *Report of Cases in the Orthopedic
    Infirmary of the City of Boston*,
    1: *120*
  surgical appointments, 1: 96–97
Brown, John Warren, 1: 97
Brown, Larry, 4: 364
Brown, Lloyd T. (1880–1961), 4: *81*
  on body mechanics and rheumatoid disease, 4: 82–83
  Boston Children's Hospital and,
    4: 82

Boston City Hospital and, 4: 406
Burrage Hospital and, 4: 226
Children's Island Sanitorium and,
  4: 87
chronic disease treatment and,
  4: 52
club foot treatment, 4: 84
congenital club foot and,
  4: 81–82, *83*, 87
death of, 4: 39, 87b
education and training, 4: 81–82
HMS appointment, 2: 223;
  4: 60, 86
hospital appointments, 4: 83
marriage and family, 4: 83, 87
medical officer teaching, 4: 84
MGH and, 4: 82, 84, 86
military surgeon training and,
  2: 42
orthopaedics surgery and, 2: 66;
  3: 268
Orthopedics and Body Mechanics
  Committee, 4: 235
posture research and, 4: 84, *84*,
  85–86, 233
private medical practice, 4: 82
professional memberships, 4: 87,
  87b
publications and research,
  2: 297; 3: 91; 4: 82–84, 87
RBBH and, 3: 257; 4: vii, 25,
  31–34, 36, 45, 79, 86–87, 93,
  111, 406
RBBH Emergency Campaign
  speech, 4: 32, 32b
rehabilitation of soldiers and,
  4: 444
retirement and, 4: 36
Brown, Marian Epes Wigglesworth,
  4: 83
Brown, Percy E., 2: 16, 54; 3: 99
Brown, Rebecca Warren, 1: 96, 98
Brown, Sarah Alvord Newcomb,
  1: 107
Brown, Sarah Tyler Meigs, 3: 257,
  263
Brown, T., 3: 209, 214
Brown, Thornton (1913–2000),
  1: *203*; 3: *257*, 263, 461
  as AOA president, 3: 262, *262*,
    263
  back pain research and, 3: 257–
    258, *258*, 259–260
  on Boston and orthopaedics,
    1: 93; 2: 324
  on changes at MGH Orthopaedic
    Service, 3: 453b–458b
  Children's Hospital/MGH combined program and, 3: 257
  death of, 3: 263

early life, 3: 257
education and training, 3: 257
Journal of Bone and Joint Surgery
  editor, 3: 260–262, 346
marriage and family, 3: 257
*Massachusetts General Hospital,
  1955–1980, The*, 3: 299
as MGH orthopaedics chief,
  3: 11b, 202, 227, *259*, 459
MGH residents and, 3: *259*, 260,
  459
as MGH surgeon, 3: 257, 398b
Milton Hospital and, 3: 257
on Mt. Sinai Hospital,
  4: 201–202
Norton-Brown spinal brace,
  3: 317–319
"Orthopaedics at Harvard,"
  1: 195; 2: 271
private medical practice, 1: 203
publications and research,
  3: 257–260, 317, 455b
RBBH and, 4: 37, 40
World War II service, 3: 257
Brown University Medical School,
  3: 400–401
Browne, Hablot Knight, 1: *21*
Browne & Nichols School, 2: 83, 97
Brubacher, Jacob W., 3: 463b
Brugler, Guy, 2: 214
Brunschwig, Hieronymus, 4: 469
Bruschart, Thomas, 3: 431
Bryant, Henry, 3: 30
Bryant, Thomas, 1: 83
Buchanan, J. Robert, 3: 391
Buchbinder, Rachelle, 3: 437
Buchman, Frank N. D., 4: 57
Buchmanism, 4: 57
Bucholz, Carl Hermann (1874–unk.),
  3: *264*
  back pain research and, 3: 203
  education and training, 3: 264
  on exercise treatment of paralysis,
    3: 265
  HMS appointment, 3: 265
  legacy of, 3: 269
  as MGH surgeon, 3: 268
  publications and research,
    2: 136, 297
  Therapeutic Exercise and Massage,
    3: 269
  World War I and, 3: 268
  Zander's medico-mechanical
    department and, 3: 71,
    264–266, 266t, 267, 268b
Buck, Emily Jane, 2: 220
Buck's traction, 1: 80
Budd, J. W., 4: 102
Bulfinch, Charles, 1: 28, 41;
  3: 10–11

Bulfinch Building (MGH), 1: *41*;
    3: *9, 13*, 15, *16*, 22, *60*, 70*b*
Bull, Charles, 3: 77
Bullard, S. E., 2: 244
Bunker Hill Monument Committee,
    1: 68
Bunnin, Beverly D., 4: 101
Burgess, Earnest M., 3: 248
Burke, Dennis W., 3: 398, 460*b*,
    464*b*
Burke, John, 3: 62, 253, 458*b*
burn care, 3: 336
Burne, F., 2: 98
Burnett, Joseph H. (1892–1963)
    BCH Bone and Joint Service,
        4: 307, 328, 369, 371
    Boston City Hospital and,
        4: 347, 368, 370–371
    Boston University Medical School
        appointment, 4: 368
    carpal scaphoid fracture case,
        4: 368
    death of, 4: 371
    education and training, 4: 368
    football injury research, 4: 370,
        370
    HMS appointment, 4: 368
    marriage and, 4: 371
    professional memberships, 4: 371
    publications and research,
        4: 368–370, *370*
    scaphoid fracture research,
        4: 360, 368–369
    sports medicine and, 4: 368–370
Burnett, Margaret Rogers, 4: 371
Burns, Frances, 2: 260, 264
Burns, John, 3: *458*
Burns, Mary, 2: 214
Burrage Hospital, 4: 226, *227*
Burrell, Herbert L., 4: 298–299,
    299, 300–301, 307
Burrell-Cotton operation, 4: 329
Burwell, C. Sidney, 1: 131, 158,
    179, 272; 4: 362
Burwell, Sterling, 4: 472
Buschenfeldt, Karl W., 3: 317
Butler, Allan M., 3: 301
Butler, Fergus A., 4: 53
BWH. *See* Brigham and Women's
    Hospital (BWH)
Bygrave, Elizabeth Clark, 2: 92, 97
Byrne, John, 2: 250
Byrne, John J., 4: 303

C

Cabot, Arthur Tracy, 2: 11;
    3: 53–54, 56
Cabot, Richard C., 2: 320
Cabot, Samuel, 3: 25, *31*

Cadet Nursing Corps, 4: 467
calcaneal apophysitis (Sever's Disease)
    case study of, 2: 89
    characteristics of, 2: 89
    heel pain in children, 2: 89
    Sever's study of, 2: 88–90, 100
    x-ray appearance of, 2: *88*
calcaneovalgus deformity, 2: 92
calcar femorale, 3: 39, *39*
Calderwood, Carmelita, 3: 303
Calderwood's Orthopedic Nursing
    (Larson and Gould), 3: 303
Caldwell, Guy A., 1: 162; 2: 183
Calhoun, John C., 1: 307
Calvé, Jacques, 2: 103–104
Cambridge Hospital, 1: 220;
    3: 396–397, 399
Camp, Walter, 1: 248, *248*
Camp Blanding Station Hospital,
    4: 475
Camp Devens (Mass.), 4: 426, 437,
    452
Camp Kilmer (N.J.), 4: 475
Camp Taylor (Kentucky), 4: 452
Camp Wikoff (Montauk Point, LI),
    4: 310–311
Campbell, Crawford J., 1: 216;
    3: 385–386, 392, 461, *462*
Campbell, Douglas, 3: 431
Campbell, W., 2: 91
Campbell, Willis, 2: 105, 294
Campbell Clinic, 4: 356
Canadian Board of Certification for
    Prosthetics and Orthotics, 2: 347
Canadian Orthopaedic Association,
    2: 137, 183
Canadian Orthopaedic Research
    Society, 3: 262
Cannon, Bradford, 3: 336
Cannon, Walter B., 4: 6, 299, 420
Cannon, Walter W., 3: 97
capitellocondylar total elbow prosthesis, 4: 145, *145*, 146–147
carbolic acid treatment, 1: 82–83, *84*
CareGroup, 1: 233; 4: 281, 284
Carlos Otis Stratton Mountain
    Clinic, 3: 311
Carnett, John B., 4: 235–236
Carney Hospital, 3: *78*
    adult orthopaedic clinic at,
        2: 101; 3: 78
    Goldthwait and, 3: 78, 80; 4: 45
    internships at, 1: 186, 189
    Lovett and, 2: 49
    MacAusland and, 3: 308; 4: 45
    orthopaedics residencies, 4: 378
    Painter and, 4: 44–45, 224
    posture clinic at, 4: 86
    Rogers (Mark) and, 4: 224
    Sullivan and, 4: 343

testing of foot strength apparatus,
    2: 102
treatment of adults and children
    in, 2: 4
Tufts clinical instruction at, 4: 45
Carothers, Charles O., 4: 356
carpal bones, 3: 101–102
carpal tunnel syndrome
    computer use and, 4: 186
    familial bilateral, 3: 321
    genetics in, 4: 186
    research in, 2: 375; 3: 402
    self-assessment of, 4: 184–185
    wrist position and, 3: 403
Carpenter, G. K., 2: 438
Carr, Charles F., 3: 363–364
Carrie M. Hall Nurses Residence,
    4: 20
Carroll, Norris, 2: 305
Carroll, Robert, 2: 251
Carter, Dennis, 3: 397
cartilage transplantation, 2: 294
Case Western Reserve University
    School of Medicine, 3: 337
Casemyr, Natalie E.J., 3: 463*b*
Casino Boulogne-sur-Mer, 4: *426*,
    427, *428*
Caspari, Richard B., 2: 279
Casscells, Ward, 3: 446
Cassella, Mickey, 2: 178–180, 182
Castle, A. C., 1: 314–317
Castleman, Benjamin, 2: 320;
    3: 205, 259
Catastrophe, The, 1: *78*
Catharina Ormandy Professorship,
    2: 438, 439*b*
Cats-Baril, William L., 3: 379, *379*
Cattell, Richard B., 4: 275–276
Cave, Edwin F. (1896–1976),
    1: *270*;
    3: *270*, 271, *273*; 4: *491*
    on Achilles tendon injury, 3: 272
    AOA presidential address and,
        3: 274, *274*
    Bankart procedure and, 3: 351,
        351
    on Barr's orthopaedic research,
        3: 211
    Children's Hospital/MGH combined program and, 3: 270
    death of, 3: 276, 448
    early life, 3: 270
    education and training, 3: 270
    endowed lectures and, 3: 275
    femoral neck fracture treatment,
        3: 185–186, *186*
    5th General Hospital and, 4: 484
    as Fracture Clinic chief, 3: 60*b*,
        241, 272

Index

Fractures and Other Injuries,
  3: 273, *273*; 4: 356
hip nailing and, 3: 237
HMS appointment, 2: 223;
  3: 272; 4: 60–61
Joint Committee for the Study of
  Surgical Materials and, 3: 210
knee arthrotomy research, 3: 351
marriage and family, 3: 271, 276
on measuring and recording joint
  function, 3: 270
as MGH surgeon, 3: 187, 192,
  270–271
New England Peabody Home for
  Crippled Children and, 2: 270
105th General Hospital and,
  4: 489
orthopaedics education and,
  3: 272–274
private medical practice,
  3: 271–272
professional honors, 3: 275*b*,
  276
publications and research,
  2: 297; 3: 270, 272, 366
Scudder Oration on Trauma,
  3: 63
Smith-Petersen and, 3: 270
34th Infantry Division and,
  4: 484
torn ligaments in the knee
  research, 3: 272
on trauma, 3: 275–276
Trauma Management, 3: 62,
  253, 273
on Van Gorder, 3: 368
World War II service, 1: 270;
  3: 271; 4: 17
Cave, Joan Tozzer Lincoln, 3: 276
Cave, Louise Fessenden, 3: 271, 276
cavus feet, 2: 228–229
CDH. *See* congenital dislocated hips
  (CDH)
celastic body jackets, 2: 178
Center for Human Simulation,
  4: 173
Center of Healing Arts, 3: 423
Central States Orthopedic Club,
  4: 393
cerebral palsy
  Banks and, 2: 196–200
  Boston Children's Hospital and,
    2: 171–172
  children and, 2: 171–172,
    196–198, 300–301
  experimental approaches to,
    3: 164
  foot surgery in, 2: 229
  Green and, 2: 171–172, 196–200
  Grice procedure and, 2: 212

hamstring lengthening and,
  2: 172
Lovett and, 2: 51
research in, 2: 196, 401
sensory deficits in children's
  hands, 2: 300–301, *301*
spinal deformities in, 2: 370
surgery for, 2: 197–198
treatment of, 2: 172, 196–200,
  300–301
triple arthrodesis (Hoke type)
  and, 2: 172
Cerebral Palsy and Spasticity Center
  (Children's Hospital), 2: 406
Cerebral Palsy Clinic (Children's
  Hospital), 2: 402, 406, 409
cerebrospinal meningitis, 2: 4
"Certain Aspects of Infantile Paralysis" (Lovett and Martin), 2: *70*
Cervical Spine Research Society,
  3: *249*, 321; 4: 265, 269
Chandler, Betsy McCombs, 3: 280
Chandler, Fremont A., 2: 176, 183
Chandler, Hugh P. (1931–2014),
  3: *277–278*, 280, *461*
  Aufranc Fellowship and, 3: 277
  *Bone Stock Deficiency in Total Hip
    Replacement*, 3: 278–279
  Children's Hospital/MGH com-
    bined program and, 3: 277
  death of, 3: 280
  direct lateral approach to the hip
    and, 3: 277–278, *278*
  early life, 3: 277
  education and training, 3: 277
  marriage and family, 3: 280
  as MGH surgeon, 3: 244, 277,
    398*b*
  pelvic osteolysis with acetabular
    replacement case, 3: 279
  publications and research, 3: 278
  recognition of, 3: 279–280
  sailing and, 3: 280
Channing, Walter, 1: 296, 299, 302
Chanoff, David, 4: *265*
Chapin, Mrs. Henry B., 1: 129
Chaplan, Ronald N., 4: 163, 193
Chapman, Earle, 3: 241
Chapman, Mabel C., 3: 304
Charcot, Jean-Martin, 3: 142
Charitable Surgical Institution, 3: 30
Charleston Naval Hospital, 3: 191;
  4: 246
Charnley, John, 2: 239
Charnley, Sir John, 3: 218–220
Chase, Henry, 3: 101
Cheal, Edward, 4: 263
Cheever, Charles A., 1: 96
Cheever, David W., 4: *297*
  on Bigelow, 3: 39, 44

Boston City Hospital and, 4: 298,
  303–304
as Boston City Hospital surgeon-
  in-chief, 4: 298, 306–307
British Expeditionary Forces and,
  4: 9–10
on Goldthwait, 3: 79
HMS appointment, 3: 94;
  4: 298, 307
PBBH and, 4: 5, 10–11, 17
Chelsea Memorial Hospital, 2: 102;
  3: 314
Chelsea Naval Hospital, 4: 47–48,
  97
chemotherapy, 2: 422–423
Chen, Chien-Min, 3: 368
Chernack, Robert, 4: 194, 195*b*
Cheselden, William, 1: 6, 36
Chessler, Robert, 1: xxii
Chest Wall and Spinal Deformity
  Study Group, 2: 361–362
Cheyne, W. Watson, 1: *83*
Chicago Polyclinic, 2: 50
Chicago Shriner's Hospital, 2: 355
Chicago University, 3: 175
Chickahominy fever, 3: 44
Child, C. Gardner, 4: 303
children
  bone granuloma and, 2: 171
  cerebral palsy and, 2: 171–172,
    196–198, 300–301
  club foot and, 1: xxii, 118–119;
    2: 12*t*, 15*t*, 22–23, 145
  development of hospitals for,
    2: 3–4
  early treatment of, 1: xxii
  growth disturbances with chronic
    arthritis, 4: 56
  heel pain in, 2: 89
  hip disease and, 2: 52
  juvenile idiopathic arthritis and,
    2: 164, 171, 350
  kyphosis and, 2: 343–345
  mortality, 2: 4–5, 15
  muscle atrophy in, 2: 110
  national health initiatives,
    4: 235–236
  orthopaedic rehabilitation and,
    1: 107, 121
  osteochondritis dissecans in,
    2: 194–195
  osteomyelitis in, 2: 169
  physical therapy and, 2: 61, 107
  poliomyelitis and, 1: 191; 2: 61,
    189–191, 210, 213
  posture and, 4: 233–234, *234*,
    235, *236*
  rheumatic heart disease and,
    1: 130

schools for disabled, 2: 36–39, 97
spinal deformities and, 1: xxi, xxii, 97–98, 123
spinal tuberculosis and, 1: 108
Sprengel deformity, 2: 195, *196*
state clinics for crippled, 2: 107, 221
trauma and, 2: 359, 365, 368, 378, 385
use of ether, 1: 63
children, disabled. *See* disabled children
Children's Convalescent Home, 2: 84
Children's Hospital (Boston, Mass.), 2: 4–16. *See also* Boston Children's Hospital (BCH)
Children's Hospital Medical Center, 4: 113–114. *See also* Boston Children's Hospital (BCH)
Children's Hospital of Philadelphia (CHOP), 2: 3–5, 424
Children's Infirmary, 2: 3
Children's Island Sanitorium, 4: 87
Children's Medical Center (Wellesley), 2: 314
Children's Memorial Hospital (Chicago), 2: 302
Children's Sports Injury Prevention Fund, 2: 439*b*
Children's Sunlight Hospital (Scituate), 3: 307
Childress, Harold M., 4: 335
Chiodo, Christopher, 4: 190*b*, 194
Chipman, W. W., 3: 113*b*
chloroform, 1: 62–63, 82; 3: 15, 31
Choate, Rufus, 1: 307
Choate Hospital, 2: 256
cholera epidemic, 1: 295; 4: 293
chondrocytes, 3: 327, 442, 444–445, 449
chondrodysplasia, 4: 218–220
chondrosarcoma, 2: 237; 3: 390, 406
Christian, Henry A., 1: 173–174, 176; 4: 4, 6, 9, 16, 79, 104
Christophe, Kenneth, 4: 40, 89
chronic diseases
anatomy and, 3: 91
body mechanics and, 3: 81, 91
bone and joint disorders, 1: 153; 3: 85, 90
faulty body mechanics and, 3: 91
Goldthwait and, 4: 39*b*, 52
orthopaedic surgeons and, 4: 46, 53
posture and, 4: 52, 86
prevention of, 3: 90

RBBH and, 4: 25*b*, 27, 30, 30*b*, 32*b*, 33, 36, 39*b*, 45, 86
rheumatoid arthritis and, 4: 36
travel abroad and, 1: 72
chronic regional pain syndrome (CRPS), 2: 68
Chronicle of Boston Jewry, A (Ehrenfried), 4: 220
Chuinard, Eldon G., 1: 162
Chung, Kevin C., 3: 410
Church, Benjamin, 1: 15–16
Churchill, Edward D., 1: 198–199; 2: 322; 3: 1; 4: 302, 470–471, *472*
Churchill, Edward H., 2: 79
Churchill, Winston, 4: 479
chymopapain, 3: 254–255, 397, 419, *421*
Civale, Jean, 3: 41
Clark, Charles, 4: 174
Clark, Dean A., 4: 158
Clark, H. G., 3: *31*
Clark, John G., 3: 113*b*, 122, 355
Clarke, Joseph Taylor, 4: 448
Clay, Lucius D., 2: 260, 264
Clayton, Mack, 4: 243
cleidocranial dysostosis, 2: 254
Cleveland, Grover, 2: 72
Cleveland, Mather, 3: 196
Clifford, John H., 1: 307
Clifton Springs Sanatorium, 3: 88; 4: 52–53
Cline, Henry, 1: 33–34, 37
Clinical Biomechanics of the Spine (White and Panjabi), 4: 262
Clinical Congress of Surgeons in North America, 3: 116, 123
Clinical Orthopaedic Examination (McRae), 1: 167
Cloos, David W., 4: 163, 193
clover leaf rod, 3: 272
club foot
apparatus for, 1: 98, 100, 106; 2: 23, 24; 4: *83*
Bradford and, 2: 22–24, 28–29
correction of, 1: *98*, 100, *100*, *101*, 106; 2: 36
correction of bilateral, 2: *29*
Denis Browne splint, 2: 208
early diagnosis and treatment for, 1: 100; 2: 28–29
medial deltoid ligament release, 2: 145
nonoperative treatment of, 2: 28; 4: 216
Ober and, 2: 145
osteotomies and, 2: 29
pathological findings and, 3: 54
plantar fasciotomy and, 2: 24

Stromeyer's subcutaneous tenotomy for, 1: 118, *118*
tarsectomy and, 2: 23
tenotomy and, 1: 106, 118; 2: 25–26
Cobb, John, 2: 225–226
Cochran, Robert C., 4: 438–439
Cochrane, William A., 3: 244, 302, 371, *371*, 372
Codman, Amory, 2: 182
Codman, Catherine, 1: 50, *129*, 130
Codman, Elizabeth Hand, 3: 93
Codman, Ernest A. (1869–1940), 3: *93*, *103*, *105*, *115*, *143*
abdominal surgery and, 3: 108
as anatomy assistant at HMS, 2: 114
anesthesia and, 3: 95, *95*, 96
bone sarcomas and, 3: 136–140, 140*b*, 141–142, 145; 4: 102
on brachial plexus injury, 2: 96
Camp Taylor base hospital and, 4: 452
cartoon of Back Bay public, 3: 121, *121*, 122, *122*
clinical congress meeting, 3: 116
Committee on Standardization of Hospitals and, 3: 112, 113*b*, 115–116, 123–124
death of, 2: 116; 3: 145–146
dedication of headstone, 3: *145*, 146
on diagnosis with x-rays, 3: 99
duodenal ulcer and, 3: 108
early life, 3: 93
education and training, 3: 93–95
End-Result Idea, 1: 194; 2: 135; 3: 110–111, *111*, 112, 114, 116, *116*, 118–119, 119*b*, 120, 122–126, *126*, 127*b*, 128–131, 136; 4: 12, 141
fluoroscope and, 2: 307
forward-thinking of, 3: 135–136
Fracture Course and, 3: 62
fracture treatment and, 3: 101–102
Halifax Harbor explosion and, 3: 132–135
Harvard Medical Association letter, 3: 119*b*
HMS appointment, 3: 96, 99
Hospital Efficiency meeting, 3: 120–122
interest in hunting and fishing, 3: 94, 143–145
interest in sprains, 3: 100–102
interest in subacromial bursitis, 3: 104–105, 107–109

Index

interest in subdeltoid bursa, 3: 95, 98, 103–104, *104*, 105, 108
legacy of, 3: 145–146
life history chart, 3: *106*
marriage and, 3: 142–143
memberships and, 3: 65
MGH internship and, 3: 95–96
as MGH surgeon, 1: 190, 194; 3: 99, 112, 118, 142, 266
on monetary value of surgeon services, 3: 129–130
operating in the Bigelow Amphitheatre, 3: *107*
personal case documentation, 3: 126, 128–130
Philadelphia Medical Society address, 3: 117*b*–118*b*
private hospital ideals, 3: 114*b*, 115
private hospital of, 3: 112, 114, 116, 118, 135
private practice and, 3: 136
publication of x-rays, 3: 97, *97*, 98, *99*
publications and research, 3: 99–104, *104*, 108–112, 115–116, 125, 136, 139–142
resolution honoring, 3: 144*b*, 146
on safety of x-rays, 3: 99–100
Shoulder, 2: 239; 3: 105, 115, 122, 140*b*
shoulder and, 3: 103–105, 107–110, 354
as skiagrapher at BCH, 2: 16, 114; 3: 96–99, 142
Study in Hospital Efficiency, 3: 125, *125*, 127*b*, 128–131
surgical scissor design, 3: *138*
Treatment of Fractures, 3: 56
World War I and, 3: 132, 135
Codman, John, 3: 94, 108, 142
Codman, Katherine Bowditch, 3: 142–143, 144*b*, 145
Codman, William Combs, 3: 93
Codman Center for Clinical Effectiveness in Surgery, 3: 146
Codman Hospital, 3: 112, 114, 116, 118, *126*, 135
Codman's Paradox, 3: 105
Cohen, Jonathan, 1: 114
Cohen, Jonathan (1915–2003), 2: *179*
as assistant pathologist, 2: 234
on Barr, 3: 206–207
bone irradiation research, 2: 237, *237*
bone lesions and tumor research, 2: 236
book reviews by, 2: 239, 240*b*
Boston Children's Hospital and, 2: 233–236, 301; 4: 126, 245
Boston Orthopedic Institution and, 1: 121
death of, 2: 241
education and training, 2: 231
Farber and, 2: 235–236
Fourth Portable Surgical Hospital (4PSH) and, 2: 232–233
Fourth Portable Surgical Hospital's Service in the War against Japan, 2: 232–233
Green and, 2: 234–235
HMS appointment, 2: 233
Jewish Hospital (St. Louis) and, 2: 231
Journal of Bone and Joint Surgery editor, 2: 238–240; 3: 346
marriage and family, 2: 241
metal implants and, 2: 237–238
MGH and, 2: 233
mobile army surgical hospitals (MASHs) and, 2: 231
105th General Hospital and, 4: 489
orthopaedic research laboratory and, 2: 234
orthopaedic surgery and, 2: 235
professional memberships, 2: 240–241
publications and research, 2: 233–234, 236, 239, *239*; 3: *216*; 4: 102
publications of, 2: 236*b*
World War II service, 2: 231–233
Cohen, Louise Alden, 2: 241
Cohen, Mark S., 3: 431
Cohnheim, Julius, 1: 82
Coleman, Sherman, 2: 302
college athletes. *See also* Harvard athletics
Arthur L. Boland and, 1: 286
Augustus Thorndike and, 1: 274
Bill of Rights for, 1: 274, 280, 280*b*
Coller, Fred A., 2: 119; 4: 389*b*
Colles fracture, 2: 47; 3: 99
Collins, Abigail, 1: 24
Collins, John, 1: 24, 31
Collis P. Huntington Memorial Hospital for Cancer Research, 1: 87
Colonna, Paul C., 2: 183; 3: 208
Colton, Gardner Quincy, 1: 56
Colton, Theodore, 3: 253
Combat Over Corregidor (Bradford), 4: *364*
Combined Jewish Philanthropies (CJP), 4: 168
Committee F-4 on Surgical Implants, 3: 210
Committee for International Activities (POS), 2: 425
Committee of Correspondence, 1: 16
Committee of the Colonization of Society, 1: 239
Committee of Undergraduate Training (AOA), 2: 183
Committee on Education of the American Medical Association, 2: 41
Committee on Industrial Injuries, 3: 63
Committee on Recording Lateral Curvature, 2: 247
Committee on Staff Reorganization and Office Building (King Committee). *See* King Report (MGH)
Committee on Standardization of Hospitals, 3: 112, 113*b*, 115–116, 123–125, 131
Committee on Surgical Implants, 2: 238
Committee on Trauma, 2: 131; 3: 63
compartment syndrome, 2: 249–250; 3: 417–418
Compere, Edward, 2: 300
compound fractures
amputation and, 1: 54, 68
Boston City Hospital outcomes, 4: *335*, 337
Committee on Fractures and, 3: 64
fracture boxes and, 1: 80
immobilization methods, 4: 399
Lister's antisepsis dressings and, 1: 84–85; 3: 59
military orthopaedics and, 2: 120; 3: 64; 4: 391, 399, 409, 423*b*, 434
orthopaedic treatment for, 4: 464
surgery and, 4: 320, 321*b*–322*b*
computed tomography (CT), 2: 365, 389, 410–411; 3: 254
Conant, William M. (1856–1937), 1: 248
Concord, Mass., 1: 17–18
concussions
athletes and, 2: 385
football and, 1: 247, 254, 274–275
signs and symptoms of, 1: 287*t*
three knockout rule, 1: 275
treatment of, 1: 286–287
congenital dislocated hips (CDH)
Allison and, 3: 164, 175
AOA Commission on, 3: 234

Bradford and, 2: 32–34
Buckminster Brown and, 1: 108
closed manipulation, 2: 33–34
Guérin's method for, 1: 106–107
open reductions, 2: 33;
  3: 233–234
reduction procedures, 3: 234–235
reductions reviewed by the AOA
  Commission, 3: 232–233,
  233t
treatment of, 2: 32–33
use of shelf procedure, 2: 151
congenital pseudarthrosis of the tibia,
  2: 172–176
congenital torticollis, 2: 256, 258
Conn, A., 2: 334–335
Conn, Harold R., 4: 473
*Conquest of Cancer by Radium and
  Other Methods, The* (Quigley),
  1: 275
Conservational Hip Outcomes
  Research (ANCHOR) Group,
  2: 392, *393*
Constable, John D., 3: 321
Constructive Surgery of the Hip
  (Aufranc), 3: 244, *246*
Continental Hospital (Boston),
  1: 24
Converse, Elizabeth, 3: 339
Converse, Frederick S., 3: 339
Conway, James, 2: 305
Conwell, H. Earle, 3: 191
Cook, Robert J., 2: 438
Cooke, John, 3: 193*b*, 238
Cooksey, Eunice, 2: 247
Coonse, G. Kenneth (1897–1951)
  Aufranc and, 4: 372–373
  BCH Bone and Joint Service,
    4: 373
  death of, 4: 375
  education and training, 4: 371
  HMS appointment, 3: 237;
    4: 371, 373
  hospital appointments, 4: 371
  humerus fracture treatment,
    4: 372
  legacy of, 4: 375–376
  marriage and family, 4: 375
  Massachusetts Regional Fracture
    Committee, 3: 64
  MGH and, 4: 371–372
  Newton-Wellesley Hospital and,
    4: 371, 373, 375
  patellar turndown procedure,
    4: 373–374
  PBBH and, 4: 373
  professional memberships,
    4: 371, 375, 375*b*
  publications and research,
    4: 371–374

synovectomy in chronic arthritis
  research, 4: 102, 371–372
treatment of shock, 4: 373, *373*
University of Missouri appoint-
  ment, 4: 372–373
World War I service, 4: 371, 373
Coonse, Hilda Gant, 4: 375
Cooper, Maurice, 4: 373
Cooper, Reginald, 1: 234; 3: 303
Cooper, Sir Astley, 1: *34*
  anatomy lectures, 1: 34–35, 37
  Bigelow on, 3: 36
  dislocations and, 1: 44–45
  as Guy's Hospital surgeon,
    1: 35–36
  influence on John Collins Warren,
    1: 36–37
  publications of, 1: 35–36
  surgical advances by, 1: 35
  *Treatise on Dislocations and Frac-
    tures of Joints*, 1: *35, 42, 43*
Cooper, William, 1: 33–34
Coordinating Council on Medical
  Education (CCME), 1: 211
Cope, Oliver, 3: 336
Cope, Stuart, 4: 116, 128, 163, 193
Copel, Joseph W. (1917–1985),
  4: *88*
  Beth Israel Hospital and, 4: 89,
    247, 262
  Boston University appointment,
    4: 89
  Brigham and Women's Hospital,
    4: 163
  death of, 4: 89
  education and training, 4: 88
  HMS appointment, 4: 89
  marriage and family, 4: 88–89
  private medical practice, 4: 89
  publications and research,
    4: 88–89
  RBBH and, 4: 35, 38, 68, 89, 93
  US Army and, 4: 88
Copel, Marcia Kagno, 4: 89
Copley, John Singleton, 1: *3, 11*
Corey Hill Hospital, 3: *88,* 89;
  4: 224
Corkery, Paul J., 4: 295
Corliss, Julie, 4: 183
Cornell Medical School, 4: 109
Cornwall, Andrew P., 3: 268
Cotrel, Yves, 2: 342
Cotting, Benjamin E., 2: 10
Cotting, Frances J., 2: 38
Cotting, W. F., 4: 338
Cotting, W. P., 2: 438
Cotting School, 2: 38, 308, *312*;
  3: 151; 4: 367
Cotton, Frederic J. (1869–1938),
  1: *202*; 4: *309, 323, 331*

ACS founder, 4: 324
ankle fractures and, 4: 313–315
bacteriology research, 4: 310
BCH Bone and Joint Service,
  4: 307, 328, 333, 380*b*
BCH residencies and, 4: 377
Beth Israel Hospital and, 4: 207,
  220
board certification efforts, 4: 324
bone and joint treatment,
  4: 313, 323, 328
book of x-ray photographs and,
  3: 57
Boston Children's Hospital and,
  4: 311
Boston Children's Hospital
  skiagrapher, 3: 56
Boston City Hospital and,
  4: 217, 242, 307, 312–313,
  328
Boston Dispensary and, 4: 311
bubble bottle anesthesia method,
  4: 323
calcaneus fracture treatment,
  4: 313, *313,* 314*b*
clinical congress meeting, 3: 116
as consulting surgeon,
  4: 323–324
Cotton's fracture and, 4: 313–
  315, *315*, 316
death of, 4: 330
Dislocations and Joint Fractures,
  3: 371; 4: 307, 314, 316–317,
  317, 318
education and training, 4: 309
on fracture management, 4: 320,
  320, 321*b*–322*b*, 339*b*–340*b*
George W. Gay Lecture, 4: 324
hip fracture treatment,
  4: 318–320
HMS appointments, 4: 323,
  323*b*, 329
honors and awards, 4: 312, 324,
  329
on industrial accidents, 4: 325–
  327, 338
lectures of, 4: 329
legacy of, 4: 329–331
marriage and family, 4: 330
Massachusetts Regional Fracture
  Committee, 3: 64
medical illustration, 3: 56, *58*
as mentor, 3: 237
MGH and, 4: 310
military reconstruction hospitals
  and, 4: 444–445, 449–451
Mt. Sinai Hospital and, 4: 204,
  220, 312
named procedures, 4: 329

Index

461

New England Regional Committee on Fractures, 4: 341
orthopaedics education and, 4: 323
Orthopedic Surgery, 4: 318
os calcis fracture research, 4: 313
PBBH teaching and, 4: 10
Physicians' Art Society and, 4: 329–330
professional memberships, 4: 324, 329–330
publications and research, 4: 310–313, 316–320, 323, 325–326, 329
Reverdin method and, 4: 216
roentgenology and, 2: 56
sling device to reduce kyphosis, 4: *317*
Spanish American War service, 4: 310–311
test to determine ankle instability, 4: *317*, 318
Treatment of Fractures, 4: 312
trigger knee research, 4: 311–312
Tufts Medical School appointment, 4: 329
US General Hospital No. 10 and, 4: 452
worker health care advocacy, 4: 325–327
workers' compensation advocacy, 4: 325, 444
World War I service, 4: 327
Cotton, Isabella Cole, 4: 309
Cotton, Jane Baldwin, 4: 330
Cotton, Jean, 4: 330
Cotton, Joseph Potter, 4: 309, 316
Cotton advancement operation, 4: 329
Cotton osteotomy, 4: 329
Cotton-Boothby anesthesia apparatus, 4: *320*, 323
Cotton's Fracture, 4: 313–315, *315*, 316
Cotton's Hammer, 4: *319*, 320
Council of Medical Specialty Societies, 1: 211
Council of Musculoskeletal Specialty Societies (AAOS), 4: 186
Councilman, William T., 2: 32; 4: 4, *6*
Coventry, Mark, 3: 261–262, 433
Cowell, Henry, 2: 239
Cox, Edith I., 4: 389*b*
coxa plana, 2: 102–106. *See also* Legg-Calvé-Perthes disease
Cozen, Lewis N., 3: 70*b*, 74, 187; 4: 383, 471
Cracchiolo, Andrea, 2: 317

Craig, John, 2: 234
Crandon, LeRoi G., 4: 207, 216, *217*
Crane, Carl C., 3: 266
craniotomy, 2: 24–25
Crawford, Alvin, 4: 246, 266*b*
Crawford, Dorothy, 2: 313
Crenshaw, Andrew H., Jr., 4: 168, 356
crew, 1: 250–251, 258
Crile, George, 3: 104
Crippled Children's Clinics (Massachusetts Dept. of Health), 2: 221, 230, 287, 299, 314; 4: 376
Crippled Children's Service (Vermont Dept. of Health), 2: 208, 220–221; 3: 209
Crockett, David C., 2: 322; 3: 259
Cronkhite, Leonard, 2: 285
Crosby, L. M., 3: 133
Crotched Mountain Foundation, 2: 221
Crothers, Bronson, 2: 171–172
Crowninshield, Annie, 1: 76
cubitus varus deformity, 2: 229
Cudworth, Alden L., 2: 326
Cullis Consumptive Home, 4: 275
curative workshops
  King Manuel II and, 4: 400–403
  rehabilitation of soldiers and, 4: 401–403, *403*, 404, 442, 448, *448*, 449
  Shepherd's Bush Military Hospital and, 4: 399, 401
  trades practiced in, 4: 402*b*
  US Army and, 4: 403–404
Curley, James M., 3: 120
Curran, J. A., 1: 185
Curtis, Burr, 2: 351
Curtiss, Paul H., Jr., 2: 238; 3: 398*b*, 461, *461–462*
Cushing, Ernest W., 4: 23
Cushing, Harvey W., 3: *180*
  American Ambulance Hospital and, 4: 9–10, *388*, 389*b*, *390*
  anesthesia charting and, 3: 96
  Base Hospital No. 5 and, 4: 420, 420*t*, 422*b*, *422*
  Boston Children's Hospital and, 2: 12
  Codman and, 3: 94–95
  on Dane's foot plate, 2: 245
  development of orthopaedics department, 1: 177
  Harvard Unit and, 2: 119, 125; 3: 369, *370*; 4: 419
  honors and awards, 3: 94
  as MGH surgeon, 3: 95
  on organization of surgery, 4: 13–14

PBBH and, 1: 174, 204; 2: 168, 269; 4: 4–6, *6*, 8–9, 12–13, 16, 79
Quigley and, 1: 276
Sever and, 2: 92
Surgeon's Journal, 3: 369
Thorndike and, 1: 263
Cutler, Elliott C., 4: *106*, *472*
  American Ambulance Hospital and, 4: 389*b*, 390–391
  Base Hospital No. 5 and, 4: 420, 422*b*
  Carl Walter and, 4: 104–105
  death of, 4: 18
  Harvard Unit and, 2: 119; 4: 17
  HMS appointment, 1: 179
  on medical education, 4: 16
  Moseley Professor of Surgery, 1: 268
  as PBBH chief of surgery, 1: 269–270; 4: 8, 10, 15–16, 18, 79, 110
  publications and research, 1: 153–154
  specialty clinics and, 4: 15–16
  support for orthopaedic surgery specialization, 4: 16–17
  Surgical Research Laboratory, 3: 237
  on wounded soldier care, 4: 389–390
  as WWII surgery specialist, 4: 471
Cutler, Robert, 4: 20
Cutler Army Hospital (Fort Devens), 2: 358

D

Dabuzhaky, Leonard, 4: 279
Daland, Florence, 3: 159, 347
Dalton, John Call, Jr., 1: 60
Dana Farber Cancer Institute, 1: 91; 2: 331
Dandy, Walter, 3: 204
Dane, Eunice Cooksey, 2: 247
Dane, John H. (1865-1939), 2: *241*
  Boston Children's Hospital and, 2: 242, 307
  Boston Dispensary and, 2: 247
  Boston Infant's Hospital and, 2: 242
  clinical congress meeting, 3: 118
  death of, 2: 247
  education and training, 2: 241–242
  flat feet research and treatment, 2: 242, *242*, 243, *243*, 244–246
  foot plate, 2: 244–246

HMS appointment, 2: 242, 247
House of the Good Samaritan
and, 2: 242
Lovett and, 2: 242, 246–247
Marcella Street Home and,
2: 242, 247
marriage and family, 2: 247
professional memberships, 2: 246
publications of, 2: 246–247
Thomas splint modification,
2: 247, *247*
US General Hospital No. 2 and,
4: 452
World War I service, 2: 247
Dane, John H., Jr., 2: 247
Danforth, Murray S.
on importance of examination
and diagnosis, 3: 185
Journal of Bone and Joint Surgery
editor, 3: 161, 344; 4: 50
MGH and, 3: 268
military orthopaedics and,
4: 406, 444
publications and research,
2: 136, 297
rehabilitation of soldiers and,
4: 444
Walter Reed General Hospital
and, 4: 452
Danforth, Samuel, 1: 15, 25, 40
D'Angio, G. J., 2: 237
Darling, Eugene A. (1868–1934),
1: 250–251
Darrach, William, 4: 473
Darrach procedure, 3: 191
Darrow, Clarence, 1: 276
*Dartmouth Atlas of Health Care in
Virginia, The* (Wennberg et al.),
2: 374, *374*, 375
Dartmouth Medical School, 2: 371;
3: 363
Dartmouth-Hitchcock Medical Center, 2: 371
David S. Grice Annual Lecture,
2: 215–216, 216t
Davies, John A. K., 4: 194, 195b,
263
Davies, Robert, 4: 262
Davis, Arthur G., 3: 344
Davis, G. Gwilym, 3: 157; 4: 406
Davis, Henry G., 2: 22–23, 26
Davis, Joseph, 2: 219
Davis, Robert, 4: 286
Davy, Sir Humphrey, 1: 56
Dawbarn, Robert H. M., 3: 105
Dawes, William, 1: 17
Dawson, Clyde W., 3: 74
Dawson, David M., 4: 168
Day, Charles, 1: 169; 4: 287
Day, George, 4: 307

Day Nursery (Holyoke), 2: 256
De Forest, R., 3: 210
De Machinamentis of Oribasius,
3: *149*
De Ville, Kenneth Allen, 1: 47
Deaconess Home and Training
School, 4: 273
Deaconess term, 4: 274b
dead arm syndrome, 3: 359–360
*Death of General Warren at the Battle
of Bunker's Hill, The* (Trumbull),
1: *19*
Deaver, George, 4: 76
DeBakey, Michael, 4: 469
debarkation hospitals, 4: 451–452
deep vein thrombosis (DVT),
3: 218; 4: 251–252
DeHaven, Ken, 3: 448
Deland, F. Stanton, Jr., 4: 114, 120
Deland, Jonathan, 1: 217b
Delano, Frederick, 2: 72
DeLorme, Eleanor Person, 3: 281,
287
DeLorme, Thomas I., Jr. (1917–
2003), 3: *281*, 285
awards and, 3: 281–282
blood perfusion research, 3: 287
Children's Hospital/MGH combined program and, 3: 285
death of, 3: 287
early life, 3: 281
education and training, 3: 281
Elgin table and, 3: *287*
expansion of MGH orthopaedics
and, 3: 286
Fracture course and, 3: *273*
Gardiner Hospital and, 3: 282,
284
heavy-/progressive resistance
exercises and, 3: 282, *282*,
283–286
HMS appointment, 3: 287
legacy of, 3: 287
Legon of Merit medal, 3: 284,
284
as Liberty Mutual Insurance
Company medical director,
3: 286–287
Marlborough Medical Associates
and, 2: 146, 269, 299
marriage and family, 3: 281
as MGH surgeon, 3: 285
Milton Hospital and, 3: 287
physical therapy and, 3: 284
PRE (Progressive Resistance Exercise), 3: *286*
publications and research,
3: 282–283, 285–286; 4: 91
rehabilitation and, 3: 459, 461

resistance training in recovery,
3: 282
spinal surgeries and, 3: 287
US Army Medical Corps and,
3: 282
weightlifting and, 3: 281
West Roxbury Veterans Hospital
and, 3: 285
DeLorme table, 3: 284
Delpech, Jacques-Mathieu, 1: xxiii,
106
Delta Upsilon fraternity, 4: 258, *258*
Denis Browne splint, 2: 208
dentistry, 1: 56–57
Denucé, Maurice, 3: 233–235
Derby, George, 4: 307
Description of a Skeleton of the Mastodon Giganteus of North America
(J. C. Warren), 1: *52*
Deshmukh, R. V., 4: 178
Detmold, William Ludwig, 1: 100–
101; 2: 25–26
DeWolfe, C. W., 3: 133
Dexter, Aaron, 1: 25, 95–96
Deyo, Richard, 2: 371
diabetes, 3: 408, 413, 438
Diagnosis in Joint Disease (Allison
and Ghormley), 3: 175, 289, *290*
Diao, Edward, 1: 217b
diarrheal disease, 2: 4
diastematomyelia, 2: 236, 399–400
Dickinson, Robert L., 3: 120, 123
Dickson, Frank D., 2: 78
Dickson, Fred, 2: 77
Dieffenbach, Johann Friedrich, 1: 76
Digby, Kenelm H., 2: 170
Diggs, Lucy, 4: 492
Dignan, Beth A., 2: 277
Dillon Field House, 1: 274, *284*,
285
Dines, Robert, 4: 247
Dingle, J., 4: 127
diphtheria, 2: 4
disabled adults
back problems and, 3: 207
hip disease and, 2: 294; 3: 155
MGH rehabilitation clinic and,
1: 273; 3: 455
orthopaedic care for, 2: 132
polio and, 3: 286
soldiers and veterans, 1: 271–
273; 2: 65, 67; 3: 44
disabled children. *See also* cerebral
palsy; club foot
advocacy for, 1: 107
Crippled Children's Clinic and,
2: 221
House of the Good Samaritan
and, 1: 123
industrial training and, 2: 97

Index

orthopaedic care for, 2: 132
polio and, 2: 191
schools for, 2: 36–41, 67–68, 97, 308, 310–311, *312*
"Discourse on Self-Limited Diseases, A" (Bigelow), 3: 12–13
Diseases of the Bones and Joints (Osgood, Goldthwait and Painter), 2: 117; 3: 81–82; 4: 45
dislocations. *See also* congenital dislocated hips (CDH); hip dislocations
chronic posterior elbow, 3: 366
patella and, 2: 294–296; 3: 79, 79*b*, 80, *81*
shoulders and, 3: 352, *352*, 353, 355–356, *356*
Treatise on Dislocations and Fractures of Joints, 1: 35, 42, *43*
use of ether, 1: 62
voluntary, 3: 355–356, *356*
Dislocations and Joint Fractures (Cotton), 3: 371; 4: 307, 314, 316–317, *317*, 318
distal humerus, 2: 250
Division of Orthopaedic Surgery in the A.E.F., The (Goldthwait), 4: 473
Dixon, Frank D., 3: 173
Dixon, Robert B., 4: 23
Doctor's Hospital, 1: 276
Dodd, Walter J., 2: 114, 116; 3: 20, *20*, 21, 96, 99, 192, 266; 4: 389*b*
Dodson, Tom, 3: 1
Donaghy, R. M., 3: 205
Doppelt, Samuel, 1: 167; 3: 386, 396, 398, 440, 460*b*, *461*
Dowling, John Joseph, 4: 420*t*, 438
Down syndrome, 2: 368, 370
Dr. John Ball Brown (Harding), 1: *95*
Dr. Robert K. Rosenthal Cerebral Palsy Fund in Orthopaedics, 2: 439*b*
Draper, George, 2: 72, 75–76, 78
Drew, Michael A., 4: 163, 193, 279
Drinker, C. K., 2: 81
Drinker, Philip, 2: 78, *78*, 191
Dubousset, Jean, 2: 342
Dudley, H. Robert, 4: 102
Duggal, Navan, 4: 288
Duhamel, Henri-Louis, 1: xxi
Dukakis, Kitty, 3: 419
Dukakis, Michael, 3: 419, 423
Dunlop, George, 4: 279
Dunn, Beryl, 2: 180–181
Dunn, Naughton, 2: 92–94, 150, 181
Dunphy, J. Englebert, 2: 220; 4: 303
Dunster House (Harvard University), 2: *388*
Duocondylar prostheses, 4: 178

duodenal ulcer, 3: 108
duopatellar prosthesis, 4: 130
Dupuytren, Guillaume, 1: 73–75
Duthie, J. J. R., 4: 33
Dwight, Edwin, 4: *302*
Dwight, Thomas, 1: 87–88, 127; 2: *97*, 247, 296; 3: 33, 94, 231; 4: 82, 310
Dwyer, Allen, 2: 336
Dwyer instrumentation, 2: 336, *336*, 342
Dwyer procedure, 2: 328
Dyer, George, 4: 190*b*

E

Eames, Charles, 4: *470*
Eames, Ray, 4: *470*
Eames molded plywood leg splint, 4: *470*
early onset scoliosis (EOS), 2: 360–361
Early Orthopaedic Surgeons of America, The (Shands), 1: 114
Earp, Brandon, 3: 410; 4: 190*b*
Easley, Walter, 3: 282
East Boston Relief Station, 2: 254
Eastern States Orthopaedic Club, 4: 87
Eaton, Richard G. (1929–), 2: *200*, 249
animal model of compartment syndrome, 2: 248
Boston Children's Hospital and, 2: 248, 250
Children's Hospital/MGH combined program and, 2: 248
education and training, 2: 248
hand surgery education, 2: 248, 250–251
HMS appointment, 2: 248
on ischemia-edema cycle, 2: 200–201, *201*
Joint Injuries of the Hand, 2: 250, *250*
Peter Bent Brigham Hospital and, 4: 22
professional memberships, 2: 251
publications and research, 2: 248–250; 3: 309
Roosevelt Hospital and, 2: 248, 250–251
US Army active duty, 2: 248
Ebert, Robert H., 1: 210–211; 2: 203; 4: 113, 119, 123
École de Médicine (University of Paris), 1: 73
Eddy, Chauncey, 1: 103
Edison, Thomas, 3: 96

Edith M. Ashley Professorship, 3: 202, 464*b*
Edsall, David L., 4: *6*
Allison and, 1: 152
Beth Israel Hospital and, 4: 213
clinical research at MGH and, 3: 211
as dean of HMS, 1: 174–177; 2: 81–82; 4: 213, 275, 297, 302
on departmental organization, 1: 176–178
on faculty governance, 1: 175–178
on faculty rank, 1: 178
HMS reforms and, 1: 147
on MGH and HMS relations, 1: 174
postgraduate education and, 2: 160
Edwards, Thomas, 4: 262–263
Effects of Chloroform and of Strong Chloric Ether as Narcotic Agents (J. C. Warren), 1: 62
Ehrenfried, Albert (1880–1951), 4: *215*
attempts at resignation from Beth Israel, 4: 209, 209*b*, 210
Beth Israel Hospital and, 4: 205–210, 220
Boston Children's Hospital and, 4: 215
Boston City Hospital and, 4: 217–218
Chronicle of Boston Jewry, 4: 220
civic and professional engagements, 4: 221*b*
clinical congress meeting, 3: 116
club foot research and, 4: 216
death of, 4: 221
education and training, 4: 215
hereditary deforming chondrodysplasia research, 4: 218–219, *219*, 220
HMS appointment, 4: 218
insufflation anesthesia apparatus, 4: 215–216
Jewish Memorial Hospital and, 4: 215
on military service, 4: 220–221
military surgeon training and, 4: 218
Mt. Sinai Hospital and, 4: 202–205, 215
on need for total Jewish hospital, 4: 205
publications and research, 4: 216–219, *219*, 220–221
pulmonary tuberculosis treatment, 4: 215

Reverdin method and,
4: 216–217
Surgical After-Treatment,
4: 217, *217*
vascular anastomosis and, 4: 216
Ehrenfried, George, 4: 215, 220
Ehrenfried, Rachel Blauspan, 4: 215
Ehrenfried's disease (hereditary deforming chondrodysplasia),
4: 218–220
Ehrlich, Christopher, 3: 401
Ehrlich, Michael G. (1939–2018),
3: *400*, *461*
Brown University Medical School appointment, 3: 400–401
death of, 3: 401
early life, 3: 400
education and training, 3: 400
gait laboratory and, 3: 397
honors and awards, 3: 400
idiopathic subluxation of the radial head case, 3: 401
marriage and family, 3: 401
as MGH surgeon, 3: 385–386, 395, 398*b*, 413
Miriam Hospital and, 3: 401
pediatric orthopaedics and,
3: 388*t*, 400–401, 460*b*
publications and research,
3: 400–401
Rhode Island Hospital and,
3: 401
Ehrlich, Nancy Band, 3: 401
Ehrlich, Timothy, 3: 401
Ehrlichman, Lauren, 3: 463*b*
Eiselsberg, Anton, 1: 264
elbow
arthroplasty of, 3: 64, 341;
4: 63
basket plaster treatment, 2: *122*
brachioradialis transfer and,
2: 153
capitellocondylar total prosthesis, 4: 145, *145*, 146–147
chronic posterior dislocations,
3: 366
early arthrogram of, 3: *99*
excision of, 3: 34, 309, 368
external epicondyle fracture of,
2: 46
flexion contracture of, 2: 418
fusion and, 3: 368
hinged prostheses, 4: 147
idiopathic subluxation of the radial head, 3: 401
intra-articular radial nerve entrapment, 3: 410–411
nonconstrained total prosthesis,
4: 145

non-hinged metal–polyethylene prosthesis, 4: 145–146
total replacement of, 4: 129
electromyogram, 3: 320
electron microscopes, 2: 323, *324*, 325
Elgin table, 3: *287*
Eliot, Charles W., 1: *139*
educational reforms and, 1: 139, 140*b*, 146–147; 2: 19, 41;
3: 44–45, 94
medical education and, 1: 141;
4: 2
on medical faculty organization,
1: 173
on medical leadership, 4: 4
on medical student caliber,
1: 131, 140
opposition to football, 1: 253
Elks' Reconstruction Hospital,
4: 447–448
Ellen and Melvin Gordon Professor of Medical Education, 4: 264
Elliott, J. W., 2: 306
Elliott G. Brackett Fund, 3: 161
Ellis, Daniel S., 3: 241
Elliston, Harriet Hammond, 4: 90, 92
Elliston, William A. (1904–1984),
4: 41*b*, *90*
Boston Children's Hospital and,
2: 313
Brigham and Women's Hospital and, 4: 193
death of, 4: 92
education and training, 4: 90
hip arthroplasty follow-up, 4: 40
HMS appointment, 4: 90
life and community service in Weston, 4: 91–92
marriage and family, 4: 90, 92
on nylon arthroplasty of the knee,
4: 91
PBBH and, 4: 18, 20
publications and research,
4: 90–91
RBBH and, 4: 32, 35, 38, 41, 68, 89–90, 93, 132
US Army Medical Corps and,
4: 90
Veterans Administration Hospital and, 4: 90–91
Elliston, William Rowley, 4: 90
Emans, John (1944–), 2: *357*
Boston brace and, 2: 358–359,
359
Boston Children's Hospital and,
2: 338, 354, 358–359
Brigham and Women's Hospital and, 4: 163, 193

Chest Wall and Spinal Deformity Study Group, 2: 361–362
Core Curriculum Committee and, 1: 216
Cutler Army Hospital and,
2: 358
education and training, 2: 358, 388
Hall and, 2: 347, 358
HMS appointment, 2: 358
honors and awards, 2: 363
Myelodysplasia Program, 2: 359
nutritional status research,
2: 361–362
Parker Hill Hospital and, 2: 358
professional memberships,
2: 363, 363*b*
publications and research, 2: *358*, 359–363
scoliosis treatment, 2: 339, 344
Spinal Surgery Service, 2: 359
embarkation hospitals, 4: 451–452
Emergency Care and Transportation of the Sick and Injured (MacAusland), 3: 310, *311*
Emerson, Ralph Waldo, 1: 57
Emerson, Roger, 3: 396, 399
Emerson Hospital, 3: 317, 319
Emmons, Nathaniel H., 2: 6
Enders, John, 2: 189
End-Result Idea (Codman)
accountability and, 3: 119*b*
bone sarcomas and, 3: 136–138
Boston Children's Hospital and,
1: 194
cards recording outcomes,
3: *111*, 113*b*
Codman Hospital and, 3: 112, 114, *126*
Codman's personal cases, 3: 126, 128–129
Codman's promotion of, 3: 126
as experiment, 3: 119–120
filing system for, 3: *116*
Halifax YMCA Emergency Hospital and, 3: 134
hospital efficiency and, 3: 127*b*
opposition to, 3: 118–120, 122–123
PBBH and, 4: 12
performance-based promotions and, 3: 123–124
promotion of, 3: 116, 118, 123
Robert Osgood and, 2: 135
spread of, 3: 125
treatment outcomes reporting,
3: 110–111
young surgeons and, 3: 130–131

Enneking, William, 1: 218–220; 3: 382
Entrapment Neuropathies (Dawson, et al.), 4: 168
Epidemic Aid Team, 2: 260
epiphyseal arrest, 2: 170–171, 192, 192*t*, *192*, 193
epiphyseal injuries, 2: 321; 4: 350–351, *351*, 352, 355
Erickson, A. Ingrid, 1: 217*b*
Ernest A. Codman Award, 3: 146
Ernst, Harold C., 1: 171; 4: *6*
Erving, W. G., 4: 394
Esposito, Phil, 3: 357, 357*b*
Essentials of Body Mechanics (Goldthwait et al.), 3: *90*, 91
Estok, Dan M., II, 4: 193, 195*b*
ether
    asthma and, 1: 56
    commemoration of first use, 1: *61*, *64*, *65*; 3: *32*
    composition of, 1: 61
    deaths and, 3: 31
    discovery rights of, 1: 60
    ethical use of, 1: 58
    Morton's inhaler, 1: *58*
    use as anesthesia, 1: 55–62, *63*, 64–65, 82
    use at MGH, 1: 57–63, 85; 3: 15, 22, 27–28, 28*b*, 29, 29*b*, 30–34
    use at social events, 1: 56
    use on children, 1: 63
    use outside the U.S., 1: 59
Ether Day 1846 (Prosperi and Prosperi), 1: *59*
Ether Dome (MGH), 1: *59*, *63*, *84*; 3: *14*, 16
Ether Monument, 1: *64*, *65*; 3: *32*, 32*b*
Etherization (J. C. Warren), 1: 62, *62*; 3: 33
Evans, Christopher, 2: 82, 166; 3: 462; 4: 194, 195*b*
Evans, D. K., 2: 211
Evans, Frances, 4: 41*b*
Evarts, C. M. "Mac," 1: 234
Ewald, Frederick C. (1933–), 4: *144*
    Brigham and Women's Hospital, 4: 163
    Brigham Orthopedic Associates (BOA) and, 4: 123
    capitellocondylar total elbow prosthesis, 4: 145, *145*, 146, *146*, 147
    Children's Hospital/MGH combined program and, 4: 144
    education and training, 4: 144
    giant cell synovitis case, 4: 148
    Helen Fay Hunter orthopaedic research fellowship, 4: 144
    HMS appointment, 4: 144
    Knee Society president, 4: 150
    legacy of, 4: 150
    PBBH and, 4: 116, 129, 144–145, 161
    professional memberships, 4: 150
    publications and research, 4: 130, *130*, 134, 144–146, *146*, 147, *147*, 148–149, *149*, 150, 189
    RBBH and, 4: 129, 132, 144–145, 150
    roentgenographic total knee arthroplasty-scoring system, 4: 150
    total knee arthroplasty and, 4: 130–131, 131*t*, 145
    total knee prosthesis research, 4: 147–148, *148*, 149–150
    West Roxbury Veterans Administration Hospital and, 4: 144
Ewing, James, 3: 137
Experience in the Management of Fractures and Dislocations (Wilson), 3: 376
"Extra-Articular Arthrodesis of the Subastragalar Joint" (Grice), 2: *208*, 209
extracorporeal shockwave therapy (ESWT), 3: 437–438

F

Fahey, Robert, 4: 341
Fallon, Anne, 2: 260, *260*
Falmouth Hospital, 4: 89
Faraday, Michael, 1: 56
Farber, Sidney, 2: 171, 215, 234–236; 4: 72
Farnsworth, Dana, 1: 277, 284
fasciotomies, 1: 35; 2: 201, 250; 3: 417–418. *See also* Ober-Yount fasciotomy
fat embolism syndrome, 2: 397, *397*, 398
Faulkner Hospital, 3: 248, 314, 331; 4: 194, *194*
Faxon, Henry H., 4: 482
Faxon, John, 1: 42, 44
Faxon, Nathaniel W., 3: 70*b*; 4: 475, 482
Fearing, Albert, 2: 5
Federated Jewish Charities, 4: 205
Federation of Jewish Charities, 4: 200
Federation of Spine Associations, 4: 265
Federation of State Medical Boards (FSMB), 3: 424
Felch, L. P., 3: 269
Feldon, Paul, 4: 98
Fell, Honor B., 4: 126
femoral heads
    acetabular dysplasia case, 2: 390
    acetabular replacement and, 3: 279
    avascular necrosis of, 4: 154–156, 238
    blood supply to, 1: 36; 2: 392
    bone allografts and, 3: 442
    excision of, 3: 155
    flattening of, 2: *103*
    fractures of, 1: 49; 3: 38–39
    hip dislocations and, 2: 352–353, 401, 418
    hip joint excision and, 3: 34
    histologic-histochemical grading system for, 3: 384
    Legg-Calvé-Perthes disease, 2: 105, 351
    osteoarthritis and, 3: 221
    osteonecrosis of, 2: 328–329, 394; 3: 434; 4: 156–157
    palpating, 1: 48
    replacement of, 3: 213
    sclerosis of, 3: 441
    slipped capital femoral epiphysis (SCFE) and, 2: 176
    tuberculosis and, 2: 108
    wear on, 3: 224
femoral neck fractures. *See also* hip fractures
    AAOS study of, 3: 191
    Bigelow and, 3: 38–39
    calcar femorale and, 3: 39, *39*
    experience among AAOS members, 3: 190*t*
    fracture research and, 3: 377
    osteoarthritis and, 3: 383–384
    roentgenology and, 3: 377
    Smith-Petersen and, 3: 62, 181, 185–186, *186*, 189, 189*b*, 190
    tissue response at, 4: 76
    treatment of, 3: 367
    triflanged nail for, 3: 62, 185–186, *186*, 189, 189*b*, 190
femoral spurs, 3: 39
femoroacetabular impingement, 3: 188–189
femur fractures
    Buck's traction and, 1: 80
    Gaucher's disease, 3: 434
    growth disturbances in, 2: 400
    immediate reamed nailings of, 3: 416
    malunions, 3: *42*

sepsis after intramedullary fixation, 2: 248; 3: 309–310
triflanged nail for, 3: 62, 185, *186*, 189, 189*b*
wartime treatment of, 4: 408
Ferguson, Albert B., Jr. (1919–2014), 4: *109*
death of, 4: 111
education and training, 4: 110
HMS appointment, 4: 111
muscle dynamics research, 4: 111
Orthopaedic Surgery in Infancy and Childhood, 2: 188, 239, 303
PBBH and, 1: 204; 2: 188; 4: 19, 21, 36, 79, 110–111
professional memberships, 4: 111
publications and research, 4: 102
RBBH and, 4: 93, 111
spiral femur fracture case, 4: 110
University of Pittsburgh appointment, 2: 188; 3: 382–383; 4: 73*b*, 111
US Marine Corps and, 4: 110
Ferguson, Albert B., Sr., 4: 109–110
Ferguson, Jeremiah, 4: 109
Fernandez, Diego L., 3: 409, 431
Fessenden, Louise, 3: 271
Fifth Portable Surgical Hospital, 4: 489
Fine, Jacob, 4: 283*t*
Fink, Edward, 4: 279–280
Fink, Mitchell P., 4: 283*t*
Finkelstein, Clara, 2: 319
Finney, John M. T., 4: 324
Finton, Frederick P., 1: *80*
First Operation Under Ether (Hinckley), 1: *55*, 59
Fischer, Josef E., 4: 287, 289*b*
Fisher, Bob, 1: 255
Fisher, Josef E., 1: 234; 2: 397
Fisher, Roland F., 3: 167
Fisher, Thomas J., 3: 431
Fiske, Eben W., 4: 389*b*, 394
Fiske, Edith, 2: 42
Fiske Prize, 2: 52
Fitchet, Seth M. (1887–1939), 2: *252*
Boston Children's Hospital and, 2: 222, 252, 274; 4: 338
cleidocranial dysostosis, 2: 254
death of, 2: 254
education and training, 2: 251
Harvard Department of Hygiene and, 2: 253
HMS appointment, 2: 252
MGH and, 2: 252
military service, 2: 251
Morris and, 2: 282
private medical practice, 2: 252

public health and, 2: 253
publications and research, 1: 263; 2: 253–254
ruptures of the serratus anterior, 2: 253
Stillman Infirmary and, 2: 253
Fitton-Jackson, Sylvia, 4: 126
Fitz, Reginald Heber, 1: 179; 3: 94
Fitz, Wolfgang, 4: 194
FitzSimmons, Elizabeth Grace Rogers, 2: 258
FitzSimmons, Henry J. (1880–1935), 1: *187*; 2: *254*, *255*, 258
on atypical multiple bone tuberculosis, 2: 257
Boston Children's Hospital and, 1: 187; 2: 252, 254–256, 258, 274, 282; 4: 338
Boston University and, 2: 258
Camp Devens base hospital and, 4: 452
congenital torticollis research, 2: 256, 258
death of, 2: 258
East Boston Relief Station and, 2: 254
education and training, 2: 254
European medical studies, 2: 255
HMS appointment, 2: 223, 256, 258; 4: 59–60
marriage and family, 2: 258
military surgeon training and, 2: 42
Ober on, 2: 256, 258
orthopaedics internship under Bradford, 2: 255
orthopaedics internship under Lovett, 2: 144
Osgood on, 2: 258–259
professional memberships, 2: 258, 258*b*
publications and research, 2: 256, 258
ton Children's Hospital and, 1: 188
World War I service, 2: 258
5005th USAF Hospital (Elmendorf), 3: 215
Flagg, Elisha, 3: 67
Flatt, Adrian, 4: 97
Fleisher, Leon, 3: 414
Flexner, Abraham, 1: 146–147; 3: 165
Flexner Report, 1: 146–147
flexor carpi ulnaris transfer procedure, 2: 172, 188, 198–199, *199*, 200
Fliedner, Theodor, 4: 274*b*
Flier, Jeffrey, 1: 242
Floating Hospital for Children, 2: 306, 370

flow cytometry, 3: 388
Floyd, W. Emerson, 3: 410
Floyd, W., III, 2: 417
Flugstad, Daniel, 3: 433
fluoroscope, 2: 307; 3: 96–97
Flynn, John, 3: 433
Foley, T. M., 4: 451
Folkman, Judah, 4: 182
Foot and Ankle, The (Trott and Bateman), 2: 317
foot problems. *See also* club foot
ankle valgus, 2: 212
arches and, 2: 317
arthritis and, 4: 61
astragalectomy (Whitman's operation), 2: 92–93
athletes and, 3: 348
Batchelor technique, 2: 212
Brewster and, 2: 228–229
calcaneovalgus deformity, 2: 92–93
cavus feet, 2: 229
cerebral palsy treatment, 2: 229
congenital flatfoot, 4: 63
correction of fixed deformities, 4: 62, 62*t*, 63
countersinking the talus, 2: 228–229, 283
Dane and, 2: 242–246
design of shoes for, 2: 54–56
evaluation through glass, 2: 54–55, *55*
extra-articular arthrodesis of the subtalar joint, 2: 210–211, *211*, 212
flat feet, 2: 54–56, 101–102, 107–108, 242–243, *243*, 244–246
gait analysis and, 2: 407
Green-Grice procedure, 2: 212
heel cord contractures, 2: 265
hindfoot pain, 4: 188
Hoke's stabilization requirements, 2: 282–283
John Brown's device for, 1: 106
Lambrinudi stabilization, 2: 229
Morton's neuroma, 2: 287
nurses and, 2: 54–56
Osgood on, 2: 123–124
paralytic flat foot deformities, 2: 210–212
planovalgus deformity, 4: 188
poliomyelitis and, 2: 210
radiography and, 2: 56
rheumatoid arthritis and, 4: 188
shoe fit and design, 2: 293, 317, 407
skeletal anatomy and, 2: 247
sling procedure and, 3: 294, *294*, 295, 296*b*–297*b*

stabilization of, 2: 282–284
treatment of, 2: 54–56, 107–108
triple arthrodesis, 2: 172, 228–229
valgus deformity treatment, 2: 197, 209–212
weakness/paralysis in, 2: 150–151
wire drop foot splints, 2: *123*
football
acromioclavicular joint dislocation in, 1: 268, 277
athletic training and, 1: 248, 250–253, 255–256, 258
Bloody Monday game, 1: 245
Boston Game, 1: 247
collegiate reform and, 1: 253–254
concussions in, 1: 247, 254, 274–275
establishment of rules in, 1: 247–248
Hampden Park, Springfield, 1: *249*
Harvard game, 1906, 1: *257*
Harvard Rose Bowl game, 1920, 1: *259*
injuries in, 1: 247–248, 252–255, 255t, 256, 258–262, 288
preventative strappings, 1: *269*
protective padding and helmets in, 1: 255, *267*
ruptures of the serratus anterior, 2: 253
secondary school injuries in, 4: 370, *370*
sports medicine and, 1: 248, 250, 254–256
team photo, 1890, 1: *249*
Forbes, A. Mackenzie, 2: 87–88; 3: 231; 4: 233, 394
Forbes, Andrew, 3: 437
Forbes, Elliot, 2: 277
Fort Bragg (Fayetteville, N.C.), 4: 484
Fort Leonard Wood (Missouri), 3: 432
Fort Oglethorpe (Georgia), 4: 338
Fort Ord US Army Hospital, 4: 259
Fort Riley (Kansas), 4: 452–453
Fort Totten (Queens, NY), 4: *422*
Fort Warren (Mass.), 1: 20
Foster, Charles C., 1: 109, 111
Foster, Charles H. W., 3: 123
Foster, Helen, 3: 228
Foultz, W. S., 2: 237
Fourth Portable Surgical Hospital (4PSH), 2: 232–233; 4: 489
Fourth Portable Surgical Hospital's Service in the War against Japan, The (Cohen), 2: 232–233

fracture boxes, 1: 80–81
Fracture Clinic (MGH), 2: 130; 3: 60, 60b, 61–62, 241–242, 245, 273, *273*, 313–315, 371, 373, 378, 456b
Fracture Committee of the American College of Surgeons, 2: 131; 3: 61
fractures. *See also* compound fractures; femoral neck fractures; femur fractures; hip fractures
amputations and, 1: 50, 54
ankle, 4: 313–315, *315*, 316
Austin Moore prosthesis, 3: 213
bandaging care and, 1: 76
basket plasters for, 2: *122*
bilateral comminuted patellar, 3: 56b
birth, 1: 264
calcaneus treatment by impaction, 4: *313*, 314b
cervical spine, 3: 340–341
clinics for, 2: 130–131
conference on treatment for, 2: 131
Cotton's, 4: 313–315, *315*, 316
displaced supracondylar humerus, 2: 379
distal femoral physeal, 2: 400
distal radius treatment, 3: 408–409
elderly patients and, 3: 353, 354, 354b; 4: 341
fender, 4: 242
Gartland type 3 supracondylar humeral, 2: 368
general and orthopaedic surgeon collaboration on, 4: 463–465
hip nailing and, 3: 237
hips and, 3: 213; 4: 74–75, 159b–160b, 318–320, 341
of the humerus, 3: 323–324; 4: 372
impaction treatment for, 4: 319–320
increase in, 1: 63
intercondylar T humeral, 2: 397, *397*
intra-articular, 3: 408
lateral tibial plateau, 4: *312*
leg length and, 2: 350
long-bone, 3: 60–61
malpractice suits and, 1: 50–51; 3: 63
managing pediatric, 2: 379
metastatic breast disease and, 2: 411
metastatic pathological, 3: *376*, 377–378
olecranon, 3: 309

open anterior lumbosacral dislocation, 3: 420
open treatment of, 3: 55–56, 58–62, 64
open-bone, 4: *400*
orthopaedic treatment of, 4: 463
os calcis, 4: 313, 314b, 335–336
outcomes of, 1: 50; 3: 339
plaster casts for, 2: *122*
portable traction device, 2: 297
Pott's, 4: *317*, 318
proximal humerus, 2: 96, *122*
pseudofracture of tibia, 3: 341, *342*
of the radial head, 2: 396–397; 3: 322–323
risk prediction research, 2: 411, *411*
scaphoid, 3: 101–102; 4: 359–361
scientific study of, 1: 264
shoulders, 3: 339
supracondylar humerus, 2: 229, 345, 379
Swiss method of treating, 2: 406
table for, 2: *121*
tibial spine, 4: 365
tibial tuberosity, 2: 91
total disability following joint, 3: *373*
traction treatment for, 2: 23
treatment for compound, 4: *335*, 337, *392*
treatment of, 1: 80–81; 3: 35, 60, 101; 4: 339b–340b, 362
triflanged nail for, 3: 62, 185–186, *186*, 189, 189b
ununited, 3: 34–35
vanadium steel plates and, 4: 340, *342*
wire arm splint for, 2: *122*
Fractures (Wilson), 3: 315
Fractures and Dislocations (Stimson), 1: 147
Fractures and Dislocations (Wilson and Cochrane), 3: 371, *371*
Fractures and Other Injuries (Cave), 3: 273, *273*; 4: 356
Fractures of the Distal Radius (Fernandez and Jupiter), 3: 409, *409*
Francis A. Countway Library of Medicine, 1: 59, 66; 2: 271; 4: 20
Frank R. Ober Research Fund, 2: 165
Franklin, Benjamin, 1: 12, 14
Fraser, Somers, 4: 438–439
Frazier, Charles H., 4: 299
Frederick and Joan Brengle Learning Center, 3: 463

Frederick W. and Jane M. Ilfeld Professorship, 2: 438, 439*b*
Fredericks, G. R., 3: 442
Free Hospital for Women, 4: 113–114
Freedman, K. B., 1: 168
Frei, Emil, III, 2: 422
Freiberg, Albert H., 2: 77–78, 87; 3: 157, 229; 4: 406, 451
Freiberg, Joseph A., 1: 193; 2: 79; 4: 59
Friedenberg, Z., 2: 214
Friedlaender, Gary, 3: 393, 440; 4: 266*b*
Friedman, Richard, 1: 217*b*
Frost, Eben H., 1: 60
Frost, Gilbert, 3: 97
frozen shoulder, 1: 277–278
Frymoyer, J. W., 3: 205
Fuldner, Russell, 3: 74
Fundamentals of Orthopaedic Surgery in General Medicine and Surgery (Osgood and Allison), 2: 135–136
Funsten, Robert, 3: 303
Furbush, C. L., 4: 439, 440*b*

G

Gage, M., 3: 210
Gage, Thomas, 1: 16
gait
    backpack loads and, 2: 408
    cerebral palsy and, 2: 406–407
    clinical analysis and, 2: 408
    hip abductor weakness and, 2: 33
    impact of shoes on, 2: 293, 407
    low back disorders and, 2: 408
    nonmechanical treatment of, 2: 244
    nonoperative treatment of, 2: 271
    Ober-Yount fasciotomy and, 2: 153
    physical therapy and, 2: 107
    shelf procedure and, 2: 151
    stroke and, 2: 408
    total knee replacement and, 2: 408
    Trendelenburg, 2: 33, 108, 151
    use of cameras to analyze, 2: 406
gait laboratory, 2: 107, 406, 424; 3: 397
Galante, Jorge, 3: 220, 222
Galeazzi method, 2: 227
Gall, Edward, 3: 331
Gallie, William E., 1: 197; 2: 160; 4: 443
Galloway, Herbert P. H., 3: 233; 4: 411, 426, 454, 464
Gambrill, Howard, Jr., 4: 40

Gandhi, Mohandas Karamchand, 4: 262
Ganz, Reinhold, 2: 390–392
Garbino, Peter, 2: 438
Gardiner Hospital, 3: 282, 284
Gardner, George E., 2: 215
Garg, Sumeet, 2: 378
Garland, Joseph E., 3: 12
Garrey, W. E., 1: 267
Gartland, John, 3: 308–309
Gates, Frank D. (1925–2011), 2: *218*
    Boston Children's Hospital and, 2: 218
    death of, 2: 218–219
    education and training, 2: 218
    HMS appointment, 2: 218
Gates, Frederick T., 1: 146
Gatton Agricultural College, 4: 489, *489*
Gaucher's disease, 3: 433–434
Gauvain, Sir Henry, 4: 363, 367
Gay, George H., 1: 308; 3: *31*
Gay, George W., 4: 324
Gay, Martin, 1: 306
Gay, Warren F., 3: 68, 266
Gaynor, David, 3: 463
Gebhardt, Mark C.
    as Beth Israel chief of orthopaedics, 4: 289*b*
    as BIDMC chief of orthopaedics, 4: 287
    Boston Children's Hospital and, 2: 439*b*
    Boston Pathology Course and, 1: 216
    Frederick W. and Jane M. Ilfeld Professorship, 2: 439*b*
    HCORP and, 1: 218, 224–225, 227
    on Mankin, 3: 393
    as MGH clinical faculty, 3: 464*b*
    orthopaedic chair at BIDMC, 1: 234, 242
    orthopaedic oncology and, 3: 460*b*
    publications and research, 3: 433
    tumor treatment and, 3: 397
Geiger, Ronald, 2: 277, 290
Gelberman, Richard H. (1943–), 3: *402*
    avascular necrosis of the lunate case, 3: 403
    Core Curriculum Committee and, 1: 216
    education and training, 3: 402
    flexor tendon research, 3: 403, *403*
    hand and microvascular service, 3: 402–403

    HCORP and, 3: 403–404
    HMS appointment, 3: 403
    honors and awards, 3: 403–405
    as MGH chief of Hand Service, 3: 403
    as MGH surgeon, 3: 399
    Operative Nerve Repair and Reconstruction, 3: 404
    publications and research, 3: 402, *402*, 403–404
    Smith Day lectures, 3: 431
    tissue fluid pressures research, 3: 404, *404*
    University of California in San Diego and, 3: 402
    Washington University School of Medicine and, 3: 404–405
gene therapy, 2: 82
General Leonard Wood Army Community Hospital, 3: 432
General Leonard Wood Gold Medal, 4: 337
genu valgum, 1: *117*
genu varum, 1: *117*
George III, King, 1: 11
George W. Gay Lecture, 4: 324
George Washington University, 2: 351
Georgia Warm Springs Foundation, 2: 77–78, 107, 264, *264*, 270
Gerald, Park, 2: 234
Gerbino, Peter, 2: 439*b*
Gerhart, Tobin, 1: 217*b*; 4: 251, 262–263, 286, 288
German Orthopaedic Association, 2: 43
Ghivizzani, Steve, 4: 194
Ghogawala, Zoher, 4: 272*b*
Ghormley, Jean McDougall, 3: 288, 290
Ghormley, Ralph K. (1893–1959), 3: *288*
    death of, 3: 290
    Diagnosis in Joint Disease, 3: 175, 289, *290*
    early life, 3: 288
    education and training, 3: 288
    HMS appointment, 3: 288; 4: 59
    on joint disease, 3: 288–289, *289*
    as joint tuberculosis expert, 3: 289
    leadership of, 3: 289–290
    marriage and family, 3: 288
    Mayo Clinic and, 3: 289
    memberships and, 3: 290, 290*b*
    as MGH surgeon, 3: 288
    military orthopaedics and, 4: 453

Index

New England Peabody Home for Crippled Children and, 2: 270; 3: 288
private medical practice, 2: 146; 3: 288
publications and research, 3: 288–289
triple arthrodesis and, 2: 150
tuberculosis research and, 3: 288–289
US Army Medical Corps and, 3: 288
Giannestras, Nicholas, 2: 317; 3: *293*
Gibney, Virgil P., 2: 27, 43, 48, 52; 4: 463
Gilbreth, Frank B., 3: 120
Gill, A. Bruce, 2: 78, 183
Gill, Madeline K., 4: 59
Gill, Thomas J., 1: 167; 3: 462, 464*b*
Gilles, Hamish G., 4: 163, 193
Giza, Eric, 1: 217*b*
glanders, 2: 46
Glaser, Robert J., 4: 113
Glazer, Paul, 4: 286
Gleich operation, 4: 313
glenohumeral deformity, 2: 418–419, 419*t*
Glick, Hyman, 4: 251, 262–263, 286, 288
Glickel, Steven Z., 3: 430
Glimcher, Aaron, 2: 319
Glimcher, Clara Finkelstein, 2: 319
Glimcher, Laurie, 2: 330–331
Glimcher, Melvin J. (1925–2014), 1: *208, 210, 285*; 2: *319, 320, 330*; 3: *455*
　activating transcription factor-2 (ATF-2) and, 2: 330
　BIH Board of Consultants, 4: 262–263
　bone research, 2: 321–330
　Boston Arm development, 2: 326
　Boston Children's Hospital and, 1: 180; 2: 320, 327, 329; 4: 127
　Brigham and Women's Hospital and, 4: 163, 193
　Children's Hospital/MGH combined program and, 2: 320
　as Children's orthopaedic surgeon-in-chief, 2: 15*b*, 286, 326–327, 337, 406, 422, 434
　death of, 2: 331
　on DeLorme's blood perfusion research, 3: 287
　as Edith M. Ashley Professor, 3: 464*b*

education and training, 2: 319–321
electron microscopes and, 2: 323, *324*, 325
epiphyseal injuries after frostbite case, 2: 321–323
gait laboratory, 2: 406
Hall and, 2: 336
as Harriet M. Peabody Professor, 2: 327, 337, 439*b*
HCORP and, 4: 247
HMS appointment, 2: 321, 327
as honorary orthopaedic surgeon, 3: 398*b*
honors and awards, 2: 319, 324–325, 327–331
leadership of, 3: 453, 455*b*–457*b*
legacy of, 2: 330–331; 3: 458*b*
marriage and family, 2: 331
MGH Orthopaedic Research Laboratories and, 2: 321–324
as MGH orthopaedics chief, 1: 210; 2: 325; 3: 11*b*, 202, 228, 245, 385, 458*b*, 459; 4: 126
MGH residents and, 2: *327*; 3: *457*
orthopaedic research and, 3: 211
orthopaedics curriculum and, 1: 164; 3: 457*b*
osteonecrosis of the femoral head research, 2: 328, *328*, 329; 4: 156
PBBH and, 4: 163
professional memberships, 2: 329, 331
publications and research, 2: 321, *321*, 322, 324–330
research laboratories, 2: 434, 439; 3: 455*b*, 458*b*
Glowacki, Julie, 4: 194, 195*b*
gluteus maximus
　modification of use of sacrospinalis, 2: 146–147
　Ober operation and, 2: 148, 153
　paralysis of, 2: 146–147
　posterior approach to the hips, 2: 353
Goddu, Louis A. O., 3: 268; 4: 204
Godfrey, Ambrose, 1: 56
Godfrey, Arthur, 3: 198–199
Goethals, Thomas R., 4: 474, 482*b*
Goetjes, D. H., 2: 91
Goff, C. F., 4: 313
Gokaslan, Ziya L., 4: 272*b*
Goldberg, Michael, 2: 368
Goldring, Steve, 4: 280
Goldstone, Melissa, 3: 328
Goldthwait, Ellen W. R., 4: 27
Goldthwait, Francis Saltonstall, 3: 89

Goldthwait, Jessie Sophia Rand, 3: 79, 89
Goldthwait, Joel C., 4: 37–38
Goldthwait, Joel E. (1866–1961), 3: *77, 89, 91*; 4: *24, 398*
　adult orthopaedics and, 2: 101; 3: 78–79
　AOA preparedness committee, 4: 394
　back pain research and, 3: 203–204
　Beth Israel Hospital and, 4: 247
　Body Mechanics in Health and Disease, 3: 91
　Boston Children's Hospital and, 1: 187; 2: 13, 40, 247; 3: 78
　Boston City Hospital and, 1: 187; 4: 305*b*
　Boston School of Physical Education and, 3: 84
　Brigham Hospital and, 3: 81, 84, 91–92
　Carney Hospital and, 3: 78, 80; 4: 45, 86
　chronic disease treatment and, 4: 52
　clinical congress meeting, 3: 118
　Corey Hill Hospital and, 3: 89; 4: 224
　curative workshops and, 4: 402–403
　death of, 3: 92; 4: 38
　Diseases of the Bones and Joints, 2: 117; 3: 81–82
　dislocation of the patella case, 3: 79, 79*b*, 80, *81*
　Division of Orthopedic Surgery in the A.E.F., 4: 473
　early life, 3: 77
　education and training, 3: 77–78
　Essentials of Body Mechanics, 3: 90, 91
　etiology of orthopaedic impairments and diseases, 3: 81–82
　on faulty body mechanics, 3: 91
　founding of AAOS, 3: 90
　on hip disease, 2: 52, *52*
　HMS appointment, 3: 80, 84
　Hospital Efficiency meeting, 3: 120
　House of the Good Samaritan and, 2: 114; 3: 78
　on importance of posture, 3: 81, 83, 87–89; 4: 53, 62, 82, 233
　interest in visceroptosis, 3: 83–84, 84*b*, 86–88
　iron bars, 3: 89, *89, 149*
　legacy of, 3: 91–92
　Marcella Street Home and, 2: 247

marriage and family, 3: 79, 89
on medical research, 3: 2
memberships and, 3: 92
MGH biochemistry laboratory,
  2: 322; 3: 455b–456b
as MGH orthopaedics chief,
  3: 11b, 67–68, 80–81, 227
military orthopaedics and,
  2: 127–128; 3: 156; 4: 406,
  443
military reconstruction hospitals
  and, 4: 440, 444–445
military surgeon training and,
  2: 65
New England Deaconess Hospital
  and, 3: 78; 4: 274
orthopaedic surgery, 2: 116
patellar tendon transfer, 2: 294
on patient evaluation, 3: 90
on polio, 2: 77
private medical practice, 4: 62
publications and research,
  3: 78–84, 90, 90, 91
RBBH and, 3: 81, 84, 91–92;
  4: 23–25, 25b, 26–28, 31,
  36–38, 39b, 79, 93, 111
rehabilitation of soldiers and,
  4: 396, 402, 411
resolution in honor of, 4: 38,
  39b
Robert Jones Lecture, 3: 90
Shattuck Lecture, 3: 84–85, 85,
  86
surgical records from, 2: 115b
US Army Distinguished Service
  Medal, 3: 83, 83
US Medical Reserve Corps, 3: 89
on variations in human anatomy,
  3: 85–86, 86t
World War I and, 2: 124–125;
  4: 402–403
World War I volunteer orthopae-
  dic surgeons and, 4: 398–399,
  399, 404, 406–407, 411
Goldthwait, Mary Lydia Pitman,
  3: 77
Goldthwait, Thomas, 3: 77
Goldthwait, William Johnson, 3: 77
Goldthwait Research Fund, 4: 27–28
Goldthwait Reservation, 3: 92, 92
Good Samaritan Hospital, 1: 107.
  See also House of the Good
  Samaritan
Goodnow, Elisha, 4: 293
Goodridge, Frederick J., 3: 266
Goodsir, John, 1: xxii
Gordon, Leonard, 3: 431
Gordon Hall, 1: 86

Gordon Research Conference on
  Bioengineering and Orthopaedic
  Sciences, 3: 445, 445
Gorforth, Helen R., 3: 365
Gorgas, William C., 4: 411, 429,
  447
Gould, Augustus Addison, 1: 60
Gould, Marjorie, 3: 303
Gould, Nathaniel D., 1: 309; 3: 293
Grabias, Stanley L., 1: 217b;
  3: 460b
Graffman, Gary, 3: 414
Graham, Henry, 2: 168
Grand Palais (Paris), 4: 401
Grandlay, J., 3: 210
Great Britain, 1: 11–16; 4: 393,
  399, 432, 476. See also British
  Expeditionary Forces (BEF); Brit-
  ish hospitals
Great Ormond Street Hospital, 2: 5
Greater Boston Bikur Cholim Hospi-
  tal, 4: 212
Greater Hartford Tuberculosis Respi-
  ratory Disease Association, 2: 267
Green, Daniel, 4: 239
Green, David, 4: 98
Green, Elizabeth, 2: 168
Green, Gladys Griffith, 2: 168
Green, Janet, 2: 168
Green, Jean, 2: 167
Green, Neil, 2: 351, 351
Green, Robert M., 1: 89
Green, Samuel A., 3: 46
Green, William T. (1901–1986),
  1: 200, 204, 207; 2: 167, 169, 177,
  179, 180, 204
  as AAOS president, 2: 201–202,
    202, 203
  on arthritis, 2: 171
  birth palsies research, 2: 415,
    417
  on bone granuloma, 2: 171
  on bone growth and leg length
    discrepancy, 2: 170, 191–193
  Boston Children's Hospital and,
    1: 158, 179–180; 2: 168–169,
    176–178, 191, 274, 301;
    3: 277, 293; 4: 72
  CDH treatment, 3: 235
  cerebral palsy treatment, 2: 171–
    172, 196–200, 229
  Children's Hospital/MGH com-
    bined program and, 4: 68, 158
  on clinical staff, 1: 201
  Cohen and, 2: 234–235
  on congenital pseudarthrosis of
    the tibia, 2: 172–176
  contributions to pediatric ortho-
    paedics, 2: 168

Crippled Children's Clinic and,
  2: 287
death of, 2: 205
early life, 2: 167
education and training,
  2: 167–168
Epidemic Aid Team, 2: 260
as first Harriet M. Peabody Professor, 2: 183, 203, 439b
flexor carpi ulnaris transfer procedure, 2: 172, 188, 198–200
grand rounds and, 2: 178–181,
  181, 182, 230, 271
on Grice, 2: 215
Growth Study, 2: 193, 193, 194,
  304, 432
hamstring contractures and,
  2: 198
Harriet M. Peabody Professor of
  Orthopaedic Surgery, 3: 202
Harvard Infantile Paralysis Clinic
  and, 2: 176, 188
HCORP and, 1: 200–210
HMS appointment, 2: 168, 176,
  183, 223, 270; 4: 61
honorary degrees, 2: 203
Infantile Paralysis Clinic and,
  2: 79
on Kuhns, 4: 66
legacy of, 2: 203–205
marriage and family, 2: 168
McGinty and, 2: 279
meticulousness and, 2: 178–179,
  182–183
on muscle grades, 2: 180
Ober and, 2: 163, 168
as orthopaedic chair, 2: 15b
orthopaedic research laboratory
  and, 2: 234
on orthopaedics curriculum,
  1: 159, 162–164, 200–201;
  2: 202
orthopaedics education and,
  2: 183–186, 188, 203, 205
orthopaedics leadership, 2: 176–
  178, 191, 197
on osteochondritis dissecans,
  2: 194–195
on osteomyelitis, 2: 169–170
PBBH and, 4: 16, 18–22, 73b,
  79, 108, 110
as PBBH chief of orthopaedic
  surgery, 4: 196b
Pediatric Orthopaedic Society
  and, 2: 351
polio research and, 2: 189–190;
  3: 332
polio treatment, 2: 188–191
private medical practice and,
  1: 179; 2: 313

Index

professional memberships, 2: 204
as professor of orthopaedic surgery, 1: 158, 176, 198; 2: 176
publications and research, 2: 169, 188, 194–200, 229, 249, 264, 350
RBBH and, 4: 40, 68
rehabilitation planning and, 1: 272
on residency program, 1: 208
resident training by, 1: 199, 202–203, *203*, 204–206
on slipped capital femoral epiphysis (SCFE), 2: 176
on Sprengel deformity, 2: 195
surgery techniques, 2: 177
Tachdjian and, 2: 301–304
tibial osteoperiosteal graft method, 2: *228*
Trott and, 2: 317–318
Unit for Epidemic Aid in Infantile Paralysis (NFP), 2: 188–189
on Volkmann ischemic contracture, 2: 200–201, *201*
Green, William T., Jr., 2: 168, 182, 204–205
Green Dragon Tavern, 1: *11*, 12, *12*, 17, 24
Green-Andersen growth charts, 2: 193, *193*, 194, 304
Greenberg, B. E., 4: 199
Green-Grice procedure, 2: 212
Greenough, Francis, 2: 9
Greenough, Robert B., 2: 119, 157–158; 3: 118; 4: 389*b*
Greer, James A., 3: 398*b*
Gregory, Ernest, 4: 226
Grenfell, Sir William, 3: 91
Grenfell Mission, 2: 111
Grice, David S. (1914–1960), 2: *207*
  AAOS and, 2: 215
  Banks and, 1: 202, 205
  Boston Children's Hospital and, 2: 208, 299
  club foot treatment, 2: 208
  education and training, 2: 207–208
  extra-articular arthrodesis of the subtalar joint, 2: *208*, 209–212
  HMS appointment, 2: 208, 210, 213
  legacy of, 2: 214–216
  marriage and family, 2: 214
  Massachusetts Infantile Paralysis Clinic and, 2: 208, 212, 314
  memorial funds for, 2: 215
  orthopaedics education and, 2: 213–214
  orthopaedics leadership, 2: 191
  paralytic flat foot operative technique, 2: 210–212
  PBBH and, 2: 208; 4: 18–19, 110
  poliomyelitis treatment, 2: 208, 212–213, 213*b*, 315
  private medical practice and, 2: 313
  professional memberships, 2: 215
  publications of, 2: 189, 208, 220
  residency training by, 2: 213–214
  Simmons College and, 2: 213
  University of Pennsylvania and, 2: 213–214
  University of Vermont and, 2: 208
  valgus deformity treatment, 2: 198, 209–210
Grice, Elizabeth Fry, 2: 207
Grice, John, 2: 207
Grice, Mary Burns, 2: 214
Griffin, Bertha Mae Dail, 2: 349
Griffin, Jesse Christopher, 2: 349
Griffin, Margaret Braswell, 2: 349
Griffin, Paul P. (1927–2018), 2: *349*, *350*, *356*
  arthritis treatment, 2: 350
  BIH Board of Consultants, 4: 262
  Boston Children's Hospital and, 2: 301, 338, 349, 351, 354–355, 434
  Chicago Shriner's Hospital and, 2: 355
  Crippled Children's Clinic and, 2: 314
  death of, 2: 356
  education and training, 2: 349
  George Washington University and, 2: 351
  HMS appointment, 2: 349–351, 354
  Laboratory for Skeletal Disorders and Rehabilitation and, 2: 413
  as orthopaedic chair, 2: 15*b*, 286
  orthopaedics appointments, 2: 351
  PBBH and, 4: 20, 22
  Pediatric Orthopaedic International Seminars program, 2: 304
  Pediatric Orthopaedic Society and, 2: 351
  pediatric orthopaedics, 2: 354–355
  private medical practice and, 2: 313
  publications and research, 2: 349–351, *351*, *354*
  traumatic hip dislocation case, 2: 352–353
Griffith, Gladys, 2: 168
Griffiths, Maurice, 4: 92
Grillo, Hermes C., 1: 184
Gritti-Stokes amputation, 3: 374
Gross, Richard, 2: 354–355, 438
Gross, Robert E., 2: 215
Gross, Samuel D., 1: 79
Gross, Samuel W., 3: 142
Groves, Ernest W. Hey, 2: 91; 3: 209
Gucker, Harriet, 2: 266
Gucker, Thomas III (1915–1986), 2: *259*, *260*
  Berlin polio epidemic and, 2: 260, 264
  Boston Children's Hospital and, 2: 260, 264
  contributions to orthopaedic rehabilitation, 2: 266
  death of, 2: 266
  education and training, 2: 259–260
  Georgia Warm Springs Foundation and, 2: 264
  marriage and family, 2: 266
  on patient reaction to polio, 2: 261*b*–263*b*
  poliomyelitis and, 2: 259, 264, 266
  professional memberships, 2: 264–265
  publications and research, 2: 264–266
  on pulmonary function, 2: 265–266
  tendon transfers and, 2: 265
  University of Pennsylvania and, 2: 265
  University of Southern California and, 2: 266
Guérin, Jules, 1: 54, 98, 106; 3: 26
gunshot injuries, 2: 66, 119, 161, 233; 3: 43, 156, 156*b*; 4: 437, 441
Gupta, Amit, 3: 431
Guthrie, Douglas, 1: 183
Guy's and Old St. Thomas hospitals, 1: *34*
Guy's Hospital (London), 1: 6, 33–35, 37, 83

H

Haggert, G. Edmund, 2: 165; 4: 344–345, 378
Hale, Worth, 1: 176–177
Hale Hospital, 3: 331

Halifax Harbor explosion, 3: 132, *132*, 133–135
Halifax YMCA Emergency Hospital, 3: *133*, 134
Hall, Caroline Doane, 2: 267
Hall, Col. John, 3: 282, 284
Hall, Emmett Matthew, 2: 333
Hall, Francis C., 3: 338
Hall, Francis N. Walsh, 2: 333, 337, 348
Hall, H. J., 2: *55*
Hall, Isabelle Mary Parker, 2: 333
Hall, John E. (1925–2018), 2: *333*, 346
    as BCH Orthopaedic chair, 2: 15*b*, 338–339, 384, 434, 436
    BIH Board of Consultants, 4: 262
    Boston Children's Hospital and, 2: 61, 279, 337–339, 399, 439*b*
    Brigham and Women's Hospital and, 2: 337; 4: 163, 193
    Cerebral Palsy Clinic and, 2: 402
    as clinical chief, 2: 286, 422
    death of, 2: 348
    Dwyer instrumentation and, 2: 342
    education and training, 2: 333
    Harrington Lecture, 2: 344, *344*
    Hospital for Sick Children and, 2: 334–336
    kyphosis and, 2: 343–345
    marriage and family, 2: 333, 337
    as mentor, 2: 345–347
    military service, 2: 333
    New England Baptist Hospital and, 2: 338
    orthopaedics leadership, 2: 347
    orthopaedics residents and, 2: *413*
    PBBH and, 4: 163
    pediatric orthopaedics, 2: 345, *345*
    private medical practice, 2: 338
    professional memberships, 2: 347
    Prosthetic Research and Development Unit, 2: 335
    publications and research, 2: *336*, 340–344, *344*, 345, 385, 391–392
    Relton-Hall frame, 2: 334–335, *335*
    Royal National Orthopaedic Hospital and, 2: 333–334
    scoliosis treatment, 2: 328, 334–336, 339–340, *340*, 341–345; 4: 127
    Seal of Chevalier du Tastevin, 2: 348
    spinal surgery at BCH and, 2: 337–338
    sports medicine and, 2: 287
    Tachdjian and, 2: 304
    Toronto General Hospital and, 2: 334
Hall, Leland, 3: 364
Hall, Llewellyn (ca.1899–1969), 2: 267, *267*
Hall, Marshall, 1: xxii
Hallett, Mark, 4: 168
hallux valgus deformities, 4: 40, 94
Halo Vest, The (Pierce and Barr), 3: 321
halo-vest apparatus, 4: 153
Halsted, William, 1: 185–186; 4: 105
Hamann, Carl A., 3: 104
Hamilton, Alice, 3: 142
Hamilton, F. A., 4: 204
Hamilton, Frank H., 1: 50–51
Hamilton, Steward, 4: 482*b*
Hamilton Air Force Base, 3: 337
Hammersmith Hospital, 4: *398*, 401
Hammond, Franklin, 4: 90
Hammond, George, 3: 275
Hammond, Harriet, 4: 90
Hampden Park (Springfield, Mass.), 1: *249*
hamstring contractures, 2: 197–198, *198*
Hancock, John, 1: 17–18
Hand, The (Marble), 3: 316
Hand Division of the Pan American Medical Association, 2: 251
Hand Forum, 3: 411
Handbook of Anatomy Adapted for Dissecting and Clinical References from Original Dissections by John Warren (Green), 1: 89
Handbook of Anatomy (Aitken), 1: *89*
hands. *See also* wrists
    arthritis and, 4: 96
    boutonniere deformities, 4: 98
    epiphyseal injuries after frostbite, 2: 321–323
    extensor tendon ruptures, 4: 97
    factitious lymphedema of, 3: 429
    focal scleroderma of, 4: 183
    IP joint hyperextension, 4: 97
    neuromas in, 2: 248
    opera-glass deformity, 4: 99
    osteochondritis in a finger, 3: 363
    pianists and, 3: 414
    proximal interphalangeal joint and, 2: 251
    reconstructive surgery of, 4: 98–99
    rheumatoid arthritis and, 4: 96–98, *98*
    sarcoidosis, 4: 98
    soft tissues and, 4: 98
    swan neck deformity, 4: 98
    systemic lupus erythematosus (SLE), 4: 98
    systemic sclerosis, 4: 98
    tendon transfers and, 3: 428
    treatment of, 2: 248
    volar plate arthroplasty and, 2: 248
Hands (Simmons), 4: 183
Hand-Schüller-Christian disease, 2: 171
Hanelin, Joseph, 3: 294; 4: 91, 237–238
Hanley, Daniel F., 2: 372
Hanley, Edward, 3: 249
Hannah, John, 3: 357
Hansen, Robert L., 3: 258, 317
Hansen, Sigvard T., 3: 416
Hansjörg Wyss/AO Foundation Professor of Orthopaedic Surgery, 3: 409, 464*b*
Harborview Medical Center, 3: 416
Harding, Chester, 1: *95*
Harmer, Torr W., 1: 264; 3: 60; 4: 208
Harold and Anna Snider Ullian Orthopaedic Fund, 2: 439*b*
Harrast, J. J., 4: 173
Harriet M. Peabody Professor of Orthopaedic Surgery (HMS), 2: 183, 203, 327, 337, 438, 439*b*; 3: 202
Harrington, F. B., 2: 245; 3: 96, 110–111
Harrington, Paul, 2: 316, 335
Harrington, T. F., 1: 23
Harrington rods, 2: 316, *317*, 325, 335, 340
Harris, C. K., 2: 285
Harris, Mathew, 2: 439
Harris, Mitchel, 4: 194
Harris, Robert, 1: 204
Harris, W. Robert, 4: 351, 355–356
Harris, William H. (1927–), 3: *215*, 217
    adult reconstruction and, 3: 460*b*
    AMTI and, 3: 224
    as Alan Gerry Clinical Professor of Orthopaedic Surgery, 3: 464*b*
    awards and, 3: 224, 224*b*
    biomechanics laboratory director, 3: 464*b*

Index

biomechanics research and, 3: 220
bone-ingrowth type prostheses, 3: 222–223
Children's Hospital/MGH combined program and, 3: 215
early life, 3: 215
education and training, 3: 215
fellowships and, 3: 216, 218
Harris Hip Score and, 3: 219, *219*
on Haversian systems in bone, 2: 241; 3: *216*
hip research and surgery, 3: 217–225, 244, 388*t*
HMS appointment, 3: 216–217, 219–220, 224
innovation and, 3: 216–217, 224
knee arthroplasty and, 4: 129
Knee Biomechanics and Biomaterials Laboratory, 3: 464*b*
legacy of, 3: 224–225
memberships and, 3: 224–225
as MGH clinical faculty, 3: 464*b*
as MGH surgeon, 3: 216, 219–220, 398*b*; 4: 126
MIT appointment, 3: 219–220
mold arthroplasty and, 3: 218–219
on osteolysis after hip replacement, 3: 220, *220*, 221
publications and research, 3: 215–216, 218–220, 243, 398; 4: 135, *135*
on Smith-Petersen, 3: 216–217
Vanishing Bone, 3: 225, *225*
Harris Hip Score, 3: 219, *219*
Harris Orthopaedic Biomechanics and Biomaterials Laboratory, 3: 220, 463
Harris S. Yett Prize in Orthopedic Surgery, 4: 251
Harris-Galante Prosthesis (HGP), 3: 222
Hartwell, Harry F., 3: 68
Harvard Athletic Association, 1: 253, 258–259, 263
Harvard Athletic Committee, 1: 250; 4: 85
Harvard athletics
athlete heart size, 1: 262, 267, 288
Athlete's Bill of Rights and, 1: 279, 280*b*, 281
basketball and, 1: 285–286
crew team, 1: 250–251, 258
dieticians and, 1: 258
fatigue and, 1: 264–265
football development, 1: 245, 247–248
football injuries and, 1: 247–248, 252–262
football team, 1: *249*, 251, *257*
ice hockey, 1: 275, 286
injury prevention and, 1: 279, 285–286
knee joint injuries in, 1: 267–268, 268*t*
musculoskeletal injuries, 1: 288
physical therapy and, 1: 258
protective padding and helmets in, 1: 255, *267*, 275
sports medicine and, 1: 245–269, 274–282, 284–286; 2: 287; 3: 399
Varsity Club logo, 1: *274*
women athletes, 1: 285–286
Harvard Cancer Commission, 1: 256
Harvard Club, 1: 181, *181*
Harvard College. *See also* Harvard University
anatomical society at, 1: 21, 133
faculty in 1806, 1: 40
football at, 1: 245
medical examination of freshmen, 4: 84
normal and abnormal posture in freshmen, 4: *84*
Spunkers and, 1: 21, 32, 133
vote to send Harvard Medical School surgeons to WWI service, 4: 386
Harvard Combined Orthopaedic Residency Program (HCORP)
accreditation of, 1: 232–233, 239–241
ACGME Orthopaedic RRC Committee review of, 1: 217–220
Beth Israel Deaconess Medical Center and, 4: 284, 288
Boston Pathology Course, 1: 216, 218
Boston Prosthetics Course, 1: 220
case sessions in, 1: 229*t*
clinical curriculum, 1: 223–225
combined grand rounds, 1: 232
conference schedule for, 1: 221*t*
core curriculum and, 1: 215–217, 227–232, 241–242
development of, 1: 192–200
directors of, 1: 243*b*
distribution of residents and staff, 1: 227*t*
diversity in, 1: 239
early surgical training, 1: 183–186
educational resources for, 1: 217
evolution of, 1: 183
funding for, 1: 206
Green and, 1: 200–210
growth of, 1: *240*
Herndon and restructuring, 1: 222–243
independent review of, 1: 234–237
leadership of, 1: 181, 210–211
Mankin and, 1: 211–220, 239; 3: 387, 397
orthopaedic research in, 1: 218
Pappas and, 1: 208–209
program length and size, 1: 214–215, 218–220, 222–223, 239
program review, 1: 238, 242–243
reorganization of, 1: 211–216
resident evaluations and, 1: 237–238
resident salaries, 1: 206
rotation schedule, 1: 225–226, 226*t*, 227, 227*t*
specialty blocks in, 1: 228, 229*t*
weekly program director's conference, 1: 230*b*
women in, 1: 239; 3: 208
Harvard Community Health Physicians at Beth Israel Hospital, 4: 263
Harvard Community Health Plan, 1: 225
Harvard Corporation, 1: 25, 27, 40, 133, 178; 3: 4
Harvard Department of Hygiene, 2: 253
Harvard Fifth Surgical Service, 4: 275, 277, 279, 297, 302–303, 305–306
Harvard Fourth Medical Service, 4: 296
Harvard Hall, 1: *25*, 134, *135*
Harvard Health Services, 3: 310
Harvard Infantile Paralysis Clinic, 2: 79, 107, 109, 176, 191, 432
Harvard Infantile Paralysis Commission, 2: 68, 70, 72, 99, 189
Harvard Medical Alumni Association, 1: 264; 2: 306
Harvard Medical Association, 3: 116, 119*b*
Harvard Medical Faculty Physicians (HMFP), 4: 214
Harvard Medical Meetings, 1: 174
Harvard Medical School (HMS), 1: *135*, *298*. *See also* Holden Chapel; orthopaedics curriculum
admission requirements, 1: 138, 141
admission tickets to lectures, 1: *27*, *300*
Almshouse and, 3: 4

attendance certificates, 1: *28*
Beth Israel Hospital and, 4: 213–214
Bigelow and, 1: 137; 3: 34, 42–44
Boylston Medical Society, 3: 25–26
Brigham Orthopaedic Foundation staff and, 4: 192
budget and, 1: 158, 174
calendar reform, 1: 140
Cheever Professor of Surgery, 4: 303
classes and faculty, 1834, 1: *297*
clinical courses at BCH, 4: 380*t*–381*t*
Coll Warren and, 1: 85
construction in 1904, 1: *86*
continuing medical education and, 3: 396
curricular reform, 1: 140
deans of, 1: 68–69
departmental organization, 1: 172–175
diversity in, 1: 239
educational reforms and, 1: 139, 140*b*, 141, 146–147; 2: 41; 3: 44–45, 94
Ellen and Melvin Gordon Professor of Medical Education, 4: 264, 266
Epidemic Aid Team, 2: 260
faculty at, 1: 40, 176
faculty salaries, 1: 178–179
financial structure reform, 1: 140
floor plan, 1: *304*
founding of, 1: 6, 25–29, 133–134
George W. Gay Lecture, 4: 324
human dissections and, 1: 26, 38
Jack Warren and, 1: 21, 25–29, 40
John Ball and Buckminster Brown chair, 2: 63–64
John Collins Warren and, 1: 38–40, 66, 68–69; 3: 30
John Homans Professor of Surgery, 4: 298
Laboratory for Skeletal Disorders and Rehabilitation, 2: 413
Laboratory of Surgical Pathology and, 2: 90
locations of, 1: 134*t*, *135*, 141
military hospitals and, 1: 270
military orthopaedic surgery course, 4: 455–462
military surgeon training at, 2: 42, 65–66
minority admissions to, 1: 138*b*

move from Cambridge to Boston, 1: 40–41; 2: 3
musculoskeletal medicine in, 1: 169
nose and throat clinic, 2: 40–41
orthopaedic clinic, 1: 173–174
orthopaedic curriculum, 1: 133–170
orthopaedic research and, 1: 193
orthopaedics as specialty course, 1: 141–143
PBBH and, 4: 1–4, 12, *12*, 13–14
postgraduate education and, 2: 157
preclinical and clinical departments, 1: 182*b*
qualifications for professors, 1: 26
radiology at, 2: 16
School for Health Officers, 2: 42, 65–66
Sears Surgical Laboratory, 4: 303
student evaluation of curricula, 1: 157–158, 167
surgery curriculum, 1: 140–141
surgical illustrations and, 3: 25
Surgical Research Laboratory, 4: 105, *106*, 107–108
teaching departments, 1: 157
Warren family and, 1: 71
women students and, 1: 138, 138*b*, 239; 3: 44
World War I volunteer orthopaedic surgeons, 2: 117–119, 124–127, 145; 3: *180*
World War II surgeons, 2: 232
Harvard Medical School (HMS). Department of Orthopaedic Surgery. *See also* Harvard Combined Orthopaedic Residency Program (HCORP)
advisory councils, 1: 182
as branch of Division of Surgery, 1: 171
chairperson of, 1: 180–182
curricular reform and, 1: 177
evolution of, 1: 171–182
faculty governance and, 1: 175–178
faculty rank and, 1: 178
faculty salaries, 1: 178–180
Harriet M. Peabody Professor of Orthopaedic Surgery, 2: 183, 203, 327, 337
John Ball and Buckminster Brown Chair of Orthopaedic Surgery, 1: 111, 177; 2: 63–64

John E. Hall Professorship in Orthopaedic Surgery, 2: 347
Lovett as chief of, 2: 64
organization of, 1: 171–182, 182*b*
teaching hospitals and, 1: 172–176, 180–181
Harvard Orthopaedic Journal, 1: 231–232
Harvard Orthopaedic Residency Program, 1: 167
Harvard Second Medical Service, 4: 296
Harvard Unit (1st), 3: 180, *180*
Harvard Unit (5th General Hospital), 1: 270, 277; 3: 271; 4: 17, *17*, 484–485
Harvard Unit (105th General Hospital), 1: 270–271; 2: 231–232; 3: 271, 351; 4: 488–489
Harvard Unit (American Ambulance Hospital), 2: 119–121, 123–124; 3: *180*, *369*, *370*; 4: 388, *388*, 389*b*, *390*, 391, 393. *See also* American Ambulance Hospital (Neuilly, France)
Harvard Unit (Base Hospital No. 5), 1: 270; 2: 125, 145; 4: 405, 419–421, 421*b*, *421*, 422–424, *428*
Harvard Unit (Walter Reed General Hospital), 4: 488
Harvard University. *See also* Harvard athletics; Harvard College
Dunster House, 2: *388*
establishment of medical school, 1: 6, 25–29, 133–134
Kirkland House, 2: 358, *358*
posture research and, 4: 84, *84*, 85–86, 234, *234*
public service ideal and, 2: 64
World War I and, 2: 64
Harvard University Health Services, 1: 274, 277, 284; 3: 450
Harvard Vanguard Medical Associates, 4: 194, 195*b*, 288
Harvard Varsity Club, 1: *272*, *282*, 289
Harvard/MGH Sports Medicine Fellowship Program, 3: 448
Hasty Pudding Club, 1: 32
Hatcher, Howard, 3: 382
Hatt, R. Nelson, 3: 368; 4: 378
Hauck, Charles, 4: 41*b*
Haus, Brian, 3: 409
Haverhill Clinic, 2: 107
Haversian system, 1: xxii
Hawkes, Micajah, 1: 42, 44, 49
Hayes, Helen, 2: 315
Hayes, Mabel, 4: 97

Index

Hayes, Wilson C. (Toby), 4: 262–264, 271, 284–285
Hayward, George, 1: 54, 60, *60*, 61–62, 65, 137, 296, 302; 3: 12, 27, 34, 112
HCORP. *See* Harvard Combined Orthopaedic Residency Program (HCORP)
Head, William, 4: 116, 129, 161–162, 193
head surgery, 3: 18
Health, William, 1: 18
health care
    disparities for minorities, 4: 264–265
    humanitarianism and, 2: 413, 421
    injured workers and, 4: 327
    issues in, 2: 375
    managed care movement, 3: 397
    medical costs, 3: 379, 379t
    physician profiling and, 2: 373–374
    policy and, 2: 371
    polio courses for, 2: 189
    prospective payment system (PPS), 3: 397
    resource utilization, 2: 372
Health Security Act, 2: 374–375
Heard, J. Theodore, 4: 23
Heary, Robert F., 4: 272b
heavy-resistance exercise, 3: 282, *282*, 283–285
Hebraic debility, 4: 203
Heckman, James, 1: 233; 2: 240; 3: 463, 464b; 4: 173–174
Hedequest, Daniel, 2: 344
Hektoen, Ludvig, 2: 78
Helems, Don, 4: 129
Helen Hallett Thompson Fund, 2: 107
Helmers, Sandra, 2: 342
Henderson, M. S., 3: 166; 4: 394
Hendren, Hardy, 2: 182, 399
Henry, William B., Jr., 3: 398b
Henry Ford Hospital, 2: 167–168; 3: 328
Henry J. Bigelow Medal, 2: 69; 3: 135
Henry J. Bigelow Operating Theater, 1: 84
Henry J. Mankin Orthopaedic Research Professorship, 3: 392
Hensinger, Robert, 2: 302
heparin, 3: 362
Hérard, Françoise, 3: 48
Herder, Lindsay, 3: 410
Hermann, Otto J. (1884–1973), 4: *334*
    AAOS and, 4: 337

BCH Bone and Joint Service, 4: 307, 328, 333–334, 337, 380b
BCH compound fracture therapy research, 4: *335*, 337
BCH residencies and, 4: 377–378
Boston City Hospital and, 3: 237; 4: 242, 333–334
Boston University Medical School appointment, 4: 335
Cotton and, 4: 334
death of, 4: 337
education and training, 4: 333
HMS appointment, 4: 334–335
honors and awards, 4: 337
lectures and presentations, 4: 334–335, 337
Massachusetts Regional Fracture Committee, 3: 64
New England Regional Committee on Fractures, 4: 341
os calcis fractures research, 4: 335–336
professional memberships, 4: 334
publications and research, 4: 335, *335*, 337
Scudder Oration on Trauma, 3: 63
Tufts Medical School appointment, 4: 335
Herndon, Charles, 2: 195
Herndon, James H., 1: *222*
Brigham and Women's Hospital and, 4: 195b
congenital kyphosis case, 2: 399
dedication of Codman's headstone, 3: *145*
fat embolism syndrome research, 2: 397
on Frank R. Ober, 2: 149
on Glimcher, 2: 325
on Hall, 2: 347
Harvard Orthopaedic Journal, 1: 232
leadership of, 1: 236
as MGH clinical faculty, 3: 464b
military service, 2: 399
Pittsburgh Orthopaedic Journal, 1: 232
as residency program director, 1: 222
restructuring of HCORP, 1: 222–243
on Riseborough, 2: 398–399
Scoliosis and Other Deformities of the Axial Skeleton, 2: 398, *398*
Smith Day lectures, 3: 431
on Watts, 2: 421–422
William H. and Johanna A. Harris Professor, 3: 464b

on William T. Green, 2: 169, 178–179
Herndon, William, 2: 359
Herodicus Society, 2: *387*
Herring, Tony, 2: 346, 438
Hersey, Ezekiel, 1: 25, 133
Heuter, Carl, 3: 181
Hey, William, 1: xxii
Heymann, Emil, 4: 215
Heywood, Charles Frederick, 1: 60
Hibbs, Russell A., 3: 155, 203; 4: 343, 394
Hibbs spinal fusion procedure, 2: 164; 3: 155; 4: 343
Hickling, Harriet Fredrica, 1: 299
Hildreth, Dr., 1: 97
Hilibrand, Alan S., 4: 266b
Hill, Walter, 4: 401
Hillman, J. William, 1: 162
Hinckley, Robert C., 1: 55, 59; 3: *30*
hip abduction splint, 1: *127*
hip dislocations. *See also* congenital dislocated hips (CDH)
    bilateral, 1: 126–127; 3: 235
    diagnosis of, 1: 46
    Henry J. Bigelow and, 3: 34–36
    hip joint excision, 3: 34
    J. Mason Warren and, 1: 75
    John Collins Warren and, 1: 42, 44–46, *46*, 47–50, 68; 3: 13, 13b, 36
    Lorenz technique and, 3: 164
    relaxing the Y-ligament, 3: 35–36, 38
    traction treatment for, 1: 108, *108*; 2: 32
    traumatic hip dislocation case, 2: 352–353
    treatment of, 1: 68, 74–75
hip disorders. *See also* total hip replacement
    abduction contracture, 2: 153, *153*
    acetabular dysplasia, 2: 389, *389*, 390
    anterior supra-articular subperiosteal approach to, 3: 181, 182b
    antisepsis technique, 2: 52
    bacterial infections and, 2: 108
    bilateral bony ankylosis, 3: *196*
    biomechanics research, 2: 407
    Bradford and, 2: 21–22, 32
    congenital hip dysplasia, 2: 302
    direct anterior approach to, 3: 181
    direct lateral approach and, 3: 277–278
    displacement of proximal femoral epiphysis, 3: 372

Down syndrome and, 2: 368
fascia lata arthroplasty and,
  3: 181
femoroacetabular impingement,
  3: 188–189
flexion/adduction contractures,
  2: 293–294
hip abductor paralysis treatment,
  2: 149–150
hip fusion for severe disabling
  arthritis, 3: 156b
importance of anticoagulation in,
  3: 218
lateral approach, 3: 219
Legg-Calvé-Perthes disease,
  2: 351
Lovett and, 2: 32, 53
Lovett and Shaffer's paper on,
  2: 49, 49, 52
metastatic malignant melanoma
  fracture case, 4: 77–78
Millis and, 2: 392
mold arthroplasty and, 3: 196,
  218–219, 241, 244
nailing fractured, 3: 237
Ober-Yount fasciotomy, 2: 172
osteoarthritis and, 2: 389;
  3: 155, 222
poliomyelitis contracture treatment, 2: 294, 295b
posterior approach to, 2: 146
prophylactic antibiotics in surgery, 3: 253
prostheses and, 2: 407
radiography in, 2: 54
septic arthritis of, 2: 380
slipped capital femoral epiphysis
  (SCFE), 2: 176
splints for, 2: 247
subtrochanteric osteotomy,
  2: 293–294
traction treatment for, 2: 21–22,
  53, 54; 3: 148
transient synovitis of, 2: 380
Trendelenburg gait and, 2: 33
Trumble technique for fusion of,
  3: 367
tuberculosis and, 2: 21–22,
  52–53, 54; 3: 148
vastus slide and, 3: 278
hip fractures. See also femoral neck
  fractures
  antibiotic use, 3: 253, 255
  anticoagulation in, 3: 218
  Austin Moore prosthesis for,
    3: 213
  Banks and, 4: 74–75
  Britten hip fusion technique,
    4: 363
  elderly patients and, 4: 341

hospitalization for, 2: 372
MGH approach to,
  4: 159b–160b
mold arthroplasty and, 3: 218
pathophysiology and treatment
  of, 4: 43
reduction and impaction of,
  4: 318–320, 322b
Hip Society, 2: 407; 3: 224; 4: 141
Hippocratic Oath, 2: 1
Hirohashi, Kenji, 4: 145
Hirsch, Carl, 4: 259–260
History of the Massachusetts General
  Hospital (Bowditch), 3: 15
History of the Orthopedic Department
  at Children's Hospital (Lovett),
  2: 247
HMS. See Harvard Medical School
  (HMS)
Ho, Sandy, 2: 405
Hochberg, Fred, 3: 414
Hodge, Andrew, 3: 397–398
Hodgen, John T., 1: 188
Hodges, Richard M., 3: 44, 51
Hodgkins, Lyman, 2: 244
Hodgson, Arthur R., 2: 336, 398
Hoffa, Albert, 2: 33
Hogan, Daniel E., 4: 263
Hoke, Michael, 2: 77–78, 282–283
Holden Chapel, 1: 135
  anatomy lectures in, 1: 26, 29,
    38
  floor plan, 1: 26
  human dissections and, 1: 26, 38
  medical instruction in, 1: 134
Holland, Daniel, 3: 241
Holmes, Donald, 4: 117
Holmes, George, 3: 192
Holmes, Oliver Wendell, 1: 291
  as anatomy professor at HMS,
    1: 66; 4: 298
  on anesthesia, 1: 56, 61
  on Bigelow, 3: 13, 27, 38, 51
  Boston Dispensary and, 2: 306
  European medical studies, 1: 73
  on George Hayward, 1: 302
  on George Parkman, 1: 291,
    294, 296
  on hip dislocation case, 1: 46
  on invention of stethoscope,
    1: 74
  on J. Mason Warren, 1: 77
  on John Warren, 1: 27, 69;
    3: 33–34
  on medical studies, 1: 138
  as MGH consulting surgeon,
    3: 14
  as MGH surgeon emeritus, 3: 46
  on need for clinics, 3: 3

reform of HMS and, 1: 139–
  140; 3: 45
Tremont Street Medical School,
  3: 42
trial of John Webster and,
  1: 308–309
Holmes, Timothy, 1: 81, 83
Holyoke, Augustus, 1: 95
Holyoke, Edward A., 1: 21
Homans, John, 2: 10, 306; 3: 38,
  94, 118, 145; 4: 5, 9
Hooton, Elizabeth, 1: 9
Hoover, Herbert, 4: 235
Hôpital de Bicêtre, 1: 73
Hôpital de la Charité, 1: 37, 73–74
Hôpital de la Pitié, 1: 73–74
Hôpital de la Salpêtrière, 1: 73
Hôpital des Enfants Malades, 1: 73,
  106
Hôpital Saint-Louis, 1: 73, 82
Hormell, Robert S. (1917–2006),
  4: 92
  Boston Children's Hospital and,
    4: 93
  chronic arthritis research,
    4: 92–93
  on congenital scoliosis, 4: 65, 93
  death of, 4: 94
  education and training, 4: 92
  HMS appointment, 4: 93
  knee arthroplasty and, 4: 93–94
  PBBH and, 4: 35
  publications and research,
    4: 92–94
  RBBH and, 4: 38, 41b, 68, 89,
    93–94
  study of hallux valgus, 4: 40, 94
Horn, Carl E., 2: 271
Hornicek, Francis J., 3: 390, 462,
  464b
Hosea, Timothy, 4: 262
Hospital for Joint Diseases, 3: 382–
  383, 385, 389, 413, 427
Hospital for Sick Children (Toronto),
  2: 334–336
Hospital for Special Surgery, 1: 89;
  2: 27; 3: 376; 4: 130, 134
Hospital for the Ruptured and
  Crippled, 2: 27, 43, 52, 225–226;
  3: 376
Hospital of the University of Pennsylvania, 4: 465
hospitals. See also base hospitals; military reconstruction hospitals
  Boston development of, 3: 3–7,
    9–12
  consolidation of, 4: 20
  debarkation, 4: 451–452
  embarkation, 4: 451–452
  end results concept, 1: 112

Index

exclusion of poor women from, 1: 123
F.H. Brown on construction of, 2: 5
government and, 2: 138b–139b
internships in, 1: 186
military field, 1: 272; 2: 118; 4: *414*, 468
military hospitals in Australia, 4: 488–489
mobile army surgical hospitals (MASHs), 2: 231–232; 4: 468–469, *470*
orthopaedics services in, 4: 451
portable surgical, 4: 468–469, 489
prejudice against Jewish physicians in, 1: 158
reserve units for army service, 4: 429
standardization of, 3: 112, 113b, 115–116, 123–125, 131
unpopularity of, 1: 41
Hôtel-Dieu, 1: 37, 73–74, 82
Hough, Garry de N., Jr., 2: 230
House of Providence, 2: 256
House of the Good Samaritan, 1: *128*; 2: 4
　Anne Smith Robbins and, 1: 123–125; 2: 114
　attraction of patients from the U.S. and abroad, 1: 125
　BCH merger, 1: 130; 2: 433
　Bradford and, 2: 21, 25, 28–29
　Buckminster Brown and, 1: 107, 121–122, 125–128; 2: 28
　Children's Ward, 1: *123*
　closure of orthopaedic wards, 1: 129–130
　disabled children and, 2: 306
　founding of, 1: 123–124
　hip disease treatment at, 1: 128–129
　Lovett and, 2: 49
　orthopaedic wards in, 1: 123, 125–126, 129; 2: 20
　orthopaedics residencies, 1: 186
　Osgood and, 2: 114
　poor women and, 1: 123–124
　rheumatic heart disease treatment at, 1: 130
　surgical records from, 2: 114, 115b
　training of orthopaedic surgeons, 1: 127, 129
　treatment of adults and children in, 2: 4
house pupils (pups), 1: 80, 184, *185*; 2: 20; 3: 4, 16
Howard, Herbert B., 3: 120

Howard University, 1: 239
Howorth procedure, 4: 243
Hresko, M. Timothy (1954–), 2: *364*
　Boston Children's Hospital and, 2: 364, 366–368, 439b
　education and training, 2: 364
　HMS appointment, 2: 364
　latent psoas abscess case, 2: 365
　Medical Student Undergraduate Education Committee, 1: 166
　orthopaedics appointments, 2: 364
　orthopaedics curriculum, 1: 167
　pediatric orthopaedics, 2: 365
　publications and research, 2: 366, *366*, 367, *367*, 368
　scoliosis and spinal deformity research, 2: 364–367
　on trauma in children, 2: 365, 368
　University of Massachusetts and, 2: 364
Hse, John, 2: 266
Hsu, Hu-Ping, 4: 194
Hubbard, Leroy W., 2: 77–78
Huddleston, James, 3: 254, 256
Huffaker, Stephen, 4: 190b
Hugenberger, Arthur, 2: 268
Hugenberger, Elizabeth, 2: 268
Hugenberger, Franklin, 2: 268
Hugenberger, Gordon, 2: 272
Hugenberger, Helen, 2: 268
Hugenberger, Herman, 2: 268
Hugenberger, Janet McMullin, 2: 272
Hugenberger, Joan, 2: 269, 271–272
Hugenberger, Paul W. (1903–1996), 2: *268*, *271*
　Boston Children's Hospital and, 2: 233, 269–272, 301
　Boston City Hospital and, 2: 269
　donations to Boston Medical Library, 2: 271
　education and training, 2: 268
　famous patients of, 2: 271–272
　Georgia Warm Springs Foundation and, 2: 270
　grand rounds and, 2: 271
　HMS appointment, 2: 269–270
　Marlborough Medical Associates and, 2: 146, 269, 299
　marriage and family, 2: 272
　MGH and, 2: 268
　New England Peabody Home for Crippled Children and, 2: 269–270
　Ober and, 2: 269, 271
　orthopaedics appointments, 2: 270

　orthopaedics internships, 2: 269
　PBBH and, 2: 269; 4: 16, 18–20, 22, 110, 116, 128
　private medical practice, 2: 269
　professional memberships, 2: 270, 272
　publications and research, 2: 268–269, 271
　Salem Hospital and, 2: 270–272
Hugenberger Orthopaedic Library, 2: 272
Huggins Hospital (Wolfeboro, NH), 2: 218
Hughes, Mable, 3: 362
human anatomy
　anatomical atlas and, 1: 89
　Astley Cooper and, 1: 34
　Harvard courses in, 1: 6, 25, 133–134, 136–138, 140–141
　HMS courses in, 1: *229*, 230
　legalization of human dissection, 1: 52
　military surgeon training and, 2: 66
　orthopaedic chronic disease and, 3: 85
　skeleton, 1: *136*
　variations in, 3: 85–86, 86t
human dissections
　grave robbing and, 1: 32, 34
　legalization of, 1: 52
　in medical education, 1: 26–27, 34, 38, 40, 51–52
　in military hospitals, 1: 24
Human Limbs and Their Substitutes (Wilson and Klopsteg), 3: 376
humeral fractures
　displaced supracondylar, 2: 379
　Gartland type 3 supracondylar, 2: 368
　intercondylar T fractures, 2: 397, *397*
　nonunion of the humerus, 2: 96, *96*, 250
　pins used in, 2: 379
　proximal, 2: 96, *122*
　resorption of the humerus, 2: 97, *97*
　supracondylar, 2: 229, 345, 379
Hunter, John, 1: xxi, 33, 36–37
Hunter, William, 1: 6, *133*
Hussey, Phyllis Ann, 4: 153
Hussey, Robert W. (1936–1992), 4: *151*
　Brigham and Women's Hospital, 4: 163
　Children's Hospital/MGH combined program and, 4: 151
　death of, 4: 153
　education and training, 4: 151

HMS appointment, 4: 152
marriage and family, 4: 153
Medical College of Virginia
    appointment, 4: 153
PBBH and, 4: 116, 128–129,
    151, 163
publications and research, 4: *151*,
    152–153
Rancho Los Amigos fellowship,
    4: 129, 151
spinal cord injury research and
    treatment, 4: 151, *151*,
    152–153
US Navy and, 4: 151
VA Medical Center (Richmond,
    VA), 4: 153
West Roxbury Veterans Administration Hospital and, 4: 129,
    152
Hutchinson, Thomas, 1: 16
Hyatt, George, 3: 439
hydroxylysine, 2: 327–328
Hylamer metal-backed polyethylene
    acetabular components, 4: 172
Hynes, John, 4: 303
hypnosis, 1: 56

I

ice hockey, 1: 275, 286
Ida C. Smith ward (BCH), 2: 431
Ilfeld, Fred, 3: 317
iliofemoral ligament, 3: 35–36, 38
iliotibial band
    ACL reconstruction and, 2: 378–
        379, *386*; 3: 448
    contractures and, 3: 209
    hip abductor paralysis treatment,
        2: 149–150
    knee flexion contracture and,
        3: 374
    modification of sacrospinalis and,
        2: 147
    Ober Operation and, 2: 153
    tendon transplantations and,
        2: 109
    tightness in, 2: 151–152
IMSuRT. *See* International Medical-
    Surgical Response Team (IMSuRT)
inclinometers, 2: 366, *367*
industrial accidents
    back disabilities and, 2: 92;
        4: 358
    BCH Relief Station and, 4: 305,
        305
    carpal tunnel syndrome and,
        4: 184–186
    Cotton and, 4: 323, 325, 327
    defects in patient care, 4: 325,
        352–354

fracture care and, 4: 338,
    339*b*–340*b*
insurance and, 2: 92; 4: 325,
    339*b*, 341
intervertebral disc surgery in,
    3: 316
kineplastic forearm amputation
    case, 4: 360
Maria Hospital (Stockholm) and,
    1: 263
os calcis fractures and, 4: 325
ruptured intervertebral discs and,
    4: 352
Sever and, 2: 92
workers' compensation issues,
    4: 184–186, 253, 325,
    352–353
Industrial School for Crippled and
    Deformed Children (Boston),
    2: 36–37, *37*, 38, 97, 308; 3: 151,
    161
Industrial School for Crippled Children (Boston), 2: 38, *38*
infantile paralysis (poliomyelitis). *See*
    poliomyelitis
infections
    allografts and, 3: 435, 440, 442
    amputations and, 1: 23, 74, 84
    antisepsis dressings and,
        1: 84–85
    carbolic acid treatment,
        1: 82–83, *83*, *84*
    hand-washing policy and, 1: 193
    infantile paralysis (poliomyelitis)
        and, 2: 261
    mortality due to, 1: 74, 81, 84
    postoperative, 3: 253
    resection and, 1: 81
    Revolutionary War deaths and,
        1: 22
    tubercular cows and, 2: 16
    use of ultraviolet light for,
        4: 164, 164*t*
infectious diseases, 1: 7–9; 2: 4–5,
    15
influenza, 1: 4, 7; 3: 135
Ingalls, William, 1: 32; 2: 5, 9, 11
Ingersoll, Robert, 4: 376
Ingraham, Frank, 2: 215
Insal, John, 4: 130
insane, 3: 3–4, 6
"Insensibility During Surgical Operations Produced by Inhalation"
    (Bigelow), 3: 27, *27*
Inside Brigham and Women's Hospital, 4: *123*
Institute for Children with Thalidomide Induced Limb Deformation,
    2: 413
Institute Pasteur, 1: 91

institutional racism, 3: 15–16
Instituto Buon Pastore, 4: *480*, 481
insufflation anesthesia apparatus,
    4: 215–216
"Interior of a Hospital Tent, The"
    (Sargent), 4: *424*
International Arthroscopic Association, 3: 422
International Association of Industrial Accident Boards and Commission, 2: 92
International Federation of Societies
    for Surgery of the Hand, 2: 251
International Hip Society, 3: 224
*International Journal of Orthopaedic
    Surgery*, 2: 80
International Knee Documentation
    Committee (IKDC), 1: 287;
    2: 381
International Medical-Surgical
    Response Team (IMSuRT),
    3: 417–418
International Pediatric Orthopedic
    Think Tank (IPOTT), 2: 304, *304*
International Society of Orthopaedic Surgery and Traumatology
    (SICOT), 2: 80–81, *81*, 137
interpedicular segmental fixation (ISF) pedicle screw plate,
    3: 420–421
Interurban Orthopaedic Club,
    2: 230
Ioli, James, 4: 193, 195*b*
Iowa Hip Score, 3: 219
Ireland, Robert, 1: 317
iron lung, 2: 79
    Berlin polio epidemic and,
        2: 260, 264
    Boston polio epidemic and,
        2: 314
    Drinker and, 2: 78, *78*
    infantile paralysis (poliomyelitis)
        and, 2: 261*b*–262*b*, 266
    invention of, 2: 191
    Massachusetts Infantile Paralysis
        Clinic and, 2: 212
    poliomyelitis and, 2: 78, *190*
ischemia-edema cycle, 2: 200–201,
    201
ISOLA implants, 2: *370*, 371
Isola Study Group, 2: 371
Istituto Ortopedico Rizzoli (Bologna, Italy), 3: 435–436

J

J. Collins Warren Laboratory, 1: 87
J. Robert Gladden Orthopaedic Society, 4: *265*
Jackson, Charles T., 1: 57, 60, 306

Index

Jackson, G. H., 3: 35
Jackson, George H., Jr., 2: 140
Jackson, Henry, 2: 20
Jackson, J. B. S., 1: 67
Jackson, James
    founding of MGH, 1: 31, 40–42; 3: 5, *5*, *6b–7b*, 12–13
    on George Hayward, 1: 302
    George Parkman and, 1: 296
    Harvard Medical teaching, 1: 299
    John Collins Warren and, 1: 37, 40, 66
    medical studies in London, 1: 37
    publications of, 1: 38–39
    support for House of the Good Samaritan, 1: 124
Jackson, James, Jr., 1: 73
Jackson, Robert W., 2: 279; 3: 446
Jaffe, Henry, 3: 382, 385, 392
Jaffe, Norman, 2: 422
Jagger, Thomas A., 3: 338
James, J. I. P., 2: 333–335, 399
James H. Herndon Resident Teaching and Mentoring Award, 3: 463
James Lawrence Kernan Hospital, 4: 157
Janeway, Charles A., 2: 215
Jasty, Murali, 3: 398, *460b*, *464b*
JDW (Jigme Dorji Wangchuk) National Referral Hospital, 3: 418
Jeffries, John, 1: 292
Jenkins, Roger, 4: 281
Jennings, Ellen Osgood, 2: 138
Jennings, L. Candace (1949–)
    cancer fatigue and, 3: 405–406
    education and training, 3: 405
    HCORP and, 3: 405
    Hospice and Palliative Medicine fellowship, 3: 407
    as MGH surgeon, 3: 405
    orthopaedic oncology and, 3: 405, *460b*
    publications and research, 3: 405–406
    ulnar nerve compression case, 3: 405–406
Jette, Alan, 3: 391
Jewish Hospital (St. Louis), 2: 231
Jewish Memorial Hospital and Rehabilitation Center, 4: 212
Jewish Memorial Hospital (Boston), 4: 212, 215
Jewish patients
    "Hebraic Debility" and, 4: 202, *203b*, *203*
    hospital formation for, 4: 200–202, 223
    limited medical care for, 4: 199–200
    in-patient care for observant, 4: 199, 204–206
Johansson, S., 3: 189
John Ball and Buckminster Brown Clinical Professor of Orthopaedic Surgery, 1: 111, 177; 2: 63–64, *64*, 133, 147, 157; 3: 202, *464b*; 4: *195b*
John E. Hall Professorship in Orthopaedic Surgery (HMS), 2: 347, 438, *439b*
Johns Hopkins Base Hospital Unit, 2: 221; 3: 288, 291
Johns Hopkins Hospital, 1: 185; 4: 429
Johns Hopkins Medical School
    departmental organization at, 1: 175–176
    Flexner Report and, 1: 146–147
    governance and, 1: 177
    trust for, 4: 1, 3
Johnson, Howard, 2: 272
Johnson, J. A., 2: 77–78
Johnson, Lanny, 3: 446
Johnson, Robert W., Jr., 4: 239
Joint Commission on Accreditation of Healthcare Organizations (JCAHO), 3: 146
Joint Commission on Hospital Accreditation, 3: 131
joint disease. *See* bone and joint disorders
Joint Injuries of the Hand (Eaton), 2: 250, *250*
Joint Kinematics Laboratory, 3: 463, *464b*
Jones, Arlene MacFarlane, 3: 291
Jones, Daniel F., 3: *60b*, 313, 371; 4: 274–276
Jones, Deryk, 4: *190b*
Jones, Ezra A., 2: 78
Jones, Howard, 4: 347
Jones, Neil, 3: 431
Jones, Sir Robert, 4: *394*
    on active motion, 2: 68
    BEF Director of Military Orthopedics, 4: 405
    on femur fracture treatment, 4: 408
    on importance of American surgeons, 4: *412b–413b*
    Lovett and, 2: 63, 80–81
    MGH and, 3: 299
    military orthopaedics and, 2: 124, 127; 4: 392–394, 401, 407
    Notes on Military Orthopaedics, 4: 442, *442*, 443
    orthopaedic surgery and, 4: 463
    Orthopedic Surgery, 2: 69, *69*
    Osgood and, 2: 116, 124–125, *125*, 126
    on prevention of deformity, 4: 409
    request for American orthopaedic surgeons, 4: 393, 398
    SICOT and, 2: 81
Jones, William N. (1916–1991), 3: *291*, 461
    death of, 3: 293
    early life, 3: 291
    education and training, 3: 291
    evolution of the Vitallium mold, 3: *292b*, 293
    "Fracture of the Month" column, 3: 243, 291
    as MGH surgeon, 3: *398b*
    mold arthroplasty and, 3: 291–292
    orthopedic arthritis service, 3: *388t*
    publications and research, 3: 291; 4: 187
    US Army Medical Corps and, 3: 291
Jones splints, 4: 389, 411
Joplin, Robert J. (1902–1983), 3: *293*
    AOFS and, 3: 295, 298
    Boston Children's Hospital and, 2: 274; 3: 293
    Boston VA Hospital and, 3: 298
    death of, 3: 298
    early life, 3: 293
    education and training, 3: 293
    on epiphyseal injuries, 4: 356
    foot surgery and, 3: 294–295, *296b–297b*, 298
    HMS appointment, 3: 293, 298
    legacy of, 3: 298
    memberships and, 3: 298
    as MGH surgeon, 3: 293–294, 298
    publications and research, 3: 293–294, *294*, 295, 341; 4: 63
    RBBH and, 3: 293; 4: 36, 93, 111
    sling procedure and, 3: 294, *294*, 295, *296b–297b*
    Slipped Capital Femoral Epiphysis, 3: 294, 333
    slipped capital femoral epiphysis research, 4: 237–238
Jorevinroux, P., 2: 340
Joseph O'Donnell Family Chair in Orthopedic Sports Medicine, 2: 438, *439b*
Joseph S. Barr Memorial Fund, 3: 214

Joseph S. Barr Visiting Consultantship, 3: 213
Joseph Warren, about 1765 (Copley), 1: *3, 11*
Josiah B. Thomas Hospital, 2: 252
Joslin, Elliott P., 4: 274
Joslin and Overholt Clinic, 4: 279
Journal of Bone and Joint Surgery (JBJS)
   American issues of, 3: 345, 347
   Annual Bibliography of Orthopaedic Surgery, 3: 261
   as British Orthopaedic Association's official publication, 3: 345
   budget deficits and, 3: 345–346
   Charles Painter as acting editor, 4: 50
   David Grice as associate editor, 2: 214
   Elliott Brackett as editor, 2: 130; 3: 157–159, 160*b*, 161
   expansion of editorial board positions, 3: 345
   Frank Ober as associate editor, 2: 165
   H. Winnett Orr as editor, 2: 125
   James Heckman as editor, 1: 233; 2: 240
   John Bell as associate editor, 2: 221
   Jonathan Cohen as editor, 2: 238–239
   as the journal of record, 3: 261–262
   logo for, 3: *261*
   name changes of, 1: xxiv
   ownership reorganization, 3: 346–347
   standards for, 3: 261
   Thornton Brown as editor, 3: 260–262
   Zabdiel Adams as associate editor, 3: 235
Journal of Pediatrics, 2: 7
Joyce, Michael, 1: 217*b*; 4: 189
Judet hip prosthesis, 3: 293
Junghanns, Herbert, 4: 262
Jupiter, Beryl, 3: 411
Jupiter, Jesse B. (1946–), 3: *407, 461*
   Cave Traveling Fellowship and, 1: 217*b*
   Children's Hospital/MGH combined program and, 3: 408
   education and training, 3: 407–408
   fracture treatment and, 3: 408–409

   Fractures of the Distal Radius, 3: 409, *409*
   Hand Forum president, 3: 411
   as Hansjorg Wyss/AO Foundation Professor, 3: 464*b*
   HMS appointment, 3: 408–409
   honors and awards, 3: 409
   intra-articular radial nerve entrapment case, 3: 410–411
   memberships and, 3: 411
   as MGH clinical faculty, 3: 464*b*
   MGH hand service and, 3: 396, 410, 460*b*
   as MGH surgeon, 3: 408
   MGH trauma unit and, 3: 399, 408
   named lectures and, 3: 410–411
   public health service and, 3: 408
   publications and research, 3: 408–411
   WRIST and, 3: 410
juvenile rheumatoid arthritis, 2: 171

K

Kaden, D. A., 4: 171
Kadiyala, Rajendra, 4: 190*b*
Kadzielski, John J., 3: 463*b*
Kagno, Marcia, 4: 89
Kanavel, Allan B., 3: 113*b*
Kaplan, Ronald K., 4: 89
Karlin, Lawrence I. (1945–), 2: *369*
   Boston Children's Hospital and, 2: 369–371
   education and training, 2: 369
   HMS appointment, 2: 370
   ISOLA implants and, 2: 371
   Isola Study Group, 2: 371
   orthopaedics appointments, 2: 369
   pediatric orthopaedics, 2: 370
   professional memberships, 2: 370
   publications of, 2: 371
   Scheuermann kyphosis treatment, 2: 371
   Tufts Medical School and, 2: 369
Karp, Evelyn Gerstein, 4: 241
Karp, Meier G. (1904–1962), 4: *240*
   as Beth Israel chief of orthopaedics, 4: 241, 289*b*
   Beth Israel Hospital and, 4: 240
   Boston Children's Hospital and, 4: 240
   death of, 4: 241
   education and training, 4: 240
   HMS appointment, 4: 240–241
   marriage and family, 4: 241
   PBBH and, 4: 18–20, 110, 240
   private medical practice, 2: 313; 4: 240

   professional memberships, 4: 241
   publications and research, 2: 229; 4: 240–241
   Thayer General Hospital and, 4: 241
   US Army and, 4: 241
   West Roxbury Veterans Administration Hospital and, 4: 240
Kasser, James
   Boston Children's Hospital and, 2: 354, 364, 434, 439*b*
   Catharina Ormandy Professorship, 2: 439*b*
   on Griffin, 2: 354
   HCORP and, 1: 224–225
   John E. Hall Professorship in Orthopaedic Surgery, 2: 439*b*
   Karlin and, 2: 369
   as orthopaedic chair, 2: 15*b*, 436
   publications of, 2: 368, 380
   on Zeke Zimbler, 4: 249
Kast, Thomas, 1: 25
Katz, Eton P., 2: 324
Katz, Jeffrey N., 2: 375; 4: 184–186, 195*b*, 269
Katzeff, Miriam (1899–1989), 2: *273*
   arthrogryposis multiplex congenita case, 2: 274–275
   Boston Children's Hospital and, 2: 222, 252, 273–275
   death of, 2: 275
   education and training, 2: 273
   as first female orthopaedic surgeon in Mass., 1: 239; 2: 275
   New England Hospital for Women and Children and, 2: 274
   orthopaedics appointments, 2: 274
   Osgood tribute, 2: 275
   professional memberships, 2: 275
   publications of, 2: 275
Kawalek, Thaddeus, 3: 282
Keats, John, 1: 36
Keely, John L., 2: 220
Keen, William W., 2: 72, *73*; 3: 103; 4: 411
Keep, Nathan C., 1: 308
Keeting, Mr., 1: 97
Kehinde, Olaniyi, 4: 169
Keith, Arthur, 2: 39
Keller, Joseph Black, 2: 126
Keller, Robert B. (ca. 1937–), 2: *371*
   Boston Children's Hospital and, 2: 286, 371
   Brigham and Women's Hospital and, 4: 193
   carpal tunnel syndrome research, 2: 375; 4: 184–185

Dartmouth Atlas of Health Care in Virginia, The, 2: 375
Dartmouth-Hitchcock Medical Center and, 2: 371
education and training, 2: 371
Harrington rods and, 2: 316, 371
health care policy and, 2: 371–376
Health Security Act and, 2: 374–375
HMS appointment, 2: 371
low-back pain research, 2: 371–372
Maine Carpal Tunnel Study, 2: 375
Maine Lumbar Spine Study Group, 2: 373, *373*
Maine Medical Assessment Foundation, 2: 372
Maine Medical Practice of Neurosurgery and Spine, 2: 376
MGH/Children's Hospital residency, 2: 371
PBBH and, 4: 22, 116, 128
private medical practice, 2: 371, 376
professional memberships, 2: 371, 376
publications of, 2: 372, *372*, 374–375, *375*, 376
scoliosis and spine surgery, 2: 371–374
University of Massachusetts and, 2: 371
Keller, William L., 3: 168; 4: 416
Kellogg, E. H., 1: 307
Kelly, Robert P., 4: 158
Kelsey, Jennifer, 4: 264
Kennedy, Edward, 3: 275
Kennedy, John F., 3: 191
Kennedy, Robert H., 4: 473
Kennedy Institute of Rheumatology, 4: 268, *268*
Kenzora, John E. (1940–)
 avascular necrosis of the femoral head research, 4: 154–156, *156*
 Beth Israel Hospital and, 4: 154
 Boston Children's Hospital and, 4: 154, 157
 Children's Hospital/MGH combined program and, 4: 154
 education and training, 4: 153
 HMS appointment, 4: 157
 hospital appointments, 4: 157
 hydroxylysine-deficient collagen disease case, 4: 155
 as MGH research fellow, 2: 328; 4: 153–154

 osteonecrosis of the femoral head research, 4: 156–157
 PBBH and, 4: 154, 157, 163
 publications and research, 2: 328, *328*; 4: *153*, 154–156, *156*, 157
 RBBH and, 4: 154
 University of Maryland appointment, 4: 157
Keogh, Alfred, 2: 68
Kermond, Evelyn Conway, 3: 299
Kermond, William L. (1928-2012), 3: *298*, 461
 death of, 3: 299
 early life, 3: 298
 education and training, 3: 298–299
 HMS appointment, 3: 299
 marriage and family, 3: 299
 as MGH surgeon, 3: 299, 398*b*
 mold arthroplasty and, 3: 292*b*
 Por Cristo volunteerism, 3: 299
 private medical practice, 1: 284; 4: 169
 publications and research, 3: 299
 White 9 Rehabilitation Unit and, 3: 299
 Winchester Hospital and, 3: 299
Kettyle, William M., 2: 277
Kevy, Shervin, 2: 234
Key, Einer, 1: 263
Key, John Albert, 1: 189; 2: 171; 4: 237, 453, 473
Kibler, Alison, 3: 328
Kidner, Frederick C., 2: 78; 4: 473
Kilfoyle, Richard, 1: 202; 2: 314; 4: 341, 378
Kim, S., 4: 251
Kim, Saechin, 4: 286
Kim, Young-Jo, 2: 390, 439*b*
Kinematic knee prosthesis, 4: 138–139, 147, 149–150
Kiner, Ralph, 4: 342
King, Donald S., 2: 195; 3: 301
King, Graham J.W., 3: 431
King, Martin Luther, Jr., 4: 262
King, Thomas V., 1: 217*b*
King Faisal Specialist Hospital, 2: 424, *425*
King Report (MGH), 3: 301–302
King's College (Nova Scotia), 2: 284, *284*
Kirk, Norman T., 4: 471, 472*b*, 473
Kirkby, Eleanor, 3: 246
Kirkland House (Harvard University), 2: 358
Kite, J. Hiram, 4: 158
Klein, Armin (1892-1954), 4: *231*
 as Beth Israel chief of orthopaedics, 4: 236, 239, 289*b*

 Beth Israel Hospital and, 4: 208*b*
 Chelsea Survey of posture, 4: 234–235
 death of, 4: 239
 education and training, 4: 231
 histology laboratory and, 2: 322
 HMS appointment, 4: 236
 Klein's Line, 4: 238–239, *239*
 legacy of, 4: 239
 MGH and, 4: 231, 236
 as MGH surgeon, 3: 375, 456*b*
 Orthopedics and Body Mechanics Committee, 4: 236
 posture research and, 4: 84, 233–235, *235–236*
 private medical practice, 4: 231
 professional memberships, 4: 239, 239*b*
 publications and research, 2: 136–137; 4: 231–233, *236*, *237*, 239
 scoliosis research and, 4: 231–233
 Slipped Capital Femoral Epiphysis, 3: 294; 4: 238
 slipped capital femoral epiphysis research, 3: 331, 333; 4: 237–239
 Tufts Medical School appointment, 4: 236
 US Army Medical Corps and, 4: 231
 US General Hospital No. 3 and, 4: 452
Kleinert, Harold E., 3: 408
Klein's Line, 4: 238–239, *239*
Kleweno, Conor, 4: 190*b*
Kloen, Peter, 4: 190*b*
Klopsteg, Paul E., 3: 376
Klumpke paralysis, 2: 90
Knee Biomechanics and Biomaterials Laboratory, 3: 463, 464*b*
knee flexion contracture
 before and after treatment, 1: *99*, *125*
 apparatus for, 1: *98*, 107
 Bradford's appliance for, 2: *20*, *21*
 iliotibial band and, 3: 374
 iron extension hinge for, 2: *123*
 leg brace for, 1: *124*
 osteotomies for, 2: 117
 physical therapy and, 3: 375
 plaster shells for, 2: 265
 prevention and, 4: 61
 surgical approach to, 3: 374–375, *375*
 treatment of, 1: 126–127
Knee Society, 4: 150
knees. *See also* total knee replacement

ACL injuries, 1: 277–278, 285–286
amputations and, 1: 61, 65, 84
ankylosis, 4: 64
arthroplasty of, 4: 64, 70*b*–71*b*, 103, 129–130, 131*t*, 179*t*
arthroscopic simulator, 4: 173
arthroscopy and, 1: 279; 4: 129
arthrotomy and, 3: 165, 165*b*, 166, 351
bilateral knee valgus deformities, 1: *125*
bone tumors and, 3: 389
cautery and, 1: 73
central-graft operation, 3: 368
discoid medial meniscus tear, 3: 422
dislocated patella treatment, 2: 294–296; 3: 79, 79*b*, 80, *81*
gait and, 2: 408
hamstring lengthening and, 2: 172
internal derangement of, 1: xxii; 4: 48
joint injuries in Harvard sports, 1: 268*t*
lateral tibial plateau fracture, 4: *312*
ligament rupture treatment, 1: 278
meniscectomy and, 1: 279
mold arthroplasty and, 3: 291–292
nylon arthroplasty in arthritic, 4: *65*, 66, 66*b*, 69, 91, 93–94
Osgood-Schlatter disease and, 2: 115
outcomes with duopatellar prostheses, 4: 180*t*
patella dislocations, 2: 294–296; 3: 79, 79*b*, 80, *81*
patella fractures, 4: 320
patellar turndown procedure, 4: 373–374
pes anserinus transplant, 1: 279
posterior cruciate ligament (PCL) deficiency, 3: 450
resection and, 1: 81
rheumatoid arthritis and, 4: 188–189
splint for knock, 2: 247
sports medicine and, 1: 267–268, 287; 2: 387
synovectomy in rheumatoid arthritis, 4: 40, 102–103
torn ligaments in, 3: 272
torn meniscus, 1: 278
treatment of sports injuries, 1: 277–279
trigger/jerking, 4: 311–312

tuberculosis and, 1: 73; 4: 225
valgus deformity, 2: *21*
Kneisel, John J., 4: 489
Knirk, Jerry L., 3: 409; 4: 194, 195*b*, 262–263
Kocher, Mininder S. (1966–), 2: *376*
  ACL research, 2: 378–379
  Beth Israel Deaconess Medical Center (BIDMC) and, 2: 377
  Boston Children's Hospital and, 2: 377, 379, 439*b*
  Brigham and Women's Hospital and, 2: 377
  clinical research grants, 2: 377–378
  education and training, 2: 377
  on ethics of ghost surgery, 2: *380*, 381
  on ethics of orthopaedic research, 2: 381, *381*
  HCORP and, 2: 377
  hip research, 2: 380
  HMS appointment, 2: 377
  honors and awards, 2: 377, 377*b*, 381
  humeral fracture research, 2: 368, 379
  New England Baptist Hospital and, 2: 377
  outcomes research, 2: 379–380
  professional memberships, 2: 382*b*
  publications and research, 2: 378, *378*, 379–381
  sports medicine and, 2: 377–378
  team physician positions, 2: 382*b*
Kocher, Theodor, 2: 146
Kocher approach, 2: 347
Köhler's disease, 4: 240
Kopta, Joseph, 1: 232
Korean War
  deferment during, 4: 125, 221
  physician volunteers and, 4: 220–221
  US Army physicians, 2: 218
Koris, Mark J., 4: 193, 195*b*
Kornack, Fulton C., 1: 217; 3: 460*b*, 464*b*
Krag, Martin, 3: 249
Kramer, D. L., 3: 420
Krane, Stephen, 2: 321; 3: 458*b*
Krause, Fedor, 4: 215
Krebs, David E., 3: 460*b*, 464*b*
Kreb's School, 2: 38
Krida, Arthur, 2: 111
Krisher, James, 4: 40
Kronenberg, Henry, 2: 330
Krukenberg procedure, 2: 425
Kubik, Charles, 3: *203*, 204
Kuhn, George H., 2: 5

Kühne, Willy, 3: 142
Kuhns, Jane Roper, 4: 66
Kuhns, John G. (1898–1969), 4: *59*
  amputations research, 3: 373, *373*; 4: 60
  arthritis research and, 4: 60–61, *61*, 63
  Body Mechanics in Health and Disease, 3: *90*, 91; 4: 62
  Boston Children's Hospital and, 2: 222, 274; 4: 59–61
  on congenital flatfoot, 4: 63
  correction of fixed foot deformities, 4: 62, 62*t*, 63
  death of, 4: 66
  education and training, 4: 59
  end-results clinic, 1: 194
  on Goldthwait, 3: 82, 92
  HMS appointment, 2: 223; 4: 59–61
  HMS medical student teaching, 4: 35
  knee arthroplasty and, 4: 64
  lymphatic supply of joints research, 1: 193; 4: 59–60
  marriage and family, 4: 66
  on medical education, 1: 93
  on nylon arthroplasty in arthritis, 4: *65*, 65, 66, 66*b*, 69
  private medical practice, 4: 62
  professional memberships, 4: 66
  publications and research, 4: 60–66, 93
  RBBH and, 3: 91, 293; 4: 31–32, 35, 38, 60–62
  as RBBH chief of orthopaedics, 4: 63–66, 79, 89, 196*b*
  on roentgenotherapy for arthritis, 4: 64, *64*
  scoliosis treatment, 2: 223; 4: 62, 65
  on Swaim, 4: 58
Küntscher, Gerhard, 3: 272
Küntscher femoral rod, 3: 272
Kurth, Harold, 4: 360
kyphoscoliosis, 1: 97, 105; 4: 155
kyphosis, 2: 343–345, 359, 366; 3: 239–240; 4: *317*

L

La Coeur's triple osteotomy, 2: 390
Laboratory for Skeletal Disorders and Rehabilitation (HMS), 2: 413
Ladd, William E., 1: 264; 3: 64
Laënnec, René, 1: 74
Lahey, Frank, 4: 275–276, 277*b*
Lahey Clinic, 4: 275–277, 281, 378
Lahey Clinic Integrated Orthopaedic Program, 4: 378–379

Lahey Clinic Medical Center, 4: 279
Lahey Hospital and Medical Center, 4: 214
Laing, Matthew, 2: 371
Lakeville State Hospital, 4: 378
Lakeville State Sanatorium, 2: 102; 3: 235, 365, 367
LaMarche, W. J., 3: 269
Lambert, Alexander, 4: 416
Lambert, Alfred, 1: 60
Lambrinudi stabilization, 2: 229
laminectomy, 3: 204, 206–208
Landfried, M., 3: 433
Landsteiner, Karl, 3: 313
Lane, Timothy, 1: 217*b*
Lange, Thomas, 3: 390
Langenbeck, Bernhard von, 1: 82; 2: 146
Langmaid, S. G., 2: 6, 9
Langnecker, Henry L., 3: 266
laparotomy, 3: 55
LaPrade, Robert F., 1: 287
Larson, Carroll B. (1909–1978), 3: *300, 303*
   AAOS subcommittee on undergraduate teaching, 1: 162
   Calderwood's Orthopedic Nursing, 3: 303
   Children's Hospital/MGH combined program and, 3: 301
   death of, 3: 303
   early life, 3: 300
   education and training, 3: 300
   foot deformity treatment, 2: 229
   hip arthroplasty research, 3: 302
   hip surgery and, 3: 238, 240
   Iowa Hip Score, 3: 219
   King Report and, 3: 301–302
   kyphosis treatment, 3: 239
   legacy of, 3: 303
   marriage and family, 3: 300
   as MGH surgeon, 3: 74, 192, 302
   mold arthroplasty and, 3: 238–239, 241, 302
   nursing education and, 3: 302–303
   private medical practice, 3: 301
   professional roles, 3: 303, 303*b*
   publications and research, 3: 239, 241–242, 244, 302–303
   Santa Clara County Hospital and, 3: 300
   septic wounds in osteomyelitis case, 3: 301
   Smith-Petersen and, 3: 237
   University of Iowa orthopaedics chair, 3: 303
   US Army ROTC and, 3: 300
   World War II service, 3: 301
Larson, Charles Bernard, 3: 300
Larson, Ida Caroline, 3: 300
Larson, Nadine West Townsend, 3: 300
Larson, Robert L., 1: 279
Lateral Curvature of the Spine and Round Shoulders (Lovett), 2: 79, *79*, 227
Lattvin, Maggie, 4: 80
Latvian Medical Foundation, 3: 451
laudanum, 1: 10
Laurencin, Cato T., 4: 266*b*
Lavine, Leroy S., 3: 386, 388, 462, *463*
Law, W. Alexander, 3: 192, 199
law of osteoblasts, 1: xxiii
Lawrence, Amos, 2: 3–4
Lawrence, John, 2: 425
Lawrence, William P., 2: 3
Le, Hai V., 3: 463*b*; 4: 190*b*
Leach, Robert E., 4: 89, *342*, 379
Leadbetter, Guy W., 4: 473
Lee, Henry, 3: 24
Lee, Olivia, 4: 190*b*
Lee, Roger I., 4: 84, *84*, 233–234, 420
Lee, Sang-Gil P., 3: 460*b*, 464*b*
Leffert, Adam, 3: 415
Leffert, Linda Garelik, 3: 415
Leffert, Lisa, 3: 415
Leffert, Robert D. (1923–2008), 3: *412, 461*
   Brachial Plexus Injuries, 3: 414
   brachial plexus injuries and, 3: 412, *412*, 413–414
   death of, 3: 415
   diabetes presenting as peripheral neuropathy case, 3: 413
   education and training, 3: 412
   HMS appointment, 3: 413, 415
   Hospital for Joint Diseases and, 3: 413
   memberships and, 3: 415
   as MGH clinical faculty, 3: 464*b*
   as MGH surgeon, 3: 320–321, 385, 395, 398*b*, 413
   Mount Sinai Medical School and, 3: 413
   orthopaedics education and, 3: 415
   pianist hand treatment and, 3: 414
   publications and research, 3: 412–415
   rehabilitation and, 3: 386, 388*t*, 413, 461
   shoulder treatment and, 3: 386, 412–414, 460*b*
   thoracic outlet syndrome treatment, 3: 415
   US Navy and, 3: 412
leg length
   discrepancy in, 2: 170, 191, 193, 350
   distal femoral physeal fractures, 2: 400
   effects of irradiation on epiphyseal growth, 3: 331
   epiphyseal arrest, 2: 170–171
   fractures and, 2: 350
   lengthening procedures, 2: 110
   muscle strength and, 3: 332
   prediction techniques for, 2: 193
   research in, 2: 191, 350
   teleroentgenography and, 2: 170, 170*t*
   use of sympathetic ganglionectomy, 3: 332
Legg, Allen, 2: 101
Legg, Arthur T. (1874–1939), 2: *84, 105*, 255
   Boston Children's Hospital and, 2: 13, 40, 101–102, 106, 252, 274, 282; 4: 338
   Clinics for Crippled Children and, 2: 230
   as consulting orthopaedic surgeon, 2: 102
   on coxa plana research, 3: 166
   death of, 2: 112
   education and training, 2: 101
   foot research, 2: 107–108
   gait laboratory, 2: 107
   Georgia Warm Springs Foundation board and, 2: 78
   Harvard Infantile Paralysis Clinic director, 2: 107, 188
   on hip disease, 2: 108
   HMS appointment, 2: 102; 4: 59–60
   identification of coxa plana, 2: 102–106; 3: 165
   on joint disease, 2: 110
   leg lengthening and, 2: 110
   marriage and, 2: 111–112
   military surgeon training and, 2: 42, 66; 4: 396
   on muscle atrophy in children, 2: 110
   orthopaedic surgery advances, 2: 79
   pediatric orthopaedics and, 2: 101, 106–107
   Physical Therapy in Infantile Paralysis, 2: 107
   poliomyelitis treatment, 2: 107, 109

professional memberships,
    2: 110–111
public health and, 2: 107
publications of, 2: 107
Section for Orthopedic Surgery
    (AMA), 2: 110–111
on tendon transplantation,
    2: 108, *108*, 109
testing of foot strength apparatus,
    2: 102
Tufts appointment, 2: 102
Legg, Charles Edmund, 2: 101
Legg, Emily Harding, 2: 101
Legg, Marie L. Robinson,
    2: 111–112
Legg-Calvé-Perthes disease
    case reports, 2: 103, *103*, 104
    epiphyseal extrusion measurement, 2: *354*
    etiology of, 2: 104
    identification of, 2: 13, 102, *102*, 103–106
    long-term study of, 2: 425
    research in, 2: 351; 3: 165–166
    treatment of, 2: 105
Legg-Perthes Study Group, 2: 425;
    4: 250
legs. *See also* leg length
    acute thigh compartment syndrome, 3: 417–418
    correction of bowleg, 1: *101*;
        2: 247
    fasciotomies, 3: 417
    limb deformities, 2: 23, 334,
        354, 413; 3: 58
    limb-salvage procedure, 2: 422,
        423*b*
    radiculitis in, 3: 204
Lehigh Valley Hospital, 3: 407
Leidholt, John, 2: 314
Leinonen, Edwin, 4: 244
Leland, Adams, 3: 313
Leland, George A., 1: 154; 3: 60;
    4: 433
Lemuel Shattuck Hospital, 3: 246,
    253
Leonard, Ralph D., 4: *359*
L'Episcopo, James B., 2: 90, 96, 417
LeRoy, Abbott, 2: 78
Lest We Forget (Rowe), 3: 61, 70*b*,
    187, 347, *357*, 360
"Letter to the Honorable Isaac
    Parker" (J.C. Warren), 1: *45*
Letterman Army Hospital, 3: 336
Letterman General Hospital, 4: 451
LeVay, David, 4: 383
Levine, Leroy, 3: 397, 398*b*, 461
Levine, Philip T., 2: 324
Lewinnek, George, 4: 262
Lewis, Frances West, 2: 4

Lewis, William H., 1: 252
Lewis, Winslow, Jr., 1: 308
Lewis H. Millender Community of
    Excellence Award, 4: 168
Lewis H. Millender Occupational
    Medicine Conference, 4: 168
Lexington, Mass., 1: 17–18
Lhowe, David W. (1951–), 3: *416*
    acute thigh compartment syndrome research, 3: 417, *417*, 418
    Cambridge Hospital clinic and,
        3: 399, 416
    education and training, 3: 416
    Harborview Medical Center and,
        3: 416
    HCORP and, 3: 416
    HMS appointment, 3: 416
    hospital appointments, 3: 416
    humanitarian work and,
        3: 416–418
    IMSuRT and, 3: 417–418
    as MGH clinical faculty, 3: 464*b*
    as MGH surgeon, 3: 416
    Pristina Hospital (Kosovo) and,
        3: 416–417
    Project HOPE and, 3: 417
    publications and research, 3: 416
    trauma care and, 3: 399, 416–418, 460*b*
    Winchester Hospital and, 3: 417
Li, Guoan, 3: 462
Liaison Committee on Graduate
    Medical Education (LCGME),
    1: 210–212
Liang, M. H., 4: 26
Liberating Technologies, Inc.,
    2: 326
Liberty Mutual Insurance Company,
    3: 287; 4: 352–353
Liberty Mutual Research Center,
    2: 326
Lidge, Ralph, 3: 448
Life of John Collins Warren, The
    (Edward Warren), 1: 46
Lifeso, Robert, 2: 424
ligatures, 1: 10, 55, 85
limb deformities
    internal fixation of fractures to
        prevent, 3: 58
    pediatric orthopaedics and,
        2: 334, 354
    thalidomide and, 2: 413
    traction treatment for, 2: 23
limb salvage surgery, 3: 390–391,
    433
Lincoln, Joan Tozzer, 3: 276
Lindbergh, Charles, 2: 232
Linenthal, Arthur J., 4: 210
Lingley, James, 3: 331

Linker, Beth, 4: 233
Linn, Frank C., 3: 324–325
Lippiello, Louis, 3: 383, 385–386
Lippman, Walter, 4: 469
Lipson, Jenifer Burns, 4: 271
Lipson, Stephen J. (1946–2013),
    4: 116*b*, 163, *267*
    on back surgery, 4: 270
    Berg-Sloat Traveling Fellowship
        and, 4: 268
    as Beth Israel chief of orthopaedics, 1: 233; 4: 223, 268,
        270, 289*b*
    as BIDMC chief of orthopaedics,
        4: 268, 270–271, 281, 289*b*
    BIDMC teaching program and,
        1: 166–167, 220, 224, 226;
        4: 286
    Cave Traveling Fellowship and,
        1: 217*b*
    death of, 4: 271
    development of multiple sclerosis,
        4: 271
    education and training, 4: 267
    HCORP and, 4: 267
    HMS appointment, 4: 271
    honors and awards, 4: 268, 272
    Kennedy Institute of Rheumatology and, 4: 268
    legacy of, 4: 271–272
    Mankin on, 4: 267–268
    marriage and family, 4: 271
    MGH and, 4: 267
    PBBH and, 4: 268
    publications and research,
        4: 268–269, *269*, 270–271
    spinal stenosis due to epidural
        lipomatosis case, 4: 269
    spine research, 4: 268–271
Lisfranc, Jacque, 1: 73–74
Lister, Joseph
    antisepsis principles, 1: 55, 81,
        84–85; 3: 45
    carbolic acid treatment,
        1: 82–83, *83*, 85
    treatment of compound fractures,
        1: 84
Liston, Robert, 1: 76, 84
litholapaxy, 3: 41
lithotrite, 3: 41
Litterer-Siewe disease, 2: 171
Little, Moses, 1: 95
Little, Muirhead, 4: 402
Little, William John, 1: xxiii, 98,
    106; 2: 26; 3: 54
Little Orthopaedic Club, 4: 74
Littlefield, Ephraim, 1: 303, *303*,
    304, 309
Littler, J. William, 2: 248, 250
Lloyd, James, 1: 6, 8, 10

Index 485

Lloyd Alpern–Dr. Rosenthal Physical Therapy Fund, 2: 439*b*
Locke, Edward, 4: 296
Locke, Joseph, 4: 100, *100*
Loder, Halsey B., 4: 438
Loh, Y. C., 3: 317
Long, Crawford W., 1: 56–57, 60, 63
Long Island Hospital, 2: 284
Longfellow, Frances (Fannie), 1: 297, 306
Longfellow, Henry Wadsworth, 1: 297, 302, 306
Longwood Medical Building Trust, 1: 264
Lord, J. F., 1: 177
Lorenz, Adolf, 2: 34, 242; 3: 234
Lorenz, Hans, 1: 264
Los Angeles Orthopaedic Hospital, 2: 266
Losina, Elena, 4: 195*b*
Loskin, Albert, 4: 280
Louis, Dean, 4: 168, 183
Louis, Pierre Charles Alexander, 1: 73–74
Louise and Edwin F. Cave Traveling Fellowship, 1: 217, 217*b*; 3: 274
Lovell General Hospital, 4: 482*b*
Lovett, Elizabeth Moorfield Storey, 2: 80, 230
Lovett, John Dyson, 2: 45
Lovett, Mary Elizabeth Williamson, 2: 45
Lovett, Robert Williamson (1859–1924), 1: *190*; 2: 45
   address to the American Orthopaedic Association, 2: 51
   Advisory Orthopedic Board and, 3: 157
   AOA and, 2: 48, *48*
   on astragalectomy, 2: 93–94
   Beth Israel Hospital and, 4: 208, 208*b*, 223
   birth palsies research, 2: 415
   Boston Children's Hospital and, 1: 188, 190–192; 2: 1, 10, 12–13, 40, 49, 54, *62*, 64, 68
   Boston City Hospital and, 1: 141, 143; 2: 45–47; 4: 298, 305*b*
   Boston Dispensary and, 2: 49
   Bradford and, 2: 49
   Brigham and Women's Hospital and, 4: 195*b*
   "Case of Glanders," 2: 46
   cerebral palsy cases, 2: 51
   "Certain Aspects of Infantile Paralysis," 2: *70*
   clinical surgery teaching and, 1: 141, 143
   Dane and, 2: 242, 246–247
   death of, 2: 80–81
   Department for Military Orthopedics and, 4: 406
   on departmental organization, 1: 176
   diaries of, 2: 45–46, *46*, 47, *47*, 48
   on disabled soldiers, 2: 67–68
   donations to Boston Medical Library, 2: 271
   early life, 2: 45
   education and training, 2: 45
   endowment in memory of, 2: 81–82
   Fiske Prize, 2: 52
   FitzSimmons and, 2: 144
   foot treatment, 2: 54–55, *55*, 56
   Harvard orthopaedic clinic and, 1: 174
   hip disease treatment and research, 2: 32, 49, *49*, 52, *52*, 53–54
   History of the Orthopedic Department at Children's Hospital, 2: 247
   as HMS chief of orthopaedics, 2: 64, 68
   House of the Good Samaritan and, 2: 49
   on incision and drainage of psoas abscesses, 2: 53–54
   Infantile Paralysis Commission, 2: 68, 99, 107
   John Ball and Buckminster Brown Professorship, 2: 63–64, *64*; 4: 195*b*
   Lateral Curvature of the Spine and Round Shoulders, 2: 79, *79*, 227
   legacy of, 2: 80
   Lovett Board, 2: *59*
   marriage and family, 2: 80, 230
   Mellon Lecture (Univ. of Pittsburgh), 2: 66–67
   military surgeon training by, 2: 42, 65–69
   New England Peabody Home for Crippled Children and, 2: 270
   at New York Orthopaedic Dispensary and Hospital, 2: 47–48
   obituary, 1: 93
   orthopaedic apprenticeship, 1: 186
   as orthopaedic chair, 2: 15*b*
   orthopaedic surgery, 2: 34, 51
   orthopaedics contributions, 2: 69–71
   Orthopedic Surgery, 2: 69, *69*; 4: 318
   PBBH and, 4: 10, 12
   pedagogy and, 2: 68–69
   as physician to Franklin D. Roosevelt, 2: 71–73, *73*, 74, *74*, 75, *75*, 76–77, 271
   poliomyelitis treatment, 2: 61–63, *63*, 70–79, 147–148, 264
   private medical practice and, 1: 176
   professional memberships, 2: 80, 80*b*
   as professor of orthopaedic surgery, 1: 147, 151, 171
   public health and, 2: 61
   publications and research, 2: 223, 246; 4: 259, 310
   scoliosis treatment, 2: 56–61, 79–80, 86, 223–225
   SICOT and, 2: 80
   social events and, 2: 49
   spina bifida treatment, 2: 51–52
   spring muscle test, 2: 70–71
   study of spine mechanics, 2: 57, *57*, 58, *58*, 59
   Surgery of Joints, The, 2: 52
   teaching hospitals and, 1: 187
   tracheostomy results, 2: 49, 51
   Treatise on Orthopaedic Surgery, A, 1: 108, 143; 2: 29–30, 43, 50, *50*, 51
   tuberculosis treatment, 2: 32
   turnbuckle jacket and, 2: 80, 224, *224*, 225
   US Army Medical Reserve Corps and, 2: 66
   use of radiographs, 2: 54
Lovett Board, 2: *59*, 86
Lovett Fund Committee, 2: 81–82
Low, Harry C. (1871–1943)
   acetonuria associated with death after anesthesia case, 3: 305
   Boston Children's Hospital and, 3: 304
   Boston City Hospital and, 3: 304
   Burrage Hospital and, 4: 226
   Children's Sunlight Hospital and, 3: 307
   Committee on Occupational Therapy chair, 3: 304–306
   death of, 3: 307
   early life, 3: 304
   education and training, 3: 304
   European medical studies, 3: 304
   marriage and, 3: 304
   on the MGH orthopaedic outpatient clinic, 3: 304, *304*, 306*b*–307*b*

as MGH surgeon, 3: 269, 304, 306
New England Home for Little Wanderers and, 3: 307
as poliomyelitis surgeon, 3: 306–307
"Progress in Orthopaedic Surgery" series, 2: 297
publications and research, 3: 304
Low, Mabel C. Chapman, 3: 304
Lowell, Abbott Lawrence, 1: 174, 176; 2: 41–42, 64
Lowell, Charles
hip dislocation case, 1: 42, 44–49, 49b, 50; 3: 13, 13b, 36
hip dislocation close-up, 1: 49
letter of support for, 1: 45
malpractice suit against John Collins, 1: 44, 50–51, 68
x-ray of pelvis and hips, 1: 49
Lowell, J. Drennan (1922–1987), 4: *158*, 161
bladder fistula case, 4: 162
Boston Children's Hospital and, 2: 384
as BWH assistant chief of orthopaedic surgery, 4: 163
BWH medical staff president, 4: 163
Children's Hospital/MGH combined program and, 4: 158
death of, 4: 164
education and training, 4: 158
Emory University Hospital and, 4: 158
Fracture course and, 3: *273*
hip fracture research, 4: *160*
HMS appointment, 4: 162
marriage and family, 4: 164
MGH and, 3: 244; 4: 158–159
on MGH approach to hip fractures, 4: 159b–160b
PBBH and, 4: 116, 116b, 128–129
as PBBH chief of clinical orthopaedics, 4: 161–163
private medical practice, 4: 158
professional memberships, 4: 162–163, 163b
publications and research, 4: 159, 161–164
RBBH and, 4: 114
reconstructive hip surgery and, 4: 159
train hobby and, 4: 160
US Army and, 4: 158
on use of ultraviolet light, 4: 162–163, *163*, 164
Lowell, Olivia, 1: 263
Lowell, Ruth, 4: 164

Lowell General Hospital, 4: 243
Lower Extremity Amputations for Arterial Insufficiency (Warren and Record), 1: 90; 3: 330
Lowry, Robert, 4: 277
LTI Digital™ Arm Systems for Adults, 2: 326
lubrication, 3: 324–325
Lucas-Championniere, Just, 1: xxiii
Ludmerer, Kenneth, 1: 146
lumbago, 3: 203
lumbar spinal stenosis, 2: 373–374
lunate dislocation, 3: 101–102
Lund, F. B., 4: 331
Lund, Fred, 4: 220
Lycée Pasteur Hospital, 4: 388, 389b, 390
Lynch, Peter, 2: 414
Lynn General Hospital, 3: 253
Lyon, Mary, 2: 276
Lysholm Knee Scoring Scale, 2: 380

M

MacArthur, Douglas, 2: 232
MacAusland, Andrew R., 3: 308
MacAusland, Dorothy Brayton, 3: 308
MacAusland, Frances Prescott Baker, 3: 308
MacAusland, William R., Jr. (1922–2004), 3: *308*
as AAOS president, 3: 311, *311*, 312
ABC traveling fellowship and, 3: 309
Carlos Otis Stratton Mountain Clinic and, 3: 311
Carney Hospital and, 3: 308; 4: 45
death of, 3: 312
early life, 3: 308
education and training, 3: 308
Emergency Care and Transportation of the Sick and Injured, 3: 310, *311*
emergency responder training and, 3: 310–311
HMS appointment, 3: 308
knee arthroplasty and, 4: 64
love of skiing and, 3: 311
marriage and family, 3: 308, 312
memberships and, 3: 309
as MGH surgeon, 3: 266, 398b
Orthopaedics, 3: 310
Orthopaedics Overseas and, 3: 310
private medical practice, 3: 308, 310

publications and research, 2: 248; 3: 308–310, *376*, 377–378
Rocky Mountain Trauma Society and, 3: 311
on sepsis after intramedullary fixation of femoral fractures, 3: 309–310
trauma research and, 3: 309
as Tufts University professor, 3: 308
US Air Force and, 3: 308
West Roxbury Veterans Administration Hospital and, 3: 312
MacAusland, William R., Sr., 3: 308
Macdonald, Ian, 4: 102
MacEwen, Dean, 2: 304
Macewen, William, 1: xxiii
MacFarlane, Arlene, 3: 291
MacFarlane, J. A., 4: 468–469, 471
MacIntosh prothesis, 4: 69, 71b, 129, 188
Mackin, Evelyn J., 4: 168
Macknight, Jane, 1: 289
Maddox, Robert, 2: *121*
Magee, James, 4: 471
Magill, H. Kelvin, 4: 376
magnetic resonance imaging (MRI), 3: 255
Magnuson, Paul B., 4: 473
Maine Carpal Tunnel Study (Keller, et al.), 2: 375, *375*
Maine Carpal Tunnel Syndrome Study, 4: 184
Maine Lumbar Spine Study Group, 2: 373, *373*, 374
Maine Medical Assessment Foundation, 2: 372, 374; 4: 184–185
Maine Medical Association, 2: 372
Maine Medical Practice of Neurosurgery and Spine, 2: 376
Maine Medical Society, 1: 49
Maisonneuve, Jacques, 1: 82
malaria treatment, 4: 491
Malchau, Henrik, 3: 219
Malenfant, J., 3: 45
Mallon, William J., 3: 143, *145*
Mallory, Tracy B., 2: 254
malpractice suits
Charles Lowell and, 1: 44, 50
early concerns about, 1: 24
fractures and, 1: 50–51; 3: 63
increase in, 1: 50–51
insurance and, 1: 51
Joseph Warren on, 1: 12
orthopaedics and, 1: 50; 3: 378–379
Malt, Ronald, 3: 217
Management of Fractures and Dislocations (Wilson), 3: 62, 273

Mankin, Allison, 3: 393
Mankin, Carole J. Pinkney, 1: 218; 3: 382, 385, 393
Mankin, David, 3: 393
Mankin, Henry J. (1928–2018), 1: *210, 212*; 3: *381, 386, 393, 461*
  AAOS and, 3: 388
  articular cartilage research, 3: 383, *383*, 384, *385*, 388, 442
  BIH Board of Consultants, 4: 262–263
  breakfast meetings with residents, 1: 213, *214*
  on Chandler, 3: 279
  chordoma of the spinal column and, 3: 390
  core curriculum and, 1: 215
  death of, 3: 393
  early life, 3: 381
  Edith M. Ashley Professor, 3: 464*b*
  education and training, 3: 381–382
  establishment of the Institute of Health Professions, 3: 391–392
  femoral allograft transplantation, 3: 389, *389*, 390
  HCORP and, 1: 210–221, 239; 3: 387, 397
  histologic-histochemical grading system, 3: 384, 384*t*, 385
  HMS appointment, 3: 385
  honors and awards, 3: 392, 393*b*
  Hospital for Joint Diseases and, 3: 382–383, 385, 389
  Korean War and, 3: 382
  limb salvage surgery and, 3: 390–391
  on Lipson, 4: 267–268
  marriage and family, 3: 382, 385
  memberships and, 3: 392
  MGH Bone Bank and, 3: 386, 388, 396, 439
  as MGH clinical faculty, 3: 464*b*
  MGH operations improvement and, 3: 387, 395–399
  as MGH orthopaedics chief, 1: 180; 3: 11*b*, 219, 228, 320, 378, 385–388, 395–399, 459, 461
  MGH residents and, 3: *387, 460*
  Mount Sinai Medical School and, 3: 383, 385
  NIH and, 3: 383, 387–388, 392
  Orthopaedic Biology and Oncology Laboratories, 3: 464*b*
  orthopaedic oncology and, 3: 386, 388, 388*t*, 390, 392–393, 460*b*
  orthopaedic research support, 1: 218
  orthopaedics education and, 3: 386
  pathology course and, 3: 396
  Pathophysiology of Orthopaedic Diseases, 4: 226
  publications and research, 3: 383–385, 387–392, 433, 440
  as residency program director, 1: 181, 210–211, 213–221
  on rickets and osteomalacia, 3: 388
  on Rowe, 3: 360
  specialty services at MGH under, 3: 388*t*, 459, 460*t*, 461–462
  on sports medicine clinic, 2: 384
  Such a Joy for a Yiddish Boy, 3: 392, *392*
  University of Chicago clinics and, 3: 382
  University of Pittsburgh appointment, 3: 382–383
  US Navy and, 3: 382
Mankin, Hymie, 3: 381
Mankin, Keith, 3: 392, *392*, 393, 398*b*, 401, 460*b*, 464*b*
Mankin, Mary, 3: 381
Mankin System, 3: 384, 384*t*, 385
Mann, Robert W., 2: 326; 3: 397, 398*b*
Mansfield, Frederick L. (1947–), 3: *419*
  education and training, 3: 419
  HCORP and, 3: 419
  HMS appointment, 3: 419
  memberships and, 3: 421
  as MGH clinical faculty, 3: 464*b*
  as MGH surgeon, 3: 419
  open anterior lumbosacral fracture dislocation case, 3: 420
  orthopaedics education and, 3: 421
  publications and research, 3: 419–421
  sciatica treatment and, 3: 254
  spine surgery and, 3: 397, 419–421, 460*b*
  use of chymopapain, 3: 254, 419, *421*
Manson, Anne, 2: 277
Manson, James G. (1931–2009)
  Boston Children's Hospital and, 2: 276–277
  death of, 2: 277
  early life, 2: 275
  education and training, 2: 276
  hemophilia clinic, 2: 276
  HMS appointment, 2: 276
  marriage and family, 2: 276–277
  MGH residency, 2: *276*
  MIT Medical and, 2: 276–277, 290
  Mount Auburn Hospital and, 2: 276
  PBBH and, 4: 22
Manson, Mary Lyon, 2: 276
Manual of Bandaging, Strapping and Splinting, A (Thorndike), 1: 268
Manual of Chemistry (Webster), 1: 299, 301
Manual of Orthopedic Surgery, A (Thorndike), 2: 311, *312*
Manual of Orthopedic Surgery (Bigelow), 3: 25–26, *26*
Manuel II, King, 4: 399–401, *401*, 402–403, 442
marathon runners, 1: 250
Marble, Alice Ingram, 3: 316
Marble, Henry C. (1885–1965), 3: *312*
  AAST and, 3: 315, *315*
  American Mutual Liability Insurance Company and, 3: 314, 316
  American Society for Surgery of the Hand and, 3: 316
  anatomy education and, 3: 314
  Base Hospital No. 6 and, 4: 433–434, 436
  Bedford Veterans Administration Hospital and, 3: 314
  blood transfusion work, 3: 313
  Chelsea Memorial Hospital and, 3: 314
  death of, 3: 316
  early life, 3: 312
  education and training, 3: 312–313
  Faulkner Hospital and, 3: 314
  as Fracture Clinic chief, 3: 60*b*
  fracture research and, 3: 340
  Fractures, 3: 315
  Hand, The, 3: 316
  HMS appointment, 3: 313
  legacy of, 3: 316
  marriage and family, 3: 316
  Massachusetts Regional Fracture Committee, 3: 64
  memberships and, 3: 316
  MGH Fracture Clinic and, 3: 60, 313–315
  MGH Hand Clinic and, 3: 314
  as MGH surgeon, 3: 313–315
  orthopaedics education and, 3: 315

publications and research, 3: 314–316
Scudder Oration on Trauma, 3: 63
Surgical Treatment of the Motor-Skeletal System, 3: 316
US Army Medical Corps and, 3: 313
US General Hospital No. 3 and, 4: 452
Marcella Street Home, 2: 242, 247
March of Dimes, 2: 315
Marcove, Ralph, 3: 382
Margliot, Z., 3: 409
Marian Ropes Award, 4: 100
Marie-Strumpell disease, 3: 239
Marion B. Gebbie Research Fellowship, 4: 127
Marjoua, Youssra, 4: 190*b*
Marlborough Medical Associates, 2: 146, 269, 299
Marmor modular design prosthesis, 4: 130
Marnoy, Samuel L., 4: 208*b*
Marshall, H. W., 3: 155
Martin, Edward, 3: 112, 113*b*
Martin, Ernest, 2: 70, 70, 71
Martin, Franklin H., 3: 113*b*; 4: 324
Martin, Geraldine, 4: 389*b*
Martin, Joseph, 1: 181, 232–234; 4: 284–285
Martin, Scott D., 1: 230; 4: 193, 195*b*
Martin, Tamara, 4: 193
Marvin, Frank W., 4: 407
Mary Alley Hospital, 2: 269
Mary Hitchcock Memorial Hospital, 3: 363–364
Mary Horrigan Conner's Center for Women's Health, 4: *194*
Mary MacArthur Memorial Respiratory Unit (Wellesley Hospital), 2: 189, 315
Maslin, Robert, 2: 354
Mason, Jonathan, 1: 38
Mason, Susan Powell, 1: 37–38, 72
Masons, 1: 10–12, 29
Mass General Brigham (MGB), 3: 462
Massachusetts Agricultural Society, 1: 29
Massachusetts Arthritis Foundation, 4: 100
Massachusetts Board of Registration in Medicine, 3: 423
Massachusetts Eye and Ear Infirmary, 2: 252; 3: 331, 339; 4: 113–114

Massachusetts General Hospital, 1955–1980, The (Brown), 3: 299
Massachusetts General Hospital, Its Development, 1900–1935, The (Washburn), 3: 1
Massachusetts General Hospital (MGH)
  apothecary position, 1: 184
  arthritis research program at, 2: 82
  Base Hospital No. 6 and, 4: 420*t*, 429–432
  blood transfusions at, 3: 313
  clinical surgery curricula at, 1: 151
  End-Result Idea, 3: 112, 114
  expansion of staff, 3: 14–15
  faculty model at, 1: 174, 176
  fee structures, 3: 16, 21–22
  first orthopaedic case at, 1: 42, 44
  first patients at, 1: 42; 3: 11
  General Hospital No. 6 and, 3: 239, 362; 4: 474, 485*b*
  HMS clinical teaching at, 3: 13
  house physicians/surgeons, 1: 184
  house pupils (pups) at, 1: 80, 184, *185*; 2: 20
  impact of World War II on, 4: 467
  innovation at, 3: 216–217
  institutional racism and, 3: 15–16
  internes/externs, 1: 184–185
  James Jackson and, 1: 31, 41–42; 3: 5, *5*, 6*b*–7*b*, 12–13
  John Ball Brown and, 3: 12
  John Collins Warren and, 1: 31, 41–42, 52–55, 57–58; 3: 5, *5*, 6*b*–7*b*, 12–13
  King Report, 3: 301–302
  military surgeon training at, 4: 396
  modernization of, 3: 453
  nursing school at, 4: 467
  occupational rehabilitation and, 4: 444
  105th General Hospital and, 4: 493
  ophthalmology service at, 3: 13
  performance-based promotions at, 3: 123–124
  postgraduate education and, 2: 157–159
  rehabilitation clinic and, 1: 273
  reserve units for army service, 4: 429–430
  roentgenology department, 3: 21
  surgical residencies, 1: 184, *185*

surgical volume due to ether use, 1: 63, 64*t*
treatment categories, 1: 54, 54*t*
treatment of children in, 2: 4, 8
treatment of soldiers, 3: 21
treatment outcomes reporting, 1: 54; 3: 112
treatments and techniques at, 3: 20–22
use of ether anesthesia, 1: 57–63, 85; 3: 15, 22, 27–28, 28*b*, 29, 29*b*, 30–34
use of ligatures, 1: 85
use of radiographs, 2: 54
visiting surgeons at, 3: *31*
Warren family and, 1: 71
women surgeons at, 1: 239
World War II and, 4: 493
x-rays and, 3: 20, *20*
Massachusetts General Hospital. Facilities
  Allen Street House, 3: 17–18
  Ambulatory Care, 3: 396, 399
  Baker Memorial, 3: *73*, 75
  Bigelow Building, 3: 15–17
  Bulfinch Building, 1: *41*; 3: *9*, *13*, 15, *16*, 22, *60*, 70*b*
  Children's Ward, 3: *71*
  East Wing, 3: *14*, 15, *60*
  Ellison Tower, 3: 75
  Ether Dome, 1: *59*, *63*, 84; 3: *14*, 16
  expansion of, 3: 14, *14*, 15, *15*, 16–18, 18*b*, 20–21, 74–75
  Gay Ward (outpatient building), 3: *19*, 265
  Henry J. Bigelow Operating Theater, 1: 84
  medical school, 3: *15*
  Moseley Memorial Building, 3: 70*b*, 75
  Nerve Room, 3: 20
  Out-Patient Department, 3: 75
  pathological laboratory, 3: 21
  Patient Ward, 3: *74*
  Pavilion Wards, 3: *17*
  Phillips House, 1: 86, 204; 3: *72*, *73*, 75
  Physical Therapy Department, 3: 269
  plot plans for, 3: *10*, *17*, *22*, *71*, *72*, *461*
  Treadwell Library, 3: 70*b*
  view in 1840, 1: *54*
  Wang ACC building, 3: 75
  Ward 5, 1: 203
  Ward A (Warren), 3: 17, *17*, *18*
  Ward B (Jackson), 3: 17, *17*
  Ward C (Bigelow), 3: 17–18
  Ward D (Townsend), 3: 18, *18*

Ward E (Bradlee), 3: 18–19, *19*
Ward F (George A. Gardner building), 3: 19
wards in, 3: *12*
Warren Building, 3: 17
West Wing, 3: 15, *60*
White Building (George Robert White), 3: *74*, 75
Massachusetts General Hospital. Founding of
 advocacy for, 1: 41; 3: 3–5, *5*, 6, 6*b*–7*b*
 Almshouse site, 1: 41
 Bulfinch design for, 1: 41; 3: 10–11
 construction of, 3: 9–10
 funding for, 1: 41–42; 3: 6–7, 9, 14, 18–19, 21
 grand opening of, 3: 11–12
 Province House and, 3: 6–7, 9
 seal of, 3: *10*, 11, *11*
 state charter authorizing, 3: 6–7, *8*
Massachusetts General Hospital. Orthopaedics Department
 adults and, 2: 157
 approach to hip fractures, 4: 159*b*–160*b*
 Biomaterials and Innovative Technologies Laboratory, 3: 463
 Biomotion Laboratory, 3: 463, 464*b*
 bone bank for allografts and, 3: 388, 396, 440–441, 443
 Cambridge Hospital clinic, 3: 396, 399
 Clinical and Research Programs, 3: 464*b*
 clinical faculty, 3: 464*b*
 clinical service rotations, 1: 198
 continuing medical education and, 3: 396
 creation of, 3: 67–69
 expansion of, 3: 286
 facilities for, 3: 68–69, 70*b*, 71, *72*, 73, *73*, 75, 80
 femoral replacement prosthesis, 4: 129
 Fracture Clinic at, 2: 130; 3: 60, 60*b*, 62, 241–242, 245, 273, *273*, 313–315, 371, 373, 378, 456*b*; 4: 464
 Fracture Course at, 3: 62
 Frederick and Joan Brengle Learning Center, 3: 463
 gait laboratory and, 3: 397
 growth in, 3: 227–228
 Hand Clinic at, 3: 314
 Harris Orthopaedic and Biomaterials laboratory, 3: 463
 HCORP and, 1: 213–215
 house officers at, 1: 189
 internships at, 1: 196
 Joint Kinematics Laboratory, 3: 463, 464*b*
 Joseph S. Barr and, 3: 453, 453*b*–456*b*
 Knee Biomechanics and Biomaterials Laboratory, 3: 463, 464*b*
 Melvin J. Glimcher and, 3: 453, 455*b*–458*b*
 opening of, 3: 68
 Orthopaedic Biochemistry and Osteoarthritis Therapy Laboratory, 3: 464*b*
 Orthopaedic Biology and Oncology Laboratories, 3: 463, 464*b*
 Orthopaedic Biomechanics and Biomaterials Laboratory, 3: 464*b*
 orthopaedic chairpersons at, 3: 11*b*
 Orthopaedic Oncology Unit, 3: 440
 orthopaedic rehabilitation and, 3: 459
 Orthopaedic Research Laboratories, 2: 321–324; 3: 211–212
 orthopaedic specialties, 3: 459, 460*b*, 461–462
 orthopaedic staff in 1984, 3: 398*b*
 orthopaedic surgery department, 1: 171, 180
 orthopaedics curriculum and, 1: 136–137, 157–158, 167
 orthopaedics fellowships, 1: 241
 orthopaedics instruction at, 1: 190
 orthopaedics residencies, 1: 186, 199, 204, 207, 217–218, 221–225, 241–242; 2: *249*, *278*, *290*, *320*, *327*; 3: 74
 Orthopedic Biomechanics Laboratory, 3: 463
 outpatient services and, 3: 80, 227, 304, 306*b*–307*b*
 pediatric orthopaedics and, 3: 388*t*, 400
 physical therapy and, 3: 454*b*
 podiatry service and, 3: 396–398
 Problem Back Clinic, 3: 254
 professorships, 3: 464*b*
 research activities, 3: 455*b*, 458*b*
 Research Building, 3: *454*
 Research Laboratory Centers, 3: 464*b*
 Sarcoma Molecular Biology Laboratory, 3: 464*b*
 specialty services under Mankin, 3: 388*t*, 396–398
 sports medicine and, 3: 397
 Sports Medicine Service, 3: 356, 448
 surgeon-scholars at, 3: 228, 395–398, 398*b*, 399, *461*
 surgical appliance shop, 3: 73
 surgical residencies, 1: 198; 3: 455*b*, 457*b*–458*b*
 Thornton Brown on changes at, 3: 453*b*–458*b*
 transition in, 3: 461–463
 Ward 1, 1: 273; 2: 116; 3: *67*, 68, *68*, 70*b*, 74–75, *80*
 White 9 Rehabilitation Unit, 3: 286, 299, 455*b*, 459, 461
 Zander Room (Medico-Mechanical Department), 3: 71, 227, 264–268
Massachusetts General Hospital Physicians Organization (MGPO), 3: 256
Massachusetts General Orthopaedic Group, 3: 246
Massachusetts General/Boston Children's Hospital residency program, 1: 210; 2: 144
Massachusetts Homeopathic Hospital, 3: 120
Massachusetts Hospital Life Insurance Company, 3: 9
Massachusetts Hospital School for Crippled Children, 2: 38–39, *39*, 384; 3: 319–320
Massachusetts Humane Society, 1: 29
Massachusetts Industrial Accident Board, 2: 92; 4: 325, 327
Massachusetts Infantile Paralysis Clinic, 2: 188–189, 191, 208, 212, 314
Massachusetts Institute of Technology (MIT), 2: 321; 4: 152
Massachusetts Medical Association, 1: 184
Massachusetts Medical College of Harvard University, 1: 6, 40, *40*, 41, *135*; 3: 35, 38
Massachusetts Medical Society, 1: 25–26, 29, 38, 99, 272–273, 277; 2: 164, 208, 230; 3: 35; 4: 162, 366*b*, 367, 367*b*
Massachusetts Memorial Hospital, 4: 347
Massachusetts Orthopaedic Association (MOA), 3: 421; 4: 253

Massachusetts Regional Fracture Committee, 3: 64
Massachusetts Rehabilitation Hospital, 3: 387, 396
Massachusetts Services for Crippled Children, 2: 208
Massachusetts Society of Examining Physicians, 4: 324
Massachusetts State Board of Health, 2: 61
Massachusetts State Hospital, 2: 102
Massachusetts Volunteer Aid Association, 2: 43
Massachusetts Women's Hospital, 4: 447–448
Massachusetts Workingmen's Compensation Law, 4: 325
massage
    avoidance of tender muscles, 1: 267; 2: 73
    congenital dislocated hips (CDH) and, 2: 178
    foot problems and, 2: 56, 245
    injured soldiers and, 2: 56, 67, 118, 120
    obstetrical paralysis and, 2: 90, 94
    physical therapy and, 1: 100; 3: 266, 297
    poliomyelitis and, 2: 62, 73, 109
    therapeutic, 3: 264–266
Massage (Böhm), 3: 266
Matson, Donald, 2: 301
Matza, R. A., 2: 279, 280*b*
Mayer, Leo, 1: 1, 107, 114; 2: 24, 33, 51, 70, 99, 165; 3: 156*b*, 196; 4: 291, 463
Mayfield, F. H., 3: 210
Mayo, Charles W., 4: 411
Mayo, Richard, 3: 310
Mayo, William J., 2: 69; 3: 40–41, 44–45, 50, 113*b*
Mayo Clinic, 3: 50, 289
McBride, Earl D., 3: 295
McCabe, Charles, 1: 167
McCall, M. G., 2: 212
McCall, Samuel W., 3: 134
McCarroll, H. Relton, 1: 162; 4: 237
McCarthy, Clare, 2: 178–180, 182, 204, 230, 287–288
McCarthy, E. A., 2: 230
McCarthy, Eddie, 3: 97
McCarthy, Joseph, 2: 368
McCarthy, Ralph, 4: 342
McCharen, Littleton L., 4: 489
McClellan, George, 3: 43
McCombs, Betsy, 3: 280
McCord, David, 4: 3, 9, 20

McDermott, Leo J., 2: 171–172, 229, 299, 438; 3: 74
McDermott, William, Jr., 4: 277–279, 303
McDonagh, Eileen, 1: 285
McDonald, John L., 2: 183
McDougall, Jean, 3: 288
McGibbon, Chris, 3: 460*b*
McGill University School of Medicine, 3: 253
McGinty, Beth A. Dignan, 2: 277–278
McGinty, John B. (1930–2019), 2: 278, 281
    AAOS chairman, 2: 281
    Arthroscopic Surgery Update, 2: 279
    arthroscopy and, 2: 279, 280*b*, 281; 3: 448
    Boston Children's Hospital and, 2: 278–279; 4: 22
    Brigham and Women's Hospital and, 4: 163, 193
    death of, 2: 281
    education and training, 2: 277
    Green and, 2: 178, 205, 279
    marriage and family, 2: 277–278
    Medical University of South Carolina and, 2: 281
    MGH and, 2: 278
    MGH/Children's Hospital residency, 2: 278
    military service, 2: 278–279
    Newton-Wellesley Hospital and, 2: 279
    Operative Arthroscopy, 2: 279
    Orthopaedics Today editor, 2: 281
    PBBH and, 2: 278–279; 4: 22, 116, 128, 163
    professional memberships, 2: 281
    publications and research, 2: 279
    Tufts University and, 2: 279
    Valley Forge Army Hospital and, 2: 279
    Veterans Administration Hospital and, 2: 279; 4: 22
McIndoe Memorial Research Unit, 2: 422, *422*
McKay, Douglas, 2: 304, 351
McKeever, Duncan, 4: 40
McKeever prosthesis, 4: 40, 69, 70*b*–71*b*, 129–130, 177, 188–189
McKittrick, Leland S., 3: 301; 4: 276, 277*b*
McLaughlin, F. L., 3: 210
McLean, Franklin C., 3: 211
McLean Hospital, 1: 294
McMahon, Mark S., 3: 449
McMahon, Vince, 4: 252
McRae, Ronald, 1: 167

Meals, Roy, 3: 431
measles, 1: 7; 2: 4
Mechanic, Gerald L., 2: 324
Mechanism of Dislocation and Fracture of the Hip, The (Bigelow), 3: 35, *35*, 38
Medearis, Donald N., 3: 397
Medical and Orthopaedic Management of Chronic Arthritis, The (Osgood and Pemperton), 4: 32
Medical College of Virginia, 4: 153
medical degrees, 1: 6–7
medical education. *See also* Harvard Medical School (HMS); orthopaedics residencies
    admission requirements, 1: 146
    American, 1: 138, 142, 146–147
    apprenticeships and, 1: 6, 8, 15
    approved teaching hospitals, 1: 196, 198
    clinical facilities for, 1: 40
    curricular reform, 1: 169
    development of medical schools, 1: 25–28
    dressers, 1: 6, 33, 36–37
    early orthopaedic surgery training, 1: 186–189
    early surgical training, 1: 183–186
    in Edinburgh, 1: 7, 37, 76
    in England, 1: 6, 33, 37, 73, 142
    examinations for physicians, 1: 15, 21, 29
    Flexner Report and, 1: 146–147
    governance and, 1: 177
    graduate education, 1: 196, 196*b*, 197–199, 213
    graduate orthopaedic surgery, 2: 160–162, 162*b*
    hospitals and, 1: 41, 52
    human dissections and, 1: 21, 24, 26–27, 32, 34, 38, 52
    impact of World War II on, 4: 467
    inclusiveness in, 2: 146
    internships and, 1: 189–190
    leaders of, 1: 147
    military hospitals and, 1: 24
    musculoskeletal medicine in, 1: 168–170
    orthopaedics curriculum in, 1: 153–155, 159–162; 2: 183–184, 184*b*, 185, 185*b*, 186
    in Paris, 1: 34, 37, 73–76
    postgraduate, 2: 157–160
    reform of, 1: 139–140
    regulation of, 1: 196–200, 211–213
    regulations and milestones of, 1: 196*b*

specialization in, 1: 189;
4: 300–301
supervised training in,
1: 198–199
surgery in, 1: 29, 33–36
teaching program in, 1: 40; 4: 3
treating and teaching of fractures
in, 1: 161
use of audio-visual aids in, 1: 161
Veterans Administration hospitals
and, 1: 91
walkers, 1: 33
Medical Institution of Harvard
College (1782–1816), 1: 25–26.
See also Harvard Medical School
(HMS)
Medical Institution of Liverpool,
2: 135
*Medical Malpractice in Nineteenth-
Century America* (De Ville), 1: 47
Medical Research Council of Great
Britain, 2: 71
Medical University of South Carolina, 2: 281
*Medical War Manual No. 4 Military
Orthopaedic Surgery*, 4: 473, *474*
Meeks, Berneda, 4: 255
Meeks, Laura, 4: 256
Meeks, Louis W. (1937–2015),
4: *254*
   as Beth Israel acting chief of orthopaedics, 4: 223, 255, 289*b*
   as Beth Israel chief of sports medicine, 4: 255
   Beth Israel Hospital and, 4: 263
   BIDMC teaching program and,
4: 286–287
   community organizations and,
4: 255, 256*b*
   death of, 4: 256
   education and training, 4: 254
   HCORP and, 4: 255
   HMS appointment, 4: 263
   marriage and family, 4: 255
   orthopaedics education and,
4: 254–255
   outpatient arthroscopic ACL
reconstructions, 4: 255
   private medical practice, 4: 254
   publications and research, 4: 255
   US Army and, 4: 254
Meigs, Joe V., 2: 254
Meigs, Sarah Tyler, 3: 257
Meisenbach, Roland O., 4: 188
Mellon, William, 3: 135
Mellon Lecture (Univ. of Pittsburgh),
2: 66–67
Melrose Hospital, 4: 343
Meltzer, S. J., 3: 212
Merrick, Phiny, 1: 307

Merrill, Ed, 3: 224
Merrill, Janet, 2: 107; 4: 60, 396
Messner, Marie Blais, 2: 170, 191,
193–194
metal implants, 2: 237–238
metatarsalgia, 4: 188
Metcalf, Carleton R., 4: 440–441,
441*b*
methylmethacrylate (bone cement),
3: 220, 222; 4: 133, 171
Meyer, George von L., 2: 432
Meyerding, Henry W., 3: 340
MGH. *See* Massachusetts General
Hospital (MGH)
MGH Institute of Health Professions, 3: 391, *391*, 392, 397
MGH School of Nursing, 3: 302,
391
MGH Staff Associates, 3: 241
MGH Surgical Society Newsletter, 3: 1
Michael G. Ehrlich, MD, Fund for
Orthopedic Research, 3: 401
Micheli, Lyle J. (1940–), 2: *383*
   on ACL reconstruction in young
athletes, 2: 385, *385*, 386, *386*
   athletic spine problems and,
2: 385
   as Boston Ballet attending physician, 2: 384
   Boston Children's Hospital and,
2: 354, 383–385, 436, 439*b*
   Brigham and Women's Hospital
and, 4: 163, 193
   education and training, 2: 383
   HMS appointment, 2: 383–384
   honors and awards, 2: 387*b*
   Joseph O'Donnell Family Chair
in Orthopedic Sports Medicine,
2: 439*b*
   Massachusetts Hospital School
and, 2: 384
   MGH/Children's Hospital residency, 2: 383
   military service, 2: 383
   New England Deaconess Hospital
and, 4: 280
   orthopaedics appointments,
2: 384
   orthopaedics leadership, 2: 387
   PBBH and, 4: 163
   private medical practice, 2: 338
   publications and research,
2: 359, 378–379, 385
   rugby and, 2: 383–385
   sports medicine and, 2: 287,
384–385, 387
*Sports Medicine Bible for Young
Adults, The*, 2: 385
Sports Medicine Bible, The,
2: 385, *385*

Middlesex Central District Medical
Society, 3: 319
Miegel, Robert, 4: 194, 195*b*
Mignon, M. Alfred, 4: 102
Milch, R. A., 4: 21
Milgram, Joseph, 3: 382
Military Orthopaedic Surgery (Orthopaedic Council), 2: 68, 69
military orthopaedics. *See also* base
hospitals
   amputations and, 1: 23;
4: 418–419
   bone and joint injuries, 4: 419
   camp work, 2: 258; 4: 452–453
   casualty clearing stations (CCS),
4: 414, *415*, 421, 424–425
   compound fractures and, 4: 391,
392
   curative workshops and, 4: 399–
403, *403*, 404, 442, 448, *448*,
449
   documentation and, 4: 407–408
   evacuation hospital care,
4: 417–418
   expanded role of orthopaedists
and, 4: 453–454
   facilities for, 4: 414–416
   Goldthwait and, 2: 127–128;
4: 443
   Goldthwait units, 4: 440
   Harvard Medical School surgery
course, 4: 455–462
   manual of splints and appliances
for, 2: 126
   massage and, 2: 56, 67, 120, 188
   medical categories for,
4: 412–414
   Medical Officer instructions for,
4: 410*b*
   necessary equipment for, 4: 393*b*
   nerve lesions and, 4: 392
   open-bone fractures, 4: *400*
   Orthopaedic Centers and, 2: 127
   Osgood and, 2: 120–128;
4: 423*b*
   patient flow process and,
4: 435–436
   reconstruction and occupational
aides, 4: 436*b*
   reconstruction hospitals and,
4: 439–443, 447–449
   rehabilitation and, 1: 270–272;
2: 121, 127; 3: 232; 4: 411,
454
   standardization of equipment for,
2: 124
   Thomas splint and, 2: 20
   Thorndike and, 1: 270–272
   trauma surgery and, 3: 274, 301;
4: 393

use of splints in, 2: 120; 4: 389, *391*, 408–409, 411, 416–417
war injuries and, 2: 124, 126, 128; 4: 391
World War I volunteer orthopaedic surgeons, 2: 117–119, 124–127, 145; 4: 386–396, 398–399, *399*, 402, 404, 406–409, 412*b*–413*b*, 425, 452
World War II and, 4: 463–464, 473, 485, 493
wound treatment and, 4: 392–393, 435–436

Military Orthopedics for the Expeditionary Forces, 3: 156

military reconstruction hospitals. *See also* Reconstruction Base Hospital No. 1 (Parker Hill, Boston)
amputation services, 4: 451
Canadian, 4: 443
Cotton on, 4: 449–451
gyms in, 4: 444
Harvard orthopaedic surgeons and, 4: 452
as models for civilian hospitals, 4: 450–451
occupational rehabilitation and, 4: 444
organization of British, 4: 441*b*
orthopaedics services in, 4: 439, 451
rehabilitation of wounded soldiers and, 4: 439–444, 447–450
in the United Kingdom, 4: 440–441

Millender, Bonnie Cobert, 4: 168

Millender, Lewis H. (1937–1996), 4: *165*
Beth Israel Hospital and, 4: 262
Brigham and Women's Hospital, 4: 163, 167
death of, 4: 168
education and training, 4: 165
Entrapment Neuropathies, 4: 168
hand therapy and, 4: 97–98, 132, 165, 168
HMS appointment, 4: 165
honors and awards, 4: 168
hospital appointments, 4: 167
marriage and family, 4: 168
Nalebuff on, 4: 167
New England Baptist Hospital and, 4: 165, 167
Occupational Disorders of the Upper Extremity, 4: 168, 183
occupational medicine and, 4: 167–168
PBBH and, 4: 116, 129, 161, 163
posterior interosseous syndrome case, 4: 165–166
publications and research, 4: 165, *165*, 166–167, *167*
RBBH and, 4: 132, 165, 167
Tufts appointment, 4: 167
US Public Health Service and, 4: 165
West Roxbury Veterans Administration Hospital and, 4: 167

Miller, Bill, 2: 339, 358, *359*
Miller, Richard H., 3: 60; 4: 475
Millet, Peter, 4: 194
Milligan, E. T. C., 4: 385
Millis, Michael B. (1944–), 2: *388*
acetabular dysplasia case, 2: 389, *389*, 390
Boston Children's Hospital and, 2: 338, 354, 388–389
Boston Concept and, 2: 391, *391*
Brigham and Women's Hospital and, 4: 163, 193
computer-simulated planning and, 2: 389
education and training, 2: 358, 388
Hall and, 2: 347, 388
HCORP and, 2: 388
hip and pelvis research, 2: 389–394
HMS appointment, 2: 388–389
honors and awards, 2: 388, 390
metacarpal phalangeal joint replacement, 4: 132
military service, 2: 388
orthopaedics appointments, 2: 389
orthopaedics education and, 2: 394
on Pappas, 2: 289
pediatric orthopaedics, 2: 394
periacetabular osteotomy research, 2: 390–394
professional memberships, 2: 392–393
publications and research, 2: 389–394

Milton Hospital, 1: 264; 3: 257, 287
Milwaukee Brace, 2: 265–266, 336
Minas, Thomas, 4: 193, 195*b*
Minot, Charles S., 3: 94; 4: 2–3, 6
Miriam Hospital, 3: 401
MIT Medical, 2: 276–277, 290
Mital, Mohinder A., 2: 234; 3: 320
Mitchell, William, Jr., 4: 286
Mixter, Charles G., 4: 283*t*, 468
Mixter, Samuel J., 2: 117; 3: *19*, 184
Mixter, William J.
back pain research and, 3: 203, *203*, 204–207
Beth Israel Hospital and, 1: 158
publications and research, 3: 302
ruptured intervertebral disc research, 3: 204; 4: 352–353
Mizuno, Schuichi, 4: 194
mobile army surgical hospitals (MASHs), 2: 231, *232*; 4: 468–469, *470*
Mock, Harry, 1: 271
Moe, John, 2: 335
Moellering, Robert, 4: 279
Mohan, Alice, 1: 62
Molasses Act, 1: 11
mold arthroplasty
evolution of the Vitallium, 3: 292, 292*b*, 293
hip surgery and, 3: 218, 242, *242*, 243–244
historical evolution of, 3: *194*
knee and, 3: 291–292
original design of, 3: 193*b*
postoperative roentgenogram, 3: *195*, *196*
preoperative roentgenogram, 3: *196*
problems with cup, 3: 241
results of, 3: 242*t*, 243*b*
Smith-Petersen and, 3: 181, 182*b*, 183, 192, *192*, 193–196, 198
Vitallium, 3: 193*b*, *195*, *196*, 238–239, 243*b*
Molloy, Maureen K., 1: 239; 3: 208
mononucleosis, 3: 324–325
Monson State Hospital, 4: 350
Montgomery, James B., 4: 407
Moody, Dwight, 4: 257
Moody, Ellsworth, 3: 165–166
Moore, Belveridge H., 2: 78, 172
Moore, Francis D.
on Banks, 4: 72
burn care and, 3: 336
as BWH chief of surgery, 3: 135
family of, 1: 90
as Moseley Professor of Surgery, 2: 421
PBBH 50th anniversary report, 4: 21*b*
PBBH and, 4: 79
as PBBH chief of surgery, 4: 8, 18, 22, 74*b*, 75
on Sledge, 4: 114
on surgery residents, 4: 19
Moore, Howard, 4: 372
Moral Re-Armament program (Oxford Group), 4: 57
Morales, Teresa, 3: 462, 464*b*
Moratoglu, Orhun, 3: 460*b*

Index

Morgan, John, 1: 23
Morris, Katherine, 2: 284
Morris, Miriam Morss, 2: 282
Morris, Richard B., 1: 317
Morris, Robert H. (1892–1971), 2: *283*
   on arthrodesis procedures, 2: 282–283
   BCH Bone and Joint Service, 4: 380*b*
   Boston Children's Hospital and, 1: 194; 2: 222, 231, 252, 274, 284
   death of, 2: 284
   education and training, 2: 282
   Fitchet and, 2: 282
   on foot stabilization, 2: 282–284
   HMS appointment, 2: 223, 282; 4: 60–61
   King's College and, 2: 284
   Long Island Hospital and, 2: 284
   marriage and family, 2: 282, 284
   professional memberships, 2: 284
   publications of, 2: 282
   RBBH and, 4: 36, 93, 111
   World War I service, 2: 282
Morrison, Gordon M. (1896–1955), 4: *346*
   AAST president, 4: 349
   Boston City Hospital and, 4: 347
   boxing and, 4: 347
   Cotton and, 4: 330
   death of, 4: 349
   education and training, 4: 346–347
   football coaching and, 4: 347
   hip fracture treatment, 4: 319
   hospital appointments, 4: 347
   ischaemic paralysis case, 4: 348
   Joseph H. Shortell Fracture Unit, 4: 307
   Massachusetts Regional Fracture Committee, 3: 64
   New England Society of Bone and Joint Surgery, 4: 347
   professional memberships, 4: 347–349
   publications and research, 4: 316, 347
   Royal Flying Corps and, 4: 346–347
   on trauma treatment, 4: 349
Morrison, H., 4: 202, 203*b*, *203*
Morrison, Sidney L., 4: 64, *64*
Morrissey, Raymond, 2: 438
Morrow, Edward R., 2: 272
Morss, Miriam, 2: 282
Morton, William T. G., 1: *57*
   ether composition, 1: 61
   ether inhaler, 1: *58*, 63
   ether patent and, 1: 60
   ether use, 1: 55, 57–60, 62; 3: 27–29, 32–33
   as witness for Webster, 1: 310
Morton's neuroma, 2: 287
Moseley, William, 3: 74
Moseley's growth charts, 2: 194, *194*
Moss, H. L., 4: 261–262
Moss, William L., 3: 313
Mott, Valentine, 1: xxiv
Mount Auburn Cemetery, 3: 23; 4: 2
Mount Auburn Hospital, 2: 276; 3: 327
Mount Sinai Monthly magazine, 4: *201*, 202
Moyer, Carl, 4: 125
Mt. Sinai Hospital (Boston)
   Chambers Street location, 4: 201*b*, 202, *202*
   closing of, 4: 205, 223
   Compton Street location, 4: 201*b*, 202, *202*
   financial difficulties, 4: 203–205
   fundraising for, 4: 202
   Jewish patients at, 4: 199–200, 202
   Jewish physicians and, 4: 202, 204
   non-discrimination and, 4: 199, 201
   orthopaedic treatment at, 4: 202, 204, 204*t*
   outpatient services at, 4: 203–204
   planning for, 4: 200–201
   Staniford Street location, 4: 202
Mt. Sinai Hospital (New York)
   Jewish patients at, 4: 200
   orthopaedics residencies and, 4: 88
   World War II and, 4: 88
Mt. Sinai Hospital Society of Boston, 4: 200–201
Mt. Sinai Medical School, 3: 383, 385, 413, 435
Mueller, Maurice, 4: 263
Mueller Professorship, 4: 263
Muir, Helen, 4: 116*b*, 268
Multicenter Arthroscopy of the Hip Outcomes Research Network (MAHORN), 2: 380
multiple cartilaginous exostoses, 4: 218–219, *219*, 220
Mumford, E. B., 4: 452
Mumford, James, 4: 52
Muratoglu, Orhun, 3: 224
Muro, Felipe, 2: 309
Murphy, Eugene, 3: 317
Murphy, Steven, 2: 389–392; 4: 286
Murray, Martha, 2: 439
Murray S. Danforth Oration of Rhode Island Hospital, 3: 275
Muscle Function (Wright), 2: 70
muscle training
   heavy-resistance exercise, 3: 282–285
   poliomyelitis and, 2: 62–63, 78, 109; 3: 284–285
   progressive resistance exercises, 3: 285
Muscular Dystrophy Association of America, 2: 266
Musculoskeletal Imaging Fund, 2: 439*b*
musculoskeletal medicine
   apparatus for, 2: 27
   biomechanics and, 2: 410
   disease and, 2: 439
   early treatment, 1: xxiii
   in medical education, 1: 168–170
   orthopaedics curriculum and, 1: 168–170; 2: 184–186
   orthopaedics research and, 2: 439
   pathology and, 3: 432
   sarcomas and, 2: 424
   spinal disorders and, 2: 337
   sports injuries and, 1: 288
   surgery advances for, 2: 36
   tissue banks for, 3: 442–443
   tumors and, 3: 432–433, 436
Musculoskeletal Outcome Data Evaluation and Management System (MODEMS), 4: 186
Musculoskeletal Tissue Banking (Tomford), 3: 443
Musculoskeletal Tumor Society, 3: 390, 436, *436*
Musnick, Henry, 4: 91
Myelodysplasia Clinic (Children's Hospital), 2: 359, 402
Myers, Grace Whiting, 3: 10
myositis ossificans, 1: 266–267

N

Nachemson, Alf, 2: 373; 4: 262
Nadas, Alex, 2: 234
Nalebuff, Edward A. (1928–2018), 4: *94*
   art glass collection, 4: 100, *100*
   Boston Children's Hospital and, 4: 95
   Brigham and Women's Hospital, 4: 163
   death of, 4: 100

education and training, 4: 94–95
hand surgery and, 4: 96, 98–100
hand surgery fellowship, 4: 95–96
HMS appointment, 4: 97–98
hospital appointments, 4: 99
implant arthroplasty research, 4: 99–100
Marian Ropes Award, 4: 100
marriage of, 4: 100
metacarpal phalangeal joint replacement, 4: 132
MGH and, 4: 95
New England Baptist Hospital and, 4: 99
PBBH and, 4: 95, 116, 129, 161, 163
professional memberships, 4: 100
publications and research, 4: 40, 95–99, 99, 166, 167
RBBH and, 4: 38, 41b, 42, 68–69, 95–97, 100, 102, 116b, 131
RBBH hand clinic and, 4: 42
as RBBH hand service chief, 4: 97–98
rheumatoid arthritis of the hand research and surgery, 4: 96, 96, 97–98, 98, 131
rheumatoid thumb deformity classification, 4: 97
surgical procedures performed, 4: 131t
Tufts appointment, 4: 98
Tufts hand fellowship, 2: 250; 4: 98–99
US Air Force and, 4: 95
Veterans Administration Hospital and, 4: 95
Nalebuff, Marcia, 4: 100
Nathan, David, 2: 234
"Nation and the Hospital, The" (Osgood), 2: 137–138, 138b–139b
National Academy of Medicine, 3: 405
National Academy of Sciences, 3: 405
National Birth Defects Center, 2: 370
National Collegiate Athletic Association (NCAA), 1: 248, 253
National Foundation for Infantile Paralysis, 2: 188–189, 191, 260
National Foundation for Poliomyelitis, 2: 188, 191
National Institute of Arthritis and Metabolic Diseases, 3: 323
National Institutes of Health (NIH), 3: 383, 387–388, 392; 4: 38–39

National Intercollegiate Football, 1: 253
National Rehabilitation Association, 2: 266
National Research Council, 2: 215–216
Natural History of Cerebral Palsy, The (Crothers and Paine), 2: 172
Naval Fleet Hospital No. 109, 4: 490
Naval Medical Research Institute, 3: 439, 440
Navy Regional Medical Center (Guam), 3: 446
necks, 2: 256
Nélaton, Auguste, 1: 82
nerve injuries, 2: 67, 120, 140, 393; 3: 157, 353
Nerve Injuries Committee (Medical Research Council of Great Britain), 2: 71
Nesson, H. Richard, 2: 272
Nestler, Steven P., 1: 215, 218, 220, 232–233; 3: 435–436, 436
neuritis, 3: 324–325
neurofibromatosis, 2: 172, 174–175
Neusner, Jacob, 4: 220
New England Baptist Hospital (NEBH)
    affiliation with BIDMC, 4: 214
    affiliation with New England Deaconess Hospital, 4: 280
    Aufranc and, 3: 246–247
    Ben Bierbaum and, 1: 233–234, 236
    Bone and Joint Institute Basic Science Laboratory, 4: 271, 286
    Brackett and, 3: 153
    Edward Kennedy and, 3: 275
    Emans and, 2: 358
    Fitchet and, 2: 252
    Hall and, 2: 338
    Hresko and, 2: 364
    Kocher and, 2: 377
    Morris and, 2: 284
    Nalebuff and, 4: 98–100
    New England Bone and Joint Institute, 4: 280
    orthopaedics residencies, 3: 247
    Painter and, 4: 47
    Pathway Health Network and, 4: 280
    Pedlow and, 3: 426
    Potter and, 4: 69, 116
    purchase of RBBH buildings and land, 4: 26, 114, 121
    reconstructive hip surgery and, 3: 246
    Runyon and, 2: 290
    Schiller and, 2: 369

    Smith-Petersen and, 3: 362
    Swaim and, 4: 58
New England Bone and Joint Institute, 4: 280
New England Deaconess Association, 2: 219–220
New England Deaconess Home and Training School, 4: 273
New England Deaconess Hospital (NEDH), 4: 273, 274, 275
    admissions and occupancy at, 4: 279
    bed allocation at, 4: 277t
    early history of, 4: 275, 276t
    foot and ankle service, 4: 279
    founding of, 4: 273
    Harvard Fifth Surgical Service and, 4: 279
    Lahey Clinic and, 4: 275–277
    long-range planning at, 4: 278b
    maps of, 4: 276
    medical and surgical (sub) specialties in, 4: 274
    merger with Beth Israel Hospital, 4: 214, 223, 270, 281, 283
    orthopaedics department at, 4: 279–280
    Palmer Memorial Hospital and, 4: 275–276
    Pathway Health Network and, 4: 280
    physician affiliations at, 4: 277, 277t, 278
    relationship with HMS, 4: 277–279
    as a specialized tertiary-care facility, 4: 279
New England Dressings Committee (Red Cross Auxiliary), 4: 10
New England Female Medical College, 2: 273; 4: 296
New England Home for Little Wanderers, 3: 307
New England Hospital for Women and Children, 2: 274
New England Journal of Medicine, 1: 39
New England Medical Center, 4: 249, 311
New England Medical Council, 2: 157–158
New England Muscular Dystrophy Association Clinic Directors, 2: 403
New England Organ Bank, 3: 443
New England Orthopedic Society, 3: 319
New England Patriots, 3: 348, 397, 399, 448

Index

New England Peabody Home for Crippled Children, 2: 37, 165, 183, 191, 230–231, 269–270; 3: 174, 202, 209, 329, 362
New England Pediatric Society, 2: 13
New England Regional Committee on Fractures, 4: 341, 347
New England Rehabilitation Center, 1: 272
New England Revolution, 3: 348, 450
New England Society of Bone and Joint Surgery, 4: 347
New England Surgical Society, 1: 90; 2: 136; 3: 63
New York Bellevue Hospital, 2: 111
New York Hospital for the Ruptured and Crippled, 1: 89
New York Orthopaedic Dispensary and Hospital, 2: 20, 47–48
New York Orthopaedic Hospital, 2: 47
Newcomb, Sarah Alvord, 1: 107
Newhall, Harvey F., 3: 266
Newhauser, E. B. D., 2: 215
Newman, Erik T., 3: 463*b*; 4: 190*b*
Newton-Wellesley Hospital (NWH), 1: 225; 2: 279; 3: 240, 331, 334, 426
Nichol, Vern, 3: 248
Nichols, Edward H. (1864–1922), 1: *252*; 4: *302*
   Base Hospital No. 7 and, 1: 256; 4: 301–302, 438–439
   Boston Children's Hospital and, 2: 247, 307
   Boston City Hospital and, 1: 174, 252; 4: 301–302
   death of, 1: 256–257
   as football team surgeon, 1: 252–256
   Harvard baseball team and, 1: 251–252
   HMS appointment, 4: 302
   HMS Laboratory of Surgical Pathology and, 2: 90
   legacy of, 1: 257
   offices of, 4: *302*
   orthopaedic research and, 1: 252
   osteomyelitis research and, 4: 301
   PBBH teaching and, 4: 10, 12
   as professor of surgery, 1: 174
   study of football injuries, 1: 254–256
   Surgery of Joints, The, 2: 52
   tuberculosis treatment, 2: 32
   vascular anastomosis and, 4: 216
   World War I medical unit, 1: 256; 4: 391
Nichols, Emma, 4: 438
Nickel, Vernon, 2: 315; 3: 249, 319, 321
Nightingale, Florence, 2: 5; 4: 274*b*
nitrous oxide, 1: 56–59, 63; 3: 15
Noall, Lawrence, 3: 208
Noble, Nick, 3: 94
non-hinged metal–polyethylene prosthesis, 4: 145–146
Nordby, Eugene J., 3: 255
North Charles General Hospital, 4: 157
North Shore Children's Hospital, 2: 269
Northwestern University, 2: 302
Norton, Margaret, 3: 320
Norton, Paul L. (1903–1986)
   adjustable reamer and, 3: 317
   Children's Hospital/MGH combined program and, 3: 317
   Clinics for Crippled Children and, 2: 230; 3: 317
   death of, 3: 320
   early life, 3: 317
   education and training, 3: 317
   Emerson Hospital and, 3: 317, 319
   HMS appointment, 3: 317
   as honorary orthopaedic surgeon, 3: 398*b*
   legacy of, 3: 320
   marriage and family, 3: 320
   Massachusetts Hospital School and, 3: 319–320; 4: 378
   memberships and, 3: 319
   as MGH surgeon, 3: 70*b*, 192, 317
   New England Orthopedic Society president, 3: 319
   Norton-Brown spinal brace, 3: 317–319
   paraplegia research and, 3: 319
   publications and research, 3: 258–259, 317–320, 455*b*; 4: 95
Norton-Brown spinal brace, 3: 317–319
Norwalk train wreck, 1: 77, *78*
nose reconstructions, 1: 71, 75–76
Notes on Military Orthopaedics (Jones), 4: 442, *442*, 443
Nuffield Orthopaedic Centre (Oxford), 3: 412
Nursery and Child's Hospital (New York), 2: 3, 5
Nursery for Children (New York), 2: 3
nursing
   Cadet Nursing Corps, 4: 467
   Children's Island Sanitorium and, 4: 87
   Deaconess training and, 4: 274*b*
   early training in, 1: 41; 2: 6–8, 13–14
   foot problems, 2: 54–56
   impact of World War II on, 4: 467
   for Jewish women, 4: 208
   Larson and, 3: 302–303
   MGH School of Nursing and, 3: 302, 391
   New England Deaconess Hospital and, 4: 273
   reforms in, 3: 142
nutrition, 2: 361–362
Nydegger, Rogert C., 4: 489

O

Ober, Ernest, 2: 144, 166
Ober, Frank R. (1881–1960), 1: *188*, *195*; 2: *143*, *147*, 255
   AAOS and, 4: 337
   as AOA president, 2: 161
   "Back Strains and Sciatica," 2: 151–152
   Barr and, 3: 201
   Base Hospital No. 5 and, 4: 420, *422*
   Bell and, 2: 220
   on biceps-triceps transplant, 2: 154
   Boston Children's Hospital and, 1: 153, 155, 158, 178, 188, 195–196, 198–199; 2: *143*, 144–147, 149, 163, 217, 252, 274, 282; 4: 338, 468
   brachioradialis transfer for triceps weakness, 2: 153–154, *154*
   Brigham and Women's Hospital and, 4: 195*b*
   Children's Hospital/MGH combined program and, 1: 210
   club foot treatment, 2: 145
   death of, 2: 166
   on diagnosis, 2: 155–156
   education and training, 2: 143–144
   expert testimony and, 2: 164–165
   on FitzSimmons, 2: 256, 258
   Georgia Warm Springs Foundation board and, 2: 78, 165
   graduate education in orthopaedic surgery and, 2: 160–162, 162*b*
   graduate education review, 1: 196–197

Green and, 2: 168
Harvard Unit and, 4: 419
HCORP and, 1: 192, 195–199
Hibbs spinal fusion procedure, 2: 164
hip abductor paralysis treatment, 2: 149–150
hip and knee contractures, 2: 153, *153*
HMS appointment, 2: 144, 146–147, 156; 4: 59
honorary degrees, 2: 165
Hugenberger and, 2: 269, 271
iliotibial band tightness and, 2: 151–152
John Ball and Buckminster Brown Professorship, 2: 147, 157; 4: 195*b*
Journal of Bone and Joint Surgery editor, 2: 165
lectures at Tuskegee Institute, 2: 146
Lovett and, 2: 144
Lovett Fund Committee and, 2: 82
Marlborough Medical Associates and, 2: 299
marriage and, 2: 144
Massachusetts Medical Society and, 2: 164
Massachusetts Regional Fracture Committee, 3: 64
medical education, 2: 155
military orthopaedics and, 4: 473
military surgeon training and, 2: 42
modification of use of sacrospinalis, 2: 146–147
Mount Desert Island practice, 2: 143–145
New England Peabody Home for Crippled Children and, 2: 270
as orthopaedic chair, 2: 15*b*
on orthopaedic problems in children, 2: 164
orthopaedics education and, 2: 155–157, 163
on orthopaedics training at Harvard, 1: 195–196
Orthopedic Surgery revisions, 2: 166
on Osgood, 2: 148
on paralysis of the serratus anterior, 2: 154–155
PBBH and, 4: 18
poliomyelitis treatment, 2: 147–148, 154–155
posterior approach to the hip joint approach, 2: 146
postgraduate education and, 2: 157–159, 164
private medical practice and, 1: 176; 2: 146, 313; 3: 454*b*
professional memberships, 2: 165
publications of, 2: 227
RBBH and, 4: 15
rehabilitation planning and, 1: 273
Roosevelt and, 2: 77
surgery techniques, 2: 177
teaching department plan, 1: 157
on tendon transplantation, 2: 108, 147–148, *148*, 149
triple arthrodesis and, 2: 149
use of shelf procedure for CDH, 2: 151
Vermont poliomyelitis rehabilitation program, 2: 149
on wartime medical education, 4: 397
weakness/paralysis of the foot and ankle treatment, 2: 150–151
World War I and, 2: 125–126
"Your Brain is Your Invested Capital" speech, 2: 156, 158*b*–159*b*
Ober, Ina Spurling, 2: 144, 166
Ober, Melita J. Roberts, 2: 143
Ober, Otis Meriam, 2: 143
Ober abduction sign, 2: 151
Ober Research Fund, 2: 436
Ober Test, 2: 151–152
Ober-Yount fasciotomy, 2: 153, 172
Objective Structure Clinical Examination (OSCE), 1: 168
O'Brien, Michael, 4: 287
O'Brien, Paul, 4: 333, 378
obstetrical paralysis
brachial plexus injuries, 2: 91, *91*
Lange's theory, 2: 91
massage and exercise for, 2: 90
Sever-L'Episcopo procedure, 2: 90, 100
Sever's study of, 2: 90, *90*, 94–96
subscapularis tendon, 2: 95, *95*
tendon transfers and, 2: 96
treatment of, 2: 89–90, 94–95, *95*, 96
Occupational Disorders of the Upper Extremity (Millender et al.), 4: 168, 183
occupational therapy, 4: 28, 29, 358–359
O'Connor, Frank, 4: 116*b*
O'Connor, Mary I., 4: 266*b*
O'Connor, Richard, 3: 446
O'Donoghue, Don, 3: 272
O'Donovan, T., 4: 167
Ogden, John, 2: 302
O'Hara, Dwight, 1: 273
Ohio State Medical Association, 3: 58
Ohio State University School of Medicine, 2: 407–408
O'Holleran, James, 4: 190*b*
Okike, Kanu, 2: *381*
Olcott, Christopher W., 4: 180
Oliver, Henry K., 1: 47, 49–50
Oliver Wendell Holmes Society, 4: 264
Ollier, Louis Xavier Edouard Leopold, 1: xxiii
O'Malley, Peter, 4: 264
O'Meara, John W., 2: 230
Omni Med, 3: 379
Oneida Football Club, 1: 247
O'Neil, Edward, Jr., 3: 379
O'Neil, Eugene, 4: 371
O'Neill, Eugene, 2: 272
Ontario Crippled Children's Center, 2: 334–335
opera-glass hand deformity, 4: 99
Operative Arthroscopy (McGinty et al.), 2: 279
Operative Hand Surgery (Green), 4: 98
Operative Nerve Repair and Reconstruction (Gelberman), 3: 404
ophthalmology, 1: 138; 3: 13
optical coherence tomography (OCT), 4: 194
Order of St. John of Jerusalem in England, 4: 401
Orr, Bobby, 3: 357, 357*b*
Orr, H. Winnett, 2: 125; 3: 159, 235, 340; 4: 383, 393, 400, 409
Orthopaedia (Andry), 1: xxi
Orthopaedic Biochemistry and Osteoarthritis Therapy Laboratory, 3: 464*b*
Orthopaedic Biology and Oncology Laboratories, 3: 463, 464*b*
Orthopaedic Biomechanics and Biomaterials Laboratory, 3: 464*b*
Orthopaedic Centers (Great Britain), 2: 127, 127*b*
Orthopaedic Fellow Education Fund, 2: 439*b*
Orthopaedic In-Service Training Exam (OITE), 1: 231
Orthopaedic Journal at Harvard Medical School, The, 1: 231–232
Orthopaedic Journal Club, 3: 369
orthopaedic oncology
allografts and, 3: 389
bone sarcomas and, 3: 136–137, 137*t*, 138–140, 140*b*, 141–142

chondrosarcoma of bone, 3: 406
data digitization and, 3: 392–393
flow cytometry and, 3: 388
giant-cell tumors and, 3: 390
limb salvage surgery and, 3: 390–391
Mankin and, 3: 386, 388
osteosarcoma and, 2: 422; 3: 391
sacrococcygeal chordoma, 3: 390
Orthopaedic Research and Education Foundation, 2: 241; 3: 213, 215, 360
Orthopaedic Research Laboratories (MGH), 2: 321–324; 3: 211–212
Orthopaedic Research Society, 2: 240, 316, 327; 3: 262
orthopaedic surgeons
  advancement of the field, 2: 26, 50, 81, 99
  assistive technology and, 2: 408
  blue blazers and, 3: 30
  board certification of, 4: 324, 377
  diagnostic skills, 2: 155–156
  education and training, 2: 133–135
  evaluation and treatment, 2: 48
  extremity injuries and, 2: 122
  fracture care and, 4: 463–464
  general surgery foundations and, 2: 24
  graduate education and, 1: 197–199
  on hip disease, 2: 52
  interest in visceroptosis, 3: 83–84, 84*b*, 86–88
  logical thinking and, 2: 155
  military and, 2: 42, 65–68, 118–120
  minimum requirements for, 2: 134
  observational skills, 2: 155
  orthopaedic physician versus, 4: 47*b*
  recruitment of, 2: 39–40
  scientific study and, 2: 32
  as surgeon-scholars, 2: 217, 357; 3: 228, 395; 4: 43, 79, 143, 163, 193–194, 195*b*
  transformation of profession, 2: 130*b*–131*b*
  volunteer wartime, 2: 124–127
  war injuries and, 2: 124
  x-rays and, 2: 56
orthopaedic surgery
  advances in, 2: 14–15, 20, 25–28
  approved teaching hospitals, 1: 198

Boylston Medical School and, 1: 138
certification in, 1: 189, 196–198, 200, 231
characteristics of, 2: 132
computer-simulated planning, 2: 389
conditions for, 4: 451
development of, 2: 78
early 20th century, 2: 36
early training in, 1: 186–189
founding of, 1: xxiii; 2: 26–27
growth-sparing, 2: 360–361
Harvard athletics and, 1: 284
knee joint resections, 1: 81
in London, 1: 106
minimal requirements for specialization, 1: 191–192
naming of, 1: xxiv
orthopaedics curriculum and, 1: 141, 143, 147, 158, 162
outcomes of, 2: 372
personalities in early, 2: 99
public reporting of, 1: 102
rehabilitation and, 2: 172
residencies, 1: 186–187, 198–199; 2: 160–161
seminal text on, 2: 29–30, 50
tracing of deformities, 2: *53*
traction treatment for, 2: 21–23, 25, 27
training in, 1: 101
transformation of, 2: 130*b*–131*b*
trauma and, 3: 275; 4: 393
in the United States, 1: 100–101, 107; 2: 23; 4: 393
use of traction, 2: 27
women in, 1: 200, 239
World War I and, 2: 119–126
World War II and, 4: 463–464, 473, 485, 493
Orthopaedic Surgery at Tufts University (Banks), 4: 77
Orthopaedic Surgery in Infancy and Childhood (Ferguson), 2: 188, 303
"Orthopaedic Surgery in the United States of America" (Mayer), 1: 114
Orthopaedic Surgical Advancement Fund, 2: 439*b*
Orthopaedic Trauma Association Visiting Scholars Program, 3: 418
orthopaedic wards
  Boston Children's Hospital and, 1: 205
  Boston City Hospital and, 2: 24
  House of the Good Samaritan, 1: 123, 125–130; 2: 25

Massachusetts General Hospital and, 1: 193, 203, 273; 2: 116, 322; 3: 62, 68, 272, 304, 343
"Orthopaedic Work in a War Hospital" (Osgood), 2: 120
orthopaedics
  18th century history of, 1: xxi, xxii
  19th century history of, 1: xxii, xxiii, xxiv
  20th century specialty of, 1: 189–192
  advances in, 4: 466–467
  diversity initiatives in, 4: 264–265
  established as separate specialty, 1: 83, 95–96, 98–99, 119
  first case at MGH, 1: 42, 44
  impact of World War I on, 4: 453–454, 463–464
  impact of World War II on, 4: 473, 493
  malpractice suits and, 1: 50
  mechanical devices and, 1: 107–108, *108*
  opening of first specialty hospital, 1: 99
  radiology and, 2: 16–17
  rehabilitation and, 4: 454
  respect for field, 4: 453, 463–464
  scientific study of, 2: 51
  specialization in, 1: 187, 193; 4: 300–301
  as specialty course at HMS, 1: 141–143
  spelling of, 1: xxiv, xxv, 177
  standards of practice and, 4: 463–464
Orthopaedics (MacAusland and Mayo), 3: 310
orthopaedics apparatus
  Abbott Frame, 4: 232, *232*
  Adam's machine, 2: 86
  adjustable reamer, 3: 317
  Austin Moore prosthesis, 3: 213
  Balkan Frame, 3: 317, 357*b*
  basket plasters, 2: *122*
  Boston Arm, 2: 326, *326*; 3: 287
  Boston brace, 2: 339–340, 358–359, *360*, 361, 423
  brace shop, 2: *22*
  braces, 3: 318–319
  Bradford Frame, 2: 27, *27*, 30–31, *31*, 32
  Bradford's method of reducing the gibbus, 3: *149*
  Buckminster Brown and, 1: 105–107

celastic body jackets, 2: 178
celluloid jackets, 2: 85
charitable surgical appliances, 2: 14
clover leaf rod, 3: 272
club foot device, 1: 98, 100, 106; 2: 23, 23, 24
De Machinamentis of Oribasius, 3: 149
Denis Browne splint, 2: 208
fluoroscope, 2: 307
foot strength tester, 2: 101–102
fracture table, 2: 121
Goldthwait irons, 3: 89, 89, 149
Harrington rods, 2: 316, 317, 325, 335
hyperextension cast, 3: 69
inclinometers, 2: 366, 367
interpedicular segmental fixation (ISF) pedicle screw plate, 3: 420
iron extension hinge, 2: 123
iron lung, 2: 78, 79, 190, 191, 260, 264, 314
ISOLA implants, 2: 370
Jewett nail-plate, 3: 320
knee flexion contracture appliance, 2: 20
Küntscher femoral rod, 3: 272
Lovett Board, 2: 59, 86
MacIntosh prothesis, 4: 69, 71b
McKeever prothesis, 4: 40, 69, 70b–71b
McLaughlin side plate, 3: 320
metal implants, 2: 237–238
Milwaukee Brace, 2: 265–266, 336
Norton-Brown spinal brace, 3: 317–319
pedicle screws, 2: 343; 3: 420
pelvic machine design, 2: 86
Pierce Collar, 3: 321
Pierce Fusion, 3: 321
Pierce Graft, 3: 321
plaster casts, 2: 122–123
portable traction device, 2: 297
pressure correction apparatus (Hoffa-Schede), 3: 151, 152
Relton-Hall frame, 2: 334–335, 335
Risser cast, 2: 178
rocking beds, 2: 314, 315
Sayre jacket, 1: 107
for scoliosis, 2: 35, 35, 36, 36, 296
scoliosis jackets, 2: 59–61, 85–87
scoliosometer, 2: 36
Smith-Petersen Vitallium mold, 3: 195, 196

for spinal deformities, 1: 107; 2: 31
splints, 3: 167, 167, 168
spring muscle test, 2: 70
Steinmann pin, 2: 237–238
surgical scissors, 3: 138
Taylor back brace, 2: 247
Thomas splint, 2: 123, 247; 3: 168
triflanged nail, 3: 62, 185–186, 186, 187, 189, 189b, 190, 320
turnbuckle jacket, 2: 80, 223–224, 224, 225, 225, 226–227, 316, 336; 3: 209
VEPTR (Vertical Expandable Prosthetic Titanium Rib), 2: 360, 362
wire arm splints, 2: 122
wire drop foot splints, 2: 123
World War I and, 2: 124
Zander chair, 3: 153
Zander tilt table, 3: 152
Zander's medico-mechanical equipment, 3: 69, 71, 264, 264, 265, 265, 266–267, 267, 268b
"Orthopaedics at Harvard" (Brown), 1: 195
orthopaedics curriculum
Allison on, 2: 134; 3: 171–173
anatomy lectures in, 1: 134, 136
cadaver dissection, 1: 142
case method and, 4: 299
case-based discussions, 1: 167
competency examinations, 1: 168
development of, 1: 140–141
early medical instruction, 1: 134, 136–138
electives in, 1: 143, 144t, 148–151, 164–166
evolution of, 1: 143, 147, 148b–151b, 152–170
examination questions, 1: 140–141, 144b
fractures in, 1: 154
graduate training, 2: 187b
Jack Warren and, 1: 40, 134
John Collins Warren and, 1: 40, 136–137
Massachusetts General Hospital (MGH) and, 1: 136–137
medical education and, 2: 183–184, 184b, 185, 185b, 186
military orthopaedic surgery course, 4: 455–462
musculoskeletal medicine in, 1: 168–170; 2: 184–186
ophthalmology and, 1: 138

orthopaedic clerkship in, 1: 167–169
orthopaedic surgery in, 1: 141, 143, 147, 158, 162
recommendations for, 1: 162–163
reform of, 1: 140
required courses, 1: 143
sample curriculum for, 1: 159–161
sports medicine elective, 1: 165–166
surgical pedagogy, 1: 137–138
teaching clinics, 1: 155–157, 163, 170, 194
teaching modalities, 3: 172
for third- and fourth-year students, 1: 144t–146t
undergraduate, 2: 183–186, 202
Orthopaedics Overseas, 3: 310
orthopaedics residencies. See also Harvard Combined Orthopaedic Residency Program (HCORP)
ABOS board and, 4: 377–379
AOA survey on, 2: 160–161
approved hospitals for, 1: 196–200
BCH and, 2: 413; 4: 377–379
BCH Bone and Joint Service, 4: 377
Carney Hospital and, 4: 378
certification examinations and, 1: 198, 231
core competencies in, 1: 238–239
examinations for, 1: 210, 231
grand rounds, 1: 189, 203, 203, 204, 204, 205, 218, 232
history of, 1: 183–186
hospital internships and, 1: 186–188
internal review of, 1: 239
Lahey Clinic and, 4: 378
Lakeville State Hospital and, 4: 378
Massachusetts General/Boston Children's Hospital residency program, 1: 210; 2: 144
MGH and, 2: 249, 276, 278, 290, 320, 327
minimum surgical case requirements for, 3: 435–436, 436
pediatric, 1: 210–211
program length and, 1: 215–216, 218–220, 222–223
restructuring at MGH, 1: 198–199
RRC for, 1: 211–213, 215, 217–220, 224, 232–233, 241–242

Index

West Roxbury Veterans Administration Hospital and, 4: 378–379
Orthopaedics Today, 2: 281
Orthopedic Nursing (Funsten and Calderwood), 3: 303
Orthopedic Surgery (Bradford and Lovett), 4: 318
Orthopedic Surgery (Jones and Lovett), 2: 69, *69*, 166
Orthopedic Treatment of Gunshot Injuries, The (Mayer), 3: 156*b*
L'Orthopédie (Andry), 3: 90
orthoroentgenograms, 2: 171
os calcis fractures, 4: 313, 314*b*, 335–336
Osgood, John Christopher, 2: 113
Osgood, Margaret Louisa, 2: 138
Osgood, Martha E. Whipple, 2: 113
Osgood, Robert B. (1873–1956), 1: *193*, *194*; 2: 113, 118, 125, 140, 222, 255; 4: *404*, 417
  adult orthopaedics and, 2: 157
  on AEF medical care organization, 4: 417
  AEF splint board, 4: 416
  American Ambulance Hospital and, 2: 117–123; 4: 386, 389*b*, *390*, 392–393
  on Andry's *Orthopaedia*, 1: xxii
  AOA preparedness committee, 4: 394
  on arthritis and rheumatic disease, 4: 58
  back pain research and, 3: 203
  Base Hospital No. 5 and, 4: 420, 421*b*, 422, 422*b*, *422*
  Beth Israel Hospital and, 4: 208*b*, 247
  Boston Children's Hospital and, 1: 192; 2: 16, 40–41, 114, 132–133, 140, 247, 274, 282; 3: 99
  Brigham and Women's Hospital and, 4: 195*b*
  British Expeditionary Forces and, 4: 420
  Burrage Hospital and, 4: 226
  Carney Hospital and, 2: 116
  as chief at MGH, 1: 151, 192
  chronic disease treatment and, 4: 52
  as clinical professor, 1: 158
  curative workshops and, 4: 403–404
  death of, 2: 140
  Department for Military Orthopedics and, 4: 405
  Diseases of the Bones and Joints, 2: 117; 3: 81–82
  education and training, 2: 113–114
  on Edward H. Bradford, 2: 44
  elegance and, 2: 138–140
  end-results clinics and, 1: 194
  European medical studies, 2: 116
  faculty salary, 1: 177, 179
  on FitzSimmons, 2: 258–259
  on foot problems, 2: 56, 123–124
  foot strength apparatus and, 2: 101–102
  Fundamentals of Orthopaedic Surgery in General Medicine and Surgery, 2: 135–136
  George W. Gay Lecture, 4: 324
  Georgia Warm Springs Foundation and, 2: 78
  hand-washing policy, 1: 193
  Harvard Unit and, 2: 119–121, 123–124; 3: *180*, 369, *370*; 4: 386–387, 421*b*
  HCORP and, 1: 192–195
  as head of HMS orthopaedic surgery department, 1: 174–175, 177, 192
  HMS appointment, 2: 116, 133–135
  honorary degrees, 2: 137
  House of the Good Samaritan and, 2: 113–114
  identification of Osgood-Schlatter disease, 2: 115, *116*, 117
  John Ball and Buckminster Brown Professorship, 2: 133; 4: 195*b*
  Journal of Bone and Joint Surgery editor, 2: 130
  Katzeff and, 2: 275
  King Manuel II and, 4: 401
  on Legg-Calve-Perthes disease, 2: 105
  Lovett Fund and, 2: 82
  marriage and family, 2: 138
  MGH and, 2: 116–117, 129–134; 3: 67
  MGH crystal laboratory, 2: 322
  MGH Fracture Clinic and, 3: 313; 4: 464
  as MGH orthopaedics chief, 3: 11*b*, 227, 266, 268; 4: 472*b*
  MGH surgical intern, 1: 189
  military orthopaedics and, 2: 124–128; 4: 403, 406–407, 412, 417–419, 423*b*, 453
  on mobilization of stiffened joints, 4: 27*b*
  "Nation and the Hospital, The," 2: 137–138, 138*b*–139*b*
  New England Surgical Society president, 2: 136
  Ober on, 2: 148
  as orthopaedic chair, 2: 15*b*
  orthopaedic research support, 1: 193, 195
  orthopaedic surgery and, 1: xxiii; 2: 79, 106, 116–117, 132, 140
  "Orthopaedic Work in a War Hospital," 2: 120
  orthopaedics education and, 1: 152; 2: 133–136
  Orthopedics and Body Mechanics Committee, 4: 235
  poetry of, 2: 128–129, 129*b*, 140
  poliomyelitis treatment, 2: 77, 264
  on preventative measures, 2: 122–123
  private medical practice and, 1: 176; 3: 338
  professional memberships, 2: 136–137
  as professor of orthopaedic surgery, 1: 172
  "Progress in Orthopaedic Surgery" series, 2: 43, 297
  publications and research, 2: 135–137; 4: 32, 65, 421*b*
  as radiologist, 2: 114–115
  RBBH and, 4: 25–26, 28, 31, 56
  on rehabilitation of wounded soldiers, 4: 451
  roentgenograms and, 2: 54, 116
  on sacroiliac joint fusion, 3: 184–185
  scoliosis treatment, 2: 87
  on synovial fluid diagnosis, 3: 175
  on transformation of orthopaedic surgeons, 2: 130*b*–131*b*, 132
  treatment of fractures, 3: 61
  US Army Medical Corps and, 3: 61
  on visceroptosis, 3: 87–88
  war injury studies and, 2: 128–129
  World War I and, 2: 65, 117–128; 3: 157, 166; 4: 403, 406–407, 412, 417, 421*b*
  World War II volunteers and, 4: 363
Osgood Visiting Professors, 2: 141*b*
Osgood-Schlatter disease, 2: 89, 115, *116*, 117
Osler, Sir William, 1: 1, 185, 275; 3: 2; 4: vii, *6*
osteoarthritis

articular cartilage structure
research, 3: 383–384, *385*
bilateral, 3: 244, 279
biomechanical factors in, 3: 322,
326–328, 383
etiology of, 3: 327
femoral neck fractures and,
3: 383–384
hip surgery and, 3: 155
histologic-histochemical grading
systems, 3: 384, 384*t*, 385
knee arthroplasty and,
4: 70*b*–71*b*
Mankin System and, 3: 384,
384*t*
mold arthroplasty and,
3: 195–196
nylon arthroplasty in, 4: 65
periacetabular osteotomy and,
2: 389
total hip replacement and,
3: 221, *222*
total knee replacement and,
4: 177
Osteoarthritis Cartilage Histopathology Assessment System (OARSI),
3: 384–385
osteoarthrosis, 3: 328
osteochondritis, 3: 363
osteochondritis deformans juvenilis,
2: 103–104. *See also* Legg-Calvé-
Perthes disease
osteochondritis dissecans,
2: 194–195
osteogenic sarcoma, 4: 102
osteolysis
after total hip replacement,
3: 220, *220*, 221–222, *222*,
223, 225
associated with acetabular
replacement, 3: 279
rapid postoperative in Paget Disease, 3: 441
osteomalacia, 3: 388
osteomyelitis
in children, 2: 169
following intramedullary nailing of femoral shaft fractures,
2: 249
Green and, 2: 169–170
in infants, 2: 169–170
of the metatarsals and phalanges,
1: 120
orthopaedic research and,
1: 193, 252, 256
pyogenic spinal, 3: 254
radical removal of diseased bone
and, 1: 252
septic wounds in, 3: 301
Staphylococcus and, 2: 169

Streptococcus and, 2: 169
treatment of, 2: 169–170
osteonecrosis
acetabular, 2: 392–394
of the femoral head, 2: 328–329;
3: 434; 4: 156–157
osteoarticular allografts and,
3: 433
pinning of the contralateral hip
and, 2: 380
osteosarcoma
adjuvant therapy and, 3: 432
allografts and, 3: 433
amputations and, 3: 136, 391,
432
chemotherapy and, 2: 422
hip disarticulation for, 1: 78
limb salvage surgery and, 3: 391,
432–433
of the proximal humerus, 2: 398
wide surgical margin and, 3: 433
osteotomies
Bernese periacetabular,
2: 391–392
Boston Concept, 2: 391–392
Chiari, 2: 345
club foot and, 2: 28–29, 36
Cotton, 4: 329
derotation, 2: 34
derotational humeral, 2: 419
femoral derotation for anteversion, 2: 33–34
hips and, 4: 171
innominate, 2: 345
for knee flexion contractures,
2: 117
knee stabilization and, 1: 279
kyphosis and, 3: 239–240
La Coeur's triple, 2: 390
lateral epicondyle, 3: 441
leg lengthening and, 2: 110
Meisenbach's procedure, 4: 188
metatarsal, 4: 188
paralytic flat foot deformities,
2: 210
periacetabular, 2: 389–394
Salter innominate, 2: 390–391
scoliosis treatment, 2: 342
subtrochanteric femur, 1: 68
subtrochanteric hip, 2: 293
total hip replacement and, 3: 221
trochanteric, 4: 133, 145
Van Nes rotational, 2: 345
VCR procedure, 2: 362
Wagner spherical, 2: 390–392
Osterman, A. Lee, 3: 431
Otis, James, 1: 13, 15
Ottemo, Anita, 4: 266
Otto Aufranc Award, 3: 224

Outline of Practical Anatomy, An
(John Warren), 1: 88
Oxland, Thomas R., 4: 266*b*
Ozuna, Richard, 1: 230; 4: 193,
195*b*

P

Pace, James, 2: 379
Paget, James, 1: 81; 2: 172, 194;
3: 25
Paget Disease, 3: 441
Paine, R. S., 2: 172
Painter, Charles F. (1869–1947),
4: 44
as AOA president, 2: 64;
4: 46–47
back pain research and, 3: 203
Beth Israel Hospital and, 4: 208*b*
bone and joint disorders, 3: 82
on Brackett, 3: 150, 161
Burrage Hospital and, 4: 226
Carney Hospital and, 2: 102;
4: 44–45
clinical congress meeting, 3: 116
death of, 4: 51
Diseases of the Bones and Joints,
2: 117; 3: 81; 4: 45
education and training, 4: 44
HMS appointment, 4: 44
hospital appointments, 4: 48
internal derangement of knee-
joints case, 4: 48
Journal of Bone and Joint Surgery
editor, 3: 161, 344; 4: 50
Massage, 3: 266
on medical education, 4: 49,
49*b*, 49, 50
MGH and, 4: 45
on orthopaedic surgeon versus
physician, 4: 47*b*
on physical therapy, 3: 266*b*
private medical practice, 2: 116
professional memberships,
4: 50*b*, 51
publications and research,
4: 44–46, 48, 50
RBBH and, 4: 25–26, 28, 31,
39*b*, 45, 56, 79, 406
as RBBH chief of orthopaedics,
4: 45–48, 79, 196*b*
rehabilitation of soldiers and,
4: 444
sacroiliac joint treatment, 3: 183
Tufts Medical School appointment, 4: 44–45, 48
World War I and, 4: 47
Paley multiplier method, 2: 194
Palmer Memorial Hospital, 2: 219,
219, 220; 4: 275, *275*, 276

Index

Panagakos, Panos G., 4: 22, 116, 128, 193
Pancoast, Joseph, 1: 79
Panjabi, Manohar M., 4: 260–262
Papin, Edouard, 3: 233–234
Pappano, Laura, 1: 285
Pappas, Alex, 2: 285
Pappas, Arthur M. (1931–2016), 2: *286, 288*
   athletic injury clinic and, 2: 287
   "Biomechanics of Baseball Pitching," 2: *288*
   Boston Children's Hospital and, 2: 277, 285–287
   Boston Red Sox and, 2: 288
   Brigham and Women's Hospital and, 4: 193
   on combined residency program, 1: 192, 210
   community organizations and, 2: 289
   Crippled Children's Clinic and, 2: 287
   death of, 2: 289
   education and training, 2: 285
   famous patients of, 2: 288
   as interim orthopaedic surgeon-in-chief, 2: 285–286
   MGH/Children's Hospital residency, 2: 285
   military service, 2: 285
   as orthopaedic chair, 2: 15*b*, 371
   Pappas Rehabilitation Hospital, 2: 39
   PBBH and, 2: 285; 4: 22, 116, 128
   private medical practice and, 2: 313
   professional leadership positions, 2: 289, 289*b*
   publications of, 2: 285, *287*, 288, 368
   on residency program, 1: 208
   sports medicine and, 2: 287–288
   on sports medicine clinic, 2: 384
   University of Massachusetts and, 2: 286–288, 371
   Upper Extremity Injuries in the Athlete, 2: 288
Pappas, Athena, 2: 285
Pappas, Martha, 2: 289
Pappas Rehabilitation Hospital, 2: 39
paralysis. *See also* obstetrical paralysis; poliomyelitis
   brachial plexus, 2: 96
   Bradford frame and, 2: 30
   of the deltoid muscle, 2: 148, 230
   exercise treatment for, 3: 265
   foot and ankle treatment, 2: 150–151
   of the gluteus maximus, 2: 146
   hip abductor treatment, 2: 149–150
   nerve lesions and, 2: 120
   Pott's Disease and, 3: 148–149
   radial nerve, 3: 64
   Roosevelt and, 2: 71–78
   spinal cord injury, 3: 347
   spinal tuberculosis and, 2: 309
   treatment of spastic, 2: 36, 172, 196
Paraplegia Hospital (Ahmadabad, India), 3: 423
Paré, Ambrose, 1: 55; 3: 48
Parfouru-Porel, Germaine, 3: 369–370
Park Prewett Hospital, 4: 363
Parker, Isaac, 1: 45–46
Parker Hill, 4: 23*b*, 24, *35*
Parker Hill Hospital, 2: 358; 4: 327, *328*
Parkman, Francis, 1: 298, 307
Parkman, George (1790–1849), 1: *292*
   care of the mentally ill, 1: 293–295
   dental cast, 1: *308*
   disappearance of, 1: 298, 303–304
   education and training, 1: 292–293
   Harvard Medical School and, 1: 296
   home of, 1: *313*
   on John Collins Warren, 1: 296
   John Webster and, 1: 302–303
   money-lending and, 1: 297, 302–303
   murder of, 1: 291, 304–312, 315, *315*, 318; 3: 40
   philanthropy and, 1: 295–297
   remains found, 1: 304, *305*, 306, *306*, 307–308
Parkman, George F., 1: *313*, 314
Parkman, Samuel (businessman), 1: 292
Parkman, Samuel (surgeon), 1: 60, 62; 3: 15
Parkman Bandstand, 1: *313*, 314
Parks, Helen, 4: 389*b*
Parran, Thomas, Jr., 4: 467
Parsons, Langdon, 3: 301
Partners Department of Orthopaedic Surgery, 1: 181
Partners Healthcare, 3: 462; 4: 192–194
Partners Orthopaedics, 4: 284
Partridge, Oliver, 1: 13

Pasteur, Louis, 1: 82
Patel, Dinesh G. (1936–), 3: *421, 424, 461*
   arthroscopic surgery and, 3: 422–423, 448
   Center of Healing Arts and, 3: 423
   Children's Hospital/MGH combined program and, 3: 422
   discoid medial meniscus tear case, 3: 422
   early life, 3: 421
   education and training, 3: 422
   HCORP and, 1: 230; 3: 423
   HMS appointment, 3: 422, 424
   honors and awards, 3: 424
   hospital appointments, 3: 422
   Massachusetts Board of Registration in Medicine and, 3: 423
   as MGH clinical faculty, 3: 464*b*
   as MGH surgeon, 3: 398*b*, 423
   Patient Care Assessment (PCA) Committee, 3: 423
   professional memberships and, 3: 422–423
   publications and research, 3: 424
   sports medicine and, 3: 388*t*, 396, 422, 448, 460*b*
Patel, Shaun, 4: 190*b*
patella. *See* knees
Pathophysiology of Orthopaedic Diseases (Mankin), 4: 226
Pathway Health Network, 4: 280
Patient Care Assessment (PCA) Committee, 3: 423
patient-reported outcomes (PRO), 4: 186
Patton, George S., 4: 478
pauciarticular arthritis, 2: 171, 350
Paul, Igor, 2: 407; 3: 326–328
Pauli, C., 3: 384
Payson, George, 3: 237
PBBH. *See* Peter Bent Brigham Hospital (PBBH)
Peabody, Francis, 2: 72; 3: 244; 4: 297
Peale, Rembrandt, 1: 23
Pearson, Ruth Elizabeth, 1: 276
Pediatric Orthopaedic International Seminars program, 2: 304
Pediatric Orthopaedic Society (POS), 2: 304, 351
Pediatric Orthopaedic Study Group (POSG), 2: 351, 425
pediatric orthopaedics. *See also* Boston Children's Hospital (BCH)
   ACL reconstruction and, 2: 385–386
   Bradford Frame and, 2: 30

children's convalescence and,
2: 9
children's hospitals and, 2: 3–9
congenital dislocated hips (CDH)
and, 2: 34
congenital kyphosis and, 2: 366
"Dark Ages" of, 2: 15
early medical literature on, 2: 7
flat feet treatment, 2: 107–108
Goldthwait and, 2: 101
Green and, 2: 168
hip disease and, 2: 108
Hresko and, 2: 365
infant and neonatal mortality,
2: 15
Karlin and, 2: 370
leg lengthening and, 2: 110
Legg and, 2: 101, 106–107
managing fractures, 2: 379
polio treatment, 2: 109–110
societies for, 2: 351
sports injuries and, 2: 287,
385–387
Tachdjian and, 2: 300–304
trauma and, 2: 365, 368, 385
tuberculosis of the spine and,
2: 11
valgus deformity treatment,
2: 209
Pediatric Orthopedic Deformities
(Shapiro), 2: 403, *404*
Pediatric Orthopedic Society of
North America (POSNA), 2: *346*,
347, 351, *351*, 363, *363*, 364, 403,
425
Pediatric Orthopedics (Tachdjian),
2: 188, 303, *303*
pedicle screws, 2: 343; 3: 420
Pedlow, Francis X, Jr. (1959–),
3: *424*
anterior vertebral reconstruction
with allograft research, 3: 426,
426
early life, 3: 424–425
education and training, 3: 425
HCORP and, 3: 426
HMS appointment, 3: 426
as MGH clinical faculty, 3: 464*b*
as MGH surgeon, 3: 426
open anterior lumbosacral fracture dislocation case, 3: 425
professional memberships and,
3: 426
publications and research, 3: 426
spinal surgeries and, 3: 425–426,
460*b*
Pedlow, Francis X, Sr., 3: 424
Pedlow, Marie T. Baranello, 3: 424
Pedrick, Katherine F., 3: 154

Peking Union Medical College,
3: 365
Pellicci, Paul, 4: 134–135
Peltier, L. F., 1: 106
Pemperton, Ralph, 4: 32
Peninsular Base Station (PBS),
4: 481–482
Pennsylvania Hospital, 1: 183
periacetabular osteotomy,
2: 389–391
Perkins, Leroy, 2: 159–160
Perkins Institution and the Massachusetts School for the Blind,
1: 273
Perlmutter, Gary S., 1: 166–167;
3: 415, 460*b*, 464*b*
Perry, Jacqueline, 3: 248
Pershing, John J., 3: 168
Person, Eleanor, 3: 281
Perthes, George, 2: 103, 105;
3: 165
Perthes disease. *See* Legg-Calvé-
Perthes disease
Peter Bent Brigham Hospital Corporation, 4: 2–3
Peter Bent Brigham Hospital
(PBBH), 4: *2, 7, 8, 9, 11, 15, 117*
Administrative Building, 4: *115,
191*
advancement of medicine and,
4: 5
affiliation with RBBH, 4: 34,
36, 39
annual reports, 4: 6, 16, 18
Banks on, 4: 73*b*–74*b*
Base Hospital No. 5 and, 4: 420*t*
blood bank, 4: 107
board of overseers, 4: 132
bone and joint cases, 4: *16*
Boston Children's Hospital and,
4: 10, 14
Brigham Anesthesia Associates,
4: 22
cerebral palsy cases, 2: 172
Clinical Research Center floor
plan, 4: *21*
construction of, 4: *4*, *4*, 5
faculty group practice, 4: 13,
21–22
faculty model at, 1: 176
50th anniversary, 4: 20–21, 21*b*
founding of, 2: 42; 4: 2–3
fracture treatment and, 4: 18–19,
22, 108
Francis Street Lobby, 4: *119*
general surgery service at,
4: 8–10, 14, 16
grand rounds and, 4: 118
growth of, 4: 20, 22
history of, 4: 1

HMS and, 4: 1–4, 12, *12*, 13–14
Industrial Accident Clinic,
4: 21–22
industrial accidents and, 4: 19, 21
internships at, 1: 189, 196
leadership of, 4: 4–5, 9–11,
14–19, 22, 99, 127
opening of, 4: *6*
orthopaedic service chiefs at, 4: 43
orthopaedic surgeons at,
4: 116–117
orthopaedic surgery at, 1: 171;
4: 8, 11, 16–18, 22, 115–116
orthopaedics as specialty at, 4: 1,
18
orthopaedics diagnoses at, 4: 6–8
orthopaedics residencies, 1: 199,
204, 207; 4: 19
outpatient services at, 1: 173;
4: 5–6, 14, 20, 22
patient volume at, 4: 124*t*, 129
Pavilion C (Ward I), 4: *8*
Pavilion F, 4: *7*
Pavilion Wards, 4: *115*
plans for, 4: *7*
professors of surgery at, 1: 174
report of bone diseases, 4: 13, 13*t*
research program at, 4: 75*b*
Spanish Flu at, 4: *11*
staffing of, 4: 5, 9, 18–19,
21–22, 128–129, 161–163
surgeon-scholars at, 4: 43, 79
surgery specialization at,
4: 10–12, 15–16, 18–20
surgical research laboratory, 4: 12,
12
surgical residencies, 1: 90
teaching clinics at, 1: 155,
157–158, 194; 4: 14
transition to Brigham and
Women's Hospital, 4: 42, 69,
113–114, 116, 116*b*, 117–119,
121, 127, 132
trust for, 4: 1, 3
World War I and, 4: 9–10, 79
World War II and, 4: 17–18
Zander Room at, 4: 14
Peter Bent Brigham Hospital Surgical
Associates, 4: 21–22
Peters, Jessica, 3: 328
Petersdorf, Robert G., 4: 121
Peterson, L., 3: 210
Petit Lycée de Talence, 4: *429, 430,*
432
Pfahler, George E., 3: 142
Pharmacopoeia of the United States,
1: 300
Phelps, A. M., 2: 99
Phelps, Abel, 4: 463
Phelps, Winthrop M., 1: 193; 2: 294

Index

Phemister, D. B., 2: 170–171, *192*
Phillips, William, 1: 41; 3: 5, 75
Phillips House (MGH), 1: 86, 204; 3: *72*, *73*, 75
phocomelia, 2: 334
Phoenix Mutual Insurance Company, 2: 267
phrenicectomy, 4: 215
physical therapy
    athletic training and, 1: 258, 266; 3: 348
    DeLorme table and, 3: 284
    early 20th century status of, 3: 266, 266*b*
    Elgin table, 3: 284, *287*
    knee flexion contracture and, 3: 375
    Legg and, 2: 107
    massage and, 1: 100; 3: 266, 297
    medical schools and, 4: 396–397
    for paralyzed children, 2: 61, 107
    RBBH patient in, 4: *28*, *29*
    rehabilitation equipment for, 2: 107
    Roosevelt and, 2: 74
    sports medicine and, 2: 287
    tenotomy and, 1: 100
    Zander's medico-mechanical equipment, 3: 71, *71*
Physical Therapy in Infantile Paralysis (Legg and Merrill), 2: 107
physicians
    bleeding and, 1: 9
    board certification of, 4: 324, 377
    18th century demand for, 1: 7–8
    examinations for, 1: 15, 21, 29
    Jewish, 1: 158; 4: 199–200, 202
    licensing of, 1: 184, 190
    medical degrees and, 1: 6–7, 26–28
    standards for, 1: 26
    surgical training and, 1: 184
Physicians' Art Society of Boston, 4: 329–330
Pierce, Donald S. (1930–), 3: *461*
    Amputees and Their Prostheses, 3: 320
    Cervical Spine Research Society president, 3: 321
    early life, 3: 320
    education and training, 3: 320
    electromyogram use, 3: 320
    familial bilateral carpal tunnel syndrome case, 3: 321
    Halo Vest, 3: 321
    HMS appointment, 3: 320
    marriage and, 3: 321
    as MGH clinical faculty, 3: 464*b*
    as MGH surgeon, 3: 248, 320, 398*b*
    orthopaedics treatment tools and, 3: 321
    on pressure sores management, 3: 321
    publications and research, 3: 320–321, 355
    rehabilitation and, 3: 388*t*, 459, 461
    spine surgery and, 3: 460*b*
    Total Care of Spinal Cord Injuries, The, 3: 321
Pierce, F. Richard, 1: 264
Pierce, Janet, 3: 321
Pierce, R. Wendell, 1: 284; 3: 299
Pierce, Wallace L., 4: 39*b*
Pierce Collar, 3: 321
Pierce Fusion, 3: 321
Pierce Graft, 3: 321
Pierson, Abel Lawrence, 1: 60, 62
Pilcher, Lewis S., 4: 318
Pinel, Philippe, 1: 293–294
Pinkney, Carole, 3: 382
Pio Istituto Rachitici, 2: 36
Pittsburgh Orthopaedic Journal, 1: 232
plantar fasciitis, 3: 437–438
plantar fasciotomy, 2: 24
Plaster-of-Paris Technique in the Treatment of Fractures (Quigley), 1: 277
plastic surgery
    development of, 1: 76
    introduction to the U.S., 1: 71–72, 77
    orthopaedics curriculum and, 1: 150, 218
Plath, Sylvia, 2: 272
Platt, Sir Harry, 1: 114; 3: 369; 4: 464
Ploetz, J. E., 3: 440
pneumonia, 1: 74; 2: 4, 306
Poehling, Gary G., 2: 279
Polavarapu, H. V., 1: 186
poliomyelitis
    Berlin epidemic of, 2: 260, 264
    Boston epidemic of, 2: 213, 314–315
    calcaneus deformity, 2: 189–190
    children's hospitals and, 3: 307
    circulatory changes in, 2: 316
    electricity and, 2: 62
    epidemics of, 1: 191; 2: 61
    ganglionectomy in, 3: 332
    Green and, 2: 188–191
    Grice and, 2: 208
    Harrington rods, 2: 316, *317*
    heavy-resistance exercise and, 3: 284–285
    hip contracture treatment, 2: 294, 295*b*
    hot pack treatment, 2: 264
    importance of rest in, 2: 63, *63*
    intraspinal serum, 2: 72
    iron lung and, 2: 78, *190*, 191, 260, 264, 314
    Legg and, 2: 107, 109
    Lovett and, 2: 61–63, *63*, 70–72, 74–75, 77, 147–148
    massage treatment for, 2: 62, 73
    moist heat treatment for, 2: 264
    muscle training for, 2: 62–63, 78
    muscle transfers, 2: 154
    nonstandard treatments and, 2: 77
    Ober and, 2: 147–148
    orthopaedic treatment for, 2: 78
    paralysis of the serratus anterior, 2: 154–155
    paralytic flat foot deformities, 2: 210–212
    patient evaluation, 2: 315
    patient reaction to, 2: 261*b*–263*b*
    prevention of contractures, 2: 78
    research in, 3: 209
    rocking beds, 2: 314, *315*
    Roosevelt and, 2: 71–78
    second attacks of, 1: 276
    shoulder arthrodesis, 2: 154
    spinal taps and, 2: 72, 78
    spring muscle test, 2: 70, *70*, 71
    study of, 2: 61–62
    tendon transfers and, 2: 96, 108, *108*, 109, 147–149; 3: 332–333
    treatment of, 2: 61–63, 71–79, 109–110, 188–191
    Trott and, 2: 314, *314*, 315
    unequal limb length and, 3: 331–332
    vaccine development, 2: 189, 191, 264, 315
    Vermont epidemic of, 2: 61–62, 71
Polivy, Kenneth, 3: 254
Pongor, Paul, 4: 279
Pool, Eugene H., 3: 338
Pope, Malcolm, 2: 371
Porter, C. A., 3: 313
Porter, Charles A., 3: 116
Porter, G. A., 1: 174
Porter, John L., 2: 78; 3: 157; 4: 406, 464
Porter, W. T., 4: 216
Poss, Anita, 4: 174
Poss, Robert (1936–), 4: *169*
    ABOS board and, 4: 173

Ames Test and, 4: 171
Brigham and Women's Hospital
and, 4: 163, 172, 193, 195*b*
Brigham Orthopaedic Foundation (BOF) and, 4: 172
Brigham Orthopedic Associates
(BOA) and, 4: 123, 172
as BWH orthopaedics chief,
4: 143, 193, 196*b*
Children's Hospital/MGH combined program and, 4: 169
Deputy Editor for Electronic
Media at *JBJS*, 4: 173–174
education and training, 4: 169
hip arthritis research, 4: 170
hip osteotomy research, 2: 390;
4: 171
HMS appointment, 4: 171–172
on Hylamer acetabular liner complications, 4: *171*, 172
marriage and family, 4: 174
MIT postdoctoral biology fellowship, 4: 169–170
PBBH and, 4: 163
private medical practice, 4: 169
professional memberships, 4: 174
publications and research,
4: 169–170, *170*, 171–172,
174
RBBH and, 4: 132, 134,
169–171
on total hip arthroplasty, 3: 223;
4: 134, 170–172, 174
US Navy and, 4: 169
Post, Abner, 4: 307
posterior cruciate ligament (PCL)
avulsion of, 2: 386
biomechanical effects of injury
and repair, 3: 448
pediatric orthopaedics and,
2: 381
retention in total knee replacement, 4: 130, 138–139, 147,
180–181
robotics-assisted research, 3: 450
posterior interosseous syndrome,
4: 165–166
posterior segment fixator (PSF),
3: 420
posture. *See also* body mechanics
body types and, 4: 235, *236*
Bradford on, 2: 36
chart of normal and abnormal,
4: *84*, *234*
Chelsea Survey of, 4: 234–235
children and, 2: 36; 3: 83
contracted iliotibial band and,
2: 152
Goldthwait and, 3: 80–81, 83,
85–91; 4: 53

Harvard study in, 4: 84, *84*,
85–86, 234, *234*
high-heeled shoes and, 2: 317
impact on military draft, 4: 233
medical conflict and, 3: 83
Ober operation and, 2: 153
research in, 4: 233–235, *235*
school children and, 4: 233–234,
234, 235, *236*
scoliosis and, 1: 109
standards for, 4: *236*
Swaim on, 4: 52–54
types of, 4: 85–86
Potter, Constance, 4: 69
Potter, Theodore A. (1912–1995),
4: *67*
arthritis treatment, 4: 67
Boston University appointment,
4: 67
Children's Hospital/MGH combined program and, 4: 68
death of, 4: 69
education and training, 4: 67
HMS appointment, 4: 69
knee arthroplasty and, 4: 64, *65*,
68–69, 70*b*–71*b*
marriage and family, 4: 69
on McKeever and MacIntosh
prostheses, 4: 189
nylon arthroplasty in arthritic
knees, 4: 65–66, 69
orthopaedic research and, 4: 38
private medical practice, 4: 67
professional memberships, 4: 69
publications and research, 4: 67,
68, 69, 96
RBBH and, 4: 35, 37–38,
67–68, 89, 93, 116*b*, 187
as RBBH chief of orthopaedics,
4: 40, 41*b*, 63, 66–69, 79, 102,
196*b*
Tufts appointment, 4: 69
Pott's Disease, 1: xxiii, 97, *97*, 105,
108–109; 2: 25, *31*, 247; 3: 148,
149, *154*, *155*
Pott's fracture, 4: *317*, 318
Prabhakar, M. M., 3: 423
*Practical Biomechanics for the
Orthopedic Surgeon* (Radin et al.),
3: 328
PRE (*Progressive Resistance Exercise*)
(DeLorme and Watkins), 3: *286*
Presbyterian Hospital, 2: 74–75
Prescott, William, 1: 18
press-fit condylar knee (PFC),
4: 180, 180*t*
pressure correction apparatus (Hoffa-Schede), 3: *151*, 152
pressure sores, 3: 321
Preston, Thomas, 1: 14

Price, Mark, 4: 190*b*
Price, Mark D., 3: 463*b*
Priestley, Joseph, 1: 56
*Principles of Orthopedic Surgery for
Nurses, The* (Sever), 2: 92, *93*
Principles of Orthopedic Surgery
(Sever), 2: 92, *93*
Pristina Hospital (Kosovo),
3: 416–417
Pritchett, Henry S., 1: 147
Problem Back Clinic (MGH), 3: 254
"Progress in Orthopaedic Surgery"
series, 2: 43, 297
progressive resistance exercises,
3: 285–286
Project HOPE, 3: 417, *417*
prospective payment system (PPS),
3: 397
Prosperi, Lucia, 1: *59*
Prosperi, Warren, 1: *59*
Prosser, W.C.H., 4: 482*b*
prostheses
all-plastic tibial, 4: 148
Austin Moore, 3: 213, 241, 354*b*
biomechanical aspects of hip,
2: 407
bone ingrowth, 3: 220–223
Brigham and Women's Hospital
and, 4: 122
Buchholz shoulder, 2: 423
capitellocondylar total elbow,
4: 145, *145*, 146–147
Cohen and patents for, 2: 237
distal humerus, 2: 250
Duocondylar, 4: 178
duopatellar, 4: 130, 180*t*
electromyographic (EMG) signals
and, 2: 326
femoral replacement, 4: 69
femoral stem, 3: *293*
hinged elbow, 4: 147
hip replacement, 2: 407
internal, 2: 423
Judet hip, 3: 293
Kinematic knee, 4: 138–139,
147, 149–150
knee arthroplasty and, 3: 292
LTI Digital™ Arm Systems for
Adults, 2: 326
MacIntosh, 4: 69, 71*b*, 129, 188
Marmor modular design, 4: 130
McKeever, 4: 40, 69, 70*b*–71*b*,
129–130, 177, 188–189
metal and polyethylene, 4: 148
metallic, 3: 433
myoelectric, 2: 326
nonconstrained total elbow,
4: 145
non-hinged metal–polyethylene,
4: 145–146

Index

PFC unicompartmental knee, 4: 177
press-fit condylar knee (PFC), 4: 180, 180t
suction socket, 1: 273
temporary, 3: 374
total condylar, 4: 130
total knee, 4: 137
unicompartmental, 4: 176, 178
used in knee arthroplasty, 4: 179t
Prosthetic Research and Development Unit (Ontario Crippled Children's Center), 2: 335
Province House, 3: 6–7, 9, 9
psoas abscesses, 2: 53–54; 4: 225
psoriatic arthritis, 4: 99
Ptasznik, Ronnie, 3: 437
public health, 2: 61, 107, 425
Pugh, J., 3: 327
pulmonary embolism (PE), 3: 196, 218, 362
pulmonary function
    anterior and posterior procedures, 2: 360
    corrective casts and, 2: 265
    Milwaukee Brace and, 2: 265–266
    scoliosis and, 2: 343
    spine fusion and, 2: 265
    thromboembolism pathophysiology, 1: 82
pulmonary tuberculosis, 1: 56; 2: 9, 16; 3: 25, 128
Pulvertaft, Guy, 3: 427; 4: 95
Putnam, George, 1: 312–313, 317
Putnam, Israel, 1: 18
Putnam, James Jackson, 2: 20
Putti, Vittorio, 2: 80; 3: 203; 4: 14, 65
pyloric stenosis, 3: 49–50

Q

Quain, Jones, 2: 242
Quain's Anatomy (Quain et al.), 2: 242
Queen Victoria Hospital, 2: 421, 422
quiet necrosis, 2: 194
Quigley, Daniel Thomas, 1: 275
Quigley, Ruth Elizabeth Pearson, 1: 276, 282
Quigley, Thomas B. (1908–1982), 1: 275, 281; 4: 342
    on acromioclavicular joint dislocation in football, 1: 268
    AMA Committee on the Medical Aspects of Sports, 1: 280
    Athlete's Bill of Rights and, 1: 280–281
    athletic injury clinic and, 2: 287
    Boston City Hospital and, 4: 297
    on Dr. Nichols, 1: 257
    education and training, 1: 276
    5th General Hospital and, 4: 484
    Harvard athletics surgeon, 1: 276–279
    Harvard University Health Service and, 1: 277
    as HMS professor, 1: 277
    legacy of, 1: 282–283
    PBBH and, 1: 204, 276–277; 2: 279; 4: 18–21, 116
    pes anserinus transplant, 1: 279
    Plaster-of-Paris Technique in the Treatment of Fractures, 1: 277
    publications of, 1: 268, 276–282; 2: 220
    sports medicine and, 1: 277–283
    US General Hospital No. 5 and, 4: 485
    WWII active duty and, 1: 270, 277; 4: 17
Quinby, William, 4: 11
Quincy, Josiah, 1: 14
Quincy City Hospital, 2: 256

R

Rabkin, Mitchell, 4: 255, 281
radiation synovectomy, 4: 64, 136
Radin, Crete Boord, 3: 328
Radin, Eric L. (1934–2020), 3: 322, 323, 328
    Beth Israel Hospital and, 3: 325
    biomechanics research, 3: 326–328
    Boston Children's Hospital and, 3: 325
    Children's Hospital/MGH combined program and, 3: 322
    death of, 3: 328
    early life, 3: 322
    education and training, 3: 322
    fracture research and, 3: 322–324
    on Glimcher, 2: 326
    on Green, 2: 177
    Henry Ford Hospital and, 3: 328
    HMS appointment, 3: 325, 327
    joint lubrication research, 3: 324–325, 325, 326, 326, 327
    marriages and family, 3: 328
    MIT appointment, 3: 325
    Mount Auburn Hospital and, 3: 327
    neuritis with infectious mononucleosis case, 3: 324–325
    Practical Biomechanics for the Orthopedic Surgeon, 3: 328
    publications and research, 2: 396, 396, 397, 406; 3: 322–326, 326, 327–328
    subchondral bone research, 3: 326–327, 327
    Tufts Medical School and, 3: 328
    University of Michigan appointment, 3: 328
    US Air Force Hospital and, 3: 323
    West Virginia University School of Medicine and, 3: 328
Radin, Tova, 3: 328
radiography
    diagnostic value of, 2: 56
    growth calculation and, 2: 194
    Harvard Athletic Association and, 1: 258
    in hip disease, 2: 54
    leg-length discrepancy and, 3: 299
    scoliosis treatment, 2: 366
radiology. *See also* roentgenograms
    Boston Children's Hospital and, 2: 16, 16, 17, 17t
    HMS and, 2: 16
    Osgood and, 2: 114–116
Radius Management Services, 4: 212
Radius Specialty Hospital, 4: 212
Ragaswamy, Leela, 2: 439b
Ralph K. Ghormley Traveling Scholarship, 3: 290
Ramappa, Arun, 4: 287
Ranawat, Chit, 4: 130, 134
Rancho Los Amigos, 4: 129, 151, 151
Rand, Frank, 4: 279–280
Rand, Isaacs, 1: 25
Rand, Jessie Sophia, 3: 79
Ranvier, Louis Antoine, 1: 82; 3: 142
Rappleye, W. C., 1: 189
Ratshesky, Abraham, 3: 134–135
Ray, Robert D., 1: 162
RBBH. *See* Robert Breck Brigham Hospital (RBBH)
Ready, John, 1: 167
Ready, John E., 4: 193, 195b
Rechtine, G. R., 3: 420
Reconstruction Base Hospital No. 1 (Parker Hill, Boston), 4: 328, 445, 446. *See also* US General Hospital No. 10
    Benevolent Order of Elks funding for, 4: 447
    development of, 4: 444–445
    physiotherapy at, 4: 447
    RBBH and, 4: 447–448

rehabilitation goals and, 4: 446–447
Record, Emily, 3: 330
Record, Eugene E. (ca.1910–2004), 3: *329*
   as AAOS fellow, 2: 215
   amputation research, 3: 330
   ankle arthrodesis case, 3: 330
   Boston Children's Hospital and, 2: 299; 3: 329
   Children's Hospital/MGH combined program and, 3: 329
   death of, 3: 330
   early life, 3: 329
   education and training, 3: 329
   Lower Extremity Amputations for Arterial Insufficiency, 1: 90; 3: 330
   Marlborough Medical Associates and, 2: 269
   marriage and family, 3: 330
   as MGH surgeon, 1: 203; 3: 329
   New England Peabody Home for Crippled Children and, 3: 329
   private medical practice, 2: 146; 3: 329
   publications and research, 3: 330
   US Army Reserve and, 3: 329
Record, Eugene E., Jr., 3: 329
Redfern, Peter, 1: xxii
Reed, John, 1: 307; 3: 347
reflex sympathetic dystrophy, 2: 68. *See also* chronic regional pain syndrome (CRPS)
Registry of Bone Sarcoma, 3: 136–142
Rehabilitation Engineering and Assistive Technology Society of North America (RESNA), 2: 408, *408*
Rehabilitation Engineering Research Center, 2: 406
Reid, Bill, 1: 252–253, 255
Reidy, Alice Sherburne, 3: 334
Reidy, John A. (1910–1987)
   early life, 3: 331
   education and training, 3: 331
   effects of irradiation on epiphyseal growth, 3: 331
   Faulkner Hospital and, 3: 331
   fracture research and, 3: 334
   ganglionectomy in polio patient case, 3: 332
   as honorary orthopaedic surgeon, 3: 398*b*
   marriage and family, 3: 334
   as MGH surgeon, 3: 74, 331
   Newton-Wellesley Hospital and, 3: 331
   polio research, 3: 331–333

   professional memberships and, 3: 334
   publications and research, 3: 209, 331–334
   RBBH and, 4: 35, 38, 89, 93
   Slipped Capital Femoral Epiphysis, 3: 294, 333
   slipped capital femoral epiphysis research, 3: 331, 333–334; 4: 237–238
   on tendon transfers in lower extremities, 3: 332–333, *333*
Reilly, Donald, 4: 286
Reinertsen, James L., 4: 283
Reitman, Charles A., 4: 272*b*
Relton, J. E. S., 2: 334–335, *335*
Relton-Hall frame, 2: 334, *335*
Remarks on the Operation for the Cure of Club Feet with Cases (Brown), 1: 100
Remembrances (Coll Warren), 1: 83
Report of Cases in the Orthopedic Infirmary of the City of Boston (J.B. Brown), 1: *120*
Reports of Cases Treated at the Boston Orthopedic Institution (Brown and Brown), 1: *120*
Residency Review Committee (RRC), 1: 211
RESNA. *See* Rehabilitation Engineering and Assistive Technology Society of North America (RESNA)
Resurrectionists (Browne), 1: *21*
Reverdin, Jaques-Louis, 4: 216
Revere, Anne, 2: 272
Revere, John, 1: 293
Revere, Paul, 1: 8, 13–17, 19–20, 22, 28, *28*; 2: 272
Reynolds, Edward, 3: 42
Reynolds, Fred, 4: 125
Reynolds, Fred C., 1: 162
rheumatic fever, 2: 171
Rheumatism Foundation Hospital, 4: 96
rheumatoid arthritis
   body mechanics and, 4: 82–83
   boutonniere deformities of the hand, 4: 98
   children and, 2: 164, 171, 350
   foot surgery and, 4: 188, *188*
   gene therapy and, 2: 82
   genetics in, 4: 169
   of the hand, 4: 96–98, *98*
   hindfoot pain, 4: 188, *189*
   knee arthroplasty and, 4: 70*b*–71*b*
   MacIntosh prothesis and, 4: 188
   McKeever prothesis and, 4: 188–189

   metacarpophalangeal arthroplasty, 4: 97
   mold arthroplasty and, 3: 239
   nylon arthroplasty in, 4: *65*
   opera-glass hand deformity, 4: 99
   radiation synovectomy and, 4: 136
   release of contractures in arthroplasty, 4: 166
   swan neck deformity, 4: 98
   synovectomy of the knee in, 4: 102
   thumb deformities, 4: 97
   total hip replacement and, 4: 134
   total knee replacement and, 4: 181
   treatment for, 4: 97, 138
   upper extremities and, 2: 137
   wrist joint damage in, 4: 166–167, *168*
rheumatoid synovitis, 4: 166
rheumatology, 2: 321
Rhinelander, Frederic W., Jr. (1906–1990), 3: *335*
   Boston Children's Hospital and, 3: 335
   burn care and, 3: 336
   Case Western Reserve University School of Medicine and, 3: 337
   death of, 3: 337
   early life, 3: 335
   education and training, 3: 335
   HMS appointment, 3: 335
   honors and awards, 3: 337, 337*b*
   Letterman Army Hospital and, 3: 336
   marriage and family, 3: 337
   as MGH surgeon, 3: 74, 335
   private medical practice, 3: 336
   publications and research, 3: 335–336, *336*, 337
   Shriners Hospital for Children and, 3: 335
   University of Arkansas College of Medicine and, 3: 337
   University of California Hospital and, 3: 336–337
   US Army and, 3: 336
   US Army Legion of Merit, 3: *337*
Rhinelander, Julie, 3: 337
Rhinelander, Philip Mercer, 3: 335
Rhode Island Hospital, 3: 401
Rhodes, Jonathan, 1: 90
Richard J. Smith Lecture, 3: 431
Richards, Thomas K. (1892–1965)
   Boston City Hospital and, 1: 258
   as football team physician, 1: 258–262

as Harvard athletics surgeon, 1: 258, 262; 4: 303
Harvard Fifth Surgical Service and, 4: 303
on physician's role, 1: 259–262
scientific studies, 1: 262
as team physician for the Boston Red Sox, 1: 258
Richardson, Frank, 1: 255
Richardson, Lars C., 4: 287
Richardson, Mary R., 3: 75
Richardson, Maurice H., 3: 18, 94; 4: 274–275
Richardson, William, 4: 3
rickets, 1: 129; 2: 36, 114; 3: 83, 388
Riley, Donald, 1: 225; 4: 193
Riley, Maureen, 2: 414
Ring, David, 1: 167; 3: 410, 463
Riseborough, Bruce, 2: 400
Riseborough, Edward J. (1925–1985), 2: *395*
   Boston Children's Hospital and, 2: 286, 399; 4: 127
   Brigham and Women's Hospital and, 4: 163, 193
   congenital kyphosis case, 2: 399–400
   death of, 2: 400
   distal femoral physeal fractures research, 2: 400
   education and training, 2: 395
   fat embolism syndrome research, 2: 397, *397*, 398
   HMS appointment, 2: 395, 399
   intercondylar fractures of the humerus research, 2: 397, *397*
   marriage and family, 2: 400
   MGH and, 2: 395; 4: 127
   orthopaedics appointments, 2: 399
   orthopaedics education and, 2: 398–399
   PBBH and, 4: 163
   professional memberships, 2: 400
   publications and research, 2: 385, 396, *396*, 397, 399–400, *400*; 3: 322–323
   rugby and, 2: 385, 400
   Scoliosis and Other Deformities of the Axial Skeleton, 2: 398, *398*
   scoliosis research, 2: 395–396, 399–400, *400*; 4: 127
   trauma research, 2: 396, *396*, 397, 399
Riseborough, Jennifer, 2: 400
Risser, Joseph, 2: 335
Risser cast, 2: 178
RMS *Aurania*, 4: 431

Robbins, Anne Smith, 1: 123–125; 2: 114
Robbins, Chandler, 2: 5
Robert Breck Brigham Hospital Corporation, 4: 23–24, 25*b*
Robert Breck Brigham Hospital for Incurables, 4: 22, 23*b*, 30, 36
Robert Breck Brigham Hospital (RBBH), 4: *26, 28, 31, 35, 37, 40, 42*
   affiliation with PBBH, 4: 34, 36, 39
   annual reports, 4: *37*
   arthritis clinic and, 3: 371; 4: 36
   arthroplasties at, 4: 64
   board of overseers, 4: 132
   Chief of Orthopedic Service report, 4: 41*b*
   chronic disease treatment at, 4: 23*b*, 25*b*, 27–28, 30, 30*b*, 32, 32*b*, 33, 36, 39*b*, 46
   as Clinical Research Center, 4: 38, 40
   clinical teaching at, 4: 32–33
   Emergency Campaign speech, 4: 32, 32*b*
   financial difficulties, 4: 25–26, 28–29, 31–32, 34, 35*b*, 37, 42
   founding of, 4: 22–24
   Goldthwait and, 3: 81, 84, 91–92; 4: 24–25, 25*b*, 26–28, 31, 36–38, 39*b*
   Goldthwait Research Fund, 4: 27
   grand rounds and, 4: 118
   growth in patient volume, 4: 124*t*
   history of, 4: 1
   HMS students and, 4: 30, 69
   laboratory at, 4: *35*
   lawsuit on hospital mission, 4: 29–30, 30*b*
   leadership of, 4: 31–33, 35–36, 38, 39*b*, 40, 41*b*, 42, 99, 127
   Lloyd T. Brown and, 3: 257; 4: 25, 30–34, 36
   military reconstruction hospital and, 4: 443–444
   occupational therapy department, 4: 28, *29*
   orthopaedic advancements at, 4: 40
   orthopaedic research and, 4: 38, 41*b*
   orthopaedic service chiefs at, 4: 43
   orthopaedic surgery at, 1: 171; 4: 28, 31, 40, 41*b*, 115
   orthopaedics and arthritis at, 4: 26–28, 43
   orthopaedics as specialty at, 4: 1

   orthopaedics instruction at, 1: 157; 4: 41*b*, 68
   orthopaedics residencies, 1: 207–208; 4: 30, 40, 131
   patient conditions and outcomes, 4: 29*t*
   patient outcomes, 4: 31*t*
   physical therapy and, 4: *28, 29*
   professorship in orthopedic surgery, 4: 114
   Reconstruction Base Hospital No. 1 and, 4: 445, 447–448
   rehabilitation service at, 4: 37, *38*
   research at, 4: 33, 42, 117, 132
   residencies at, 4: 34–35, 39–40, 42
   rheumatic disease treatment, 4: 47, 136, 188
   as specialty arthritis hospital, 4: 122–123
   staffing of, 4: 25, 28, 32, *34*, 35–38, 45, 68, 131–132
   statistics, 1945, 4: 34*t*
   surgeon-scholars at, 4: 43, 79
   surgery at, 4: *132*
   surgical caseloads at, 4: 131, 131*t*, 132
   total knee arthroplasty and, 4: 129–130, 131*t*
   transition to Brigham and Women's Hospital, 4: 42, 69, 113–114, 116, 116*b*, 117–119, 121, 127, 132
   World War I and, 4: 25–26, 79
   World War II and, 4: 33
Robert Brigham Multipurpose Arthritis and Musculoskeletal Disease Center, 4: 184
Robert C. Hinckley and the Recreation of The First Operation Under Ether (Wolfe), 1: 59
Robert Jones and Agnes Hunt Orthopaedic Hospital, 3: 426
Robert Jones Orthopaedic Society, 2: 132
Robert Leffert Memorial Fund, 3: 415
Robert Salter Award, 2: 415
Robert W. Lovett Memorial Unit for the Study of Crippling Diseases, 2: 82
Robert W. Lovett Professorship, 2: 166; 4: 195*b*
Roberts, Ada Mead, 3: 338
Roberts, Elizabeth Converse, 3: 339
Roberts, Melita Josephine, 2: 143
Roberts, Odin, 3: 338
Roberts, Sumner N. (1898–1939), 3: *338*

cervical spine fracture research, 3: 340–341, *341*
Children's Hospital/MGH combined program and, 3: 338
congenital absence of the odontoid process case, 3: 340
death of, 3: 342
early life, 3: 338
education and training, 3: 338
fracture research and, 3: 339–341, *342*
HMS appointment, 2: 223; 3: 338–339; 4: 61
marriage and family, 3: 339
Massachusetts Eye and Ear Infirmary and, 3: 339
as MGH surgeon, 3: 187, 270, 339
private medical practice, 3: 338
professional memberships and, 3: 341–342
publications and research, 3: 339–341; 4: 63
RBBH and, 3: 339; 4: 31, 60
World War I and, 3: 338
Robinson, James, 1: 248
Robinson, Marie L., 2: 111–112
Robson, A. W. Mayo, 2: 91
Rockefeller Foundation, 1: 147
Rockefeller Institute, 2: 72
rocking beds, 2: *315*
Rocky Mountain Trauma Society, 3: 311
Rodriguez, Edward, 3: 410
Rodriquez, Ken, 4: 287
Roentgen Diagnosis of the Extremities and Spine (Ferguson), 4: 110
Roentgen Method in Pediatrics, The (Rotch), 2: 170
roentgenograms. *See also* x-rays
arthritis and, 4: 64, *64*
in curriculum, 1: 161
diagnosis and, 2: 155; 3: 99
discovery of, 2: 24, 54; 3: 57, 96
MGH and, 3: 20–21
Osgood and Dodd on, 2: 116
slipped capital femoral epiphysis and, 4: 238
total knee arthroplasty-scoring system, 4: 150
ROFEH International, 2: 363, *363*
Rogers, Carolyn, 1: 239
Rogers, Elizabeth Grace, 2: 258
Rogers, Emily, 3: 350
Rogers, Emily Ross, 4: 230
Rogers, Fred A., 1: 180
Rogers, Horatio, 4: 475
Rogers, Margaret, 4: 371

Rogers, Mark H. (1877–1941), 4: *224*
American Journal of Orthopedic Surgery editor, 4: 226
AOA resolution on orthopaedics, 4: 227
as Beth Israel chief of orthopaedics, 4: 220, 223, 228–230, 289*b*
Beth Israel Hospital and, 4: 208*b*
as Boston and Maine Railroad orthopaedic surgeon, 4: 225
Boston City Hospital and, 4: 229–230, 328
Burrage Hospital and, 4: 226
Clinics for Crippled Children and, 2: 230
education and training, 4: 224
Fort Riley base hospital and, 4: 452–453
HMS appointment, 4: 226, 226*b*
legacy of, 4: 230
marriage and family, 4: 230
Massachusetts Regional Fracture Committee, 3: 64
MGH orthopaedics and, 1: 189; 3: 266, 268; 4: 224, 226, 226*b*
as MGH orthopaedics chief, 3: 11*b*, 173, 227
New England Deaconess Hospital and, 4: 225
New England Regional Committee on Fractures, 4: 341
orthopaedics education and, 4: 228–230
professional memberships and roles, 4: 229*b*
psoas abscess in the lumbar retroperitoneal lymph glands case, 4: 225
publications and research, 4: 224–225, *225*, 226, 228–229, 242
RBBH and, 4: 406
rehabilitation of soldiers and, 4: 444
Trumbull Hospital and, 4: 225
tuberculosis research and, 4: 224–226
Tufts appointment, 4: 226, 226*b*
US Army Medical Corps and, 4: 226–227
Rogers, Orville F., Jr., 2: 119; 4: 389*b*
Rogers, Oscar H., 3: 343
Rogers, W. B., 3: 420
Rogers, William A. (1892–1975), 3: *343*

closed reduction of lumbar spine facture-dislocation case, 3: 347
death of, 3: 350
early life, 3: 343
education and training, 3: 343
fracture research and, 3: 343, 347–348
HMS appointment, 2: 223; 4: 60–61
honors and awards, 3: 350
Journal of Bone and Joint Surgery editor, 2: 165; 3: 161, 260, 344–347
legacy of, 3: 349
marriage and family, 3: 349–350
on mental attitude and spine fractures, 3: 349*b*
as MGH surgeon, 1: 158; 3: 187, 192, 270, 343–344, 348, 375
publications and research, 2: 297; 3: 184–185, 294, 347–349
RBBH and, 4: 31, 36, 93, 111
sacroiliac joint arthrodesis and, 3: 184–185
sling procedure for the foot and, 3: 294
spinal fusion and, 3: 321, 344
spinal research and, 3: 343–344, 347–349, *349*
Rogers, William Allen, 4: *200*
Roi Albert I Anglo-Belgian Hospital, 4: 401
Rokitanasky, Karl, 1: 82
Romney, Mitt, 3: 424
Roosevelt, Eleanor, 2: 72
Roosevelt, Franklin D.
chair lift design, 2: 76, *76*
Lovett and, 2: 72, *73*, *74*, *75*–76, 271
Lovett's diagram of muscle exam, 2: *75*
nonstandard treatments and, 2: 77
onset of poliomyelitis, 2: 71–72
poliomyelitis treatment, 2: 72–78
suggestions on treatment, 2: 76–77
and Warm Springs Foundation, 2: 77–78
World War II and, 4: 465–466, *466*
Roosevelt, James, 2: 72
Roosevelt, Theodore, 1: 248, 253; 4: 361
Roosevelt Hospital, 2: 248, 250–251
Root, Howard F., 4: 229
Roper, Jane, 4: 66
Ropes, Marian W., 3: 336

Rose, P., 3: 327
Rose, Robert M., 2: 407; 3: 327–328
Rosenau, Milton J., 4: 6, 210
Rosenberg, Benjamin, 2: 368
Rosenthal, Robert K. (1936–2021), 2: *401*
    Boston Children's Hospital and, 2: 401–402
    Brigham and Women's Hospital and, 4: 163, 193
    Cerebral Palsy Clinic and, 2: 402
    cerebral palsy research, 2: 401, *401*, 402
    education and training, 2: 401
    HMS appointment, 2: 401
    PBBH and, 4: 163
    professional memberships, 2: 402
    publications and research, 2: 401–402
Rossier, Alain B., 4: 152
Rotch, Thomas Morgan, 2: 13–14, 170
Roussimoff, André (Andre the Giant), 4: *251*, 252–253
Rowe, Carter R. (1906–2001), 3: *350*, *359*, *360*, *361*, *447*, *461*; 4: *491*
    as AOA president, 3: 355, 355*b*, 360
    Bankart procedure and, 3: 351, *351*, 352–354, 357–359, *359*, 360
    Children's Hospital/MGH combined program and, 3: 237
    dead arm syndrome and, 3: 359–360
    death of, 3: 361
    early life, 3: 350
    education and training, 3: 350–351
    on Ernest Codman, 3: 143
    on Eugene Record, 3: 330
    Fracture course and, 3: *273*
    fracture research and, 3: 354
    on fractures in elderly patients, 3: *353*, 354, 354*b*
    Harvard Unit and, 1: 270, *270*
    HMS appointment, 3: 354, 360
    on Klein, 4: 236
    knee arthrotomy research, 3: 351
    legacy of, 3: 360–361
    Lest We Forget, 3: 61, 187, 257, 347, *357*, 360
    on Mankin, 3: 387
    marriage and family, 3: 361
    MGH Fracture Clinic and, 4: 464
    as MGH surgeon, 3: 354, 360, 398*b*
    MGH Ward 1 and, 3: 70*b*, 74
    105th General Hospital and, 3: 351; 4: 489, 490*b*–491*b*
    as orthopaedic surgeon for the Boston Bruins, 3: 356–357, 357*b*
    private medical practice, 3: 271, 448
    professional memberships and, 3: 354–355, 360
    publications and research, 3: 350–359, 448–449
    Shoulder, The, 3: 360
    shoulder dislocations and, 3: 352, *352*, 353, 355–356, *356*
    shoulder surgery and, 3: 352–354, 356
    on Smith-Petersen, 3: 187
    sports medicine and, 3: 356, 388*t*
    34th Infantry Division and, 4: 484
    on Thornton Brown, 3: 257
    US Army Medical Corps and, 3: 351
    voluntary shoulder dislocation case, 3: 355–356
    on William Kermond, 3: 299
    on William Rogers, 3: 347, 349
    World War II service, 4: 17
Rowe, George, 4: 3
Rowe, Mary, 3: 361, *361*
Roxbury Clinical Record Club (R.C.R.C.), 3: 161
Roxbury Ladies' Bikur Cholim Association, 4: 212
Roxbury Latin School, 1: 6, 20
Royal National Orthopaedic Hospital (London), 1: 106; 2: 333–334, *334*; 3: 412, 426
Royal Orthopaedic Hospital (Birmingham, England), 2: 181
Rozental, Tamara D., 3: 410; 4: 288
RRC. *See* Residency Review Committee (RRC)
Rubash, Harry E.
    Edith M. Ashley Professor, 3: 464*b*
    HCORP and, 1: 224–225
    Knee Biomechanics and Biomaterials Laboratory, 3: 464*b*
    as MGH clinical faculty, 3: 464*b*
    as MGH orthopaedics chief, 3: 11*b*, 228, 399, 462–463
Rubidge, J. W., 1: *34*
Rubin, S. H., 4: 199
Ruby, Leonard, 2: 250; 4: 99
Rudman, Warren, 2: 414

Rudo, Nathan, 2: 173, 175–176, 438
Ruggles, Timothy, 1: 13
Ruggles-Fayerweather House, 1: 22, *22*
Rugh, J. T., 3: 158
Rumford, Count Benjamin, 1: 292–293
Runyon, Lucia, 2: 291
Runyon, Robert C. (1928–2012), 2: *290–291*
    Boston Children's Hospital and, 2: 289–290
    death of, 2: 291
    education and training, 2: 289
    marriage and family, 2: 291
    MGH/Children's Hospital residency, 2: 289
    MIT Medical and, 2: 277, 290–291
    private medical practice, 2: 289
    publications of, 2: 291
    sports medicine and, 2: 290
Runyon, Scott, 2: 291
Rush, Benjamin, 1: 25, 293; 3: 23
Russell, Stuart, 3: 364
Ruth Jackson Orthopaedic Society, 2: 413, *414*
Ryerson, Edwin W., 1: 197; 2: 160; 4: 394
Ryerson, W. E., 2: 105

S

Sabatini, Coleen, 4: 190*b*
Sabin, Albert, 2: 191, 264, 315
sacrococcygeal chordoma, 3: 390
sacroiliac joint
    arthrodesis of, 3: 183–185
    fusion for arthritis, 3: 184–185
    fusion for tuberculosis, 3: 185
    ligamentous strain of, 3: 191
    low-back and leg pain, 3: 184
    orthopaedic surgeon opinions on fusion of, 3: 184–185
sacrospinalis, 2: 146–147
Saint Joseph Hospital, 4: 157
Salem Hospital, 1: 220, 224–225; 2: 270–272
Salib, Philip, 3: *238*, 239, 460*b*
Salk, Jonas, 2: 189
Salter, Robert B., 1: 167; 2: 209, 302, 334–335; 4: 351, 355–356
Salter innominate osteotomy, 2: 390–391
Salter–Harris classification system, 4: 351, 355–356
Saltonstall, Francis A. F. Sherwood, 3: 89
Salvati, Eduardo, 4: 134

Salve Regina College, 1: 216
Salzler, Matthew, 3: 463*b*
Salzman, Edwin W., 4: 251
Samilson, Robert, 3: *293*
San Diego Naval Center, 4: 246
Sancta Maria Hospital, 4: 342, 346
Sandell, L. J., 3: 445
Sanders, Charles, 3: 391
Sanders, James, 2: 378
Sanderson, Eric R., 4: 489
Sanderson, Marguerite, 4: 444
Sanhedrin, Mishnah, 4: 197
Santa Clara County Hospital, 3: 300
Santore, R. F., 4: 176, *176*, 177
Santurjian, D. N., 1: *179*
sarcoidosis, 4: 98
Sarcoma Molecular Biology Laboratory, 3: 464*b*
Sargent, John Singer, 4: *424*
Sarmiento, Augusto, 3: 249
Sarni, James, 3: 463, 464*b*
Sarokhan, Alan, 2: 249
Sayre, Lewis A., 1: 119; 2: 26, 30, 48, 50–51, 63, *227*
Sayre, Reginald H., 2: 52
Scannell, David D., 4: 207, 439
scaphoid fracture, 3: 101–102; 4: 359–361, 368–369
Scardina, Robert J., 3: 396, 398*b*, 460*b*, 464*b*
scarlet fever, 1: 7; 2: 4, 52
Scarlet Key Society (McGill), 3: 253, *253*
Schaffer, Jonathan L., 4: 193, 195*b*
Schaffer, Newton M., 2: 47–48
Schaller, Bill, 4: 284
Scheuermann kyphosis, 2: 343, 359
Schiller, Arnold, 2: 369
Schlatter, Carl B., 2: 115
Schlens, Robert D., 2: 266
Schmitt, Francis O., 2: 321, 323; 3: 248, 455*b*
Schmorl, Georg, 3: 204; 4: 262
Schneider, Bryan, 2: 439*b*
School for Health Officers (HMS), 2: 42, 65–66
Schurko, Brian, 4: 190*b*
Schussele, Christian, 1: *57*
Schwab, Robert, 3: 286
Schwab, Sidney I., 3: 164
Schwamm, Lee, 3: 412–413
Schwartz, Felix, 4: 489
Schwartz, Forrest, 3: 463*b*
sciatica
  herniated disc as cause of, 3: 184
  laminectomy and, 3: 204, 206
  low-back pain research, 2: 396; 3: 184, 203–206
  nonoperative treatment of, 2: 373–374

ruptured intervertebral disc and, 3: 205–207, *207*
surgery for, 2: 373–374, 396
treatment of, 2: 152–153; 3: 203
use of chymopapain, 3: 254–255, 419, *421*
scoliosis
  Abbott Frame, 4: 232, *232*
  Adam's machine, 2: 86
  Boston brace, 2: 339–340, 358–359
  brace management of, 2: 339–340, 367
  Bradford and, 2: 35, *35*, *36*, 58
  Brewster and, 2: 223–228
  cadaver studies, 2: 56, 58, *58*
  celluloid jackets, 2: *85*
  collagen and, 2: 328
  congenital, 4: 62, 65
  devices for, 2: 35, *35*, *36*, 296–297, *297*
  diastematomyelia in, 2: 399–400
  Dwyer instrumentation, 2: 336
  Dwyer procedure, 2: 328
  early onset (EOS), 2: 360–361
  exercises for, 2: 59
  Forbes method of correction, 2: 87, *87*; 3: 229; 4: 232, *232*
  forward flexion test, 2: *367*
  Galeazzi method, 2: 227
  genetic background and, 2: 399, 400
  growth-sparing surgery, 2: 360–361
  Hall and, 2: 334–335
  Harrington rods, 2: 316, 325, 335, 340
  Hibbs spinal fusion procedure, 2: 164
  idiopathic, 1: xxiii; 2: 334, 339, 341, 343, 358–359, 366–367, 399
  jackets for, 2: 59, *59*, 60, *60*, 61, 85–87
  kyphoscoliosis, 1: 97, 105
  latent psoas abscess case, 2: 365
  Lovett and, 2: 56–61, 79, 86, 223–225
  Lovett Board, 2: *59*, 86
  Lovett-Sever method, 2: 87
  measurement methods, 2: 366, *367*
  Milwaukee Brace, 2: 336
  pedicle screws, 2: 343
  pelvic machine design, 2: 86
  photography and, 2: 247
  posterior spinal fusion, 2: 341
  pressure correction apparatus (Hoffa-Schede), 3: *151*, *152*

Relton-Hall frame, 2: 334
right dorsal, 3: *229*
self-correction of, 2: *297*
Sever and, 2: 84–86
Soutter and, 2: 296
spinal surgery and, 2: 334–335, 337–338, 340–343
surgical procedures for, 2: *369*
suspension and, 2: *336*
tibial osteoperiosteal grafts, 2: 316
treatment of, 1: xxi, xxii, 100, 106, 109, *116*; 2: 35, 84–88, 296, 316, 334, 366–367, 396; 3: 208–209, 229; 4: 232–233
turnbuckle jacket, 2: 80, 223–226, 226*b*, 227, 227*b*, 316, *336*; 3: 209
use of photographs, 2: 84
vertebral transverse process case, 3: 229–230
x-rays and, 2: 79
Zander apparatus for, 3: *152*, *153*
Scoliosis and Other Deformities of the Axial Skeleton (Riseborough and Herndon), 2: 398, *398*
Scoliosis Research Society (SRS), 2: 338, 342, 347, 370, 400, 411, *411*
scoliosometer, 2: 36
Scollay, Mercy, 1: 19
Scott, Catherine, 4: 175
Scott, Dick, 1: 167
Scott, Richard D. (1943–), 4: *175*
  Brigham and Women's Hospital and, 4: 163, 181, 193
  CHMC and, 4: 176
  education and training, 4: 175
  HCORP and, 4: 175
  hip and knee reconstructions, 4: 175–178
  HMS appointment, 4: 176, 178
  honors and awards, 4: 180
  on importance of PCL preservation, 4: 181
  on metal tibial wedges, 4: 180, *180*
  metallic tibial tray fracture case, 4: 177
  MGH and, 4: 175
  New England Baptist Hospital and, 4: 181
  New England Deaconess Hospital and, 4: 280
  PBBH and, 4: 163
  PFC unicompartmental knee prothesis, 4: 177
  publications and research, 4: 176, *176*, 177–178, *178*, 180, *180*, 181, *181*, 189
  RBBH and, 4: 132, 175–176

Index

Total Knee Arthroplasty, 4: 176
  on total knee replacement outcomes, 4: 178, 180–181
  unicompartmental prothesis and, 4: 176
Scott, S. M., 2: 212
Scudder, Abigail Taylor Seelye, 3: 55
Scudder, Charles L. (1860–1949), 3: *53, 57, 63, 65*
  ACS Committee on Fractures, 3: 64
  American College of Surgeons Board of Regents and, 3: 62–63
  Boston Children's Hospital and, 2: 438; 3: 54
  Boston Dispensary and, 2: 306
  clinical congress meeting, 3: 118
  club foot research and, 3: 54
  "Coll" Warren and, 3: 54–55
  death of, 3: 65
  early life, 3: 53
  education and training, 3: 53–54
  fracture treatment and, 3: 55–56, 56*b*, 58–65; 4: 340*b*
  HMS appointment, 3: 58, 61
  legacy of, 3: 64–65
  marriage and family, 3: 55, 64
  at MGH case presentation, 3: *54*
  MGH Fracture Clinic and, 2: 130; 3: 60, 60*b*, 371; 4: 464
  as MGH house officer, 1: 189; 3: 54
  as MGH surgeon, 3: 54, 58, 64, 266; 4: 472*b*
  New England Deaconess Hospital and, 4: 274
  professional memberships and, 3: 65
  publications and research, 1: 264; 3: 55–58, 64–65; 4: 335
  Treatment of Fractures, 1: 147; 3: 55–56, *57, 58,* 64, 99; 4: 312, 350
  Tumors of the Jaws, 3: 64
Scudder, Evarts, 3: 53
Scudder, Sarah Patch Lamson, 3: 53
Scudder Oration on Trauma, 3: 63
Scutter, Charles L., 2: 66
Seal of Chevalier du Tastevin, 2: 348, *348*
Sears, George, 4: 303
Seattle Children's Hospital, 4: 250
Section for Orthopedic Surgery (AMA), 2: 110–111, 176
Seddon, Herbert, 2: 135, 140; 3: 412
Sedgwick, Cornelius, 4: 276–277, 279

Seeing Patients (White and Chanoff), 4: *265*
Seelye, Abigail Taylor, 3: 55
Segond, Paul, 2: 91
Seider, Christopher, 1: 14
Sell, Kenneth, 3: 439
Selva, Julius, 2: 31
Semmelweis, Ignaz, 1: 81, 84, 193
sepsis. *See also* antisepsis
  amputations and, 3: 373
  ankle arthrodesis case, 3: 330
  following intramedullary fixation of femoral fractures, 2: 248; 3: 309–310
  hip fractures and, 3: 218
  infectious research and, 1: 91
  recurrence of, 3: 196, 301
septic arthritis, 2: 79
Sevenson, Orvar, 2: 302
Sever, Charles W., 2: 83
Sever, Elizabeth Bygrave, 2: 92, 97
Sever, James T., 2: 252
Sever, James W. (1878–1964), 2: *84, 98, 255*
  on astragalectomy, 2: 92–93
  on back disabilities, 2: 92
  birth palsies research, 2: 415, 417
  Boston Children's Hospital and, 1: 187; 2: 13, 40, 84, 90, 92, 274, 282, 296; 4: 338
  Boston City Hospital and, 4: 305*b*, 307–308, 308*b*, 328
  brachial plexus injury study, 2: 90, 96
  on Bradford, 2: 44, 92
  as Browne & Nichols School trustee, 2: 97
  calcaneal apophysitis study, 2: 88–90, 100
  clinical congress meeting, 3: 116
  death of, 2: 100
  early life, 2: 83
  foot research, 2: 107
  fracture research, 3: 340
  HMS appointment, 2: 92, 97; 4: 59
  HMS Laboratory of Surgical Pathology and, 2: 90
  on improvement of medicine, 2: 98
  marriage and family, 2: 92, 97
  Massachusetts Industrial Accident Board examiner, 2: 92
  Massachusetts Regional Fracture Committee, 3: 64
  medical appointments, 2: 84
  as medical director of the Industrial School, 2: 97
  medical education, 2: 83

  military surgeon training and, 4: 396
  New England Regional Committee on Fractures, 4: 341
  obstetrical paralysis study, 2: 89–90, *90,* 91, 94–96, 100
  on occupational therapy, 4: 359
  on orthopaedic surgery advances, 2: 99–100
  pelvic machine design, 2: 86
  Principles of Orthopedic Surgery, 2: 92, *93*
  Principles of Orthopedic Surgery for Nurses, The, 2: 92, *93*
  professional memberships, 2: 97–98
  publications of, 2: 84, 92, 223
  schools for disabled children, 2: 97
  scoliosis treatment, 2: 59, 61, 84–86
  Textbook of Orthopedic Surgery for Students of Medicine, 2: 92, *93*
  tibial tuberosity fracture treatment, 2: 91, 96–97
Sever, Josephine Abbott, 2: 97
Sever, Mary Caroline Webber, 2: 83
Sever procedure, 2: 90
Sever-L'Episcopo procedure, 2: 90, 100, 417
Sever's disease. *See* calcaneal apophysitis (Sever's Disease)
Seymour, N., 2: 211
Shaffer, Newton M., 2: 43, 48, *49,* 57, 99
Shanbhag, Arun, 3: 462, 464*b*
Shands, Alfred, 1: 99, 114, 180
Shands, Alfred R., Jr., 2: 165, 183; 3: 208, 290
Shands Hospital, 3: 432
Shapiro, Frederic (1942–), 2: *402*
  Boston Children's Hospital and, 2: 354, 403, 403*b*, 439*b*; 4: 280
  education and training, 2: 402–403
  HMS appointment, 2: 403, 403*b*
  honors and awards, 2: 403–404
  Pediatric Orthopedic Deformities, 2: 403, *404*
  professional memberships, 2: 403–405
  publications and research, 2: 400, 403–404, *404*
Sharpey, William, 1: 84
Sharpey-Schafer, Edward A., 2: 242
Shattuck, Frederick C., 2: 20, 39, 43; 3: 94
Shattuck, George Cheever, 4: 414–415

Shaw, A., 2: 115
Shaw, Amy, 1: 85
Shaw, Benjamin S., 2: 8
Shaw, Lemuel, 1: 302, 307, 310–311
Shaw, Robert Gould, 1: 303, 308
Shaw, Robert S., 3: 287
Shea, William D., 4: 163
Sheehan, Diane, 1: 239
Sheltering Arms (New York), 2: 5
Shephard, Margaret, 3: 219
Shepherd's Bush Military Hospital, 4: 398, *398*, 399, 402, 411, 444
Shepherd's Bush Orthopaedic Hospital, 3: 365
Sherman, Henry M., 3: 234
Sherman, William O'Neill, 3: 60–61; 4: 338, 339*b*, 340, 340*b*, *342*
Sherrill, Henry Knox, 3: 1
Shields, Lawrence R., 4: 116, 116*b*, 117, 128, 163
Shippen, William, 1: 25
shock, 4: 373
Shortell, Joseph H. (1891–1951), 4: *338*
   AAOS and, 4: 337
   American Expeditionary Forces and, 4: 338
   athletic injury treatment, 4: 342
   BCH Bone and Joint Service, 4: 307, 328, 333–334, 341, 380*b*
   BCH residencies and, 4: 377
   Boston Bruins and, 4: 342
   Boston Children's Hospital and, 2: 252, 274; 4: 338
   Boston City Hospital and, 1: 199; 3: 64; 4: 242, 338, 341
   death of, 4: 342
   education and training, 4: 338
   fracture treatment and, 4: 339*b*, 342
   hip fractures in elderly case, 4: 341
   HMS appointment, 4: 338, 341
   on industrial accidents, 4: 338, 341
   New England Regional Committee on Fractures, 4: 341
   professional memberships, 4: 341
   publications and research, 4: 338, 341
   Ted Williams and, 4: 342
Shortkroff, Sonya, 4: 136, 194
Shoulder, The (Codman), 2: 239; 3: 105, *105*, 115, 122, 140*b*
Shoulder, The (Rowe), 3: 360
shoulders
   acromioclavicular dislocation, 3: 449
   amputations, 1: 23
   anterior subluxation of, 3: 360
   arthrodesis outcomes, 2: 154
   Bankart procedure, 3: 351–354, 357–358, *359*, 450
   Bankart procedure rating sheet, 3: 358*t*
   brachial plexus injuries, 2: 90–91, 96; 3: 412, *412*, 413–414
   cleidocranial dysostosis, 2: 254
   Codman's Paradox, 3: 105
   dislocations and, 3: 352, *352*, 353, 355–356, *356*
   fracture treatment and, 3: 339
   frozen shoulder, 1: 277–278
   glenoid labrum composition, 3: 449
   instability and, 3: 352, 448–450, *450*
   posterior dislocations, 2: 417–418
   ruptures of the serratus anterior, 2: 253
   sports injuries and, 2: 288
   subacromial bursitis, 3: 104–105, 107–109
   subdeltoid bursa, 3: 95, 98, 103–105, 108
   supraspinatus tendon, 3: 108–109
   surgery, 1: 29
   transfers for, 2: 154
   transient subluxation of, 3: 359
   treatment of, 3: 107–110
Shriners Hospital for Crippled Children, 4: 378
Shriners Hospitals for Children, 2: 110, 212, 424; 3: 335
Sibley, John, 1: 307
sickle cell disease, 3: 403
SICOT. *See* International Society of Orthopaedic Surgery and Traumatology (SICOT)
Siffert, R. S., 1: 126
Silen, William, 1: 167; 4: 262, 283, 283*t*
silicone flexible implants, 4: 132, 166–167, *167*
Siliski, John M., 1: 217*b*; 3: 399, 460*b*, 464*b*
Silver, David, 2: 31, 64, 67, 87; 3: 87, 156, 158, 375; 4: 405, 412, 451
Simcock, Xavier C., 3: 463*b*; 4: 190*b*
Simmons, Barry P. (1939–), 4: *182*
   AO trauma fellowship, 4: 182
   Beth Israel Hospital and, 4: 182, 262
   Brigham and Women's Hospital and, 2: 375; 4: 163, 183, 193, 195*b*
   carpal tunnel syndrome research, 2: 375; 4: 183–184, *184*, 185, *185*, 186
   Children's Hospital/MGH combined program and, 4: 182
   CHMC and, 4: 182
   education and training, 4: 182
   focal scleroderma of the hand case, 4: 183
   hand surgery fellowship, 4: 116*b*, 182
   Hands, 4: 183
   Harvard University Athletics Department and, 4: 183
   HMS appointment, 4: 183
   honors and awards, 4: 186
   New England Baptist Hospital and, 4: 183
   Occupational Disorders of the Upper Extremity, 4: 168, 183
   orthopaedics education and, 4: 186
   outcomes movement and, 4: 186
   PBBH and, 4: 163, 182
   professional memberships, 4: 186
   publications and research, 4: 182–185, *185*, 186
   RBBH and, 4: 182, 184
   residency rotations, 4: 182, 182*b*
   Richard J. Smith Lecture, 3: 431
   US Navy and, 4: 182
   West Roxbury Veterans Administration Hospital and, 4: 182–183
Simmons, C. C., 4: 102
Simmons College, 2: 213, 413
Simon, Michael A., 3: 435–436, *436*
Simon, Sheldon R. (1941–), 2: *405*
   Albert Einstein College of Medicine and, 2: 408
   Boston Children's Hospital and, 2: 406–407
   Brigham and Women's Hospital, 4: 163
   Cave Traveling Fellowship and, 1: 217*b*
   cerebral palsy research, 2: 406–407
   computer-simulated planning and, 2: 389
   education and training, 2: 405–406
   foot and ankle treatment, 2: 407
   gait research, 2: 406–408, 439
   Glimcher and, 2: 406
   HMS appointment, 2: 406–407
   honors and awards, 2: 406–407, 407*b*
   MGH and, 2: 406

Index

Ohio State University School of Medicine and, 2: 407–408
orthopaedics appointments, 2: 408
PBBH and, 4: 163
Practical Biomechanics for the Orthopedic Surgeon, 3: 328
professional memberships, 2: 407, 407*b*
publications and research, 2: 406, *406*, 407–408; 3: 326
RESNA and, 2: 408
study of Swiss method of treating fractures, 2: 406
West Roxbury Veterans Administration Hospital and, 2: 406
Simon, William H., 3: 377
Simpson, Sir James, 1: 84
69th Field Ambulance, 4: 405*b*
Skaggs, David, 2: 379
skeletogenesis, 2: 439
skiagraphy, 2: 16
Skillman, John J., 4: 251
skin grafts, 1: 75, 77; 3: 310; 4: 204, 216–217
Skoff, Hillel, 4: 263, 286
Sledge, Clement (1930–), 4: *126*, *128*, *133*
   AAOS and, 4: 139–141
   Affiliated Hospitals Center board and, 4: 119
   articular cartilage research, 4: 133, 136
   on avascular necrosis, 4: 238
   on Barr, 3: 213
   BIH Board of Consultants, 4: 262–263
   Boston Children's Hospital and, 2: 354–355
   Brigham Orthopaedic Foundation (BOF) and, 4: 123, 191
   Brigham Orthopedic Associates (BOA) and, 4: 123, 191
   BWH chair of orthopaedic surgery, 1: 180, 284; 4: 132–133, 143, 191–193, 195*b*–196*b*
   Children's Hospital/MGH combined program and, 1: 210; 4: 126
   chondrocyte metabolism in cell culture research, 4: 133
   on Codman, 4: 141
   on diastematomyelia, 2: 236
   education and training, 4: 125–127
   embryonic cartilage research, 4: 127, *127*
   Hip Society president, 4: 141
   HMS appointment, 4: 127
   honors and awards, 4: 142
   John Ball and Buckminster Brown Professorship, 3: 202; 4: 132, 195*b*
   joint replacement research and treatment, 4: 40, 133, *133*, 134–135, *135*
   knee arthroplasty and, 4: 129–130, 147, 149
   mandate to unify orthopaedics at Brigham Hospitals, 4: 116, 116*b*, 117–118
   Marion B. Gebbie Research Fellowship, 4: 127
   on merger of RBBH and PBBH, 4: 128
   as MGH honorary orthopaedic surgeon, 3: 398*b*
   MGH orthopaedics department and, 1: 210–211; 4: 127
   on orthopaedic basic and clinical research, 4: 141, *141*, 142
   as PBBH chief of orthopaedic surgery, 2: 269, 279; 4: 43, 115–117, 128–129, 132, 143, 191, 196*b*
   as PBBH orthopaedic surgery professor, 4: 43, 114–115
   publications and research, 4: 127, 129–130, *130*, 131, 133–139, *139*
   radiation synovectomy research, 4: 64, 136, *136*, 137
   RBBH board of overseers, 4: 132
   as RBBH chief of surgery, 2: 279; 4: 43, 115, 128–129, 131–132, 143, 191, 196*b*
   as RBBH orthopaedic surgery professor, 4: 43, 114–115
   as research fellow in orthopaedic surgery, 4: 126
   rheumatoid arthritis treatment, 4: 138–139
   Strangeways Research Laboratory fellowship, 4: 126
   US Navy and, 4: 125
Slipped Capital Femoral Epiphysis (Joplin et al.), 3: 294, 333
Slipped Capital Femoral Epiphysis (Klein et al.), 4: 238
slipped capital femoral epiphysis (SCFE)
   acetabular morphology in, 2: 392
   Howorth procedure and, 4: 243
   impingement treatment, 3: 189
   internal fixation of, 2: 176
   Klein's Line and, 4: 238–239, *239*
   open reduction of, 2: 168; 4: 237
   recommendations for, 2: 176
   research in, 3: 294, 331, 333; 4: 237–238, 243
   treatment of, 2: 137
   treatment outcomes, 2: 380
   use of roentgenology in, 3: 334
Slocum, Donald B., 1: 279
Slowick, Francis A., 2: 230
smallpox, 1: 8–9, 295; 2: 4
Smellie, William, 1: 6
Smith, Dale C., 4: 464
Smith, Ethan H., 3: 160*b*
Smith, Gleniss, 3: 427
Smith, H., 3: 210
Smith, H. W., 1: *31*
Smith, Homer B., 1: 253–254
Smith, Ida, 2: 431–432
Smith, J. V. C., 1: 97
Smith, Jacob, 3: 427
Smith, Job L., 2: 7
Smith, Lyman, 3: 254
Smith, Nellie, 3: 247
Smith, Richard J. (1930–1987), 3: *427*, *428*, *430*
   ASSH and, 3: 428–429, *430*
   death of, 3: 399, 429–430
   early life, 3: 427
   education and training, 3: 427
   factitious lymphedema case, 3: 429
   hand surgery and, 3: 385–386, 388*t*, 427–429, 460*b*
   HMS appointment, 3: 428
   Hospital for Joint Diseases and, 3: 413, 427
   legacy of, 3: 430–431
   Mankin on, 3: 427, 429–430
   as MGH surgeon, 3: 395, 398*b*, 413, 428
   professional memberships and, 3: 428, 430
   publications and research, 3: 427–429
   Smith Day lectures, 3: 431
   Tendon Transfers of the Hand and Forearm, 3: 428
Smith, Robert M., 2: 177, 234, 432
Smith, Rose, 3: 427
Smith, Theobold, 4: *6*
Smith-Petersen, Evelyn Leeming, 3: 362
Smith-Petersen, Hilda Dickenson, 3: 198
Smith-Petersen, Kaia Ursin, 3: 179
Smith-Petersen, Marius N. (1886–1953), 3: *174*, *179*, *197*, *198*
   AAOS and, 4: 337
   AAOS Fracture Committee and, 3: 191
   adjustable reamer and, 3: 317
   American Ambulance Hospital and, 4: *388*, 389*b*, *390*

approach to wrist during arthrodesis, 3: 191
Brackett and, 3: 180–181
death of, 3: 198
early life, 3: 179
education and training, 3: 179–181
femoral neck fracture treatment, 3: 185–186, *186*, 189, 189*b*, 190
femoral stem prothesis, 3: *293*
femoroacetabular impingement treatment, 3: 188–189
Harvard Surgical Unit and, 2: 119, 123–124; 3: 180, *180*, *370*
hip nailing and, 3: 237
hip surgery and, 3: 244
HMS appointment, 3: 183, 187, 192; 4: 59
innovation and, 3: 216–217
Knight's Cross, Royal Norwegian Order of St. Olav, 3: *198*
kyphosis treatment, 3: 239
legacy of, 3: 198–199
on Legg-Calve-Perthes disease, 2: 103
marriage and family, 3: 198
MGH Fracture Clinic and, 3: 60*b*, 315
MGH orthopaedics and, 1: 179, 189, 203–204; 2: 297; 3: 183, 269, 456*b*
as MGH orthopaedics chief, 3: 11*b*, 187–188, 191, 227, 375
MGH physical chemistry laboratory, 2: 322
military orthopaedics and, 4: 473
mold arthroplasty and, 3: 181, 183, 192, *192*, 193, 193*b*, 194, *194*, 195, *195*, 196, *196*, 198, 216, 238–239, 241, 292, 292*b*, 293
New England Rehabilitation Center and, 1: 272
orthopaedic surgery and, 1: 158
personality of, 3: 187–188
pillars of surgical care, 3: 187
private medical practice, 3: 183, 192
professional memberships and, 3: 197, 197*b*
publications and research, 2: 136; 3: 188, 192–193, 241–242, 302, 366
RBBH and, 4: 31, 36, 93, 111
sacroiliac joint treatment, 3: 183–185, 191

supra-articular subperiosteal approach to the hip, 3: 181, *181*, 182*b*
treatment of fractures, 3: 62
triflanged nail development, 3: 62, 185–186, *186*, 187, 189–190; 4: 237
World War II and, 3: 191
Smith-Petersen, Morten (1920–1999), 3: *361*
Children's Hospital/MGH combined program and, 3: 361
death of, 3: 362
early life, 3: 361
education and training, 3: 361
hip surgery and, 3: 362
HMS appointment, 3: 362
marriage and family, 3: 362
New England Baptist Hospital and, 3: 362
publications and research, 3: 362
Tufts appointment, 3: 362
US Naval Reserves and, 3: 361
Smith-Petersen, Morten, Sr., 3: 179
Smith-Petersen Foundation, 3: 198
Snedeker, Lendon, 2: 191
Snyder, Brian D. (1957–), 2: *409*
biomechanics research, 2: 410–411
Boston Children's Hospital and, 2: 409–411
Cerebral Palsy Clinic and, 2: 409
contrast-enhanced computed tomography and, 2: 411
education and training, 2: 409
fracture-risk research, 2: 411, *411*
HCORP and, 2: 409
HMS appointment, 2: 409
honors and awards, 2: 411
hospital appointments, 2: 409
modular spinal instrumentation device patents, 2: 412
orthopaedics appointments, 2: 409
professional memberships, 2: 412
publications and research, 2: 410, *410*, 411
Society for Medical Improvement, 3: 35
Society of Clinical Surgery, 3: 113*b*
Söderman, P., 3: 219
Sohier, Edward H., 1: 307, 310
Solomon, Dr., 4: 210
Soma Weiss Prize, 2: 319
somatosensory evoked potentials (SSEPs), 2: 342
Sons of Liberty, 1: 11, 13, 15–16
Soule, D., 2: 372

Southern Medical and Surgical Journal, 1: 63
Southmayd, William W., 1: 279; 4: 163, 193
Southwick, Wayne, 4: 258, 261
Soutter, Anne, 2: 292
Soutter, Charlotte Lamar, 2: 292
Soutter, D. R., 2: 34
Soutter, Helen E. Whiteside, 2: 292
Soutter, James, 2: 292
Soutter, Lamar, 2: 292, 293*b*
Soutter, Robert (1870–1933), 2: *292*, 293
Boston Children's Hospital and, 2: 34, 292; 4: 338
Boston City Hospital and, 4: 305*b*
Bradford and, 2: 292, 297
cartilage transplantation, 2: 294
critique of shoes, 2: 293
death from blood poisoning, 2: 299, *299*
dislocated patella treatment, 2: 294–296
education and training, 2: 292
hip contracture treatment, 2: 294, 295*b*
hip disease treatment, 2: 293–294
HMS appointment, 2: 223, 298; 4: 59–60
hot pack treatment, 2: 264
letter to Catherine A. Codman, 1: *129*, 130
marriage and family, 2: 292, 293*b*
military surgeon training by, 2: 42, 66
New England Peabody Home for Crippled Children and, 2: 270, 292
orthopaedic device innovations, 2: 296–297
orthopaedic surgery and, 1: 171
orthopaedics appointments, 2: 292
professional memberships, 2: 292, 292*b*
"Progress in Orthopaedic Surgery" series, 2: 297
publications of, 2: 61, 293, 297
scoliosis treatment, 2: 296
surgical procedure innovations, 2: 294–296
Technique of Operations on the Bones, Joints, Muscles and Tendons, 2: 294, 297–298, *298*
Soutter, Robert, Jr., 2: 292
Soutter, Robert, Sr., 2: 292
Spalding, James Alfred, 1: 47, 49, 49*b*, 50
Spanier, Suzanne, 3: 390

Index

Spanish American War, 4: 310–311, *311*
Spanish Flu, 4: *11*
Sparks, Jared, 1: 310
Spaulding Rehabilitation Hospital, 1: 217, 225; 3: 387–388, 396, 426, 461
Spear, Louis M., 4: 23, 26–28, 31–32, 45, 79
"Special Orthopedic Hospital–Past and Present, The" (Platt), 1: 114
Spector, Myron, 4: 194, 195*b*
Speed, Kellogg, 4: *319*
Spencer, Herbert, 4: 466–467
Spencer, Hillard, 2: 367
Spencer, Upshur, 4: 190*b*
spina bifida
    Lovett on, 2: 51–52
    research in, 2: 370
    ruptures of sac, 2: 309–310
    treatment of, 2: 51–52
    University of Massachusetts clinic, 2: 364
Spinal Deformity Study Group, 2: 365
spinal dysgenesis, 2: 366
spinal fusion wake-up test, 2: 340–342
Spinal Surgery Service (Children's Hospital), 2: 359
spinal taps, 2: 72, 78
spinal tuberculosis, 1: *109*
    operative treatment for, 4: 343
    pediatric patients, 2: 11, 308–309; 3: 289
    research in, 3: 289
    treatment of, 1: 100, 106, 108–109; 2: 308–309; 4: 225
spine. *See also* scoliosis
    advances in, 2: 338
    anterior and posterior procedures, 2: 343–345, 360, 366; 3: 426
    apparatus for, 1: 107; 2: *35, 36*
    athletes and, 2: 385
    benefits of, 2: 373
    Boston Children's Hospital and, 2: 337–338, 338*t*
    Bradford Frame and, 2: 30
    cerebral palsy and, 2: 370
    children and, 1: 123; 2: 385
    closed reduction of lumbar fracture-dislocation, 3: 347
    community-based physicians and, 2: 373
    computed tomography and, 3: 254
    congenital absence of the odontoid process, 3: 340
    degenerative stenosis, 4: 269–270
    Down syndrome and, 2: 370
    Dwyer instrumentation and, 2: 336
    for early-onset, 2: 360
    fractures and dislocations, 3: 349*b*, *349*
    fusion in tubercular, 3: 148–149, 157–158, 158*b*; 4: 343
    halo-vest apparatus, 4: *152*, 153
    Harrington rods and, 2: 316, 325, 335–336, 338
    Hibbs spinal fusion procedure, 2: 164; 3: 155
    instability of lower cervical, 4: 261
    interpedicular segmental fixation (ISF) pedicle screw plate, 3: 420–421
    lumbar spinal stenosis, 2: 373–374
    measurement of, 2: *31*
    mental attitude and, 3: 349*b*
    MRI and, 3: 255
    myelodysplasia, 2: 359
    neurologic effects after surgery, 4: 269
    nutritional status and, 2: 361–362
    open anterior lumbosacral fracture dislocation, 3: 420, 425
    paraplegia and, 3: 319
    pedicle screws in, 2: 343; 3: 420
    posterior segment fixator (PSF), 3: 420
    Pott's Disease, 1: 97, 108–109; 3: 148–150
    pressure and pain, 2: 271
    prosthetic titanium rib and, 2: 360, *362*
    research in, 2: 343
    sacrococcygeal chordoma, 3: 390
    Scheuermann kyphosis, 2: 343, 359
    somatosensory evoked potentials (SSEPs), 2: 342
    spinal dysgenesis, 2: 366
    spinal fusion, 2: 271, 334–335, *335*, 343, 369; 3: 207–208
    spinal fusion wake-up test, 2: 340–342
    spinal height increases, 2: 367
    spondylolisthesis, 3: 421
    strengthening exercises for, 1: 100
    study of, 2: 57, *57*, 58, *58*, 59
    thoracic insufficiency syndrome, 2: 360
    tibial fracture, 4: 365
    treatment of, 1: 97–98, 100, 106; 2: 359; 4: 152
    vertebral column resections (VCRs), 2: 362–363
Spine Care Medical Group, 4: 263
Spine Patient Outcomes Research Trial (SPORT), 2: 371, 373
Spitzer, Hans, 2: 80
splints
    for drop-foot deformity, 4: *418*
    Eames molded plywood leg, 4: *470*
    first aid, 4: *418*
    Jones splints, 4: 389, 411
    manufacture of, 3: *167*, 168
    military orthopaedics and, 2: 120; 4: 389, 408–409, 416–417, *418*
    standardization of, 3: 167–168
    Thomas, 2: 20, *123*, *257*; 3: *168*; 4: 389, *391*, *408*, 409, 411, 417, *418*
    use during transportation, 3: 169, 169*b*; 4: 389
sports medicine. *See also* Harvard athletics
    acromioclavicular joint dislocation in, 1: 268, 277
    acute ligament injuries, 1: 277–278
    ankle injuries and, 1: 281
    assessment and treatment in, 1: 274
    athlete heart size, 1: 262, 267, 288
    athletic training and, 1: 248, 250–251, 258, 265–266
    BCH clinic for, 2: 287, 384
    caring for athletic injuries, 1: 268
    concussions in, 1: 247, 254, 275, 286–287; 2: 385
    dieticians and, 1: 258
    fatigue and, 1: 264–265
    foot and ankle treatment, 3: 348
    football injuries and, 1: 247–248, 252–255, 255*t*, 256, 258–262, 288
    frozen shoulder, 1: 277–278
    guidelines for team physicians, 1: 287
    Harvard athletics and, 2: 287
    ice hockey and, 1: 275, 286
    injury prevention and, 1: 265, 285–286
    knee joint injuries, 1: 267–268, 268*t*, 278–279, 285–287
    knee problems and, 2: 387
    MGH and, 3: 397
    Morton's neuroma, 2: 287
    musculoskeletal injuries, 1: 288
    myositis ossificans and, 1: 266–267
    neuromusculoskeletal genius and, 1: 279

orthopaedics curriculum and, 1: 165–166
pediatric, 2: 287, 385–387
physical therapy and, 3: 348
preventative strappings, 1: *269*, 274
professional teams and, 3: 348, 356–357, 397, 399, 448, 450
progress in, 1: 267
reconditioning and, 1: 271
rehabilitation and, 1: 275
scientific study of, 1: 250–251, 254–256, 262, 267–269, 277–278
spinal problems, 2: 385
sports teams and, 1: 248, 250–251
tenosynovitis of the flexor hallucis longus, 3: 348
torn meniscus, 1: 278
women basketball players and, 1: 285–286
Sports Medicine Bible for Young Adults, The (Micheli), 2: 385
Sports Medicine Bible, The (Micheli), 2: 385, *385*
Sports Medicine Fund, 2: 439*b*
Sports Medicine Service (MGH), 3: 356
Sprengel deformity, 2: 195, *196*
spring muscle test, 2: 70, *70*, 71
Springfield, Dempsey S. (1945–), 1: *242*; 3: *431*
 allograft research and, 3: 433, 435
 Association of Bone and Joint Surgeons and, 3: 436
 education and training, 3: 431–432
 Gaucher hemorrhagic bone cyst case, 3: 434
 HCORP and, 1: 242–243; 3: 435
 HMS appointment, 3: 432
 honors and awards, 3: 431, 436
 limb salvage surgery and, 3: 433
 as MGH surgeon, 3: 432
 Mount Sinai Medical School and, 3: 435
 Musculoskeletal Tumor Society and, 3: 436
 orthopaedic oncology and, 3: 399, 432, 435, 460*b*
 orthopaedics education and, 3: 435–436
 publications and research, 3: 432–433, 435–436
 on resident surgical case requirements, 3: 435–436, *436*
 Shands Hospital and, 3: 432
 surgical treatment of osteosarcoma, 3: 432–433
 University of Florida and, 3: 432
 US Army and, 3: 432
Spunkers, 1: 21, 32, 133
Spurling, Ina, 2: 144, 166
St. Anthony Hospital, 2: 111
St. Botolph Club (Boston), 2: *284*
St. George's Hospital, 1: 81, 83, 106
St. Louis Children's Hospital, 3: 165
St. Louis Shriners Hospital for Crippled Children, 3: 173
St. Luke's Home for Convalescents, 2: *307*
St. Luke's Hospital (New York), 2: 5, 20
St. Margaret's and Mary's Infant Asylum, 2: 256
St. Mary's Hospital (Nairobi, Kenya), 3: 379
St. Thomas's Hospital, 1: 37
Stack, Herbert, 2: 249
Stagnara, P., 2: 340
Staheli, Lynn, 2: 302; 4: 250
Stamp Act, 1: 11–13
Stamp Act Congress, 1: 13
Stanish, William, 2: 423
Stanton, Edwin, 3: 43
Staples, Mable Hughes, 3: 362
Staples, Nellie E. Barnes, 3: 362
Staples, O. Sherwin (1908-2002)
 Boston Children's Hospital and, 2: 438
 Children's Hospital/MGH combined program and, 3: 362
 Dartmouth Medical School appointment, 3: 363–364
 death of, 3: 364
 early life, 3: 362
 education and training, 3: 362
 on Edwin Cave, 3: 276
 as first orthopaedic surgeon in NH, 3: 363–364
 marriage and family, 3: 362
 Mary Hitchcock Memorial Hospital and, 3: 363–364
 as MGH surgeon, 3: 74, 362
 New England Peabody Home for Crippled Children and, 3: 362
 on osteochondritis in a finger, 3: 363
 private medical practice, 3: 271, 362
 publications and research, 3: 362
 6th General Hospital and, 4: 482
 White River Junction VA Hospital, 3: 364
 World War II service, 3: 362
Staples, Oscar S., Sr., 3: 362
Star and Garter Hospital, 4: 402
State Hospital School for Children (Canton), 2: 308
Statement by Four Physicians, 2: 6, *6*, 7
Steadman, Richard, 3: 446
Steadman Hawkins Clinic, 2: 378
Stearns, Peter N., 3: 83
Steele, Glenn, 4: 279
Steele, Mrs., 4: *128*
Steindler, Arthur, 2: 94; 3: 303; 4: 362
Steiner, Mark, 1: 217*b*, 289; 4: 194, 195*b*
Steinmann pin, 2: 237–238; 4: 166
Stelling, Frank H., 2: 351; 4: 19
Stephen J. Lipson, MD Orthopaedic and Spine lectureship, 4: 272, 272*b*
Stern, Peter, 3: 431
Stern, Walter, 1: xxiv
stethoscope, 1: 74
Stevens, James H., 2: 96, 415; 3: 109
Stevens, Samuel, 1: 6
Stevens, W. L., 3: 133
Stillman, Charles F., 2: 50–51
Stillman, J. Sidney, 4: 37, 40, 79
Stillman, James, 2: 253
Stillman Infirmary, 2: 253, *254*
Still's disease, 2: 171
Stimson, Lewis A., 1: 147
Stinchfield, Allan, 3: 332
Stinchfield, Frank, 3: 275
Stirrat, Craig, 4: 194, 195*b*
Stone, James S., 2: 146, 230, 307, 438; 4: 310
Stone, James W., 1: 308
Storer, D. Humphries, 3: 42
Storey, Elizabeth Moorfield, 2: 80
Strammer, Myron A., 4: 208*b*
Strangeways Research Laboratory, 4: 126
Stromeyer, Georg Friedrich Louis, 1: xxiii, 101, 105–106
Strong, Richard P., 4: 389*b*, 422*b*
Stryker, William, 3: 249; 4: 246
Stubbs, George, 1: *136*
Study in Hospital Efficiency, A (Codman), 3: 125, *125*, 127*b*, 128–131
Sturdevant, Charles L. (b. ca. 1913)
 Boston Children's Hospital and, 2: 299
 Crippled Children's Clinic and, 2: 299
 education and training, 2: 299
 HMS appointment, 2: 299
 Marlborough Medical Associates and, 2: 146, 269, 299

Index

MGH orthopaedics residency, 3: 74
PBBH and, 4: 18–20, 110
publication contributions, 2: 300
Sturgis, Susan, 3: 30
Sturgis, William, 3: 30
subacromial bursitis, 3: 104–105, 108–109
subdeltoid bursa, 3: 95, 98, 103–105, 108
Subjective Knee Form (IKDC), 2: 381
Subjective Shoulder Scale, 2: 380
subscapularis tendon, 2: 95, *95*
subtrochanteric osteotomy, 2: 293
Such a Joy for a Yiddish Boy (Mankin), 3: 392, *392*
suction socket prosthesis, 1: 273
Suffolk District Medical Society, 3: 120–122
Sugar Act, 1: 11
Suk, Se Il, 2: 343
Sullivan, James T., 4: 233
Sullivan, Louis, 4: 266*b*
Sullivan, Patricia, 3: 460*b*
Sullivan, Robert, 1: 317
Sullivan, Russell F. (1893-1966), 4: *343*
   BCH Bone and Joint Service, 4: 343–344, 346, 380*b*
   Boston City Hospital and, 4: 307
   Boston Red Sox and, 4: 345
   Carney Hospital and, 4: 343
   death of, 4: 346
   education and training, 4: 343
   elbow joint fracture-dislocation case, 4: 345
   Lahey Clinic and, 4: 345
   marriage and family, 4: 346
   Melrose Hospital and, 4: 343
   private medical practice, 4: 344
   professional memberships, 4: 346
   publications and research, 4: 343, 344*b*
   spinal tuberculosis research, 4: 343, 344*b*
   Ted Williams and, 4: 345–346
   Tufts Medical School appointment, 4: 343
Sullivan, Thelma Cook, 4: 346
Sullivan, W. E., 3: 86
Sumner Koch Award, 2: 415
Sunnybrook Hospital, 2: 334
SUNY Downstate Medical Center, 3: 388
supraspinatus tendon, 3: 108–109
Surgeon's Journal, A (Cushing), 3: 369
surgery. *See also* orthopaedic surgery
   abdominal, 1: 81
   antisepsis principles and, 1: 85, 141
   Astley Cooper and, 1: 34, 36, 42, 44
   Clavien-Dindo classification in, 2: 393
   Coll Warren and, 1: 81–84
   early training in, 1: 183–186
   fracture care and, 4: 463–464
   general anesthesia and, 1: 141
   HMS curriculum for, 1: 140–141
   infection from dirty, 3: 60
   Jack Warren and, 1: 22–23, 25, 29, 40
   John Collins Warren and, 1: 36–37, 53, 68
   Joseph Warren and, 1: 6, 9, 15
   long-bone fractures, 3: 60–61
   pedagogy and, 1: 34, 137–138
   plastic, 1: 71, 76–77
   Richard Warren and, 1: 90
   shoulder and, 1: 29
   use of ether, 1: 55–65
Surgery (Keen), 3: 103
Surgery (Richard Warren), 1: 90
Surgery of Joints, The (Lovett and Nichols), 2: 52
Surgical After-Treatment (Crandon and Ehrenfried), 4: 217, *217*
surgical instruments, 3: 40–41
Surgical Observations with Cases and Operations (J. M. Warren), 1: 47, 75, 78
Surgical Treatment of the Motor-Skeletal System (Bancroft), 3: 316
Sutterlin, C. E., 3: 420
Sutton, Silvia Barry, 3: 259
Suzedell, Eugene, 2: 233
Swaim, Caroline Tiffany Dyer, 4: 51
Swaim, Joseph Skinner, 4: 51
Swaim, Loring T. (1882-1964), 4: *51*
   American Rheumatism Association and, 4: 57–58
   Arthritis, Medicine and the Spiritual Law, 4: 58, *58*
   back pain research and, 3: 203
   Body Mechanics in Health and Disease, 4: 53
   Buchmanism and, 4: 57
   chronic arthritis growth disturbances case, 4: 56
   chronic arthritis treatment and, 4: 54–58
   chronic disease treatment and, 4: 52–53
   Clifton Springs Sanatorium and, 3: 88; 4: 52–53
   death of, 4: 40, 59
   early life, 4: 51
   education and training, 4: 52
   HMS appointment, 2: 223; 4: 57, 59–60
   on importance of posture, 4: 52–54
   marriage and family, 4: 59
   MGH and, 3: 269; 4: 52, 54
   Moral Re-Armament program and, 4: 57
   on patient care, 4: 54, 55*b*, 58
   private medical practice, 4: 53
   professional memberships, 4: 58–59
   publications and research, 2: 136, 297; 3: 91; 4: 52–55, 57–58, 60–61
   RBBH and, 4: 93, 406
   as RBBH chief of orthopaedics, 4: 48, 55–57, 79, 196*b*
   RBBH orthopaedic surgeon, 4: 28, 31, 33, 35, 63
   rehabilitation of soldiers and, 4: 444
   World War I and, 4: 54
Swaim, Madeline K. Gill, 4: 59
Swartz, R. Plato, 2: 438
Sweet, Elliot, 3: 242, 243*b*
Sweetland, Ralph, 3: 396
Swinton, Neil, 2: 232
Swiontkowski, Marc, 2: 424–425
Syme, James, 1: 56, 84
synovectomy, 4: 64, 102, 371–372
synovial fluid, 3: 174, *174*, 175
syringes, 1: 80, *80*
System of Surgery (Holmes), 1: 81
systemic lupus erythematosus (SLE), 4: 98
systemic sclerosis, 4: 98

T

Tachdjian, Jason, 2: 305
Tachdjian, Mihran O. (1927-1996), 2: *300*
   birth palsies research, 2: 417
   Boston Children's Hospital and, 2: 301–302
   cerebral palsy treatment, 2: 300–301, *301*
   Children's Memorial Hospital (Chicago) and, 2: 302
   course on congenital hip dysplasia, 2: 302
   death of, 2: 305
   education and training, 2: 300
   Green and, 2: 301–304
   honors and awards, 2: 305*b*
   intraspinal tumors in children case, 2: 301–302
   marriage and family, 2: 305

Northwestern University and,
2: 302
PBBH and, 4: 20
Pediatric Orthopaedic International Seminars program,
2: 304
Pediatric Orthopaedic Society
and, 2: 351
pediatric orthopaedics and,
2: 300–304
Pediatric Orthopedics, 2: 188,
303, *303*
professional memberships,
2: 304, 305*b*
publications and research,
2: 300–303, 303*b*, 304
Tachdjian, Vivian, 2: 305
Taft, Katherine, 4: 286
Taitsman, Lisa, 4: 190*b*
tarsectomy, 2: 23
Taylor, Charles Fayette, 1: 107;
2: 20, 22, 26, 47
Taylor back brace, 2: 247
Tea Act, 1: 15
Technique of Operations on the Bones, Joints, Muscles and Tendons (Souter), 2: 294, 297–298, *298*
Tegner Activity Scale, 2: 380
teleroentgenography, 2: 170, 170*t*
Temperance Society, 1: 40
tendon transfers
ankles and, 2: 148
flexor carpi ulnaris transfer procedure, 2: 172, 188, *199*
hands and forearms, 3: 428
iliotibial band and, 2: 109
Ober on, 2: 147–149
obstetrical paralysis and, 2: 96
patella, 2: 294
polio and, 2: 108–109
polio patient lower extremities,
2: 265; 3: 332–333
quadriplegic patient hands and,
2: 265
Trendelenburg limp and, 2: 108,
108
for wrist flexion and pronation
deformity, 2: 172
Tendon Transfers of the Hand and Forearm (Smith), 3: 428
tenosynovitis, 2: 89; 3: 315, 414,
438
tenotomy
Achilles, 1: 100–101, 106; 2: 25
club foot and, 1: 106, 118;
2: 25–26
early study of, 1: xxiii, 100
Guérin's, 1: 118
physical therapy and, 1: 100
Stromeyer's subcutaneous,
1: 118, *118*
technique for, 1: 100–101
Terrono, A., 4: 167
Textbook of Disorders and Injuries of the Musculoskeletal System (Salter),
1: 167
Textbook of Orthopedic Surgery for Students of Medicine (Sever),
2: 92, *93*
thalidomide, 2: 334, *334*
Thane, George D., 2: 242
Thayer General Hospital, 4: 241,
241
Theodore, George H. (1965–),
3: *437*
education and training, 3: 437
extracorporeal shockwave therapy (ESWT) research, 3: 437–438,
438
foot and ankle treatment,
3: 460*b*
HCORP and, 3: 437
HMS appointment, 3: 437
as MGH clinical faculty, 3: 464*b*
as MGH surgeon, 3: 348, 437
plantar fasciitis treatment,
3: 437–438
professional sports teams and,
3: 348
publications and research,
3: 437–438
Theodore, Harry, 3: 437
Theodore, Marie, 3: 437
Therapeutic Exercise and Massage (Bucholz), 3: 269
Thibodeau, Arthur, 4: 91, 95, 333,
378
Thilly, William G., 4: 171
Thomas, Charles, 4: 187
Thomas, Claudia L., 4: 266*b*
Thomas, Hugh Owen, 1: xxiii;
2: 20, 22, 116
Thomas, John Jenks, 2: 90
Thomas, Leah C., 4: *235*, 236
Thomas, Margaret, 4: 189
Thomas, William H. (1930–2011),
4: *187*
Brigham and Women's Hospital,
4: 163, 187
Brigham Orthopedic Associates
(BOA) and, 4: 123
Children's Hospital/MGH combined program and, 4: 187
death of, 4: 189
education and training, 4: 187
Florida Civil Air Patrol and,
4: 189
on foot surgery and rheumatoid
arthritis, 4: 188, *188*, 189
HMS appointment, 4: 187–188
honors and awards, 4: 189
marriage and family, 4: 189
on McKeever and MacIntosh
prostheses, 4: 188–189
MGH and, 4: 187
PBBH and, 4: 116, 128–129,
161, 163, 187
publications and research, 4: 69,
70*b*–71*b*, 134, 187–188, *189*
RBBH and, 4: 40, 68, 116*b*,
129, 131, 187–188
rheumatoid clinic and, 4: 188
West Roxbury Veterans Administration Hospital and, 4: 187
Thomas B. Quigley Society, 1: *282*,
283
Thomas splint, 2: 20, *123*, *247*;
3: *168*; 4: 389, *391*, *408*, 409,
411, 417, *418*
Thompson, Milton, 3: 192
Thompson, Sandra J. (1937–2003),
2: *412*, 413
arthritis clinic and, 2: 413
Boston Children's Hospital and,
2: 413
death of, 2: 414
education and training,
2: 412–413
HMS appointment, 2: 413
humanitarianism and, 2: 413
Laboratory for Skeletal Disorders
and Rehabilitation and, 2: 413
pediatric orthopaedics and, 2: 414
professional memberships,
2: 413–414
prosthetic clinic and, 2: 413
publications of, 2: 414
Ruth Jackson Orthopaedic Society and, 2: 413
Simmons College and, 2: 413
Thomson, Elihu, 2: 114; 3: 97–98
Thomson, Helen, 1: 317
thoracic insufficiency syndrome,
2: 360
thoracic outlet syndrome, 3: 415
thoracic spine, 4: 259–260
thoracostomy, 2: 360
Thorn, George W., 4: 79
Thorndike, Alice, 2: 312
Thorndike, Augustus (1863–1940),
2: *305*
address to the American Orthopaedic Association, 2: 311
Bar Harbor Medical and Surgical
Hospital and, 2: 312
Boston Children's Hospital and,
2: 34, 40, 307
Boston Dispensary and, 2: 306

Index

Boston Lying-in-Hospital and, 2: 306
death of, 2: 312
disabled children and, 2: 307–308
education and training, 2: 305–306
hip infection treatment, 2: 108
HMS appointment, 2: 307
House of the Good Samaritan and, 2: 114, 115b, 306
Manual of Orthopedic Surgery, A, 2: 311, *312*
marriage and family, 2: 312
MGH and, 2: 306
on orthopaedic supervision in schools and sports, 2: 310
orthopaedic surgery and, 1: 171; 2: 311
poliomyelitis treatment, 2: 264
professional memberships, 2: 306–307, 312
publications and research, 2: 61, 308–309
rupture of the spina bifida sac case, 2: 309–310
schools for disabled children, 2: 36, 38, 308, 310–311; 3: 151
St. Luke's Home for Convalescents, 2: 307
tuberculosis treatment, 2: 308
Thorndike, Augustus, Jr. (1896–1986), 1: *263*, *270*; 3: *450*; 4: *491*
on acromioclavicular joint dislocation in football, 1: 268
AMA Committee on the Medical Aspects of Sports, 1: 274, 280
Athlete's Bill of Rights and, 1: 279–281
Athletic Injuries. Prevention, Diagnosis and Treatment, 1: 265, *266*
Boston Children's Hospital and, 1: 264
clinical congress meeting, 3: 118
education and training, 1: 263–264
5th General Hospital and, 4: 484
first aid kit, 1: *270*
Harvard Department of Hygiene and, 2: 253
Harvard football team and, 1: 259, 263
Harvard University Health Service and, 1: 274, 277
legacy of, 1: 274–275
Manual of Bandaging, Strapping and Splinting, A, 1: 268
Massachusetts Regional Fracture Committee, 3: 64

military orthopaedics and, 1: 270–272
New England Regional Committee on Fractures, 4: 341
105th General Hospital and, 4: 489–491
preventative strappings, 1: *269*, 274
publications of, 1: 263–268, 271–274, 280–281
rehabilitation and, 1: 271–274
sports medicine and, 1: 264–269, 274–275
study of fracture treatment, 1: 264
suction socket prosthesis and, 1: 273
34th Infantry Division and, 4: 484
World War II active duty and, 1: 270–272; 2: 232; 4: 17
World War II civilian defense and, 1: 269–270
Thorndike, Charles, 3: 338
Thorndike, George, 4: 297
Thorndike, Olivia Lowell, 1: 263
Thorndike, William, 4: 297
Thornhill, Thomas S.
Brigham and Women's Hospital and, 4: 143, 163, 193–194, 195b
as BWH orthopaedics chief, 4: 172, 196b
John Ball and Buckminster Brown Professorship, 4: 195b
New England Deaconess Hospital and, 4: 280
PFC unicompartmental knee prothesis and, 4: 176–177
publications and research, 4: 180, *180*
Thrasher, Elliott, 2: 277, 290
Three Star Medal of Honour, 3: 451, *451*
thrombocytopenia, 3: 434
tibia
anterolateral bowing of, 2: 173
congenital pseudarthrosis of, 2: 173–176
pseudofracture of, 3: 341, *342*
tibial tubercle
lesions during adolescence, 2: 115, *116*, 117
nonunion of the humerus, 2: 96, *96*, 97, *97*
Osgood-Schlatter disease and, 2: 115, *116*, 117
Sever's study of, 2: 91, 96–97
treatment of, 2: 91, 96
Ticker, Jonathan B., 3: *145*

Tobin, William J., 3: 74
Toby, William, 4: 266b
Toldt, C., 2: 170
Tomaselli, Rosario, 4: 41b
Tomford, William W. (1945–), 3: *439*, 461
adult reconstruction and, 3: 460b
articular cartilage preservation research, 3: 442, *442*
on bone bank procedures, 3: 440–441, *442*
Children's Hospital/MGH combined program and, 3: 439
early life, 3: 439
education and training, 3: 439
HMS appointments, 3: 440, 440b
leadership of, 3: 443
MGH Bone Bank and, 3: 396, 439–441, 443
as MGH clinical faculty, 3: 464b
as MGH orthopaedics chief, 3: 11b, 228, 399, 443
as MGH surgeon, 3: 398b, 440, 440b
Musculoskeletal Tissue Banking, 3: 443
Naval Medical Research Institute and, 3: 439
orthopaedic oncology and, 3: 440
orthopaedic tumor fellowship program and, 3: 388
publications and research, 3: 440–443
rapid postoperative osteolysis in Paget Disease case, 3: 441
tissue banks and, 3: 386
transmission of disease through allografts research, 3: 442–443, *443*
US Navy and, 3: 439
Toom, Robert E., 2: 408
Toronto General Hospital, 2: 334
torticollis brace, 1: *99*, 100, *124*
Tosteson, Daniel, 4: 119
Total Care of Spinal Cord Injuries, The (Pierce and Nickel), 3: 321
total condylar prosthesis, 4: 130
total hip replacement
bladder fistula after, 4: 162
bone stock deficiency in, 3: 279
cemented/uncemented, 3: 223–224
Charnley and, 3: 218–219
Gibson posterior approach, 4: 170
Harris and hybrid, 3: 220
Hylamer acetabular liner complications, 4: *171*, 172
infections and, 4: 170
introduction to the U.S., 3: 218

osteoarthritis and, 3: 221, *222*
osteolysis after, 3: 220, *220*, 221–222, *222*, 223, 225
patient outcomes, 4: 134–135
pelvic osteolysis with acetabular replacement, 3: 279
radiographs of uncemented, 3: *223*
RBBH and, 4: 129
renal transplant infarction case, 4: 252–253
rheumatoid arthritis complications, 4: 134
sensitivity to heparin and, 3: 362
surgeon preferences in, 4: 170*b*
trochanteric osteotomy in, 4: 133–134
ultraviolet light and, 4: 162
use of bone ingrowth type prostheses, 3: 222–223
use of methylmethacrylate (bone cement), 3: 220, 222; 4: 129, 133, 171
total joint replacement
BWH registry for, 4: 141, *172*, 173
continuing medical education and, 3: 225
implant design, 4: 137–138
infection rates, 4: 164
metals for use in, 2: 234
patellofemoral joint, 4: 137
patient outcomes and, 3: 277; 4: 134
proximal femoral grafts and, 3: 435
research in, 3: 326; 4: 133–134, 136
tibial component fixation, 4: 137, 148
ultraviolet light and, 4: 164
Total Knee Arthroplasty (Scott), 4: 176
total knee replacement
Duocondylar prostheses and, 4: 178
duopatellar prosthesis, 4: 180*t*
gait and, 2: 408
giant cell synovitis case, 4: 148
inflammatory reactions, 3: 223
kinematic, 4: 138–139
Kinematic prosthesis, 4: 138–139, *139*, 147, 149–150
Maine Medical Assessment Foundation, 2: 372
McKeever prothesis, 4: 40, 130
metal and polyethylene prosthesis, 4: 147–148, *148*
metallic tibial tray fracture, 4: 177

osteoarthritis and, 4: 177
preservation of PCL, 4: 130, 138–139, 147, 180–181
press-fit condylar knee (PFC), 4: 180, 180*t*
prosthesis development, 4: 137, 179*t*
at RBBH, 1950–1978, 4: 131*t*
research in, 4: 133, 135
roentgenographic arthroplasty-scoring system, 4: 150
soft tissue balancing and, 4: 139
tibial component fixation, 4: 148
tourniquet, 1: 55
Towle, Chris, 3: 386
Townsend, Nadine West, 3: 300
Townsend, Solomon Davis, 1: 59; 3: 14, 18, *31*
Townshend, Charles, 1: 13
Townshend Acts, 1: 13–15
tracheostomy, 2: 49, 51
traction
Buck's, 1: 80
continuous, 1: 108; 2: 32
femoral neck fractures and, 3: 186, 189–190
flexion injuries and, 3: 348–349
for fractures and limb deformities, 2: 23, 25
halo-femoral, 2: 342, 344, 399
hip disease and, 2: 21–22, 32–33, 52–54; 3: 148
lumbar fracture-dislocation and, 3: 347
modification of, 2: 27
reductions of dislocations and, 1: 10, *43*, 44, 52, 68
scoliosis and, 2: 35, 296–297
slipped capital femoral epiphysis (SCFE) and, 2: 176
Sprengel deformity and, 2: 195–196
Thomas splint, 3: *168*, 169
Tracy, Edward A., 4: 204
Trahan, Carol, 3: 386, 392
Training Administrators of Graduate Medical Education (TAGME), 1: 238
transmetatarsal amputation, 4: 276
trauma
acute compartment syndrome of the thigh and, 3: 417
amputations and, 3: 373
bone cysts and, 2: 236
cartilaginous labrum and, 3: 352
in children, 2: 359, 365, 368, 378, 385
coxa plana, 2: 104
to the epiphysis, 2: 176, 193

fracture treatment and, 4: 339*b*–340*b*
fractures of the radial head and, 2: 396–397
hip dislocations, 2: 352–353
ischemia-edema cycle and, 2: 200
laparotomy and, 3: 55
lesions of the atlas and axis, 2: 117
military orthopaedics and, 3: 274, 301; 4: 393
olecranon fractures and, 3: 309
orthopaedic surgery and, 3: 220, 275, 376, 416; 4: 393
paralysis and, 2: 71
Sever's disease and, 2: 88–89
sports injuries and, 2: 279, 385
thoracic spine and, 4: 259
tibial tubercle and, 2: 115
treatment deficiencies, 4: 349
Trauma Management (Cave, et al.), 3: 62, 253, 273
Travis, Dorothy F., 2: 324
Travis Air Force Base, 3: 337
Treadwell, Ben, 3: 386
Treatise on Dislocations and Fractures of Joints, A (Cooper), 1: *35*, 36, *42*, 43
Treatise on Orthopaedic Surgery, A (Bradford and Lovett), 1: 108; 2: 29–30, *30*, 43, 50, *50*, 51
Treatise on the Disease of Infancy and Childhood (Smith), 2: 7
Treatment of Fractures, The (Scudder), 1: 147; 3: 55–56, *57*, *58*, 64, 99; 4: 312, 350
"Treatment of Infantile Paralysis, The" (Lovett), 2: 71
Tremont Street Medical School, 3: 26, 42
Trendelenburg limp, 2: 33, 108, *108*, 151
triceps
brachioradialis transfer for weakness, 2: 148, 153–154, *154*
tendon repair, 3: 309
transfers for deltoid muscle paralysis, 2: 230
triflanged nail, 3: 62, 185–186, *186*, 187, 189, 189*b*, 190; 4: 237
triple arthrodesis
foot deformities and, 2: 197, 228–229
heel-cord lengthening and, 2: 172
modification of, 2: 180–181
Ober and, 2: 149
stabilization of polio patients by, 2: 265

tendon transplantations and,
  3: 333
 weakness/paralysis of the foot
  and ankle, 2: 150–151
Trippel, Stephen B. (1948–), 3: *444*
 adult reconstruction and,
  3: 460*b*
 articular cartilage research,
  3: 445
 Cave Traveling Fellowship and,
  1: 217*b*
 education and training, 3: 444
 Gordon Research Conference
  and, 3: 445
 growth-plate chondrocytes
  research, 3: *444*, 445
 HCORP and, 3: 444
 HMS appointment, 3: 444–445
 as MGH clinical faculty, 3: 464*b*
 as MGH surgeon, 3: 444–445
 professional memberships and,
  3: 445
 publications and research,
  3: 444–445
 University of Indiana School of
  Medicine and, 3: 445
trochanteric osteotomy, 4: 133, 145
Trott, Arthur W. (1920–2002),
  2: *179, 313–314*
 AAOS and, 2: 314
 Boston Children's Hospital and,
  2: 233, 301, 313–316
 Boston polio epidemic and,
  2: 314–315
 Brigham and Women's Hospital
  and, 4: 163, 193
 on circulatory changes in poliomyelitis, 2: 264
 Crippled Children's Clinic and,
  2: 314
 death of, 2: 318
 education and training, 2: 313
 Foot and Ankle, The, 2: 317
 foot and ankle treatment,
  2: 316–317
 Green and, 2: 177, 286, 317–318
 on Grice, 2: 214
 Korean War and, 2: 313
 March of Dimes and, 2: 315
 marriage and family, 2: 313
 military service, 2: 313
 as naval hospital surgical consultant, 2: 313–314
 PBBH and, 2: 313; 4: 19–20,
  22, 116, 128, 163
 poliomyelitis research and
  treatment, 2: 190, 314, *314*,
  315–316
 private medical practice and,
  2: 313

 publications and research, 4: 243
 publications of, 2: 316–317
Trott, Dorothy Crawford, 2: 313,
  318
Trout, S., 2: 417
Trowbridge, William, 2: 114
Truax, R., 1: 15
Trumble, Hugh C., 3: 367
Trumble, Thomas E., 3: 431
Trumbull, John, 1: *19*
Trumbull Hospital, 4: 225
Truslow, Walter, 2: 84; 3: 229
Tseng, Victor, 1: 217*b*
tuberculosis. *See also* spinal
  tuberculosis
 amputations and, 3: 374
 bone and joint, 2: 11, 16, 25,
  308–309; 3: 148, 166
 decline due to milk pasteuriza-
  tion, 2: 16
 hip disease and, 2: 21–22
 of hips, 2: 52–53, *54*
 infected joints and, 1: 61, 73,
  75, 81; 4: 225
 of the knee, 1: 73; 4: 225
 mortality due to, 2: 4
 open-air treatment of, 4: 363,
  367
 pulmonary, 1: 56; 2: 16
 sacroiliac joint fusion for, 3: 185
 spinal, 1: 100, 106, 108–109,
  109; 2: 11; 3: 289; 4: 225
 synovial joints and, 4: 226
 treatment advances in, 2: 32
Tubiana, Raoul, 4: 182
Tucker, Sarah, 1: 4
Tufts Medical Center Hospital,
  2: 306; 4: *311*
Tufts University School of Medicine
 affiliation with Beth Israel Hospital, 4: 213–214, 214*b*, 228
 affiliation with Boston City Hospital, 4: 228, 296–297
 Aufranc and, 3: 247
 Boston Pathology Course at,
  1: 230
 Fitchet and, 2: 252
 hand fellowships and, 2: 250
 Karlin and, 2: 369–370
 Legg and, 2: 102
 Lovett and, 2: 64
 MacAusland and, 3: 308
 Ober and, 2: 165
 orthopaedics residencies,
  4: 377–379
 Painter and, 3: 266
 Radin and, 3: 328
 Smith-Petersen and, 3: 362
 Webber and, 2: 9
Tukey, Marshall, 1: 304, 309

tumors
 Barr and Mixter on, 3: 204
 bone irradiation and, 2: 237
 Codman on, 3: 110
 femoral allograft transplantation,
  3: 389–390
 giant-cell, 3: 390
 intraspinal in children, 2: 301–302
 knee fusion with allografts, 3: 435
 musculoskeletal, 3: 433, 435
 research in, 2: 236–237
 sacrococcygeal chordoma, 3: 390
Tumors of the Jaws (Scudder), 3: 64
turnbuckle jacket, 2: 80, 223–224,
  224, 225, *225*, 226, 226*b*, 227,
  227*b*, 316, *336*; 3: 209
Turner, Henry G., 4: 434
Turner, Roderick H., 2: 397;
  3: 246; 4: 187
Tyler, Charles H., 4: 303
typhoid fever, 2: 4

U

Ulin, Dorothy Lewenberg, 4: 244
Ulin, Kenneth, 4: 244
Ulin, Robert (1903–1978), 4: *242*
 BCH surgeon-in-chief, 4: 333
 as Beth Israel chief of orthopaedics, 4: 243–244, 289*b*
 Beth Israel Hospital and, 4: 242,
  247
 Boston City Hospital and, 4: 242
 Boston VA Hospital and, 4: 242
 death of, 4: 244
 education and training, 4: 242
 Faulkner Hospital and, 4: 242
 fender fracture case, 4: 242
 HMS appointment, 4: 244
 Lowell General Hospital and,
  4: 243
 marriage and family, 4: 244
 private medical practice,
  4: 242–243
 professional memberships, 4: 244
 publications and research,
  4: 229, 242–243
 silverwork by, 4: *242*, *243*, 244,
  244
 slipped capital femoral epiphysis
  research, 4: 243
 subdeltoid bursitis research,
  4: 243
 Tufts Medical School appointment, 4: 242, 244
 US Army and, 4: 242–243
ultraviolet light, 4: 162–164, 164*t*
unicompartmental prothesis, 4: 176,
  178

Unit for Epidemic Aid in Infantile Paralysis (NFP), 2: 188–189
United Cerebral Palsy Association, 2: 401
United States General Hospital (Readville, Mass.), 2: 5
University of Arkansas College of Medicine, 3: 337
University of California Hospital, 3: 336–337
University of California in San Diego (UCSD), 3: 402
University of Chicago, 3: 382
University of Edinburgh, 1: 7
University of Florida, 3: 432
University of Indiana School of Medicine, 3: 445
University of Iowa, 3: 303
University of Maryland Health Center, 4: 263–264
University of Maryland Medical Center, 4: 157
University of Massachusetts, 2: 286–288, 364
University of Massachusetts Medical School, 2: 293, 371
University of Miami Tissue Bank, 3: 442
University of Michigan Medical Center, 4: 254–255
University of Missouri, 4: 372
University of Pennsylvania Medical School, 1: 7; 2: 424
University of Pittsburgh School of Medicine, 3: 382–383, 385; 4: 111
University of Southern California, 2: 266
Upper Extremity Injuries in the Athlete (Pappas and Walzer), 2: 288
Upton, Joseph, III, 3: 431
Urist, Marshall R., 3: 433
US Air Force Hospital, 3: 323
US Army
    Boston-derived base hospitals, 4: 420*t*
    curative workshops and, 4: 403
    Division of Orthopedic Surgery, 2: 65; 4: 411–412
    Harvard Unit and, 1: 270
    hospital reconditioning program, 1: 271–272
    Hospital Train, 4: *414*
    levels of medical care by distance, 4: 475*t*
    Medical Officer instructions for, 4: 410*b*
    recruiting poster, 4: *397*
    staffing of ambulances with medics, 4: 387

US Army 3rd General Hospital (Mt. Sinai), 4: 88
US Army 3rd Southern General Hospital (Oxford), 3: 365
US Army 7th General Hospital (St. Alban's, England), 4: 90
US Army 11th General Hospital, 4: 420, 422*b*, 424–425
US Army 13th General Hospital (Boulogne, France), 4: 422*b*
US Army 22nd General Hospital, 4: 415
US Army 42nd General Hospital, 4: 488, 490
US Army 105th General Hospital, 4: *490*
    Biak Island deployment, 4: 491, 491*b*, 492, *492*
    camaraderie at, 4: 492
    Cave and, 3: 271; 4: 489
    closing of, 4: 493
    construction of, 4: 489
    in Gatton, Australia, 1: 270; 4: 488–489, *489*
    Harvard Unit and, 1: 270–271; 2: 231–232; 4: 484, 487–489
    hospital beds at, 4: 490
    malaria treatment and, 4: 491
    MGH and, 4: 493
    orthopaedic staff at, 4: 489–490
    patient rehabilitation and, 1: 271; 4: 490–491
    plaque commemorating, 4: *492*
    Rowe and, 3: 351; 4: 489, 490*b*–491*b*
    Sheldon Hall Surgical Building, 4: *490*
    tent ward, 4: *491*
    Thorndike and, 4: 489–491
US Army 118th General Hospital, 4: 488
US Army 153rd Station Hospital (Queensland), 4: 488
US Army Base Hospital No. 5 (Boulogne, France), 4: *424*, *426*
    commemoration of Harvard Unit, 4: *428*
    Cushing and, 4: 420, 420*t*, 422–423
    demobilization of, 4: 426
    first two years at, 4: 422*b*
    Harvard Unit and, 1: 270; 4: 420, 423–424, *428*
    hazards and mortality rate at, 4: 424–425
    map of, 4: *427*
    Ober and, 2: 145
    officers of, 4: *422*
    operating room at, 4: *427*

    Osgood and, 2: 125; 4: 405, 421*b*, 422
    patient ward in, 4: *428*
    PBBH and, 4: 420*t*
    training in, 4: 420–421
    US and British medical staff in, 4: 422–423, 425
US Army Base Hospital No. 6 (Talence, France)
    Adams and, 3: 232; 4: 433–434
    buildings at, 4: *432*
    demobilization of, 4: 437
    expansion of, 4: 433–434
    map of, 4: *429*
    MGH orthopaedists and, 3: 313; 4: 420*t*, 429–432
    operating room at, 4: *431*
    patient census at, 4: 436, 436*t*, 437
    patient flow process at, 4: 435–436
    patients treated at, 4: *434*
    reconstruction and occupational aides, 4: 436*b*
    release of equipment to Base Hospital No. 208, 4: 437
    surgical & orthopaedic wards, 4: *431*
    surgical ward at, 4: *433*
    use of the Petit Lycée de Talence, 4: *429*, 432
    Ward in Lycée building, 4: *430*
    WWII reactivation of, 4: 474
US Army Base Hospital No. 7 (Tours, France), 4: *438*
    Boston City Hospital and, 1: 256; 4: 420*t*, 438–439
    Harvard Unit and, 4: 437–439
    Nichols and, 4: 438–439
    Ward 6, 4: *437*
US Army Base Hospital No. 8 (Savenay, France), 3: 365
US Army Base Hospital No. 9 (Chateauroux, France), 4: 409
US Army Base Hospital No. 10 (Roxbury, Mass.), 2: 258
US Army Base Hospital No. 18 (Bazoilles-sur-Meuse, France), 2: 221–222
US Army Base Hospital No. 114 (Beau-Desert, France), 3: 232
US Army Base Hospital No. 208, 4: 437
US Army Evacuation Hospital No. 110 (Argonne), 4: 439
US Army Hospital (Landstuhl, Germany), 3: 418
US Army 34th Infantry Division, 4: 484

US Army Medical Board, 2: 124; 3: 168
US Army Medical Corps, 2: 124, 130, 220, 222; 3: 282, 288, 291, 313, 351, 365, 370; 4: 387, 420
US Army Medical Reserve Corps, 2: 66, 268; 3: 61, 89, 232
US Army Mobile Unit No. 6 (Argonne), 4: 426
US Army Nurse Corps, 4: 492
US Army ROTC, 3: 300
US Food and Drug Administration (FDA), 3: 249
US General Hospital No. 2 (Fort McHenry, Maryland), 4: 452
US General Hospital No. 3 (Camp Shanks, Orangeburg, New York), 4: 88
US General Hospital No. 3 (Colonia, N.J.), 4: 452
US General Hospital No. 5, 4: *487*
    in Belfast, Ireland, 4: 484–485
    closing of, 4: 487
    construction of, 4: *486*
    facilities at, 4: 485–486
    Fort Bragg and, 4: 484
    Harvard Unit and, 1: 270, 277; 3: 271; 4: 484
    in Normandy, France, 4: 486, *486*, 487
    nursing at, 4: *487*
    in Odstock, England, 4: 486
    operating room at, 4: *487*
    personnel and training, 4: 484
    ward tent, 4: *486*
US General Hospital No. 6
    Aufranc and, 3: 239, 240*b*
    bivouac and staging area in Maddaloni, Italy, 4: *479*
    in Bologna, Italy, 4: *481*, 482
    Camp Blanding and, 4: 474–475
    Camp Kilmer and, 4: 475
    in Casablanca, 4: 476–477, *477*, 480*b*
    closing of, 4: 482, 484
    commendation for, 4: 485*b*
    experiences at, 4: 483*b*
    hospital ward in Naples, 4: *479*
    Instituto Buon Pastore and, 4: *480*, 481
    leadership of, 4: 482*b*
    main entrance, 4: *481*
    medical staff, 4: *476*
    MGH and, 3: 239, 362; 4: 474, 485*b*
    mobilization of, 4: 475–476
    operating room at, 4: *481*
    organization of, 4: 477
    orthopaedics section of, 4: 482, 483*b*
    Peninsular Base Station and, 4: 481–482
    personnel and training, 4: 474–475
    prisoners of war and, 4: 484
    relocation of, 4: 479, 481
    in Rome, Italy, 4: 481–482
    surgical services at, 4: 478, *478*
    temporary camp in Italy, 4: *480*
    wards at, 4: *478*
US General Hospital No. 10, 4: *328*, *445*, *446*
    Cotton and, 4: 452
    Elks' Reconstruction Hospital and, 4: 447–448
    Massachusetts Women's Hospital and, 4: 447–448
    as a model for civilian hospitals, 4: 450–451
    RBBH and, 4: 447–448
    West Roxbury plant (Boston City Hospital), 4: 447–448
US Medical Department, 4: 439
US Naval Hospital, 3: 201, 207
US Naval Medical Corps, 3: 248
US Navy Tissue Bank, 3: 439–440, 442
US Public Health Service, 4: 165
US War Department, 4: 474
USS *Arizona*, 4: 465
USS *Okinawa*, 3: 446, *447*
USS *West Point*, 4: 488

V

Vail Valley Medical Center, 3: 446
Vainio, Kauko, 4: 96
Valley Forge Army Hospital, 2: 279
Van Dessel, Arthur, 1: 193
Van Gorder, George W. (1888–1969), 3: *364*
    arthrodesis procedures, 3: 368, *368*
    Brackett and, 3: 365
    Cave on, 3: 368
    chronic posterior elbow dislocation case, 3: 366
    Clinics for Crippled Children and, 2: 230; 3: 365
    death of, 3: 368
    early life, 3: 364
    education and training, 3: 364–365
    femoral neck fracture research and treatment, 3: 185–186, *186*, 367, *367*
    fracture research and, 3: 334, 366–367
    hip nailing and, 3: 237
    HMS appointment, 3: 365
    hospital appointments, 3: 365
    marriage and family, 3: 365
    MGH Fracture Clinic and, 3: 60*b*, 314, 366
    as MGH house officer, 1: 189
    as MGH orthopaedics chief, 1: 199; 3: 11*b*
    as MGH surgeon, 3: 187, 192, 365, 367–368
    Peking Union Medical College and, 3: 365
    private medical practice, 3: 365
    professional memberships and, 3: 368
    publications and research, 3: 365–368
    Trumble technique for hip fusion and, 3: 367, *367*
    US Army Medical Corps and, 3: 365
    World War I volunteer orthopaedics, 4: 407
Van Gorder, Helen R. Gorforth, 3: 365
Vanguard, The, 4: *421*
Vanishing Bone (Harris), 3: 225, *225*
vascular anastomosis, 4: 216
vastus slide, 3: 278
Vauzelle, C., 2: 340
Venel, Jean-Andrew, 1: xxii
VEPTR (Vertical Expandable Prosthetic Titanium Rib), 2: 360, *362*
Verdan, Claude, 4: 96
Vermont Department of Health, 2: 221
Vermont Medical Association, 2: 221
Vermont State Medical Society, 2: 147
vertebral column resections (VCRs), 2: 362–363
Veterans Administration Hospital (La Jolla, Calif.), 3: 402
Veterans Administration Medical Center (Richmond, Virginia), 4: 153
Veterans Administration Prosthetic and Sensory Aids Service, 1: 273
Veterans Administration Rehabilitation Research and Development Programs, 4: 152
Vincent, Beth, 2: 119; 4: 389*b*
Virchow, Rudolf, 1: 82
visceroptosis, 3: 83–84, 84*b*, 86–88
Vogt, E. C., 3: 341, *342*
Vogt, Paul, 2: 115
volar plate arthroplasty, 2: 248
Volkmann ischemic contracture, 2: 200–201, *201*, 249–250

Volunteer Aid Association, 3: 152–153
Von Kessler, Kirby, 2: 325
Vose, Robert H., 4: 389*b*
Vrahas, Mark, 1: 167, 235; 3: 462, 464*b*; 4: 194
Vresilovic, Edward J., Jr., 4: 288

W

Wacker, Warren E.C., 4: 132
Wagner, Katiri, 3: 410
Wagner spherical osteotomy, 2: 390–392
Waite, Frederick C., 4: 50
Waldenström, Johann H., 2: 104
Waldo County General Hospital, 2: 371
Walford, Edward, 1: *34*
Walker, C. B., 4: 10
Walker, Irving, 4: 305
Walker, Peter, 4: 130, 137–138, 147, 152, 176, 178
Walker, Thomas, 3: 132–133
Wallis, Oscar, 3: 25
Walsh, Francis Norma, 2: 333
Walter, Alice, 4: 109
Walter, Carl, 4: 109
Walter, Carl Frederick, 4: 104
Walter, Carl W. (1905–1992), 4: *104, 106, 108*
   aseptic technique interest, 4: 105–106
   Aseptic Treatment of Wounds, 4: 106, *106*, 107*b*
   blood storage bag, 4: 107, *107*, 108
   canine surgical scenarios and, 4: 105
   death of, 4: 109
   education and training, 4: 104
   fracture treatment and, 1: 204; 4: 16, 18
   HMS appointment, 4: 105, 107*b*
   HMS Surgical Research Laboratory, 4: 105, *106*, 107–108
   marriage and family, 4: 109
   medical device development, 4: 107–108
   PBBH and, 4: 16, 18–20, 79, 104–105
   PBBH blood bank and, 4: 107–108
   PBBH fracture service, 4: 108–109
   professional memberships, 4: 109
   publications and research, 4: 106
   renal dialysis machine modification, 4: 108
   on ultraviolet light use, 4: 164
Walter, David, 4: 109
Walter, Leda Agatha, 4: 104
Walter, Linda, 4: 109
Walter, Margaret, 4: 109
Walter, Margaret Davis, 4: 109
Walter, Martha, 4: 109
Walter Reed General Hospital, 3: 168; 4: 327, *450*, 451, 488, *488*
Walzer, Janet, 2: 288
War of 1812, 1: 40–41
Ware, John, 1: 296, 299, 302
Warman, Matthew, 2: 439, 439*b*
Warner, Jon J. P., 3: *145*, 462, 464*b*; 4: 194, 195*b*
Warren, Abigail Collins, 1: 24, 28, 31
Warren, Amy Shaw, 1: 85, 87
Warren, Anne Winthrop, 1: 55
Warren, Annie Crowninshield, 1: 76–78
Warren, Edward (author), 1: 46, 68
Warren, Edward (son of Jack), 1: 24, 28, 31
Warren, Elizabeth, 1: 4
Warren, Elizabeth Hooton, 1: 9, 15, 21
Warren, Gideon, 1: 4
Warren, Howland (1910–2003), 1: 90–91
Warren, Howland Shaw, Jr. (1951–), 1: 71, 91
Warren, John (1874–1928), 1: *88*
   anatomical atlas and, 1: 88–89
   anatomy instruction at Harvard Medical School, 1: 71, 88; 2: 296; 4: 82
   enlistment in WWI, 1: 88
   injury and death of, 1: 89
   medical education, 1: 87–88
   Outline of Practical Anatomy, An, 1: 88
Warren, John (ca. 1630), 1: 4
Warren, John Collins (1778–1856), 1: *31, 33, 67, 68*
   American mastodon skeleton and, 1: 51, *51*, 52
   amputations and, 1: 52–53, 61
   apprenticeship with father, 1: 33
   birth of, 1: 24, 31
   on chloroform, 3: 31
   community organizations and, 1: 69
   daily routine of, 1: 39
   death of, 1: 66–67, 77
   diagnostic skills, 1: 52–53
   dislocated hip treatment, 3: 13, 13*b*
   donation of anatomical museum, 1: 66
   early life, 1: 31
   educational organizations and, 1: 38–39
   Etherization, 1: 62, *62*; 3: 33
   European medical studies, 1: 33–37, 54
   on father's death, 1: 29–30
   first use of ether at MGH, 1: 56–59, *59*, 60–62, *63*, 64–65, 77; 3: 27–28, 28*b*, 29, 29*b*, 30, 32–34
   founding of Boston Medical Association, 1: 38
   founding of MGH, 1: 31, 41–42, 71; 3: 5, *5*, 6*b*–7*b*, 12–13
   fundraising for hospital in Boston, 1: 41
   Genealogy of Warren, 1: 4
   at Harvard College, 1: 31–32
   Harvard Medical School and, 1: 38–40, 66, 68–69, 299; 3: 30, 94
   as Hersey Professor of Anatomy and Surgery, 1: 29, 66, 68
   hip dislocation case, 1: 42, 44–46, *46*, 47–50, 68; 3: 36
   home of, 1: *38*, 51
   influence of Astley Cooper on, 1: 36–37
   influence on Mason, 1: 72, 75
   interest in exercise, 1: 54
   John Ball Brown and, 1: 97–99
   legacy of, 1: 68–69
   "Letter to the Honorable Isaac Parker," 1: 45, *45*
   marriage to Anne Winthrop, 1: 55
   marriage to Susan Powell Mason, 1: 37–38
   medical and surgical practice, 1: 37–39, 51–55, 66
   medical studies at Harvard, 1: 32–33
   orthopaedics curriculum and, 1: 136–137
   orthopaedics specialty and, 1: 99–100, 119
   Parkman on, 1: 296
   postsurgical treatment and, 1: 52–53
   publications of, 1: 46, 52, *52*, 53, 62, *62*, 69*b*
   reputation of, 1: 51–53
   retirement and, 1: 65–66
   Spunkers and bodysnatching, 1: 32–33
   surgical apprenticeship, 1: 33–37
   surgical practice at MGH, 1: 52–55, 57–58, 65
   Temperance Society and, 1: 40
   thumping skills, 1: 37

Index

Warren, John Collins "Coll" (1842–1927), 1: *79, 80, 82*; 3: *19*
   antisepsis principles and, 1: 85–86; 3: 45
   Charles L. Scudder and, 3: 54–55
   as Civil War hospital surgeon, 1: 79–80
   death of, 1: 87
   European medical studies, 1: 81–84
   fundraising for cancer research, 1: 87
   fundraising for Harvard Medical School, 1: 85, 87; 4: 3
   Harvard Medical School campus and, 1: 87
   Henry Bowditch and, 1: 82
   honorary degrees, 1: 87
   as house pupil at MGH, 1: 80–81
   influence of father on, 1: 80
   influence of Lister on, 1: 84
   Lowell hip dislocation and, 1: 49
   medical and surgical practice, 1: 84–85, *85*, 86; 2: 3
   medical education, 1: 79–81
   professorship at Harvard Medical School, 1: 87; 2: 32
   publications of, 1: 87
   Remembrances, 1: 83
   research laboratory at MGH, 1: 71
   study of tumors, 1: 85
   as supervisor at MGH, 2: 20
   surgical training, 1: 81–84
   treatment of tumors and, 1: 82
Warren, John "Jack" (1753–1815), 1: 23
   admission tickets to lectures, 1: *27*
   anatomical studies, 1: 22–25
   anatomy lectures, 1: 24, 26–29
   anti-slavery sentiment, 1: 24
   apprenticeships by, 1: 15, 21, 25, 33
   attendance certificates, 1: *28*
   community affairs and, 1: 29
   death of, 1: 29–30, 41
   early life, 1: 21
   establishment of medical board, 1: 29
   father's death and, 1: 3–4
   founding of Boston Medical Association, 1: 25
   founding of Harvard Medical School, 1: 21, 25–29, 40, 71
   at Harvard College, 1: 21
   institutionalization of Boston medicine and, 1: 30
   marriage and family, 1: 24, 28, 31
   Masons and, 1: 29
   medical studies at Harvard, 1: 6
   military service, 1: 22
   orthopaedics curriculum and, 1: 134
   as pioneer of shoulder surgery, 1: 29
   private medical practice, 1: 22, 24, 28
   publications of, 1: 29
   as senior surgeon for Continental Army, 1: 22–24
   smallpox inoculations and, 1: 9, 29
   Spunkers and bodysnatching, 1: 21
Warren, Jonathan Mason (1811–1867), 1: *71, 76*
   birth of, 1: 38
   chronic illness, 1: 72, 76–78
   European medical studies, 1: 53, 73–76
   fracture care and, 1: 76
   influence of father on, 1: 72, 75
   influence on Coll, 1: 80
   instrument case, 1: *77*
   introduction of plastic surgery to the U.S., 1: 71–72, 77
   legacy of, 1: 78–79
   on Lowell's autopsy, 1: 47–50
   medical practice with father, 1: 76–77
   medical studies at Harvard, 1: 72
   MGH and, 1: 53; 3: 15, *31*
   Norwalk train accident and, 1: 77
   orthopaedic surgery and, 1: 81
   plastic surgery techniques, 1: 76–77
   publications of, 1: 78
   scientific method and, 1: 71, 74
   support for House of the Good Samaritan, 1: 124
   Surgical Observations with Cases and Operations, 1: 47, 75, 78
   use of ether, 1: 57, 63
   as visiting surgeon at MGH, 1: 77
   Warren Triennial Prize and, 1: 78
Warren, Joseph (1663–1729), 1: 4
Warren, Joseph (1696–1755), 1: 3–4
Warren, Joseph (1741–1775), 1: *3, 11*, 18
   apprenticeships by, 1: 15
   Boston Massacre oration, 1: 15–16
   Boston Massacre report, 1: 14
   Bunker Hill battle, 1: 18–19
   command of militia, 1: 18
   death at Bunker Hill, 1: 3, 19, *19*, 20, 22
   early career, 1: 6
   father's death and, 1: 3–4
   as founder of medical education in Boston, 1: 15
   marriage to Elizabeth Hooten, 1: 9
   Masons and, 1: 10–12
   medical studies at Harvard, 1: 6
   Mercy Scollay and, 1: 19
   obstetrics and, 1: 9
   orthopaedic practice and, 1: 10
   physician apprenticeship, 1: 6, 8
   as physician to the Almshouse, 1: 15
   as president of the Third Provincial Congress, 1: 18
   private medical practice, 1: 8–10, 15
   publications and, 1: 12
   as Revolutionary War leader, 1: 10–20
   smallpox inoculations and, 1: 8–9
   Suffolk Resolves and, 1: 16
   tea party protest and, 1: 16
Warren, Joseph (1876–1942), 1: 87, 90
Warren, Margaret, 1: 4
Warren, Martha Constance Williams, 1: 90
Warren, Mary, 1: 19
Warren, Mary Stevens (1713–1803), 1: 3–4, 10
Warren, Peter, 1: 4
Warren, Rebecca, 1: 96
Warren, Richard (1907–1999), 1: 71, 90–91, 270; 3: 330; 4: 20
Warren, Richard (d. 1628), 1: 4
Warren, Shields, 4: *277b*
Warren, Susan Powell Mason, 1: 37–38, 72
Warren Anatomical Museum, 1: 28, 49–50, 52, 66; 3: 38
Warren family
   early years in Boston, 1: 4
   Harvard Medical School (HMS) and, 1: 71
   history of, 1: *4b*
   lineage of physicians in, 1: 3, *5*, 6, 71
   Massachusetts General Hospital (MGH) and, 1: 71
Warren Russet (Roxbury) apples, 1: 3, *4*
Warren Triennial Prize, 1: 78
Warren's Atlas, 1: 89
Warshaw, Andrew, 3: 146

Washburn, Frederick A., 1: 188;
3: 1, 70*b*, 174; 4: 420*t*, 429–430,
432, 433
Washington, George, 1: 19, 22–23
Washington University, 3: 163–165
Washington University Base Hospital
No. 21, 3: 166
Washington University School of
Medicine, 3: 165, 170, 404–405
Watanabi, Masaki, 2: 279
Waterhouse, Benjamin, 1: 25, 40
Waters, Peter (1955–), 2: *414*
birth palsies research, 2: 415,
417, *417*, 418–419, *419*, 420
Boston Children's Hospital and,
2: 415, 415*b*, 420, 439*b*
education and training, 2: 414
hand surgery and, 2: 414–415
hand trauma research, 2: 415
HMS appointment, 2: 415, 415*b*
honors and awards, 2: 415
John E. Hall Professorship in
Orthopaedic Surgery, 2: 439*b*
as orthopaedic chair, 2: 15*b*
orthopaedics curriculum and,
1: 216, 225
orthopaedics education and,
2: 416*b*
posterior shoulder dislocation
case, 2: 417–418
professional memberships,
2: 416*b*
publications and research,
2: 415, 417, *417*, 418–420
radiographic classification of glenohumeral deformity, 2: 419*t*
on Simmons, 4: 186
visiting professorships and lectures, 2: 415, 416*b*
Watkins, Arthur L., 1: 273; 3: 269,
285–286, *286*, 454*b*
Watts, Hugh G. (1934–), 2: *420*
Boston brace and, 2: 423–424,
424
Boston Children's Hospital and,
2: 422–423
Brigham and Women's Hospital
and, 4: 193
Children's Hospital of Philadelphia and, 2: 424
education and training, 2: 420
on gait laboratories, 2: 424
global public health and, 2: 421,
424–425
HMS appointment, 2: 422
humanitarianism and, 2: 421
on the Krukenberg procedure,
2: 425
limb-salvage procedure by,
2: 422, 423*b*

McIndoe Memorial Research
Unit and, 2: 422
PBBH and, 4: 163
on pediatric orthopaedics,
2: 303–304
professional memberships, 2: 425
publications and research,
2: 421–422, *422*, 423–424,
424, 425
scoliosis research, 2: 423
University of California and,
2: 425
University of Pennsylvania and,
2: 424
Wayne County Medical Society,
2: 135
Weaver, Michael J., 3: 463*b*
Webber, S. G., 2: 5, 9
Webster, Daniel, 1: 54, 307
Webster, Hannah White, 1: 298
Webster, Harriet Fredrica Hickling,
1: 299
Webster, John W., 1: *299*
confession of, 1: 312–313
debt and, 1: 302–303
detection of arsenic poisoning,
1: 301–302
education and training, 1: 299
Ephraim Littlefield and,
1: 303–304
execution of, 1: *313*, 314
on guilt of, 1: 314–318
HMS chemistry professorship,
1: 296, 298–301
home of, 1: *302*
letters on behalf of, 1: 309, *309*,
310–311
Manual of Chemistry, 1: 299,
301
murder of George Parkman,
1: 305–312, 315, *315*, 318
publications of, 1: 299–301
trial of, 1: 307, *307*, 308–311,
314–316; 3: 40
Webster, Redford, 1: 298
Weed, Frank E., 4: 409
Weigel, Louis A., 2: 56
weight training, 3: 281–282
Weiland, Andrew J., 3: 431
Weiner, David, 2: 436
Weiner, Norbert, 2: 326
Weinfeld, Beverly D. Bunnin,
4: 101, 103
Weinfeld, Marvin S. (1930–1986),
4: *101*
Beth Israel Hospital and, 4: 247
Brigham and Women's Hospital,
4: 163
death of, 4: 103
education and training, 4: 101

HMS appointment, 4: 102–103
hospital appointments, 4: 102
knee arthroplasty evaluation,
4: 103
marriage and family, 4: 101, 103
on McKeever and MacIntosh
prostheses, 4: 189
MGH and, 4: 101
osteogenic sarcoma research,
4: 102
PBBH and, 4: 163
private medical practice, 4: 102
professional memberships, 4: 103
publications and research,
4: 102–103
RBBH and, 4: 41*b*, 68, 80,
102–103, 116*b*, 131
synovectomy of the knee research,
4: 40, 102–103
total elbow replacement and,
4: 129
US Army Medical Corps and,
4: 101
Weinstein, James N., 2: 371;
4: 266*b*
Weiss, Charles, 3: 385–386, 395,
413, 460*b*
Weiss, Soma, 3: 350; 4: 79
Weissbach, Lawrence, 3: 460*b*
Weld, William, 3: 424
Weller, Thomas, 2: 234
Wellesley Convalescent Home, 2: 9,
189, 191
Wellington, William Williamson,
1: 59
Wells, Horace, 1: 56–57, 60
Welsh, William H., 1: 185
Wenger, Dennis, 2: 403
Wennberg, Jack, 2: 372, 374, *374*
Wennberg, John, 4: 185
Wesselhoeft, Walter, 3: 120
West Roxbury Veterans Administra-
tion Hospital
DeLorme and, 3: 285
Ewald and, 4: 144
HCORP residencies and,
1: 199–200, 206–208, 218,
220, 224–225
MacAusland and, 3: 312
McGinty and, 2: 279; 4: 22
orthopaedic biomechanics labora-
tory, 4: 137
orthopaedics residencies, 4: 378
RBBH and, 4: 36
Simon and, 2: 406
spinal cord injury research and
treatment, 4: 152
Spinal Cord Injury Service,
4: 152–153
training program at, 4: 117

Index

West Virginia University School of Medicine, 3: 328
Weston, Craig, 1: 217*b*
Weston, G. Wilbur, 2: 438
Weston, Nathan, 1: 44–45, 50
Weston Forest and Trail Association, 4: 91, *91*
Whipple, John Adams, 1: *31*
Whipple, Martha Ellen, 2: 113
White, Anita Ottemo, 4: 266
White, Arthur H., 4: 263
White, Augustus A., III (1936–), 4: *257*, *263*
   "Analysis of the Mechanics of the Thoracic Spine in Man," 4: 259, *259*
   AOA Alfred R. Shands Jr. lecture, 4: 264
   back pain research and, 4: 258
   as Beth Israel chief of orthopaedics, 4: 262–264, 289*b*
   as Beth Israel chief of surgery, 4: 223, 255
   BIDMC teaching program and, 4: 286
   BIH annual reports, 4: 262–263
   biomechanics research, 4: 260–261
   Brigham and Women's Hospital and, 4: 163, 193
   Cervical Spine Research Society president, 4: 265
   Clinical Biomechanics of the Spine, 4: 262
   clinical research protocols at BIH and, 4: 262
   Delta Upsilon fraternity and, 4: 258
   diversity initiatives in orthopaedics, 4: 264–265
   education and training, 4: 257–258
   Ellen and Melvin Gordon Professor of Medical Education, 4: 264, 266
   Federation of Spine Associations president, 4: 265
   Fort Ord US Army Hospital and, 4: 259
   HMS appointment, 4: 262, 264, 266
   honors and awards, 4: 264–265
   legacy of, 4: 265–266
   marriage and family, 4: 266
   MGH and, 3: 398*b*
   nonunion of a hangman's fracture case, 4: 261
   Oliver Wendell Holmes Society and, 4: 264
   orthopaedic biomechanics doctorate, 4: 259
   professional memberships and activities, 4: 265
   publications and research, 4: 259–262, 264
   Seeing Patients, 4: 265
   spine fellowship program and, 4: 263
   spine research, 4: 259–261, *261*, 262, 264
   University of Maryland Health Center presidency offer, 4: 263–264
   US Army Medical Corps and, 4: 258–259
   Yale University School of Medicine and, 4: 259–260, 262
White, D., 1: 258
White, George Robert, 3: 75
White, Hannah, 1: 298
White, J. Warren, 2: 197
White, John, 3: 191
White, Kevin, 4: 379
White, Paul Dudley, 4: 431
Whitehill, W. M., 2: 11
White's Apothecary Shop, 1: 39–40
Whiteside, Helen E., 2: 292
Whitman, Armitage, 4: 233
Whitman, Royal, 2: 31, 93
Whitman's foot plate, 2: 244–245
Whitman's operation (astragalectomy), 2: 92–94
Whittemore, Wyman, 4: 211, 283*t*
whooping cough, 2: 4
Wickham, Thomas W., 4: 371
Wiggin, Sidney C., 4: 330
Wigglesworth, George, 3: 124
Wigglesworth, Marian Epes, 4: 83
Wilcox, C. A., 3: 34
Wilcox, Oliver D., 3: 34
Wild, Charles, 1: 96
Wilensky, Charles F., 1: 158
Wilkins, Early, 3: 448
Willard, DeForest P., 1: 197; 2: 78, 160
Willard, Joseph, 1: 25
Willard Parker Hospital, 1: 276
Willert, H. G., 3: 220
William H. and Johanna A. Harris Professorship, 3: 464*b*
William H. Thomas Award, 4: 189, 190*b*
William T. Green Fund, 2: 436
William Wood and Company, 2: 50–51
Williams, Harold, 1: 250
Williams, Henry W., 1: 138
Williams, Ted, 1: 258; 4: 342, 345–346
Wilson, Edward, 3: 369
Wilson, George, 1: 56
Wilson, Germaine Parfouru-Porel, 3: 370
Wilson, H. Augustus, 3: 234
Wilson, James L., 2: 78, 191
Wilson, John C., Sr., 1: 189
Wilson, Louis T., 4: 313
Wilson, Marion, 4: 389*b*
Wilson, Michael G., 3: 248; 4: 193–194, 195*b*
Wilson, Philip D., Sr. (1886–1969), 3: *369*, *375*
   American Ambulance Hospital and, 4: 389*b*, *390*
   American Appreciation, An, 3: 369
   amputation expertise, 3: 371, 373–374; 4: 472*b*
   arthroplasty of the elbow, 4: 63
   back pain research and, 3: 204
   on Cobb, 2: 225–226
   death of, 3: 376
   displacement of proximal femoral epiphysis case, 3: 372
   early life, 3: 369
   education and training, 3: 369
   Experience in the Management of Fractures and Dislocations, 3: 376
   fracture research and, 3: 371–373
   Fractures, 3: 315
   Fractures and Dislocations, 3: 371, *371*
   Harvard Unit and, 2: 119, 123; 3: *180*, 369
   HMS appointment, 3: 371
   Hospital for the Ruptured and Crippled, 3: 376
   Human Limbs and Their Substitutes, 3: 376
   knee flexion contracture approach, 3: 374–375, *375*
   Management of Fractures and Dislocations, 3: 62, 273
   marriage and family, 3: 370
   MGH Fracture Clinic and, 3: 60*b*, 61, 314, 371, 373, 376
   as MGH house officer, 1: 189
   as MGH surgeon, 3: 187, 269, 370
   military orthopaedics and, 4: 473
   New York Hospital for the Ruptured and Crippled and, 1: 89
   on Osgood, 2: 138
   private medical practice, 3: 338
   professional memberships and, 3: 376

publications and research, 2: 136, 297; 3: 371–373, *373*, 374–376; 4: 60, 363
RBBH and, 4: 28, 31, 55
Robert Breck Brigham Hospital and, 3: 370
Scudder Oration on Trauma, 3: 63
slipped capital femoral epiphysis treatment, 4: 237
US Army Medical Corps, 3: 370
World War II volunteers and, 4: 363
Wilson, Philip, Jr., 4: 134
Wiltse, Leon, 3: 249
Wimberly, David, 1: 233
Winchester Hospital, 2: 218–219; 3: 299, 417; 4: 169, 214
Winter, R. B., 2: 343
Winthrop, Anne, 1: 55
Winthrop Group, 2: 317
Wirth, Michael, 2: 288
Wislocki, George B., 1: 179
Wistar, Casper, 1: 39
Wittenborg, Dick, 2: 234
Wojtys, Edward, 1: 286
Wolbach, S. Burt, 2: 234; 4: *6*
Wolcott, J. Huntington, 2: 5
Wolfe, Richard J., 1: 59
Wolff, Julius, 1: xxiii
women
 ACL injuries, 1: 285–286
 admission to HMS, 1: 138, 138*b*, 239
 chronic illness treatment, 1: 123–124, 129
 as MGH house officers, 1: 239
 nursing training, 1: 41; 2: 7–8; 4: 208
 opposition to medical studies by, 3: 44
women orthopaedic surgeons
 first HCORP resident, 1: 239
 limited teaching residencies for, 1: 200
 Ruth Jackson Orthopaedic Society and, 2: 413
Wong, David A., 4: 272*b*
Wood, Bruce T., 4: 117, 129, 163, 193
Wood, Edward Stickney, 3: 94
Wood, G. W., 3: 420
Wood, Leonard, 4: 337
Woodhouse, Charles, 4: 378
Woods, Archie S., 2: 82
Worcester, Alfred, 1: 259, 262–263
workers' compensation
 Aitken and, 4: 353–354
 carpal tunnel syndrome and, 2: 375; 4: 186

Cotton and, 4: 325, 444
major medical problems and, 3: *379*
rehabilitation goals and, 4: 354
surgical interventions and, 2: 373; 4: 352
treatment protocols and, 4: 353–354
Yett and, 4: 253
World Health Organization, 1: 168
World War I. *See also* American Expeditionary Forces (AEF); British Expeditionary Forces (BEF)
 American Ambulance Hospital (Neuilly, France), 2: 117–119, *119*, 120; 3: 166, 180, *180*; 4: 9, 386, *386*, 387, *387*
 American base hospitals, 4: 419–420
 American Expeditionary Forces, 2: 126, 128, 221
 American experience in, 4: 405*b*
 American Field Service Ambulance, 4: 386, *386*, 387, *387*, 388
 American medical volunteers, 1: 256; 2: 117–119; 4: 387–396, 398–399, *399*, 402, 404, 406–409, 412*b*–413*b*, 425
 AOA and orthopaedic hospitals, 2: 64
 British Expeditionary Forces, 4: 10
 curative workshops, 4: 399–403, *403*
 end of, 4: *453*
 facilities for wounded soldiers, 4: 414–416
 femur fracture treatment, 4: 408
 field ambulances, 4: 414–415, *415*
 field hospital equipment, 4: 393*b*
 field hospitals, 4: *414*
 First Goldthwait Unit, 4: *399*
 Harvard Medical School and, 2: 41, 64, 117–120, 125, 145
 hospital trains, 4: *414*, *416*
 impact of posture-related conditions, 4: 233
 impact on medical education, 4: 397
 impact on orthopaedics, 4: 453–454, 463–464
 impact on US economy, 4: 465
 military hospitals and, 1: 270
 military reconstruction hospitals and, 4: 439–441
 military surgeon training and, 1: 148; 2: 65–69

 New England Dressings Committee (Red Cross Auxiliary), 4: *10*
 orthopaedic contributions before, 2: 50–63
 orthopaedic surgery, 2: 119–126
 postural treatments and, 3: 83
 recruiting poster, 4: 397
 rehabilitation of soldiers and, 2: 67–68; 4: 396
 scheme of British hospitals, 4: *414*
 splints and, 3: 167–169, 169*b*; 4: 389, *391*, *408*, 409, 411, 416–417
 standardization of equipment, 2: 124; 3: 167–168
 transport of injured, 3: 169, 169*b*, *170*
 trench warfare in, 4: 385, 389, *390*
 US Army Hospital Train, 4: *414*
 US declaration of war on Germany, 4: *396*
 US entry into, 4: 409
 wound treatment during, 4: 385, 389, *390*, 391, 395–396, 407, 471
World War II
 American medical volunteers, 4: 363
 bombing of Pearl Harbor, 4: *465*, 466
 civilian defense and, 1: 269–270
 civilian surgery specialists, 4: 471–472
 field hospitals and, 4: 468
 Fifth Portable Surgical Hospital, 4: 489
 Fourth Portable Surgical Hospital (4PSH), 2: 232–233; 4: 489
 Harvard Unit (5th General Hospital), 1: 270, 277; 3: 271; 4: 17, 484
 Harvard Unit (105th General Hospital), 1: 270–271; 2: 231–232; 4: 488–489
 HMS surgeons and, 1: 270; 2: 232
 Hospital Trains, 4: *478*
 impact on training programs, 4: 467
 impact on US economy, 4: 465
 impact on US hospitals, 4: 467–468
 military hospitals in Australia, 4: 488–489
 military surgery and, 4: 469–470
 mobile army surgical hospitals (MASHs), 2: 231–232, *232*, 233; 4: 468–469, *470*
 mobile warfare in, 4: 468–469

Index

orthopaedic surgery and, 4: 463, 473, 493
physician preparation for war injury treatment, 3: 367
US Army 5th General Hospital, 4: 484–487
US Army 6th General Hospital, 4: 474–478, *478*, 479, 480*b*, 481–482, 483*b*, 484, 484*b*
US Army 105th General Hospital, 1: 270; 2: 232; 3: 351; 4: 487–493
US Army levels of medical care, 4: 475*t*
US entry into, 4: *466*, 467
wound management and, 3: 274; 4: 469, 469*b*, 470–473
wound management
  amputations, 4: *469*
  aseptic treatment of, 4: 107*b*, 469
  changes from WWI to WWII, 4: 471, 473
  evidence-based practices and, 2: 379
  gunshot injuries, 2: 66, 119, 161, 233; 3: 43; 4: 437, 441
  impact of World War II on, 3: 274; 4: 469, 469*b*, 470–472
  military orthopaedics and, 2: 121, 128, 233; 3: 43
  in osteomyelitis, 3: 301
  standardization of, 4: 470
  wounded soldiers and, 4: 385, 391, 398–399, 432, 434–435, 437, 451
  WWI Medical Officer instructions for, 4: 410*b*
Wright, John, 1: 216, 224–225; 2: 378
Wright, R. John, 4: 193, 195*b*
Wright, Wilhelmine, 2: 70
Wrist and Radius Injury Surgical Trial (WRIST), 3: 409–410
wrists. *See also* hands
  arthrodesis procedures, 3: 191, 239; 4: 166–167
  avascular necrosis case, 3: 403
  carpal injuries, 3: 101–102
  distal radius fractures, 3: 408–409
  flexor carpi ulnaris transfer procedure, 2: 172, 188, 198–199, *199*, 200
  fusion and, 2: 198, 200; 4: 167
  lunate dislocation, 3: 101–102
  reconstruction of, 2: 248
  rheumatoid arthritis and, 4: 166–167, *167–168*
  scaphoid fracture, 4: 361

  tendon transfers and, 2: 172
  ulnar nerve compression and, 3: 405–406
  vascularity and, 3: 403
Wry neck, 2: 256
Wulfsberg, Karen M., 1: 231
Wyman, Edwin T., Jr. (1930–2005), 3: *377*, *378*, *380*, *461*
  Children's Hospital/MGH combined program and, 3: 376
  death of, 3: 380
  education and training, 3: 376
  fracture research and, 3: 376–378
  fracture service and, 3: 388*t*
  HMS appointment, 3: 380
  medical cost research, 3: 379, 379*t*
  metastatic pathological fracture case, 3: *376*, 377–378
  as MGH clinical faculty, 3: 464*b*
  MGH Fracture Clinic and, 3: 378
  MGH operations improvement and, 3: 378–379
  as MGH surgeon, 3: 376, 398*b*
  MGH trauma unit and, 3: 396, 399, 460*b*
  Omni Med and, 3: 379
  orthopaedics education and, 3: 378
  private medical practice, 3: 310
  publications and research, 3: *376*, 377–379, *379*
Wyman, James, 1: 308
Wyman, Jeffries, 1: 306, *306*; 3: 25
Wyman, Stanley, 3: 241
Wynne-Davies, Ruth, 2: 399, *400*

X

x-rays. *See also* roentgenograms
  accidental burns, 3: 100
  American Surgical Association on, 3: 58
  bone disease diagnosis and, 3: 101–103
  bone lesions and, 4: 110
  of bullet fragments, 3: *98*
  calcaneal apophysitis (Sever's Disease) and, 2: *88*
  clinical use of, 3: 97, 99–100
  discovery of, 3: 58
  Dodd and, 3: 20, *20*, 21, 96, 99
  experiments with, 3: 96
  fluoroscope and, 3: 96–97
  MGH and, 3: 20
  orthopaedic surgeons and, 2: 56
  publication of, 3: 97, *97*, 98, *99*
  safety of, 3: 99–100
  scoliosis and, 2: 79

  skin injury and, 3: 97–98

Y

Yale University School of Medicine, 4: 259–260
Yanch, Jacquelyn C., 4: 136
Yee, Lester B. K., 3: 351; 4: 489
Yett, Harris S. (ca. 1934–), 4: *250*
  Andre the Giant and, 4: 252–253
  as Beth Israel chief of orthopaedics, 4: 251, 289*b*
  Beth Israel Hospital and, 4: 248, 251, 253, 262–263
  BIDMC and, 4: 253
  BIDMC teaching program and, 4: 286–287
  Boston Orthopaedic Group, 4: 251
  Children's Hospital/MGH combined program and, 4: 250–251
  deep vein thrombosis research, 4: 251–252
  education and training, 4: 250
  HMS appointment, 4: 251
  honors and awards, 4: 251
  hospital appointments, 4: 251
  MGH and, 4: 251
  professional memberships, 4: 253
  publications and research, 4: 251–253
  renal transplant infarction case, 4: 252–253
Y-ligament, 3: 35–36, 38
Yoo, Won Joon, 2: 379
Yorra, Alvin, 3: 258
Yosifon, David, 3: 83
Young, E. B., 2: 115
Young, Thomas, 1: 14
Yount, Carl, 2: 153, 294
youth sports, 2: 384–385, *385*, 386
Yovicsin, John, 1: 275
Yun, Andrew, 1: 217*b*

Z

Zaleske, David J., 3: 401, 460*b*, 464*b*
Zander, Gustav, 3: *69*, *71*, *152*, 264–265
Zarins, Antra, 3: 383, 386
Zarins, Bertram (1942–), 3: *359*, 388*t*, *446–447*, *461*
  anterior interosseous nerve palsy case, 3: 449
  arthroscopic surgery and, 3: 422, 446, 448
  as Augustus Thorndike Professor, 3: 464*b*

Cave Traveling Fellowship and, 1: 217*b*
Children's Hospital/MGH combined program and, 3: 446
early life, 3: 446
education and training, 3: 446
glenoid labrum composition research, 3: 449
Harvard University Health Services and, 3: 450
HMS appointment, 3: 448, 450
honors and awards, 3: 450–451
Latvian Medical Foundation and, 3: 451
leadership roles, 3: 451*b*
as MGH clinical faculty, 3: 464*b*
as MGH surgeon, 3: 398*b*, 450
posterior cruciate ligament (PCL) research, 3: 450
private medical practice, 3: 448
professional sports teams and, 3: 448, 450
publications and research, 3: 359, 448–450, *450*
shoulder surgery and research, 3: 448–450
sports medicine and, 3: 396, 399, 422, 446, 448, 450, 460*b*
sports medicine fellowship program director, 3: 448
Three Star Medal of Honour and, 3: 451
US Navy and, 3: 446
Vail Valley Medical Center and, 3: 446
as Winter Olympics head physician, 3: 448
Zausmer, Elizabeth, 2: 260, *260*
Zechino, Vincent, 2: 299
Zeiss, Fred Ralph, 2: 438
Zeleski, David, 1: 225
Zevas, Nicholas T., 3: 420
Zilberfarb, Jeffrey, 4: 286–287
Zimbler, Seymour "Zeke" (ca. 1932–2021), 4: *245*, *247*
  as Beth Israel chief of orthopaedics, 4: 247–249, 251, 289*b*
  Beth Israel Hospital and, 4: 246–247
  Boston Children's Hospital and, 2: 279, 439*b*; 4: 245–250
  breast carcinoma and chondrosarcoma case, 4: 247–249
  Charleston Naval Hospital and, 4: 246
  Children's Hospital/MGH combined program and, 4: 245
  education and training, 4: 245
  on Green, 2: 182
  HCORP and, 4: 247–248
  HMS appointment, 4: 247
  Legg-Perthes Study Group and, 2: 425; 4: 250
  MGH and, 3: 401; 4: 250
  New England Medical Center and, 4: 249
  pediatric orthopaedics and, 4: 248–250
  private medical practice, 4: 247, 249
  publications and research, 4: 246–247, 250
  on shoes with correctives, 4: 250
  Simmons College physical therapy lectures, 4: 246
  Tufts Medical School appointment, 4: 248–249
  US Navy and, 4: 246
Zimmerman, C., 4: 253
Zurakowski, D., 2: 380